General Surgical Operations

We dedicate this book
with affection to our wives,
Peggy and Judy, and our families.

General Surgical Operations

EDITED BY

R M Kirk MS FRCS
Consultant Surgeon, The Royal Free Hospital, London, UK

R C N Williamson MA MD MChir FRCS
Professor of Surgery, Bristol Royal Infirmary, Bristol, UK

SECOND EDITION

CHURCHILL LIVINGSTONE
EDINBURGH LONDON MELBOURNE AND NEW YORK 1987

CHURCHILL LIVINGSTONE
Medical Division of Longman Group UK Limited

Distributed in the United States of America by Churchill
Livingstone Inc., 1560 Broadway, New York, N.Y. 10036, and
by associated companies, branches and representatives
throughout the world.

First edition 1978
Second edition 1987

ISBN 0 443 02787 0

British Library Cataloguing in Publication Data
General surgical operations. — 2nd ed.
  1. Surgery, Operative
  I. Kirk, R.M.   II. Williamson, Robin C.N.
  617′.91   RD32

Library of Congress Cataloging in Publication Data
  Main entry under title:

  General surgical operations.

  Includes bibliographies and index.
  1. Surgery, Operative.   I. Kirk, R.M. (Raymond
Maurice).   II. Williamson, Robin C.N. (Robin Charles
Noel) [DNLM: 1. Surgery, Operative. WO 500 G3245]
RD32.G43   1986   617′.91   85–15197

Produced by Longman Singapore Publishers (Pte) Ltd.
Printed in Singapore

Preface

Experience acquired in the eight years since the first edition and the appointment of a co-editor has generated a fresh appraisal of the aims and content of this book. Many contributors to the first edition have generously relinquished their chapters so that the major ones have been completely re-written.

The book is intended primarily as a practical manual for the general surgeon about to carry out an operation. The operations are those that the surgeon performs in his everyday practice and those that he may be called upon to carry out in an emergency or because he works in isolation from specialist colleagues. As a rule a single, safe, well-tried operation is given. Alternative techniques are described for selected operations and to cover the requirements of examinations for Fellowship of the Royal Colleges of Surgeons and for the American Board of Surgery.

Each specialist contributor has been asked to describe those operations in his field that a general surgeon should know or might need to perform in special circumstances. With this in mind the selected specialist operations are life-saving, commonly performed or minor.

Those operations that the surgeon meets early in his career are explained in detail. Descriptions of more extensive operations contain fewer details since the surgeon who performs them is generally more experienced. Some sophisticated major operations are described in outline for the benefit of assistants and for those preparing for examinations. These operations should be studied by reading original descriptions and by watching the masters of our profession; many of them demand not only technical skill but also proper selection of patients and trained teamwork to achieve success.

In order to give the book unity, our contributors have courteously adopted a direct style and, as far as possible standard headings. Sections entitled 'Appraise' and 'Aftercare' have been added to the 'Access', 'Assess' and 'Action' of the first edition.

The indications for surgical treatment and for the selection of an appropriate procedure are not always clearcut and are properly discussed in general surgical texts rather than in operation manuals. For this reason they were excluded in the first edition. We have, however, decided to include them in the second edition. This gives the author the opportunity to give relative indications, contra-indications, mention of alternatives and caveats. The emphasis remains mainly in describing the operations themselves, concentrating on the decisions that must be made in the operating theatre. We have placed a greater emphasis than is usual on describing the difficulties and dangers instead of outlining idealized operations that are rarely encountered in practice.

Before attempting specific operations an aspiring surgeon must acquire basic skills and familiarity with materials and instruments used during surgical procedures. These first steps are described in *Basic Surgical Techniques*, also published by Churchill Livingstone.

Success in surgical operations is measured by restoring patients to health and activity, not by the speed and virtuosity of the procedure. We have described well-tried techniques but unless they are used carefully, in the correct circumstances, they will fail. Always keep in mind the succinct American aphorism 'Choose well, cut well, get well'. Unfortunately the effects of all the factors involved, such as selection and preparation of the patient, the timing, and the choice of procedure are not yet known. Consequently a patient may survive following a badly chosen and performed operation, and this appears to be a success. Conversely a patient may succumb following a carefully selected and well-performed procedure and this is a failure. There is still an element of luck in surgery but successful surgeons overall tend to be thoughtful, discriminating and assiduous.

We would like to thank our publishers, Churchill Livingstone, for their strong support throughout the production of this book and also Mr Stephen McAllister who has produced the large numbers of new and revised illustrations. We wish to thank our secretaries, Mrs Geeta Wynne and Mrs Susan McCall, for their outstanding help.

We sadly report that Professor Cyril Conway has died. He saw his chapter through to page proof but was unable to see the completed book.

London & Bristol
1987

R.M.K.
R.C.N.W

Contributors

D Abrams MA DM FRCS DO
Consultant Ophthalmic Surgeon, The Royal Free Hospital, London and Honorary Consultant Ophthalmic Surgeon, Hospital of St. John and St. Elizabeth, London

M Baum ChM FRCS
Professor of Surgery, King's College Hospital Medical School, London

R J Brereton FRCS
Senior Lecturer in Paediatric Surgery, Institute of Child Health, University of London and Honorary Consultant Surgeon, Hospital for Sick Children, Great Ormond Street and Queen Elizabeth's Hospital for Children, London

M D Brough MA MB BChir FRCS
Consultant Plastic Surgeon, University College Hospital, The Royal Free Hospital, Whittington Hospital and The Royal Northern Hospital, London

K G Burnand MS FRCS
Consultant Surgeon, St Thomas' Hospital, London

C M Conway MB BS FFARCS
Professor of Anaesthetics, Charing Cross and Westminster Hospital Medical School, London and Honorary Consultant Anaesthetist, Westminster Hospital, London

N J Fiddian MA FRCS
Consultant Orthopaedic Surgeon, Poole and Christchurch Hospitals, Dorset

J Groves MB BS FRCS
Consultant ENT Surgeon, The Royal Free Hospital, London

P R Hawley MS FRCS
Consultant Surgeon, St Mark's Hospital, London

K E F Hobbs MB BS ChM FRCS
Professor of Surgery, The Royal Free Hospital, London

M Hobsley TD PhD MChir FRCS
Professor of Surgery, Middlesex Hospital, London

R M Kirk MS FRCS
Consultant Surgeon, The Royal Free Hospital, London

I M Laws TD MB ChB FDSRCS
Consultant Oral Surgeon, Whittington Hospital, London

A W F Lettin MS MB BSc(Hons) FRCS
Senior Consultant Orthopaedic Surgeon, St Bartholomew's Hospital, London and Consultant Orthopaedic Surgeon, The Royal National Orthopaedic Hospital, London

P S London FRCS MBE MFOM FACEM (Hon)
Senior Surgeon, The Accident Hospital, Birmingham

A R Makey MS FRCS
Consultant Cardiothoracic Surgeon, Charing Cross Hospital and West Middlesex University Hospital, London and Civil Consultant in Thoracic Surgery to the Royal Air Force

A Marston MA DM MCh (Oxon) FRCS MD (Nice)
Consultant Surgeon, Middlesex and University College Hospitals, London and Senior Lecturer in Surgery, University of London

R S Maurice-Williams MA MB BChir MRCP FRCS
Consultant Neurosurgeon, The Royal Free Hospital, London

J G Mosley BSc MD MRCP FRCS
Consultant Surgeon, Leigh Infirmary, Leigh, Lancashire

P R Riddle MS FRCS
Consultant Urologist, St George's and St Peter's Hospitals, London and Senior Lecturer, Institute of Urology, University of London

M E Setchell FRCS MRCOG
Consultant Obstetrician and Gynaecologist, St Bartholomew's Hospital, London

L Spitz MB ChB PhD FRCS FRCS (Edin)
Nuffield Professor of Paediatric Surgery, Institute of Child Health, University of London and Consultant Paediatric Surgeon, Hospital for Sick Children, Great Ormond Street, London

J P S Thomson MS FRCS
Consultant Surgeon, St Mark's Hospital, London, Consultant Surgeon, Hackney Hospital, London, Honorary Consultant Surgeon, St Mary's Hospital, London, Honorary Lecturer in Surgery, The Medical College of St Bartholomew's Hospital, London and Civil Consultant in Surgery (Rectal) to the Royal Air Force

A J Webb ChM FRCS FIAC
Consultant Surgeon, Bristol Royal Infirmary, Bristol

R C N Williamson MA MD MChir FRCS
Professor of Surgery, Bristol Royal Infirmary, Bristol

Contents

Introduction

In surgery, as in other occupations requiring expertise, it is difficult to decide how much depends upon technical skill and how much upon the materials and methods used. It is important to operate in the best conditions, with the best anaesthetist, assistants, nurses, theatre, instruments and materials. A surgeon who carries out operations within the limits of his skill, but which are too demanding upon the resources of the rest of his team or upon the equipment available, is not acting in the best interests of the patient. On the other hand, the most highly skilled team, the most superbly equipped theatre, will not make up for an unskilful, unenlightened, indecisive or impatient surgeon.

The surgeon's competence stems from an intimate knowledge of the materials that he handles. The supremely important surgical material is the patient's body. Each tissue is unique in appearance, texture and strength. Similar tissues vary from patient to patient, in health and disease. A firm pull may be tolerated in a young slim patient, but the presence of fat, disease, or old age, calls for gentleness. The skillful surgeon recognizes structures although they may be diseased or distorted.

However, skill is not an end in itself. Surgeons are sometimes compared, wrongly, with musicians. A violinist cannot create fine music without mastering technique; but a surgeon can carry out a successful operation with limited technical skill, provided he has good judgement. Keep in mind at all times that you are not operating to impress any-

body, but to carry out the simplest procedure that will safely achieve the results you seek. When you contemplate a risky procedure, knowing that others would be less ambitious, ask yourself how you will react if the patient has serious complications or dies. Will you spend a sleepless night? Of course, you cannot always protect yourself from soulsearching. Overconfidence is a dangerous thing in this profession. Fortunately, surgeons tend to be resilient and optimistic, and our patients would suffer if we were oppressed by failure to the point of losing our nerve. We must have the courage to seize the occasional chance of curing a patient when boldness is required.

PRE-OPERATIVE ASSESSMENT

1. Apart from thorough clinical examination, a number of tests may be carried out on patients before operation. The selection of tests depends on the age and fitness of the patient, the condition for which operation is to be performed, and the clinical findings. Blood haemoglobin estimation, blood grouping, serum electrolytes and urea, and chest X-ray are often ordered routinely. The value of routine tests has been questioned, since abnormal findings are excessively low in patients in whom no clinical suspicion is raised.

2. Do not hesitate to seek the advice of the anaesthetist and of specialist physicians when high-risk factors are discovered. In some hospitals, outpatient anaesthetic assessment can be arranged but in complex cases, be prepared to bring the patient into hospital 2–3 days before operation for full assessment and correction.

3. Review the patient's medical treatment on admission. It is usual to stop antihypertensive drugs over the period of operation. Take note in particular of treatment with digoxin, coronary artery vasodilators, diuretics, corticosteroids, antidiabetic drugs, and antibiotics, in regard to the anaesthetic, but also because of what they reveal of underlying medical conditions.

4. Assess respiratory function clinically and by chest X-ray but carry out pulmonary function tests when there is

clinical suspicion, and before operations that will impair respiratory function. Order pre-operative physiotherapy, steam inhalations and bronchodilator drugs if necessary. If possible stop patients smoking before operation. This may be difficult and the attitude of surgeons varies — some totally forbid it, others segregate smokers and some accept the need of inveterate smokers to continue.

5. Evaluate myocardial disease clinically, with chest X-ray and electrocardiography. Elderly patients, arteriopaths and those who have suffered previous cardiac disease require careful monitoring before and during operation. Avoid elective surgery on patients who have recently suffered from cardiac infarction and wait 3 months if possible.

6. Make sure the patient is not anaemic. Do not hesitate to ask for a blood haemoglobin estimation before even trivial operations if you suspect it will be low and always check it before more major procedures. If the patient is anaemic, postpone an elective operation if possible. If the patient is be postponed, correct the anaemia, if necessary by infusing blood or packed cells, especially if the procedure is likely to cause bleeding. If bleeding is likely at operation, send blood for grouping and ask for the serum to be saved. Crossmatch blood for major operations but since this is expensive and time-consuming, do not order it routinely for straightforward operations on fit patients who are not anaemic.

7. Exclude blood diseases that could result in unexpected bleeding at operation. Order a sickle-cell test on all negroes, those from the Indian subcontinent, eastern Mediterranean, including Arabs and Greeks. If it is positive, warn the anaesthetist. Before major operations take expert advice on the likely benefits of partial exchange transfusion in such a patient. If the patient is jaundiced or suffering from liver disease, check the prothrombin time. Give vitamin K analogue by intramuscular injection, 10 mg three times a day, to correct an abnormal prothrombin time. Stop anticoagulant treatment or switch temporarily to heparin which can be rapidly reversed. Exclude other possible causes of bleeding, such as platelet deficiency, haemophilia and capillary abnormalities and seek advice from the haematologist about possible correction and precautions.

8. Ensure that there is no impairment of renal function and no urinary tract obstruction. Carry out urinalysis, check the level of blood urea and if necessary the creatinine clearance.

9. Make sure the patient does not suffer from known, or undetected, diabetes. Test the urine for sugar and ketones. Always stabilize the patient before operation. Set up an intravenous infusion so that dextrose solution can be given, and convert the treatment to soluble insulin over the period of operation. Remember that diabetes increases the risk of postoperative infection.

10. If the patient is under treatment with corticosteroids, assess the reasons for this. Always give a perioperative boost to those who have taken steroids within the previous 2 years before operation. Consider giving an ACTH stimulation test. After operation plan to gradually tail off treatment with steroids.

11. Jaundiced patients are at risk in a number of ways. Hypoprothrombinaemia increases bleeding tendency while hypoalbuminaemia and other deficiencies impair wound healing and increase the risk of sepsis. Correct the bleeding tendency by giving vitamin K analogue beforehand.

12. Many patients are undernourished because they have not taken sufficient food, or digested and absorbed it, or because of the catabolic effects of their disease. Impaired wound healing and increased risk of postoperative complications is to be expected, although this is not proven. Make sure that malnourishment is corrected by oral feeding, if necessary adding specially formulated or proprietorial feeds. Administer fluid feeds to patients who cannot swallow by nasogastric tube, into a gastrostomy or a jejunostomy.

When enteral feeding is not possible, insert a central venous catheter under strict aseptic precautions through which can be infused aminoacids, glucose and emulsified fat solutions. Parenteral feeding carries severe risks of producing infection and many techniques are used in the hope of reducing this including subcutaneous tunnelling of the catheter track. Undoubtedly, the greatest single improvement in management is the provision of specially trained nurses to deal with central venous catheters.

The presence of sepsis or malignancy may neutralize efforts to restore positive nutritional balance. In such cases deal with the cause as soon as practicable.

PERI-OPERATIVE PROPHYLAXIS

INFECTION

1. Although many surgeons condemn routine antibiotic prophylaxis in theory, they often practise it on slender indications. This discrepancy is understandable. Theoretical objections recede when we contemplate the hazards of sick patients developing serious infection.

2. It is accepted that antibiotic treatment is necessary if infection already exists as in operations for peritonitis, but this is scarcely prophylaxis. Similarly, operations that convey a high incidence of bacterial contamination such as those on the large bowel, should be covered. Prophylactic antibiotics are also justified in patients who are in particular jeopardy should they develop infection, such as those with severe cardiac disease and especially someone with a prosthetic heart valve, even if there is minimal risk of infection.

3. Antibiotic prophylaxis has traditionally started at the time of operation and continued for 5–7 days. Recently it has been shown that a single dose or a short course is just as effective, provided the blood level is maximal at the time of possible contamination. Thus the antibiotic should be

administered systemically at the time of induction of anaesthesia, or beforehand if it is given orally or rectally.

4. The choice of antibiotic should be suited to the likely organism. Bowel organisms are mainly Gram negative and many are anaerobic. Skin organisms are usually Gram positive. The best selection changes as new antibiotics are introduced and it is wise to consult the microbiologists regularly rather than persist in using familiar combinations that are no longer appropriate.

SELF-INOCULATION

Australia antigen

1. There is a relatively low risk of hepatitis 'B' positive patients in Britain, northern Europe, North America and Australasia, with intermediate risk in patients from Mediterranean countries, the Middle East, Central America and South Africa. There is high risk in the Indian subcontinent, tropical Africa, South America and the Orient. Test patients from moderate — or high-risk areas routinely, all obstetric patients, haemophiliacs, those with renal failure, liver disease, leukaemia and seriously ill patients in intensive therapy units. In addition test suspected drug addicts and homosexuals. Warn the operating theatre staff 24 hours before an elective operation on an Australia antigen positive patient, so that the theatre can be emptied of inessential equipment.

2. Theatre staff wear disposable gloves, aprons and overshoes. The patient is brought to the anaesthetic room on his bed. After everyone has entered the theatre the doors are closed and towels soaked in 1% sodium hypochlorite solution are placed on the floor inside all the doors. No one should enter or leave except in an emergency.

3. During the operation, all cutting instruments such as knives, scissors and needles are kept in a kidney dish which is handed to the surgeon so that he can take them out and replace them himself. Used swabs are placed in a specially marked plastic bag for disposal.

4. Take great care to avoid cutting yourself or your operating theatre colleagues. Whenever possible adopt a no-touch technique to guard against coming into contact with the sharp end of cutting instruments.

5. Postoperatively, allow the patient to recover from the anaesthetic in the theatre then return him directly to the ward.

6. The instruments are collected together in the table cover and sent for double sterilization. All the operators dip their gloved hands in methylene blue solution, then carefully remove the gloves, watching for staining of the skin, denoting glove punctures. Sites of glove punctures are examined for bleeding.

7. The whole team leaves through the exit door where arrangements have already been made for them to remove all their clothes including disposable aprons and overshoes, which are placed in special bags for disposal. Clean replacement clothing is donned so that the staff can reach the changing rooms where each member takes a hot shower before dressing.

8. If any member of the team has pricked the skin, however minutely, inform the Control of Infection Officer. A blood sample is taken to determine if he is antigen positive and if he is not, then potent gamma globulin is given prophylactically. Ideally he should not take part in an operation on an antigen positive patient for 2 months.

Acquired Immunodeficiency Syndrome (AIDS)

This appears to be a communicable disease although there are no reports of hospital staff contracting it from patients. Seek advice regarding homosexuals, drug addicts, Hiati nationals and haemophiliacs and especially members of these groups suffering from Kaposi's sarcoma. Precautions are similar to those for hepatitis B.

PHLEBOTHROMBOSIS

1. The fear of deep leg vein thrombosis occuring at or following operations, with the subsequent possibility of pulmonary embolism, still remains in spite of intensive research.

2. Thrombosis occurs much more frequently than is clinically detectable. It is particularly associated with elderly patients, those who are inactive, obese, those with malignant disease, polycythaemia or a past history of thromboembolism, women taking the contraceptive pill and specific operations such as those on the hip joint or within the pelvis.

3. The association of the contraceptive pill with thromboembolism has led many surgeons to advise patients to stop taking the pill for 1 month before elective operation. There is no evidence that this policy is beneficial and it may be thwarted by an unplanned conception. In any case oral contraceptives are believed to exert a thrombogenic effect for up to 3 months.

4. Thrombosis develops on the operating table in almost half the patients. Methods have been developed for mechanically massaging the legs or moving the ankle joints or electrically stimulating the calf muscles during the operation, to prevent stagnation of blood in the legs. They have not been generally adopted, and in most operating theatres the legs are slightly elevated and the calf muscles are protected from compression against the table by placing a rubber cushion beneath the Achilles tendon.

5. The risk of deep venous thrombosis and embolism can be reduced by giving prophylactic anticoagulation treatment. Patients over the age of 40 years, those with malignant disease, and those with diabetes, obesity, varicose veins or a history of previous thrombosis are treated

in addition to women who have recently been taking the contraceptive pill. Calcium heparin in a dose of 5000 units is given subcutaneously with the premedication drugs, followed by a similar dose 8 hourly for 7 days thereafter. Alternatively 500 ml of dextran 70 may be infused intravenously during the operation and a further 500 ml is given during the next 24 hours.

OPERATIVE CHECKS

CORRECT PATIENT? CORRECT OPERATION?

1. It must be every surgeon's nightmare that he will perform the wrong operation on a patient. For various reasons the order of operating lists may be changed. The theatre technicians bring a patient to the anaesthetist, and the masked, unconscious patient is placed before a surgeon who is expecting to perform a particular operation and has the appropriate instruments at hand. Perhaps his assiduous assistant has prepared the skin, applied the towels, and even made the incision. There is no absolute safeguard except by maintaining a high level of anxious attention to the danger and never allowing it to sink. You have entered a demanding profession and this is but one of the many anxieties you will have to sustain.

2. The only way to be sure is to see and talk to every patient beforehand and discuss the operation. If the procedure is unilateral, make your own mark on the appropriate side and instruct the patient to let no one erase it. In the anaesthetic room and the theatre, look at the patient again. You are the surgeon, it is your responsibility and you must trust no one. Having accepted that it is your sole final responsibility, involve everyone else in helping you to avoid mistakes. Your surgical assistants, the anaesthetists, the technician who fetches the patients, the theatre and ward nurses, must all feel responsibility for seeing that the correct patient has the correct operation. Only by this means will you hope to cover your occasional and human lapse of absolute care.

ROUTINES

1. Sterile techniques in theatre have been worked out over many years. Those who enter the operating theatre for the first time feel uneasy because they fear they may inadvertently offend against the rules. More experienced people carry out the correct procedures instinctively. In such circumstances it is wise to accept the need to follow strict routines and so be free to concentrate on other aspects of the operation. Question the routines from time to time to decide if they are really valuable. Discuss them with other surgeons and with the theatre sister, whose teaching of

nurses may be undermined by thoughtless disparagement of a routine.

2. The technique of carrying out surgical operations is fairly standardized by the pooling of the experience of many surgeons. At the beginning of your career adopt the accepted and orthodox procedures and the procedures followed by your chief. In this way you will at least have the consolation if anything goes wrong that you can justify your routine. Later in your career you may question certain points of technique and have the courage to adopt unorthodox methods. Wait until you are confident enough to face your own conscience if disaster follows. Surgeons are very conservative. We follow well-tried methods because experience has shown that in our hands they work.

SWAB AND INSTRUMENT COUNT

1. There is no single once-and-for-all action to prevent articles being left in the wound, bringing distress and often tragedy for the patient and surgeon alike. You must worry about the possibility without a moment's let-up, and accept full responsibility. Check everything yourself every time. Do not let your acceptance of responsibility, however, prevent you from involving as many others as possible in the check. They may save you from a momentary lapse.

2. Use as few swabs at a time as possible. Always use the largest swabs compatible with the task. Avoid burying all the swab or pack in a wound; leave a portion protruding to be clipped to the wound towels, or use packs with tapes that can be clipped or ringed. Even when you have removed every pack and the count is correct, check the wound yourself before closing it.

3. Everyone is conscious of the danger of leaving swabs, but fewer surgeons are aware of the dangers of leaving instruments. These are sometimes less assiduously counted by the theatre sister. For this reason, use as few instruments as possible at any one time. Never use short-handled instruments in a deep wound, and always ensure that the handles protrude or never leave your grasp. Check the wound before closing.

MATERIALS

A short account of the threads and needles is given here, but no attempt is made to describe the use of the many surgical instruments that are available. As an apprentice, use the materials and methods of your master. One of the greatest benefits of working with a number of teachers is that you are able to have first-hand knowledge of many methods: take advantage of it, so that when you are free to choose for yourself, you can select confidently the method most suited to your own practice.

LIGATURES AND SUTURE MATERIALS

Absorbable materials

1. Catgut is the prepared submucous coat of the sheep's (and, more recently, cow's) intestine. Plain catgut is selected for fine sutures and ligatures where rapid digestion is no disadvantage. Chromicized catgut has been treated to delay digestion in the tissues. It is usually not absorbed until healing has progressed enough to prevent the tissues from separating. The catgut is standardized by its rate of absorption in animals. The site and local conditions affect the rate of absorption in humans.

2. Polyglycolic acid sutures are synthetic filaments of polymerized hydroacetic acid, which is degraded by hydrolysis in the tissues.

3. Polyglactin 910 maintains its strength for longer than the other absorbable sutures. It is eventually broken down to glycolic acid and lactic acid in the tissues.

Non-absorbable materials

1. Silk is a partially absorbable material of great strength and suppleness. It is used most frequently as a twisted or braided thread. Floss silk is loosely twisted to encourage cellular infiltration between filaments, with subsequent collagen deposition.

2. Linen and cotton threads have similar handling properties to silk.

3. Nylon is a plastic synthetic material which is relatively inert in the tissues. Monofilament nylon is somewhat stiff, springy and smooth-surfaced, so that multiple throws are necessary to knot it securely. The bristly ends should be buried when suturing near the skin to prevent sinus formation. Braided nylon is soft and easy to use. Floss nylon is also available.

4. Other plastics such as polyesters, polyethylene and polypropylene are similarly well tolerated in the tissues.

5. Inert metal sutures are useful in certain situations. Stainless steel is strong, either as a monofilament or as braided thread. Silver, tantalum and aluminium can also be used. When using metallic threads make sure they do not kink, by ensuring that each loop is controlled as it is pulled through the tissues. After knotting them, turn the spiky ends of wires underneath to bury them.

Sizes

Although attempts have been made to introduce metric sizes from the European Pharmacopoeia (EP), most British surgeons adhere to the US Pharmacopeoia sizes (USP). Since the metric sizes will probably gain popularity in the future, a table of comparisons is given. Unless specified, all the sizes in this book are USP, except that linen and silk threads are still frequently given in the old-fashioned but popular thread sizes.

Knots (Fig. 1.1)

1. Generally use a triple throw knot, each half hitch forming a reef knot with the contiguous hitch. When tightening the first half hitch, do not cross the threads. When tying ligatures, make sure that clamps or forceps are relaxed, so that the enclosed tissue can be compressed within the encircling thread. Apply equal tension to each end of the ligature.

Table 1.1 Thread sizes

USP Nonabsorbable and synthetic absorbable	Absorbable	EP	Diameter (mm)
8/0	7/0	0.5	0.05–0.069
7/0	6/0	0.7	0.07–0.099
6/0	5/0	1	0.10–0.14
5/0	4/0	1.5	0.15–0.19
4/0	3/0	2	0.20–0.24
3/0	2/0	2	0.25–0.29
2/0	0	3	0.30–0.39
0	1	4	0.40–0.49
1	2	5	0.50–0.59
2	3	6	0.60–0.69
3	4	7	0.70–0.79

2. Tie the second half hitch tightly on to the first.

3. If it is important that the first hitch does not slip while tying the second, tie a surgeon's knot, or cross the threads so that they jam, while tying the second half hitch.

4. Now tie a third half hitch so that it forms a reef knot with the second half hitch.

5. Do not try to tie knots 'cleverly'. When possible empty your hands of instruments and tie two-handed knots

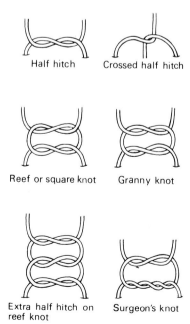

Half hitch   Crossed half hitch

Reef or square knot   Granny knot

Extra half hitch on reef knot   Surgeon's knot

Fig. 1.1 Knots used in surgery.

as though tying shoe laces. These are quicker in the end than repeated fumblings at 'one-handed' knots or knots tied with forceps. A competent surgeon is recognized by the safety, not the rapidity, of his knot tying.

6. When tying knots within a cavity, you cannot pull both threads towards the surface of the wound. If it is not possible to pull them apart in the depths of the wound, push one thread deeper into the cavity, while pulling upon the second one.

7. Do not waste time trying to tie threads that are too short.

8. Have the ends cut 2–3 mm long beyond the knot when tying fine catgut, linen or silk thread. For thick catgut and monofilament nylon, have the threads cut about 5 mm long.

Stitches (Fig. 1.2)

1. If you are a beginner, discover the methods used by your chief and use them.

2. The bowel is usually closed in two layers. For the inner, all-coats stitch, use 00 chromic catgut, preferably mounted on an eyeless needle. The outer seromuscular stitch may be 00 chromic catgut, 00 silk, 90 or 100 linen thread. There is no particular advantage in using non-absorbable material, since this suture is intended only to appose the peritoneal surfaces.

3. The peritoneum and the posterior rectus sheath where present, are sutured with continuous 0 or 1 chromic catgut, or 0 or 1 nylon. The pleura is closed in a similar fashion. Make sure the sutures are inserted at least 1 cm from the edges.

4. Muscles are sutured with interrupted 0 or 1 chromic catgut. Do not pull the sutures tight, or they will merely cut through the muscles.

5. Aponeurotic sheaths are sutured with continuous or interrupted stitches of 1 chromic catgut, 00 or 0 silk or nylon, 60 or 40 linen thread, or 35 swg stainless steel wire. Place the stitches at least 1 cm from the edges.

6. Subcutaneous tissues are apposed with 00 plain catgut stitches.

7. Skin stitches may be of silk, nylon, polypropylene or polyglycolic acid. Use coloured thread, since it is easily seen. The stitches may be simple, interrupted, or longitudinal mattress. Clean wounds may be closed using simple continuous, blanket or subcuticular stitches. In subcuticular stitching, a continuous thread picks up alternate sides of the wound just beneath the surface.

8. Deep tension stitches must of smooth-surfaced thread if they include the skin and will, therefore, be removed; 0 silk or nylon, 40 linen thread or 35 s.w.g. stainless steel wire are suitable.

Needles (Fig. 1.3)

1. Use round-bodied needles when stitching bowel, blood vessels, peritoneum and muscles.

2. Use cutting needles for sewing the skin, aponeuroses and scarred tissues.

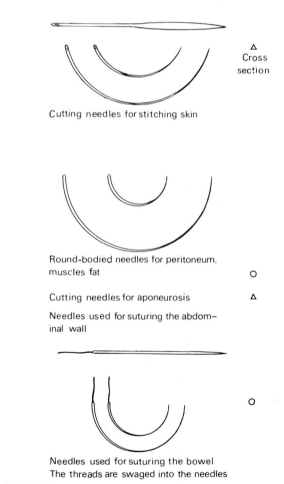

Fig. 1.3 Needles.

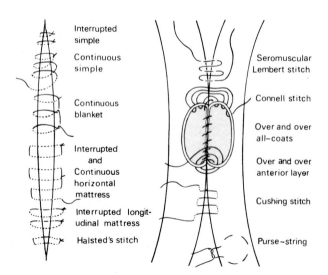

Fig. 1.2 Stitches. Left, some stitches used in surgery. Right, stitches used for hollow viscera.

3. When they are available, use eyeless needles for stitching delicate tissues like blood vessels and bowel.

4. Try straight and curved needles; try small needles held by means of forceps and large needles held in the hands.

MECHANICAL LIGATURES AND SUTURES

A number of superbly designed and useful instruments have become available to assist the surgeon. In some circumstances they are invaluable. As a trainee, do not use them constantly in preference to traditional methods of haemostasis and suturing, since the older methods are more versatile. However, take the opportunity to try them and appreciate their use when manual methods would be difficult, or in saving time during long procedures.

Ligatures

1. Haemostatic metal clips can be applied to occlude small tubes including blood vessels in specially constructed forceps. Using such methods, haemostasis can be achieved easily in circumstances where it would be difficult to insert a suture or tie a ligature. The clips, which are radio-opaque, are usefully applied, mark a deep site for subsequent study or to plan radiotherapy. Recently introduced models have a magazine so that a series of clips can be applied seriatim.

2. The LDS machine applies two clips side by side across a small piece of tissue and at the same time an enclosed knife blade cuts the tissue between the two clips. This offers a rapid method of dissecting through vascular tissues. A disposable powered model is marketed.

Sutures

1. Michel clips have been used for skin closure for many years. One pair of toothed dissecting forceps has a gallery on which are arranged metal clips with fine teeth at each end. A second pair of dissecting forceps has grooved tips that grip either the skin or the clips. Right-handed people hold the forceps with the clips in the left hand, the grooved-tipped forceps in the right hand. Starting at the right hand end of the wound, the skin edges are apposed accurately, held with the left hand forceps while a clip is removed, applied across the edges, and while still held, the clipped skin is drawn to the right to stretch it while the left hand forceps is released and gains a fresh grip to the left. The right hand forceps are released as the left hand draws the skin edges to the left. The released right hand forceps removes a clip from the gallery and applies it to the left of the previous one, retaining a grip as it is drawn to the right. The sequence is repeated along the length of the wound. Skin clips are usually removed earlier than stitches

and there are special forceps designed to facilitate this by opening out the clips to detach the teeth.

2. Individual metal clips can be inserted to appose aponeuroses or skin edges by instruments that work in a similar manner to industrial staplers. Disposable powered staplers are available.

3. Straight double rows of staples can be applied to occlude tubes using disposable staplers. These are available in 30, 55 and 90 mm sizes. The flattened tube is held between the jaws of the instrument. When it is actuated the staples are pushed through both layers of the flat tube, strike the shaped anvil so the ends are turned over and closed. It is usually unnecessary to reinforce the closure with sutures.

4. The GIA Autosuture stapler inserts four parallel, linear rows of staples and at the same time cuts between the two middle rows. The instrument separates into two parts, and can be used to unite two tubes, producing a stoma between them (Fig. 1.4). Lay the tubes together. Make a hole in each tube so that the separated jaws of the GIA stapler can be inserted, and laid parallel to each other. Lock the two halves together after ensuring that no extraneous tissue is inadvertently trapped. Actuate the stapler, then separate the two halves and withdraw them. Check that the edges are correctly united, if necessary inserting reinforcing sutures. It only remains now to close the single hole, through which the machine was withdrawn. From within the hole, identify and pick up the ends of the staple lines with tissue forceps. Separate the forceps to create a linear defect. Close the defect either with sutures, or conveniently apply a straight double stapler of suitable length, such as a TA30.

5. There are a number of circular staplers available for uniting tubes such as bowel or other viscera (Fig. 1.5). A single, or double concentric row of metal staples is held in a circular cartridge. This is apposed to a circular anvil with the edges to be united trapped between them. When the stapler is actuated, a single or double ring of staples is extruded from the cartridge, the ends pierce the layers of both viscera, strike the anvil beyond and are bent over and

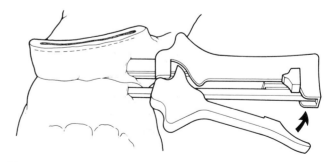

Fig. 1.4 Creating a side-to-side anastomosis using the GIA stapler. One link has been passed into each viscus through an entry hole. The two handles are about to be locked together. The push bar will be actuated, the limbs separated and withdrawn. The now fused entry hole will be closed.

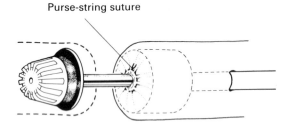

Purse-string suture

Fig. 1.5 Joining the ends of two cylindrical viscera using a circular stapling device. The opened device is inserted into one viscus, protrudes from the end which is then drawn over the staple cartridge with a purse-string suture. The end of the second viscus is drawn over the anvil with a purse-string stitch. The anvil is then closed onto the cartridge, the device is actuated, opened and withdrawn. The entry hole in then closed.

closed. At the same time a circular knife blade cuts off excess tissue, creating a circular lumen between the two viscera.

When the ends of tubes are to be united, first ensure that the safety catch is applied so that the instrument will not be inadvertently actuated. Insert the cartridge through a convenient orifice or create one which will be closed later. Separate the anvil from the cartridge. Insert a purse-string suture of monofilament fine plastic around the edges of the tube and tie the purse-string to draw the edges over the cartridge towards the spindle. A special clamp is available to insert the purse string but it is not essential. Draw the end of the second tube over the anvil and insert a similar purse-string suture to hold the end against the spindle. Appose the anvil and cartridge to trap the double layers of tube ends between them. Check that no extraneous tissues are inadvertently trapped. Release the safety catch and actuate the stapler. The two ends are united by the staples and the excess tissue is trimmed off. Separate the anvil from the cartridge and with a gentle twisting motion withdraw the stapler. Ensure that the circular staple line is intact and if necessary reinforce it with sutures. Remove the anvil and confirm that two intact toroidal 'doughnuts' of tissue can be seen on the spindle, confirming that the circular anastomosis is complete. If a hole has been specially created to insert the stapler, close it with sutures or use a straight stapler.

Side anastomoses can be created using a slightly different technique. Remove the anvil. Introduce the spindle and cartridge into the viscus and press the spindle end against the far wall. Make a small incision through which the spindle end can be pushed until the cartridge comes into contact with the wall. It is not necessary to insert a purse string suture. Replace the anvil and insert this into the second viscus, drawing the edges over the anvil surface with a purse string suture. Appose the anvil and cartridge, actuate the machine, separate the anvil and cartridge and withdraw it.

HAEMOSTASIS

1. Operative surgery is inevitably associated with damage to blood vessels and consequent bleeding. In addition, surgeons must operate to control spontaneous bleeding resulting from local disease or a generalized bleeding tendency and the bleeding that follows trauma. Although most arteries and veins are capable of contracting to stop bleeding and capillaries collapse if the inflow pressure falls below a critical point, blood vessels are not always cleanly transected and effective contraction may not occur. In addition the clotting mechanism may be defective and the platelet function of vascular plugging may fail.

2. As a rule simple pressure over a bleeding point kept up for a few minutes will suffice to control most bleeding at operation. Maintain the pressure with a hand placed over a gauze pack or arrange the pack so that its position is maintained without manual pressure.

3. Anticipate oozing from raw surfaces and consider injecting into the tissues to be cut a solution of 1 : 250 000 adrenaline (epinephrine) in physiological saline solution. This manoeuvre constricts the vessels and decreases oozing.

4. Anticipate localized bleeding from cut vessels and apply haemostatic forceps on each side of the intended cut beforehand, subsequently ligate the tissue grasped within the forceps. Use fine catgut near the skin, otherwise use fine silk or linen thread. Alternatively pass ligatures around the tissue on either side using an aneurysm needle, tie the ligatures and cut between them.

6. Control general oozing whenever possible by picking up individual vessels and ligating them or coagulating them with diathermy current. Try applying gauze packs wrung out in a saline solution that is just uncomfortably hot to the touch, for 5 minutes by the clock. Sometimes small areas can be covered with gelatin foam. If this fails, can the raw surface be safely folded and stitched in apposition to compress and seal it? If no other method controls general oozing, consider inserting a pack and leave it for 24–48 hours (see p. 9). Of course surface wounds are particularly amenable to this method of haemostatic control.

7. The cautery is infrequently used in general surgery. The electric cautery has a resistance element built into its tip that heats up when current is passed through it. The heated element is then touched against tissues to coagulate bleeding vessels.

DIATHERMY

1. Body tissues are heated when a high-frequency oscillating current is passed through them. The diathermy machine provides a suitable current.

2. An indifferent electrode, now usually disposable, must be bandaged closely to the patient's thigh to provide

a wide area of skin contact. Make sure the wire lead is firmly attached.

3. The active electrode, sterilized with its wire lead, may be a rod, point or forceps. The handle is insulated; even so it should be kept within a rubber sheath when not in use.

4. The steady oscillating current is disruptive and is used for cutting tissues. The machine can be switched to produce a damped current, which coagulates without disrupting the tissues.

5. The machine is controlled from a foot switch by the surgeon.

6. The smaller the area of tissue in contact with either electrode, the greater the heating effect. Therefore the indifferent lead must contact a large area. The active electrode must contact a small area and must not be used in a pool of blood where the current is dissipated. Try to pick up individual vessels for coagulation. The resulting dead tissue then compares favourably with the volume of tissue strangled by a ligature. Do not rely upon diathermy coagulation for control of anything but minor vessels.

7. The cutting current is applied through a needle electrode or special knife blade. The cutting effect is accompanied by local tissue heating which decreases bleeding. Cutting diathermy is particularly useful when dividing muscles, although some surgeons prefer to proceed more slowly using a coagulating current.

8. Coagulation diathermy can be provided with current flow confined to the tissues enclosed between the tips of the forceps, each tip being a separate electrode.

9. It is well known that diathermy must not be used in the presence of inflammable anaesthetic gases or explosive bowel gases, as in the colon. It is not so well known that spirit-containing skin sterilizing preparations may explode, especially if atmospheric oxygen tension is raised.

10. Diathermy must be used with care close to the skin, because superficial diathermy burns often take weeks to heal. Accidental burns occur when the indifferent electrode does not make proper contact, or if current flows inadvertently through other metals such as drip stands, anaesthetic or surgical appliances in contact with the patient. If the indifferent contact is lost or its wire breaks, current flows through alternative pathways to earth. Therefore test the leads and circuitry before using the machine each time. Isolated circuitry is intended to avoid the dangers of leakage to earth, but the instruments in use are not universally reliable in this respect.

PACKING

1. Occasionally wounds must be packed, the pack acting as an obturator. If bleeding within a cavity cannot be controlled by any other method, packing may be the only possible manoeuvre. Do not think this problem will never confront you. Sooner or later you may open into a haemorrhagic tumour that cannot be excised, or attempt a simple operation only to find that the anatomy is not what you expected and that you have damaged an inaccessible source of bleeding. You may also meet the problem when dealing with casualties.

2. Take one end of a large sterile gauze roll down to the bottom of the cavity with forceps, then feed the gauze in layers, back and forth, packing it like a 'jumping jack' firecracker, so that it can later be removed easily. In deciding how tightly to pack it, remember the presence of major blood vessels or ducts that could be occluded. When inserting packs within the abdomen remember that a high pack may restrict diaphragmatic movements. Bring out the end of the roll through the wound and cover it with a large sterile dressing. Determine to leave the pack for 4–5 days, then remove it gently and carry out delayed primary suture of the wound if it is uninfected.

3. Occasionally, after removing a large tumour, primary closure cannot be accomplished. An example is failure to close the peritoneum of the pelvic floor following synchronous combined abdominoperineal resection of the rectum. A temporary obturator can be made by inserting the central portion of a sheet of sterile plastic material or oiled silk from the perineal aspect and packing the under surface of the domed sheet with sterile gauze roll. Remove the packing and sheet after 5–7 days when a fibrinous floor has formed.

DRAINS

1. A drain forms a channel along which fluids can reach the surface while allowing the main wound to be closed. The drain itself may form the channel when it is tubular, or it may form a channel in the tissues when it is a sheet or ribbon.

2. Do not expect too much from the use of drains. Some of the blood, exudate or other fluid may find its way along the provided path, but it is equally likely that the fluid will remain to form a collection or track in another direction. Certainly do not expect the insertion of a drain to be any protection against future leakage of fluids following secondary haemorrhage or leakage from an anastomosis. On the other hand, a well-placed drain inserted when the calamity has occurred may be lifesaving, provided the cause is also properly dealt with.

3. Drains may be inserted within hollow organs or ducts. The common bile duct, urinary bladder or the stomach may be drained along a normal or abnormal track to the surface, while healing takes place after operation. Such drainage prevents the accumulation of contents leaking from suture lines.

4. A drain may be inserted into an abnormal channel such as a fistula to drain the effluent conveniently into a

receptacle, thereby reducing contact of the fluid with surrounding skin and other tissues.

5. A drain may be inserted into an existing cavity to keep it empty and allow it to shrink, for example when an abscess or haematoma is drained.

6. Corrugated rubber or plastic strips have been used for many years. Thin Paul's tubing, with or without an internal wick of gauze, is soft and unlikely to produce pressure necrosis of delicate tissues or suture lines. Various rubber and plastic tubes with specially shaped tips, side holes or gutters are useful in particular circumstances. Provided the fluids can be encouraged or sucked into tubular drains, they can be channelled away and so prevented from returning to the source.

7. Whenever possible, use drains that incorporate radioopaque markers that enable them to be traced if they are displaced.

8. Preferably insert drains through separate stab wounds rather than through the main wound, which may otherwise become contaminated by the discharging fluid. However, small tubular drains can sometimes be led out at the extremity of the main wound.

9. Fix the drain so that it can neither be lost into the depths, nor be pulled out accidentally. Transfix and suture to the skin a corrugated drain, and insert a safety pin through it. Fix a closed tubular drain by inserting a skin stitch, tie this loosely then encircle the tube once or a number of times with ligatures. Stitch a flexible tubular drain to the skin one or more times to prevent external tension from pulling it out.

10. It is controversial whether contamination often occurs through an open drain, but certainly emerging material may contaminate other areas. In consequence the modern tendency is towards closed drainage systems, utilizing a tube drain emptying into a closed container. In the past glass bottles were used, but disposable plastic collection bags with sealed-in tubing are more convenient.

11. A closed system must be used when draining the pleural cavity to prevent air entering with consequent collapse of the lung. However, air and fluid must be able to drain to the exterior. A tube drain is led through a stab wound in the chest wall down into a bottle by the bedside, partially filled with sterile water. The tubing is led through the bung and beneath the water, so that the sucking action that occurs on inspiration tends to draw water up the tube, thus creating a vacuum in the system equivalent to the height of the column of water in the tubing. When intrapleural pressure exceeds atmospheric pressure, retained air is expelled underwater and bubbles to the surface, escaping from the bottle through a second short, angled tube that also pierces the bung. Alternatively, the chest drain may be connected to a disposable rubber flutter valve that allows fluids to escape into a closed collecting vessel. The valve collapses and seals when intrapleural pressure falls below atmospheric pressure.

12. Closed drainage systems can incorporate vacuum drainage. The drainage tube, or the air escape tube of an underwater sealed drain, can be connected to a centralized system or to an electrically driven suction pump. The emerging fluids are collected in a closed vessel placed between the drain tube and the vacuum pump.

Special bottles evacuated of air with a suction pump can be attached to drainage tubing to exert suction drainage. These bottles incorporate indicators to show when the pressure within them has risen to atmospheric and they must then be replaced.

Suction drainage can be accomplished very simply when only small amounts of fluid are expected to escape. A syringe with a plastic or rubber bulb that tends to re-expand when it is forcibly compressed may be emptied, attached to the drainage tube, and then released. The syringe maintains suction and gradually fills with any free fluid from the drained area. From time to time it must be detached, emptied, reconnected and released.

Suction must be gentle, otherwise surrounding tissues tend to be drawn into the holes of the tube and seal them, so that they become ineffective.

Suction drains are very useful in helping to close cavities caused by an abscess or haematoma and in preventing cavities from forming by keeping the tissues in contact. Tubing attached to a form of suction drain apparatus can be placed subcutaneously to replace external compression dressings following surgical procedures.

13. A disadvantage of suction drains is that if the holes are blocked by sucked-in tissues, they cease to function. This possibility can be partially overcome by using sump drainage. A large drainage tube creates a cavity within the tissues; being perforated, it allows fluids to seep into the sump it provides. Lying loosely within it is a suction tube that removes the collected fluid. The sump drain and interior suction tube must be inserted so that they are dependent and reach the lowest part of the cavity. Sump drains are now available with filters that prevent bacteria from being drawn into the cavity by the air flowing into the suction tube. Alternatively, a leaky system of suction can be incorporated so that the vacuum is never sufficient to trap tissues in the drain tubing. This is accomplished by placing a small open tube alongside the drain tube to conduct air to the depths, or by using a special suction pump that intermittently allows the pressure to rise to atmospheric.

14. Whenever you insert a drain, record it in the notes and instruct the nurses how to manage it. As a rule, determine to remove the drain after 48 hours unless it is discharging fluid. In the case of a chest drain, determine to remove it 24 hours after the water in the tubing stops oscillating with respirations.

15. Intraperitoneal drains are of doubtful benefit, although most surgeons use them following operations such as cholecystectomy. They are usually partially effective in

letting out fluids already present or flowing continuously, but cannot be relied upon as monitoring devices to warn of future bleeding or anastomotic leakage. It is generally safer to drain the fluid within a sutured viscus or duct, such as stomach, bile duct or urinary bladder, rather than place an external intraperitoneal drain to protect a suture line.

16. The ineffectiveness of intraperitoneal drainage in generalized peritonitis has led to trials of peritoneal lavage. Sterile physiological saline at body temperature may simply be poured into the peritoneal cavity, left to penetrate everywhere and then be aspirated; the manoeuvre is repeated until the aspirate is quite clear. To the lavage fluid may be added an antiseptic such as noxythiolin 1% or dilute povidine-iodine solution. Alternatively antibiotic solutions may be instilled into the peritoneal cavity. These solutions are all poured in, allowed to percolate throughout the cavity and are then sucked out.

Another method of managing generalized peritonitis is to insert a small inflow catheter through a stab wound in the upper abdomen and a sump drain in the pelvis. The abdomen is closed, and subsequently sterile fluid is instilled through the inflow catheter and syphoned or sucked out through the sump catheter for a few days until the drainage fluid is crystal clear and sterile on culture. Various lavage fluids can be tried.

Whichever method you use, remember that the most important safeguards are to gently remove all debris and dead and doubtful material from the peritoneal cavity and take the greatest care to prevent further soiling.

CONTAMINATED WOUNDS

1. Do not lightly close a wound that is contaminated, that has ischaemic tissues within it forming a potential source of infection or if body fluids are likely to collect that will form good culture material for micro-organisms. Always take swabs and specimens of fluid for aerobic and anaerobic culture, and determination of antibiotic sensitivites.

2. If there is considerable swelling and tension of the deep tissues, do not hesitate to debride the wound by laying open the constricting tissues, taking care to avoid damage to important structures. In the limbs, this is accomplished by making longitudinal incisions through the skin and if necessary through the deep fascia (see Ch. 27).

3. Excise from traumatized wounds all dead or dying tissue, in particular muscle that has been crushed, is ischaemic, or has been devitalized by the close passage of a high velocity missile. Remove all foreign material since it is potentially infected. Preserve important structures such as major blood vessels and nerves, remembering that they may be displaced following injury. Do not remove attached bone fragments unless they are grossly displaced. Do not

over-aggressively excise damaged skin especially of the face and hands.

4. If contamination of the subcutaneous tissues is minimal consider instilling an antibiotic or chemotherapeutic agent into the wound and closing it with or without a drain. This regimen has long been popular both in surgery of trauma and in abdominal surgery but the benefits are arguable. Antibiotics instilled routinely into abdominal wounds may reduce wound infection rates.

5. Delayed primary suture allows the tissues to reject necrotic cells, organisms and collected fluids and prevents anaerobic organisms from flourishing. Leave the wound open until it appears clean, healthy and safe to close.

Delayed primary suture has long been practised in military surgery and in civilian trauma surgery, especially when the injury has occurred more than 6–8 hours before operation, or in the presence of compound fractures. It has become increasingly popular in abdominal surgery when contamination has occurred, although the peritoneum is usually closed.

After excising all dead tissues and ensuring haemostasis, lay in a single layer of sterile non-adherent plastic net or tulle gras. Pack the wound with gauze dressings. Provided the patient's general condition is satisfactory, leave the wound for 4–5 days, then inspect it with a view to closing the skin by mobilizing the edges, or by laying in split skin grafts.

6. Systemic antibiotics given prophylactically, either as a single dose or in a short course, have potential benefits. Do not, though, expect antibiotics to make up for inadequate surgical management.

7. The peritoneum is remarkably capable of dealing with residual infection provided the source is adequately dealt with and gross particles and fluid are removed. It is sometimes safe to close the peritoneum and drain or leave open the rest of the abdominal wall for delayed primary closure. Peritoneal lavage (see above) may also be used during and after operation.

DRESSINGS

1. If wounds are carefully closed and haemostasis has been perfect, they need no dressing. A scab of dried blood adheres to the suture line and remains until the stitches are taken out. Small skin wounds can be left alone after closure or sealed with Whitehead's varnish or a plastic spray. A number of proprietary self-adherent dressings are now available that allow moisture to evaporate through them so that wounds do not become macerated. They are useful to seal the wound against infection, inspection and interference.

2. Unfortunately more major wounds cannot be relied upon to remain absolutely free from discharge. More elaborate dressings are often required. Make sure that each

dressing you apply has a well-defined purpose and will fulfil that purpose.

3. Clean, open wounds that are to be allowed to granulate should be covered with a single layer of non-adherent net or tulle gras, followed by an absorbent layer of sterile gauze sufficiently thick to soak up all the likely discharge until the next change of dressing. Cavities may be packed with gauze soaked in flavine emulsion.

4. Infected or oozing open wounds may be covered with a single layer of non-adherent net, followed by a thick pad of gauze to soak up the profuse discharge that can be expected. Make sure you have taken a swab for culture of the organisms. Local antiseptics, antibiotics or chemotherapeutic agents may then be applied to combat infection although they are often ineffective. Very infected and sloughing wounds may be dressed with gauze soaked in eusol solution, salicylic acid solution 0.006 per cent, or hydrogen peroxide solution. It is beneficial to vary these solutions to change the milieu and discourage bacteria. If *Pseudomonas aeruginosa* is suspected, apply 1% acetic acid solution.

The separation of the slough can be aided by coating the wound with small spheres of a dextranomer, or applying local proteolytic and fibrinolytic enzyme preparations.

5. Extensive wounds that leave potential cavities frequently result in the cavities filling with blood and exudate to produce a haematoma, which may then become infected. The collection of fluid is best prevented either by compressing the wound or by keeping the potential cavity emptied by suction drainage.

6. If compression is employed, it must be distributed evenly over the wound. This goal is best accomplished in most cases by applying a layer of dry cotton wool before bandaging. Do not use the cotton wool as an extra absorbent layer or it will form a hard and useless cake. Instead, apply sufficient gauze beneath it to act as an efficient absorber. As an alternative to cotton wool, use natural or artificial sponge or an inflatable air cushion. A cavity can be conveniently filled using silicone elastomer foam as an alternative to conventional packing.

7. Some form of bandaging must now be applied to hold the dressings in place and exert compression. An evenly applied, encircling bandage such as crepe bandage is ideal; it is particularly useful for limb wounds, but always encase the limb with bandage from the extremity up to the site of the wound, to prevent the garter effect of a firm bandage applied only proximally. Whenever possible when bandaging a limb, let the tips of fingers and toes remain visible so that cyanosis can be seen if the bandages are too tight. For abdominal dressings, disposable elastic corsets are available to provide compression. When an encircling bandage cannot be applied, compression can be achieved by using strips of elastic adhesive, but do not stretch these too tightly or they tend to drag off the skin where they adhere to it.

8. Place separate absorbent gauze dressings around open drain sites so that they can be changed without disturbing the main wound.

9. Compression dressings are often difficult to apply and restricting for the patient and retained exudate is offensive and potentially infective. In addition, they make inspection of the wound difficult for the surgeon. Consequently, suction drainage may be preferable (see p. 10). Multiple tubes may be used following extensive surgical procedures, and they can be joined together for connection to a single source of suction.

POSTOPERATIVE CARE

1. At the end of the operation you should have done everything possible to leave the operation site perfectly safe. In particular there should be no source of continuing bleeding or residual nidus of infection, and no ischaemic tissue. The anaesthetist has taken care throughout the operation to maintain the patient's general condition stable and avoid respiratory and cardiovascular complications in particular.

2. Subsequently ensure by your postoperative care that the operation site and the patient as a whole are allowed to recover quickly and without complication. Careful and frequent monitoring reveals early changes that can often be corrected to avert trouble.

3. Keep the part or system that has been operated upon at rest as far as possible. If necessary assist the function if it must continue, as following operations upon the heart or lungs.

4. Many operations produce pain. Control or alleviate it, preferably using small repeated doses of analgesics or continuous controlled infusion.

5. In appropriate patients call on the help of physiotherapists to aid the patient after operation, both in maintaining satisfactory respiratory function but also in mobilizing the part operated upon, and to help the patient to get about and return to an optimistic outlook.

6. Do not forget the presence of pre-existing conditions in causing postoperative complications and the development of complications from undiagnosed or totally new conditions.

7. Local complications are dealt with at appropriate places in the text

8. The eventual aim of surgery is to restore the patient and the operation site to as near as possible full function.

REMINDERS

BEFORE OPERATION

When operation is decided upon, check the following points:

1. Has the operation consent form been signed?

2. Is the premedication ordered?
3. Has the patient an empty bladder and has the urine been tested?
4. Has the patient had a recent meal?
5. Has the anaesthetist been informed and theatre staff alerted?
6. Is an intravenous drip or blood transfusion necessary?
7. Should the patient have an orogastric or nastogastric tube?
8. Should you notify your chief?

In the anaesthetic room, ask if this is the correct patient.

In the theatre, the patient is placed on the operating table lying flat on his back, except when stated otherwise. Before making the incision, ask yourself again if this is the correct patient and, if this is a unilateral operation, is this the correct side?

AFTER OPERATION

1. The patient's condition should be checked with the anaesthetist.
2. Operation notes should be completed. Specimens preserved for laboratory examination must be labelled.
3. Tell the nurses what operation was performed and how to manage the patient.
4. Order analgesics, antibiotics and any other drugs required.
5. Plan a postoperative visit to the patient.

Further reading

Altemeier W A 1982 W A Sepsis in surgery. Archives of Surgery 117: 107–112

Atik M, Hanson B, Isla F, Harkess J W 1969 Pulmonary embolism: a preventable complication. American Surgeon 34: 888–894

Davis J M, Wolff B, Cunningham T F, Drusin L, Dineen P 1982 Delayed wound infection: an 11 year Cornell University Medical Center survey. Archives of Surgery 117: 113–117

Douglas D M 1949 Tensile strength of sutures. I. The B.P C. method test. Lancet 2: 497–499

Dudley H A F (ed) 1977 Hamilton Bailey's Emergency Surgery, 10th edn. Wright, Bristol.

Fraenkel G J, Ludbrook J, Dudley H A F 1978 Guide to house surgeons in the surgical unit 6th edn. Heinemann, London

Hardy J D 1981 Complications in surgery and their management, 4th edn Saunders; Eastbourne

Hill G L, Church J 1984 Energy and protein requirements of general surgical patients requiring intravenous nutrition. British Journal of Surgery. 71: 1–9

Hoffbrand A V, Pettit J E 1980 Essential haematology. Blackwell, Oxford.

Irvin T T 1981 Wound healing: principles and practice. Chapman and Hall, London

Jacobson J H, Bush H S Jr 1964 More foreign material with continuous or interrupted suture technique? Surgery 55: 418–420

Keighley M R B, Burdon D W 1979 Antimicrobial prophylaxis in surgery. Pitman, London

Kirk R M 1978 Basic surgical techniques, 2nd edn. Churchill Livingstone Edinburgh

Kirk R M, Stoddard C J, 1986 Complications of surgery of the upper gastrointestinal tract. Baillière Tindall, *London*.

Kyle J, Hardy J D 1981 Scientific foundations of surgery, 3rd edn. Heinemann, London

Mervine T B, Goracci A F, Nicholl G S 1973 The handling of contaminated wounds. Surgical Clinics of North America 53: 611–615

Mitchell J P, Lumb G N, Dobbie A K 1978 A handbook of surgical diathermy. Wrights, Bristol.

Nicholaides A N, DuPont P A, Desai S T et al 1972 Small doses of subcutaneous sodium heparin in preventing deep venous thrombosis after major surgery. Lancet 2: 890–893

Spencer F C 1983 Observations on the teaching of operative technique. Bulletin of the American College of Surgeons. 68: 3–6

Rob C, Smith R 1983 Operative surgery, 4th edn. Vol 1. Butterworths London

Turk J L 1978 Immunology in clinical medicine, 3rd edn. Heinemann, London

Yates J L 1905 An experimental study on the local effects of peritoneal drainage. Surgery, Gynecology and Obstetrics, 1: 473–480

Anaesthesia: related techniques

Respiration
Shock
Local Anaesthesia

Certain techniques commonly undertaken by the anaesthetist should be within the competence of the surgeon. These
include control of a patient's airway and the initial treatment of acute hypovolaemia. As many minor and peripheral surgical procedures can be performed under local
anaesthesia, the surgeon should have some knowledge of
the available local anaesthetic agents, and the scope and
limitations of local anaesthetic techniques.

RESPIRATION

TRACHEAL INTUBATION

Appraise

1. Tracheal intubation, widely practised during anaesthesia, is also indicated in many other situations. Because
it can be lifesaving it should be within the capabilities of
every doctor. Effective endotracheal intubation guarantees
the integrity of the upper airway.

2. It overcomes upper airway obstruction, from haemorrhage or following trauma.

3. It prevents entry of blood, gastric contents, secretions
and other foreign matter into the tracheobronchial tree.

4. It permits effective ventilation.

5. It facilitates tracheobronchial toilet in severe debility
and postoperative atelectasis.

6. Intubation may be lifesaving in unconscious states,
such as following head injury, depressant poisoning, or
when there is inadequate spontaneous breathing, as in cardiac arrest, following chest injury, or after a severe drug
overdosage.

Prepare

1. Laryngoscope. The Macintosh pattern curved laryngoscope blade is popular and the easiest to learn to use.
The standard adult Macintosh blade is suitable for most
patients over 10 years of age. Check the laryngoscope bulb.

2. Tracheal tube. Use disposable plastic tracheal tubes,
available in a full range of sizes, for emergency intubation.
These tubes are marked to show their internal diameter in
millimetres. Use cuffed tubes in adults. Select a 9 mm internal diameter tube for adult males and an 8 mm tube for
adult females. Children below the age of 10 require non-
cuffed tubes. A convenient guide to the likely tube diameter in children is

$$\text{internal diameter(mm)} = \frac{\text{age in years}}{4} + 4.5$$

Additionally in children have available tubes 0.5 mm larger
and 0.5 mm smaller than the calculated tube size. Tube
length is important, especially in children. Tubes for
emergency use in adults should be precut to a length of
22–24 cm. An approximate formula for tube length in children is

$$\text{length (cm)} = \frac{\text{age in years}}{2} + 12$$

Test the cuff of the tube and then apply water-miscible
lubricant to the tube.

3. Connections (Fig. 2.1) Plastic disposable connectors
have two male ends. One of these fits into the proximal end
of the endotracheal tube. These connectors are available in the
same range of sizes as for tracheal tubes. Carefully choose
the correct size of connector for the selected tube. The
other end of the connector is of standard size to fit a universal angle piece. Use a corrugated rubber catheter mount
to connect the angle piece to an anaesthetic machine, resuscitation device or ventilator. Assemble the connection
to the tracheal tube.

4. Have a 20 ml syringe and a clamp to inflate and seal
the cuff.

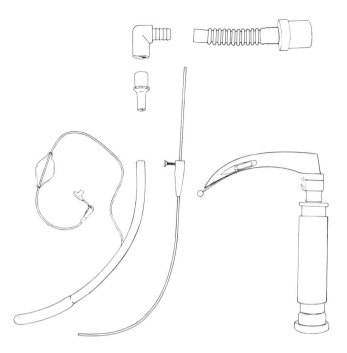

Fig. 2.1 Tracheal intubation equipment: cuffed endotracheal tube (disposable); introducing stylet; two-part angle piece; catheter mount; Macintosh laryngoscope.

5. Have a curved malleable metal stylet or a long gum-elastic bougie to assist in difficult intubation.

6. Position the patient. Correct posture is essential. Moderately flex the cervical spine by raising the head on one pillow, and then extend the atlanto-occipital joint by fully extending the head on the neck.

7. Inspect the teeth. Remove any dentures. Look for any loose teeth, crowns or bridges, especially in the upper incisor area, so as to avoid damage or dislodgement during intubation.

Action

1. Hold the laryngoscope handle in the left hand and insert the blade into the right side of the mouth. Slide the blade along the right hand side of the tongue, initially directing the blade slightly towards the left tonsil. When the blade has passed the bulk of the tongue move the blade into the midline, thus holding the tongue out of the line of vision and over to the left. Continue advancing the blade in the saggital plane until you see the epiglottis. Then pass the blade anterior to the epiglottis, between it and the base of the tongue, and lodge the tip firmly in the vallecula. The vocal cords may be visible at this time. More usually in order to visualize the glottis it is necessary to displace the tongue by lifting the laryngoscope in the direction of the handle. Do not use the upper teeth or gums as a fulcrum. This causes damage and will not give an adequate view of the glottis.

2. If the epiglottis is not visualized either the laryngo-scope blade is not in the midline or it has passed down the oesophagus. Withdraw the blade to about midway along the tongue and then readvance it.

3. When the glottis is visualized, take the endotracheal tube in the right hand with the concavity of its curve upwards, and pass it via the right hand side of the mouth, aiming it medially so that the tip comes into the midline immediately in front of the glottis. Insert the bevel between the vocal cords and slide the tube onwards through the larynx. Withdraw the laryngoscope and secure the protruding end of the tube with adhesive strapping to the patient's face or by means of a loop of tape or bandage around the neck.

4. Check that the tube is in the correct position. Press sharply on the subject's chest. A puff of air emerging from the tube indicates that it has entered the trachea (rather than the oesophagus). Connect to a ventilating apparatus and apply positive pressure. Uniform expansion of the chest indicates correct placement. If one side of the chest (usually the right) expands more than the other then the tube has been passed too far and has entered a main bronchus. Withdraw the tube until chest expansion is uniform. Confirm correct placement by auscultatation during ventilation.

5. The commonest difficulty encountered is in obtaining a sufficiently anterior view to expose the glottis fully and in persuading the tube to take the necessary curve behind the epiglottis so as to enter the larynx. Pass a lubricated malleable metal stylet into the tube to about 1 cm from the tip, and angulate the tube more sharply. Alternatively, pass a long gum elastic bougie through the tube so that it protrudes for a few centimetres and angulate the end of this to aid laryngeal entry. In difficult cases pass a gum elastic bougie alone and 'railroad' the tracheal tube along the bougie into the trachea.

6. If a cuffed tube has been passed then ventilate the patient's lungs and slowly inflate the cuff until audible leakage during inspiration ceases. Clamp the distal end of the cuff-inflating tube.

7. When deciding whether an unconscious patient requires intubation in order to safeguard the airway, be guided by the state of the laryngeal reflexes and the degree of muscle tone. If these are such that intubation is likely to be possible without great difficulty, then it should be carried out.

8. Acquire skill in tracheal intubation by practice under supervision during induction of anaesthesia for routine surgery or practice on an intubation training simulator.

ARTIFICAL VENTILATION

Institute intermittent positive pressure ventilation without delay whenever spontaneous breathing is absent or inadequate. Do not attempt to compensate for deficient ventilation by giving oxygen. Hypoxia may be temporarily corrected but carbon dioxide will continue to accumulate until depressant levels are reached and sudden respiratory arrest occurs.

Methods range from emergency expired air resuscitation (mouth to mouth, mouth to nose, mouth to tracheal tube), to the use of self-inflating ventilating bags (Ambu, Laerdal) or of automatic lung ventilators. Detailed consideration of techniques and equipment is not appropriate here, but some general points will be made.

Airway

1. A clear airway is essential. Remove any dentures and clear the pharynx and mouth of any gross contamination by blood, gastric contents or other foreign matter.

2. Fully extend the head on the neck and elevate the jaw — best done by applying pressure from behind the angles of the mandible. This opens the airway in nearly all cases. Insert an oropharyngeal airway if necessary.

3. Intubate the trachea (see p. 14) if prolonged respiratory support is needed or if the patient is deeply unconscious. Consider tracheostomy and insertion of a cuffed tracheostomy tube if prolonged tracheal intubation is envisaged. This is best performed as an elective procedure after tracheal intubation.

Ventilation

1. Underventilation is harmful, overventilation rarely so. Aim for a minute volume of 8–9 litres in an adult.

2. Ventilate at a rate of 12–15 per minute. Inflate the lungs over 1–1.5 seconds and allow 2–2.5 seconds for expiration to occur passively.

3. Use an automatic lung ventilator for prolonged ventilation, monitoring arterial oxygen and carbon dioxide levels to control ventilation level and inspired oxygen concentration.

4. Persistence of some degree of (invariably inadequate) efforts at spontaneous breathing is harmful. It may indicate inadequate artificial ventilation or the presence of excessive secretions. If no cause is apparent the spontaneous efforts can be abolished by incremental doses of 1 mg of phenoperidine intravenously. If control is difficult it may be necessary to use a neuromuscular blocking agent such as pancuronium.

Secretions

Tracheobronchial toilet will be necessary during prolonged artificial ventilation. Sterility is important. Sterile disposable whistle-tip catheters are suitable. Choose a size of suction catheter less than half the diameter of the tracheal or tracheostomy tube and use only once. Avoid catheters having a single aperture as these stick to the tracheal wall and are both difficult to advance and traumatic. Insert the catheter using sterile gloves or forceps, and apply suction in-

termittently during its withdrawal. Avoid prolonged suction as this causes hypoxia. Repeat tracheo-bronchial toilet as often as is indicated by the quantity of secretions aspirated.

OXYGEN THERAPY

Indications

In general, oxygen is used to restore a deficient cellular oxygen supply to normal. Specific indications relevant to surgery include:

1. All acute hypoxic states, such as chest injury and pulmonary oedema.

2. In the immediate postoperative period, especially after upper abdominal surgery and in older subjects.

3. Shock of all types, in order to compensate for the reduced cardiac output, impaired pulmonary function, reduced oxygen carrying capacity of the circulation and impaired tissue perfusion.

4. Hypermetabolic states such as thyroid crisis or hyperthermia, to satisfy an increased tissue oxygen requirement.

5. To hasten nitrogen elimination from distended bowel, pneumothorax and pneumoperitoneum and in decompression sickness.

6. Hyperbaric oxygen therapy has been used to treat gas gangrene and to improve the viability of skin flaps.

Action

1. For routine oxygen therapy use a disposable plastic face mask such as the Edinburgh or Hudson type. These are semi-rigid and perforated, and are thus safe in the event of oxygen failure, as the patient is then free to breathe atmospheric air.

2. Alternatively use a nasal catheter which is less cumbersome and more acceptable to the patient for long term use. Specially designed catheters are available or an ordinary 10 or 12 FG disposable suction catheter can be used. The catheter need only be inserted a short distance into the nose. Humidification is needed if a nasal catheter is to be used for more than a few hours or if an oxygen flow of more than 4 litres per minute is to be given.

3. Use an oxygen flow of about 4 litres per minute. This results in an inspired oxygen concentration in the range of 30–60%.

4. Never give patients with acute-on-chronic respiratory failure high oxygen concentrations to breathe from a mask. These patients commonly depend upon a certain degree of hypoxic respiratory drive and dire effects can result from the abolition of hypoxia under these circumstances. Provide oxygen therapy in such patients with a 'fixed performance' device, such as the Vickers Ventimask, which supplies a high flow of constant composition oxygen-enriched air. Start treatment with a 24% mask and as long

as no further respiratory depression occurs you can change to masks delivering progressively higher oxygen concentrations.

5. If 100% oxygen is required, it is necessary to use a close-fitting mask and a reservoir bag, and to supply a high flow of oxygen. This is best achieved using an anaesthetic machine and patient breathing system, with an oxygen flow of 8–10 litres per minute.

Dangers

1. Risk of fires and explosions.

2. Risk of producing respiratory depression in patients with chronic respiratory disease.

3. Complete atelectasis may rapidly develop in any portion of the lung served by a bronchus which becomes blocked (usually by retained secretions) when a patient is breathing high oxygen concentrations. This is because of the rapid absorption of oxygen in the isolated lung segment.

4. Oxygen toxicity. Exposure to high oxygen concentrations over several days or exposure to hyperbaric levels of oxygen for more than a few hours may produce a clinical picture similar to that of bronchopneumonia, with cough, retrosternal pain, and bronchiolar and alveolar exudates. Oxygen toxicity is never a problem in the initial stages of acute respiratory resuscitation.

SHOCK

Shock can be defined as a generalised impairment of vital organ function due to acute circulatory failure. The main types of shock are hypovolaemic, cardiogenic, septic and anaphylactic. Of these hypovolaemic shock following trauma is the variety of most importance to the surgeon.

Other conditions can produce a shock-like state. These include:

1. A restricted venous return from tension pneumothorax or cardiac tamponade.

2. Adrenocortical failure from adrenal disease or sudden withdrawal of steroid therapy.

3. Loss of vasomotor tone caused by spinal cord transection.

4. Psychological reactions to pain and emotion.

Be careful to recognize these entities since treatment appropriate to hypovolaemic shock may here be inappropriate or even harmful.

MANAGEMENT OF TRAUMATIC SHOCK

Appraise

1. The cornerstone of management is the early restoration of adequate tissue oxygenation by intravenous fluid therapy. Untreated or severe shock can lead to major organ failure of which the most important are cardiac failure and renal failure.

2. Problems can arise if there is associated intracranial damage from head injuries, unrecognized continued bleeding from closed abdominal trauma and hyperkalaemia from massive tissue damage and release of intracellular potassium.

Emergency (First Aid) treatment

1. Establish an airway (see p. 16).
2. Stop any considerable bleeding using local pressure of tourniquets.
3. Give 100% oxygen by mask.
4. Position the patient in the lateral position if unconscious or bleeding into the nasopharynx.
5. Set up an intravenous infusion, initially giving readily available crystalloid.
6. Take blood for grouping and crossmatch.
7. If control of the airway is in doubt pass an endotracheal tube (see p. 14).
8. Institute positive pressure ventilation if spontaneous breathing is inadequate.
9. Control pain with small doses of intravenous morphine, or (if available) pre-mixed 50% nitrous oxide in oxygen (Entonox).

Assess

1. Assess the degree of shock on the basis of the history and clinical examination, estimated blood loss, central venous pressure (see below for assessment of blood loss, and page 21 for central venous pressure measurement).

2. Take a venous blood sample for electrolyte estimation.

3. Examine the patient carefully for associated injuries. Order X-ray if appropriate and if the patient's condition permits.

Action

1. Early and energetic intravenous replacement therapy is essential. Aim first to restore plasma volume, then treat extracellular fluid and intracellular fluid losses. The choice of replacement fluid depends on the nature of the fluid lost and the availability of the desired fluids (see p. 18).

2. If larger volumes of fluid are to be infused warm it to body temperature.

3. In severe shock monitor central venous pressure and insert a urinary catheter to monitor renal function.

4. In severe shock give sodium bicarbonate, 1–1.5 mmol per kg body weight to counter acidosis from tissue hypoxia.

5. Chart all treatment and monitored information.

6. Carry out corrective surgery as soon as possible following resuscitation.

Failure to respond

1. The commonest and most important reason for failure to respond to adequate replacement therapy is the presence of unrecognized continued blood loss from closed injuries. Inexplicable failure to respond to therapy is often an indication for urgent surgical abdominal exploration.

2. Impaired myocardial function as evidenced by hypotension, oliguria, cold extremities may necessitate the use of beta-adrenergic agonists.

(a) Isoprenaline has both beta-1 and beta-2 actions, and produces an increase in myocardial contractility and heart rate together with a reduction in peripheral resistance. Renal blood flow may fall. The dose is $0.02–0.2$ μg/kg/min.

(b) Dopamine in doses of $0.5–2$ μ/kg/min. increases renal blood flow and glomerular filtration without any direct cardiac effects being evident. At infusion rates of $2–10$ μg/kg/min myocardial contractility and heart rate are increased and peripheral resistance is either lowered or unchanged. Infusion rates above 20 μg/kg/min cause an increase in peripheral resistance and a reduction in renal blood flow. Dobutamine resembles dopamine in its actions and is given in similar doses, but has a lesser vasoconstrictor effect at high doses. When inotropic agents are needed in shock states isoprenaline should be used if there is a bradycardia. Otherwise dopamine is the agent of choice. High infusion rates may be necessary initially to maintain a good systolic pressure. Lower the dose rate as soon as possible so as to reduce left ventricular work and improve renal function.

3. Persistent peripheral vasoconstriction in the presence of a raised central venous pressure may respond to judicious use of an alpha-adrenergic blocking agent such as chlorpromazine in a dose of 1 mg intravenously repeated cautiously until the desired effect is attained. The major hazard of this approach is the sudden production of profound hypotension. Fluids may have to be infused rapidly as the drug begins to take effect and the constricted circulation 'opens up'.

4. Persistent poor peripheral perfusion in spite of adequate fluid therapy and a normal central venous pressure may respond to digoxin if it results from hypoxic heart failure. Administer cardiac glycosides with great caution in shocked patients because they have a long half-life.

5. Plasma potassium concentration may rise to high levels in traumatic shock from potassium release from damaged cells. Severe hyperkalaemia should be treated with intravenous dextrose and insulin (25 units of soluble insulin per litre of 5% dextrose).

ASSESS BLOOD LOSS

1. Severity of the injury. Table 2.1 indicates the levels of blood loss likely with moderate to severe injuries to various parts of the body.

Table 2.1 Blood loss and site of injury

Injured area	Probable blood loss
Arm	500–1000 ml
Lower leg	500–2000 ml
Thigh	1000–3000 ml
Pelvis	1000–4000 ml
Thorax	1000–4000 ml
Abdomen	1000–5000 ml

2. 'Hands' method. Evaluate the area or volume of tissue trauma in relationship to the size of the patient's hand or fist. A full-thickness skin loss of an area equivalent to the patient's flat hand, or severe damage to tissue of a bulk equivalent to the clenched fist each result in a loss of about 10% of circulating blood volume.

3. Measurement of blood loss. Estimate directly blood loss during the period of resuscitation and surgery. Swab weighing is the simplest and best method. Subtract the weight of a batch of clean and dry swabs from their weight after use and equate the weight gain in grams to blood loss in millilitres. Include loss into suction bottles and allow for loss in drapes. More elaborate methods of blood loss estimation, such as colorimetric examination or conductivity measurements of washings from swabs are rarely appropriate in shock. Blood volume estimation by indicator dilution techniques is not very accurate in fit patients and may give gravely erroneous results in the presence of active bleeding or fluid replacement therapy.

4. Clinical methods. Observe colour, skin temperature, capillary refill time, and presence of sweating. Chart blood pressure and heart rate. Blood pressure per se is not a good indicator of the degree of shock — up to 35% of blood volume may be lost without any changes in blood pressure. Tachycardia is an earlier and more reliable sign of shock. Monitor urine output. An output below 0.5 ml/kg/hr indicates reduced renal function.

INTRAVENOUS FLUIDS

Normal adults have a blood volume in the order of 70 ml per kg body weight. Replacement therapy is needed when about 20% of the blood volume the been lost. Children have blood volumes of up to 85 ml per kg, and require urgent replacement therapy when 10% of this has been lost. The choice of replacement fluid rests between blood, plasma and plasma substitutes and crystalloids and has to take account of the availability of various fluids. Restoration of circulating volume is initially of greater importance than restoring the total red cell mass. Resuscitation is commonly started with readily available crystalloid solutions. In acute situations large volumes of crystalloid alone have been shown to be valuable for initial resuscitation. In all forms of shock considerable extracellular and intracellular fluid defects arise. Although crystalloids have a limited duration of residence in the circulation, they are useful in making up extravascular fluid losses. The commonest pat-

Table 2.2 Plasma and plasma substitutes

	Advantages	Disadvantages
PPF(plasma protein fraction)	Shelf life 2 years; no risk of serum hepatitis; physiological volume expander	Must be refrigerated; expensive; contains no fibrinogen
Dextran Polysaccharide; available as dextran 40, 70 & 110 in dextrose or saline; dextran 70 stays in circulation 8–12 hours	Long shelf life; cheap; reduces viscosity; lowers incidence of thromboembolism	May interfere with crossmatching; dextran 40 can cause renal failure; occasional hypersensitivity reactions; contains no clotting factors
Haemaccel Gelatin preparation	Long shelf life; cheap; no interference with cross-matching	Short plasma life (4–6 hours); hypersensitivity reactions more common than with dextrans; no clotting factors

tern of fluid therapy in shock is initially to give a litre or so of crystalloid solution such as Ringer-lactate (Hartmann's solution) and then continue with a suitable colloid solution.

1. Blood. Stored blood suffers from a number of defects. Blood is stored at a temperature of 4°C, and large infusions can cause marked hypothermia. Stored blood is deficient in Factors V, VIII, IX, X and XI. Bank blood has a low pH, partly because of the acid composition of the anticoagulants used and partly because of continued anaerobic red cell metabolism. Blood infusion thus induces some degree of metabolic acidosis, but later metabolism of citrate to bicarbonate produces and alkalosis. Stored blood may have a plasma potassium level as high as 30 mmol per litre, and hyperkelaemia can be induced if cold blood is given rapidly in large volumes. Stored blood, especially CPD blood, contains a large amount of aggregated debris which is filtered out by the pulmonary capillaries and may play a part in the later production of 'shock lung'. If possible when blood is given it should previously be fully crossmatched. When patients need to receive uncrossmatched blood, give blood of their own group if known or group O rhesus negative blood. When more than 2 units are to be given, pass the blood through a warming device to heat it to close to body temperature and use a suitable 40 micron filter to remove debris.

2. Plasma and plasma substitutes. Dried pooled plasma is rarely used nowadays. Its reconstitution with water is time-consuming, and its use is associated with a risk of serum hepatites. The commonly used plasma expanders are shown in Table 2.2

SETTING UP AN INTRAVENOUS INFUSION

Appraise

For a high-capacity, trouble free infusion there is no substitute for a large cannula in a large vein. Venepuncture for

this purpose should be a methodical technique. Prepare carefully and do not rush at any stage. In any one patient your first attempt at venepuncture should offer the best chance of success.

Equipment

For the ordinary percutaneous technique, have ready:
1. An infusion stand bearing the container of the chosen fluid to which had been attached an intravenous fluid administration set primed to remove air.
2. A venous occlusion tourniquet.
3. Swabs for skin cleaning.
4. A suitable infusion needle/cannula assembly (see below).
5. A 2 ml syringe fitted with an intradermal needle and containing 0.5 ml of 1% lignocaine without adrenaline.
6. A small sterile disposable scalpel blade.
7. A good source of light.
8. Adhesive strapping to fix the cannula once inserted.

Action

1. Explain to the patient what is to be done and reassure him that discomfort will be minimal.

2. Select a suitable vein. The best sites are in the upper limb. Veins of the lower limb are more difficult to enter, more capable of spasm, and more liable to thrombosis. If possible avoid veins overlying the wrist and elbow joints. There is usually a straight segment of vein well supported by subcutaneous tissues on the radial side of the forearm just proximal to the wrist.

3. Apply a suitable tourniquet to distend the vein. Milk blood from the periphery into the chosen segment. Provide good illumination, preferably from one side rather than from directly above. If necessary shave the skin over the selected vein. Clean the skin with a suitable cleaning solution such as surgical spirits, isopropyl alcohol or chlorhexidine.

4. In a conscious patient always use a local anaesthetic. This involves intradermal injection of a minute quantity of local anaesthetic, and greatly facilitates venepuncture.

5. The point of skin penetration should be 0.5–1 cm distal to the point of entry to the vein itself. Select this skin site and inject the local anaesthetic intradermally so as to raise a weal about 4 mm diameter. Allow a short time for the local anaesthetic to work and then penetrate this weal with the tip of a small scalpel blade held vertically. This small skin incision prevents the cannula from being gripped by the skin during insertion and allows more precise entry into the vein.

6. For ordinary purposes choose one of the many proprietary needle-inside cannula devices (Fig. 2.2), such as the Abbocath or Medicut. These are disposable and are supplied in a variety of sizes. They all consist of a flexible blunt-ended plastic cannula, fitting snugly over an inner

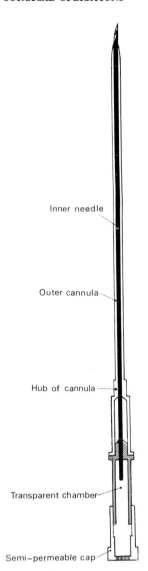

Inner needle

Outer cannula

Hub of cannula

Transparent chamber

Semi-permeable cap

Fig. 2.2 Percutaneous intravenous cannula placement unit

steel needle of slightly greater length, so that the tip of the needle projects slightly from the end of the cannula. The hub of the inner needle is commonly fitted with a plug that allows air (but not fluid) to be displaced when blood enters the inner needle and thus allows visual confirmation of successful venepuncture. Alternatively, attach a 2 ml syringe to the hub of the needle and confirm venepuncture by aspirating blood.

7. Select a cannula/needle assembly of a size appropriate to the size of the chosen vein, the type of fluid to be infused and the desired rate of infusion. For treatment of acute hypovolaemia in adults use a 16 gauge unit (colour code grey).

8. Hold the hub of the unit with the bevel of the needle upwards and insert it at a shallow angle through the small skin incision. Use the thumb of the other hand to stretch the skin distal to the point of insertion so as to keep the vein straight and taut. Run the tip of the needle up to the vein, keeping in the long axis of the vein and enter it from its superficial aspect. Entry is confirmed by the passage of blood back along the needle. Advance the unit a further 0.5 cm along the vein to ensure that the tip of the cannula is well into the lumen. Hold the hub of the needle steady relative to the skin and slide the cannula down the needle and into the vein.

9. Remove the venous tourniquet. Completely withdraw the needle from the cannula, applying pressure over the vein at the level of the cannula tip to prevent blood loss. Attach the infusion set to the cannula and ensure that fluid can flow freely. Secure the infusion assembly with a strip of adhesive tape placed over the hub of the cannula and adjacent tubing. A splint is not usually needed but may be required if the site of venepuncture is at the level of a joint. In chidren, use a plaster of Paris back slab. Do not bandage to a splint or back-slab so tightly as to impede venous return.

10. With careful and methodical technique it is rarely necessary to use the cut-down method. If this is required use the cephalic vein on the lateral aspect of the upper arm. It is constant, large and leaves the patient free to move his arms and use both hands. Avoid the saphenous vein at the ankle. It is long, has muscular walls and is particularly prone to venospasm.

11. For intravenous feeding insert a catheter into the superior vena cava via the cephalic vein in the arm, or (less desirably) into the inferior vena cava via the saphenous vein at the groin. Prolonged parenteral nutrition is an indication for insertion of a central line into the superior vena cava or right atrium via the subclavian vein under fully sterile conditions, with the distal end of the catheter led out through a subcutaneous tunnel to pass through the skin some distance from the site of venepuncture.

12. To increase the rate of infusion raise the fluid container as high as possible, use an infusion pump or, if the fluid container is collapsible, apply external pressure to it with a sphygmomanometer cuff or one of the specially designed pressure bags. Avoid pressurization of rigid containers by injection of air into them. There is a high risk of air embolus associated with this manoeuvre. When large volumes of fluid have to be infused rapidly use two or even three separate infusion sites.

13. To avoid thrombophlebitis when prolonged infusion is necessary:
(a) Use a strict aseptic technique during venepuncture.
(b) Change the site of infusion every 24 hours.
(c) Use non-irritant (Teflon) cannulae in large veins in the upper rather than lower limbs.
(d) When possible avoid dextrose containing solutions.

MEASUREMENT OF CENTRAL VENOUS PRESSURE (CVP)

Appraise

1. Monitoring of CVP is a quick and useful method of assessing the state of the circulation. It involves placing a catheter into the right atrium or adjacent vena cava.
2. Indications.
(a) In the management of shock of all varieties.
(b) To regulate large volume whole blood transfusions.
(c) In acute circulatory failure or instability.
3. Avoid unnecessary CVP monitoring. Complications are common, particularly sepsis. If bacteraemia exists the catheter may provide a focus for continued infection. Local trauma from the catheter insertion needle may occur and catheter embolism is possible.
4. The vein. For access, use a large vein of the upper arm or antecubital fossa, or the internal jugular vein in the neck. Venepuncture is easier in the upper limb, but correct catheter placement is more likely if the internal jugular vein is used. Access to the right atrium via the subclavian vein is more hazardous than other routes.
5. The catheter. Many special catheters are available. They usually consist of a long radio-opaque catheter which can be inserted in a non-touch manner through a needle or cannula inserted through the skin into a suitable vein (e.g. Argyle Intramedicut, Abbott Drum Cartridge catheter). If the internal jugular vein is used it is possible to insert one of the many short disposable percutaneous cannulae designed for intravenous infusions, since no valves intervene between this vessel and the heart. Alternatively a short large-bore cannula can be inserted into the internal jugular vein and a longer and finer catheter passed through this into a central position.

Internal jugular vein catheterization

1. With the head turned to the opposite side the surface markings of the internal jugular vein can be represented as a broad line drawn from the lobe of the ear to the medial end of the clavicle. The vein lies posterior to the external carotid artery in the upper third of the neck, lateral to the common carotid in the middle third and anterolateral to it in the lower third. The sternomastoid muscle overlaps the vein in its upper course. Lower down in the neck the vein lies deep and just lateral to the medial edge of the clavicular head of the sternomastoid muscle. The right internal jugular vein is used more commonly than the left, as on this side the internal jugular vein, innominate vein and superior vena cava are almost in line. There is some risk of injuring the thoracic duct if the left side is used.
2. Tilt the patient head-down 20–30° in order to distend the vein and reduce the risk of air embolus. Turn the head to side opposite to that of the proposed cannulation. It may be possible to palpate the vein deep to the sternomastoid muscle.
3. Thoroughly clean the skin. Sepsis involving CVP catheters may be dangerous.
4. Raise an intradermal weal with a small amount of local anaesthetic just lateral to the carotid artery midway between the ear lobe and the medial end of the clavicle. Make a small skin incision with the point of a scalpel blade.
5. Use the fingers of the left hand to displace the carotid artery medially, insert the needle at an angle of about 35° to the skin, aiming for the sternal end of the clavicle. A 'give' is felt as the deep fascia is pierced and another as the vein is entered. Reflux of venous blood confirms entry. Advance along the vein for a further 1 cm and then withdraw the needle from the cannula. Either advance the cannula for its full length into the vein, or pass a catheter through the cannula into the superior vena cava and withdraw the cannula.

Antecubital fossa catheterization

1. It is easier to pass a catheter centrally from the cephalic rather than the basilic vein. Enter the needle-catheter assembly into the vein as for routine venous cannulation. Once the needle has fully entered the vein advance the catheter through it.
2. Difficulties often arise as the catheter traverses fascial layers at the shoulder and root of the neck. Try abducting the arm to aid passage of the catheter into the thorax. A frequent cause of failure when this route is used for central venous catheterization is persistent passage of the catheter into the internal jugular vein.

Correct placement of CVP catheters

1. The tip of the catheter should lie in or near the right atrium. Pressure readings must fluctuate with respiration and blood must flow freely back along the catheter on aspiration.
2. Appearance of a sudden high pressure in the catheter indicates entry into the right ventricle, as may the appearance of extrasystoles. The catheter should be withdrawn until the high pressure disappears and then for a further 2–3 cm.
3. Confirm that the catheter is correctly placed with a chest X-ray, since these catheters are radio-opaque.

Care of CVP catheters

1. A central venous line provides a first class route for the entry of bacteria into the circulation.
2. Observe strict sterile precautions during insertion of the line, and also when infusion fluids and administration sets are changed.

3. Inject any drugs slowly through a central line to prevent bolus effects on the heart.

Measurement

1. Connect the CVP catheter to a simple saline manometer, using a three-way tap so that a slow infusion of crystalloid runs through the catheter at all times except when measurements are being recorded.

2. Adjust the height of the fluid level in the manometer so it is level with the patient's mid-axillary line, or 10 cm below the sternal angle. Use a rod bearing a spirit level or a simple optical sight. Remember that changing the position of the patient will affect the zero reading of the CVP manometer.

3. To measure CVP use the three-way tap to raise the level of fluid in the manometer above the predicted CVP level. Then turn the tap to connect the manometer directly to the catheter and allow the fluid level to fall to the correct level.

Significance of the CVP

1. The 'normal' CVP is in the range of 2–10 cm saline. Limited reliance can be placed upon isolated CVP readings as, in clinical circumstances, there is often uncertainty as to the exact position of the catheter tip and the zero reference point is usually an arbitrary one. A very low CVP reading probably indicates hypovolaemia, whilst a high reading may result from either fluid overload or right heart failure.

2. A useful application of the CVP during fluid replacement therapy is to observe the response to a rapid infusion of 50–100 ml of saline. In the normal circulation the response to this manoeuvre is a rise of CVP of a few cm of saline and a fall to the initial levels within a few minutes. Failure of the CVP to rise or a very brief pressure rise indicates hypovolaemia. A sustained pressure rise indicates either fluid overload or heart failure. CVP measurements give semi-quantitative information on the ability of the right side of the heart to cope with the load being presented to it.

3. If, during resuscitation, the interpretation of CVP measurements is difficult, and there are doubts as to the patient's true cardiac state, it may be necessary to catheterize the pulmonary artery. Flow-directed catheters can be placed in the pulmonary artery without X-ray control. The 'wedge' pressure obtained by wedging the tip of the catheter into a pulmonary arteriole reflects left atrial pressure and thus gives an indication of left ventricular function.

LOCAL ANAESTHESIA
Appraise

1. Virtually every surgical procedure that is normally performed under general anaesthesia can be carried out using local anaesthetic techniques. However, it must not be thought that because a patient is not asleep that local techniques are necessarily safer than general ones. All local anaesthetic agents have toxic effects. Some local anaesthetic techniques require the use of high doses of local anaesthetic agents. Local anaesthetic techniques do not prevent the physiological disturbances of body function which are a consequence of most surgical procedures.

2. Local anaesthetic techniques can be dangerous. Many patients have died because of these agents. The morbidity and mortality associated with local anaesthetic techniques is invariably related not to the operator's inability to perform a particular nerve block but to his inability to rapidly and effectively counter unexpected toxic effects. Do not use local anaesthetic techniques until you are well versed in the relevant aspects of resuscitation.

3. The commonest applications of local techniques used by a surgeon are the removal of small superficial non-infected lesions and minor surgery on the hands.

Methods

1. *Topical anaesthesia* — application of local anaesthetics to the mucous membranes of the conjunctival sac, nose, tracheobronchial tree or urethra.

2. *Local infiltration* — direct injection of the anaesthetic into the operative site.

3. *Field block* — injection of local anaesthetic around the operative site so as to create an analgesic zone.

4. *Regional intravenous anaesthesia* — injection of a large volume of diluted local anaesthetic into a previously exsanguinated limb.

5. *Regional blocks* — injection of local anaesthetic around the nerve or nerves specifically supplying the region to be operated upon:
(a) Peripheral nerve blocks
(b) Extradural blockade — injection of local anaesthetic into the extradural (or caudal) space affects the nerves in that space or the agent can diffuse out through the intervertebral foramina
(c) Spinal anaesthesia — insertion of local anaesthetic drugs into the subarachnoid space.

Drugs

1. A large number of local anaesthetic agents are available. Only a few will be detailed here. Most local anaesthetics are used as the soluble hydrochlorides. Before they can act in the body they must dissociate to liberate the free base and dissociation is inhibited in an acid medium. This is the reason why poor anaesthesia usually results when local anaesthetics are injected into inflamed tissues.

2. The duration and intensity of action of local anaesthetics is increased if they are combined with vasoconstrictors such as adrenaline. By retarding absorption vasoconstrictors will also reduce the toxicity of local anaesthetics. For infiltration concentrations of 1 in 250 000 of adrenaline may be used (by the addition of 1 mg of ad-

renaline tartrate to 250 ml of local anaesthetic solution). There are no advantages in using higher concentrations than this. The total amount of adrenaline injected should not exceed 0.5 mg. Do not add adrenaline to local anaesthetics which are to be injected into areas supplied by end arteries, such as the fingers, toes and penis, as prolonged ischaemia may here lead to tissue necrosis. Addition of adrenaline is usually unnecessary and probably unwise in outpatients undergoing minor surgery.

3. Lignocaine. This is probably the most widely used local anaesthetic. It is stable, only moderately toxic, produces no vasodilatation, has a relatively rapid onset of action and a duration of 60–90 minutes. It is used in concentrations of 4 per cent for topical anaesthesia and concentrations of 0.5–2% for infiltration and nerve blocks. The maximum safe dose is 3 mg per kg body weight when used without adrenaline and 7 mg per kg used with adrenaline.

4. Prilocaine. Chemically related to lignocaine, prilocaine is less toxic but also less potent. Duration of action is less influenced by the addition of adrenaline than is the case with lignocaine. Prilocaine is used as a 4% solution for topical anaesthesia and in concentrations of 1–3% for nerve blocks. The maximum safe dose is in the order of 10 mg per kg. Excessive doses of prilocaine produce methaemoglobinaemia which may cause cyanosis. Hypoxia results from administration of more than 15 mg per kg.

5. Bupivicaine. The major advantage of bupivicaine over other local anaesthetics is the prolonged duration of anaesthesia it produces, which varies between 5 and 16 hours. Bupivicaine is about four times as potent as lignocaine. It is used in concentrations of 0.25–0.5%, and the maximum dose is 2 mg per kg.

Toxicity

1. All local anaesthetics exert toxic effects when given in excessive doses. Inadvertent intravascular administration even in small doses can cause toxic actions. The important toxic actions manifest themselves in the central nervous and cardiovascular systems resulting in restlessness, convulsions, hypotension, bradycardia, and in extreme cases, respiratory and cardiac arrest.

2. Management of these toxic effects includes the use of oxygen therapy, anticonvulsants and pressor agents. Endotracheal intubation and artificial ventilation may be necessary. It is for this reason that resuscitative equipment must always be available when local anaesthetics are used.

TECHNIQUE

Appraise

It is outside the scope of this book to desribe all of the various local anaesthetic techniques that can be employed during surgery. In this section I shall describe the general approach to the use of local anaesthesia and describe infiltration anaesthesia for surgery of small superficial lesions, digital nerve block and intravenous regional anaesthesia. Details of other uses of local anaesthesia can be found in textbooks devoted to the subject. It is not difficult to learn how to execute most local blocks. Two important warnings must be given about the use of local anaesthesia:

1. No matter how apparently trivial a local block is, always have means of resuscitation available. Dire effects can result from very small amounts of local anaesthetic agents inadvertently injected into the wrong place.

2. Never perform any but the most trivial blocks singlehanded. Toxic effects of local anaesthetic drugs can develop insidiously. A single-handed operator-anaesthetist who is engrossed in the surgery he is performing is not in a good position to observe the patient or to treat untoward reactions.

Prepare

1. Apply skin cleansing fluid and suitable drapes. 2% iodine in spirit or 70% alcohol are widely used for skin sterilization.

2. Have 10 ml and 2 ml syringes. Use 25 swg needles (colour code orange) for the initial intradermal injections and 23 swg needles (colour code blue) for infiltration. Use a separate wide-bore needle to draw up local anaesthetic solutions from ampoules.

3. Choose local anaesthetic drugs. 0.5 or 1% lignocaine or prilocaine without adrenaline is suitable for most nerve blocks or infiltrations. Calculate the maximum allowed dose before starting the block. For instance, in a 70 kg adult the maximum dose of lignocaine (without adrenaline) is 210 mg. 1% lignocaine contains 10 mg per ml, therefore do not use more than 21 ml.

4. Check the resuscitation equipment. This need not be very elaborate. The minimum resuscitation equipment consists of a means of ventilating a patient with high concentrations of oxygen, drugs to deal with convulsions and means of combating sudden circulatory failure. A cylinder of oxygen with a reducing valve, a resuscitating bag such as the Ambu, Air Viva or Laerdal, thiopentone (as an anticonvulsant) and an ampoule of metaraminol will thus suffice for resuscitation during simple blocks.

Action

1. Explain to the patient what is going to happen. Stress that he will feel no pain, but he may still feel touch.

2. Study the landmarks of the area before scrubbing up.

3. Treat this as a sterile procedure. Scrub up and wear a gown and gloves. Fully prepare the skin and cover with suitable drapes.

4. Use a small amount of local anaesthetic from a 2 ml syringe to raise skin blebs, using a fine needle for the purpose.

5. When infiltrating local anaesthetic inject as the needle is being moved. When injecting round specific nerves aspirate before injecting. These precautions will minimize the likelihood of intravascular injection.

6. Be on the constant lookout for untoward reactions to the local anaesthetic. Drowsiness and slurring of speech are early signs of central nervous system toxicity. If you see these prodromal signs, stop injecting local anaesthetic and be prepared to initiate urgent treatment.

7. Wait for 10–15 minutes after the block is completed for the local anaesthetic to take full effect. Be careful in testing whether a block is working that you or the patient do not confuse the sensation of pain with that of touch.

8. Operations performed under local anaesthesia must be carried out in a quiet atmosphere. Keep casual non-relevant conversation to a minimum.

9. Warn the patient that he may feel some discomfort after 1–2 hours when the block begins to wear off.

INFILTRATION ANAESTHESIA

1. Infiltration of a local anaesthetic agent is useful for providing good operating conditions for the removal of small superficial lesions, such as sebaceous cysts and lipomata.

2. Do not use infiltration anaesthesia for the removal of infected lesions, as adequate sensory block is unlikely to be achieved.

3. Follow the general advice on equipment and actions as detailed above, raise a small skin bleb adjacent to the lesion and then infiltrate though this bleb, attempting to place the local anaesthetic so that it spreads along tissue planes and the lesion 'floats' in an anaesthetized area.

4. Allow an adequate time for the local anaesthetic to take effect before commencing surgery.

DIGITAL NERVE BLOCK

1. This block is frequently used in casualty departments for minor operations on the fingers.

2. Do no use it for the incision of an infected finger — local anaesthetics may not work effectively in tissues adjacent to an infected area and there are dangers of spreading the infection.

3. Never add adrenaline to the local anaesthetic used for this block. The prolonged ischaemia that this may cause can lead to gangrene of the finger.

4. The digital nerves pass along the anterolateral line of the finger. Raise a skin bleb over the dorsum of the proximal phalanx. Pass a 23 swg needle through this to deposit about 2 ml of 1% lignocaine on either side of the phalanx.

5. Up to 20 minutes may be needed before analgesia is complete.

INTRAVENOUS REGIONAL ANAESTHESIA

Appraise

1. In this technique dilute local anaesthetic is injected into the venous system of a limb which has been exsanguinated and is kept isolated from the rest of the circulation. The block is commonly known as a 'Bier's block', having been initially described by Bier in 1908.

2. The local anaesthetic exerts its action by diffusing from the vascular system into the tissues and thus affecting the terminal branches of sensory nerves. This is a very useful but potentially very dangerous block.

3. Never perform this block single-handed. The main danger is failure of the occluding tourniquet and the sudden release of a large amount of local anaesthetic into the circulation. For this reason it is essential for one suitably trained and qualified person to be responsible for the block whilst another performs the necessary surgery.

4. This block works best in the upper limb. It can be used in the leg, but the larger doses of local anaesthetic needed make its use for this purpose more dangerous.

Action

1. Insert an indwelling 23 swg 'butterfly' needle into a suitable vein not adjacent to the operation site.

2. Apply two pneumatic tourniquets to the upper arm. A special double cuffed tourniquet is also available.

3. Exsanguinate the arm, using an Esmarch rubber bandage, elevation for 3 minutes or an inflatable splint.

4. Inflate the upper tourniquet cuff to above systolic blood pressure, then remove the Esmarch bandage or inflatable splint.

5. Inject local anaesthetic through the indwelling needle. Use 0.5% prilocaine. The average volume needed for the upper arm of an adult is 40 ml. Do not exceed 3 mg per kg. The local anaesthetic will start to take effect within 5 minutes.

6. After 10 minutes inflate the lower cuff to above systolic pressure and then release the upper cuff. By this time the arm beneath the lower cuff will be anaesthetized and the patient will not experience tourniquet pain.

7. Throughout the procedure pay constant attention to the degree of inflation of the cuffs. Pneumatic tourniquet cuffs commonly leak. Confusion can arise if the same pump or inflating system is used to inflate both cuffs.

8. At the end of the procedure deflate the cuff. Sensation will not be totally restored immediately as the local anaesthetic has diffused from the circulation into the tissues.

9. Do not deflate the cuff until at least 20 minutes has elapsed from the time of injection of local anaesthetic. This allows adequate time for anaesthetic to diffuse from the vessels, and reduces the chance of a large bolus of anaesthetic being released into the circulation.

Further reading

Eriksson E 1979 Illustrated handbook in local anaesthesia, 2nd edn. Munksgaard, Copenhagen
Wilson F, Park W G 1980 Basic resuscitation. MTP Press, Lancaster

Surgery of the abdominal wall

INGUINAL HERNIA

Appraise

1. In the past indirect hernias were usually repaired, diffuse direct hernias were treated with a truss. Now it is customary to operate on most inguinal hernias.

2. In a very obese patient with a large, diffuse direct hernia, defer operation until the patient has lost weight.

3. Trusses are rarely prescribed. Most patients have operations and the few who do not are usually better left without a truss, which often requires considerable skill to manage.

4. In Britain, surgical repair of inguinal hernias is usually performed under general anaesthesia but in patients with cardiovascular or respiratory disease, epidural or local anaesthesia can be used. At the Shouldice Clinic in Toronto, the vast majority of hernias are repaired under local anaesthesia. There are economic pressures for hernia repairs to be carried out on a short stay basis. Local anaesthesia is therefore increasingly used.

5. Never fail to see the hernia yourself and mark the side with indelible skin marker. Check again that you have the correct patient and are sure which side you will repair.

6. Bilateral hernias may be repaired at the same time but the results are not quite so good as when they are repaired separately. Do not hesitate to repair a severe hernia on one side, deferring repair of a minor hernia on the other side until later.

7. If this is a recurrent hernia and repair will be difficult, will it be necessary, in a male patient, to replace the testis in the abdomen or remove it? If so, discuss it with the patient and obtain written consent.

8. Many surgeons accept the challenge of repairing recurrent diffuse hernias in obese patients with stretched, fat-infiltrated tissues or with chronic coughs. I am reluctant to do so. These patients are not at risk of strangulation and recurrence is likely following repair. As a trainee, do not embark on these operations.

Local anaesthesia

1. Make up sterile dilute lignocaine, 100 ml 0.25% to which is added 0.5 ml 1 in 1000 adrenaline (epinephrine). Mix well and inject 20 ml along the line of the proposed incision using a fine needle to raise a continuous bleb within the epidermis.

2. Replace the needle with a larger one to inject deeper and along the same line superficial to the anterior wall of the canal.

3. Inject a pool of fluid laterally into and through the external oblique aponeurosis to block the iliohypogastric and ilio-inguinal nerves.

4. Reserve about half the anaesthetic to inject around the neck of the sac and into other sensitive areas during the operation.

Access

1. Make an incision 2 cm above the medial two-thirds of the inguinal ligament, after identifying the pubic

tubercle and anterior superior iliac spine. Cut through the fascia to expose the external oblique aponeurosis, ligating and dividing two or three veins which cross the line of the incision. Avoid cutting into the hernial sac and spermatic cord at the medial end of the incision.

2. Apply wound towels to the skin edges.

3. With a gauze swab, sweep the superficial fascia from the external oblique aponeurosis on each side of the line of the inguinal canal to expose the glistening fibres.

4. Identify the external inguinal ring and the line of the inguinal canal. Make a short split with a knife in the line of the fibres of the external oblique aponeurosis over the inguinal canal. Enlarge the split medially and laterally by pushing the half-closed blades of the scissors in the line of the fibres. At the medial end of the split, the external inguinal ring will be opened.

5. Apply artery forceps to the edges of the aponeurosis and gently elevate each side. As the upper leaf is turned back, look for the arching lower border of internal oblique muscle, with the cord below it. As the lower leaf is everted, sweep loose tissue from the deep surface of the inguinal ligament.

HERNIAL SAC

Indirect sac

1. Pick up the cord where it crosses the pubic tubercle. There is a 'mesentery' of fascia which must be broken through posteriorly, then the cord may be enclosed in ring forceps.

2. With the left thumb in front, gently stretch the cord over the left index finger, which is placed behind the cord. Make a short split with a knife, in the line of the cord, through the cremasteric and internal spermatic fascial layers. Continue the split in the fascial layers proximally to the internal ring using scissors, first with their blades on the flat, separating fascia from deeper layers, then splitting the fascia.

3. Look for the sac. A white curved edge may be seen if the hernial sac is small (Fig. 3.1); if it is large it will be obvious as the fascial layers are separated. If the vas and vessels are seen with no intervening sac, and can be followed back to the internal ring, look for a direct sac or a femoral hernia.

4. Pick up the sac with two artery forceps and open it between the forceps with a knife. Note any contents of the sac and return them to the peritoneal cavity.

5. Pass the little finger through the neck if it will slip through easily; ensure that the finger reaches the main peritoneal cavity and can be moved in all directions. Feel the posterior wall of the inguinal canal and the femoral canal from inside the abdomen.

6. Grasp the emptied sac with three or four artery for-

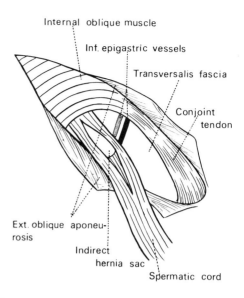

Internal oblique muscle

Inf. epigastric vessels

Transversalis fascia

Conjoint tendon

Ext. oblique aponeurosis

Indirect hernia sac

Spermatic cord

Fig. 3.1 Exposure of the right inguinal canal. The cremasteric fascia of the cord is split to show an indirect hernial sac.

ceps and isolate it up to the neck by gently wiping off the other structures with a gauze swab, snipping firm attachments with scissors. Keep the dissection close to the sac to avoid damaging other structures in the cord.

7. While the empty sac is held vertically by means of the artery forceps, transfix its neck with a suture of chromic catgut mounted on a round-bodied needle. Tie the ends of the suture-ligature into a half hitch, completely encircle the neck of the sac and tie a triple throw knot. Ligate the neck of the sac.

8. Do not let your assistant cut the catgut. First excise the sac 1 cm distal to the ligature. Examine the cut end to ensure that only sac is seen, then cut the ligature yourself.

Large sac

1. Complete hernias, or scrotal funicular hernias, have no distal edge to the sac as seen at the level of the pubic tubercle. Attempts to dissect out the whole sac cause the scrotal part of the sac and the testis to be drawn into the wound.

2. The sac should be purposefully divided straight across at the level of the pubic tubercle. Isolate the proximal portion up to the internal ring, and leave the distal portion open. In this way the dissection is kept to a minimum.

3. After opening the sac in front, place artery forceps at intervals round the inside as markers. Lift up two forceps, stretch the portion of sac between them, separate the sac from the other structures and cut it distal to the forceps. Take the next two forceps and repeat the manoeuvre. Continue in this manner until the proximal circum-

ference of the sac is completely sectioned, with the edges still held in the forceps.

4. After stripping the proximal part of the sac to the inguinal ring, transfix and ligate the neck.

5. Leave the distal part of the sac open.

SLIDING HERNIA

1. In some hernias, abdominal retroperitoneal structures slide down to form part of the sac wall. The caecum, sigmoid colon or bladder are most commonly found.

3. The organ lying outside the sac is discovered when an attempt is made to empty and free the sac.

3. If the sac is intact, do not open it if it is small.

4. If the sac has been opened, mark the fringe of peritoneum on the viscus with artery forceps and close the sac. Ensure that closure is complete.

5. Before replacing the viscus inside the abdomen, make sure that neither the organ nor its blood supply was damaged before the true situation was recognized. If the bladder was damaged, repair the wall and remember to insert an indwelling urethral catheter at the end of the operation.

6. Replace the viscus, together with the sac, in the abdomen.

7. Carry out the best possible repair of the posterior wall of the inguinal canal. If a sound repair cannot be achieved in any other way it may be necessary to divide the cord so that there is no gap in the repair. When a sliding hernia is suspected before operation, discuss the possibility with the patient and where necessary obtain written permission to cut the spermatic cord, and if need be, remove the testis.

HERNIA IN INFANTS

1. Infants' tissues are not suitable for handling by impatient or rough surgeons.

2. Exposure is difficult if the pubic fat is thick. The well-developed deep fascia is easily mistaken for the external aponeurosis.

3. The internal and external rings are superimposed at this age and it is therefore unnecessary to split the external oblique aponeurosis.

4. Isolate the cord just distal to the external ring, open the external fascial layers of the cord and look for the sac. Pick up each layer with two pairs of fine artery forceps and open it between the forceps in the line of the cord. A short sac can be recognized by the white curved distal edge. The easy movement of the slippery internal surfaces of a large sac helps in identifying it. Make sure you are in the correct layer. When the sac is opened, the inner wall is shiny and slippery and the tips of the forceps can be passed into the peritoneal cavity.

5. Take great care in dissecting the fragile sac proximally. Avoid tearing or splitting it. Avoid damaging the inconspicuous and adherent vas deferens. At the external ring, transfix, ligate and divide the neck of the sac. Do not twist the sac, because the vas may be inadvertently twisted with it and damaged.

6. Narrow the external ring with one or two chromic catgut stitches if it has been stretched by a large hernia. No other repair is usually necessary in an infant.

HERNIA IN WOMEN

1. The approach is similar to that employed in men

2. The round ligament of the ovary lies in the position of the male spermatic cord.

3. Recognize and isolate the sac, then transfix, ligate and divide it at its neck.

4. If the hernial sac is small, herniotomy is sufficient. Repair a larger hernia by Bassini's method (see p. 29) and divide and ligate the round ligament at the level of the internal ring so that the posterior wall of the inguinal canal can be completely closed.

DIRECT HERNIA

1. Always look for an indirect sac first.

2. Elevate the cord to expose the posterior wall of the inguinal canal and look for the direct sac.

3. If the sac is funicular, resulting from a localized defect in the posterior wall, isolate it, empty it, then transfix, ligate and divide it at the neck. Define the margins of the posterior wall defect. If the hole is small and it can be closed without tension, suture it now, with non-absorbable material on a fine, curved, round-bodied needle.

4. If the sac is diffuse and associated with a general weakness of the posterior wall, do not open it unless it is so big that a portion must be excised. Remember that the urinary bladder is frequently drawn into the medial wall of the hernia.

5. If the sac is to be left unopened, push it inwards and maintain the invagination by a running suture carried across the wide neck. The sutures must not bite deeply or the bowel or bladder may be damaged. Use chromic catgut size 0 on an eyeless needle.

6. Carry out a suitable repair of the posterior wall of the canal.

Difficulty?

1. If you cannot find the sac or recognize the tissues first find the vas deferens which can be felt as a string-like structure towards the back of the cord. The testicular vessels lie near the vas and once these are separated, the rest

of the cord may be cautiously divided, starting at the front, while keeping in mind that abdominal organs may be encountered. If a structure seems to be the sac, cautiously open it after tenting a portion between two artery forceps. Look for a glistening inner surface and insert a finger to determine if the sac communicates with the peritoneal cavity.

2. Torn neck of sac? Carefully free peritoneum from the abdomen to form a new neck.

3. Sometimes large lipomatous masses of extraperitoneal fat are found. Isolate them and divide them with care, ligating the proximal ends. Ensure that there is no peritoneal sac in any of them.

4. If the neck of the hernial sac passes below the inguinal ligament, this is a femoral hernia. The repair can be successfully carried out through the inguinal canal.

REPAIR

1. In an infant, a child or young adult with a small indirect hernia, herniotomy is all that is required.

2. If the margins of the internal ring have been stretched by an indirect hernia, narrow the gap in the posterior wall using a non-absorbable suture, such as 00 silk or nylon, or 60 linen thread, mounted on a fine curved needle.

3. If the hernia is direct, re-examine the posterior wall of the inguinal canal to see if anything further can be done to leave a firm, flat wall. Sometimes a few sutures may plicate a weak, bulging area, leaving it stronger.

4. Further repairs to the posterior wall in general use are of two types which may be used separately, or combined (Fig. 3.2).

(a) Tissues are brought in from the margins to strengthen the posterior wall. In the Bassini repair, the lower fibres of the internal oblique and transversus abdominis muscles, with their medial aponeurosis, are sutured to the inguinal ligament behind the cord. In the Halsted repair, the external oblique aponeurosis is also repaired behind the cord.

(b) Natural or artificial material may be inserted as a sheet to bridge the defect. The insert must be large enough to reach firm tissue on all sides, otherwise the repair will fail, however strong the implanted sheet.

Bassini's repair

1. Evert the lowest leaf of the external oblique aponeurosis. Identify the inner surface of the inguinal ligament from the pubic tubercle to the internal ring.

2. Evert the upper leaf and identify the arching muscle and aponeurosis of internal oblique and transversus muscles. Firm tissue is best identified by feel rather than by sight.

3. Suture the aponeurosis and muscles to the inguinal

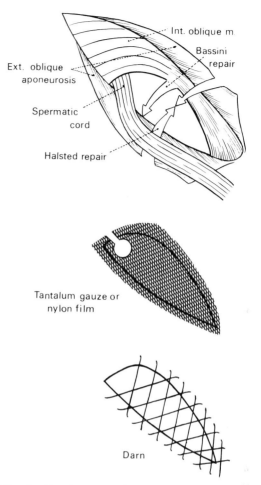

Fig. 3.2 Repair of inguinal hernia. The defect may be closed by drawing the edges together, by inserting a sheet of material, or by means of a darn.

ligament, starting medially, taking a good bite of the aponeurosis and of the periosteum over the pubic tubercle. Carry the union laterally, behind the cord as far as the internal ring, where the emerging cord is enclosed snugly. The sutures may be of 0 or 1 chromic catgut (although absorbable stitches are out of favour), 00 silk, 60 linen, 00 monofilament nylon or other synthetic material. The stitches may be interrupted single, mattress 'X' or 'N', or may be continuous running or locked. A fine needle is essential, preferably an eyeless type, since the stitch holes are potential sites of weakness.

4. Two modifications may be used where appropriate:

(a) Tanner 'slide'

(i) Apposition of the conjoint tendon to the inguinal ligament may result in tension. A relaxing incision prevents this.

(ii) Separate the upper leaf of external oblique aponeurosis from the aponeuroses of the internal oblique and transversus abdominis muscles, starting at the level of the pubic tubercle as far medially as possible. Extend the incision upwards for a hand's breadth, then curve it laterally to within 2 cm of the lateral edge of the rectus muscle.

(iii) The conjoint tendon now slides down towards the inguinal ligament without tension, opening up a gap at the relaxing incision through which the rectus muscle is seen.

(iv) Suture the lower margin of the gap to the rectus muscle, to prevent the edge rolling downwards.

(b) Complete closure of the inguinal canal

(i) If the spermatic cord is divided the conjoint tendon can be completely approximated to the inguinal ligament. The testis sometimes survives, but it is usually safer to perform orchidectomy. Make sure you obtained written permission before operation.

(ii) Many patients, even when elderly, do not wish to have an orchidectomy. An alternative is to mobilize the testis and cord and tuck them laterally, deep to the origin of the lowest fibres of transversus abdominis muscle, so that the canal can be closed in front of them. If the testis is placed within the abdomen the risk of malignant change occurring is increased to equal the risk of a normal woman developing malignant change in her intra-abdominal ovaries. It can be ignored in elderly men with difficult and recurrent hernias.

Darn

1. This may be used alone to fill the gap between the conjoint tendon and the inguinal ligament. It may also be used to overlay and reinforce sutures which pull the margins together.

2. Use two layers; the threads of the second layer are angled in a different direction from those of the first layer. Size 00 silk or monofilament nylon or 60 linen thread are satisfactory; braided or floss nylon, floss silk, strips of fascia lata and other materials have also been successfully used. The author deprecates the use of fascia lata strips; the stitch holes are so large that they form good starting places for recurrences.

Implants

1. Natural or synthetic materials in sheet form enjoyed a vogue for repairing large defects. At different times silver filigree, tantalum gauze, stretched skin, plastic mesh have been tried for closing large defects. The author is reluctant to offer surgical repair to a patient with a large diffuse hernia and badly stretched tissues. The patient runs no risk of strangulation, repair is difficult and recurrence likely.

2. The inserted material must extend in all directions beyond the weak area, where it is stitched to firm tissues, using sutures of non-absorbable material.

Shouldice repair

1. Although this is a variant of Bassini's technique the results obtained at the Shouldice Clinic in Toronto are so outstanding that the method is increasingly used elsewhere. Hernia repairs alone are carried out at the Clinic. Many thousands of patients have been operated upon usually under local anaesthesia, as short stay patients. The same technique is used for all types of hernia and the recurrence rate for primary repairs is well below 1%.

2. Of course much credit must go to the operators who accumulate a vast experience and any operation carried out many times using an unvaried technique produces better and better results. However, other surgeons achieve comparable results using the Shouldice method.

Action

1. Isolate, elevate, open, empty, ligate the neck, and excise the sac.

2. The essential step is the repair of the transversalis fascia at the neck of the sac and along the posterior wall of the canal (Fig. 3.3). Dissect free the transversalis fascia around the medial part of the internal inguinal ring, separating it from the extraperitoneal tissues and the inferior epigastric vessels. Do not hesitate to reduce the bulk of the cord by excising loose cremasteric muscle, fascia and fat.

3. Divide the transversalis fascia from the medial edge of the internal ring along the length of the canal midway between the conjoint tendon and the inguinal ligament.

4. Elevate the upper flap.

5. Elevate the lower flap down to the inguinal ligament, doubly clamping, ligating and dividing the cremasteric vessels that arise from the inferior epigastric vessels and pierce the lower leaf.

6. The transversalis fascia will be repaired by overlapping the edges. Suture the edge of the lower flap to the under surface of the upper flap with a running stitch of metric 3 polypropylene. Deliberately insert the stitches slightly irregularly: if the depth of bite is uniform a strip of transversalis fascia may be pulled off, vitiating the repair. Lay the overlapping portion of the upper flap down over the lower flap and continue the running stitch to secure its edge to the outer surface of the lower flap. Make sure that this refashions the internal ring snugly around the emerging cord.

7. Now complete the Bassini repair by suturing the conjoint tendon down to the inguinal ligament. Use a layer of irregularly inserted, running, metric 3 polypropylene stitches to draw the deep surface of the conjoint tendon down to the inguinal ligament, followed by a second layer of

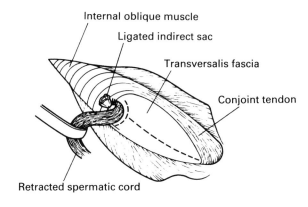

Internal oblique muscle
Ligated indirect sac
Transversalis fascia
Conjoint tendon
Retracted spermatic cord

a

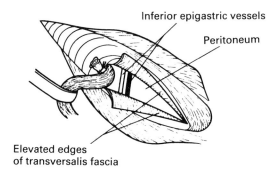

Inferior epigastric vessels
Peritoneum
Elevated edges
of transversalis fascia

b

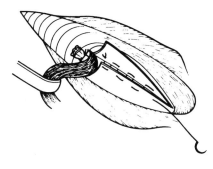

c

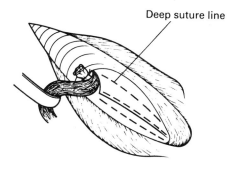

Deep suture line

d

Fig. 3.3 Shouldice repair. a) The broken line is the incision in transversalis fascia and around the internal ring ; b) The upper and lower flaps have been elevated; c) The lower flap is sutured to the under surface of the upper flap; d) The upper flap is sutured over the lower flap.

sutures uniting the lower edge of the conjoint tendon to the deep surface of the external oblique aponeurosis just above and parallel to the inguinal ligament.

8. In the Shouldice Clinic patients frequently walk on and walk off the operating table, having had the procedure performed under local anaesthesia.

Closure

1. Lay the cord in its original position.

2. Repair the split in the external oblique aponeurosis starting laterally, using a continuous suture of 0 chromic catgut mounted on a fine, curved, round-bodied needle. Refashion the external ring by closing the external oblique snugly around the emerging cord.

3. If the patient is a woman, or if the cord has been cut in a man, the external oblique aponeurosis may be completely closed.

4. Appose the subcutaneous fascia with 00 plain catgut sutures mounted on fine, curved, round-bodied needles.

5. Close the skin wound with stitches, clips or adhesive strips.

RECURRENT HERNIA

It is advisable, where appropriate, to obtain written permission from the patient to divide the cord and excise the testis if necessary.

Access

1. Excise the previous skin scar.

2. Deepen the incision at a higher level than the previous approach, so that unscarred external oblique aponeurosis is encountered.

3. Display the external oblique aponeurosis downwards to the inguinal ligament.

4. Re-open the inguinal canal through the scar in the external oblique aponeurosis. Avoid damaging the contents of the canal which may be adherent.

5. Elevate the upper and lower leaves of the external oblique aponeurosis until you reach unscarred tissue.

6. Isolate the spermatic cord below the pubic tubercle and free it up to the internal ring.

Action

Hernial sac

1. Look for an indirect recurrence. If a sac is found isolate it, empty it, then transfix, ligate and divide it at the neck.

2. Look for a direct recurrence. If the recurrence is funicular, isolate it, empty it, then transfix, ligate and divide

it at the neck. If it is a diffuse bulge, invert the sac and suture the wide neck to maintain the invagination.

Repair

1. Dissect the edges of the posterior wall of the canal until you reach firm tissue. Make a decision regarding the form of repair.

2. Is it possible to carry out any preliminary repair of the posterior wall or inguinal ring?

3. Are the margins of the defect widely separated? Will they come together, with or without a relaxing incision, or will it be necessary to bridge the defect with a darn or an insert?

4. Is it necessary to cut the cord and to remove the testis? Can the testis and cord be replaced in the abdomen?

Difficulty?

1. The procedure that has been outlined for the repair of a recurrent hernia assumes that the anatomical relationships have not been altered by previous operations. There are several findings which may perplex the surgeon.

2. In the Halsted method, the posterior wall was reinforced by closing the external oblique aponeurosis behind the cord, bringing the cord through the external oblique laterally, thus superimposing the internal and external rings. A recurrence may appear alongside the cord, leaving the rest of the repair sound. Isolate the sac, empty it, then transfix, ligate and divide it at the neck. Define the edges of the stretched ring. If appropriate, divide the spermatic cord. Narrow the ring or close it with strong sutures. Attempts to reopen the canal are difficult because the posterior wall and the external oblique aponeurosis tend to fuse. A medial recurrence is fortunately rare, but is best repaired by defining the edges and apposing them if possible; a wide darn is made to bridge the weak area.

3. The previous use of a tantalum gauze or plastic mesh insert may result in a recurrent hernia in which the tissues are matted together, making dissection difficult, because the knife or scissors encounter the rolled-up edge of the metal gauze or mesh. When the recurrence is a small one, treat it when possible as a local condition; excise the sac, clean the margins of the defect and suture them together. When the defect is large, or when there are multiple defects, excise the inserted gauze and define the edges of the total defect. Deal with the sac and perform the best possible repair with the tissues available. The layers are fused together and it is better to make a good one-layer closure than attempt to split the layers.

4. Recurrences following darns with non-absorbable material or fascia lata are usually local defects. Leave the sound parts undisturbed.

Aftercare

1. Following repair of inguinal hernia under local anaesthesia, the patient may walk immediately with help to a wheelchair to leave the operating theatre. Following a general anaesthetic the patient may walk the next day with help.

2. Some surgeons repair hernias from Day wards or from '5-Day' wards. Most patients benefit from early mobilization and discharge.

3. Sutures may be removed after 5 days either in the clinic or by arrangement with the District Nurse at home.

4. Activities should be increased gradually. A fit slim male who performs a physically demanding job should be back at work within 4–6 weeks. Sedentary workers can return to work after 1 week.

5. Many pateints ask what is the likelihood of recurrence and what can they do to avoid the possibility. There is but one way in which they can prejudice the repair and that is to increase weight, especially if this is rapid.

FEMORAL HERNIA

Appraise

1. It is usually accepted that all femoral hernias are repaired because of the fear of strangulation, but there are no absolute rules in surgery. Occasionally a patient is seen who is very old, very frail, with an incidentally discovered, longstanding femoral hernia that can reasonably be left alone.

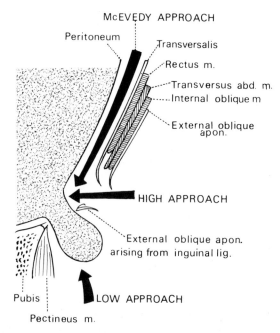

Fig. 3.4 Femoral hernia. A sagittal section through the hernial sac shows the possible approaches.

2. One of the reasons for offering surgical repair freely is that the operation can be accomplished easily using local anaesthesia.

3. Be aware of the prevascular femoral hernia. It lies in front of the vessels, so the neck is lateral to expectation.

4. Try each of the approaches for femoral hernia (Fig. 3.4). They all have merits and they are all safe, provided the operation is skilfully performed. We all eventually settle upon our favourite approach and I invariably use the lower approach.

5. Which side requires operation? Make sure you mark the side personally.

LOW APPROACH

Access

1. Make an incision 8–10 cm long in the crease of the groin, centred midway between the symphysis pubis and the anterior superior iliac spine.

2. Cut the superficial tissues over the hernia in the line of the skin incision. Look out for the small viens running into the long saphenous vein; ligate and divide them as necessary (Fig. 3.5).

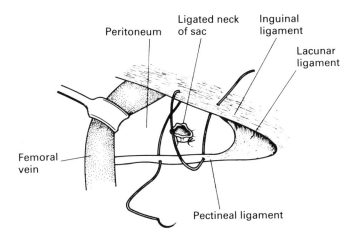

Fig. 3.5 Lower approach to right femoral hernia.

Action

Hernial sac

1. Expose the fat-covered hernial sac. Clean the sac so that it may be traced proximally beneath the inguinal ligament.

2. Cautiously open the sac by incising it while it is held up between two artery forceps. Recognize the inside of the sac by seeing free fluid, a glistening surface and contents which may be reduced into the main peritoneal cavity.

3. Pick up the open edges of the sac with three equally spaced artery forceps, then sweep away the external fat to expose the neck, lying between the inguinal ligament anteriorly and the pectineal ligament posteriorly in the same horizontal plane. Note how deeply the neck of the sac lies.

4. Identify the femoral vein lying just laterally, and preserve it from damage.

5. Empty the sac, transfix and ligate the neck with 0 chromic catgut.

6. Excise the sac 1 cm distal to the ligature.

Repair

1. The inguinal and pectineal ligaments meet medially through the arched lacunar ligament. The object of the repair is to unite the ligaments for about 1 cm laterally, without producing constriction of the femoral vein.

2. Use 00 silk or monofilament nylon, 60 linen thread or 35 swg stainless steel wire mounted on a small J-shaped needle.

3. Place the left index finger over the femoral vein to protect it and draw it laterally. Insert a stitch deeply into the inguinal ligament; a narrow retractor then draws that ligament upwards, while the needle is insinuated behind it, to take a good bite of the pectineal ligament. Avoid taking too deep a bite or the needle point will break as it strikes the pubic crest. A single stitch, two or three stitches or a recrossing 'X' or 'N' stitch may be used. As the stitches are tightened, keep a finger over the femoral vein to ensure that it is not constricted.

Difficulty?

1. Can you not identify the sac in the fatty lump? Remember that most of the lump may be preperitoneal fat. Gently and carefully incise it and separate it. When the peritoneum is incised you can usually see glistening visceral peritoneum or lobulated omental fat. If the sac contains free fluid it appears bluish and may be confused with the appearance of congested bowel. When the sac is carefully incised the fluid escapes, revealing the contents.

2. If you inadvertently tear the neck of the sac, gently free peritoneum from the peritoneal cavity so that it can be drawn down to form a new neck.

3. If the femoral vein is torn, control the bleeding with pressure from gauze packs for 5 minutes. Meanwhile, order replacement blood for the patient, arterial sutures, tapes, bulldog clamps and 3.5% citrate solution, and summon assistance. Expose the vein; do not hesitate to approach it from above and below the inguinal ligament. Apply bulldog clamps and tapes above and below the damaged segment. Insert fine 4/0 or 5/0 sutures set 1 mm apart, 1 mm from the torn edges to evert them and close the hole. Flush

with citrate solution at intervals. Release, then remove the clamps and tapes.

Closure

1. Unite the subcutaneous tissues with a few plain catgut stitches.
2. Close the skin.

HIGH APPROACH

Access

1. Make an incision 2 cm above the medial two-thirds of the inguinal ligament. As this is deepened to reach the external oblique aponeurosis, clamp, divide and ligate the veins which cross the line of the incision.
2. Expose the lower portion of the external oblique aponeurosis with the external inguinal ring and the inguinal ligament.
3. Split the fibres of the external oblique aponeurosis from the pillars of the external ring, outwards in the line of its fibres.
4. Displace the cord or round ligament upwards to expose the posterior wall of the inguinal canal just above the inguinal ligament.
5. Incise the transversalis fascia for 4–5 cm at the medial end of the posterior wall, 1 cm above and parallel to the inguinal ligament.

Action

Hernial sac

1. Identify the neck of the sac and the external iliac vein.
2. Isolate the neck of the sac and gently withdraw the fundus. If there is difficulty, have the lower skin flap retracted downwards, incise the cribriform fascia and isolate, open and empty the sac from below.
3. Ensure that the sac is empty, that the bladder is not adherent, then transfix, ligate and divide the neck of the sac.

Repair

1. With the index finger, feel the margins of the femoral canal. In front is the inguinal ligament, medially the lacunar ligament, posteriorly the pectineal ligament, and laterally the femoral vein.
2. Narrow the triangular gap by inserting non-absorbable sutures of metric 3.5 polypropylene, nylon, 2/0 silk or 60 linen thread, between the pectineal ligament and the inguinal ligament.
3. If the upper approach was selected because there is also an inguinal hernia, deal with this now.

Closure

1. Close the hole in the posterior wall of the inguinal canal using non-absorbable stitches. Sew the upper leaf of the transversalis fascia to the lower leaf and to the inguinal ligament.
2. Close the anterior wall of the inguinal canal by repairing the split external oblique aponeurosis in front of the cord, using a continuous suture of 0 chromic catgut on a round-bodied needle. Reform the external inguinal ring.
3. Re-appose the subcutaneous tissues then close the skin.

HENRY'S APPROACH

1. Make sure the bladder is empty.
2. Make an incision 8–10 cm long in the midline below the umbilicus.
3. Incise the rectus sheath on the side of the hernia in a line parallel to the skin wound.
4. Displace the rectus muscle laterally. Separate the extraperitoneal tissues downwards and laterally until the sac is reached.
5. Reduce, isolate, open and empty the sac, then transfix, ligate the divide the neck.
6. Repair the femoral canal from above.
7. Suture the two sides of the rectus sheath using 0 chromic catgut mounted on a cutting or spear-pointed needle then repair the subcutaneous tissues and the skin.

McEVEDY'S APPROACH

1. Make an incision from over the femoral canal, vertically upwards for 7–8 cm.
2. Isolate the sac in the lower part of the incision.
3. Incise the rectus sheath starting 2.5 cm above the external ring, passing obliquely upwards, keeping just above and parallel to the lower border of the rectus muscle. The sheath is in two separate layers.
4. Open the thin transversalis fascia and dissect between it and the peritoneum down to the neck of the sac.
5. Reduce the sac, manipulating it from above and below. Isolate, open and empty it, then transfix, ligate and divide the neck of the sac.
6. Repair the canal from above.
7. Close the incision in the rectus sheath with 0 chromic catgut on a round-bodied needle. Appose the subcutaneous layers and close the skin.

STRANGULATED HERNIA

Access

1. The approach is similar to that for an elective operation.

2. Some surgeons who use the lower approach for elective repair of femoral hernias eschew this for strangulated femoral hernias. They argue that bowel resection is difficult from the lower approach. I always use the same approach in all circumstances and have not regretted it, but if bowel resection proved difficult I should have no hesitation in opening the abdomen formally.

Assess

1. If the history was short, the sac will frequently be empty by the time you expose it. The relaxation produced by the premedication drugs, reinforced by the anaesthetic, often succeeds when other conservative methods have failed to reduce a hernia. There is no merit in exploring the abdomen. Repair the hernia as though this were an elective operation.

2. If bowel is present in the sac, do not let it slip back into the abdomen, but gently draw it down into the sac. The bowel is likely to have suffered the greatest damage where it was trapped at the neck of the sac.

3. Feel the margins of the neck of the sac with a fingertip.

4. In Richter's hernia, most frequently associated with femoral hernia, a knuckle of part of the bowel wall is trapped. The bowel lumen is thus not obstructed but the knuckle may become gangrenous and perforate.

5. Maydl's strangulation is very rare. Two loops lie in the sac but the blood supply to an intermediate loop within the abdomen may be prejudiced so that it is gangrenous.

Is the bowel viable?

1. If there is a sheen to the bowel wall, if it is pink or becomes pink after release, if the arteries pulsate, if peristalsis is seen, replace the bowel with confidence.

2. If the wall is black, green or purple, with no sheen, if there is no pulsation in the mesenteric vessels or it is malodorous, resect it.

3. If the bowel is congested, bluish or plum-coloured and still has a sheen, but peristalsis is not seen and vascular pulsations cannot be felt, then the viability is doubtful. Remember though, that extravasated blood in the subperitoneal layer cannot be reabsorbed immediately so the colour may not change. Cover the bowel with warm moist packs for 5 minutes and re-examine it. If it has improved in appearance, it is probably viable.

4. The critical areas are the constriction rings at the point of entrapment. These are white when the bowel is first drawn down but may be greenish or black if they are obviously necrotic. Re-examine doubtful rings after an interval to see if the blood supply returns. If it does not, the bowel must be resected.

5. Try to avoid resection of doubtful bowel in poor risk patients. Replace the bowel and determine to open the

abdomen 24–48 hours later. The patient can be resuscitated in the interval and if resection is necessary it can be carried out easily through the abdomen.

6. Experienced surgeons probably resect bowel less frequently than those who are inexperienced. The mucosa is more vulnerable that the seromuscularis to the effects of ischaemia and if the outer layers survive the mucosa may slough to leave an annular ulcer. When this heals a constriction may develop, though not inevitably. This is the intestinal stenosis of Garre. The patient presents with incipient small bowel obstruction. Provided this is anticipated a simple elective abdominal resection can be carried out.

Action

1. If the neck is constricted, place an index fingertip on each side of the contents, nails facing outwards. Gently dilate the neck of the sac (Fig. 3.6).

2. If the bowel is viable, return it to the abdomen.

3. If necessary, resect a gangrenous segment of bowel, performing an end-to-end anastomosis.

Difficulty?

1. Sometimes the bulk of tissues contained in the hernial sac makes reduction seem impossible. Provided the margins of the neck are defined, gentleness, patience and persuasion will succeed. If only a little at a time is reduced, do not despair because the reduction must get progressively easier.

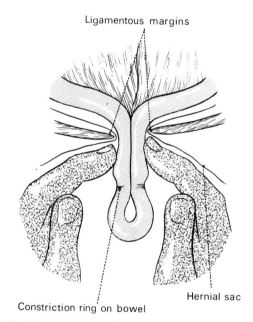

Fig. 3.6 Reducing a strangulated hernia. Healthy bowel is drawn down. The index fingers form a wedge to dilate the ligamentous margins.

2. When reducing a strangulated femoral hernia, it is often advised that a grooved director should be passed medial to the neck of the sac, followed by a bistoury to cut the lacunar ligament. The author has not yet found it necessary to use this method and indeed, finds it illogical. Failure to reduce the hernia results from a tight sac neck, not from tight ligamentous margins, which are absent laterally. The femoral vein can be emptied and displaced producing ample room to reduce the contents. Hay Groves' manoeuvre of dividing the inguinal ligament, reducing the hernia and repairing the ligament is never necessary.

3. A large mass of fibrotic greater omentum may be adherent within the sac. Do not hesitate to excise the mass, provided the neck of the sac can be isolated, the bowel is not damaged and every blood vessel is safely ligated.

4. If gangrenous bowel slips back into the abdomen and cannot be recovered, repair the hernia, then open the abdomen through a right lower paramedian incision. Find the gangrenous segment and resect it.

Repair

After opening the sac and dealing with the contents, repair the hernia as though this is an elective operation.

UMBILICAL HERNIA

ADULT UMBILICAL HERNIA

Appraise

1. Most hernias in adults are para-umbilical, protruding usually above or below the cicatrix.

2. Some adults, especially of African origin, have true umbilical hernias that have been present throughout life.

3. Umbilical hernia is conventionally treated by early operation for fear of strangulation. However, many patients are grossly obese, elderly, with cardiovascular or respiratory disability and a longstanding hernia that has not been troublesome. The authour adjures such patients to lose weight and hesitates about offering operation. Ascites may provoke umbilical hernia: find the cause and treat it but since in many cases there is extensive malignant disease, surgery is rarely indicated.

4. Operate on strangulated, painful irreducible — but not necessarily painless irreducible — hernias and painful reducible hernias, especially those with small hard margins.

Access

1. Make a curved incision in the groove below the hernia. Extend the cut transversely outwards on each side, for 2–4 cm.

2. Deepen the incision, identify the anterior rectus sheath and expose it around the lower half of the circumference of the hernia.

3. If the hernia is small, preserve the umbilical skin by dissecting it upwards as a flap. If the hernia is large, make a semicircular incision above the umbilicus so that the hernia is encircled and excise the stretched skin.

4. Expose the rectus sheath around the upper margin of the hernia.

Action

1. Cut through the thinned-out edge of rectus sheath to expose the peritoneum and gradually work round to display the whole circumference of the neck of the sac.

2. Clear the sac of fatty tissue and cut it right round, at least 2 cm distal to the neck if possible. The contents of the sac are less likely to be adherent here than in the fundus, but free them if necessary. Mark the peritoneal edges with artery forceps.

3. If the contents of the sac are free, reduce them. If they are adherent to the fundus of the sac, free them and return them to the peritoneal cavity. If there is a mass of fibrous omentum, excise it with the fundus of the sac but take care to ligate all the bleeding omental vessels and avoid damaging the transverse colon.

4. Separate the peritoneum from the undersurface of the rectus sheath all round.

5. Close the peritoneal neck of the sac with a continuous 0 chromic catgut suture, producing a transverse linear suture line.

Mayo's repair (Fig. 3.7)

1. Cut the rectus sheath laterally for 2–3 cm on each side. This allows the upper and lower edges to be overlapped.

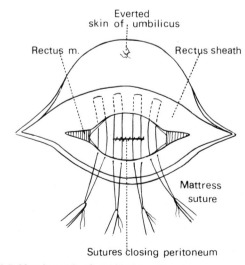

Fig. 3.7 Mayo's repair of umbilical hernia.

2. Place a series of horizontal mattress sutures of metric 3.5 polypropylene, 0 silk or nylon, or 40 linen thread, without tying them. Each stitch penetrates the upper leaf of rectus sheath 3–4 cm from the edge, passes beneath it to catch the lower leaf 1 cm from the edge and passes back beneath the upper leaf, to emerge near the entry stitch, 3–4 cm from the edge. When the stitches are tied, the lower leaf is drawn up underneath the upper leaf.

3. Sew the overlapping upper edge on to the anterior surface of the lower rectus sheath, using continuous or interrupted stitches.

Closure

1. If the skin of the fundus was excised, close the skin wound to produce a transverse suture line.

2. If the skin over the fundus was preserved, pick up the undersurface of the navel with a catgut stitch and sew it to the rectus sheath to produce an inverted umbilicus. Suture the skin as a curved line beneath the newly fashioned umbilicus.

INFANTILE UMBILICAL HERNIA

Appraise

1. Most infantile umbilical hernias protrude through the incompletely closed cicatrix. They appear to be more frequent in infants of African origin. Many of them close spontaneously without surgical repair. They were usually left for 1 year but may be left for 2 or more years. Repair them only if they increase in size.

2. Infants infrequently develop para-umbilical hernia. This is usually a supra-umbilical hernia. It is not symmetrical but droops like the trunk of a baby elephant. It will not close spontaneously, so repair it locally through a transverse incision sited directly over the defect.

Access

1. Approach the hernia through a transverse incision curved beneath the everted umbilicus.

2. Preserve the umbilical skin by turning it upwards as a flap.

Action

1. Expose the rectus sheath and the neck of the sac. The separation is much easier than in acquired hernias.

2. Open the sac, empy it, then close it by suture or transfixion ligature.

Repair

Edge-to-edge repair of the rectus sheath above and below the hernia is effective. Make sure the peritoneum is separated sufficiently to allow good bites of sheath to be taken, without piercing the peritoneum. Use stitches of fine polypropylene, 00 silk or nylon or 60 thread.

Closure

1. Suture the deep surface of the umbilical skin to the rectus sheath.

2. Close the skin to leave a curved transverse wound.

OMPHALOCELE

The operation should be carried out with the minimum delay after birth, or infection supervenes and the neonatus will die (see Ch. 32).

UMBILICAL INFECTIONS, TUMOURS, FISTULAS AND SINUSES

Appraise

1. Is infection merely the result of aggregated keratin forming an 'omphalolith' that can be lifted out of a deep umbilicus without the need of an anaesthetic? Persistent omphalitis stimulates granulation tissue, forming a 'polyp.' It was conventional treatment to apply a horsehair ligature but cauterize the stalk. Neglected or imperfectly treated umbilical sepsis, especially in infants can progess to septicaemia, distant pyogenic infections, pylephlebitis, liver suppuration and fatal jaundice.

2. An enteroteratoma is the remnant of the vitello-intestinal duct forming a raspberry tumour. Cauterize it to destroy the mucosa. Rarely, heterotopic gastric mucosa secretes acid causing excoriation of the skin.

3. An enterocystoma is persistence of the intermediate part of the vitello-intestinal duct, producing a cyst attached to the antimesenteric border of the ileum, free within the peritoneal cavity.

4. Persistent discharge from the umbilicus may be difficult to elucidate. Inject radio-opaque fluid medium and perform sinography to determine the depth of a sinus or demonstrate a connection with the bowel or bladder.

5. Congenital faecal fistula results from persistence of the whole vitello-intestinal duct. Faecal staining may be temporary if the fistula closes spontaneously. If there is atresia distally or imperforate anus then the fistula persists and the distal obstruction must be relieved at the same time as the fistula is closed.

6. Patent urachus is persistence of the allantois, usually associated with membranous obstruction of the urethra. The urinary obstruction must be dealt with at the time of closing the fistula.

7. Squamous epithelioma may develop at the umbilicus and subsequently can involve the inguinal lymph nodes.

Excise the umbilicus and if indicated, carry out bilateral block dissection of the inguinal nodes.

8. Endometrioma at the umbilicus classically bleeds at the time of the menses.

9. Secondary carcinoma from the liver or porta hepatis may reach the umbilicus along the ligamentum teres.

EPIGASTRIC HERNIA

Appraise

A small knuckle of extraperitoneal fat insinuates itself through the linea alba through a defect where blood vessels penetrate it. If the falciform ligament contains much fat there is little risk of peritoneum and intestine passing through the defect.

Action

1. Make a transverse or vertical incision through the skin and deepen it down to the herniated fat.

2. Define the margins of the defect and reduce the hernia. It is rare to find a peritoneal sac and if one is found do not open it at an elective operation but simply invaginate it into the peritoneal cavity.

3. Repair the defect using non-absorbable stitches.

4. Close the skin.

HAEMATOMA OF RECTUS SHEATH

Appraise

1. A sudden strain may rupture one of the inferior epigastric vessels entering the lower rectus abdominis muscle producing pain. Since the right side is affected more frequently than the left, the localized pain and tenderness may be misdiagnosed as appendicitis.

2. If you operate thinking the patient has appendicitis and discover a haematoma lying behind the lower rectus muscle, evacuate it. If there is a suspicion of continuing bleeding, isolate and ligate the inferior epigastric vessels in continuity.

DESMOID AND OTHER ABDOMINAL WALL TUMOURS

Appraise

1. Desmoid tumours are non-encapsulated tumours which develop in the muscle intersections. Women are usually affected, especially those who have borne children. Remove desmoids completely or they recur.

2. Carcinoma of intra-abdominal structures may secondarily invade the abdominal wall. If the tumour is otherwise resectable do not hesitate to excise a portion of the abdominal wall en bloc with the primary neoplasm.

Action

1. Concentrate on excising the tumour with adequate clear margins and depth. In the case of a desmoid tumour do not fail to cut through healthy muscle and connective tissue all the way round.

2. If the abdominal wall is invaded from its deep surface and peritoneum and the deep part of the muscle wall is excised but leaving intact the superficial muscle layer, do not attempt to repair the defect. A peritoneum-like cellular layer will develop on the deep surface of the muscle.

3. Close a small full-thickness defect layer by layer.

4. A large defect can often be closed by creating a flap of anterior rectus sheath based on its medial edge to swing to the opposite side, or a layer of lateral muscle may be swung over. The fact that the abdominal wall is composed in most areas of a number of layers allows most defects to be closed by using one of these multiple layers. Always obtain advice on the planning of such manoeuvres whenever possible.

5. If you cannot close the defect with muscle or aponeurosis, the best alternative is to use a myocutaneous flap from the chest or thigh. Unless you are skilled in preparing such flaps, obtain the help of a plastic surgical colleague.

6. When you cannot close the defect by any other means, create a large skin flap based laterally that you can slide over to cover the defect, applying split skin grafts to the donor site.

7. If you are completely unable to close the defect, consider inserting a Marlex or other plastic sheet until you can obtain help and advice.

INCISIONAL HERNIA

Appraise

1. Incisional hernia is deep disruption of the abdominal wound while the superficial layers remain intact. If the superficial layers also separate then burst abdomen results.

2. Herniation may develop early, while the patient is still in hospital or later, usually during the next few months.

3. Incisional hernias can often be avoided. They are associated with careless suturing, the use of catgut instead of unabsorbable material, haematomas and infection, the too early removal of through and through stitches, the insertion of drains through the main incision and damage to abdominal nerves. Jaundice and malnutrition, obesity,

post-operative distension and re-exploration through the same incision after a short interval are other contributory factors.

4. Incisional hernia rarely causes strangulation, therefore do not rush to re-operate. Make sure that the margins are well defined and not too widely separated. If the patient is overweight, make sure that the excess is lost before contemplating further surgery. Since straining to cough, opening the bowels or passing urine may prejudice the repair, improve the patient as much as possible before operation.

5. I am reluctant to offer repair to overweight patients with poor margins, in whom the edges cannot be reapposed satisfactorily so that some form of prosthetic mesh must be used to bridge the gap.

Access

1. Excise the old skin scar.
2. If the skin and peritoneum are fused, excise an ellipse of skin wide enough to expose subcutaneous tissue.
3. Dissect back the skin on each side until unscarred subcutaneous tissue is reached, beyond the margins of the defect.

Action

1. Deepen the incision until aponeurosis or muscle is reached, then work towards the margins of the defect.
2. Dissect the edges cleanly and separate the peritoneum from the deep surface all around.
3. Is there anything to be gained by opening and excising some of the stretched peritoneum? If possible, invaginate the sac and suture the margins together.

Repair

1. If the incision was paramedian or through several layers of muscle, it is sometimes profitable to cut into the rounded edge of the defect, so forming two layers. Do not be deluded into thinking, however, that two thinned, 'button-holed' and ragged layers are better than one intact undamaged layer. I personally leave the layers intact but ensure that there is no fat or other extraneous tissue interposed between the aponeurotic layers.
2. Meticulously stop all bleeding.
3. Appose the edges as one layer or several layers. Use metric 3.5 polypropylene, 0 silk or nylon, 40 linen thread, or 35 swg stainless steel wire. Insert the stitches set back at least 1 cm from the edges and 0.5 to 1 cm apart either interrupted or continuous, but taking irregular bites of tissue. If each bite is set back from the edge the same distance there is a danger of stripping off the edge.
4. Include the peritoneum with the aponeurotic edges.
5. Trim the skin edges as necessary, and close the wound.

Technical points

1. The particular suture material used for the repair is a matter for choice. If the anatomy is restored to normal, use the suture material which would be selected for a normal closure.

2. Do not use techniques which involve overlap unless there is spare, thinned-out aponeurosis. Any other sort of overlap involves undue tension.

3. In Maingot's 'keel' repair, the sac is inverted as a ridge. The margins of the defect are apposed using a mattress stitch of floss silk. In my hands this has given poor results. The multiple layers of suture lines add nothing to the strength of the repair which depends solely on the last row of stitches.

4. If the defect is so large that an insert of plastic polyester (Marlex) mesh, tantalum gauze or other material must be used to bridge the defect, reconsider the value of performing the operation. These materials must overlap the margins of the defect so widely that the chance of their giving way at some point is very high. An edge-to-edge repair may first be accomplished and then a sheet of mesh is laid over it and sutured to the anterior surface of the aponeurotic abdominal wall with tacking stitches of nonabsorbable stitches over the whole area of the sheet, thus reinforcing the repair. Alternatively, a sheet can be sewn extending from the edge of the defect on each side and tacked over its whole area to the aponeurotic abdominal wall. Then pick up with stitches the aponeurotic edge and the edge of the mesh together, cross to the other side and there pick up the opposite edge of aponeurosis and mesh, drawing them together as further stitches are inserted.

5. For midline incisional hernias below the umbilicus, the the lower ends of rectus muscles may be detached from the pubis and crossed over the defect. The tendon of each one is then sutured to the origin of the other. Make sure the blood supply and nerve supply to the muscles is not damaged. I have no personal knowledge of this method.

PERISTOMAL HERNIA

Appraise

1. Stomas leave weak areas in the abdominal wall. The whole area around the stoma may bulge diffusely. Segments of bowel may insinuate themselves alongside the emerging bowel to produce a swelling with deformity of the stoma, or occasionally pass between the layers as an interstitial hernia. In addition the segment of bowel itself may prolapse.

2. Some peristomal hernias can be accepted, in particular diffuse hernias that are not troublesome since they are unlikely to produce obstruction.

3. Those that have a localized defect can be repaired locally, by narrowing the channel through the musculo-aponeurotic abdominal wall.

4. Most peristomal hernias requiring surgical repair must be re-sited so that the herniated area can be closed completely. Make sure that the new site is carefully selected beforehand (see Ch. 8).

NON-HIATAL DIAPHRAGMATIC HERNIA

Appraise

1. Neonatal hiatal hernia must be repaired immediatey because the lungs cannot expand since the chest cavity is filled with abdominal viscera. There is no hernial sac because the defect is the persistent pleuroperitoneal canal and this is the hernia of Bochdalek (see Ch. 22).

2. Adults occasionally present with acute obstruction within a persistent pleuroperitoneal canal. The hernia is almost always on the left side.

3. As a rule reduction from below is easy, but when the abdominal viscera are adherent within the chest, freeing them from below may be difficult.

Persistent pleuroperitoneal canal (hernia of Bochdalek)

1. There should be no hernia sac because the defect is a canal between the abdominal and pleural cavities.
2. By whatever approach is favoured, reduce the abdominal viscera.
3. Trace out the margins of the defect and close the hole using non-absorbable sutures. The margins usually come together more easily than anticipated.

Eventration of the diaphragm

1. A thinned-out leaf of the diaphragm is found, with good muscle at the periphery.
2. Plicate the diaphragm by gathering up a fold and suturing the base of the fold. Lay the fold flat and stitch it down flat, using non-absorbable suture material.

Hernia of the foramen of Morgagni

1. An abdominal approach is best for this rare hernia, passing between the costal and xiphoid slips of the diaphragm.
2. Define and repair the defect.

Traumatic hernia

1. An abdominal approach is usually satisfactory and the viscera can be returned and correctly placed within the abdomen.
2. The margins of the defect are nearly always easy to define and repair using non-absorbable suture material.

OBTURATOR HERNIA

Appraise

1. This is rare. I have seen but one in my career. Females are six times as likely to be affected as males, they are nearly always aged more than 50 years and the right side is more frequently affected than the left.

2. Most of the patients are admitted with small bowel obstruction which is discovered to be from obturator hernia at operation, sometimes with a Richter's type of hernia. I have not seen the Howship-Romberg syndrome of pain down the inner thigh and knee, aggravated by straining and coughing but not by movements of the hip joint.

3. Rarely the hernia protrudes into the thigh between the pectineus and adductor longus muscles.

Action

1. Assuming an operation is performed for intestinal obstruction and the small bowel is found to be tethered in the region of the obturator canal, improve the access by carrying the incision down to the pubis. A catheter should already be draining the bladder.

2. Identify the canal. Remember that the nerve enters it from the anteromedial aspect, the artery is posterolateral.

3. Gently free the bowel and inspect it to determine if it is viable.

4. Make no attempt to repair the defect.

LUMBAR HERNIA

Appraise

1. This may emerge spontaneously either through the triangle of Petit bounded by the iliac crest, the posterior edge of external oblique muscle and the anterior edge of latissimus dorsi muscle or below the 12th rib under serratus posterior inferior, the lateral edge of erector spinae and above the internal oblique muscle.

2. Lumbar hernia complicates renal incisions in the loin, drainage of lumbar abscess, or paralysis of the muscles in the lumbar region.

3. Operative repair is rarely required.

GLUTEAL AND SCIATIC HERNIA

Appraise

1. Gluteal hernia emerges above or below the pyriformis muscle through the greater sciatic notch.

2. Sciatic hernia emerges through the lesser sciatic notch.

3. These hernias are usually discovered at exploratory laparotomy for intestinal obstruction and rarely produce a palpable swelling in the buttock.

PELVIC FLOOR HERNIA

As a rule they accompany a cystocele, rectocele or rectal prolapse if they are spontaneous. Pelvic herniation most frequently follows on surgery of the pelvic floor including abdominoperineal resection and hysterectomy.

INTERNAL HERNIA

Appraise

1. The majority of internal hernias follow abdominal or abdominothoracic operations. Intestine may herniate behind an anterior gastroenterostomy, through a transverse mesocolic defect following posterior gastroenterostomy, through the diaphragm following thoracoabdominal surgery or lateral to a segment of bowel passing forwards to an external abdominal stoma if the space is not sealed.

2. All surgeons hope to make a pre-operative diagnosis of herniation into the paraduodenal fossa, in the free edge of which lies the inferior mesenteric vein. Classically, a patient presents with acute intestinal obstruction and acute haemorrhoids from obstruction of the vein. I am still waiting to see one.

3. Intestine may pass through the foramen of Winslow or aditus to the less sac. Bowel trapped in the lesser sac may rupture the flimsy gastrohepatic omentum so the nature of the obstructing band containing the portal vein, hepatic artery and common bile duct may not be evident. The famous surgeon Heneage Ogilvie recounts the humbling experience of discovering this when he was about to divide the band.

Further reading

Bassini E 1890 Ueber die Behandlung des Leistenbruches. Langenbecks Archir für Klinische Chirurgie 40: 429–476

Burdick C G, Higginbotham N L 1935 Division of the spermatic cord as an aid an operating on selected types of inguinal hernia. Annals Surgery 102: 863–874

Dudley H A F 1970 Layered and mass closure of the abdominal wall — a theoretical and experimental analysis. British Journal of Surgery 57: 664–667

Glassow F 1984 Inguinal hernia repair using local anaesthesia. Annals Royal College of Surgeons of England 66: 382–387

Henry A K 1957 Extensile exposure. Livingstone, Edinburgh

Jenkins T P N 1976 The burst abdominal wound: a mechanical approach. British Journal of Surgery 131: 130–140

Kirk R M 1972 Effect of method of opening and closing the abdomen and incidnece of wound bursting. Lancet 2: 352–353

Kirk R M 1974 Intra-abdominal replacement of the testis as an aid to the repair of difficult and recurrent inguinal hernias. British Journal of Surgery 61:538–

Kirk R M 1983 Which inguinal hernia repair? British Medical Journal 287: 4–5

Lichtenstein I L, Shore J M 1976 Exploding the myths of hernia repair. American Journal of Surgery 132: 307–315

Lotheissen G 1898 Zur Radikaloperation der Schenkelhernien. Zentralblatt fur Chirurgie 21: 548–550

McEvedy P G 1950 Femoral hernia. Annals of the Royal College of Surgeons of England 7: 484–496

McVay C B, Anson B J 1949 Inguinal and femoral hernioplasty Surgery Gynecology and Obstetrics 88: 473–485

Tanner N C 1942 A 'slide' operation for inguinal and femoral hernia. British Journal of Surgery 115: 285–289

Laparotomy: elective and emergency

OPENING THE ABDOMEN

Preparation

1. Whenever possible, go and see the patient in the anaesthetic room while he or she is still awake. Check that this is the correct patient by visual identification and inspection of the identity bracelet.

2. Inspect the case notes and make sure that any relevant X-rays are available in theatre. If the lesion is unilateral, be quite certain that the operation will be carried out on the correct side (this should have been marked beforehand). It is inexcusable to neglect these elementary precautions.

3. Make sure that the anaesthetist is prepared for the operation to start. Laparotomy is nearly always performed under general anaesthesia, with endotracheal intubation and an intravenous cannula in situ.

4. Consider whether a prophylactic injection of a broad-spectrum antibiotic should be given at this stage, for example in intestinal operations.

5. Cleanse the skin of the operation area with an antiseptic solution applied on gauze held in long sponge-holding forceps. Appropriate solutions include chlorhexidine (Hibitane) 1 : 5000, cetrimide 1% and 95% white spirit. Apply the solution along the line of the incision, and continue to apply it in a centrifugal manner over a wide area. Do not use an inflammable agent, such as white spirit, if you intend to employ diathermy to the skin or immediate subcutaneous tissues.

6. Apply sterile sheets or towels, and secure them to the skin with towel clips (unless local anaesthetic is being used). Leave exposed a limited extent of the abdomen on either side of the proposed line of incision.

Types of incision (Figs. 4.1 and 4.2)

1. *Midline* incisions transgress the linea alba, the tough and relatively avascular cord that unites the anterior and posterior rectus sheaths. They therefore have the advantages of being relatively quick to make and to close and of provoking less bleeding than incisions that divide muscle fibres. Midline incisions can provide access to many ab-

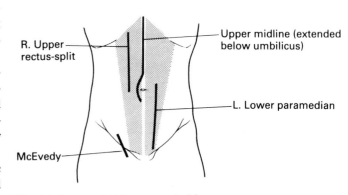

Fig. 4.1 Some vertical laparotomy incisions

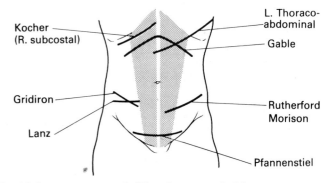

Fig. 4.2 Some transverse and oblique laparotomy incisions

Table 4.1 Incisions to expose the abdominal viscera

Midline		Upper	hiatus, oesophagus, stomach, duodenum, spleen, liver, pancreas, biliary tract
		Central	small bowel, colon
		Lower	sigmoid, rectum, ovary/tube/uterus, bladder and prostate (extraperitoneal)
		Throughout	aorta
Paramedian (incl. rectus split)		Upper	biliary tract (right), spleen (left) etc.
		Central	small bowel, colon
		Lower	pelvic viscera, lower ureter (extraperitoneal)
Oblique		Subcostal	liver and biliary tract (right), spleen (left)
		Gable	pancreas, liver, adrenals
		Gridiron	caecum-appendix (right)
		Rutherford Morison	caecum-appendix (right), sigmoid (left), ureter and external iliac vessels (extraperitoneal)
		Posterolateral	kidney and adrenal (extraperitoneal)
Transverse		Right upper quadrant	gallbladder, infant pylorus, colostomy
		Mid-abdominal	small bowel, colon, kidney, lumbar sympathetic chain, vena cava (right)
		Lanz	caecum-appendix (right)
		Pfannenstiel	ovary/tube/uterus, prostate (extraperitoneal)
Thoracoabdominal		Right	liver and portal vein
		Left	gastro-oesophageal junction, enormous spleen

dominal viscera (Table 4.1). In the upper abdomen you can avoid the falciform ligament by keeping just to one or other side of the midline when entering the peritoneal cavity. In the lower abdomen remember that the linea alba is less well developed and take corresponding care to close the wound securely. When necessary, bypass the umbilicus by curving the skin incision and bevelling the underlying cut to regain the midline of the aponeurosis.

2. *Paramedian* incisions provide very similar access to the upper, central or lower abdomen. All layers are divided in the line of the vertical skin incision, placed 2 cm to the right or left of the midline, except that the rectus muscle is dissected free and is drawn laterally, thus remaining intact. At the end of the operation the rectus muscle is allowed to fall medially to cover the line of peritoneal closure.

3. *Rectus-splitting* incisions are made 3–4 cm lateral to the midline and divide all the tissues (including the rectus muscle) in this line. They avoid the time-consuming dis-

section required to free the muscle belly. In theory the medial part of the rectus muscle is denervated and thus rendered atrophic, but in practice the wounds heal strongly. A right upper rectus-split provides good access to the gallbladder.

4. *Oblique* incisions can sometimes provide good access. Kocher's incision extends 2 cm below the right costal margin from the midline to the lateral edge of the rectus muscle and exposes the gallbladder. The equivalent left subcostal incision can be used to approach the spleen. In the lower abdomen, Rutherford Morison's incision starts just above the anterior superior iliac spine and divides all tissues in the line of the external oblique muscle and aponeurosis. The gridiron incision splits each of the three muscle layers of the abdominal wall in the line of its fibres; it thus seldom gives rise to an incisional hernia. It provides an excellent approach to the appendix and can be enlarged by extending the skin incision in either direction and by dividing the internal oblique and transversus muscles (i.e. conversion into a Rutherford Morison incision).

5. *Transverse* incisions usually leave the best cosmetic scars and provide adequate exposure, provided they are made long enough. They are therefore best suited for limited exposure in a planned procedure. Ramstedt's pyloromyotomy or transverse colostomy may be performed through a short transverse incision. Transverse laparotomy is useful in children, in certain obese patients and in the upper abdomen when the costal angle is broad. The Lanz incision is a horizontal modification of the gridiron incision for appendicectomy and provides the least obtrusive scar at the expense of slightly inferior access. Pfannenstiel's incision runs transversely above the pubis but just below the hairline. The aponeurosis is divided transversely and reflected above and below, allowing the rectus muscles to be separated vertically in the midline. Gynaecologists then open the peritoneum to gain access to the female reproductive organs, whereas urologists stay in the extraperitoneal plane for retropubic approach to the bladder and prostate.

6. *Angled* incisions provide not a mere slit, which can be pulled into an ellipse, but a space in the abdominal wall. Combined right and left subcostal incisions joining at the xiphisternum (the 'high gable' incision) enable a large flap to be turned down and provide excellent access for hepatectomy, pancreatectomy and bilateral adrenalectomy. A vertical incision with a T-shaped transverse extension (or vice versa) allows two flaps to be turned back. These incisions take longer to make and repair but can be invaluable for difficult or very extensive operations.

7. *Thoracoabdominal* incisions usually follow the line of a rib and extend obliquely into the upper abdomen. They make light of the cartilaginous cage protecting the upper abdomen. Radial incision of the diaphragm towards the oesophageal hiatus (left) or vena cava (right) throws the abdomen and thorax into one cavity and provides unparalleled access for oesophagogastrectomy and right hepatic

lobectomy. Thoracolaparotomy may be indicated for removal of an enormous tumour of the kidney, adrenal or spleen.

8. *Posterolateral* incisions for approach to the kidney, adrenal and upper ureter are described in the relevant chapters.

Making the incision

1. Incise the skin with the belly of the knife. Cut cleanly down to the aponeurosis or muscle. Discard the knife.

2. Stop the bleeding. Firmly press each bleeding site with a swab, then remove the swab quickly and pick up the vessel with the minimum surrounding tissue. Use fine toothed or non-toothed dissecting forceps, which are touched with the diathermy electrode to coagulate the vessel. Alternatively, use diathermy forceps. In either case, be careful not to burn the skin when coagulating superficial vessels. Larger vessels should be picked up with aretery forceps and ligated with plain 2/0 or 3/0 catgut. As the first half-hitch is tightened, the assistant smoothly releases the forceps. Complete a reef knot. The catgut should be cut 2–3 mm beyond the knot for small vessels, but 4–5 mm should project when larger vessels are tied with catgut.

3. Apply wound towels to the skin edges, if these are to be used. Fix the towels with clips or stitches. Wound towels help to prevent contamination of the wound by the fluid contents of abdominal viscera.

4. Incise the aponeurosis with a clean knife in the line of the skin incision.

5. Cut, split or displace the muscles of the abdominal wall.

(a) Cut the muscles with a knife or diathermy blade. When cutting the rectus muscle transversely, it helps to insinuate your index finger or a pair of curved artery forceps beneath the muscle and then divide the fibres onto the finger or forceps. The assistant picks up vessels running vertically and these are coagulated.

(b) Split the muscle, if the fibres run in the line of the incision or in the gridiron and Lanz incisions.

(c) In a paramedian approach displace the rectus muscle laterally within its sheath. Cut the tendinous intersections free from the medial part of the sheath and draw the muscle belly laterally.

6. Stop the bleeding with diathermy coagulation or fine ligatures. Control persistent muscle bleeding by inserting a 2/0 catgut stitch on a round-bodied needle. Tie the suture just tightly enough to stop the bleeding and not so tight that it cuts through the muscle.

7. Open the peritoneum (Fig. 4.3). Pick it up with toothed dissecting forceps and grip the tented portion with artery forceps. Release the artery forceps and reapply to the peritoneum. The change of grip allows the viscera to escape if they are caught by the first application of the forceps.

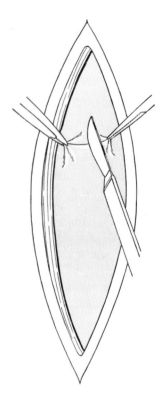

Fig. 4.3 Incising the peritoneum

Incise the peritoneum with the belly of the knife. Air enters the abdomen and the viscera fall clear. Insert your index finger and complete the peritoneal opening with scissors, taking care not to injure the abdominal contents.

RE-OPENING THE ABDOMEN

Siting the incision

1. Does the previous incision coincide with the site you would have chosen for present access? If so, reopen it. If not, ignore it and make a new incision in the correct site.

2. Remember that you may require a longer incision than would be necessary for an initial operation.

Access through the old incision

1. Make an incision down the centre of the old scar. If the scar is ugly or stretched, excise it as an elongated ellipse.

2. Do not attempt to dissect out a previous paramedian incision, but cut through all the tissues in the line of the skin wound. Do not cut too boldly, because the deeper layers may be defective, so that you may quickly enter the cavity or even the contents of the abdomen.

3. When opening the peritoneum in the line of the previous incision, remember that viscera may be adherent to

its undersurface. Entering the abdomen is greatly facilitated if the wound is extended at one end, so that unscarred peritoneum can be incised.

4. Once the abdomen is opened, carefully extend the incision little by little. Use fine scissors for this dissection and ensure that each proposed cut is clear of adherent structures.

5. Do not inexorably separate firmly fixed structures through an incomplete incision. Either skirt around them so that they now remain attached to one side of the wound, or open the other end of the wound and approach them from a different direction.

6. Have the wound edge lifted with tissue-holding forceps and encircle the adherent structures to estimate the degree of fixity and the plane of cleavage between them and the original parietal peritoneum. At intervals in the dissection allow the structures to relax, assess progress and start again, possibly from a new approach. Use a scalpel or scissors, remembering never to cut what cannot be seen.

7. Make sure that you leave the abdominal wall and, if possible, the peritoneal lining intact, so that satisfactory closure can be achieved.

Access through a new incision

1. Although this approach may be easier, remember that after a previous operation viscera may be adherent to the parietal peritoneum anywhere.

2. Once the abdomen is opened, at a distance from the previous incision, dissection of adherent viscera from the undersurface of the old scar has to be carried out beneath the elevated wound edge with only one aspect of the adhesions accessible to view. Much of the advantage of making a fresh incision may therefore be lost.

Division of adhesions

1. Adhesions may develop congenitally or result from peritoneal inflammation, but in most cases they follow previous laparotomy. When operating on the abdomen, try to minimise the likelihood of adhesions by washing off all glove powder from the outside of your gloves, and avoid leaving foreign bodies (e.g. lengths of suture material) or ischaemic tissue (e.g. omentum) within the peritoneal cavity.

2. Separation of adherent viscera from the wound edge has already been described. It can be an arduous and hazardous task, and the small bowel is particularly vulnerable to injury. If you enter the small-bowel lumen inadvertently, close the defect with two layers of catgut sutures immediately, pausing only to free the damaged loop of bowel to facilitate closure. Try and limit contamination of the wound with intestinal contents by prompt use of the sucker and gauze swabs. If contamination occurs nevertheless, consider lavage of the wound and peritoneal cavity with warm saline.

3. It is not necessary to divide every single adhesion between viscera during every laparotomy; indeed such a policy would often be counterproductive. On the other hand, when the viscera are tangled together it can be difficult to progress with the operation until the normal anatomical relationships have been restored. Learn to recognise thick fleshy band adhesions which could distort the small bowel and give rise to future symptoms. When operating for adhesion obstruction, it is usually best to take down the adhesions completely and replace the small bowel in an orderly fashion.

4. When dividing intra-abdominal adhesions, vary the point of attack but do not become aimless. Keep in mind the objects of the dissection: to allow adequate exploration, to permit safe closure without fear of damaging the viscera and to prevent subsequent kinking or herniation of the bowel.

Further reading

Ellis H, 1980 Internal overhealing: the problem of intraperitoneal adhesions. World Journal of Surgery 4: 303–306

EXPLORATORY LAPAROTOMY

Access

Choice of incision

1. Never forget that the prime function of an incision is to provide safe access. Although important, unsightliness, liability to herniation and discomfort are side issues. Remember that incisions heal from the sides and not the ends.

2. Open the abdomen over the site of the suspected lesion, so far as the costal margin and iliac crest allow. Use one of the established types of laparotomy incision (p. 42). Remember that the incision may need to be extended, particularly if you do not have a confident pre-operative diagnosis.

3. The choice of incision for a particular operation is listed in Table 4.1 and discussed in the chapter devoted to the relevant organ. The choice may vary according to circumstances. For example, some surgeons perform elective cholecystectomy through a transverse incision, which leaves an excellent scar, but prefer the greater flexibility of a vertical incision when tackling the gallbladder in an emergency or in the presence of obstructive jaundice. In emergency colonic surgery, bear in mind the possible need for an intestinal stoma when selecting the laparotomy incision.

4. In emergency laparotomy for unexplained peritonitis or abdominal trauma, use either a right paramedian incision or a midline incision that skirts the umbilicus. Place the incision more above or more below the umbilicus, depending on the probable site of disease or damage. Incisions that extend on either side of the umbilicus can readily

be extended in either direction once the pathology is revealed.

5. Midline incisions are quicker to create (and close) than paramedian incisions and should therefore be selected in cases of rapid bleeding, such as ruptured spleen or leaking aortic aneurysm.

6. Be prepared to use a previous laparotomy incision if it is conveniently placed or can readily be extended to allow appropriate access. The technique of abdominal re-entry is described in the preceding section of this chapter.

Access within the abdomen

1. If on entering the peritoneal cavity you find that the incision is likely to provide inadequate exposure, do not hesitate to extend it. If the incision proves to be inappropriate (e.g. a right Lanz incision for perforated peptic ulcer), close it and start again. Never be too proud to perform one or other of these maneuvres. Disasters tend to occur when inexperienced surgeons struggle to complete an operation through the wrong incision.

2. Figure 4.4. illustrates ways in which certain common incisions can be extended to deal with unexpected lesions or intra-operative difficulties.

3. Remember that the position of the patient on the operating table can greatly affect exposure particularly of organs at either end of the abdominal cavity. To approach the pelvic viscera ask the anaesthetist to tilt the table head down (Trendelenburg position). Have the patient tilted head up (reversed Trendelenburg) for access to the oesophagus and diaphragmatic hiatus. Rotating the table away from yourself facilitates an extraperitoneal approach to the ureter or lumbar sympthetic chain on your side. Rotation towards the surgeon operating from the patient's right may improve access to the spleen. If you anticipate steep tilts in any direction secure the patient adequately beforehand, using a pelvic strap and/or a support beneath the heels.

4. Nearly every laparotomy requires some retraction of the abdominal wall and adjacent viscera to expose the organ(s) in question. Retraction of the wound edge will assist the initial exploratory laparotomy. When you have assessed the abdominal viscera and determined your operative strategy, insert retractor(s) and instruct your assistant(s) how to hold them. Pack away 'unwanted' organs, principally small-bowel loops, using large gauze swabs to which metal rings have been sewn to minimise the risk of their being left in the abdomen during closure. These packs should be wrung out in warm physiological saline, and they are more effective at restraining the bowel if they are not completely unfolded.

5. Marshal the forces at your disposal carefully. Use of a self-retaining retractor may release an assistant to provide more direct help. Instruments of the De Bakey pattern have an optional third blade, which may help to keep the small bowel out of the pelvis. A sternal retractor is invaluable in operations on the abdominal oesophagus and upper stomach. The instrument hooks under the xiphisternum and is connected to a gantry over the patient's head.

6. Specific manoeuvres are either essential or extremely helpful in the exposure of certain organs. For access to the oesophagus and hiatus, mobilise the left lobe of liver by dividing its peritoneal attachment to the diaphragm. To examine fully the back wall of the stomach and the body of pancreas, you must enter the lesser sac, usually by dividing part of the greater omentum. For thorough examination of the duodenum, divide the peritoneum along the convexity of its loop (Kocher's manoeuvre). Displace the small bowel into the upper abdomen to approach the pelvic viscera and out of the abdominal cavity into a plastic bag for operations on the aorta.

Assess

1. Wash blood and all glove powder from the gloves. The starch lubricant is an important cause of adhesions. Deal with established adhesions as described on page 45.

2. Make sure that there are no instruments near the wound except for a retractor for your assistant and a sucker tube available for yourself. It is helpful to have someone in attendance to adjust the theatre light as necessary.

3. Carry out a methodical examination of the abdomen and its contents by feel and, whenever possible, by sight. Always follow the same sequence (Fig. 4.5):
(a) Right lobe of liver, gallbladder, left lobe of liver, spleen
(b) Diaphragmatic hiatus, abdominal oesophagus and stomach: cardia, body, lesser curve, antrum, pylorus and then duodenal bulb

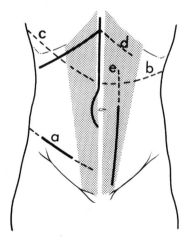

Fig. 4.4 Methods of extending certain abdominal incisions: a) gridiron incision extended laterally and (to a greater extent) medially; b) midline incision with T extension into left upper quadrant to deal with profuse splenic haemorrhage; c) midline incision with T extension into the right chest for ruptured liver; d) Kocher incision with left subcostal extension for major hepatic procedures; e) left lower paramedian incision extended upwards for mobilisation of left colic flexure.

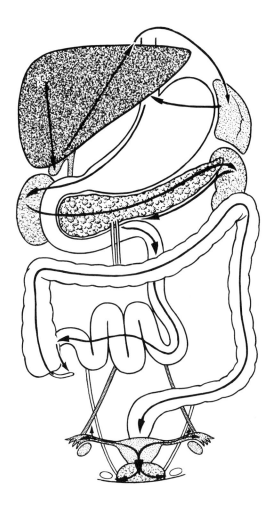

Fig. 4.5 The order of examining the abdominal contents at exploratory laparotomy.

(c) Bile ducts, right kidney, duodenal loop, head of pancreas. Now draw the transverse colon out of the wound towards the patient's head

(d) Body and tail of pancreas, left kidney

(e) Root of mesentery, superior mesenteric and middle colic vessels, aorta, inferior mesenteric artery and vein, small bowel and mesentery from ligament of Treitz to ileocaecal valve

(f) Appendix, caecum, the rest of the colon, rectum

(g) Pelvic peritoneum, uterus, tubes and ovaries in the female, bladder

(h) Hernial orifices and main iliac vessels on each side. The ureters can sometimes be seen in thin patients, or if they are dilated

4. Aim to carry out a thorough examination (as above) in most **elective** cases, and record your findings carefully and in detail. These principles are particularly important when laparotomy is the last of a series of investigations to identify the cause of symptoms. Sometimes the incision chosen precludes a complete exploration, for example in interval appendicectomy or pyloromyotomy in infancy.

Sometimes the condition found makes further exploration pointless, for example in carcinomatosis peritonei. In this circumstance make a gentle search for the primary tumour, obtain a biopsy from one of the deposits, make sure no palliative procedure (e.g. intestinal bypass) is required and close the abdomen. As a general rule do not handle a malignant tumour more than is essential for fear of dissemination.

5. In **emergency** laparotomy immediate action may be required, for example to stop bleeding or close a perforation. Thereafter, proceed to a methodical examination of the other viscera as before, unless the patient's general condition is poor or there is localised infection. Drainage of an abscess should usually be treated as a local condition. Do not forget to note the nature and amount of any free fluid, and obtain swabs for bacteriological culture of any potentially infected collection.

Action

1. In deciding the definitive procedure now to be undertaken, you will be guided by your pre-operative knowledge of the patient, the extent of disease as revealed at laparotomy and the patient's age and general condition. Options include partial or total resection of an organ, bypass, drainage, exteriorisation, closure of perforation, removal of foreign body, biopsy or perhaps no active procedure. In elderly or sick patients, control of the emergency or major elective condition should take precedence over the complete eradication of disease. Once you have formulated a plan of campaign, discuss your intentions with the anaesthetist and intimate how long you are likely to take to carry them out.

2. Be wary of tackling incidental procedures, such as prophylactic appendicectomy, without a clear indication. The chance finding of gallstones, diverticula, fibroids, ovarian cysts etc. does not automatically call for action unless they pose an immediate threat to health or offer a better explanation for symptoms than the condition originally diagnosed. By contrast, an unsuspected neoplasm should ordinarily be removed, if necessary through a separate incision, provided the patient's condition allows. Whatever course you adopt, be sure to record all your findings in the operation note.

3. Remember that the interior of the distal small bowel and the entire large bowel is unsterile. Contents of hollow viscera that are normally sterile (e.g. bile, urine, gastric juice) may also become infected as a result of inflammation and obstruction. Before opening the bowel or other potentially contaminated viscera, isolate them from contact with the wound and other organs. Consider using non-crushing clamps to occlude the lumen, and make sure that you have an efficient suction apparatus to remove any contents that spill. Pack away other structures before opening the viscus and discard the packs once it is closed. Remember that all

the instruments used on opened bowel become unsterile, therefore they must be isolated and subsequently discarded. Likewise, change your gloves before closing the abdomen.

4. The danger of infection is one of degree. The tissues can normally cope with a small number of organisms but are overwhelmed by heavy contamination or re-infection. Generally, wounds are more susceptible to infection than the peritoneal cavity itself. If there has been gross spillage of infected visceral contents, wash out the abdominal cavity with warm saline and start broad-spectrum antibiotic therapy.

5. Intestinal clamps are of two sorts: crushing and non-crushing. **Crushing** clamps are applied to seal the bowel when it is cut. Payr's powerful double-action clamps are most frequently used, but Lang Stevenson has devised a similar clamp with narrow blades. Cope's triple clamps allow the middle clamp to be removed, so that the bowel can be divided through the crushed area, leaving its ends sealed. **Non-crushing** clamps have longitudinal ridges and control the leakage of bowel contents without causing irreversible damage to the gut. Lane's twin clamps, which can be locked together, allow two pieces of gut to be occluded and held in apposition for anastomosis. Pringle's clamps hold cut ends of bowel securely and the crushed segment is so narrow that it can safely be incorporated in the anastomosis.

6. The danger of leaving articles in the abdominal cavity is ever-present but to do so is inexcusable. Unfortunately, there is no single routine that will entirely guard against this mishap. Always use the minimum number of instruments and the largest swabs, and make sure they are never out of sight. Involve all your team in guarding against leaving an instrument or swab, even though you must accept the responsibility personally. If the scrub nurse reports a missing swab or instrument while you are closing the abdomen, check the peritoneal cavity once again. If all else fails, obtain an abdominal X-ray before letting the patient awake from the anaesthetic.

Further reading

Ellis H 1984 How to do a laparotomy. British Journal of Hospital Medicine 31: 437–439
Everett W G 1974 Sutures, incisions and anastomoses. Annals of the Royal College of Surgeons of England 55: 31–38
Kirk R M 1976 Exploration of the abdomen. Annals of the Royal College of Surgeons of England 58: 452–456

CLOSING THE ABDOMEN

Assess

1. Before starting to close, make sure that the swab count and instrument count are both correct. Check for haemostasis. Decide whether you need to drain the abdo-

men (see below). Remove any odds and ends of suture material and replace the viscera in their correct anatomical position.

2. There are several different techniques for abdominal closure and three are described below. The choice depends upon the type of incision, the extent of the operation, the patient's general condition and the surgeon's preference. As you assist different surgeons you will learn various technical modifications and develop your own methods of closing the abdomen under differing circumstances. Most surgeons use a continuous suture for the deep layers of the abdominal wall.

3. It is a common error among surgical trainees to sew up the abdomen too tightly, for fear it will fall apart. Remember that wounds swell during the first 3–4 postoperative days and that oedema will make the sutures even tighter. There is a risk of tissue necrosis and subsequent dehiscence. As a general rule the length of suture material used for the aponeurotic layer(s) should be about 3 times the length of the incision. Place each suture 1 cm from the edge of the wound and 1 cm away from the previous 'bite'.

4. Select a strong non-absorbable suture material for closing the deeper (aponeurotic) layers of the abdominal wall; 1 monofilament nylon on a round-bodied needle is very satisfactory in adults. Some surgeons use a doubled length of finer material (e.g. 0 nylon) and run the first stitch through the loop to avoid having a knot at the end of the wound. With a long wound or an obese patient it may be more convenient to use two lengths of suture, starting at each end and meeting in the middle.

5. Consider using tension sutures if the abdomen is distended or obese, if the wound is infected or likely to become so, if the patient is malnourished, jaundiced, suffering from advanced cancer or has a chronic cough — in short, in any situation where you anticipate poor wound healing.

6. Remember that the abdominal wound is the only part of the operation that the patient can see, and take care to produce a neat result. Bury the knots used to tie off the deep sutures, especially in a thin patient. In an uncontaminated wound, aim for close apposition of the skin and a fine linear scar; consider the use of subcuticular sutures, therefore.

Action

Layered closure

1. Some surgeons do not bother to close the peritoneum, especially in a midline incision. Certainly there is little strength to this layer, and a new mesothelial lining apparently develops to cover the defect from within. Where the posterior rectus sheath exists as a separate layer, as in paramedian, transverse and oblique incisions in the upper abdomen, the peritoneum can also be incorporated in the deepest layer of sutures.

2. Pick up the edges of the peritoneum and posterior

rectus sheath, and apply one pair of artery forceps to these combined layers on each side of the wound. Make sure the bowel is not caught. Have the assistant hold up the artery forceps, so that the peritoneum is lifted clear of the viscera as you insert each suture.

3. Starting at one or other end of the incision, take a bite on each side close to the apex and tie the knot securely. Make sure that the needle does not pick up bowel or omentum. Take generous bites with each stitch and pull up snugly but not tightly. Having tightened the stitch, do not let it slacken. Have the assistant keep tension on the thread while the next stitch is inserted. After placing four or five stitches and tightening them, insert a finger to confirm that the bowel is free. Tie the knots securely, and do not have the ends shorter than 5 mm.

4. When muscles have been cut or split, unite them with interrupted 0 catgut sutures tied just tightly enough to appose the edges. When the rectus muscle is cut transversely, it is not necessary to repair it with sutures because the tendinous intersections limit retraction. Similarly, in a paramedian incision, the rectus muscle falls back into place after closing the peritoneum, and no sutures are required.

5. Repair the aponeurosis of external oblique or the anterior rectus sheath. After tying the knot at the end of the incision, cut the end of suture material short and take the next bite from within to without; this manoeuvre will help to bury the knot. Once again have the assistant maintain an even tension on the thread and avoid pulling up each suture so tightly that you strangle tissue.

6. Ensure that there is no oozing of blood in the superficial layers. Ligate or coagulate any vessels that are still bleeding. If the subcutaneous tissues are deep, consider using a few interrupted 2/0 or 3/0 catgut sutures to appose them.

7. Appose the skin edges, using one of several standard techniques. Interrupted sutures are preferable in a contaminated or irregular wound. Mattress sutures help to evert the skin edges slightly and bring together the deeper layers. Suitable suture materials include 2/0 black silk, 2/0 or 3/0 monofilament nylon or polypropylene; Michel clips and adhesive skin strips are alternatives. Some surgeons use a continuous over-and-over or continuous mattress suture routinely.

8. In a clean and straightforward wound, a subcuticular suture, using 2/0 polypropylene on a straight needle, can provide a very acceptable scar. Insert the needle in the line of the incision about 1 cm away from its apex and bring it out through the apex in the subcuticular plane. Now continue along the incision taking small and frequent bites of the subcutis; avoid piercing the skin. When you reach the other end, bring the needle out through the skin about 1 cm beyound the apex of the incision. Tighten the suture material to close the wound and make sure that it runs freely. Fix the suture at each end with tiny lead weights, or tie the ends in a slack loop.

Mass closure

1. The peritoneum and rectus sheaths may be closed with a single stitch, or the linea alba may be closed in one layer without suturing the peritoneum. This is a simple, rapid technique which can be used routinely or reserved for difficult cases. It is particularly useful when closing an incision through a previous scar, when the layers are often partly fused.

2. Insert a continuous running stitch of 1 monofilament nylon mounted on a large spear-pointed needle. Place the stitches 1–2 cm from the edges, catching all the included layers.

3. Tighten the stitches as you proceed, checking that the bowel is free beneath. Do not let the stitch slip afterwards by getting your assistant to follow up, but avoid undue tension. Make doubly sure the bowel is free before tightening and tying the last stitch. Cut the bristly ends of nylon short.

4. Close the skin as for layered closure.

Closure with tension sutures (Fig. 4.6)

1. Tension sutures should usually pass through all layers of the abdominal wall, including the skin. Interrupted through-and-through sutures are inserted first and tied at the end. They are used to supplement a standard closure in poor-risk patients. Some surgeons exclude the skin and leave the tension sutures buried in the tissues.

2. Use a strong non-absorbable suture material, such as 1 monofilament nylon, swaged to a curved hand needle (cutting). Take deep bites about 3 cm away from the edge of the wound and incorporating all layers. Be very careful neither to prick the bowel when inserting the stitches nor to trap it when tightening them. It is a good idea to interpose the greater omentum between the wound and the small intestine to lessen this risk.

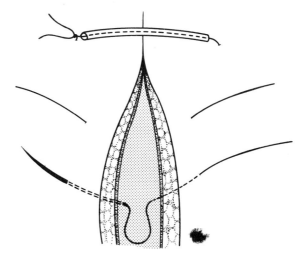

Fig. 4.6 Abdominal closure with deep tension sutures. Strong through-and-through sutures are placed 2–3 cm apart and tied over a protective polyethylene bar (after all sutures have been inserted).

3. After inserting each deep tension suture, leave an artery forceps attached to each end of the suture while closing the deeper layers of the abdominal wall. Then tie the tension sutures to appose the skin and subcutaneous tissues. Thread each suture over a length of polyethylene or rubber tubing to prevent it cutting in, and be particularly careful not to tie it too tightly. A limited number of interrupted skin sutures may be placed to complete the closure.

4. If healing proceeds satisfactorily, it is usual to remove the skin sutures 7–10 days postoperatively but to leave the tension sutures for a further 2–4 days.

Delayed closure

1. If the abdominal cavity is grossly contaminated, as in faecal peritonitis, some degree of wound sepsis is almost inevitable. One option is to close the superficial tissues lightly around a drain. Another is delayed primary suture, leaving the skin and subcutaneous tissue widely open. In either case, parenteral antibiotics should be given and the peritoneal cavity should be drained. Consider also the possibility of postoperative lavage (see below).

2. Close the musculoaponeurotic layers of the abdominal wall with a continuous monofilament nylon suture. Be particularly careful not to draw the edges together too tightly, because considerable swelling can be anticipated. Superficial to this layer, loosely pack the wound with gauze swabs wrung out in saline.

3. Change the packs and inspect the wound daily. Delayed primary suture can be performed when the patient's condition improves and any wound sepsis has abated.

Difficulty?

The deepest layer may be difficult to close because the abdominal contents keep bulging through the wound. Inadequate anaesthesia, obesity or intestinal distension are usually to blame. Even after successfully inserting your stitches, they may cut out. Be patient and do not despair.

1. Ask the anaesthetist if he can produce greater relaxation of the abdominal muscles.

2. Insert the stitches 2–3 cm from the edges, using a continuous over-and-over or mattress technique. Do not tighten the thread until you have inserted three or four stitches loosely. Now pull up slowly in the line of the incision, while the assistant compresses the abdomen from each side. The assistant should maintain the tension while you insert the next batch of sutures. As the closure proceeds it becomes easier.

3. The bowel is doubly at risk during difficult closures. Consider using a swab on a holder, a length of rubber drain or a 'shoe-horn' depressor laid in the wound to protect the bowel; remove it before completing the closure. Remember to avoid the bowel when placing the final sutures.

4. If a stitch tears out, remain phlegmatic. Insert a mattress suture from within the abdomen, 3–4 cm from the edge, taking a deep bite of tissue.

Drains and dressings

1. Tubular or corrugated drains of plastic or rubber may be inserted either through the end of the wound or through a separate stab hole in the abdominal wall. The inner end of the drain is placed in the region of the operation site to evacuate blood and any other fluid contents from the peritoneal cavity. Fine-bore polyethylene tube drains are now available, which can be screwed to a special trocar for insertion through the abdominal wall. They have many tiny drainage holes, all of which should be placed within the peritoneum, and they can be connected to a vacuum bottle or bag to maintain suction down the tube.

2. Other tube drains can be used to drain certain viscera to the exterior during the postoperative period. Again, these should usually be inserted through a separate stab incision. Examples are a T-tube into the bile duct, a gastrostomy or suprapubic cystostomy catheter and a feeding jejunostomy tube.

3. Stitch the drain to the skin. When possible, insert a large safety pin through the drain to prevent any possibility of it being lost within the abdomen. If a drainage tube is attached to a closed bag or suction apparatus, tie the stitch securely around the tube.

4. Apply dressings to seal the main wound, with separate dressings over the drain wound. The drain may then be re-dressed, shortened and removed, without disturbing the main wound.

5. Opinions differ widely concerning the use of drains following laparotomy. Drains rarely do harm when properly inserted, provided they are removed after about 48 hours if there is no discharge. A closed drainage system should not introduce infection. Insertion of a drainage tube is no substitute for good operative technique, however. Some generally accepted indications for draining the peritoneal cavity are as follows:

(a) Routinely after operations on the gallbladder, bile duct on pancreas, in case there is leakage of bile or pancreatic juice.

(b) When there is a localized abscess.

(c) After suture of a perforated viscus, such as stomach, duodenum or colonic diverticulum, when the tissues are friable. Consider if another operative manoeuvre would give greater safety.

(d) When there is a large raw area from which oozing can occur. Do not make insertion of a drain an excuse for failure to control bleeding, however.

(e) Sometimes after operations for general peritonitis, even if you have removed the cause.

6. Wound drains are occasionally indicated in very obese

patients or grossly contaminated wounds. A thin corrugated drain or a tube suction drain is inserted deep to the skin and subcutaneous tissues and removed after 2–3 days or when it ceases to discharge.

7. Dressings are also controversial. From a bacteriological standpoint it probably makes little difference whether the wound is occluded by a dressing or left open to the atmosphere. Transparent adhesive dressings have the advantage of allowing the surgeon to inspect the wound repeatedly without disturbing the dressing. If a good deal of discharge is anticipated, use dressing gauze and wool. Remember that some patients are sensitive to adhesive strapping.

Lavage

1. The peritoneal cavity has a remarkable ability to combat sepsis. Nonetheless, spillage of contaminated contents, such as faeces or infected bile, may lead to early septicaemia and late abdominal abscess.

2. Where local peritonitis is marked, it is important to remove all pus and debris from that part of the abdomen. We usually wash out the area with aliquots of warm saline (ca. 500 ml in toto), sucking out the fluid and inserting a drain. The theoretical risk of disseminating the infection through the peritoneal cavity does not appear to hold true in practice.

3. In generalised peritonitis the abdomen should be thoroughly cleansed with warm saline (1–2 l) at the end of the operation. In very severe cases (e.g. pancreatic necrosis, faecal peritonitis), consider inserting 1 or 2 delivery tubes and 1 or 2 drainage tubes for postoperative lavage. One drainage tube is placed in the abscess cavity and one in the pelvis; soft, wide-bore, silicone tubes or sump drains are appropriate. We use warmed peritoneal dialysis fluid (Dialaflex 61) with added potassium for lavage, irrigating between 50–500 ml per hour depending on the extent of sepsis. Try and obtain a watertight closure of the abdominal wound and start with small amounts of dialysate (50 ml/hour) overnight, until the peritoneum seals the defects. Postoperative lavage is well tolerated and does not seem to interfere with intestinal motility. Continue the treatment for up to 2 weeks and remove the drains when the return fluid becomes clear.

Further reading

Dudley HAF 1970 Layered and mass closure of the abdominal wall. British Journal of Surgery 57: 664–667

Hubbard TB Jr, Rever WB Jr 1972 Retention sutures in the closure of abdominal incisions. American Journal of Surgery 124: 378–380

Jenkins T P N 1976 The burst abdominal wound: a mechanical approach. British Journal of Surgery 63: 873–876

Penninckx FM, Poelmans SV, Kerremans RP, Beckers JP 1979 Abdominal wound dehiscence in gastroenterological surgery. Annals of Surgery 189: 345–352

RESUTURE OF BURST ABDOMEN

Access

1. Have the dressings removed, and make sure they are kept separate from the swabs. Have any skin sutures that remain in place removed.

2. Open up the whole wound after preparing the skin and towelling off the area. Remove all suture material.

Assess

1. Why has this wound broken down? Collect a bacteriological specimen for aerobic and anaerobic culture. Examine the suture material and the suture holes. Is the peritoneum partly intact? Where are its edges?

2. Are the abdominal contents normal? Make sure that the underlying small bowel is intact. If free fluid or pus are present or if the bowel is grossly dilated, check the cause.

Action

1. Dissect the skin and subcutaneous tissues from the aponeurotic layer on each side to clear 2 cm of aponeurosis (or muscle). Similarly, free the omentum and bowel for a short distance on the deep aspect of the wound on each side.

2. Insert deep tension sutures, as described in the previous section. Each suture should pass through all layers of the abdominal wall, including the skin. Allow 3–4 cm between tension sutures.

3. Now proceed with mass closure of the peritoneum and rectus sheath or the linea alba. Be certain to take deep bites of tissue, using plenty of suture material, and again avoid excessive tension on the wound. Some surgeons prefer to use interrupted stitches of a strong non-absorbable material.

4. Whether continuous or interrupted sutures are employed, take great care not to incorporate the viscera in any of the stitches.

5. Close the skin fairly loosely and consider using a superficial wound drain.

6. A many-tailed bandage or an elastic corset provides extra support.

LAPAROTOMY FOR ABDOMINAL TRAUMA

Appraise

1. Resuscitate a shocked patient, but do not delay laparotomy longer than necessary if you suspect active intraperitoneal bleeding. Exsanguinating haemorrhage from rupture of the spleen or liver can only be controlled by prompt intervention.

2. In blunt abdominal trauma, exploration may be indicated by increasing abdominal tenderness and girth, persisting hypovolaemia despite replacement therapy and diagnostic paracentesis confirming haemoperitoneum. Rupture of a hollow viscus such as the small bowel may present more slowly with failure of symptoms and signs to improve as the injury recedes in time.

3. In open injuries, exploration may be indicated by evidence of peritonism, a bloody tap on needling the abdomen or penetration confirmed by sinography or exploration of the wound under local anaesthetic.

4. Paracentesis may be quickly peformed by inserting a needle into each of the four abdominal quadrants in turn and aspirating with a syringe. A more reliable method of confirming a haemoperitoneum is to insert an intravenous cannula into the peritoneal cavity through a small nick in the skin, about 5 cm below the umbilicus in the midline. One litre of warm saline is rapidly instilled and allowed to drain back by gravity.Use local anaesthetic for either technique in a conscious patient.

5. If there is any chance of renal injury, try to obtain an emergency intravenous urogram before opening the abdomen.

Access

1. If the site of injury is uncertain or the damage is likely to be widespread, open the abdomen through a 15–20 cm midline or right paramedian incision placed half above and half below the umbilicus. In a bleeding patient select the midline incision, which is quicker.

2. If there is a local penetrating injury of the abdomen in a convenient position, excise the wound and extend it to allow full exploration.

3. Do not hesitate to extend the wound quickly to gain control of haemorrhage. A T-shaped extension into the left hypochondrium is occasionally necessary in ruptured spleen, and extension into the right chest may be required in ruptured liver.

Assess

1. The commonest causes of traumatic haemoperitoneum are ruptured spleen, ruptured liver and a mesenteric tear, in that order. Feel the spleen and liver in turn. Remove clot, suck out blood and gain control of the bleeding.

2. Proceed to a methodical examination of the abdominal contents, including the abdominal wall and retroperitoneum. Remember that more than one organ may be injured. In appropriate cases, search for foreign bodies, such as bullets.

Action

1. If the spleen is injured try and staunch the bleeding and determine whether any splenic tissue can be salvaged (p. 216). If the organ is severely lacerated or pulped, deliver it quickly and remove it after ligation of the pedicle.

2. If the liver is injured decide whether to suture it, excise the damaged portion or, if all else fails, pack the wound. Enlist senior support if possible.

3. Remove a ruptured gallbladder. Repair ruptured bile ducts with fine catgut sutures, leaving a T-tube to splint the anastomosis.

4. Examine the gut, its mesenteries and vessels from oesophagus to rectum. Oversew bruised areas or partial tears. Suture holes in two layers and avoid narrowing the lumen. Remember that bullet holes come in multiples of two. Excise portions of bowel that are grossly damaged or have an impaired blood supply, e.g. from a torn mesentery. Inspect haematomas of the mesentery to see if they are spreading or the bowel is ischaemic; if in any doubt incise the overlying peritoneum, shell out the clot and identify and ligate the bleeding points. Colonic injuries demand extreme caution. It is safest to exteriorise the perforation as a colostomy or to defunction repaired segments with a proximal colostomy. Again after partial resection, do not hesitate to exteriorize the ends for anatomosis at a later date.

5. A retroperitoneal haematoma in the upper abdomen suggests the possibility of duodenal or pancreatic injury and should be actively pursued. Mobilise the duodenum by Kocher's manoeuvre and explore its posterior surface. Enter the lesser sac to expose the pancreas. Repair superficial lacerations, but if the gland is fractured where its neck crosses the vertebral column, proceed to distal pancreatectomy.

6. A retroperitoneal haematoma in the lower abdomen can be left alone with greater safety, provided it is not obviously expanding. The haematoma may have resulted from renal contusion or a fractured pelvis, and opening the retroperitoneum may encourage the bleeding to continue. Most renal injuries should be treated conservatively. Avulsion of the vascular pedicle will probably necessitate nephrectomy, but it is mandatory to show satisfactory function of the opposite kidney. Lesser injuries may be amenable to suture or partial nephrectomy.

7. Repair a divided ureter with fine sutures and leave a stenting tube in situ. If the injury is low down, reimplantation into the bladder may be a better option. Repair an intraperitoneal rupture of the bladder in two layers and insert a urethral catheter at the end of the operation. If the bladder is clearly completely disconnected from the prostate at laparotomy (complete rupture of the urethra), perform suprapubic cystostomy and try to 'railroad' a catheter across the defect.

8. If possible repair the damaged ovaries, tubes and uterus of a young woman, but excise them in a woman who has passed the menopause.

9. Examine the aorta, the inferior vena cava and the abdominal wall, before closing the abdomen.

10. Insert a drain if there has been extensive damage, oozing or established infection. Always drain injuries to the liver or pancreas

Further reading

Bewes PC 1983 Open and closed abdominal injuries. British Journal of Hospital Medicine 29: 402–410
Johnstone GW, Kennedy TL 1976 Limb and abdominal injuries: principles of treatment. British Journal of Surgery 63: 738–741

LAPAROTOMY FOR GENERAL PERITONITIS

Appraise

1. Generalized peritonitis usually follows fairly rapid perforation of an inflamed hollow viscus, as in acute appendicitis or an anterior duodenal ulcer; the abdominal cavity is flooded with infected contents. A similar clinical picture occurs with intraperitoneal haemorrhage, e.g. from blunt abdominal trauma, acute pancreatitis or ruptured ectopic pregnancy, but these patients may exhibit pallor and shock as well as abdominal tenderness and rigidity. If perforation occurs slowly, as in some cases of cholecystitis and sigmoid diverticulitis, the greater omentum and adjacent organs may be able to localize the inflammation, but there is always a risk that the resultant abscess will burst into the general peritoneal cavity.

2. Very occasionally generalised peritonitis develops in the absence of any overt visceral disease. Primary peritonitis can occur spontaneously in children and seems to be commoner in patients with ascites or nephrotic syndrome. The pneumococcus is one of the commoner infecting organisms.

3. Consider starting antibiotic therapy pre-operatively once you have made the decision to operate for generalized peritonitis. Parenteral administration of a cephalosporin or an aminoglycoside plus an anaerobicide (e.g. metronidazole) will provide broad-spectrum cover.

Access

1. If there are no localizing signs, use a midline or right paramedian incision placed half above and half below the umbilicus. Be prepared to extend it in either direction once the lesion is revealed. Examination of the abdomen under anaesthetic may reveal an unsuspected mass, which helps you to site the incision correctly in the first place.

2. Since acute appendicitis is the commonest cause of peritonitis, use a Lanz or gridiron incision if the diagnosis seems at all likely. The incision can be extended medially or laterally to deal with nearby conditions if the diagnosis proves wrong, or it may be closed and a fresh incision made.

3. Remember that irritant fluids, such as gastric juice, blood and bile may track around the abdomen. Make sure you establish where the pain first started.

4. If peritonitis follows a recent operation, reopen the previous incision (p. 44).

Assess

1. Note any free fluid, and save a specimen for laboratory examination.

2. After a rapid preliminary examination of the abdomen, carry out a methodical exploration.

Action

1. Make sure that the incision, the assistance and the instruments available are adequate for the proposed procedure.

2. Resect an inflamed appendix, gallbladder, segment of gangrenous or damaged bowel, perforated neoplasm or Meckel's diverticulum.

3. Repair ruptured small bowel or a leaking suture line from a previous operation. Close a perforated peptic ulcer, but consider definitive procedures such as vagotomy or gastrectomy in appropriate patients with a long history of indigestion.

4. Resect a specimen of perforated colon, but be very cautious about restoring intestinal continuity without a proximal diverting colostomy. Resection with exteriorisation of the bowel ends is an even safer option. Closure of a perforated sigmoid diverticulum with or without transverse colostomy may be appropriate in selected cases, but perforated carcinomas should be resected if possible.

5. Remove any foreign bodies from the peritoneal cavity. Consider saline lavage and postoperative drainage if there is gross infection or contamination with intestinal contents. Drain an abscess.

6. Normally take no definitive action if you encounter acute pancreatitis, acute salpingitis, uncomplicated ileitis or primary peritonitis. Consider whether a biopsy (e.g. of a lymph node in Crohn's disease) or bacteriological culture swab (e.g. of the uterine tube) might provide useful information. Pancreatitis is recognised by a bloodstained effusion, discolouration of the retroperitoneum and the presence of whiteish patches of fat necrosis. In salpingitis, both uterine tubes are reddened, swollen and oedematous, often discharging pus from the abdominal ostia. Regional ileitis produces an inflamed, thickened bowel and mesentery, often covered with exudate. In primary peritonitis no cause can be found; the pus tends to be odourless and a gram film may reveal cocci.

Further reading

Armitage TG, Williamson RCN 1983 Primary peritonitis in children and adults. Postgraduate Medical Journal 59: 21–24
Editorial 1980 Peritonitis today. British Medical Journal 280: 1095–1096
Silen W 1979 Cope's Early diagnosis of the acute abdomen, 15th edn. Oxford University Press, London

LAPAROTOMY FOR INTESTINAL OBSTRUCTION

Appraise

1. Before proceeding to laparotomy make sure that the patient is adequately rehydrated with intravenous fluids (usually at least two litres are required) and pass a nasogastric tube to decompress the gut. Consider prescribing an enema to overcome an incomplete obstruction.

2. Inspect the erect and supine abdominal X-rays to determine the level of obstruction. Dilated caecum indicates that the obstructing lesion lies in the large intestine. The commonest cause is carcinoma and some of these can be reached by sigmoidoscopy or even digital examination of the rectum. Adhesions and strangulated external hernia are the commonest causes of small-bowel obstruction; look for scars and a lump in the groin.

3. Continuing pain, tachycardia and local tenderness suggest strangulation. Proceed to laparotomy with the minimum of delay.

Access

1. Make a midline incision half above and half below the umbilicus and at least 15 cm long, unless the site of obstruction is known (e.g. strangulated femoral hernia: see p. 33). Alternatively, use a right paramedian incision of similar length.

2. If the patient has had a previous operation, incise through the old scar, if it is convenient. Extend one end of the incision so that the peritoneum can be opened where it is unlikely to be adherent.

Assess

1. Aspirate any free fluid after obtaining a bacteriological specimen.

2. Insert your hand and gently explore the abdomen. Identify the caecum; if it is collapsed, the obstruction lies within the small bowel.

3. If the abdomen is grossly distended, lift out all the dilated loops of bowel and wrap them in warm, moist packs. Avoid any drag on the mesentery which could render the exteriorised bowel ischaemic. Have the assistant support the heavy distended coils of bowel.

4. Trace the dilated bowel distally to identify the cause of the obstruction, dividing any major adhesions that you encounter.

Action

Small-bowel obstruction

1. Release the obstruction if possible. Divide adhesions and bands. Reduce an internal hernia or overlooked external hernia or volvulus of the small bowel.

2. Pause, if strangulated bowel has been released. If it recovers, close the abdomen. If it does not recover, resect the ischaemic segment and perform an end-to-end anastomosis (p. 108).

3. Sometimes a knuckle of small bowel that has been trapped in an internal or external hernia will spontaneously reduce itself. If you observe constriction rings, look for the possible site of hernia and try to close the defect. Constriction rings that remain slightly ischaemic may be invaginated by Lembert sutures.

4. Resect the obstructed bowel if there is a neoplasm or if the bowel or its blood supply are damaged. Massive resection may be necessary if the main vessels are blocked; consider embolectomy in selected patients (p. 120).

5. Bypass the obstruction if it cannot be removed. Gastroenterostomy relieves pyloric or duodenal obstruction. Duodenojejunostomy bypasses annular pancreas or duodenal atresia. An enteroanastomosis short-circuits an irresectable primary or secondary tumour of the jejunum or ileum (p. 114). Obtain a biopsy specimen in all irresectable cases.

6. Break up, push on or remove intraluminal obstructions such as a food bolus, gallstone or collection or worms.

7. Reduce an intussusception (p. 120). Resect a polyp or other pathological lesion at the apex of the intussusception (usually in adults).

8. Consider stricturoplasty, akin to Heineke-Mikulicz pyloroplasty (p. 77), for the rare ischaemic stricture or a localised, quiescent Crohn's stricture.

9. Create a proximal stoma if no other relief can be given. Jejunostomy is rarely appropriate, but ileostomy is occasionally necessary as a short-term measure.

10. The management of neonatal obstruction is detailed in Chapter 32.

11. For recurrent adhesion obstruction consider Noble's plication. Lay the small bowel back and forth and unite contiguous loops with catgut sutures. Alternatively, use a long intraluminal tube left in situ for 7–10 days postoperatively.

Large-bowel obstruction

1. Release an external cause of obstruction.

2. Resect an obstructing carcinoma of the caecum, ascending colon or transverse colon; restore continuity with end-to-end ileocolostomy. An extended right hemicolectomy may also be appropriate for obstructing carcinoma of the descending colon. Distal to this segment (sigmoid colon, rectum) the best option is probably to resect the lesion and exteriorise both ends of bowel, merely oversewing the distal cut end if it cannot be brought to the surface of the abdomen. In a favourable case with limited distension of the bowel, consider resection and primary anastomosis, with or without defunctioning loop transverse colostomy (or caecostomy). In an unfavourable case, loop transverse

colostomy alone will at least overcome the obstruction. Consider caecostomy if the caecum is in danger of perforating owing to distal obstruction.

3. Bypass an irresectable carcinoma of the right colon by ileotransverse colostomy. Bypass an irresectable carcinoma of the left colon by colocolostomy, if possible. Bypass an irresectable carcinoma of the sigmoid colon or rectum by pelvic loop or terminal colostomy. Obtain a biopsy specimen from all lesions that are not resected.

4. Untwist a volvulus. Prevent future twisting by stitching the bowel to the parietes. If the sigmoid colon is gangrenous, exteriorize it for resection by the Paul-Mikulicz method (p. 145).

5. Move on, break up or remove intraluminal obstructions such as faecaliths.

6. Resection with colostomy or primary anastomosis may be needed for other obstructing lesions such as diverticulitis, Crohn's colitis and ischaemic colitis.

Difficulty?

1. In the presence of grossly distended bowel, do not flounder within the abdomen through an inadequate incision. Extend the incision and gently deliver the entire small bowel. Consider decompressing the small bowel by means of a special sucker (p. 117). Decompress the upper small bowel by milking contents back up to within reach of the nasogastric tube, and try to manoeuvre this tube through the pylorus into the duodenum or jejunum.

2. Sometimes adhesions prevent easy delivery of the small bowel or produce an apparently inextricable tangle. Such cases can be very testing. Settle down to a prolonged dissection. Make sure that the incision is adequate for you to visualise the restraining bands, which should then be divided. Patiently disentangle all adherent loops and run the whole small bowel through your hands to make sure it is unravelled.

Closure

This can be difficult if the abdomen is distended. Take care to avoid injuring dilated loops of small bowel. Consider inserting tension sutures if abdominal distension is gross.

Further reading

Kirk RM 1970 The management of intestinal obstruction in the adult. Annals of the Royal College of Surgeons of England 46: 147–158
Munro A, Jones PF 1978 Operative intubation in the treatment of complicated small bowel obstruction. British Journal of Surgery 65: 123–127
Stewardson RH, Bombeck CT, Nyhus LM 1978 Critical operative management of small bowel obstruction. Annals of Surgery 187: 189–193

LAPAROTOMY FOR GASTROINTESTINAL BLEEDING

Appraise

1. The development of flexible endoscopy and angiography have made it exceptional to have to embark upon a 'blind' laparotomy for gastrointestinal haemorrhage. Indeed, you should spare no effort to obtain a pre-operative diagnosis. Occasionally catastrophic haematemesis or haematochezia (bleeding per rectum) demand urgent operation, but even here you should exclude conditions for which laparotomy can be inappropriate: perform oesophagoscopy to exclude varices or proctosigmoidoscopy to exclude an anorectal source for bleeding.

2. The nature of the bleeding provides a helpful but not infallible guide to its likely source. Haematemesis suggests oesophageal varices, erosive gastritis, gastric ulcer or duodenal ulcer, but the blood may be coming from the small bowel. Oesophagogastro-duodenoscopy should reveal the cause, but you may need to wash out the clot from the stomach to obtain a satisfactory view. Melaena suggests an upper gastrointestinal source but can accompany bleeding from the right colon. Undertake upper endoscopy; consider colonoscopy and visceral angiography if negative. The passage of bright blood per rectum usually indicates a lesion of the left colon or rectum but can follow brisk bleeding from the small bowel. Carry out sigmoidoscopy, colonoscopy or angiography. Barium studies and abdominal scintiscanning with radiolabelled erythrocytes can reveal bleeding sites otherwise missed.

3. Resuscitate the patient as you assess and investigate him and before operation. Order further units of crossmatched blood to cover the operation. Set up a cental venous pressure line and replenish clotting factors if a major transfusion is required (e.g. >5 units of blood).

4. These are not operations to be carried out by inexperienced surgeons or anaesthetists if there is any possibility of more senior help.

Access

Make a midline or right paramedian incision, sited in the upper or lower abdomen according to the preoperative diagnosis or midway if this is uncertain.

Assess

1. Blood in the lumen can be recognised from without owing to the bluish-black colouration of the gut. The distribution of blood in the stomach, small bowel and colon may roughly localise the site of bleeding, but remember that blood can travel for a considerable distance proximal as well as distal to the lesion.

2. Inspect and palpate the alimentary canal from oesophagus to rectum. Note any abnormality, particularly an

ulcer crater, tumour, inflammation, petechiae, scarring or a local increase in vascularity. Examine the liver and spleen. Cirrhosis raises the possibility of variceal haemorrhage; splenomegaly might be associated with a clotting defect. If the gut appears normal, remember that haemobilia and pancreatic cysts are rare causes of gastrointestinal haemorrhage.

Action

1. If there is evidence of *upper* gastrointestinal bleeding, concentrate on the stomach, duodenum and jejunum.
(a) Enter the lesser sac to examine the posterior surface of the stomach. Consider an anterior gastrotomy in the body of the stomach, which can be extended to allow inspection of the entire gastric mucosa. Under-run any bleeding vessels. Options for gastric ulcer include biopsy or local resection plus vagotomy and drainage, and (in fit patients) partial gastrectomy.
(b) Closely inspect the anterior surface of the pylorus and duodenal cap for petechial haemorrhage and scarring, consistent with active duodenal ulcer disease. A duodenotomy may need to be extended across the pyloric ring to allow adequate exposure of an ulcer crater. Under-run the bleeding ulcer with stout non-absorbable sutures (e.g. 0 silk) and make sure that haemorrhage is fully controlled. Truncal vagotomy and pyloroplasty is the simplest option thereafter.
(c) If the stomach and duodenal bulb seem normal, turn your attention to the rest of the duodenal loop, duodenojejunal flexure and jejunum. Look for tumours and diverticula in particular. Consider mobilising the duodenal loop by Kocher's manoeuvre and taking down the ligament of Treitz. Resect the segment of small bowel bearing a bleeding lesion.

2. If there is evidence of *lower* gastrointestinal bleeding, concentrate on the colon and ileum. The site of bleeding can be difficult to identify in the intestine.
(a) Look for obvious lesions in the colon, including diverticula, arteriovenous malformations and tumours. Sigmoid diverticula are common in the elderly and cannot necessarily be assumed to explain the haemorrhage. Colonoscopy performed by yourself or a colleague during laparotomy may help to reveal a small mucosal lesion. Resect the segment of large bowel bearing a bleeding lesion. If all else fails, consider transverse colostomy; any future episodes of bleeding can then at least be localised to the right or left colon.
(b) Examine the entire small bowel from ligament of Treitz to ileocaecal valve. Look in particular for Meckel's diverticulum, acquired diverticula of the jejunum or ileum, tumours and ulcers. If examination is negative but you strongly suspect a small-bowel source of bleeding, consider making a mid-enterotomy and passing a flexible colonoscope up and down the small bowel from

this point. By inspecting the transilluminated bowel from without and the mucosal surface from within, you may be able to detect a small vascular lesion.

Further Reading

Cotton P B, Russell R C G 1977 Haematemesis and melaena. British Medical Journal 1: 37–39
Fiddian-Green R G, Turcotte J C 1980 Gastrointestinal Hemorrhage. Grune and Stratton, New York
Wright H K, Pellicia O, Higgins E R Jr, Sreenivas V, Gupta A 1980 Controlled, semielective, segmental resection for massive colonic hemorrhage. American Journal of Surgery 139: 535–538

LAPAROTOMY FOR POST-OPERATIVE COMPLICATIONS

Appraise

1. Most surgeons find this the most daunting operation in the repertoire. Reopening the abdomen is associated with a sense of guilt and failure. We feel that if the first operation had been done better, a second operation would not be necessary. Alternatively, we may feel that if our best efforts did not succeed originally, we cannot hope to surmount the difficulties from a less advantageous start. Do not feel defeated before you begin. True, this is a testing procedure but a successful outcome will be the greater accomplishment.

2. Reasons for reoperation include wound dehiscence (p. 51), anastomotic leakage and other types of fistula, reactive or secondary haemorrhage, intra-abdominal sepsis and intestinal obstruction. If you are a surgical trainee, discuss the patient in detail with your chief. Reoperation is a heavy responsibility and he may wish to share the burden of decision with you.

3. Determine to start the operation with the patient in the best possible condition and with the best help and equipment. Set aside plenty of time so that you do not feel rushed.

Access

1. Have the dressings and skin sutures removed. Alternatively, wear two pairs of sterile gloves and discard the outer pair after removing the skin sutures yourself.

2. After cleansing the skin separate the wound edges, using the handle of a scalpel. Seek and remove the deep stitches.

3. Open up the peritoneal cavity with care, using a fingertip to break through the partially sealed peritoneal edges.

Assess

1. Note any gas, blood or other fluid, and save a specimen for subsequent microscopy and culture.

2. Display the area of the previous operation to detect bleeding, mechanical obstruction, anastomotic breakdown, infection, ischaemia or necrosis.

3. Continuing haemorrhage demands immediate control. All other conditions are best considered carefully to determine the best course of action. The patient is more likely to succumb to hurried, ineffectual surgery than to deliberate and well-planned corrective measures.

4. Remember why you have re-entered the abdomen. Plan to carry out the simplest effective procedures that will allow the patient to recover. Do not become sidetracked by minor issues.

5. Consider what you reaction would be if the patient does not recover satisfactorily. Will you wish that you had chosen another procedure? If so, why are you not planning to carry out that procedure now?

Action

1. Control bleeding in the most effective way possible and ensure that it will not recur.

2. Consider why an anastomosis has leaked: tension, inadequate blood supply, poor technique, a continuing disease process, impaired wound healing or a combination of factors? Sometimes it is possible to insert a few sutures to repair a limited leak. Usually it is necessary to re-do the anastomosis completely, perhaps after resecting devitalised tissue and carrying out further mobilisation to avoid tension. Leaking ureteric or biliary anastomoses are best repaired over a stenting tube. If a colonic anastomosis leaks, it is better to bring out each end of bowel as a stoma (or oversew the rectum) than attempt another primary anastomosis. Sometimes a bypass procedure will help to protect a resutured anastomosis, for example gastrojejunostomy to bypass a duodenal leak.

3. Correct mechanical obstruction as if this were a first operation. It is particularly important to avoid any distal obstruction (e.g. from adhesions) after refashioning a gastrointestinal anastomosis.

4. Seek the source of infection and control it if possible.

Avoid spreading the infection if it is localised. If local sepsis fully explains the complication, it may be best to limit yourself to dealing with it and avoiding further exploration. Be careful not to disturb anastomoses that appear to be healing satisfactorily.

5. Evacuate any residual blood, pus or other intra-abdominal fluid and provide adequate drainage to the operation site.

Check list

1. Have you dealt adequately with the complication?

2. Check the area of the operation thoroughly to ensure that all is well. Memorize exactly your findings and procedure so that you can record the details straight after the operation.

3. It is usually best to explore the whole abdomen to make certain that no other condition is missed, particularly if the local findings do not fully explain the original complications.

4. Replace the viscera in their anatomical position to prevent future mechanical complications.

Closure

1. It is usually best to drain the peritoneal cavity, preferably through a separate stab incision.

2. Use the simplest and most effective means of closing the abdomen. Many surgeons close these wounds like a burst abdomen, using deep tension sutures. Fortunately, like burst abdomens, reopened wounds seldom break down completely, though superficial separation may complicate infection.

Further reading

Irving M H 1983 Abdominal complications following gastrointestinal surgery. In: Irving M H Beart R W Jr (eds) Gastroenterological Surgery. Butterworths, London p. 242–260
White T T, Harrison R C 1973 Reoperative gastrointestinal surgery. Little, Brown & Company, Boston.

Gastroduodenal surgery

ENDOSCOPY

Appraise

1. Diagnostic endoscopy using flexible fibre-optic endoscopes has become so easy that even inexperienced clinicians can safely pass the instrument and interpret most abnormalities. Certainly all gastrointestinal operators should be familiar with the use of the endoscope.

2. Endoscopy does not compete with radiology but is complementary to it. Consider endoscopy whenever there is any possibility of a lesion lying within its scope. It often provides authoritative diagnosis because of the facility to remove guided biopsy specimens or cytological brushings.

3. It is no longer ethical practice to operate on a patient for suspected oesophago-gastro-duodenal disease without carrying out endoscopy when this is available, even when the diagnosis seems certain. Occasionally, diagnoses by radiology and other means prove to be fallacious, or other, unsuspected lesions are discovered in addition to or instead of the expected one. Conversely, many patients are spared operations because an expected condition is excluded.

4. Endoscopy is mandatory before operations for gastrointestinal bleeding. Even when the exact site of bleeding is not seen, it is often possible to exclude suspected lesions.

5. Following previous gastric surgery, radiology may be difficult to interpret and endoscopy allows the mucosa to be studied visually and by histology of biopsy specimens.

6. During an operation when an unexpected diagnostic difficulty is encountered, an endoscope can be passed down to allow examination of the interior of the upper gastrointestinal tract by the surgeon or a colleague.

7. When strictures are encountered they may be dilated before passing the endoscope through them to view the viscus beyond. If necessary a splinting tube may be impacted in the stricture to prevent it from recurring.

8. Polyps may be snared and the base can be coagulated with diathermy current. With some double-channelled instruments, the polyp can be steadied with forceps while the snare is accurately placed.

9. With specially designed instruments it is possible to cannulate the ampulla of Vater for biliary and pancreatic duct radiology after injecting radio-opaque medium, or aspirate fluid for cytology. A diathermy wire can be used to perform sphincterotomy at the ampulla. Stones can be removed using a modified Dormia basket and the bile duct can be dilated and cannulated with an indwelling drainage tube leading through an obstruction into the duodenum. These techniques require special training and equipment.

Prepare

1. The easiest endoscope to pass is a slim end-viewing instrument originally designed for paediatric use, but other

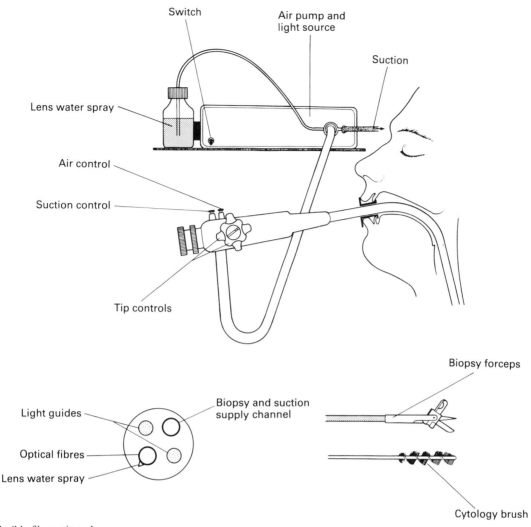

Fig. 5.1 Flexible fibreoptic endoscopy.

types offer wider suction and biopsy channels through which larger forceps can be passed for biopsy, grasping foreign bodies, or snaring polyps. The very flexible ends of end-viewing endoscopes make them very versatile but side-viewing instruments are of value in special circumstances, notably when cannulating the ampulla of Vater. (Fig. 5.1).

2. Make sure that the instrument, light source, suction apparatus, biopsy forceps, and air insufflation pump all work satisfactorily and that the instrument has been sterilized according to the manufacturer's recommendations.

3. Obtain written, informed consent from the patient.

4. The patient takes no food or fluids overnight before a morning endoscopy but may be allowed a light breakfast if the endoscopy is scheduled for the afternoon or evening. When there is no evidence of gastric delay, endoscopy is often worthwhile even when the patient has taken food or fluids within 4 hours. In an emergency attempt endoscopy even if the patient has had a recent meal, determining to remove the endoscope, pass a large gastric tube and wash out the stomach with water if necessary, using an electric sucker or Senoran's evacuator.

5. Ensure that the patient has no dentures. Anaesthetize the pharynx with an aerosol spray of 4% lignocaine or by giving amethocaine lozenges to be sucked 60 minutes and 30 minutes before the examination. The patient may be premedicated using papaveretum 20 mg with hyoscine hydrobromide 0.4 mg (Omnopon and Scopolamine) by intramuscular injection 1 hour before the procedure or a slow intravenous injection of up to 50 mg of pethidine (meperidine, Demerol). For simple diagnostic endoscopy diazepam (Valium) 10–40 mg given over a period of 3–4 minutes intravenously through an indwelling butterfly-type needle, just before the instrument is passed, is generally sufficient sedation. Other short-acting benzodiazepines, such as lorazepam may be used as alternatives. Further increments of sedative can be given and if the procedure becomes painful, small doses of pethidine can be given. If peristaltic activity is excessive, give hyoscine butylbromide (Buscopan) 20–40 mg through the indwelling butterfly needle.

6. Insert a plastic mouthpiece between the patient's teeth or gums through which the instrument will slide easily. Smear the endoscope shaft with water-soluble lubricant. Secretion and mucus are less likely to adhere to the lens if it is smeared with silicone liquid and lightly polished to leave a thin film.

7. The patient may be laid on his left side, with no pillow but with the head steadied by an assistant who maintains neck flexion, discouraging the patient from extending his neck which tends to make the instrument pass into the larynx. The patient's pronated left hand lies on the right chest, the right hand grasps the edge of the bed. Both knees and hips are flexed. Alternatively, the patient may lie supine but with the head of the bed raised. Stoical patients can be examined while they sit on a chair provided they are given minimal or no sedation and provided the instrument is passed with great skill and gentleness.

8. Before passing the instrument carefully inspect any barium meal radiographs to assess potential difficulties and pinpoint areas requiring special attention.

Access

1. Slightly flex the tip of the instrument. Pass it through the mouthpiece, over the tongue, keeping the flexed tip strictly in the midline pointing towards the cricopharyngeal sphincter. As the tip reaches the sphincter there is a hold up. Ask the patient to swallow. The tip will be slightly extruded and do not resist this but suddenly the obstruction disappears as the sphincter relaxes and the instrument can be smoothly passed into the stomach after unflexing the tip.

2. If there is any difficulty, insert the index and middle fingers of the left hand alongside the mouthpiece to guide and control the tip of the endoscope to the correct place. **DO NOT USE FORCE.**

3. Look down the instrument and concentrate on safely passing the instrument through the oesophagus, stomach and into the duodenum, noting incidentally if there is any abnormality. Insufflate the minimum of air to open up the passage. Hold the eyepiece with the left hand, adjusting the tip controls with the left thumb. Hold the shaft of the endoscope with the right hand close to the patient's mouth, advancing, withdrawing and rotating it as necessary. When the gastric angulus is passed, flex the tip to identify the pylorus. Advance the tip, keeping the pylorus in the centre of the field until the tip slips through.

4. The side-viewing endoscope has a rounded tip that makes it easier to negotiate the pharynx. If there is any doubt about the free passage, always examine the patient first with an end-viewing endoscope. Become familiar with the tip control and angle of view before passing it. When it has passed into the stomach, rotate it to bring into view the relatively smooth, straight lesser curve which ends

below at the arch of the angulus below which can be seen the pylorus in the distance. Angle the instrument up towards the roof of the angulus while advancing the instrument. The view of the pylorus is lost momentarily as the tip slips through into the duodenum. Paradoxically, if the shaft is slightly withdrawn the instrument is straightened and the tip advances further into the duodenum. Rotate the shaft to bring the medial duodenal wall into view and as the instrument enters the second part of the duodenum the ampulla of Vater is usually seen as a nipple, often with a hooded mucosal fold above it.

Assess

1. Withdraw the end-viewing instrument in a spiral fashion to bring into view the whole circumference of the duodenum and stomach. Withdraw the side-viewing endoscope whilst rotating it 180° either side to view the whole circumference. Do not overinflate the stomach and duodenum with air. In the duodenum and distal stomach, keep the endoscope still and watch the peristaltic waves form and pass distally, to estimate the suppleness of the walls and exclude rigidity from infiltration or disease. With the tip of the end-viewing instrument lying in the body of the stomach, flex it fully while gently advancing the shaft to bring the fundus and cardia into view. Flex the side-viewing instrument to produce the same view. From just above the cardia the end-viewing instrument displays the pinchcock action of the diaphragmatic crura at each inspiration. If gastric mucosa is seen above this, there is a sliding hiatal hernia. The gastric mucosa is pink and shiny: at the crenated transition to the thinner and more opaque oesophageal squamous mucosa, the colour becomes paler and sometimes slightly bluish.

2. If the view disappears, withdraw the instrument and insufflate a little air. If the lens is obscured, clean it with the water jet or wipe it against the mucosa to free it of adherent mucosa.

3. Look out for inflammation in duodenitis, gastritis and oesophagitis. As a rule the mucosa appears florid and reddened but endoscopy is uncertain and biopsy specimens should be removed when in doubt. In atrophic gastritis the distal mucosa is thinned and translucent so that submucosal vessels are visible through it. In gastric atrophy, associated with pernicious anaemia, the fundic mucosa is particularly affected being flat and featureless. Menetrier's hypertrophic gastritis results in strikingly florid mucosal folds, as may the fundic mucosa in the Zollinger-Ellison syndrome and also in lymphomas.

4. Peptic ulcers usually display a basal slough but adherent mucosa may simulate a crater. Healed ulcers typically appear flat and white, with radiating mucosal folds. Diverticula, seen usually high on the gastric lesser curve, have healthy mucosa entering the mouth of the diverticu-

lum. Mallory-Weiss tears show a ragged, often bleeding edge in the mucosa at the cardia.

5. Tumours are typically elevated and malignant ulcers have raised, everted edges. Gastric polyps may be single or multiple, and can be mucosal or submucosal, such as leiomyomas and leiomyosarcomas, which frequently have healthy mucosa overlying them. Lymphomas often produce only hypertrophic mucosal folds which display no histological abnormality. By the time tumours become obvious they are usually well advanced and the best time to recognise them is in the early pre-invasive stage. Any slight irregularity of the mucosa is suspicious, whether it is a localized depression, plateau, cobblestone irregularity or ulcer — especially if this is an unusual site for a peptic ulcer. Never fail to remove cytology brushings and biopsy specimens for examination.

6. Oesophageal varices, seen in portal venous hypertension, appear as tortuous, sometimes bluish projections into the lumen of the lower oesophagus and may continue into the gastric fundus or are occasionally visible only in the upper stomach. Do not assume in patients who have gastrointestinal bleeding that visible varices are necessarily the site of bleeding (see p. 281).

7. Pyloric stenosis may prevent the passage of the instrument into the duodenum and it is sometimes impossible to assess whether the obstruction is from benign duodenal ulceration, a mucosal diaphragm in the distal stomach or from neoplastic infiltration.

8. Previous gastric surgery distorts the anatomy and preliminary radiological examination is helpful. A stoma or pyloroplasty allows bile to reflux into the stomach. The mucosa around a stoma is often florid. Stomal ulcers usually develop just distal to the anastomosis and the instrument can be passed through it to view them. Recurrent gastric and duodenal ulcers are usually easy to see but remember that carcinoma appears to occur more frequently following previous gastric surgery for peptic ulceration. Occasionally an ulcerating nonabsorbable suture is seen, hanging like a green stalactite into the lumen and amenable to removal with alligator forceps.

9. Bleeding from the upper gastrointestinal tract can often be localized at endoscopy. If possible use an instrument with a wide-bore channel through which efficient suction can be applied. Be willing to withdraw the instrument, pass a large-bore gastric tube and aspirate the stomach or wash it out with water, emptying it by syphon action, with a Senoran's evacuator or an electric suction pump. Reinsert the instrument and if necessary rotate the patient to bring the site of bleeding uppermost, so that it is not hidden at the bottom of a pool of blood and other gastroduodenal contents. If the source of bleeding cannot be found, remember that the examination can be repeated. If an operation is to be performed, this can be carried out just prior to surgery or during the operation when the abdomen is opened.

Action

1. Remove biopsy specimens under vision from any suspicious sites, including tumours, the edges of ulcers, irregularities of the mucosa and suspected inflammation. Take specimens from different places, preferably from each quadrant of an ulcer. Place the specimens in carefully labelled separate pots containing formol saline fixative for histological examination.

2. Cytological diagnosis is extremely helpful: pass the brush through the biopsy channel and rotate it against the suspicious area. Withdraw it and wipe it against clean glass slides which are sprayed with fixative or placed in special jars containing fixative. The brush may be agitated in a separate jar of fixative — this will be subsequently centrifuged and the cells stained and examined.

3. Polypoid lesions can be caught in a snare for removal and histological examination. If the polyp has a broad base ensure that this is completely caught and if bleeding is likely, coagulate the base with the diathermy before it is removed.

4. Foreign bodies can be grasped with forceps, snared or caught in a modified Dormia basket for withdrawal. An external tube may be slid over and pushed beyond the endoscope tip to enclose a sharp foreign body as it is withdrawn to protect the mucosa from damage.

5. Oeosphageal varices can be injected under direct vision, using sclerosant solution injected through a long needle passed down the biopsy channel (see p. 281). Bleeding ulcers may be coagulated by spraying on thrombogenic substances or using the diathermy point. Laser beam coagulation is under trial.

6. A cannula can be passed through a special side-viewing endoscope for insertion in the bile and pancreatic ducts to obtain radiographic pictures following the injection of radio-opaque medium. The ampulla and lower bile duct can be slit with a diathermy wire, stones can be removed with a modified Dormia basket. A stricture can be dilated from below followed by the insertion of a prosthetic indwelling plastic tube to maintain a passage. These techniques require special training and equipment.

Post-operative

1. If the patient is heavily sedated, lay him on his left side, slightly face down, under the care of a trained nurse who will watch him until he recovers fully. If he has any respiratory obstruction this must be overcome: chest physiotherapy will help him to cough up his retained secretions. Do not allow any fluids or foods to be given until the patient is fully recovered and until the effect of pharyngeal anaesthesia has worn off — usually 4 hours.

2. Carefully clean and check the instrument.

PERI-OPERATIVE CARE

Pre-operative

1. Patients are admitted the day before operation for clinical assessment and routine check of blood count, blood urea, serum electrolytes and chest X-ray. For those over 40 years of age, or if there is suspicion of cardiac disease, order an electrocardiogram.

2. Explain the intended operation to the patient and obtain informed, signed consent.

3. The prophylaxis of deep venous thrombosis is not yet fully agreed. Many surgeons administer 5000 units of calcium heparin subcutaneously before the patient goes to the operating theatre and this is repeated twice daily until the patient is fully ambulant. Approximately half the deep venous thromboses develop while the patient lies on the operating table and it is possible that controlled intravenous infusion of heparin by the anaesthetist during the operation may be more beneficial.

4. The patient receives no food or fluid following a light supper on the night before operation. If there is evidence of gastric retention, then the stomach should be emptied the day before operation by passing a nasogastric tube for aspiration. Such patients should have an intravenous infusion set up to ensure that they are not dehydrated or electrolytically depleted.

5. Patients with gross pyloric stenosis are best admitted a few days before operation to ensure that the stomach is empty. Pass a large bore gastric tube and syphon off the gastric contents. Run in 300 ml of water at a time through a funnel and syphon it off repeatedly until the efflux is clear. Repeat this daily or twice daily as necessary. Set up an intravenous infusion to replace the loss of electrolytes, correct the disturbed acid:base balance and provide nutritional support since the patient will not be able to absorb oral foods.

6. Make sure the patient is encouraged to empty his bladder before being given the premedication injection.

7. The anaesthetist usually orders the premedication but for fit adults this is usually papavaretum (Omnopon) 20 mg and hyoscine hydrobromide (Scopolamine) 0.4 mg by intramuscular injection 1 hour before operation.

8. Ask the ward sister to pass a nasogastric tube as soon as the premedication drug has begun to take effect and aspirate the stomach until it is empty. In patients who are apprehensive, defer this and ask the anaesthetist to pass the tube as soon as anaethesia is induced.

Action

1. Although the contents of the healthy stomach are virtually sterile this is not so in the presence of disease and especially if there is any gastric stasis.

2. Adopt a routine of performing as much dissection as possible before opening the stomach, then isolate the area using added towels of distinctive colour. Keep within the isolated area during the part of the operation that requires the gut to be opened and use a limited number of instruments that are kept separate. Sometimes in spite of careful pre-operative preparation and aspiration of the indwelling nasogastric tube, the stomach is distended with content. In this case, after isolating the area, make an incision into it that will just allow the sucker tube to be inserted and empty it before proceeding. Otherwise the area is likely to be flooded with foul, retained gastric content. Following this, apply noncrushing clamps to occlude the lumen to prevent further efflux. When the bowel is closed, discard the special towels and the instruments and change into fresh, sterile gloves to continue the operation.

3. The stomach is well supplied with blood and tolerates extensive mobilization without risk to its blood supply. However, this rich blood supply can lead to bleeding from the suture line so a haemostatic over-and-over stitch is preferable to a Connell type of stitch, unless the blood vessels are first picked up individually and tied.

The duodenum is fragile and does not tolerate tension or vigorous mobilization. Rather than anastomose it under tension, be prepared to close it and perform gastroenterostomy if this is possible.

Aftercare

1. Have the patient's condition monitored carefully until he recovers from the anaesthetic, in particular note his colour, respiration, pulse rate and blood pressure. The blood pressure is taken every 15 minutes for the first 3 hours and then every hour until it is stable but the other observations are checked every few minutes depending upon the patient's condition. Have the wound checked regularly to ensure that there is no bleeding.

2. See that the urinary output is checked frequently. Many patients have difficulty in passing urine whilst laying supine. Most patients can be allowed to stand up with support very early after operation. Whenever the patient is reported to be restless, check the level of the bladder. In case of doubt, pass a small catheter with strict aseptic precautions. A patient who has had a major operation such as total gastrectomy or a thoracoabdominal operation should have an indwelling catheter to ensure that urinary output is adequate. This will be removed as soon as the patient is recovered and active.

3. Order the nasogastric tube aspiration to be carried out every 15 minutes for the first 3 hours to detect postoperative intragastric bleeding. Thereafter it may be aspirated every hour for the first 24 hours. As a rule it can then be aspirated every 2 hours for a day and then every 3 hours. It will be removed when the amount aspirated is less than the oral intake and the aspirate is clear, provided the patient is comfortable, with a soft abdomen, passing flatus per anus and has bowel sounds. Try to remove the naso-

gastric tube early in patients with respiratory problems, if necessary, restricting oral fluid intake. It is very difficult to cough with a tube irritating the pharynx.

4. Order intravenous fluids remembering that sodium retention is frequent following operations and that, provided the patient started in fluid and electrolyte balance, lost electrolytes only need be replaced. Provided also that renal function is good, then if sufficient fluid is given, small imbalances will be compensated. For the 1 or 2 days that are required before adequate oral intake is achieved, a previously fit patient need be given only glucose for his metabolic needs. Establish at once an intravenous feeding regime on a previously undernourished patient or one who has required an oesophageal anastomosis and will not be able to take adequate oral feeding for several days.

5. Allow a patient who has had an operation for peptic ulcer or distal gastric carcinoma sips of water as soon as he is completely recovered from the anaesthetic. If he is adequately hydrated he will anyway swallow saliva and the gastric content can be reduced by nasogastric tube aspiration. On the morning after operation, allow 30 ml of water each hour increasing to 60 ml the second day and 90 ml the third day, when normal intake can be resumed and intravenous fluid replacement stopped. Following many operations, especially when the stomach and duodenum have not be opened, this regime may be speeded up so that the morning after operation the nasogastric tube can be removed and oral fluid intake allowed in increasing amounts depending on the patient's tolerance and general condition. Withhold oral fluids following gastric operations with oesophageal anastomosis but allow the patient to have mouthwashes. It is not possible to prevent a little fluid and saliva from being swallowed but as a rule wait for 4–5 days after operation, then check the intactness and adequacy of the anastomosis radiologically using water-soluble medium before commencing oral fluids and proceeding gradually to full diet.

6. Modern attitudes to activity following abdominal surgery are more liberal than previously. Allow the patient to sit out of bed the morning following operation and have him walking a little during the next day or two, depending upon his general condition. The help of a cheerful physiotherapist in encouraging the patient to breathe deeply, cough up retained sputum and move freely is of enormous value in preventing the patient from remaining static in bed.

ACCESS IN THE UPPER ABDOMEN

Do not attempt difficult manoeuvres in the upper abdomen unless there is an adequate view. As a rule routine exposures are satisfactory but in occasional patients the view is severely restricted.

GASTRIC CARDIA

1. Tilt the whole patient slightly head up.

2. Use an upper right or left paramedian or midline incision, opening the peritoneum to one or other side of the falciform ligament. Start the incision at/or alongside the xiphoid process and carry it vertically down for 20 cm, skirting the umbilicus.

3. Transverse and oblique incisions do not provide adequate access except in those with a wide costal margin, but they may be combined with vertical incisions to form a flap. An inverted 'V' incision offers good access since the apex of the 'V' can be folded down and sutured to the lower abdominal wall.

4. Carefully place retractors and ensure that the operating theatre light is correctly focussed and aimed.

5. Mobilize the left lobe of the liver if this interferes with the view. Insert the fully pronated left hand with the index and middle fingers passing on each side of the left triangular ligament to draw down the lobe. Cut the ligament from its free edge towards the right with long handled scissors, avoiding damage to the subphrenic vessels and left hepatic veins. Fold the lobe to the right, cover it with a gauze pack and have it held out of the way with a large curved retractor. Remember to replace it carefully at the end of the operation.

6. Carry the whole depth of the incision right up to the xiphisternum or into the angle between it and the costal margin. Do not hesitate to excise the xiphisternum using bone cutting forceps, after dissecting off the two diaphragmatic muscle slips from its under surface (Fig. 5.2).

7. In case of exceptional difficulty, split the sternum subcutaneously in the midline. First separate the skin from the lower sternum using Mayo's scissors held on the flat. Insert the left index finger between the cut xiphoid slips of diaphragm, up behind the sternum into the anterior mediastinum. Use straight bone-cutting forceps to split the sternum, keeping strictly in the midline, protecting the pericardium from damage by the deep blade of the forceps with the left index finger (Fig. 5.3). If necessary carry the split as high as the manubriosternal joint. Gently prise the two halves of sternum apart (Fig. 5.4). At the end of the operation do not attempt to repair the bony split.

KOCHER'S DUODENAL MOBILIZATION

Appraise

1. This manoeuvre (Fig. 5.5) raises the head of the pancreas contained within the duodenal loop into its embryological midline position, restrained by the structures in the free edge of the lesser omentum above, the superior mesenteric vessels below, the body and tail of the pancreas to the left.

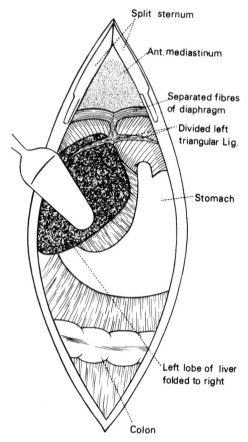

Fig. 5.2 Access in the upper adomen.

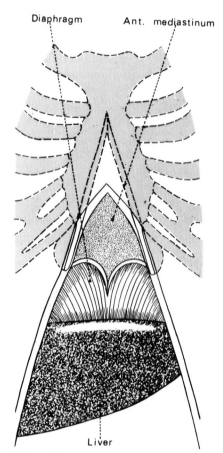

Fig. 5.4 The two halves of the sternum and xiphisternum have been separated to improve access to the upper abdomen.

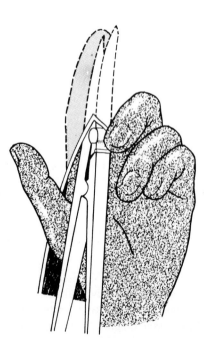

Fig. 5.3 Splitting the xiphisternum and sternum in the midline. The left index finger protects anterior mediastinal contents from injury.

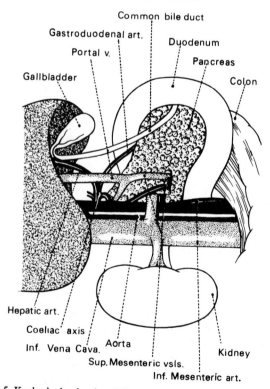

Fig. 5.5 Kocher's duodenal mobilization, as seen from the right side of the patient.

2. The head and neck of the pancreas can be examined from behind and palpated between fingers and thumb. The lower end of the common bile duct can be palpated and sometimes seen although it is usually buried within the pancreatic head. The duodenum and especially the ampullary region can be palpated. Duodenotomy allows inspection of the interior of the duodenum. If the incision is placed at the level of the ampulla this can be seen and palpated for tumours or stones. Biopsy, excision of ampullary neoplasms, sphincterotomy, sphincteroplasty, and cannulation or instrumentation of the bile and pancreatic ducts can be carried out under vision.

3. Mobilization is essential for excision of the pancreatic head and duodenal loop in Whipple's pancreato-duodenectomy.

4. Elevation of the duodenal loop and pancreatic head reveals the inferior vena cava when performing portocaval anastomosis or major hepatic resections.

5. The manoeuvre is particularly valuable in gastro-duodenal operations. Pyloroplasty can be performed easily and the extremities of the gastroduodenal incision can be brought together without tension. In gastrectomy, the proximal duodenum is easily dissected and can be closed or united to the stomach with ease. Full mobilization is an essential step when the stomach is drawn up for gastro-oesophageal or gastropharyngeal anastomosis.

Action

1. If incomplete mobilization is sufficient, as for palpating the lower end of the bile duct or the pancreatic head or for the purpose of carrying out pyloroplasty and gastrectomy by the Polya or Billroth I methods, then it may be sufficient to elevate only the superior part of the duodenal loop and pancreatic head. Insinuate a finger into the aditus to the lesser sac and gently split the floor of the foramen downwards, allowing the finger to separate the upper duodenum and pancreas from the inferior vena cava. Extend the mobilization by continuing the split with scissors downwards, just outside the convexity of the duodenal loop.

2. For full mobilization, have your assistants draw the hepatic flexure of the colon downwards, the right edge of wound outwards and the duodenal loop to the left.

3. Incise the peritoneum and underlying fascia of Toldt for 5 cm, placed 1 cm from and parallel to the convex border of the second part of the duodenum.

4. Insinuate your fingers beneath the descending duodenum and pancreatic head. A natural plane of cleavage opens up between the embryological layers which were present when the duodenum was freely suspended in the peritoneal cavity.

5. Having defined the plane, cut the peritoneum and fascia upwards, just outside the duodenal convexity, into the mouth of the aditus to the lesser sac, meanwhile lifting the proximal duodenum forward with a finger, so protecting the inferior vena cava from damage. The dissection is easy and can be carried out by splitting with the finger except in the presence of severe scarring as from severe duodenal ulceration.

6. Continue the peritoneal and fascial split below, taking care to avoid damaging the right colic vessels which must be pushed downwards with the hepatic flexure of the colon and mesocolon, to release the junction of the second and third parts of the duodenum.

7. Continue the separation of the pancreas and duodenum across the aorta where it is tethered below by the superior mesenteric artery and its pancreatic branches. The structures in the free edge of the lesser omentum restrain it superiorly.

8. When the appropriate procedure is completed, carefully check the pancreatic head, duodenal loop and the bed from which the structures have been mobilized, before laying them back in place.

EXAMINATION OF THE STOMACH AND DUODENUM

1. Did you make a firm diagnosis before operation? Mucosal lesions within hollow organs are best assessed from within the lumen by radiology and endoscopy, not by examination of the exterior at operation.

2. Feel for the lower oesophagus and diaphragmatic crura. Sometimes there is an obvious invagination of the gastric cardia through the diaphragmatic hiatus. If the normal anatomy can be restored by applying traction to the lesser curve of the stomach, this is a sliding hiatal hernia. If the cardia cannot be drawn down, there is a fixed hiatal hernia which may be primary or may be secondary to disease in the posterior mediastinum that should have been detected and assessed before carrying out this operation. There may be a gap between the crura into which the fingers can be inserted but the stomach remains fixed within the abdomen. Gently grasp the gastric cardia between finger and thumb and see if it can be slid through the hiatus into the chest. An asymptomatic hiatal hernia discovered incidentally when carrying out another procedure should be recorded but not repaired. Palpate the fundus of the stomach. If it disappears through the hiatus into the posterior mediastinum, this is a rolling hernia. These may cause obstructive symptoms and if the patient has complained of this then repair may be considered, depending upon the severity of the symptoms, the extent of herniation, the fitness of the patient and the severity of the proposed operation.

3. Examine the body and lesser curve of the stomach for evidence of ulcers and ulcers scars. Ulcers and healed scars are often palpable and visible, and former ulcers can sometimes be detected by pinching away the loose mucosa along

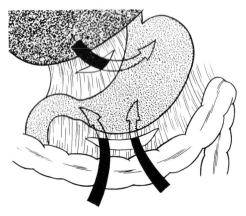

Fig. 5.6 Approaches to the posterior surfaces of the stomach and duodenal bulb, through the gastrohepatic and gastrocolic omenta.

the lesser curve — it may be tethered at the site of a healed ulcer. The stomach can be palpated most readily by making holes through avascular parts of the lesser and gastrocolic omenta so that fingers can be passed behind to feel the two layers of gastric wall against the thumb placed anteriorly (Fig. 5.6). The scar of an undetected posterior gastric ulcer may be adherent to the pancreas but there are normally flimsy adhesions across the lesser sac between the stomach and pancreas. Of course, preoperative endoscopy should have resolved the diagnosis but in case of doubt, gastroscopy may be arranged now. Sometimes a colleague can come to the operating theatre. The anaesthetist or an assistant may be asked to pass the endoscope but it is usually best to leave the operation temporarily and pass the instrument, reach a decision and re-scrub, put on a fresh sterile gown and gloves and continue the operation. If this is not possible, carry out gastrotomy, preferably in the middle of the anterior wall of the stomach at the level of the suspected ulcer or other lesion and evaginate the lesion through the gastrotomy for visual assessment, biopsy or excision. The gastrotomy may then be closed either because no further action is necessary or prior to carrying out gastrectomy if this is a hitherto unsuspected chronic gastric ulcer causing the patient's symptoms. In poor risk patients, gastric ulcer may be treated by ulcer excision and proximal gastric vagotomy or by truncal vagotomy and pyloroplasty, preferably with ulcer excision. Very high ulcers can be successfully treated by modest hemigastrectomy of Polya type, leaving the ulcer alone; this is the Kelling-Madlener operation which successfully produces ulcer healing. Gastric ulcers 'secondary' to (that is, developing later than) coexisting duodenal ulcers, usually heal together with the duodenal ulcer if proximal gastric vagotomy is carried out provided there is no associated gastric retention from duodenal ulcer scarring or from the vagotomy.

4. Look and feel for neoplasms. Carcinoma is most frequently seen although lymphosarcoma, reticulum-cell sarcoma, leiomyoma and leiomyosarcoma are not rare, and adenomatous polyps may be felt. Carcinoma may produce a tumour within the stomach, or be felt as an ulcer with raised margins. An apparently benign ulcer may have developed malignant characteristics. Extensive submucosal infiltration produces the rigid 'leather-bottle' stomach, often with penetration of the serosa producing a crystallized sugar appearance with beaded irregular bloodvessels. If carcinoma is suspected, proven or unexpectedly encountered, do not touch it but examine the pre-rectal pouch, the ovaries in the female, the remainder of the peritoneal cavity, the root of the mesentery and the liver to assess the degree of spread before palpating the primary tumour, so that malignant cells are not carried around on the gloves. Feel the local glands along the greater and lesser curves, and through holes in the avascular portions in the lesser and gastrocolic omenta, assess the degree of posterior infiltration into the pancreas, and the involvement of glands around the coeliac axis and along the superior border of the pancreas. When in some cases, the diagnosis remains in doubt, gastrotomy should be performed with the removal of a specimen for frozen section histology and then closed. On the basis of the report and the operative assessment, decide on the immediate action. If a distal carcinoma appears to be totally resectable, carry out radical distal gastrectomy. An apparently curable proximal carcinoma is ideally treated by radical total gastrectomy through a left thoracoabdominal incision and the abdominal incision can be extended to the left after the patient has been turned onto the right side, has had the skin prepared and fresh sterile towels have been applied. Mid-gastric tumours can sometimes be adequately excised by abdominal total gastrectomy. Carry out high gastroenterostomy if inoperable distal carcinoma threatens to cause obstruction.

Adenomas should be completely excised since histology may reveal malignant changes. Sometimes they are multiple and gastrectomy may be more appropriate. Benign tumours such as angioma and lipoma require merely local removal. Leiomyoma cannot be differentiated at operation, or even by frozen section histology, from leiomyosarcoma. It should be excised with a healthy margin but only time will tell whether this is benign or malignant. Leiomyoblastoma is less frequently seen and is usually benign. Lymphosarcoma and reticulum-cell sarcoma may be difficult to diagnose before operation and frozen-section histology at the time of operation may be valuable in case of doubt. Even if the tumour is extensive it is worth excising as much as possible to leave the minimum tumour bulk for subsequent radiotherapy and chemotherapy.

5. Examine the pyloroduodenal region. The pyloric ring can be picked up between the index finger and thumb of both hands, but the mucosal ring may be smaller than the muscular ring. To check this, invaginate the anterior antral wall through the pylorus on an index finger and invaginate the anterior duodenal wall back into the stomach in a similar manner. If there is obstruction, look again at the stomach. Is it dilated? Is the muscular wall hypertrophied?

Look and feel for duodenal ulcer, remembering that the majority of ulcers lie in the bulb, although they may be in the post-bulbar region or further distally, especially if the Zollinger-Ellison syndrome. Sometimes an ulcer crater can be palpated, sometimes there is gross and incontrovertible scarring and narrowing, together with pseudodiverticulum formation but there may be minimal scarring, a few petechial haemorrhages — that could be iatrogenic — or there may be nothing abnormal to see or feel. Of course the diagnosis should have been made endoscopically before operation. Occasionally endoscopy has failed because the tip of the instrument could not negotiate the narrow or distorted pyloroduodenal canal. If doubt remains, could a small endoscope be passed by the anaesthetist and the tip negotiated through manually to allow the interior to be viewed? Alternatively, create a small prepyloric gastrotomy and examine the interior with a finger, by placing small retractors within the pyloroduodenal canal, or by introducing a cystoscope to view the interior. A mucosal diaphragm which is soft and easily stretched can be dilated, or conventionally treated by pyloroplasty.

6. Diverticula of the stomach are most frequently found on the upper lesser curve, sometimes produced by traction from a leiomyoma. If no primary lesion is present leave an asymptomatic diverticulum alone. Pseudodiverticula of the duodenum develop when chronic duodenal ulcer causes distortion. The most frequent duodenal diverticulum is not seen unless it is sought for since it lies close to the ampulla, protruding into the pancreas which must be mobilized by Kocher's manoeuvre to approach from posteriorly. It rarely causes symptoms and should normally be left alone.

GASTROTOMY AND GASTRODUODENOTOMY

Appraise

1. Gastric, gastroduodenal and duodenal incision allows the interior of the bowel to be examined to confirm, biopsy or to treat a suspected lesion such as an ulcer, tumour or source of bleeding.

2. Gastrotomy allows access from below to the lower oesophagus. Strictures are often dilated more safely from below than from above. If a prosthetic tube such as Mousseau-Barbin or Celestin is to be pulled through an oesophageal stricture, it is necessary to carry out gastrotomy.

Access

1. As a rule, open the stomach on the anterior wall midway between the greater and lesser curves.

2. To recover a tube or dilate the gullet, open the proximal stomach only sufficiently to pass a finger or bougie or for the prosthetic tube to emerge.

3. For the purpose of diagnosis, start with a small incision, 3–4 cm long, the proximal end of which is 5–6 cm from the pylorus. This incision ensures that the intact pylorus or mucosal diaphragm can be examined and it may be unnecessary to destroy the pyloric muscular ring. The incision can be extended proximally or if it becomes necessary, distally through the pyloric ring onto the anterior wall of the duodenal bulb.

4. To view the interior, first aspirate all the contents. Retractors may be placed to hold open the stomach so that it can be examined by adjusting the theatre light to shine through the opening. The stomach can be manoeuvred manually to bring different parts of the interior into view. Frequently the gastric wall can be evaginated through the incision so that it can be examined and any lesion excised or biopsied. If the pylorus is not too narrow, small retractors may be placed in to to allow the duodenal bulb to be viewed, and if it is wide, an unscarred duodenal bulbar wall may be evaginated through it on a finger. If there is difficulty in viewing the duodenum to exclude or confirm disease, a cystoscope may be introduced through it. Sometimes when fibre-optic endoscopy is ineffective before operation, perhaps resulting from inability to evacuate the gastric contents, the stomach may be emptied and endoscopy can then be performed. The gastrotomy can be temporarily occluded with a clamp to allow the stomach to be inflated but as a rule the stomach can be held open to allow endoscopy to be accomplished without the need for inflation.

Closure

1. Close a gastrotomy in two layers, leaving a longitudinal suture line.

2. It is conventional practice to close a gastroduodenotomy as a Heineke-Mikulicz pyloroplasty. This may be accomplished using a single edge-to-edge row of sutures, a two-layer invaginating suture or with a row of staples. However, this destroys the pyloric metering function and if vagotomy is not carried out, it may be preferable to carefully close the incision to create a longitudinal scar, bringing the edges together without invagination in a single layer, taking care to appose the pyloric edges perfectly. Cover the suture line with a layer of omentum as an extra precaution.

3. Use ingenuity to incorporate the gastrotomy in plans for other procedures. A distal gastrotomy may be incorporated in a gastroenterostomy. The proximal part of a long gastroduodenotomy may be closed longitudinally and the distal part converted into a pyloroplasty if necessary. If gastrectomy is intended, temporarily close the gastrotomy with stitches or staples to limit soiling to a minimum.

PYLOROMYOTOMY

Appraise

1. Pyloromyotomy for infantile pyloric stenosis is described in Chapter 22.

2. Adult hypertrophic pyloric stenosis is rarely discovered as a cause of gastric retention. It is not known whether or not this represents undiagnosed infantile pyloric stenosis.

3. Following vagotomy for duodenal ulcer, pyloromyotomy may have a beneficial effect in preventing gastric retention if there is no organic stenosis, although most surgeons have not sufficient confidence in the method to employ it routinely. However, when the stomach is mobilized for anastomosis to the oesophagus in the chest or neck, gastric vagotomy is inevitably carried out. No drainage operation is necessary if the pyloric size is adequate but some surgeons perform pyloromyotomy.

Assess

Endoscopy should have been performed before operation but if this was not possible, pick up the pylorus and feel the thickness of the muscular ring. Assess the size of the mucosal channel by attempting to invaginate the anterior antral wall and the anterior duodenal wall through the pylorus on the tip of an index finger.

Action

1. Grasp the pylorus between finger and thumb of the left hand to steady it (Fig. 5.7).

2. With a scalpel, incise the seromuscularis along the middle of the anterior antral wall from 1 cm proximal to the thickened segment and carefully extend it distally across the pylorus onto the anterior duodenal wall for 1 cm. The duodenal wall at the fornix is very thin, so take care not to incise into the lumen.

3. Deepen the incision through the thickened muscle of the antrum until the mucosa bulges into the split. Make sure all the muscle fibres are divided. The final split may be accomplished by grasping the wall on each side of the split with dry gauze swabs and separating the edges, to allow mucosa to bulge freely along the whole of the incision.

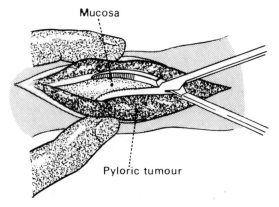

Fig. 5.7 Pyloromyotomy.

Mucosa

Pyloric tumour

4. Carry the split distally to the pylorus and carefully divide all the circular muscle fibres here, again taking care to expose but not damage the mucosa of the first part of the duodenal bulb. Lift the muscle fibres free of the mucosa with fine non-toothed dissecting forceps and then cut them.

Check

1. Make sure all the fibres have been cut.

2. Gather some gastric air into the segment with the pyloromyotomy, to distend the mucosa so that it bulges into the split. Watch carefully for any leaks. It is no disaster to find a leak and carefully close it with fine catgut stitches on eyeless needles. It may be disastrous to miss a leak.

GASTROSTOMY

Appraise

1. Gastrostomy offers a valuable method of feeding patients who are unable to swallow because of oesophageal obstruction, bulbar palsy and other causes. Patients with mechanical obstruction who will have reconstructive surgery utilizing the stomach as a conduit should not normally have a temporary gastrostomy since this will interfere with subsequent reconstructive surgery. They are better served by a jejunostomy.

2. As a rule gastrostomy is intended as a temporary measure and some surgeons consider permanent gastrostomy to be a barbaric procedure. When all else fails, do not hesitate to offer it after discussion with the patient.

3. Gastrostomy offers a means of providing gastric aspiration without nasogastric intubation, valuable in patients who have respiratory difficulties and those who cannot tolerate the presence of the tube in their pharynx, during the post-operative recovery period from gastric operations.

4. Duodenal fistula can be treated using a gastrostomy. Two tubes are passed through it. The end of one lies at the site of the leak, kept on continuous aspiration to reduce the rate of flow through the track. A second, longer tube passes into the bowel at least 30 cm beyond the fistula, for enteric feeding.

5. A number of techniques have been described. Stamm's gastrostomy is almost universally used now and shall be described below. The tube passes through the abdominal wall and enters the stomach through a small stab wound. The hole is prevented from leaking by invaginating it using a series of purse-string sutures so that it resembles a non-spill inkwell. Witzel's gastrostomy is similar but leakage is prevented by laying the emerging tube along the stomach wall and covering it by suturing over it ridges of gastric wall so that it lies in a tunnel. The Depage-Janeway

gastrostomy employs a flap of stomach formed into a tube which is brought to the skin surface to create a permanent conduit.

Access

1. Gastrostomy can be accomplished under local anaesthesia if necessary. Mix 20 ml 2% lignocaine with 80 ml of sterile water for injection. After preparing and towelling off the skin area, inject 20 ml intracutaneously along a vertical line from 1 cm above the left costal margin over the middle of the left rectus muscle, downwards for 8–10 cm. With a longer needle, inject a further 20 ml in the subcutaneous tissues and anterior rectus sheath. Now inject deeper into the posterior rectus sheath and preperitoneal tissues. When the peritoneum is pierced resistance to injection suddenly disappears. Allow a small volume to enter the peritoneal cavity.

2. Incise the skin vertically downwards from the costal margin for 6–8 cm, cutting through all the tissues into the peritoneum in the same line. Inject additional local anaesthetic into the posterior rectus sheath and preperitoneal connective tissue before incising the peritoneum.

Action

1. Insert retractors and adjust the light to identify the stomach and draw out a portion of the midstomach using tissue forceps.

2. After towelling off the area, make a stab wound as high as possible on the anterior wall, midway between the greater and lesser curves. Aspirate the gastric contents with a sucker tube. Insert the end of a 20–24 F soft latex catheter for 7–10 cm with the tip directed towards the pylorus (Fig. 5.8).

3. Insert a purse-string suture on an eyeless needle 0.5 cm from the tube, and as it is tightened and tied, push the edges of the stabwound inwards. Tie the ends of the suture around the tube to fix it. Insert a second purse-string 0.5 cm outside this to invaginate it and if necessary, a third.

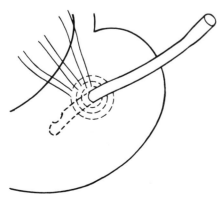

Fig. 5.8 Stamm gastrostomy.

4. Hold the edges of the upper part of the abdominal wound everted and suture the stomach around the gastrostomy to the peritoneum under the edges so that the tube emerges through the upper end of the wound.

Closure

1. Close the remainder of the wound in layers. Insert an extra skin stitch at the upper end of the wound and tie it around the emerging tube to fix it.
2. Apply wound dressings.
3. Test the patency of the gastrostomy by injecting 30 ml of sterile water, then temporarily spigot it.

PERFORATED PEPTIC ULCER

Appraise

1. Perforation of other viscera such as colon or gallbladder may be confused with gastroduodenal perforations. If you are in doubt, proceed as though this were a peptic ulcer perforation but be willing to close the incision and make a better sited one if the need arises. This is preferable to making a compromise incision.

2. Not all patients who have a perforated peptic ulcer should have operation. Ochsner showed that patients who were unfit or seen late following perforation, could be treated successfully by conservative methods. Nasogastric suction, parenteral feeding, systemic antibiotics and chest physiotherapy are instituted and operation is resorted to only if the patient fails to improve or deteriorates.

3. Is definitive surgical treatment of a perforated duodenal ulcer justified as an emergency procedure? Many papers have been written to show that definitive surgery is as safe as simple suture. However, although the proportions differ from one study to the next, it has been shown that some patients following simple suture never have any serious subsequent dyspepsia, some have recurrent dyspepsia that does not require elective surgery and some require elective or emergency surgery. No one can predict to which group an individual patient belongs when he is admitted with a perforated peptic ulcer.

In a subsequent section, the author shall advocate conservatism in offering elective surgery for uncomplicated duodenal ulcer, so there has to be good reason to carry out definitive surgery as an emergency. I believe that the only justification is if a fit patient has perforated within an hour or two of being admitted, would have been offered elective surgery for his disabling and uncontrollable symptoms before he had perforated and the operation to be carried out is the one the surgeon would choose electively as the best. In addition the surgeon, his team and the facilities available must all be of the best.

4. Most gastric ulcer perforations are successfully managed by simple suture after excising a specimen from the

edge for histology. Sometimes they are difficult to close and demand gastrectomy including the ulcer. If there is doubt about the nature of the ulcer, treat it as though it is benign, remove a biopsy specimen from the edge and if malignancy is demonstrated histologically, carry out the appropriate operation 2 weeks later as an elective procedure. If the ulcer cannot be sutured but is of doubtful origin and frozen section histology is equivocal or cannot be arranged, then carry out gastrectomy as though this is a benign ulcer and be prepared to re-operate to carry out an elective radical procedure 2 weeks later.

5. Bleeding associated with perforation demands control of both complications. Bleeding, perforated gastric ulcer is conventionally controlled by distal gastrectomy including the ulcer. Bleeding is rarely a complication of anterior perforating duodenal ulcer but if there is a co-existent bleeding posterior duodenal ulcer, the anterior perforation can be incorporated into a gastroduodenotomy. Insert non-absorbable stitches into the base of the posterior ulcer to control the bleeding and then close the gastroduodenotomy as a pyloroplasty. Complete the procedure with truncal vagotomy.

6. Perforated gastric carcinoma may be amenable to the same operation as would be carried out electively. If not, consider suturing it or plugging the defect with omentum and re-operating electively two weeks later after the patient has been brought to the best possible condition. Sometimes inadequate resection is forced upon the surgeon. If so, consider whether this can be corrected later by a more adequate operation.

Access

Use a midline or right paramedian incision from the xiphisternum to the umbilicus, 10–12 cm long.

Assess

1. Remove all instruments from the field with the exception of a retractor for your assistant and the sucker tube for yourself.

2. Aspirate any free fluid after collecting a specimen for laboratory examination. Gastric juice is usually bile stained.

3. Examine the duodenal bulb and the stomach, especially along the lesser curve. If necessary open the lesser sac of omentum through the lesser or gastrocolic omenta to view the posterior gastric wall.

4. Remember that multiple perforations can occur.

5. Always remove a biopsy specimen from the edge of a gastric ulcer.

6. If you cannot find the perforation after a diligent search, explore the whole abdomen if necessary extending the incision downwards. Examine in particular the gallbladder and sigmoid colon.

7. If you are a surgeon in training and find yourself in difficulty either because of failure to discover the cause, or indecision about the best course of action, or because the required procedure is beyond your capabilities, do not hesitate to contact your chief for advice and assistance.

8. Remember that your function at this emergency operation is to perform the simplest procedure that will correct the catastrophe. If you do more than this, will you be able to justify it to yourself and others if the patient succumbs?

Simple closure

1. Place two or three parallel sutures of chromic catgut on eyeless needles through all coats, passing in 1 cm proximal to the ulcer edge and emerging 1 cm distal to the ulcer (Fig. 5.9). Do not pick up the opposite wall as this will obstruct the lumen. When all the sutures are in place tie them just tightly enough to appose the edges.

2. If a stitch starts to cut through as you tighten it, do not continue. Pick up a convenient fold of omentum and place it over the perforation between the suture ends, and tie the suture over it to occlude the hole. Insert further stitches to reinforce the obturating action of the omentum, to make sure the hole is adequately sealed.

3. Even when closure seems secure, do not hesitate to suture omentum over it.

4. Aspirate any free fluid from above and below the liver, from within the lesser sac, the right paracolic gutter and from the pelvis.

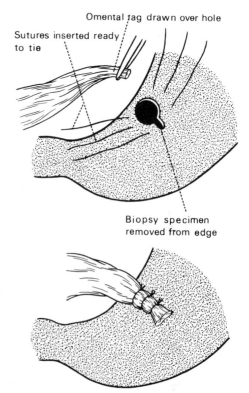

Omental tag drawn over hole

Sutures inserted ready to tie

Biopsy specimen removed from edge

Fig. 5.9 Suture of a perforated peptic ulcer.

Check list

1. Re-examine the closure of the perforation.
2. Aspirate in the collection areas once more.

Drain?

If the perforation was sutured without delay, if the closure is secure and peritoneal toilet was adequate, drainage is unnecessary. Make sure the insertion of a drain does not replace careful technique.

ELECTIVE SURGERY FOR PEPTIC ULCER

Appraise

1. Opinions about chronic peptic ulcer change constantly partly because new treatments are introduced and partly because the pattern of peptic ulcer is also changing. Before the turn of the century gastric ulcer was frequent in Europe, occurring mainly in young women. With the arrival of the twentieth century, duodenal ulcer became more frequent, principally affecting men. Surgeons operating on duodenal ulcers during the thirties and forties encountered very florid ulcers and many techniques were devised for dealing with them. During the last 20 years the severity of duodenal ulceration appears to be reduced and it is unusual to see the large active ulcers formerly seen. Chronic duodenal ulcers are frequently self-limiting so that if the patient can be tided over the years when his ulcer is active, it often becomes gradually quiescent.

2. Uncomplicated duodenal ulcer that did not respond to treatment with simple antacids, bland diet and reduction in activity was formerly treated most effectively with surgery. In the last few years, medical treatment has become increasingly effective, with more potent antacids, atropine-like drugs, liquorice extracts, mucosal coating substances, histamine H_2-receptor blocking drugs and the promising substances that act as H^+ and K^+ ATPase inhibitors. Most patients can be controlled with these powerful and safe agents and the only people who may require surgery are the minority who cannot be controlled medically or who cannot or will not take the treatment as required.

Before surgery is contemplated, the diagnosis must be firmly established. Many patients have a typically intermittent history with barium meal X-rays demonstrating distortion of the duodenal bulb 'compatible' with ulceration yet at endoscopy no ulcer or scar is seen. Operation on these patients would be totally unjustified and would merely modify the symptoms which would then be dismissed as 'postvagotomy' or 'postgastrectomy.'

The first operation for uncomplicated duodenal ulcer was gastroenterostomy alone, which diverted acid away from the ulcer but in a proportion of patients led to anastomotic ulcer at the gastroenterostomy. Partial gastrec-

tomy of Polya type replaced gastroenterostomy and this has now been replaced by some form of vagotomy. The operation that is in vogue at present is proximal gastric vagotomy, otherwise called highly selective vagotomy. An adjunctive operation to overcome gastric retention is unnecessary if there is no evidence of impending pyloroduodenal stenosis resulting from the chronic ulcer scarring. If there is, then some surgeons dilate up the canal through a prepyloric gastrotomy using a Hegar's type dilator or a finger or by invaginating the anterior duodenal wall and the anterior antral wall through the stenosed pylorus on an index finger tip — a manoeuvre first used by Jaboulay. If the stenosis is entirely in the bulb, a longitudinal incision can be made through it without impinging on the pyloric ring and it can be closed as a transverse suture line, after the manner of a pyloroplasty — hence this is called a duodenoplasty. Many surgeons prefer truncal vagotomy combined with pyloroplasty, gastroenterostomy or distal gastrectomy to improve gastric emptying. Selective gastric vagotomy is an intermediate operation that has largely been replaced by proximal gastric vagotomy. Anterior gastric seromyotomy combined with posterior truncal vagotomy is under trial. Although the combination of vagotomy and distal gastrectomy or 'antrectomy' has been popular in the USA, it is infrequently used in Britain as a primary operation since it carries a higher mortality and morbidity than the other procedures.

3. Gastric ulcer is treated more aggressively by surgeons than is duodenal ulcer. Many surgeons adopt a fixed policy of carrying out endoscopy and biopsy to confirm that this is initially a benign ulcer, then give the patient a 6–8 week course of medical treatment with an H_2-receptor blocking drug or carbenoxolone followed by a check endoscopy. If the ulcer is healed, operation is deferred. If the ulcer is not healed, or if it soon recurs, then surgical treatment is recommended. This more aggressive treatment stems partly from anxiety about the possibility of early malignancy or impending change and partly from the pragmatic knowledge that chronic gastric ulcers are less likely than chronic duodenal ulcers to become quiescent.

The operation that has stood the test of time for the cure of gastric ulcers is Billroth I partial gastrectomy including the ulcer in the specimen. Vagotomy and pyloroplasty is less certain, but proximal gastric vagotomy and excision of the ulcer has been shown to be as effective as gastrectomy. For high ulcers, a modest Polya gastrectomy leaving the ulcer undisturbed reliably results in ulcer healing — this is the Kelling-Madlener procedure.

4. Combined gastric and duodenal ulcers are seen and in this case the duodenal ulcer appears to precede the gastric ulcer, which is therefore often referred to as 'secondary'. Combined ulcers are often resistant to medical treatment and may require surgery. As a rule, an operation that is suitable for the management of duodenal ulcer will also cure the gastric ulcer, such as proximal gastric vago-

tomy, provided there is no evidence of impending pyloro-duodenal obstruction. However, many surgeons wish to remove the gastric ulcer and carry out gastrectomy, an ulcer excision combined with proximal gastric vagotomy.

5. Postbulbar duodenal ulcers are quite frequently seen in certain countries, especially southern India, but are relatively uncommon in western countries. They are often severe and stenosing so that operation may be recommended for fear of incipient obstruction. Proximal gastric vagotomy is effective if the lumen is still widely patent: if it is not, then truncal vagotomy and gastroenterostomy is the best procedure.

6. Zollinger-Ellison syndrome associated with hypergastrinaemia, usually from G-cell hyperplasia or gastrin-secreting tumour in the pancreas generally produces peptic ulcers in usual sites. If an ulcer lies in an unusual site, or if there are multiple ulcers and especially if the ulcer is in the upper jejunum, suspect the Zollinger-Ellison syndrome (see p. 102).

7. Oesophageal peptic ulceration occurs when gastric acid refluxes into the oesophagus where the squamous mucosa is unresistant to acid attack. This develops most frequently as a result of hiatal hernia but can occur in the absence of herniation of the stomach into the chest. A less frequent cause of peptic ulcer in the oesophagus is in the condition of Barrett's oesophagus. This appears to be acquired although it used to be called 'congenitally short oesophagus.' The gastric mucosa invades the oesophagus and the oesophagogastric mucosal junction moves progressively upwards and an ulcer sometimes develops just above the junction. Its treatment is described on page 292.

8. Recurrent ulcer may develop in the duodenum following proximal vagotomy, vagotomy and pyloroplasty or distal gastrectomy of Billroth I type for duodenal ulcer. Gastric ulcer may develop following vagotomy for duodenal ulcer especially if there is postoperative gastric retention. Anastomotic, stomal or jejunal ulcer all refer to the type of ulcer thast develops following gastroenterostomy or gastrectomy with gastrojejunal anastomosis for duodenal ulcer (see p. 89).

VAGOTOMY

TRUNCAL VAGOTOMY

Appraise

1. Never embark on elective vagotomy without confirming the diagnosis of peptic ulcer by endoscopy.

2. Per-hiatal truncal vagotomy is indicated for the management of uncomplicated duodenal ulcer when the full range of medical treatment has been tried and failed to control the symptoms, leaving the patient incapacitated. It is normally accompanied by distal gastrectomy (antrectomy), pyloroplasty or gastroenterostomy to improve the rate of

gastric emptying. Antrectomy has never become popular in Britain. Pyloroplasty (see p. 77) is simple to perform unless the patient is very obese with a deep abdomen and with a fixed, very scarred pylorus. Anterior juxtapyloric gastroenterostomy is convenient if pyloroplasty is difficult to perform and has the advantage that it is not irrevocable.

3. Truncal vagotomy may be used when controlling gastroduodenal bleeding from peptic ulcer. At such operations the main task is to stop the bleeding but the secondary task is to prevent bleeding from recurrent or persistent ulcer.

4. In the surgical management of recurrent peptic ulcer truncal vagotomy is best combined with partial gastrectomy.

5. Truncal vagotomy combined with a 'drainage' operation is sometimes advocated for the definitive management of a perforated duodenal ulcer. It is impossible to predict in an individual patient whether he will have further problems requiring surgery, have some symptoms controlled by medical treatment or never have further symptoms following simple repair of a perforated ulcer. The improvement in medical management of uncomplicated duodenal ulcer urges conservatism.

6. Truncal vagotomy and a drainage operation is often effective treatment for chronic gastric ulcer in an unfit patient but gastrectomy including the ulcer is preferred treatment whenever possible.

Access

1. Use the upper paramedian or midline incision 20 cm long skirting the umbilicus.

2. Excise the xiphoid process if necessary and mobilize the left lobe of the liver, folding it to the right, to obtain a good view.

3. In an obese patient with a high diaphragm try the effect of tilting the patient 25–30° head up.

Assess

1. Explore the whole abdomen. Remember that patients with proven peptic ulceration may have incidental conditions which might help to explain their symptoms.

2. Examine the stomach and duodenum and note the effects of the ulcer in distorting the duodenum and fixing it, so that you may make a decision about the easiest and safest adjunctive operation.

3. Always favour simple and safe procedures. There is little difference between the results of the various operations so do not feel that you must perform a difficult procedure regardless of other considerations.

Action

1. Make sure there is a nasogastric tube in place, as a guide to the line of the gullet at the oesophageal hiatus.

2. While an assistant grasps the lower anterior wall of

the stomach and draws it down, identify the hiatus by feeling for the nasogastric tube. Open the peritoneum transversely, avoiding the inferior phrenic vessels. Beneath this is the phreno-oesophageal ligament. Open this and enlarge the incision to 3–4 cm. You can now pass the closed scissors anterior to the gullet into the posterior mediastinum. If you cannot, you have not yet opened the phreno-oesophageal ligament.

3. Look out for the anterior vagal trunk lying in front of the oesophagus (Fig. 5.10) and separate it upwards for 5 cm and downwards to where it gives off the hepatic and gastric body branches, continuing as the anterior nerve of

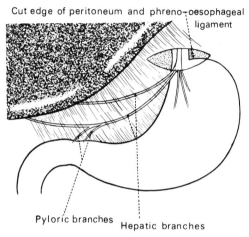

Fig. 5.10 Truncal vagotomy. Exposure of the anterior nerve; the distribution of the nerve is indicated.

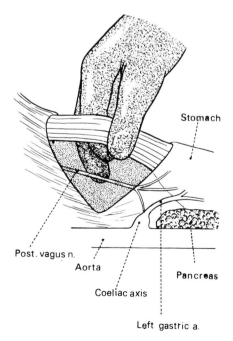

Fig. 5.11 Truncal vagotomy. Exposure of the posterior nerve as seen from the right side of the patient. While the gullet is encircled by the right thumb and forefinger, the right middle finger pushes the 'mesentery' containing the dorsal nerve to the right.

Latarjet. Transect it where it breaks up below, crushing the distal stump to occlude the small vessels running with it. Place a curved Moynihan clamp across it as high as possible and transect it just below the clamp, then remove the clamp. This is a 'vagectomy' and ensures that the whole trunk is removed.

4. Encircle the lower gullet with the right forefinger and thumb. There is a 'mesentery' behind the gullet in which lies the posterior vagal trunk (Fig. 5.11). Pass the middle finger to the left of the gullet and push this 'mesentery' to the right so that the nerve trunk can be identified. Separate the oesophagus from the vagus and burst through the mesentery behind the vagus. As the trunk is traced down, part of it passes backwards to the coeliac plexus (Fig. 5.12), part continues downwards as the posterior nerve of Latarjet and branches leave to reach the body of the stomach. Crush and cut the nerve below and again as high as possible to remove a segment of nerve to insure against leaving a separate branch intact.

5. Search for missed, separate branches around the whole circumference of the oesophageal wall. They feel like tight threads and should be divided. Make sure that there is no damage to the oesophagus and that all the bleeding is controlled.

6. Repair the horizontal defect in the hiatus using two or three non-absorbable sutures.

7. Carry out the selected adjunctive procedure of pyloroplasty, gastroenterostomy or gastrectomy.

Difficulty?

1. Access can be very difficult in obese patients. Do not proceed if you do not have an adequate view. Tilt the pa-

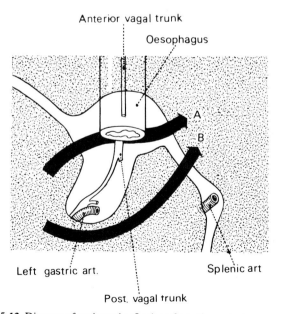

Fig. 5.12 Diagram of peritoneal reflections from the posterior abdominal wall. The posterior vagal trunk is gathered along path A but not along path B.

tient head up, remove the xiphoid process, mobilize the left lobe of the liver and fold it to the right. If the view is still restricted, do not hesitate to split the sternum in the midline. The only danger is of embarking on vagotomy without being able to see properly and control what is done.

2. The assistant's hand drawing down the stomach may be in the way. Make a hole in an avascular part of the upper lesser omentum, pass curved forceps behind the fundus of the stomach and push them through the gastrophrenic ligament near the angle of His. Draw a rubber tube through the hole as a sling to exert traction without distorting or obscuring the cardia.

3. Damage to the oesophagus? Repair the hole carefully, using all-coats sutures followed by a muscle coat stitch. Leave a nasogastric tube in the stomach.

4. Cannot find the vagi? Clumsy opening of the phreno-oesophageal ligament may lead to inadvertent anterior vagotomy. Carefully open the peritoneum and phreno-oesophageal ligament until the oesophagus can be seen encircled above by the diaphragmatic crus. The cut anterior trunk will be seen lying on the oesophagus. Alternatively you will see that the anterior trunk has been displaced to one side.

The posterior vagal trunk does not always lie close to the oesophagus. If it cannot be felt, carefully display the oesophagus emerging through the crus. The vagal trunk may be seen lying against the muscle of the crus. If you are a surgeon in training and cannot find the vagi, call for advice and assistance. Otherwise remember that more than half of patients treated surgically by gastroenterostomy will be cured of their symptoms. An experienced surgeon may carry out Polya gastrectomy in appropriate circumstances.

Technical points

1. Burge described a test for the completeness of vagotomy at operation. Atropine and similar drugs are eschewed in premedication. The lower oesophagus is encircled by a clamp carrying electrodes so that residual vagal fibres can be stimulated. This evokes gastric muscular contraction that can be measured as a rise in pressure within the stomach after closing the lumen proximally and distally with non-crushing clamps. However, the device works only if it encircles the vagi and the nerves are most frequently missed when they lie at a distance from the oesophagus. I believe the surgeons most in need of help are least likely to place the clamp correctly.

2. Grassi has described a test for completeness of vagotomy depending upon the stimulation of acid secretion as measured with a pH probe in the stomach during operation. Again the method depends upon correct placement of the clamp.

3. Staining the nerves with leucomethylene blue was also claimed to aid recognition of intact nerves but the technique is unreliable.

PROXIMAL GASTRIC VAGOTOMY

Appraise

1. This operation is otherwise known as highly selective vagotomy.

2. Proximal gastric vagotomy aims to denervate only the acid-secreting proximal part of the stomach, leaving the alkali-secreting antrum, with its muscular pumping action, still innervated. Thus gastric acid secretion is reduced but gastric emptying is usually unimpaired. The addition of a drainage operation can be dispensed with in most patients in the absence of pyloroduodenal stenosis. However, proximal gastric vagotomy is sometimes used in the presence of pyloroduodenal stenosis with the addition of dilatation with Hegar's instruments passed through a gastrotomy, by invaginating the anterior gastric antral wall through the pylorus on an index finger as originally described by Jaboulay or by carrying out duodenoplasty (see p. 78). Proximal gastric vagotomy is not justified if the pyloric metering function is destroyed or bypassed.

Access

Use an upper midline or paramedian incision, skirting the umbilicus, 20 cm long.

Action

1. Make a hole through an avascular area in the midportion of the gastrocolic omentum. While the stomach is lifted forwards, carefully and completely separate the flimsy attachments of the stomach to the pancreas, watching out for and preserving, the fold of peritoneum that contains the left gastric vessels. Separate the stomach from the posterior wall right up to the roof of the lesser sac. Occasionally you will be surprised to find the scar of an unsuspected posterior gastric ulcer.

2. Pass the right index finger through the hole in the gastrocolic omentum and grasp the gastric antrum to draw it down, so stretching the lesser curve of the stomach. In all but the most obese patients the taut anterior nerve of Latarjet can be seen running parallel to the lesser curve, separating into branches which form a 'crow's foot' pattern as they cross the curvature at the angulus, accompanied by blood vessels from the descending branch of the left gastric artery (Fig. 5.13). The posterior nerve cannot usually be seen from the front but can be displayed by looking through the hole in the gastrocolic omentum after turning the stomach forwards and upwards.

3. Carefully make a hole through the lesser omentum close to the gastric wall, just to the left of the 'crow's foot' of nerves, while protecting the posterior structures from damage with the right index finger passed through the defect in the gastrocolic omentum. Pass one end of a tape through the hole in the lesser omentum drawing it out

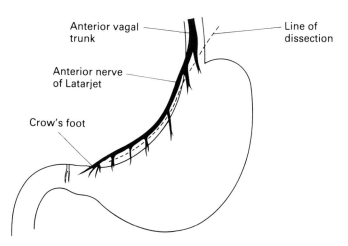

Fig. 5.13 Proximal gastric vagotomy. The anterior nerve of Latarjet, showing line of separation by dissection. The posterior nerve runs parallel to the anterior nerve.

through the hole in the gastrocolic omentum. The tape now encircles the stomach at the level of the angulus, marking the lower limit of dissection. Clip the ends of the tape together so they may by used to exert gentle downward traction on the stomach by an assistant to tauten and define the nerves of Latarjet.

4. Make a second, higher hole in the lesser curve close to the stomach just above the next visible vessels. Doubly clamp, divide and ligate the vessels and accompanying nerve filaments. Take care! The length of tissue available for double clamping between the nerve of Latarjet and the lesser curve is short. If you place the haemostats well apart you risk damaging the lesser curve, or the nerve of Latarjet or both. Alternatively, pass double ligatures with an aneurysm needle or with Lahey's fine curved forceps, tie them carefully and divide the tissue between them.

It is possible to use haemostatic clips instead of ligatures and one instrument applies two clips side by side and cuts between them : there is not usually sufficient length to use this here but it may be carefully used where the vessel and nerve length is adequate.

5. Proceed upwards step by step, dividing the vessels and nerves that cross the lesser curve, carefully preserving the nerves of Latarjet as they are separated from the stomach. Higher up on the stomach, the vessels and nerves do not tend to penetrate at the lesser curve but cross it to enter the gastric wall on the posterior or anterior wall. Take advantage of this extra length by carrying the dissection onto the anterior and posterior walls. The separation of the anterior and posterior nerves of Latarjet from the stomach now proceed independently onto the anterior and posterior gastric walls.

6. As the anterior and posterior leaves separate, slide non-toothed forceps under avascular sections and cut between the opened blades. Small vessels may be sealed with low power diathermy applied for the minimum time

through fine forceps applied well away from the main nerves.

7. At the level of the main left gastric artery and vein quite large vessels must be ligated and divided on the anterior and posterior walls, together with their accompanying nerve filaments. Above these, the lowest portion of the oesophagus can be separated from the nerves of Latarjet without dividing any large vessels.

8. As the dissection reaches the cardia, the main trunks of the vagus nerve are separated from the gullet, the nerves of Latarjet being the inferior prolongations of them. At this point temporarily stop the dissection.

9. Draw down the gastric fundus while an assistant retracts the left costal margin. Identify the angle of His between the fundus and the left edge of the lower gullet. Carefully incise the peritoneum in the angle, without damaging the stomach or oesophagus. Open up the hole gently with the right index finger and pass the right thumb through the upper part of the defect in the lesser omentum, behind the fundus of the stomach. Thumb and finger are prevented from meeting by the peritoneum of the roof of the lesser sac which can now be broken through.

10. At the level of the cardia separate, doubly ligate and divide the peritoneum, phreno-oesophageal ligament and nerve fibres across the anterior aspect of the lower oesophagus leaving the muscle coat denuded but intact.

11. Divide loose tissue and nerve fibres around the posterior aspect of the lower oesophagus, rotating it to improve the view. A troublesome fragile vein is encountered running posteriorly from the cardia. Tie it, seal it with diathermy current or apply a haemostatic clip. Do not encroach on the greater curve aspect of the gastric fundus or you will damage the short gastric vessels and the spleen.

12. Clear the whole circumference of the lower 5–7 cm of oesophagus of nerve fibres. Do not damage the longitudinal muscle coat. Catch any small veins that have retracted into the muscle coat using fine sutures if necessary (Fig. 5.14).

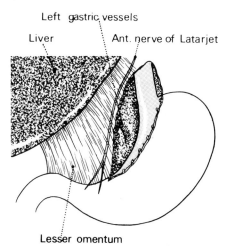

Left gastric vessels
Liver
Ant. nerve of Latarjet
Lesser omentum

Fig. 5.14 Proximal gastric vagotomy. The nerves of Latarjet have been separated from the lesser curvature of the stomach.

Difficulty?

1. Bleeding into the lesser omentum? A vessel retracts out of the ligature, continues to bleed between the layers of the omentum to form a large, spreading swelling. Do not try to grab it with large artery forceps. The ooze does not emerge directly from the vessel but trickles through the haematoma. Gently close the blades of a swab-holding forceps over the area and leave them from 5 minutes, timed by the clock. Remove the forceps. If bleeding does not recur during the remainder of the operation it is safe to leave the vessel. If oozing recurs or you are in doubt, gently dissect between the layers, identify the vessel and ligate it.

2. Thick, fatty omentum? Do not attempt to ligate it as a single layer. If you bunch it, subsequent traction on the stomach stretches the base of the bunch, and the ligature is forced off. If you are lucky, bleeding starts now. If you are unlucky, it will start later and you will miss it. Safeguard against this by picking up vessels with the minimum extraneous tissue. If necessary, perform the dissection in three separate layers, along the anterior leaf of lesser omentum, the lesser curve and the posterior leaf.

3. The operation can be difficult in an obese patient, in spite of taking steps to obtain a good view. Consider if truncal vagotomy would be easier, combined with a drainage operation. If you decide to proceed with proximal gastric vagotomy concentrate on each step, not anticipating the difficulties of the next step. Remarkably, the dissection usually becomes easier as the stomach is mobilized.

Check list

1. Examine the lesser omentum, lesser curve of stomach, lower oesophagus and upper lesser sac for signs of damage or bleeding. Have the short gastric vessels or spleen been damaged?

2. Re-examine the lower oesophagus for the presence of persistent vagal fibres and for signs of damage to the muscular coat. Finally, look again at the gastric lesser curve to ensure there is no damage.

TRANSTHORACIC TRUNCAL VAGOTOMY

Appraise

1. In his initial operations on humans, Lester Dragstedt approached the vagal trunks through the chest. This method is rarely used now because it is conventional to add some form of drainage operation to accompany truncal vagotomy and this cannot be performed through the chest.

2. In recurrent ulceration following some form of vagotomy it is usual to explore the abdomen and complete the vagotomy, followed by partial gastrectomy as a double assurance against further recurrence. If this has also failed and if the Zollinger-Ellison syndrome has been excluded

by noting that basal acid output is not raised and serum gastrin is within normal limits, then it is likely that vagotomy is still incomplete. Confirm this with an insulin test. Transthoracic vagotomy may be performed since there is less chance of failing to find and divide the trunks completely through the chest, provided no adjunctive procedure is required.

Access

1. Use the left thoracic approach through or just above the seventh or eighth rib (see p. 285).

2. Have the lower lobe of the left lung retracted upwards, dividing the pulmonary ligament, avoiding damage to the pulmonary vein.

3. Identify the descending aorta. Incise the pleura anterior to it to expose the lower oesophagus (Fig. 5.15). Gently free it, taking care not to open the right pleura.

4. Identify the vagal trunks lying anteriorly and posteriorly on the oesophageal muscle. Trace them upwards where they are formed from the anterior and posterior oesophageal plexuses and downwards to where they pass through the oesophageal hiatus.

Action

1. Elevate the nerves in turn from the oesophageal wall, taking care not to damage the longitudinal muscle coat. Free at least 5 cm of trunk, recognizing any small filaments that may leave the main trunk to run separately. Section the nerves above and below.

2. Seek and divide any further filaments around the whole circumference of the oesophagus.

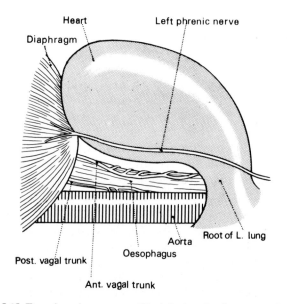

Fig. 5.15 Transthoracic vagotomy. The left chest has been opened.

Closure

1. Do not close the left mediastinal pleura.
2. Allow the anaesthetist to gently re-expand the left lower lobe.
3. Close the thoracotomy wound after inserting a basal drain attached to an underwater seal.

PYLOROPLASTY

Appraise

1. Reformation of the pylorus has the effect of increasing the size of the lumen and also destroys the pyloric sphincteric metering function. It can be used to overcome stricture of the pylorus and also to improve gastric emptying following truncal vagotomy. Following proximal gastric vagotomy, the distal stomach or 'antral pump' remains innervated so that gastric emptying is not usually prejudiced and pyloroplasty is not required.

2. Pyloroplasty is simple to perform in most circumstances and has enjoyed great popularity as an adjunctive operation with truncal vagotomy for duodenal ulcer. It may be difficult to perform if the duodenum is very scarred and adherent to the pancreas and the structures in the free edge of the lesser omentum if the abdomen is obese and deep.

3. It is probable that many postvagotomy symptoms are attributable to the drainage procedure and not to the vagotomy. Many such patients are improved if the drainage procedure is reversed. Although the pylorus can be anatomically restored to normal, the author has not been impressed with the longterm results.

4. Inevitably a number of methods of performing pyloroplasty have been described. The Heineke-Mikulicz method is the simplest but some surgeons favour the Finney pyloroplasty.

HEINEKE-MIKULICZ PYLOROPLASTY

Access

Gently mobilize the pyloroduodenal region by Kocher's manoeuvre and place a large pack behind the upper duodenal loop to bring it forwards in the wound.

Action

1. Make a longitudinal incision through all coats starting on the anterior wall of the duodenal bulb, carried through the pylorus and onto the anterior gastric antral wall (Fig. 5.16). The incision, 4–5 cm long, should be centred on the narrowest part of the pyloroduodenal canal. If there is an active anterior ulcer, encircle it so that a lozenge-shaped segment of anterior pyloroduodenal wall is excised, containing the ulcer. This 'pylorectomy' was described by Judd.

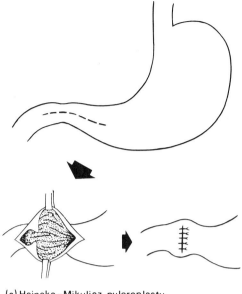

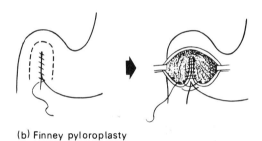

(a) Heineke–Mikulicz pyloroplasty

(b) Finney pyloroplasty

Fig. 5.16 Pyloroplasty.

2. Aspirate the contents and inspect the interior of the distal stomach and proximal duodenum. Sometimes there is a mucosal diaphragm with no evidence of ulcer in patients with typical features of pyloric stenosis in whom an endoscope would not pass. If a diaphragm is suspected, start the incision on the anterior antral wall 3–4 cm proximal to the pylorus and inspect the interior before cutting through the pyloric ring. Make sure there is not a second narrow duodenal segment distal to the pyloroplasty as may develop in postbulbar duodenal ulceration.

3. Gently apply tissue forceps to the middle of the upper and lower cut edges, and draw them apart, allowing the proximal and distal limits of the incision to come together, transforming the longitudinal cut into a transverse slit.

4. Close the incision, starting from the upper tissue forceps, ending at the lower forceps. Three methods are possible. The traditional technique is to insert an invaginating continuous all-coats layer of catgut, reinforced with a second seromuscular layer of sutures. The invaginated edges temporarily produce some hold up and many surgeons insert a single layer of all-coats sutures placed closely together, uniting the walls edge to edge without invagination. In the last few years stapling devices have gained popu-

larity and a single straight TA 55 stapler may be placed along the edges as they are held in their new position, with the opposed edges everted, close and activate the stapler. Cut off the excess tissue with a scalpel blade held in contact with the upper surface of the stapler which is then removed. Insert a reinforcing layer of seromuscular stitches if desired.

FINNEY PYLOROPLASTY

Appraise

Advocates claim that this produces a wider lumen than the Heineke-Mikulicz pyloroplasty. Of course the lumen size depends to some extent on the length of the incision. To my mind the Finney technique merely represents a generously fashioned Heineke-Mikulicz pyloroplasty with the inferior 'dog ear' pushed in.

Action

1. Gently mobilize the duodenal loop by Kocher's manoeuvre so the descending duodenum can be laid alongside the greater curve part of the gastric antrum.

2. Unite the adjacent gastric and duodenal walls with a seromuscular stitch, from above downwards, closing the angle below the pylorus.

3. Incise the full thickness of the stomach, pylorus and duodenum along an inverted horse-shoe shaped line which runs from the gastric antrum 4–5 cm proximal to the pyloric ring, through the pylorus curving through the duodenal bulb and down the descending duodenum.

4. Starting at the pylorus, unite with an all-coats stitch the adjacent walls of the stomach and duodenum. Continue the stitches round the lower limits of the incisions to unite the right duodenal cut edge to the left gastric cut edge, using an invaginating stitch.

5. Continue the seromuscular stitch to cover the anterior all-coats suture line.

DUODENOPLASTY

Appraise

1. The advent of proximal gastric vagotomy removed the need to perform an adjunctive drainage operation in the majority of patients with duodenal ulcer since in modern times most patients with incipient pyloric stenosis are operated upon before it becomes severe.

2. If pyloroplasty is necessary there is no advantage in performing proximal gastric vagotomy, since the metering action of the pylorus is lost. However, in some patients, stenosis is distal to the pylorus and can be overcome with-

out damaging the sphincteric mechanism. This is particularly true when the patient has post-bulbar duodenal ulceration. Proximal gastric vagotomy can then be justified.

Action

1. Mobilize the pyloroduodenal region by Kocher's manoeuvre and confirm that the pyloric ring itself is widely patent by invaginating the anterior antral wall through it on an index finger. The site of stenosis should have been determined before operation but this is not always easy to assess.

2. Make a longitudinal incision through the anterior duodenal wall stopping short of the pyloric ring (Fig. 5.17). This needs to be only about 1.5–2 cm long. If the ulcer and stenosis are post-bulbar remember that the distortion may draw the ampulla out of its normal place exposing it to inadvertent damage.

3. Gently apply tissue forceps to the middle of each cut edge and separate them to produce a transverse slit.

4. Close the slit transversely. Insert a single layer of closely applied stitches bringing the edges together without inversion.

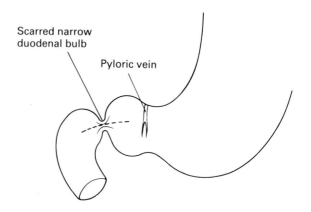

Scarred narrow duodenal bulb

Pyloric vein

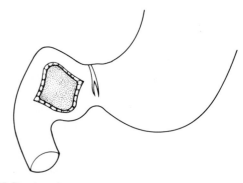

Fig. 5.17 Duodenoplasty.

GASTRODUODENOSTOMY

Appraise

1. This resembles the Finney pyloroplasty but does not include division of the pyloric ring.

2. It is an alternative method to pyloroplasty or gastroenterostomy for overcoming pyloric obstruction and may be appropriate if the descending duodenum has been opened.

Action

1. Mobilize the descending duodenum by Kocher's manoeuvre and join the descending duodenum to the anterior wall of the distal stomach with a running seromuscular stitch.

2. Incise the descending duodenum and anterior gastric walls for 5 cm, parallel and close to each side of the seromuscular stitch. Aspirate the contents and inspect the interior (Fig. 5.18).

3. Join the adjacent gastric and duodenal walls with a continuous all-coats stitch, carrying this round onto the anterior walls as an invaginating stitch to encircle the anastomosis.

4. Continue the seromuscular stitch onto the anterior wall to bury the all-coats stitch and complete the two layer anastomosis.

5. The anastomosis can be accomplished using the GIA stapler. Bring the stomach and duodenum together with a posterior seromuscular stitch. Make a stab hole in the stomach and the duodenum at the lower limit of the intended anastomosis. Pass in the separated limbs of the stapler, one into each hole, with the points towards the pylorus. Lock the limbs together so they lie just anterior

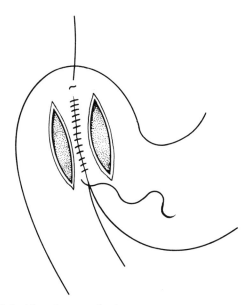

Fig. 5.18 Incisions for gastroduodenostomy.

to the seromuscular stitch line with no extraneous tissues intervening. Actuate the stapler which inserts four parallel rows of staples and cuts between the middle rows. Unlock the stapler, withdraw the limbs, inspect the completeness of the union and pick up the extremities of the staple lines through the stab wounds, which are now united, with tissue forceps. Separate the tissue forceps to draw the defect into an everted slit. Close the defect with a TA55 stapler. Check the integrity of the anastomosis and if desired continue the seromuscular stitch from the posterior suture line to bury the anterior stapled line.

GASTROENTEROSTOMY

Appraise

1. Gastroenterostomy was originally applied to the relief of pyloric obstruction from distal gastric carcinoma. It offers an important method of relief when gastrectomy cannot be carried out because the growth is locally too extensive or has already metastasized. Always place the gastroenterstomy as high on the stomach as possible to guard against the stoma becoming obstructed by advancing growth.

2. Gastroenterostomy was used for the relief of benign pyloric stenosis from duodenal ulceration but in the absence of stenosis it diverts some of the acid away from the ulcer, which usually heals. A proportion of patients eventually develop an ulcer at the stoma although this may be delayed for many years. The rate of anastomotic ulcer was unacceptable to many surgeons and it was mainly abandoned. It gained a new lease of life as a drainage operation combined with truncal vagotomy. A great advantage is that it can be carried out however severe the ulcer, since the anastomosis is to undamaged stomach. A further advantage is that if the patient subsequently has post-prandial symptoms from the drainage operation, it can be taken down quite simply provided that the pyloroduodenal canal is adequate. Gastroenterostomy for duodenal ulcer is placed as close to the pylorus as possible.

3. Gastroenterostomy may be used as a bypass in the presence of duodenal ileus or fistula. For many years surgeons argued about the merits of different techniques for gastroenterostomy. As a general rule surgeons now use only anterior juxtapyloric gastroenterostomy for benign disease (Fig. 5.19) and this will be described in detail with a note on the previously very popular posterior gastroenterostomy.

Access

Use a right upper paramedian or midline incision 15 cm long.

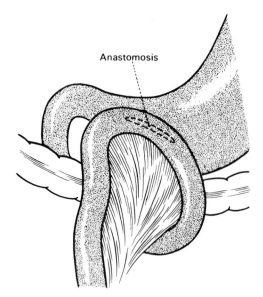

Anastomosis

Fig. 5.19 Juxtapyloric anterior gastroenterostomy.

Assess

Explore the abdomen. If the patient proves to have extensive carcinoma with no evidence of impending distal obstruction, carry out limited exploration only, but remove a biopsy specimen.

Action

1. Pick up a longitudinal fold of anterior gastric wall and grasp it with one of Lane's twin clamps. Choose a fold as close to the pylorus as possible if this is for benign pyloric obstruction or accompanies vagotomy for ulcer. Choose a fold as high as possible if this is to bypass an unresectable distal gastric carcinoma.

2. Lift up the greater omentum and transverse colon to identify the duodenojejunal junction. Draw the first loop of jejunum up over the colon and greater omentum to the stomach, with the short but not taut afferent loop against the proximal part of the clamped gastric fold and the efferent loop against the distal end of the fold. Place the second twin clamp along the apposed bowel, avoiding the mesentery, to occlude the lumen but not the blood supply. Lock the clamps together.

3. Unite the adjacent gastric and jejunal walls with a running seromuscular catgut stitch on an eyeless needle. Leave the ends long so that the stitch can be continued to encircle the anastomosis.

4. Open the stomach and jejunum parallel to the seromuscular stitch and 0.5 cm from it on each side, for 4–6 cm if this is for benign disease and for as long as possible if it is to bypass malignant obstruction.

5. Apply specially coloured towels to isolate the area and keep separate instruments during the next part of the operation when the potentially infected interior of the bowel will be exposed.

6. Unite the adjacent gastric and jejunal walls with a running all-coats stitch. Carry the stitch round the corner onto the anterior wall to complete the anastomosis. As the anterior gastric and jejunal walls are brought together, invert the edges. A Connell mattress stitch may be used as an alternative to the simple over and over stitch but take care that the blood vessels are picked up and tied along the edges, since the Connell stitch is not haemostatic.

7. Remove the twin clamps, discard and take sterile replacements for the soiled towels, instruments and gloves.

8. Carry the seromuscular stitch round the end onto the anterior wall and complete it to encircle the anastomosis, burying the all-coats stitch.

Check list

1. Examine the anastomosis and make sure it is patent.
2. Make sure there is no tension on the loop of jejunum. Draw the transverse colon and greater omentum to the right so there is no weight of bowel to drag on the anastomosis.

Difficulty?

1. The duodenum may be bound down in patients with severe duodenal ulcer. It is then difficult to make a juxtapyloric anastomosis. Make a more proximal safe and easy anastomosis.

2. It may be difficult to draw down sufficient proximal stomach to make a high anastomosis as a palliative bypass operation for obstructing distal carcinoma. Do not hesitate to enlarge the incision and abandon clamps if they are difficult to apply.

Technical points

1. The anastomosis can be fashioned using the GIA stapler. Draw the jejunum up to the stomach and attach it along the proposed line of the anastomosis with a seromuscular stitch at each end. Make stab wounds in the stomach and the jejunum close to the stitch uniting the afferent jejunal loop to the proximal stomach. Insert a sucker to empty the gastric and jejunal contents. Separate the two halves of the GIA stapler and insert one blade into each of the stab wounds, pointing towards the distally placed stitch. Lock the blades together, taking care not to include extraneous tissue. Actuate the device to insert four parallel rows of staples and cut between the central rows, forming an anastomosis between stomach and jejunum. Unlock the blades and withdraw them. Inspect the anastomosis all round from within and without, inserting sutures to reinforce doubtful areas. Pick up the ends of the staple lines on each side of the defect and draw them apart to create a linear slit. Apply a TA 55 stapling device along the everted edges of the linear defect, close the device and ac-

tuate it to seal the edges. Remove the device and examine the anastomosis to ensure it is perfect, inserting further stitches if necessary.

2. Suture material and stitches vary from surgeon to surgeon. I have described a sutured anastomosis using two layers of continuous catgut. Many surgeons insert interrupted non-absorbable stitches such as silk on the outer, seromuscular layer. It is not the material or type of stitch but the care with which they are inserted that determines whether the patient will recover without complications.

3. The use of clamps is argued about by surgeons. Certainly many successful surgeons use them routinely when they can be conveniently applied to prevent the leakage of bowel content into the wound, and to hold the stomach and bowel perfectly apposed while the anastomosis is fashioned. If you use clamps, apply them to the bowel only and not across the mesentery. Apply them sufficiently firmly to occlude the arteries as well as the veins, otherwise the bowel becomes congested and oedematous.

POSTERIOR GASTROENTEROSTOMY

1. This method was used with success for many years. From time to time it offers a convenient way of fashioning the anastomosis for benign disease. It cannot be used conveniently for high gastroenterostomy to relieve malignant distal gastric obstruction.

2. Hold up the greater omentum and transverse colon in order to inspect the mesocolon. Identify the middle colic vessels and make a conveniently placed vertical hole through the mesocolon to one or other side of them, 5–7 cm long.

3. Identify the posterior wall of the stomach through the hole and draw it down. Select a dependent and distal part of the stomach.

4. Apply the twin clamps to the protruding part of the stomach and to the first loop of jejunum beyond the ligament of Treitz. Lock the clamps and carry out the anastomosis.

5. Suture the margins of the cut mesocolon to the stomach to prevent small bowel loops from slipping through into the lesser sac and becoming obstructed.

BILLROTH I PARTIAL GASTRECTOMY

Appraise

1. Billroth I gastrectomy was originally used to resect distal gastric carcinoma but is now most frequently employed to resect gastric ulcers. It has the advantage that a high lesser curve ulcer can be included in the gastrectomy while leaving a generous amount of greater curvature. Since the duodenum is usually unscarred, gastroduodenal anastomosis is easily fashioned. The only other procedures that are equally effective are Polya gastrectomy above or below the ulcer and ulcer excision with proximal gastric vagotomy.

2. Surgery for gastric ulcer is conventionally offered if the ulcer fails to heal or rapidly recurs following treatment for 6–12 weeks with H_2-receptor blocking drugs, carbenoxolone or other demonstrably effective drugs. The decision is made following initial endoscopy with biopsy and cytology to exclude neoplasm and further endoscopy following a full course of medical treatment. Billroth I gastrectomy is employed in an emergency for the control of bleeding gastric ulcer and perforated gastric ulcer in most patients, although local control of a bleeding ulcer is sometimes attempted and suture of a perforation followed by a course of medical treatment can be tried.

3. Billroth I gastrectomy is less effective than Polya gastrectomy for the control of duodenal ulcer but combined with vagotomy, it has enjoyed a vogue in the USA.

4. Billroth I gastrectomy is still used by many surgeons to resect distal gastric carcinoma but in suitable patients radical distal gastrectomy (see p. 92) is preferred. It is important that there is adequate distal and proximal clearance otherwise the anastomosis may develop obstruction from recurrence. If there is insufficient distal clearance, it is safer to carry out Polya gastrectomy which takes the duodenum out of continuity. In addition, full width gastrojejunostomy offers better protection against anastomotic recurrence with stomal obstruction than does gastroduodenostomy.

Access

Use a right upper paramedian or midline incision about 20 cm long in the adult, skirting the umbilicus.

Assess

1. The diagnosis of gastric ulcer will have been made endoscopically but confirm this by looking for the serosal scarring, petechial haemorrhages and adhesions. Carry out a full exploration of the abdomen to exclude other conditions.

2. Gastric carcinoma will also have been confirmed endoscopically. Start the abdominal exploration in the pelvis and examine the para-aortic glands, peritoneum, liver and move centripetally towards the stomach to avoid disseminating cells around the abdomen. Now assess the degree of glandular involvement, the severity of invasion of the tumour and determine its operability. Decide upon routine Billroth I gastrectomy only if the tumour lies distally in the stomach, but the presence of metastases makes radical total (p. 92) or radical subtotal gastrectomy (p. 92) inappropriate. If the disease is so extensive that resection cannot be accomplished without cutting through growth, you may better serve the patient by choosing proximal gastroenterostomy to prevent distal gastric obstruction.

Resect

Benign disease

1. If the ulcer is adherent to the liver or pancreas, pinch it off and free the stomach. If this leaves a hole in the stomach, close it temporarily with a few stitches. Leave the healthy granulating base of the ulcer undisturbed.

2. Make a hole through an avascular part of the gastrocolic omentum to reach the lesser sac and divide any flimsy adhesions to the posterior gastric wall.

3. Isolate, doubly clamp, divide and ligate the vessels in the left part of the gastrocolic omentum outside the arcades up to and including the left gastroepiploics. It is not usually necessary to divide any of the short gastric vessels in this operation. Divide the right portion of the gastrocolic omentum down to and including the right gastroepiploic vessels. Remember that the main vessels lie only 1 cm from the middle colic vessels and avoid making holes in the transverse mesocolon.

4. Mobilize the duodenum by Kocher's manoeuvre. This makes the dissection and subsequent anastomosis easier. In thin patients it is necessary only to mobilize the upper portion of the duodenal loop.

5. Make a hole in an avascular part of the lesser omentum and isolate, doubly clamp, divide and ligate the right gastric vessels just above the pylorus.

6. It is usually necessary to divide the main left gastric vessels to mobilize the upper gastric lesser curve. This may be carried out after dividing the duodenum and turning the distal stomach upwards, but it can be carried out now before opening the viscus. Through the opening in the lesser omentum or the gastrocolic omentum identify the fold of peritoneum running forward to the upper lesser curve of the stomach and identify, isolate, doubly clamp, divide and securely ligate the left gastric artery and vein.

7. Isolate the area with specially coloured towels.

8. Place a thin crushing clamp such as Lang Stevenson's, just beyond the pylorus and a second Payr clamp parallel to and proximal to it on or just above the pylorus. Transect the duodenum just above the distal clamp, and cover both cut ends with swabs to limit the contamination.

9. Have the assistant hold the distal stomach vertically. Select the line of resection as far distally as possible on the greater curve and just above the ulcer thickening on the lesser curve. Ligate any small vessels here to leave the transection sites clean. Place a thin crushing clamp such as Lang Stevenson's crossing the greater curve at the chosen level of transection, that extends halfway across the stomach and place a second crushing clamp such as Payr's parallel and distal to it. Cut between the two clamps halfway across the stomach. From the end of this incision, apply a large curved Parker-Kerr clamp that arches upwards and crosses the lesser curve above the ulcer thickening. Place

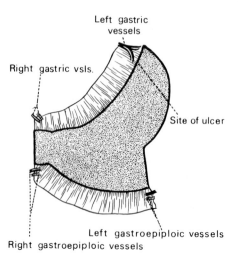

Fig. 5.20 Billroth I partial gastrectomy. The removed specimen.

a second clamp below and parallel to the first and cut between the clamps, thus removing the section which will be sent for histological examination (Fig. 5.20).

10. The lesser curve portion of stomach held in the curved Parker-Kerr clamp will form the new gastric lesser curve. Oversew it, including the clamp with a loose running stitch. Slide out the clamp, tightening up the loops seriatim to close the defect. Tie off the stitch and reinforce the suture line with a second running Lembert seromuscular stitch to invaginate the first.

Malignant disease

1. If radical resection (see p. 92) is not feasible because the growth has extended beyond its limits, resect it in the manner described for benign disease.

2. Make sure you can leave an adequate tumour free margin of 4–5 cm at each end of the specimen otherwise it is better to carry out Polya gastrectomy.

Difficulty?

1. Gastric ulcer may lie not on the lesser curve but on the anterior or posterior wall so that the curved resection to the lesser curve would have to be very high to include the ulcer. After freeing the stomach, slide the anterior and posterior walls round to bring the ulcer onto the right folded edge — a new lesser curve — before carrying out the gastrectomy. This 'rotation gastrectomy' was described by Tanner and facilitates the resection which can be more modest than resecting from the true greater and lesser curves.

2. If the ulcer lies very high on the lesser curve do not attempt to use a clamp. Make sure a nasogastric tube is in place. Start the cut from above the ulcer and start the closing suture so that as the cut continues little by little, the closing suture follows close behind. The remainder of the

stomach can be used to exert gentle traction on the upper stomach to maintain a linear defect. When the specimen is removed and the all-coats stitch is completed, tie it off and reinforce it with a second, invaginating Lembert seromuscular. If the defect extends onto the lower oesophagus, it is safer to perform a gastrojejunal anastomosis, taking the afferent loop of jejunum a little higher than the defect and suturing it around the oesophagus to reinforce the anastomosis.

3. An alternative method of dealing with a very high gastric ulcer in case of severe difficulty is to abandon ulcer resection. Instead carry out a Polya gastrectomy below the ulcer which will invariably heal. This is the Kelling-Madlener procedure. Although ulcer excision and proximal gastric vagotomy would be effective, this is as technically difficult as gastrectomy.

4. The diagnosis of benign ulcer or malignant tumour should have been made before operation but if for any reason you decide that a benign ulcer may be malignant after all, remove a specimen for frozen section histology. If this is not available, resect the ulcer as though it were benign and be prepared to carry out a radical resection when paraffin section histology demonstrates malignancy. This is better than a half-hearted radical resection.

Unite

1. Bring together the cut distal stomach and the duodenum, each held in a thin crushing clamp. The lesser curve half of stomach approximately matches the duodenum. There must be no tension. If necessary further mobilize the duodenum by Kocher's manoeuvre.

2. Unite the posterior gastric and duodenal walls with a seromuscular stitch. This is usually best accomplished by passing the needle between them while they are held apart.

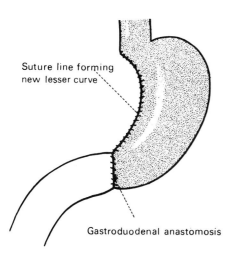

Fig. 5.21 Billroth I partial gastrectomy. The gastroduodenal anastomosis is complete, after reforming the lesser curve of the stomach.

The stitches are then tightened seriatim to draw the seromuscular layers into contact.

3. Cut across the stomach and duodenum with the knife blade held in contact with the thin clamps so that the crushed bowel is removed with the clamps.

4. Join the stomach and duodenum using a continuous all coats stitch starting on the posterior walls and turning round to the anterior wall back to the start (Fig. 5.21).

5. Discard and obtain sterile replacements for the instruments, soiled towels and gloves.

6. Complete the seromuscular suture by carrying the posterior stitch round onto the anterior walls.

7. Stapled anastomosis is not entirely satisfactory for gastroduodenal anastomosis.

POLYA PARTIAL GASTRECTOMY

Appraise

1. Polya gastrectomy is no longer routinely used alone as primary treatment for uncomplicated duodenal ulcer. Some form of vagotomy is preferred, although in vagotomy and antrectomy a distal Polya gastrectomy is carried out.

2. Polya gastrectomy is not usually employed for the cure of gastric ulcers but occasionally Polya gastrectomy below a high ulcer may be employed. The high ulcer will almost invariably heal. This is the Kelling-Madlener operation.

3. Combined gastric and duodenal ulcers may be treated by Polya gastrectomy, especially if the duodenum is scarred and narrow.

4. Recurrent ulceration following a previous duodenal ulcer operation employing some form of vagotomy is best treated by ensuring that the vagotomy is complete and carrying out Polya partial gastrectomy.

5. At an emergency operation for bleeding peptic ulcer, the most certain procedure is to excise the ulcer-bearing area. If the ulcer is duodenal then Polya gastrectomy with closure of the ulcer-bearing duodenum gives good results. At present however, the most frequently performed procedure is pyloroplasty with vagotomy and under-running of the ulcer with non-absorbable sutures. Erosive bleeding rarely demands operation but the multiple haemorrhages can only be dealth with by excision of the affected gastric wall and this involves gastrectomy. Fortunately, the bleeding is usually from the distal stomach.

6. The most frequent indication for gastrectomy is for distal carcinoma. Polya gastrectomy is now preferred to Billroth I gastrectomy because it allows a full width stoma to be constructed which is unlikely therefore to become obstructed by growth. Since the duodenum is closed and not used for anastomosis, distal spread of growth is less serious than when gastroduodenal anastomosis is used. The preferred method of resecting distal carcinoma is by radical subtotal gastrectomy (see p. 92).

Access

Make a right upper paramedian or midline incision that skirts the umbilicus, extending downwards from the xiphoid process for 20 cm. Ligate and divide the ligamentum teres and divide the falciform ligament.

Assess

1. Explore the whole abdomen. If the operation is for carcinoma, start in the pelvis and lower abdomen, para-aortic region and root of the mesentery, proceeding to the liver before touching the stomach in order to avoid carrying malignant cells around the peritoneal cavity.

2. Carefully examine the stomach and duodenum to confirm the diagnosis and assess the strategy of the operation. If necessary open the lesser omentum or gastrocolic omentum to examine the posterior wall of the stomach and contents of the lesser sac, including the glands around the coeliac axis and along the superior border of the pancreas.

Resect

Benign disease

1. Make a hole in an avascular area of the gastrocolic omentum to the left of the gastroepiploic vascular arch. Identify the posterior gastric wall and separate it from the pancreas and transverse mesocolon.

2. Clamp in sections, divide and ligate the gastrocolic omentum extending on the left up to and including the main left gastroepiploic vessels and the first one or two short gastric vessels. Avoid damaging the spleen directly or by exerting heavy traction on the stomach. To the right divide and ligate the main right gastroepiploic vessels as they lie near the inferior border of the pylorus. The separation of this vascular tissue can be accomplished rapidly using the LDS device which places two clips across the tissue and cuts between them in a single action. Avoid damaging the middle colic vessels which lie within 1 cm.

3. Clamp, divide and ligate the right gastric vessels after identifying and isolating them as they run to the left in the lesser omentum just above the duodenal bulb and pylorus. Divide the lesser omentum proximally, if possible preserving an accessory hepatic artery if one is present.

4. Free the first 1–2 cm of duodenum after applying fine artery forceps on the small vessels posteriorly, dividing and ligating them with fine ligatures. Now apply a Payr's clamp across the duodenum just beyond the pylorus. Place a second clamp just proximal to this to occlude the stomach. If there is insufficient room for this apply a non-crushing clamp across the distal stomach. Transect the duodenum just above the distal Payr clamp ensuring that no gastric mucosa remains attached to the duodenum. Cover the cut distal stomach with a swab.

5. Dissect the duodenum free for 2–3 cm so that it can be safely closed, applying fine forceps and ligatures to the vessels, keeping close to the duodenal wall. The common bile duct lies near the posterior and superior parts of the proximal duodenum and may be drawn out of its normal relationship by scar tissue. The gastroduodenal artery runs close to the medial wall of the duodenum.

6. Close the duodenal stump. First use a running over and over spiral stitch that encircles the clamp and the enclosed crushed duodenum. Gently ease out the clamp, tightening the stitches seriatim as it is withdrawn. Tie the stitch. Insert a second invaginating seromuscular suture to cover the first stitch line or insert a purse-string suture and invaginate the first suture line as it is tightened and tied. If possible insert a third stitch that picks up and draws together the ligated right gastric and right gastroepiploic vessel stumps, the anterior duodenal wall and the peritoneum over the head of the pancreas.

The duodenal stump may be closed using the TA 30 or TA 55 stapling device. This places a double row of staples across the duodenum. If it is to be used it is applied just beyond the pylorus in place of the Payr crushing clamp and a proximal clamp is placed across the distal stomach. Activate the stapling device to staple and seal the duodenum which is transected using a scalpel applied closely to the upper edge of the stapler. It is wise to invaginate the everted staple line with a layer of sutures, then cover this with the right gastric and right gastroepiploic vessel stumps sutured over it.

7. Exert a little tension on the left gastric vessels by elevating the pyloric end of the stomach. Identify the artery by feeling for the pulsations. Isolate the vessels from the lesser curve of the stomach, doubly clamp, divide and ligate them.

8. Select the line for the transection of the stomach (Fig. 5.22). When Polya gastrectomy was the standard operation for duodenal ulcer, a two-thirds gastrectomy was usually carried out. If distal gastrectomy or 'antrectomy' is to be carried out to accompany vagotomy, then only the

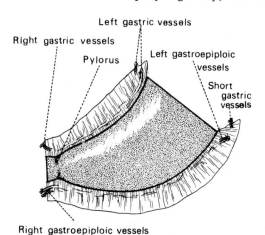

Fig. 5.22 Polya partial gastrectomy. The removed specimen.

distal third or half should be excised. If gastrectomy is for ulcer recurrence and accompanies vagotomy or completion of vagotomy, resect at least half the distal stomach. Clamp, divide and ligate the small vessels on the greater and lesser curves at the level of transection to leave them cleanly exposed.

9. Ask the anaesthetist to withdraw the nasogastric tube until the tip lies above the line of transection.

10. If gastrectomy is for peptic ulceration the medial half of the stomach may be closed so that only the greater curve half of the gastric lumen forms a stoma with the jejunum. This is a 'valved' gastrectomy designed to limit the rate of gastric emptying in the hope of preventing 'dumping.' It is debatable whether a valved stoma confers any benefit, since the rate of gastric emptying is restricted by the lumen of the efferent jejunal loop.

Malignant disease

1. Radical subtotal gastrectomy is described on page 92 but nonradical partial gastrectomy is appropriate in frail patients and in those who have a resectable carcinoma but already have metastatic deposits in the liver or elsewhere which make radical resection impossible.

2. It may not be possible to be sure that the distal resection is clear of growth but always ensure that the proximal line of resection is well clear of growth. Aim at a minimum of 5 cm apparently tumour-free margin. If the resection line cuts through tumour, the anastomotic line may break down during recovery from the operation. If it does not do so, recurrent tumour at the anastomosis may soon obstruct the lumen.

3. It is useless to carry the line of resection widely beyond the stomach so adopt the same technique as for resection for benign disease.

4. Plan to provide a full width gastroenterostomy stoma to guard against recurrent tumour causing obstruction.

Unite

1. Place one of the twin gastroenterostomy clamps across the stomach 2 cm above the proposed line of transection, from greater to lesser curve. Place a long non-crushing clamp across the stomach 3 cm distal to the twin clamp and parallel to it. The stomach will be transected just above this clamp. Fold the distal part of the stomach upwards. Reach down and identify the duodenojejunal junction. Draw up to the stomach the first loop of jejunum, with afferent loop to lesser curve with no slack but not tight. The efferent loop is placed at the greater curve. Place the second of the twin clamps across this loop of bowel, occluding only the lumen and not the mesentery. Marry and lock the clamps together.

2. Run a continuous seromuscular stitch to unite the adjacent gastric and jejunal walls.

3. If this is to be a full width stoma, incise the full width of the posterior gastric wall 0.5 cm above the clamp taking care at this time to leave the anterior wall intact. Make a parallel incision in the jejunum, 0.5 cm from the seromuscular suture line. Join the adjacent gastric and jejunal edges with an all-coats stitch of catgut on an eyeless needle. Now cut through the anterior wall of the stomach 1 cm distal to the clamp and remove the specimen of distal stomach. Continue the all-coats stitch round onto the anterior wall and along it to completely encircle the anastomosis. Remove the clamps, discard and take sterile replacements of the towels, gloves and instruments. Complete the seromuscular suture line onto the anterior wall to encircle the anastomosis.

4. When performing gastrectomy for benign disease it is conventional to close the lesser curve half of the stomach and form a small stoma between the greater curve half of the stomach and the jejunum. This is referred to as a valved anastomosis (Fig. 5.23). A different technique is used after uniting the stomach and jejunum in the twin clamps and with the posterior seromuscular stitch. Have the distal stomach held vertically and place halfway across it from the lesser curve, and 1 cm distal to the twin clamp, a short Payr's crushing clamp. Cut halfway across the stomach just distal to the Payr clamp, transecting the lesser curve half of the stomach. Oversew the clamp and contained crushed stomach edge with a running loose spiral stitch. Release and gently withdraw the clamp as the sutures are tightened seriatim. This manoeuvre leaves just the greater curve half of the stomach to be united to a matched hole made in the jejunum. The anastomosis is accomplished in a similar manner to the creation of a full width stoma. After the gloves, towels and instruments have been replaced, continue the posterior seromuscular stitch round and along the anterior wall to encircle the stoma and closed lesser curve.

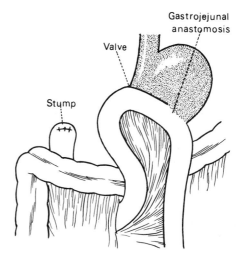

Fig. 5.23 Polya partial gastrectomy. The antecolic valved gastrojejunal anastomosis, with afferent loop joined to lesser curve, is complete. The duodenal stump is closed.

5. Alternatively the gastroenterostomy can be accomplished using stapling devices. Place and actuate a TA 90 across the stomach at the proposed line of section and cut off the distal gastric specimen with a scalpel run along the distal edge of the stapler. Remove the stapler. Bring up a proximal loop of jejunum and suture it to the posterior wall of the stomach 5 cm above the staple line, a seromuscular stitch at each end, with the afferent loop to the lesser curve, the efferent loop to the greater curve. Make a stab wound in the greater curve aspect of the posterior wall of the stomach 2 cm proximal to the staple line and make a matching stab wound in the jejunum at the origin of the efferent loop. Insert the limbs of a GIA stapler separately into the holes, with the tips pointing to the lesser curve. Ensure that there is no interposed tissue, lock the two limbs together and actuate the machine. Four lines of staples will have united stomach to jejunum and the knife will have cut a stoma between the centre rows of staples. Unlock and withdraw the stapler. Carefully check that the staple lines are perfect. Place tissue forceps at the ends of the inner and outer staple lines and separate the forceps to create an everted linear defect in the anastomosis. Place a TA 55 stapler across the everted lips of the defect, tighten and actuate it. Cut off the excess tissue, remove the stapler and check the line of closure carefully, if necessary reinforcing the whole anastomosis all round with sutures.

Difficulty?

1. It may be difficult and hazardous to dissect out and close the duodenum in the presence of extensive scarring and distortion from chronic severe duodenal ulceration. There are alternative techniques available for the elective primary treatment of duodenal ulcer and you should select one that does not carry the risk of duodenal dissection. If the ulcer is postbulbar, it is often easy to carry out a pre-ulcer closure by dissecting just as far as the ulcer, transecting the duodenum just beyond the pylorus and closing the relatively unscarred pre-ulcer segment of duodenum. If for some reason you are committed to closing the duodenum, then an alternative is to transect the gastric antrum, dissect out and excise the antral mucosa and close the cut edge of duodenal mucosa, leaving raw antral seromuscularis. Now close this using a series of internal purse-string sutures.

2. If you have committed yourself to dissecting out and closing the duodenum and now find yourself in difficulty, carefully stick close to the duodenal wall. If you encounter a large ulcer crater, this cannot be mobilized to help close the duodenum. There are three choices. The best choice is to carefully pinch off the duodenum just at the distal ulcer edge and carefully mobilize a sufficient cuff of duodenum beyond to close safely, leaving the ulcer crater undisturbed. The second choice is to leave the duodenum attached to the ulcer and mobilize the anterolateral duodenal wall so that it can be sewn down to the distal fibrotic edge of the ulcer crater, thus closing off the duodenum. If neither of these is possible or can be safely accomplished, then do not try to close the duodenum. Sew in a large tube and bring this to the surface of the abdomen. Leave it attached to a closed drainage system for 10 days and if the patient is well, gradually withdraw it. The duodenal fistula will usually heal spontaneously. Even if it does not do so, the track is so well established that there will be no intra-abdominal complications of the manoeuvre.

3. Is it difficult to mobilize the proximal stomach? The spleen may be adherent to the diaphragm and the costal margin may be narrow in an obese patient. Make sure the stomach is not adherent posteriorly through adhesions or a previously unsuspected gastric ulcer — if it is, pinch off the ulcer and if necessary, temporarily close the defect with sutures, and include the ulcer in the gastrectomy specimen.

4. In time of difficulty make sure that the light, the exposure and the assitance are all optimal.

5. Bleeding? Avoid panic measures. Control severe bleeding with local pressure while preparing to pick up the bleeding point accurately with artery forceps. Do not tie blood vessels together with large pieces of omentum or mesentery. The blood vessel may retract and quietly bleed into the closed mesentery. If the splenic capsule is torn, remove the spleen (but see p. 216).

6. Damage to the common bile duct? Correct it now, or call upon a more experienced person to do so. Ensure that you have available radiography to help in elucidating the damage. Repair the injured duct as you would at a routine biliary operation and plan to leave a 'T-tube' drain in the common duct to drain the biliary tract temporarily. Immediate and perfect repair of bile duct injuries ensure minimal disability. Missed or imperfectly repaired injuries seriously threaten the patient's well-being.

Technical points

1. The inside of the stomach and bowel are infected with micro-organisms. While fashioning anastomoses isolate the interior of the bowel from the peritoneal cavity and wound edges by using separate towels, instruments and gloves. When the bowel is repaired, discard and replace them with sterile gloves, towels, and instruments.

2. Retrocolic anastomosis may be fashioned following gastrectomy but it does not confer any benefits over the antecolic anastomosis.

3. Some surgeons avoid the use of clamps during the fashioning of gastric anastomoses. There is no evidence that clamps damage the bowel. However, every surgeon has firm ideas on techniques and should respect the convictions of others.

Check list

1. Examine the anastomosis. See that it is perfectly fashioned and intact. If necessary insert extra sutures. Ensure that you can invaginate the gastric and jejunal walls through the stoma.

2. Check each of the main vascular ligatures. Retie them if they are insecure.

3. Check the spleen. Aspirate all the blood from under the left cupola of the diaphragm and recheck it just before closing the abdomen to ensure that there has been no further collection of blood.

4. Make sure the duodenal stump is safely closed. Should you leave a drain down to it? If so, does this replace careful technique and should you therefore reclose the duodenum or reinforce the closure?

5. Examine the colon to ensure there is no damage to it, or the mesocolon or middle colic vessels. Draw the greater omentum, transverse colon and mesocolon through to the right so there is no weight of colon resting on the anastomosis.

6. Aspirate any blood from under the right cupola of the diaphragm, from under the liver and in the right pre-renal pouch. Finally, aspirate any blood that has collected in the pelvis.

GASTRODUODENAL BLEEDING

Appraise

1. Do not embark on operation for upper gastrointestinal bleeding without preliminary endoscopy. This establishes the cause in a high percentage of cases. Even if it does not, it may exclude possible sites such as oesophageal varices. If pre-operative endoscopy has failed, repeat it when anaesthesia is induced and have it available during the operation. The source of bleeding is mucosal and seeking it from within the lumen is far more successful than searching the exterior of the suspect viscera at laparotomy.

2. Are you clear that operation is indicated? The presence of shock on admission in a patient aged more than 50 years and continuing or recurrent bleeding following admission are well recognised points in favour of surgery. Endoscopic confirmation of active bleeding, the presence of a visible vessel or clot in the ulcer crater are further points, while multiple erosions are an indication for a trial of conservative management with intravenous cimetidine, resorting to surgery only if this fails.

3. Is the patient well prepared for an emergency operation? Calamitous bleeding requires surgery without delay but is infrequent. All other patients can be resuscitated and stabilized. Exclude or correct any bleeding tendency. Have sufficient crossmatched blood available for transfusion. Exclude and treat other incidental conditions. Check, and correct as far as possible, any malfunction of the body systems.

4. Obscure recurrent upper gastrointestinal bleeding often gets loosely labelled 'peptic ulcer haemorrhage.' If repeated endoscopy fails to reveal a cause do not be pressured into carrying out an operation without first obtaining a diagnosis. Such episodes rarely demand urgent surgical intervention. Localization of the bleeding site may be aided by the use of radio-active isotope labelling of red cells injected into the circulation with gamma camera monitoring of leakage into the gut. The patient can be asked to swallow a string which is attached at its upper end to the cheek; subsequently the string is withdrawn and tested along its length for the presence of blood, giving a clue to the site of bleeding. Most surgeons would now opt for angiography carried out during bleeding. This often displays the site and rate of bleeding.

5. Surgical management of severe or recurrent bleeding may be replaced by other methods although the exact indications are not yet clearcut and depend upon operator capability. Through the endoscope, bleeding points may be sprayed with clotting factors or coagulated with diathermy current or laser beam. At angiography, supplying arteries can be embolized with various substances.

Access

Make a generous upper abdominal paramedian or midline incision skirting the umbilicus, 20–25 cm long. Ligate and divide the ligamentum teres and incise the falciform ligament.

Assess

1. As the abdomen is opened blood, which appears bluish through the bowel wall, may be seen in the small or large bowel. Dilated and congested veins on the viscera with a stiff cirrhotic liver make portal venous hypertension obvious. Scarring and oedema of the stomach or duodenum may indicate the site of bleeding.

2. Remember that in Britain, most upper gastrointestinal bleeds requiring emergency surgery are from peptic ulceration or erosions but also remember that there are sometimes multiple causes and the detection of a possible site does not exclude the possibility of other causes. Therefore carry out a thorough check of the lower oesophagus, stomach and duodenum, remembering that there may be an unsuspected lesion in the small or large bowel.

3. If no cause is detected and there is no site of active bleeding, do not hesitate to repeat the endoscopy yourself or ask an experienced colleague to do so. It may be valuable first to have a large bore gastric tube passed so that the stomach can be washed out, if it contains blood or retained food.

4. Alternatively — but often less satisfactorily — perform gastrotomy or gastroduodenotomy. Make an incision through the anterior gastric wall midway between the greater and lesser curves in the distal stomach, carrying this through the pylorus into the anterior duodenal wall for 2–3 cm if necessary. Aspirate the gastric contents. Insert large-bladed retractors for your assistants, have the light adjusted to shine into the stomach and carefully examine the interior of the stomach and if necessary the duodenal bulb seeking the cause of bleeding. Sometimes the gastric wall can be evaginated through the gastric wound to allow close inspection. If the pylorus has not been incised it is often possible to insert thin-bladed retractors through it to view the duodenal bulb, or a cystoscope may be passed, offering excellent views of the bulb.

5. Do not carry out a procedure unless the cause is found. 'Blind' gastrectomy was once recommended but this merely confuses the problem and adds to the patient's risk. Make a thorough examination of the whole gastrointestinal tract including structures that could produce bleeding into it, such as the biliary tract. If there is no active bleeding and no cause is found, close the abdomen and determine to repeat the endoscopy at the first sign of rebleeding followed if necessary by other methods of detection and isolation of bleeding sites.

Action

1. Bleeding duodenal ulcer is preferably treated at present by pyloroplasty, suture of the bleeding vessels and truncal vagotomy. Create a gastroduodenotomy (p. 67) of the size that would usually be made for a pyloroplasty. Aspirate blood and clot from the ulcer base and isolate the site of bleeding. This is usually from the gastroduodenal artery. Carefully insert stitches of 2/0 silk on a round-bodied small curved eyeless needle placed transversely to pick up the artery (Fig. 5.24). Remember the common bile duct lies close, so insert the sutures carefully. Make sure the bleeding is completely controlled. Sometimes the edges of the ulcer can be brought together to form a linear suture line. Close the gastroduodotomy as a pyloroplasty. Change instruments, drapes and gloves before performing truncal vagotomy.

2. The florid duodenal ulcers that were formerly seen are less common now but occasionally the duodenal ulcer is so large, the walls so thickened and distorted that pyloroplasty will not be successful. Plan to perform Polya gastrectomy (p. 83). The difficulty will be in freeing and closing the duodenum. If the duodenum has already been opened to perform pyloroplasty before the problem is appreciated, first control the bleeding with 2/0 silk sutures. Now decide whether to dissect the duodenum distal to the ulcer sufficiently to allow it to be closed. If not, Nissen's manoeuvre may succeed: suture the anterior cut duodenal edge to the distal ulcer edge and if there is sufficient free

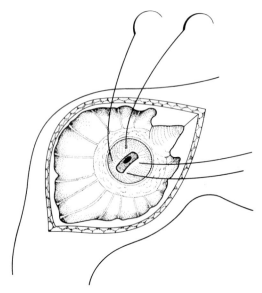

Fig. 5.24 Suture-ligature of gastroduodenal artery in the base of posterior duodenal ulcer, using 2/0 silk.

anterior duodenal wall, suture it over the ulcer to the proximal ulcer edge (see Fig. 5.25).

If the difficulty of performing pyloroplasty is appreciated early, perform Polya gastrectomy preserving as much of the anterior duodenal wall as possible, provided the ulcer base can be exposed and the bleeding controlled with sutures. This allows the closure of the duodenum to be carried out securely.

Control of the bleeding may be difficult in the presence of a large ulcer and the base may be exposed most easily by 'pinching off' the duodenum from the ulcer edge to leave the base free. Control the bleeding. The problem of closing the duodenum can now be tackled calmly, either accomplishing it in the post-ulcer segment, or closing the hole created by the ulcer defect (see p. 84).

If all else fails insert a large catheter into the duodenal defect and close the duodenum around it. Bring the catheter to the surface of the abdomen to create a controlled fistula. This can be removed after 10–14 days and nearly always closes without complication.

3. Bleeding gastric ulcer can be treated by Billroth I partial gastrectomy (see p. 81). This is a straightforward operation in most circumstances. On occasion when the stomach has been opened, excision of the ulcer or suture-ligation of the bleeding vessels may be considered with pyloroplasty and truncal vagotomy in a poor risk patient.

4. The surgical treatment of erosive gastritis is often unsatisfactory and most surgeons are conservative whenever possible. If bleeding is uncontrollably severe, then perform high gastrectomy. Billroth I reconstruction is usually appropriate.

5. Gastric carcinoma or sarcoma are rare causes of severe gastrointestinal bleeding and should have been appreciated before surgery was contemplated. Ideally the operation to

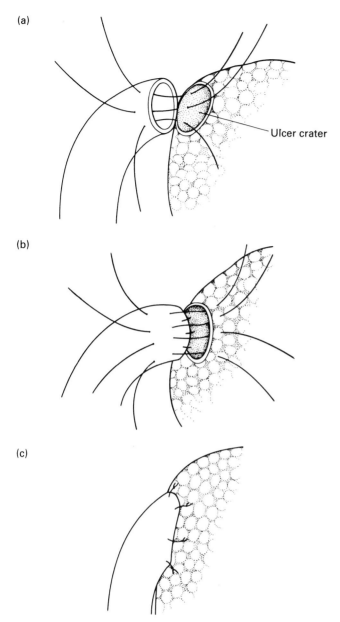

(a)

Ulcer crater

(b)

(c)

Fig. 5.25 Nissen's manoeuvre for closure of duodenal stump. The cut anterior duodenal edge is first sutured to the distal ulcer edge. The anterior duodenal wall is then sutured to the proximal ulcer edge.

be performed is the one that would be selected at an elective operation. However, as a life-saving operation, be prepared to carry out a limited resection. In suitable patients it is reasonable to plan re-operation after 2–3 weeks to carry out radical resection.

RECURRENT PEPTIC ULCER

Appraise

1. A compromise has been reached between the effectiveness of operations for peptic ulcer and the mortality and morbidity associated with them. Minimal surgery is safer but sometimes less effective in controlling peptic ulcers than more major procedures. However, provided the number of patients who develop recurrences is small, it is logical to treat all patients by the simplest and safest method, reserving more aggressive surgery for those who develop recurrent ulcers, since it is impossible at present to predict this group. Stephen Wangensteen has succintly stated, 'death is more serious than ulcer recurrence.'

2. Recurrent ulcer is an objective diagnosis based on endoscopic visualization of the ulcer. Never explore a patient with 'suspected' recurrence without first carrying out endoscopy. Test the basal, pentagastrin stimulated and insulin stimulated gastric acid secretion. High basal secretion suggests the possibility of a Zollinger-Ellison tumour in which case estimate the serum gastrin level and exclude hyperparathyroidism (see p. 102). A positive insulin test may suggest incomplete vagotomy if that was the original operation.

3. An episode of recurrent ulcer does not necessarily demand re-operation. Try the effect of an H_2-receptor blocking drug. The ulcer may heal and not recur.

4. In some patients who have had multiple operations who have high gastric acid output in spite of gastric resection, truncal vagotomy may be conveniently performed through the left chest (see p. 285). Since recurrence can be controlled medically there is usually no indication for an inexperienced surgeon to attempt re-operation.

Access

1. Explore the abdomen through the original incision unless this is unsuitably placed in which case use a long upper abdominal midline or left paramedian incision.

2. Carefully separate the adhesions to permit exploration of the whole abdomen. The stomach or remnant is often firmly adherent to the under surface of the left lobe of the liver and must be carefully separated from it.

Assess

1. Recurrent duodenal ulcer following vagotomy and pyloroplasty lies usually on the pyloroplasty suture line. Aim to complete the vagotomy and carry out hemigastrectomy with gastrojejunal anastomosis. If the distal line of transection is proximal to the ulcer there is a danger of leaving gastric antral mucosa in the duodenal stump with resultant gastric acid hypersecretion; therefore, either perform transection and closure distal to the ulcer or excise the mucosa proximal to the ulcer when performing pre-ulcer closure.

2. Recurrent duodenal ulcer following proximal gastric vagotomy is best treated by hemigastrectomy of Polya type plus truncal vagotomy. Make sure the spleen is present first. If it was removed at the first operation, the stomach will be supplied only by the right gastric and right gastro-

epiploic vessels. Distal gastrectomy will deprive the gastric remnant of its blood supply. Gastric mucosal resection is permissible because it does not demand the ligation of any major blood vessels.

3. Stomal ulcer following vagotomy and gastroenterostomy should be treated by disconnection of the gastroenterostomy followed by Polya hemigastrectomy and completion of the vagotomy.

4. Gastroenterostomy alone may have been carried out in a poor risk patient with pyloric stenosis. Such recurrence could probably be adequately controlled medically but at operation, truncal vagotomy should suffice with revision of the drainage procedure only if the ulcer has caused stomal obstruction from stenosis.

5. If this recurrent ulcer is associated with high basal gastric acid output, carefully explore the pancreas and duodenum to exclude the presence of a Zollinger-Ellison tumour (see p. 101).

6. Recurrent gastric ulcer is rare following Billroth I gastrectomy but if it does develop, carry out a higher gastrectomy, excising the ulcer. The anastomosis may once again be gastroduodenal but Polya gastrectomy is highly effective in preventing recurrence. Recurrent gastric ulcer following proximal gastric or truncal vagotomy with excision of the ulcer or a 'drainage procedure' is also best treated by gastrectomy.

7. Recurrent ulcers may develop following conversion surgery to relieve dumping, bile vomiting or diarrhoea. As a rule, the surgeon will have taken precautions to prevent recurrence but if these have failed, the basis of surgical treatment is combined truncal vagotomy and gastrectomy.

Action

1. Truncal vagotomy demands expert knowledge of the area. If the trunks were missed previously, search carefully not only around the lower oesophagus but also within the whole of the oesophageal hiatus. The posterior trunk may lie posteriorly on the right crus of the diaphragm. Remember that missed trunks may have been displaced at the first operation.

2. Partial gastrectomy is not necessarily more difficult than at a primary operation but great care is necessary to mobilize the stomach or remnant.

3. Do not leave a complicated anatomical result but prefer to take down anastomoses, leaving the anatomy simple. Blind and redundant loops of bowel endanger the patient's longterm wellbeing.

REVISIONARY SURGERY FOLLOWING PEPTIC ULCER SURGERY

Appraise

1. Inexperienced and occasional gastric surgeons should not embark on revisionary surgery for the relief of sequelae following operations for peptic ulcer. Many of the patients improve with time following reassurance, and almost all of them can be improved by adherence to simple rules such as avoiding large meals and food that they have learned is likely to be upsetting, by taking small meals separate from fluids and resting after meals and by avoiding food and drinks containing excessive sugar. In any case, it is wise to wait at least 2 years from the primary operation before contemplating a revisionary operation.

2. Bilious vomiting following the creation of a gastroenterostomy stoma is most likely to respond to anatomical revision. It is thought that the afferent loop is functionally or mechanically obstructed and distends with bile, pancreatic juice and duodenal secretions, discharging intermittently into the stomach. The gastric lining is irritated and the patient may vomit or regurgitate some of the bile-stained fluid. At endoscopy, the region of the stoma reveals florid gastritis. If bilious vomiting follows gastroenterostomy plus truncal vagotomy the anastomosis can often be simply disconnected provided the pyloroduodenal canal has an adequate lumen. If it follows Polya gastrectomy, conversion to a Roux-en-Y anastomosis (see Fig. 5.26) with drainage of the duodenal loop into the efferent limb at least 50 cm from the stomach diverts bile away from the stomach. An alternative is a Roux-19 conversion in which

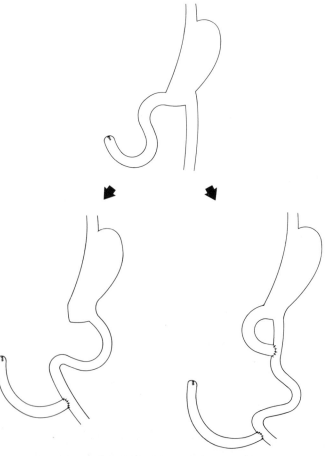

Fig. 5.26 Conversion surgery for relief of bile vomiting following Polya partial gastrectomy. Lower left is the Roux-Y operation. Lower right is the Tanner Roux-19 operation.

the afferent loop is divided and the ends are anastomosed into the efferent loop at least 50 cm apart; this procedure can be carried out without mobilizing the stomach. These operations increase the risk of stomal ulceration and if the original operation was for duodenal ulcer, it is wise to perform truncal vagotomy.

Occasionally bilious vomiting complicates Billroth I gastrectomy. A practical procedure is to isolate a 20–30 cm segment of proximal jejunum with its blood supply intact and insert this segment in an isoperistaltic fashion between the distal stomach and the duodenal bulb. Alternatively, the anastomosis can be disconnected, the duodenum closed and the stomach connected to a Roux-Y loop of jejunum

3. Dumping syndrome is named from the probability that it develops because of the destruction of pyloric metering of gastric contents into the small bowel. Thus food and fluid may be rapidly deposited into the jejunum, causing overdistension and causing discomfort usually within 30 minutes of the meal. Rapid absorption of fluid may produce circulatory disturbances, while hyperosmolar solutions attract fluid into the lumen, depleting the circulating fluid volume and at the same time overfilling the jejunal lumen. Rapid absorption of sugars may evoke hyperglycaemia stimulating insulin release, followed by rapid fall in blood glucose and the symptoms of hypoglycaemia usually 2–4 hours after meals. Proximal gastric vagotomy without drainage for duodenal ulcers appears to reduce the incidence of dumping, since the metering function of the antrum and pylorus is left intact.

Following Polya partial gastrectomy dumping may be diminished by conversion to a Billroth I anastomosis or by conversion to a Roux-en-Y, adding truncal vagotomy to protect from recurrent ulceration. Neither of these procedures is totally satisfactory in every patient. Elaborations have been recommended, usually in the form of interposed antiperistaltic or isoperistaltic jejunal segments between the gastric remnant and the duodenum or efferent loop of small bowel. As a trainee surgeon, do not attempt to perform these complicated and often ineffective operations.

Severe dumping infrequently complicates Billroth I gastrectomy but occasionally an isolated isoperistaltic or antiperistaltic loop of jejunum is interposed between the gastric remnant and the duodenum.

Dumping following vagotomy is usual only when accompanied by an adjunctive procedure to improve gastric emptying. Gastroenterostomy can be taken down if the pyloroduodenal canal is adequate and the results are usually good. Pyloroplasty can be revised so that the pylorus is restored to anatomical normality but reports are varied on the success of the procedure and in my experience it does little to improve the patient's symptoms in the longterm.

4. Gastric retention produces postprandial bloating sensation and regurgitation or vomiting of gastric contents often with eructations. It was notorious in a proportion of patients treated by truncal vagotomy alone for the cure of duodenal ulcer and was relieved or prevented by the addition of gastrectomy, gastroenterostomy or pyloroplasty. As a rule, improvement occurs with time even when there is no drainage operation. Some patients appear to develop complete gastric atony following vagotomy, including proximal gastric vagotomy, whether or not a drainage operation has been added; this also tends to slowly improve with time. If a drainage operation was not used originally then perform gastroenterostomy.

Occasionally gastric retention develops from stomal obstruction associated with adhesions trapping the efferent bowel, intussusception of the afferent loop into the stomach or prolapse of hypertrophic gastric mucosal folds into the stoma, and from stenosis following recurrent ulcer. The diagnosis is made by contrast radiography and endoscopy. Treatment is surgical relief of the obstruction or bypass.

5. In post-gastrectomy patients who swallow indigestible food without first chewing it, the bolus of food may impact in the bowel usually in the terminal ileum. Surgical relief is necessary: the bolus can usually be broken up without opening the bowel. Subsequently adjure the patient to avoid eating unchewed meat, fruit and other foods.

6. Diarrhoea may complicate peptic ulcer surgery. Make sure that the patient does not have some unrelated cause. An occult tendency to coeliac disease, colitis or irritable bowel disease may become manifest following peptic ulcer surgery. Dumping of food and fluid, especially hyperosmolar fluid, provokes intestinal hurry and diarrhoea as well as dumping syndrome and these symptoms can be controlled with simple dietary advice. Nearly all patients following gastrectomy have a tendency to steatorrhoea although this may not be clinically evident. A rare cause of diarrhoea is inadvertent gastroileostomy instead of gastrojejunostomy; this requires urgent surgical correction.

A few patients have crippling, uncontrollable diarrhoea following vagotomy and drainage for peptic ulcer. Diarrhoea is associated with dumping and can usually be alleviated by controlling the dumping. Diarrhoea alone may be controlled by reversing a 10–12 cm length of jejunum, 100 cm beyond the ligament of Treitz or an 8 cm loop of ileum 40 cm proximal to the ileocaecal valve.

7. Surgery for peptic ulcer is thought to predispose to gastric carcinoma. Do not assume that all symptoms, especially those developing late or with a changed pattern from previous symptoms are 'postpeptic ulcer surgery syndrome.' Successful resection is possible in some patients with stump carcinoma.

GASTRIC CARCINOMA

Appraise

1. At present the best hope of cure is resection. The tumours are usually resistant to radiotherapy and chemotherapy.

2. Radical surgery offers the most effective treatment including the primary tumour, likely involved glands, and intervening tissue en bloc. Other structures such as the parietes, a liver lobe, pancreas and transverse colon may be included in a radical resection if they are locally invaded. For distal tumours, radical subtotal gastrectomy can be carried out through the abdomen. For tumours of the midstomach and cardiac region radical total gastrectomy is the method of choice, usually performed through a combined left thoraco-abdominal incision but which can be performed through the abdomen in suitable subjects with carcinoma of midstomach and mobile, tumour-free cardia.

3. The awareness of early gastric cancer has been stimulated by excellent Japanese studies. Distal in situ carcinoma is treated by distal gastrectomy including the first tier of draining lymph nodes. Proximal or multiple early lesions are usually treated by total gastrectomy, again including the first tier of lymph nodes. Total gastrectomy is advisable if there is associated gastric atrophy associated with pernicious anaemia.

4. An increased incidence of gastric carcinoma is thought to be associated with previous surgery for peptic ulcer. Be aware of the possibility and do not attribute symptoms lightly to 'postpeptic ulcer operation syndrome.' Confirm the diagnosis with endoscopic biopsy. Be prepared to explore such patients since successful resection is possible.

5. Removal of the primary carcinoma is valuable even when the disease has spread beyond the limits of radical resection. Palliative total gastrectomy is appropriate for midstomach or proximal growths although proximal gastrectomy may sometimes be employed and palliative distal gastrectomy is suitable for distal growths. Try not to leave tumour at the resection lines by excising the stomach at least 2 cm and preferably 5–7 cm beyond detectable growth.

6. When resection is impracticable, try to relieve existing or impending obstruction. Distal obstruction can usually be prevented or relieved by creating a proximal gastroenterostomy but proximal obstruction may require the anastomosis of bowel to the oesophagus in the chest or the neck. When surgical bypass of a proximal obstruction is not justified, consider inserting a splinting tube of the Mousseau-Barbin type after dilating the constricting tumour.

RADICAL ABDOMINAL SUBTOTAL AND TOTAL GASTRECTOMY

Appraise

1. Radical resection for distal carcinoma will be described. It almost exactly resembles radical total gastrectomy except that a fringe of proximal stomach is retained,

provided it is well clear of the growth, to allow safe intra-abdominal gastrojejunostomy to be performed. The size of the fringe of retained stomach depends on the extent of the growth. It is carried out on patients who are sufficiently fit to withstand the procedure, who display no evidence of distant metastases and who have no local invasion into contiguous structures that cannot be resected with the stomach. Gastric carcinoma spreads proximally well beyond the limits of visible and palpable growth so that, if possible, 8–10 cm of stomach should be excised above the apparent upper limits of the growth. If this entails transecting the lower oesophagus, formal total gastrectomy through a left thoraco-abdominal incision is preferable but in slim patients, total abdominal gastrectomy is possible.

2. To a lesser extent, growth spreads distally across the pylorus and transection should be sited 5 cm clear of detectable growth.

3. Radical gastrectomy is intended to remove the gastric tumour, the lymphatics that run with the right and left gastro-epiploic arteries, the right and left gastric arteries and the short gastric arteries, together with the spleen, the omenta in contact with the stomach including the greater omentum, the lesser omentum and the gastric bed of the lesser sac. In addition, the distal pancreas, part of the left lobe of the liver, a segment of transverse colon, small bowel or part of the abdominal wall may be removed if this allows apparently total excision of the tumour with a clear margin.

4. If the patient would have detectable residual tumour still present then radical resection is not achieved and a lesser resection should be planned, similar in scope to the operation for benign disease provided the resection is well clear of the tumour proximally. If the tumour is unresectable or very extensive with metastases in the liver and elsewhere, then resection of any sort is usually inappropriate. Cytotoxic drug treatment of inoperable gastric carcinoma may be more effective the smaller the tumour mass and palliative resection is sometimes carried out to achieve this.

5. Extensive distal carcinoma that is likely to produce pyloric obstruction should be bypassed when ever possible by fashioning a proximal gastroenterostomy.

6. Lymphomas and sarcomas are often too extensive for radical resection but usually respond, at least temporarily, to radiotherapy or chemotherapy. Removal of as much tumour as possible is recommended to reduce the mass.

7. Non-radical total gastrectomy is suitable for patients with Zollinger-Ellison syndrome (see p. 101) who fail to respond to medical treatment.

Access

1. Make a long vertical paramedian or midline incision in the upper abdomen extending from alongside alongside the base of the xiphisternum, skirting the umbilicus below.

2. If necessary, excise the xiphoid process. Be prepared to mobilize the left lobe of the liver and fold it to the right.

Assess

1. Carry out a complete abdominal exploration feeling the tumour last. Start in the pelvis to exclude peritoneal deposits and in the female, ovarian seedlings. Feel the para-aortic nodes and those at the base of the mesentery and transverse mesocolon. Feel both lobes of the liver.

2. Examine the whole length of the stomach starting at the cardia, handling the tumour as little as possible. Note the size, fixity and extent of penetration of the growth. If necessary make a hole through an avascular area of the gastrocolic or lesser omentum to determine if the growth is adherent to the pancreas or other posterior structures.

3. Feel the nodes around the cardia, the coeliac and left gastric glands and those along the superior border of the pancreas. Feel the nodes above and below the pylorus and in the porta hepatis. If doubt exists whether the nodes are malignant, send a typical one for frozen section histology to decide whether to proceed with radical resection or carry out palliative resection.

Resect

1. Lift the greater omentum and dissect it from the transverse colon through the bloodless connective tissue that allows it to be split as a separate leaf from the mesocolon. Do not injure the mesocolon or its contained blood vessels. Gently strip the omental sheet as far as the posterior abdominal wall over the pancreas but leave it attached for the present.

2. Draw the spleen to the right with the left hand and cut through the peritoneum and fascia of the left leaf of the lienorenal ligament so that the spleen and tail of the pancreas can be drawn forwards.

3. Turn now to the right margin of the greater omentum and distal stomach where the right gastroepiploic vessels pass forwards from the gastroduodenal vessels. Sweep forwards all the loose tissue and lymph nodes to display the origin of the right gastroepiploic vessels, doubly ligate and divide them. Isolate the right gastric vessels above the pylorus, follow the arteries up to their origin from the hepatic artery, doubly ligate and divide them.

4. Mobilize, by Kocher's manoeuvre, the upper half of the duodenal loop so that the line of the common bile duct can be monitored and the duodenum can be safely divided and closed. Dissect the first part of the duodenum from the head of the pancreas, applying fine artery forceps close to the duodenal wall, dividing between the forceps and duodenal wall, then picking up the vessel on the duodenal wall separately before tying it. Aim to transect the duodenum at least 3 cm distal to the pylorus, so that 5–6 cm must be mobilized to allow safe closure. Isolate the area with distinctive coloured towels. Apply two pairs of thin crushing clamps such as Lang Stevenson's close together across the duodenum at the selected site and transect the duodenum

between them. Cover the proximal cut end with a swab and fold it upwards. Close the distal cut end in the manner described in the section on gastrectomy for benign disease.

5. Expose the porta hepatis and incise the peritoneum over the front of the hepatic artery, which has been identified by feeling for pulsations. Strip the peritoneum, connective tissue and lymph nodes off the hepatic artery to leave it clean. Extend the initial peritoneal incision to the left where the lesser omentum joins the liver, taking care to identify, doubly ligate and divide an accessory hepatic artery, which may run with the hepatic vagal branches. Continue the separation of the lesser omentum right up to the diaphragm, leaving it attached to the lesser curve of the stomach. The loose tissue and glands can now be stripped from the hepatic artery right up to the coeliac axis.

6. Have the distal stomach elevated by an assistant to place the left gastric vessels on stretch. The peritoneum over the neck of the pancreas has already been stripped to the coeliac axis and can now be stripped further to expose the coeliac artery and the origin of the hepatic and left gastric arteries, freeing and elevating all the nodes to leave the right side of the coeliac artery stripped. Isolate, doubly ligate and divide the left gastric vein as far posteriorly as possible. Similarly isolate, doubly ligate and divide the origin of the left gastric artery.

7. Now return to the spleen and distal pancreas. Elevate the pancreas medially, with the spleen and splenic vessels, the peritoneum and glands along the upper border. Just distal to the entry of the inferior mesenteric vein doubly ligate and divide the splenic vein, leaving the proximal splenic vein in situ. Just to the left of the midline transect the pancreatic neck after doubly ligating and dividing the small vessels entering it above and below from the right. Cut across it, picking up further small vessels within its substance and ligating them. Identify, isolate, clamp and ligate the main duct. With a running catgut suture on an eyeless needle close the raw proximal cut end with a running stitch.

8. The distal pancreas remains attached to the coeliac artery through the splenic artery. Dissect the artery, its adventitia and glands to the coeliac artery, doubly clamp, divide and ligate it at its origin.

9. The distal stomach, omenta, spleen and distal pancreas will now be removed by transecting the stomach or the whole stomach will be removed by transecting the lower oesophagus (Fig. 5.27). If the tumour invades the left lobe of the liver, parietes, the left adrenal gland, transverse colon or small intestinal loop, resect them clear of growth and repair the damage.

SUBTOTAL GASTRECTOMY

1. Select a line of transection that leaves but a fringe of stomach 2–5 cm from the cardia. Isolate, clamp, ligate and

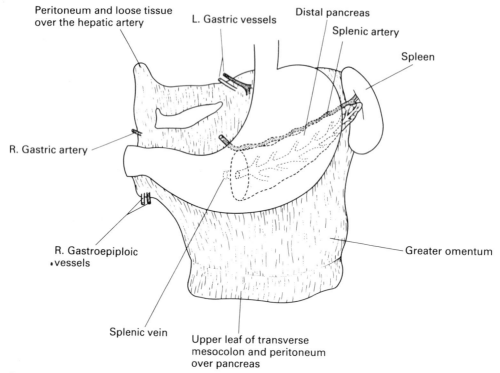

Peritoneum and loose tissue over the hepatic artery

L. Gastric vessels

Distal pancreas

Splenic artery

Spleen

R. Gastric artery

R. Gastroepiploic
·vessels

Greater omentum

Splenic vein

Upper leaf of transverse
mesocolon and peritoneum
over pancreas

Fig. 5.27 Radical total gastrectomy. The resected specimen.

divide the vessels on the greater and lesser curves at the level of transection to leave the curvatures clean and free.

2. Ask the anaesthetist to withdraw the nasogastric tube into the upper stomach and apply one of the twin gastroenterostomy clamps just above the proposed line of section, placing below and parallel to it a long crushing Payr clamp.

3. Transect the stomach just above the Payr clamp and remove the specimen. Alternatively, leave the specimen attached until the posterior gastrojejunal seromuscular stitch has been inserted and then transect it.

Unite

1. Draw up a loop of proximal jejunum in exactly the same manner as following Polya gastrectomy for benign disease (see p. 85). Apply the second of the twin gastroenterostomy clamps across the jejunum after ensuring that the afferent loop is as short as possible. Marry the twin clamps, uniting the afferent jejunal loop to the lesser curve.

2. Create a full width stoma between the cut end of the stomach and the jejunum, with two layers of catgut sutures. Discard and replace the soiled towels, instruments and gloves.

3. The anastomosis can be made using a GIA stapling device. In this case transect the stomach with a double line of staples applied with a TA90 stapler and transect it below the line of staples. Bring up the selected jejunal loop and suture it at each end to the posterior wall of the stomach. Make stab wounds through the gastric and jejunal walls close to the uniting stitch at the greater curve end of the proposed anastomosis and pass in the separate blades of the GIA stapler — one into the stomach, one into the jejunum, lying parallel to each other and pointing to the gastric lesser curve. Lock the two blades together after ensuring that there is no intervening tissue. Actuate the stapler to insert four parallel rows of staples uniting the stomach and jejunum and cutting between the middle rows to form a stoma. Unlock and remove the stapler. Inspect the interior to ensure the anastomosis is perfect. Pick up the incomplete ends of the staple lines with tissue forceps and separate them to leave a longitudinal defect. Close this with a TA 30 straight stapling device.

TOTAL GASTRECTOMY

1. Complete the gastric mobilization by dividing the lesser omentum right up to the diaphragm and dividing the gastrophrenic ligament close to the diaphragm. Posteriorly, there is a vein arching backwards from the upper stomach that must be ligated or occluded with haemostatic clips and divided.

2. The stomach is now attached only to the oesophagus. Gently free this in the hiatus. Transect the anterior and posterior vagal trunks and decide on the level of transection. Do not divide the oesophagus until either the posterior oesophago jejunal outer Lembert suture line is in place to prevent to oesophagus from retracting out of sight or

until the purse string suture has been inserted for use with a circular stapling device.

3. If a nasojejunal tube is to be used, have it drawn up into the lower oesophagus. It can be pulled down when making a sutured anastomosis when the posterior all-coats suture is in place and pushed on into the jejunum. If a stapled anastomosis is made, have the anaesthetist push it on with a twisting motion when the stapler is withdrawn.

Unite

1. Oesophagojejunostomy is preferably performed using a Roux-en-Y jejunal loop (see p. 98). Transect the jejunum close to the ligament of Treitz and divide sufficient primary vascular arcades to allow the distal portion to be taken up to the oesophagus. Transect the bowel and join the cut proximal end to be united end-to-side into the Roux loop. If a sutured anastomosis is used, close the end of the jejunum in two layers. The loop should be led up to the oesophagus posterior to the transverse mesocolon. Make sure it lies without tension or twisting. Insert a posterior running suture line of Lembert stitches joining the posterior wall of the oesophagus to the posterior wall of the Roux loop about 5 cm from the closed end. Now transect the oesophagus below the suture line and remove the specimen. Create a hole in the antimesenteric border of the jejunum exactly matching the oesophageal lumen. Insert a stitch through all-coats of the oesophagus and jejunum at each end so they can be slightly stretched. Carefully insert a circular all-coats continuous 2/0 chromic catgut stitch to produce perfect union (see p. 287). Now carry the posterior Lembert stitch onto the anterior wall to encircle the anastomosis, trying to draw up the jejunal wall to cover the inner, all-coats stitch. Discard and replace the soiled towels, instruments and gloves.

2. End-to-end Roux loop anastomosis is possible if the oesophagus is sufficiently dilated so that its lumen matches that of the cut end of the jejunum and if the jejunum can be laid straight with not too much tendency to curve at its free end. A two layer anastomosis is fashioned.

3. An intact loop of proximal jejunum may be brought up for end to side oesophagojejunostomy as an alternative technique. Theoretically, it produces the risk of alkaline oesophagitis but this is not inevitable. Some surgeons perform jejunojejunostomy between the afferent and efferent loops in the hope of diverting bile into the efferent loop. A two layer, end-to-side anastomosis is fashioned.

4. The oesophagojejunal anastomosis may be accomplished using one of the circular stapling devices. Before the oesophagus is transected an all-coats purse string suture is inserted and the specimen is then resected below it and removed. Introduce a size testing head so that the correct size of stapler can be used. If an intact loop or end-to-end anastomosis is intended, make a hole on the antimesenteric border of the jejunum 7–8 cm below the point of union, to pass in the stapling device. The device is passed into the bowel without the anvil for an end-to-side anastomosis, the spindle is pushed against the intended antimesenteric anastomotic site, a cut is made over it so that it projects and the anvil is replaced. An end-to-side Roux anastomosis does not require a separate stab since the instrument, without the anvil, can be passed in through the cut end of bowel which will be closed in two layers after it is withdrawn. In an end-to-end anastomosis the anvil remains in place but well separated from the staple cartridge and a purse-string suture is used to draw in the jejunal end over the cartridge.

Now feed the anvil head into the cut end of oesophagus, tighten and tie the purse string suture and close the anvil head onto the cartridge after ensuring there is no extraneous tissue trapped and that the oesophagus and jejunum lie without tension or twist. Release the safety catch and actuate the gun. Open it remove it, check the intactness of the anastomosis and the doughnut shaped rings on the spindle. Close the portal of entry of the device, in two layers. If the oesophageal wall is very thick, dissect back a cuff of muscularis so that it is not included in the stapler. After uniting the oesophagus to jejunum, insert a layer of stitches drawing the muscle coat onto the jejunum around the stapled anastomosis

Check

1. Stop all bleeding.
2. Ensure that the anastomoses are perfect, the bowel is a good colour, untwisted and not stretched and the mesentery lies free.
3. Check all the other structures that have been disturbed. The hiatus does not need to be repaired if total gastrectomy has been carried out. The liver must be replaced if the left lobe was folded to the right. Repair the transverse mesocolon if there is a hole through which small bowel may prolapse.

Closure

1. Most surgeons leave drain to the cut end of the pancreas, although it rarely produces a warning discharge if pancreatitis develops.
2. Close the abdomen in routine fashion.

Aftercare

1. Manage a patient following subtotal gastrectomy in the same manner as following gastrectomy for benign disease (see p. 62).
2. Following transabdominal total gastrectomy manage the patient in a similar manner to one who has had thoracoabdominal total gastrectomy (see p. 99).

RADICAL THORACO-ABDOMINAL TOTAL GASTRECTOMY

Appraise

1. Never embark upon this operation without first obtaining a tissue diagnosis with endoscopic biopsy or cytology or frozen section histology at operation. Never embark upon it without making every effort by pre-operative and operative assessment to exclude metastatic tumour.

2. As a rule, this is a radical operation undertaken for carcinoma of the middle or proximal stomach which can apparently be totally encompassed by this major resection of the stomach, lower oesophagus, omenta, spleen, body and tail of the pancreas, with all the primary lymph nodes and all those up to and including the coeliac nodes.

3. It should be accomplished through a left thoraco-abdominal incision and this will be described. It can be carried out through an upper midline abdominal incision only if the upper stomach is free of growth and in that case it is merely an extension of radical partial gastrectomy to include the upper fringe of stomach in the resection (see p. 94). Do not attempt trans-abdominal total gastrectomy if the growth extends proximally to within 5 cm of the gastric cardia since at least a 2–5 cm segment of apparently uninvolved lower oesophagus should be resected. Do not attempt it in an obese patient with a narrow coastal margin.

4. Total gastrectomy is justifiable as a palliative procedure in the presence of metastases provided the patient is expected to survive for a reasonable period. In this case the resection is as extensive longitudinally as a radical gastrectomy, but is not carried widely from the stomach.

5. Lymphoma and sarcoma of the stomach are best treated by radical gastrectomy but even if they extend beyond the scope of the operation total gastrectomy may be justified to reduce the bulk of the tumour. Radiotherapy and chemotherapy may then be more effective.

6. Non radical total gastrectomy through the abdomen was conventionally carried out on patients with Zollinger-Ellison syndrome, whether or not a gastrin-secreting tumour had been totally excised. It is now reserved for the minority of patients whose ulcer cannot be controlled medically (see p. 102).

7. This major resection is often planned for patients who are elderly, have other conditions which prejudice recovery and are also malnourished. Ensure that the nutritional state is restored by oral feeding with high calorie, high protein and vitamin rich diet, nasogastric feeding or if necessary, intravenous feeding through a centrally placed venous catheter. Organize pre-operative chest physiotherapy and check all other body systems to anticipate and prevent complications. Make sure that the patient has an indwelling urinary catheter in place during and after the operation to allow the urinary output to be monitored.

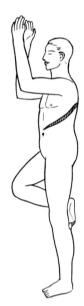

Fig. 5.28 Left thoracoabdominal approach for total gastrectomy, as seen from above the patient. The shaded section shows the extent of the incision.

Access

1. The anaesthetized, intubated patient lies on his right side (Fig. 5.28), tilted backwards 30°, right hip and knee flexed, left leg straight and separated from the right leg by a pillow. The pelvis is fixed by a wide strip of adhesive tape to prevent it from rolling backwards and a fixed post, covered with sponge, supports the left scapula posteriorly to maintain its position. The arms are brought in front of the face in the 'hornpipe' position.

2. Stand at the patient's back.

3. Open the abdomen obliquely from the midline to the costal margin in the line of the left seventh or eighth rib.

Assess

1. Note any free fluid. Feel the pelvic peritoneum for deposits, then the para-aortic and middle colic nodes, then the liver.

2. Examine the stomach and its related nodes, in particular the coeliac nodes. Note if the tumour is fixed to adjacent structures such as the liver, pancreas, colon, or abdominal wall and if partial resection of these allows radical resection to be accomplished. Decide if radical resection is feasible.

Resect

1. Extend the incision along the seventh or eighth rib as far as the lateral border of the sacrospinalis muscle. Open the chest either by resecting the rib or along the upper border of the rib. If the rib remains, remove a 2 cm length posteriorly and cut a similar piece from the next rib

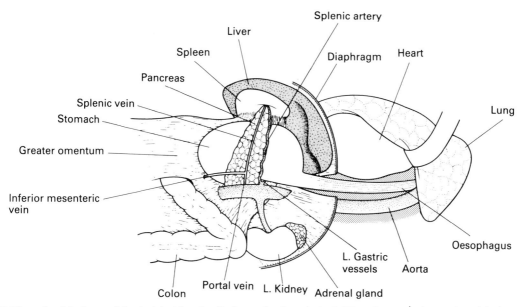

Fig. 5.29 Through a left thoracoabdominal incision the diaphragm has been incised. The spleen, splenic vessels and body and tail of the pancreas have been elevated, together with the greater curve of the stomach.

above. Isolate and divide the intercostal nerve posteriorly to prevent postoperative girdle pain.

2. Incise the diaphragm radially down towards but not into the hiatus. It may be necessarily to resect the crural part en bloc with the growth.

3. Mobilize the spleen forwards (Fig. 5.29) after incising the lienorenal ligament, lifting up the tail and body of the pancreas. When the inferior mesenteric vein is encountered, doubly ligate and divide the splenic vein distal to it and separate the proximal pancreas from the right part of the splenic vein, ligating any small vessels joining the two structures.

4. Lift up the greater omentum and separate its whole length from the transverse colon in the bloodless plane just above the colon, so that the omentum can be stripped upwards as an intact leaf from the mesocolon. Avoid damaging the mesocolon or its contained blood vessels.

5. Rotate the spleen, omentum and greater curve of stomach over to the right. At the pyloric end the right gastroepiploic vessels are taut and at the cardiac end of the stomach the left gastric vessels are tensed. Dissect out the right gastroepiploic vein on the pancreas and doubly clamp, divide and ligate it. Dissect out the origin of the right gastroepiploic artery. Doubly clamp, divide and ligate it. Above the pylorus, identify the right gastric vessels, trace the arteries up to their origin from the hepatic artery and doubly clamp, divide and ligate them. Mobilize the first part of the duodenum for at least 5–7 cm beyond the pylorus: there are small vessels connecting it to the pancreas. Clamp these close to the duodenum, divide them between the clamps and the duodenum, pick up the vessels on the duodenal wall and ligate them.

6. Isolate the area with distinctive coloured towels.

Transect the duodenum 3–5 cm beyond the pylorus between thin crushing clamps such as Lang Stevenson's. Close the distal cut end with a loose running over and over catgut stitch on an eyeless needle including the clamp. Withdraw the clamp and tighten the sutures seriatim. Insert a second layer of invaginating stitches to bury the first layer. Alternatively, close the duodenum with a TA 55 stapling device, with or without a row of reinforcing invaginating stitches.

7. Fold the distal stomach to the left. Expose the porta hepatis and incise the peritoneum over the hepatic artery, recognised by palpation. Strip the peritoneum, connective tissue and lymph nodes from the hepatic artery back to the coeliac artery. Continue the peritoneal incision in the porta hepatis to the left, keeping close to the liver, to detach the lesser omentum.

8. Have the distal stomach drawn upwards to place the left gastric vessels on stretch within their peritoneal fold. Isolate, doubly clamp, divide and ligate the vein on the posterior abdominal wall. Continue the dissection of lymph nodes and connective tissue from the hepatic artery up the coeliac artery and origin of the left gastric artery, then doubly clamp, divide and ligate the left gastric artery at its origin.

9. Just below and to the right of the coeliac axis transect the neck of the pancreas, picking up and ligating the small vessels above and below. Identify the main duct and separately ligate it. Close the raw proximal cut end of the pancreas with a running catgut stitch.

10. The right hand side of the coeliac axis has been cleared of connective tissue and nodes. Now sweep off the tissue on the left hand side to reveal the cleaned origin of the splenic artery. Doubly clamp, divide and ligate the

splenic artery at its origin. The distal splenic artery with its associated glands is now freed together with the body and tail of the pancreas and spleen.

11. The distal stomach is free. Decide whether or not to excise a cuff of diaphragmatic crura in continuity with the upper stomach and lower oesophagus. In any case, continue up the dissection of the upper stomach and lower oesophagus keeping well away from them so the loose connective tissue and lymphatics will be incorporated in the specimen.

12. Have the left lower lung held forwards with a lung retractor. Incise the pleura over the lower oesophagus. Mobilize the oesophagus above the diaphragm and dissect downwards stripping all the surrounding connective tissue, lymphatics and lymph nodes with it.

13. Extend the radial cut in the diaphragm to the crura. Now preferably dissect on either side to leave a cuff of crus still attached to the free oesophagus. If the tumour is well away it is permissible to split through the crus and dissect out all the loose tissue with the oesophagus.

14. The specimen is now attached only by the oesophagus and vagal trunks. Divide the vagi. Decide the level of oesophageal transection to be 7–10 cm clear of detectable tumour. Reconstruction will be easy if the oesophagus is cut across midway between the aortic arch and the diaphragm since the upper end will retract up to just below the arch. Do not stint on the resection, however. If necessary, the oesophagus can be freed and united on the outside of the arch, or freed up to the neck and united there. Transect the oesophagus cleanly. If a nasogastric tube was in place have it first withdrawn to just above the line of transection.

15. Scrupulously ensure total haemostasis now. It will be impossible to examine the area when the reconstructive conduit is in place.

Unite

1. Pick up the proximal jejunum. Carefully examine the vascular pattern. Create a Roux loop that will easily reach the retracted oesophagus (p. 286). Draw the loop through a hole in the mesocolon, subsequently suturing the margins of the mesocolon carefully to the loop and its mesentery to prevent other loops of bowel from herniating through.

2. The anastomosis may be end to end but the jejunum usually sits most comfortably with the oesophagus joined end to side. If this is a sutured anastomosis, close the end of the jejunum with a purse-string suture reinforced with an invaginating seromuscular stitch. Make a hole in the antimesenteric border of the jejunum to match the lumen of the oesophagus. Place stay sutures through all-coats of oesophagus and jejunum at each end and have these drawn apart to stretch the anastomotic lines. Now carefully insert an all-coats stitch uniting the adjacent oesophageal and jejunal walls, placing the sutures 2 mm apart, with 2–3 mm

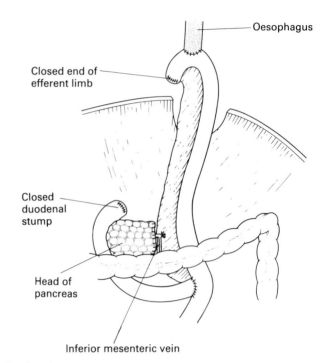

Fig. 5.30 Radical total gastrectomy. The oesophagojejunal anastomosis is complete, using a Roux loop of jejunum taken behind the mesocolon. The duodenal bulb is closed, the duodenal loop is joined end to side to the jejunum.

bites. The stitches may be continuous or interrupted, catgut, linen, silk or monofilament plastic thread. The material and method are less important than the perfection of every stitch (Fig. 5.30).

3. Many surgeons employ a single suture layer. Alternatively, a second layer may be inserted of continuous or interrupted stitches which pick up the muscularis and submucosa of the oesophagus close to the anastomosis and the seromuscularis of the jejunum 5 mm below the anastomosis so that as it is gently tightened it draws a cuff of bowel up and over the all coats suture line. The anastomosis can be rotated to allow the stitch to be inserted around the whole circumference. Now discard and replace the soiled towels, instruments and gloves.

4. The anastomosis can be fashioned using the SPTU, EEA or Proximate circular staplers. Choose a suitable cartridge size by inserting a test head into the oesophagus. Do not close the jejunal end. Apply the stapler safety catch and remove the anvil from the spindle. Introduce the spindle and cartridge through the open end of the jejunum, cut down upon the spindle end 5–7 cm from the jejunal end, on the antimesenteric border, and push the spindle through the small hole. Replace the anvil. Introduce a purse-string suture of monofilament plastic suture around the cut oesophageal end. Introduce the anvil into the oesophagus and tighten the purse-string suture, cutting off the spare thread. Close the anvil onto the cartridge with the intact purse-stringed oesophagus and jejunal wall separating them

and with no extraneous tissue caught. Release the safety catch and actuate the stapler. Separate the anvil from the cartridge and gently withdraw the instrument. Confirm that there are two intact toroidal fragments of oesophagus and jejunum on the spindle. Check the suture line. If necessary reinforce it partially or completely with sutures. Now close the cut jejunal end with two purse string sutures or use a TA 30 stapler. If the oesophagus is very thick, dissect back the muscular coat as a cuff which is not included in the stapler. After 'firing' and withdrawing the stapler, unite the oesophageal muscle to the jejunum with a continuous ring of sutures.

5. Manoeuvre the nasogastric tube through the anastomosis and if possible down to or beyond the duodenojejunal anastomosis if it is intended to use it for feeding.

Technical points

1. Radical resection may be accomplished if the tumour has invaded the abdominal wall or diaphragm provided it is possible to excise part of these en bloc with the tumour. If the body or tail of the pancreas is invaded posteriorly, this part of the gland will have been removed as a routine. The transverse colon can be resected en bloc with the stomach, and the left lobe of the liver may also be resected. If the tumour spreads distally into the duodenum or into the head of the pancreas then pancreatoduodenectomy would be necessary and this is very rarely feasible.

2. It is important to stretch the anastomosis slightly when uniting it with sutures, since the oesophagus contracts down to a narrow tube and sutures placed close together become widely separated when a bolus of food stretches it, allowing leakage to take place.

3. If the oesophagus retracts under the aortic arch gently free it until it can be brought onto the outside of the arch and complete the anastomosis there. With care this can be accomplished perfectly but occasionally it is worth creating a second, higher thoracotomy. If anastomosis cannot be safely performed, do not persist. Dissect up the oesophagus to the neck and complete it safely there, using a suitable conduit, a Roux loop of jejunum or a segment of colon (see p. 305).

4. A jejunostomy may be created (see p. 118) to allow early feeding if the patient was severely undernourished or if slow recovery is possible. Alternatively the nasal tube may be passed into the upper jejunum for feeding purposes. In patients who find the tube intolerable the upper end can be brought out in the neck as a pharyngostomy (see p. 307).

Check list

1. In the chest make sure the anastomosis is perfectly executed, that it lies without tension and is not twisted. Ensure that the lung is undamaged and that it can be re-

expanded by the anaesthetist if he has deliberately collapsed it.

2. Check all the main ligatures. Re-examine the closed neck of pancreas and duodenal stump closure. Check that there is no continuing oozing from the raw surfaces.

3. Check the duodenojejunal anastomosis, ensure that the Roux loop passes upwards without twisting, and that its blood supply is not prejudiced. Re-examine the passage of the jejunum through the mesocolon and ensure that the blood supply to the colon is not damaged.

Closure

1. Insert a left basal chest drain and connect it to an underwater seal. Insert an abdominal drain to the distal cut pancreas.

2. Close the cut diaphragm using mattress sutures of non-absorbable material. Even if a cuff of crura has been removed it will close without tension. Do not tighten the new hiatus to constrict the jejunal loop. Do not suture the bowel to the diaphragm but allow it to lie freely.

3. Close the chest in layers (see Ch. 19).

4. Close the abdomen.

Aftercare

1. Nurse the patient in the intensive therapy unit for the first 24 hours. As a rule it is valuable to keep him attached to the mechanical respirator overnight.

2. Institute physiotherapy for the chest. Remove the underwater drain after 48 hours. Order daily chest X-rays until the chest is clear. If fluid collects in the base of the left pleural cavity, aspirate it.

3. Give jejunostomy feeds or parenteral feeds. After 4–5 days examine the anastomosis radiologically after the patient has swallowed water-soluble radio-opaque medium. If leakage is excluded remove the nasogastric tube and start oral fluids proceeding to food.

PALLIATIVE OPERATIONS FOR GASTRIC CARCINOMA

Appraise

1. Palliative resection for carcinoma should be interpreted to mean apparently complete removal of the primary tumour, even though there is metastatic growth outside the scope of a radical resection. If growth is cut across in the stomach then the anastomosis may not heal so that the patient develops leakage and peritonitis, or soon develops stomal obstruction from recurrent tumour, or the growth is spread widely during the procedure. This view may need to be modified as cytotoxic chemotherapy improves since some of the agents are more effective if the tumour bulk is reduced.

2. If palliative resection is precluded, the patient can be relieved of impending or existing obstruction in many cases.

PALLIATIVE TOTAL GASTRECTOMY

Appraise

1. Fit patients with carcinoma of midstomach or proximal stomach may be given dramatic and often long-term palliation by total gastrectomy. Occasionally what appeared to be metastatic tumour proves to be reactionary changes producing enlarged lymph nodes and the patient survives indefinitely.

2. Abdominal total gastrectomy is appropriate for carcinoma of the midstomach. If palliative total gastrectomy is planned for upper gastric carcinoma, the thoracoabdominal route is preferable to avoid cutting through tumour or prejudicing the anastomosis of oesophagus in the abdomen in an obese patient with a narrow costal margin.

Action

1. Whether the abdominal or abdomino-thoracic route is used, proceed as for partial gastrectomy for peptic ulcer (p. 84), dividing the gastrocolic omentum but continuing higher so that all the short gastric vessels are doubly clamped, divided and ligated, leaving the spleen intact.

2. Distally, doubly clamp, divide and ligate the right gastro-epiploic and right gastric vessels and divide the duodenum. A wide, clear margin is not so essential here if the duodenum is to be closed. Close the distal cut end of duodenum.

3. Elevate the stomach to display the left gastric vessels and isolate, doubly clamp, divide and ligate them.

4. Gently mobilize the upper stomach and lower oesophagus and select a point of transection that is at least 5–7 cm clear of detectable growth. Cut across the gullet and vagal trunks.

5. In a small number of patients an uninvolved duodenum can be brought up to the lower oesophagus after fully mobilizing it by Kocher's manoeuvre and it can then be anastomosed end to end. As a rule it is necessary to bring up jejunum to the oesophagus. This may be a Roux loop (see p. 98) or an intact proximal loop. The intact loop has the theoretical disadvantage that bile reflux into the oesophagus may be troublesome. This is infrequent but is not, in my experience, always prevented by creating an anastomosis between the afferent and efferent loops in the hope of diverting bile away from the oesophageal stoma. These patients have a limited outlook and the simplest operation should be preferred.

PALLIATIVE PARTIAL GASTRECTOMY

Appraise

1. For distal gastric carcinomas associated with metastases outside the scope of radical surgery, distal gastrectomy may still offer good palliation. However, the proximal cut edge should be well clear of growth or the stoma will either leak or subsequently obstruct from recurrent growth.

2. If the growth is very extensive in the stomach however, it may be more damaging to perform gastrectomy than to leave the patient alone.

Action

1. Perform the gastrectomy in the same manner as for benign disease (see p. 84). Make sure that the line of proximal section is at least 5–7 cm above detectable disease.

2. Close the duodenal stump and bring up a proximal loop of jejunum and create a full width stoma to guard as far as possible against stomal obstruction if the carcinoma recurs here.

UPPER PARTIAL GASTRECTOMY

Appraise

1. This procedure may be carried out through the abdomen but is better performed through a left thoracoabdominal incision. It may be useful to palliate proximal gastric carcinoma but it is essential to transect the lower oesophagus sufficiently high to insure against local recurrence and this usually means that the transection and anastomosis must be performed in the chest.

2. Its main advantage over palliative total gastrectomy is that if the distal stomach is free of tumour, it provides a convenient conduit to unite to the gullet.

Action

1. Open the gastrocolic omentum and divide the vessels upwards including the left gastro-epiploics and the short gastrics. Alternatively, remove the spleen.

2. Distally preserve the right gastro-epiploic and right gastric vessels but mobilize the duodenal loop by Kocher's manoeuvre until the pylorus can be drawn up to the oesophageal hiatus. Ensure that there is no pyloric obstruction by invaginating the anterior gastric antral wall through the pylorus on an index finger.

3. Incise the lesser omentum proximal to its free edge to gain access to the lesser sac to the right of the stomach. Identify, isolate, doubly clamp, divide and ligate the left gastric vessels.

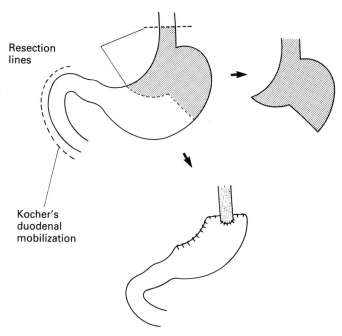

Resection
lines

Kocher's
duodenal
mobilization

Fig. 5.31 Upper partial gastrectomy.

4. Decide the upper and lower limits of the resection. Both of them should be 5–7 cm clear of detectable growth. Transect the oesophagus and vagal trunks. Transect the stomach, and remove the specimen.

5. The cut edge of the stomach may be partially closed from the lesser curve aspect to leave a hole equal in size to the oesophagus so that an end to end anastomosis can be made between the oesophagus and the greater curve part of the cut stomach. Alternatively the cut proximal edge of the stomach may be closed using a stitch or the TA 90 straight stapling device. An anastomosis can now be created between the oesophagus and the anterior or posterior wall of the greater curve portion of stomach at least 2 cm proximal to the line of closure (Fig. 5.31) This again may be sutured or created with a stapling device. To staple the anastomosis make a hole in the middle of the anterior wall of the gastric remnant and pass through it the spindle of the EEA or SPTU or Proximate stapling device after removing the anvil. Press the spindle end against the posterior wall of the stomach near the greater curvature at least 2 cm proximal to the closed end. Make a small cut to enable the spindle to emerge and replace the anvil. Place a purse-string suture around the cut end of the oesophagus, insert the anvil of the stapler into the oesophagus and tighten and tie the purse-string, cutting off the loose ends. Close the anvil down onto the cartridge and actuate the stapler. Open the device, gently withdraw it, check that there are two intact toroids of excised oesophagus and stomach. Check the anastomosis and insert reinforcing stitches if necessary.

GASTROENTEROSTOMY

Appraise

1. If a distal growth is extensive and cannot be resected or if there are gross metastases, relieve the existing or impending obstruction in the pyloric region by creating a proximal gastroenterostomy.

2. Bypass may offer as good palliation and disturb the patient less than resection that cuts through tumour.

Action

1. Reach below the transverse mesocolon and draw up the proximal jejunum, selecting the first loop that will reach easily to the upper stomach.

2. Create a high, wide stoma between the upper anterior gastric wall and the jejunum. Use twin gastroenterostomy clamps only if they facilitate the procedure.

CARDIAC OBSTRUCTION

Appraise

1. An inoperable proximal carcinoma that obstructs the cardia offers a challenge. If nothing is done the patient will starve to death.

2. Rarely it is reasonable to draw a loop of intestine or colon into the chest or neck to bypass the obstruction (see p. 305).

3. Either a Mousseau-Barbin, Celestin or Atkinson type of tube may be passed after dilating the malignant stricture. This can be achieved using the pulsion technique from above. If the abdomen is open, make a small high gastrotomy and dilate the cuff of tumour from below. Pass up a bougie and ask the anaesthetist to attach the leader of a Mousseau-Barbin or Celestin tube to it and draw it down until the tube is impacted in the malignant stricture. Cut off the excess tube and close the gastrotomy.

4. Occasionally, it is valuable to insinuate a nasogastric tube through into the stomach for feeding purposes before trying the effect of radiation therapy. In some patients, the effect is dramatic in shrinking the tumour and relieving the obstruction.

5. Many surgeons deprecate creating a gastrostomy in patients with terminal disease and attitudes are determined by one's philosophy. I do not oppose gastrostomy as an alternative to watching the patient starve to death.

ZOLLINGER-ELLISON SYNDROME

Appraise

1. The classical syndrome consists of severe and sometimes intractable peptic ulcer developing as a rule in

expected sites but sometimes distally in the duodenum and proximal jejunum, associated with gastric acid hypersecretion of marked degree. The ulcers may be multiple. There may be diarrhoea usually attributed to irritability of the bowel from contact with its high acid content. The syndrome is caused by a gastrin-secreting tumour of the pancreatic islets which may be benign or malignant, or there may be hyperplasia without tumour formation (see Ch. 10). The serum gastrin is raised and appears to act as a trophic hormone acting on gastric parietal cells which undergo hyperplasia. The gastric fundic mucosa appears hypertrophied and extends almost to the pylorus, hypersecreting acid in response to the hypergastrinaemia at basal rates approaching maximal acid output. Zollinger-Ellison syndrome may be part of a multiple endocrine neoplastic (MEN) syndrome, the parathyroid glands being particularly frequently involved. The features of hypergastrinaemia are reproduced in the absence of a pancreatic tumour when the antrum is congenitally duplicated and when it is sequestered in an alkaline medium.

2. The diagnosis is suspected when duodenal ulcer does not respond as expected to medical treatment or is multiple or ulcers occur in the stomach, distal duodenum and upper jejunum or in unexpected areas of the stomach such as the greater curvature. The suspicion is confirmed when very high basal levels of acid output are measured and maximal pentagastrin stimulation has little or no added effect. Serum gastrin is raised. Search for other endocrine abnormalities, particularly of the parathyroid glands.

3. Total gastrectomy was previously advocated but should now be reserved only for those who fail to respond to adequate treatment with H_2-receptor blocking drugs.

4. After employing scanning techniques to exclude metastases, plan to explore the abdomen and carefully examine the pancreas, duodenum, stomach, liver, and remainder of the abdomen searching for single or multiple tumours and metastases. If a solitary tumour is found in the head of the pancreas in the absence of metastases, enucleate it. If a tumour is found in the body or tail of the pancreas, excise the body and tail. If no tumour is found in the pancreas, duodenum or elsewhere, excise the body and tail of the pancreas for histological exclusion of hyperplasia.

GASTRIC OPERATIONS FOR MORBID OBESITY

Appraise

1. Patients with morbid obesity have a seriously reduced life expectancy for a number of reasons. Some have an underlying metabolic disorder, others over-eat for psychological reasons. When dietary management has failed, and attempts to restrict food intake using teeth wiring have failed to produce a longterm weight reduction, surgery is sometimes advocated on the ground that weight loss, however achieved, is just as much a lifesaving procedure as cancer surgery.

2. There are certain ethical considerations. In the first place it can be argued that in circumstances of starvation or near starvation, such as the Nazi concentration camps, morbid obesity did not occur, so that voluntary restriction of food intake by the patient will overcome even the most stubborn metabolically generated obesity. Morbid obesity is seen with greatest frequency in properous countries, especially the USA.

3. All surgeons agree that if operations for morbid obesity can be justified, they must be performed by surgeons working in conjuction with specialist colleagues so that the

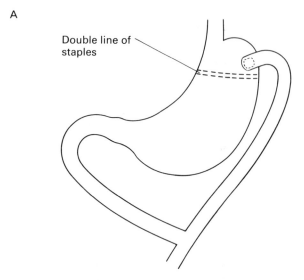

A

Double line of staples

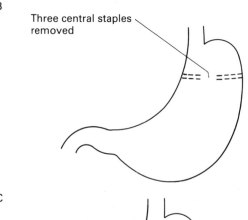

B

Three central staples removed

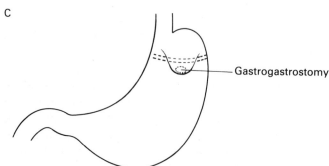

C

Gastrogastrostomy

Fig. 5.32 Some gastric operations for morbid obesity.

indications for surgery and the results can be monitored. Therefore, do not embark upon such surgery if you are in training or working in isolation.

4. The gastric operations in vogue are designed to place a restriction on the passage of food into the gastrointestinal tract. The first convenient region for this restriction beyond the teeth is the upper stomach. Most of the operations utilize the convenient TA90 stapling device that places a double row of staples through the full thickness of the gastric wall. After mobilizing the stomach two double rows of staples are placed across the upper stomach to form a small loculus. A Roux-en-Y loop of jejunum may be brought up for anastomosis to the upper loculus (Fig. 5.32) or three staples may be removed from the centre of each row to allow a limited passage into the main stomach or a small gastrogastrostomy may be fashioned to form a limited passage. Many other techniques have been devised to overcome the tendency of the small passage to stretch and become ineffective.

5. The gastric operations are not the sole method of surgically controlling morbid obesity. The majority of the small bowel may be bypassed (see p. 114).

Further reading

Akiyama H 1979 Thoracoabdominal approach for carcinoma of the cardia of the stomach. American Journal of Surgery 137: 345–349

Duthie H L, Bransom C J 1979 Highly selective vagotomy with excision of the ulcer compared with gastrectomy for gastric ulcer in a randomized trial. British Journal of Surgery 66: 43–45

Goligher J C De Dombal F T, Conyers J H, Duthie H L, Feather D B, Latchmore A J C et al 1968 Five to eight year results of Leeds/York controlled trial of elective surgery for duodenal ulcer. British Medical Journal 2: 781–787

Goligher J C, Pulvertaft C N, De Dombal F T, Clark C G, Conyers J H, Duthie H L et al 1968 Clinical comparison of vagotomy and pyloroplasty with other forms of elective surgery for duodenal ulcer. British Medical Journal 1: 787–789

Kirk R M 1975 Gastric mucosal resection in the treatment of peptic ulcers: a 1–10 year clinical follow-up. British J. Surgery 62: 608–609

Kirk R M 1983 Diagnostic upper gastrointestinal endoscopy. In: Dudley H, Pories W J, Carter D C (eds) Rob and Smith's Operative surgery, vol 1, 4th edn. Butterworths, London. p 1–7

Kirk R M 1985 Drainage procedures. In: Ellis H, Schwartz S (eds) Maingot's abdominal operations, 8th edn. Appleton Century Crofts, New York. p 821–827

Kirk R M, Jeffery P J 1981 Development of surgery for peptic ulcer: a review. Journal of the Royal Society of Medicine 74: 828–830

Kirk R M, Stoddard C J 1986 Complications of Surgery of the upper gastrointestinal tract. Baillière Tindall, London.

Kodama Y, Sugimachi K, Soejima K, Matsusak T, Inokuch K 1981 Evaluation of extensive lymph node dissection for carcinoma of the stomach. World Journal of Surgery 5: 241–248

Molina J E, Lawton B R, Myers W O, Humphrey E W 1982 Esophagogastrectomy for adenocarcinoma of the cardia: ten years' experience. Annals of Surgery 195: 146–151

Papachristou D N, Shiu M H 1981 Management by en bloc multiple organ resection of carcinoma of the stomach invading adjacent organs. Surgery Gynecology Obstetrics 152: 483–487

Taylor T V, Gunn A A, Macleod D A D, Maclennan I 1982 Anterior lesser curve seromyotomy and posterior truncal vagotomy in the treatment of chronic duodenal ulcer. Lancet 2: 846–849

Thomas W E G, Thompson M H, Williamson R C N 1982 The long-term outcome of Billroth I partial gastrectomy for benign gastric ulcer. Annals of Surgery 195: 189–195

Thompson J C, Lewis B G, Weiner I, Townsend C M Jr 1983 The role of surgery in the Zollinger-Ellison syndrome. Annals of Surgery 197: 594–607

Wyllie J H, Clark C G, Alexander-Williams J, Bell P R F

Kennedy T L, Kirk R M, Mackay C 1981 The effect of cimetidine on surgery for duodenal ulcer. Lancet 1: 1307–1308

Surgery of the small bowel

Examination of the small bowel
Intestinal anastomosis
Enterectomy (small-bowel resection)
Enteric bypass
The Roux loop
Enterotomy
Enterostomy
Miscellaneous conditions

EXAMINATION OF THE SMALL BOWEL

NORMAL APPEARANCE

1. The duodenum is 25 cm long. Apart from the proximal 2–3 cm, it is retroperitoneal. The remaining small bowel, which has a mesentery, is variable in total length (ca. 3–5 m) and difficult to measure with accuracy in vivo. It is arbitrarily divided into a proximal 40% (jejunum) and a distal 60% (ileum). On palpation the jejunal wall is thicker than that of the ileum, so that the examining fingers gain the impression of a double layer, rather like feeling a shirt through the sleeve of a jacket.

2. Examine the duodenal loop. Locate the duodenojejunal flexure by displacing the transverse colon upwards and tracing the coils of jejunum proximally to the ligament of Treitz. Pick up the small bowel at the duodenojejunal flexure and feed it through your fingers down to the ileocaecal valve. Note the diameter and contents of the bowel and the thickness and colour of its wall. In a thin person lacteals may appear as white lines crossing the jejunum and its mesentery.

3. Examine the small bowel mesentery throughout. Its thickness varies with the patient's adiposity. In a thin patient mesenteric lymph nodes can often be seen. Determine whether the nodes are enlarged or inflamed and whether the mesenteric blood vessels are normal.

ABNORMALITIES

1. *Diverticula*. These are quite common. Meckel's diverticulum, which arises from the distal ileum, is considered below. Acquired diverticula may affect the duodenum, jejunum and to a lesser extent the ileum and are frequently multiple. Do not remove incidental diverticula, but excise localized groups if they are causing symptoms, such as pain or bleeding.

2. *Inflammation*. Crohn's disease may affect any part of the alimentary canal but especially the terminal ileum. Affected segments of bowel are inflamed, thickened, narrowed and often covered with fibrinous exudate. The mesentery is thickened and encroaches on a greater proportion of the circumference of the bowel; adjacent lymph nodes are enlarged. Look for evidence of disease elsewhere in the small and large bowel. Segmental resection is usually indicated for chronic Crohn's enteritis (see below). Tuberculous and yersinial infection can produce similar changes of ileitis; if in doubt remove a gland for bacteriological and histological examination. Coeliac disease particularly affects the jejunum. The diagnosis is indicated by dilatation of subserous and mesenteric lymphatics, thinning and pigmentation of the bowel wall and splenic atrophy, and it is confirmed by full-thickness biopsy (see below). Small-bowel ulcers and strictures may occur spontaneously or follow either radiotherapy, transient strangulation in an external hernia or the ingestion of potassium tablets.

3. *Infarction*. The viability of the small bowel must be carefully checked after reduction of a strangulated hernia or untwisting of a volvulus in adhesion obstruction. Any frankly necrotic or perforated loops should be excised. If you are in doubt about the viability of a dusky segment, return it to the abdomen and wait for 5 minutes (timed by the clock). The return of a shiny, pink appearance, pulsation of the mesenteric vessels (or bleeding if pricked) and peristalsis across the affected segment indicate viability. If you are still in doubt, resect. Constriction rings

may be carefully invaginated, using interrupted seromuscular sutures.

4. *Tumours*. Serosal deposits occur in carcinomatosis peritonei and may cause kinking and obstruction of the small bowel, requiring side-to-side bypass (see p. 114). Primary neoplasms are less common. Benign tumours include adenoma, leiomyoma, lipoma and Peutz-Jeghers hamartomas; they can cause intussusception. Carcinoid tumours favour the ileum, but may be multiple and metastasizing; they are hard with a yellowish cut surface. Malignant tumours comprise adenocarcinoma, lymphoma and leiomyosarcoma in that order of prevalence. Primary neoplasms should be excised, or biopsied if irresectable.

BIOPSY

1. Multiple biopsies of duodenal and jejunal mucosa can safely be obtained by the peroral route; the patient swallows an appropriate, retrievable capsule. Operative biopsy of the small intestine is seldom indicated. It is usually possible to excise the segment of bowel in question, and intestinal biopsy should be avoided in Crohn's disease. If a full-thickness biopsy is required however, the incision should be closed in two layers just like an intestinal anastomosis.

2. Mesenteric lymph nodes can be biopsied with relative impunity. Where possible, select a node close to the bowel wall and avoid dissecting deep in the root of the mesentery. Carefully incise the peritoneum and dissect out the entire node, using diathermy to coagulate its small blood vessels.

INTESTINAL ANASTOMOSIS

GENERAL PRINCIPLES

1. Several hundred intestinal anastomoses are carried out each week in Britain, and the vast majority heal rapidly by primary intention. It is fortunate that the small bowel does heal so satisfactorily, since discharge of intestinal contents into the abdominal cavity is potentially lethal, and inability to use the gut within a few days of operation makes adequate nutrition much more difficult. Healthy large intestine heals almost as well as small intestine, with the exception of anastomoses situated in its last few centimetres, which do not enjoy serosal cover.

2. Remember that most of the intestinal canal is contaminated with bacteria, disproportionately so towards the distal end. Elaborate techniques were devised in the past to avoid exposing open bowel, but it is now accepted that a secure anastomosis is more easily achieved by opening the bowel. Take appropriate precautions against disseminating faecal organisms (p. 47) before dividing and

resuturing the bowel; clamps are usually indicated to prevent faecal spillage (p. 48). Postoperative abscess formation is likely to impair anastomotic healing.

3. The key to a successful anastomosis is the accurate union of two viable bowel ends, with complete avoidance of tension. Ensure that the bowel ends are pink and bleeding freely, and leave the mesentery attached to the bowel right up to the point of intestinal transection. If either cut end is bruised or dusky, it is usually sensible to sacrifice a few more centimetres of intestine, even if (in the case of the large bowel) this requires further mobilisation.

4. Tension puts the mesenteric vessels on stretch and tends to distract the bowel ends. It usually results from inadequate mobilisation, especially of the colon. Though readily avoidable, twisting of the mesentery can also render an anastomosis ischaemic. The mesenteric/mesocolic defect should normally be repaired after completing an intestinal anastomosis to prevent postoperative internal herniation, but take care in so doing not to compromise the vessels supplying the bowel ends.

5. Distended loops of bowel are heavy and difficult to handle. Moreover, healing is impaired, probably because the bowel wall is thinner and somewhat ischaemic. Distended small bowel may be decompressed by milking contents upwards into the reach of the nasogastric tube or by enterotomy and insertion of a sucker (p. 117). Gaseous distension of the large bowel can be relieved by introducing a needle obliquely through its wall. Try and avoid leaving hard faecal lumps proximal to a colonic anastomosis. If possible milk them beyond the site of intended colonic transection.

HAND-SUTURING TECHNIQUES

1. Traditionally, bowel is united in two layers, using catgut or another absorbable suture material for the inner, all-coats layers and an outer stitch (called after its inventor, Lembert) to join the seromuscular layers. In certain sites only a one-layered anastomosis can sometimes be achieved, e.g. colorectal and biliary-enteric anastomoses and oesophagojejunostomy.

2. Surgeons have long disputed the best suture material, the best type of stitch and the best methods of fashioning a suture line. I believe that these technical points are less important than the principle stated above: to achieve accurate and tension-free coaptation of two healthy mucosal surfaces. Nevertheless, each surgeon develops his own variations of technique, which he believes to be the most appropriate. As an assistant, therefore, follow the method of your present chief and hope to experience a number of methods before you have to select one for yourself.

3. Surgical trainees are often uncertain whether to use

continuous or interrupted sutures in a given situation. A continuous (running) stitch is undoubtedly quicker and it achieves good haemostasis. It is therefore appropriate for straightforward gastric, enteric and colonic anastomoses. Be careful to maintain the tension on the previous stitch when inserting and pulling through its successor. The assistant should keep the suture material taut until you are ready to pull up the next stitch.

4. Interrupted sutures allow slightly greater precision and may be more convenient than a continuous stitch when there is marked disparity in the size of the bowel ends to be united or the anastomosis is technically difficult. In inaccessible situations (e.g. colorectal anastomosis deep in the pelvis or hepaticojejunostomy) it may be wise to insert the entire posterior row of interrupted sutures before tying any individual stitch.

5. Many surgeons routinely use two layers of continuous catgut sutures for gastric and intestinal anastomoses. If impaired healing is anticipated, e.g. in Crohn's disease, consider whether an inner layer of continuous catgut and an outer layer of interrupted silk would provide added security. Non-absorbable sutures are usually indicated when joining small bowel (or colon) to the oesophagus, pancreas or rectum; suitable materials include silk (2/0 or 3/0), polypropylene (Prolene), monofilament nylon and stainless-steel wire.

6. Whichever type of suture and suture material you employ, take care to achieve the correct degree of tension when pulling through and tying the stitch. Insert each stitch separately and invert the bowel edges as the catgut is tightened. Once the bowel edge is inverted, prevent the suture material from slipping by getting your assistant to follow up. Alternatively, follow up yourself, using the taut suture as a means of steadying the bowel against the thrust of the needle. The objective is a snug, watertight anastomosis. Excessive tension risks strangulating the bowel incorporated in the stitch and perhaps causing subsequent leakage.

7. Do not place the sutures so close to the edge of the bowel that they might tear out nor so deep that they turn in an enormous cuff of tissue and narrow the bowel; usually 3–5 mm is about the correct depth of 'bite'. Be sure that the all-coats suture does in fact incorporate all coats of the bowel wall. The muscularis tends to retract and may escape being sutured, especially posteriorly. The best way to master these important technical points is to assist at and then perform under supervision a number of intestinal anastomoses.

8. The seromuscular stitch unites the adjacent bowel walls outside the all-coats stitch. Sometimes the posterior seromuscular layer is inserted before opening the gut, e.g. in side-to-side anastomoses (Fig. 6.1). After the all-coats stitches have been inserted, the seromuscular sutures are carried round the ends of the anastomosis and across the front wall, ultimately encircling the anastomosis so that the

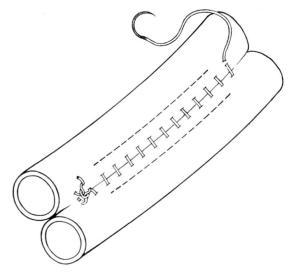

Fig. 6.1 A continuous layer of posterior seromuscular sutures has been inserted before fashioning a side-to-side anastomosis. The dotted lines indicate the lines of incision of the bowel.

all-coats stitches can no longer be seen. For end-to-end anastomoses in small and large intestine it may be simpler to complete the all-coats layer before placing any Lembert sutures. Thereafter, the seromuscular layer can be inserted all the way round by rotating the bowel.

9. The all-coats stitch is accepted as the paramount stitch for holding bowel edges, since it catches the strong submucosa. There are many ways of inserting these stitches; three popular methods are described below:

a) *Continuous over-and-over suture.* Approximate the two edges of cut bowel. Starting at one end, insert a corner stitch from outside to in, then over the adjacent edges of bowel and out through the other corner. Tie the suture and clip the short end. Pass the stitch back through the nearest bowel wall, over the contiguous cut edges and back through the full thickness of both walls. Continue over-and-over stitches to the opposite corner (Fig. 6.2). After the last stitch is inserted right into the corner, take it back through the nearest corner

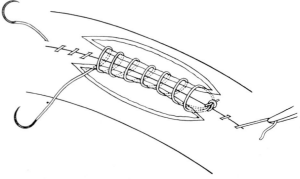

Fig. 6.2 The all-coats stitch is being inserted in a continuous over-and-over fashion. Care is taken to include mucosa and muscularis in each bite.

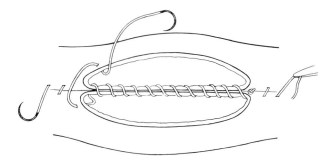

Fig. 6.3 The all-coats stitch is continued round the corner. A single loop-on-the-mucosa stitch starts the return over-and-over stitch.

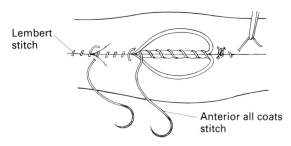

Fig. 6.4 The anterior all-coats stitch is continued; then the anterior seromuscular stitch completes the anastomosis.

leaving a loop on the mucosa so that the stitch emerges from the outer wall of the bowel (Fig. 6.3). Now sew the front walls together by passing the stitch over and over, from out to in and then from in to out (Fig. 6.4). Continue until the anastomosis has been encircled and the edges inverted, then tie off the ends of suture material. This over-and-over stitch is haemostatic.

b) *Continuous over-and-over plus Connell suture.* Commence in the middle of the posterior wall by placing a stitch between the adjacent cut edges of bowel and tying it on the luminal surface. Now continue towards one corner with over-and-over stitches. At the corner the needle passes from in to out on the nearside cut surface, then crosses to the far edge and is passed in and out to leave a loop on the mucosa (Fig. 6.5). The needle returns to the near edge and another loop-on-the-mucosa (Connell) stitch is inserted. These Connell stitches turn the corner neatly. Once you are round the corner, leave this stitch and return to the middle of the posterior wall. Use a new length of suture material, unless there is a needle at each end of the original length. Insert and tie a stitch close to the site of the original ligature, tie the two short ends of suture material and proceed towards the opposite corner, using Connell sutures to negotiate the corner again. Either continue with Connell stitches along the anterior wall from each end, or return to over-and-over stitches once you are round the corners. Tie off the ends of suture material in the middle of the anterior wall. The Connell stitch is not haemostatic, therefore all bleeding points must be secured.

c) *Interrupted suture.* Insert a stitch from out to in and in to out at each corner. If the anastomosis is easily accessible, tie each stitch at this stage. Clip the ends of suture material and get your assistant to hold the clips to exert traction on the posterior cut edges of bowel (Fig. 6.6). Insert a row of posterior sutures 2–3 mm apart, tying the knots on the luminal surface. If the anastomosis is relatively inaccessible, avoid tying any sutures until the entire posterior row has been inserted. Then approximate the bowel ends and tie the sutures snugly and in order, proceeding from one corner to the next. Now place an anterior row of interrupted sutures. It is easier to tie the knots on the outside at this stage, and inversion does not appear to be essential. Indeed, some surgeons practise edge-to-edge or eversion techniques routinely for intestinal anastomosis, preferring not to turn in a ridge of tissue that might obstruct the lumen.

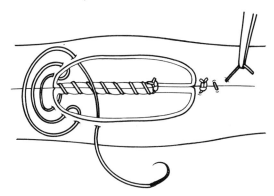

Fig. 6.5 Starting from the middle of the back wall, an over-and-over stitch has been inserted as far as the corner. Two or three Connell stitches are placed to turn the corner, followed by an anterior over-and-over stitch. A separate suture is used to fashion the other half of the anastomosis.

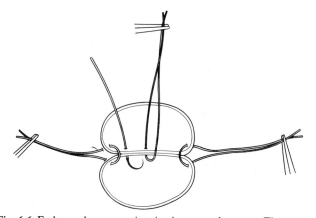

Fig. 6.6 End-to-end anastomosis using interrupted sutures. The two corner stitches are tied with the knots on the outside, but for the remainder of the posterior wall the knots are placed on the inside. If access is restricted, each suture is inserted and held in a clip before any one is tied (as shown).

MECHANICAL STAPLING TECHNIQUES

1. Stapling machines are now available to carry out most types of gastrointestinal anastomosis. For end-to-end anastomosis (e.g. colorectal, oesophagojejunal) the stapling gun (Fig. 6.7a) is introduced into the intestinal lumen downstream, brought out through the distal cut end of bowel and then insinuated into the proximal cut end. The largest anvil should be chosen that will fit comfortably into the proximal lumen. Proximal and distal gut are snugged tightly around the central rod (Fig. 6.8), using purse-string sutures, and the anvil is then approximated to the cartridge by closing the instrument. When the gun is fired, a circular double row of stainless steel staples is inserted, and at the same time a complete 5 mm rim of each bowel end (the 'doughnut') is resected. The machine is then withdrawn, the 'doughnuts' are checked and the anastomosis is complete.

2. For side-to-side anastomosis a different instrument is used, resembling a pair of scissors (Fig. 6.7b). One 'blade' is inserted into each of the two intestinal segments to be united, and the blades are closed. Firing the gun advances a knife, which divides the adjacent surfaces of bowel between two parallel rows of staples.

3. Yet another set of instruments has been designed to place a double row of staples across the end of a segment of intestine or stomach (Fig. 6.7c). The staple line can be 30, 55 or 90 mm long. After firing the staples, the instrument is left attached and used as an anvil on which to transect the gut. Some surgeons prefer to bury the staple line with a continuous Lembert suture.

4. Using a mechanical stapler does not guarantee a perfect result. It is just as important to prepare healthy bowel ends and avoid tension as it is in hand-sewn anastomoses, and a different set of technical details has to be learnt. Stapling machines reduce the time involved in fashioning an anastomosis and facilitate certain operations that can be difficult to complete by hand, such as oesophageal transection, oesopagogastrectomy (Fig. 6.8) or low anterior resection of the rectum. The introduction of disposable stapling guns obviates the need for careful maintenance of the re-usable instrument and may reduce the substantial costs involved in mechanical stapling. On the other hand there are many situations where the stapler is inappropriate (e.g. choledochojejunostomy) or unnecessary (most small-bowel anastomoses). Aim to be versatile and try to acquire experience in both methods of gastrointestinal anastomosis.

TYPES OF ANASTOMOSIS

1. End-to-end anastomosis

This is the simplest way of restoring intestinal continuity after partial enterectomy and/or colectomy. After removal of the resected specimen (see p. 111), clean and approxi-

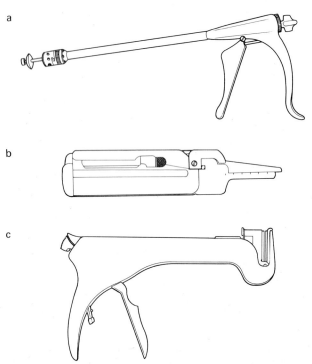

Fig. 6.7 Auto Suture ® instruments used for gastrointestinal anastomosis. (a) Model EEA is for end-to-side anastomosis; (b) Model GIA is for side-to-side anastomosis; (c) Model TA30 is for closing off the end of the bowel.

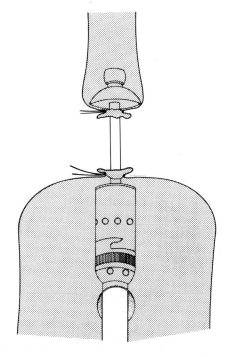

Fig. 6.8 Oesophagogastric anastomosis, using the EEA stapling gun inserted through a small gastrotomy. After tying each purse-string suture around the central rod, the anvil is approximated to the cartridge and the staples are discharged.

a

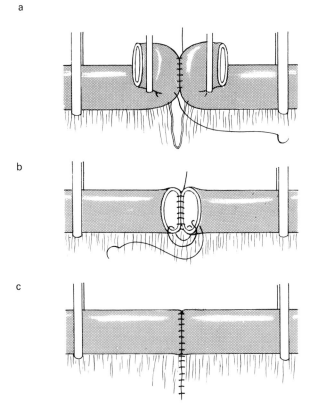

b

c

Fig. 6.9 End-to-end intestinal anastomosis. (a) and (b) Two layers of stitches being inserted; (c) The completed anastomosis with the mesentery repaired.

mate the bowel ends. The anastomosis is usually created in two layers, using a continuous 2/0 chromic catgut suture swaged onto an eyeless needle (Fig. 6.9). Insert the all-coats stitch, using one of the techniques described above or a variant that you have been shown. Remove the intestinal clamps and check that the anastomosis is airtight and watertight by gently squeezing intestinal contents across it. Now insert the circumferential seromuscular stitch, taking care not to turn in too thick a cuff of tissue. Make sure the thumb and forefinger can invaginate bowel wall on each side through the anastomosis. Some surgeons prefer to unite the bowel ends with a posterior layer of Lembert sutures before embarking on the all-coats stitch, but I only resort to this manoeuvre with end-to-end anastomosis if I anticipate subsequent difficulty in placing the posterior seromuscular layer. Lastly, unite the cut edges of mesentery and/or mesocolon on each aspect with interrupted catgut sutures, taking care to avoid damaging the vessels.

2. Oblique anastomosis

When the ends of bowel are disproportionate in size, they may be matched by incising the antimesenteric border of the narrow bowel longitudinally (Fig. 6.10a). This manoeuvre is useful in joining obstructed to collapsed

bowel or ileum to colon. In neonates with congenital intestinal atresia, the lumen of the distal bowel is particularly narrow and this type of 'end-to-back' anastomosis is necessitated. The mesentery of the proximal bowel is also disproportionately big and should be shortened with a few gathering stitches before being united to the distal cut edge of mesentery. When two segments of narrow intestine must be united, they may both be opened along their antimesenteric borders, which are then joined back-to-back (Fig. 6.10b). The mesenteries are now on opposite sides of the anastomosis and cannot always be neatly approximated. Poth has described an elegant variant of this technique, in which the end of the larger segment is sutured to the end-to-lateral aspect of the smaller segment of bowel (Fig. 6.11).

a

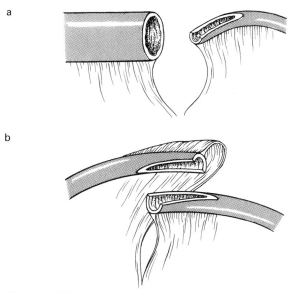

b

Fig. 6.10 Oblique anastomoses. (a) End-to-back anastomosis. The narrow bowel has been opened along its antimesenteric border so that its lumen matches the end of the wider bowel; (b) Back-to-back anastomosis. Two narrow segments of bowel have been opened along their antimesenteric borders to create a wide anastomosis.

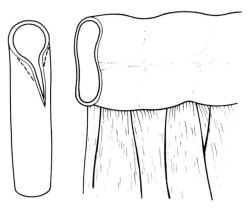

Fig. 6.11 End-to-lateral anastomosis. Poth's variation of the oblique anastomosis may be used to unite ileum to colon. The corners on the ileal segment are trimmed along the dotted lines.

3. End-to-side anastomosis

This is most commonly used when creating a Roux-en-Y anastomosis. Approximate the cut end to the side of bowel to which it will be joined, and insert a posterior seromuscular suture (Fig. 6.12). Incise the antimesenteric border of the side of bowel to accommodate the cut end. Insert the all-coats stitch as before, remove the clamps and complete the seromuscular stitch. Lastly, join the cut edge of mesentery to the side of the intact mesentery.

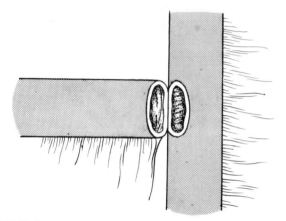

Fig. 6.12 End-to-side anastomosis

4. Side-to-side anastomosis

This can be used to join two loops of bowel without resection, or to unite intestine to stomach, bile duct etc. (Fig. 6.13). It may also be employed as an alternative to end-to-end anastomosis after intestinal resection, in which case the cut ends of bowel should first be closed and invaginated. The advantages of the side-to-side anastomosis are that the segments of bowel to be united have no interruption to their blood supply at all and that the incisions can

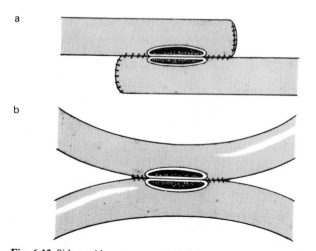

Fig. 6.13 Side-to-side anastomoses. (a) After transection of the bowel, with closure of each end; (b) Two segments are joined without dividing the bowel.

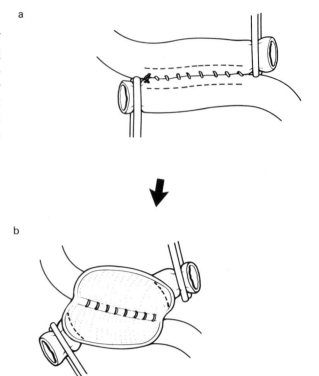

Fig. 6.14 Poth's modification of the side-to-side anastomosis. (a) The posterior seromuscular stitch has been inserted; each segment is opened along the dotted line; (b) The posterior all-coats stitch has been placed; the corners are trimmed along the dotted lines.

be made exactly congruous. The disadvantages are that there are more suture lines involved and that there may be some degree of stasis and bacterial overgrowth; Poth's adaptation of the side-to-side anastomosis may overcome these objections (Fig. 6.14).

Lay the segments to be joined side by side in contact for 8–10 cm and insert a posterior seromuscular stitch. Incise the antimesenteric borders for about 5 cm and insert an all-coats stitch. Remove the clamps and complete the anterior seromuscular layer of stitches. When side-to-side anastomosis follows bowel resection, suture the cut edge of mesentery to the adjacent intact mesentery on each side of the anastomosis.

Further reading

Orr N W M 1969 A single-layer intestinal anastomosis. British Journal of Surgery 56: 771–774
Poth E J 1950 A technique for suturing bowel. Surgery, Gynecology and Obstetrics 91: 656–659

ENTERECTOMY (SMALL-BOWEL RESECTION)

Appraise

1. Resection is often indicated for congenital lesions of the small bowel (atresia, duplication), traumatic

perforation, critical ischaemia (from mesenteric trauma, strangulation or arteriosclerosis), Crohn's disease or other cause of stricture, and tumours of the bowel or its mesentery. Resection is sometimes indicated for fistula, diverticulitis, intussusception and a symptomatic blind loop. Small portions of the duodenum and ileum are removed during partial gastrectomy and right hemicolectomy respectively.

2. There are several reasons for being conservative in the management of Crohn's disease: the indolent nature of the disease, its relapsing course and its strong tendency (>50%) to recur anywhere in the intestinal tract, but especially at and just proximal to the anastomosis. Do not resect for Crohn's ileitis discovered incidentally during laparotomy for suspected appendicitis. On the other hand most patients with chronic Crohn's enteritis eventually require resection of the affected segment because of subacute obstruction, fistula or abscess. Bypass is obsolete: the defunctioned segment is unlikely to heal, bacterial overgrowth of the blind loop may aggravate diarrhoea and there is a long-term risk of carcinoma.

3. In the presence of an obstructing lesion, ensure that the patient is adequately resuscitated before operation with nasogastric intubation and intravenous rehydration. In non-obstructed patients undergoing small-bowel operations, a nasogastric tube should be passed after induction of anaesthesia.

4. Healthy ileum has a resident bacterial flora, and in the presence of obstruction the entire small bowel may be colonised. It is sensible to cover all operations likely to involve intestinal resection with appropriate prophylactic antibiotics, e.g. a cephalosporin plus metronidazole given preoperatively by a single shot.

Access

1. Adequate exposure of the entire small bowel can be provided by a number of different incisions. I usually employ a midline incision that skirts the umbilicus and can be extended in either direction, as necessary.

2. Remember that the small bowel quite often adheres to the back of a previous laparotomy incision, and take particular care during abdominal re-entry. The chances are that an accidental perforation will not be located in a segment of bowel that you would in any case have intended to remove.

Assess

1. Expose and examine the entire small bowel (see p. 104). Continue by examining the stomach, large bowel and remaining abdominal viscera.

2. If a loop of small bowel has been strangulated in an external hernia, for example, release the obstruction and check the viability of the bowel after allowing a minimum

period of 5 minutes for possible recovery in doubtful cases (p. 35).

3. Healthy small intestine possesses both a considerable functional reserve and the capacity to adapt to partial tissue loss by compensatory villous hyperplasia of the portions that remain. Nevertheless do not gratuitously sacrifice healthy bowel, particularly terminal ileum, which has specialised transport functions. Except when operating for primary malignant tumours it is quite unnecessary to excise a deep wedge of mesentery, which might increase the extent of small bowel requiring removal. In Crohn's disease do not remove more than a few centimetres of gut on either side of the affected segment, but include any fistulae or sinuses. It is more than likely that further resection will be required in future, and microscopic inflammation of the bowel at the resection margin does not appear to increase subsequent anastomotic recurrence. Conventional right hemicolectomy is unnecessary for small-bowel Crohn's disease; conservative ileocaecal resection should be undertaken.

4. Sometimes a partial resection of small bowel can be performed, leaving the mesentery intact. Appropriate conditions include Richter's hernia, Meckel's diverticulum and small tumours arising on the antimesenteric border.

Action

1. Isolate the diseased loop of bowel from the other abdominal contents by means of large, moist packs or a special towel.

2. Hold up the bowel and examine the mesentery against the light. Note the vascular pattern.

Standard resection

1. Determine the proximal and distal sites for dividing the bowel, and select the line of vascular section in between; keep fairly close to the bowel wall (Fig. 6.15),

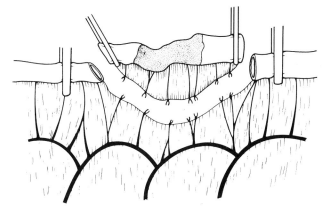

Fig. 6.15 Resection of an ischaemic segment of small bowel including a shallow wedge of mesentery. The narrower bowel end has been cut obliquely to match the wider end.

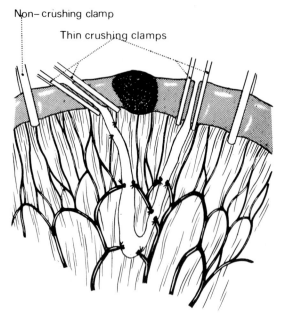

Non–crushing clamp

Thin crushing clamps

Fig. 6.16 Resection of a small bowel tumour. A deeper wedge of mesentery is included than in operations for benign disease (see Fig. 6.15). As before, the narrower segment of bowel (on the left) is transected obliquely, removing more of the mesenteric border with the specimen.

except when resecting a neoplasm (Fig. 6.16). Incise the peritoneum along this line on each aspect of the mesentery. This manoeuvre is most easily accomplished by inseting one blade of a pair of fine, curved scissors beneath the peritoneum and cutting superficially to expose the mesenteric vessels.

2. Using small artery forceps, create a small mesenteric window right next to the bowel wall at each point chosen for intestinal transection. Starting at one end, insinuate a curved artery forceps through this window and back through the mesentery (denuded of peritoneum) 1–2 cm away, thus isolating a small leash of mesentery with its contained vessels. Either doubly ligate this leash in continuity and divide between ligatures, or divide between artery forceps, ligating the mesentery beneath each pair of forceps. Proceeding in this manner, divide the mesentery right up to the bowel wall at the further end of the line of peritoneal incision. Take care in placing and tying each ligature; if the knot slips, there can be troublesome haemorrhage. I use 2/0 silk ties.

3. Apply four intestinal clamps (Fig. 6.15). The first two clamps are crushing clamps (Payr's, Lang Stevenson's or Pringle's). They should be applied obliquely at the points of intended intestinal transection, so that slightly more of the antimesenteric border is resected than of the mesenteric border; the obliquity reduces the risk of a tight anastomosis. Now apply a non-crushing clamp about 5 cm outside each crushing clamp, having milked the intervening bowel free of contents.

4. Place a clean gauze swab beneath the clamps at each end (to catch spills), and divide the bowel with a knife flush against the outer aspect of each crushing clamp. Place the specimen and the soiled knife in a separate dish, which is then removed.

5. Cleanse each bowel end, using small swabs or pledgets of gauze soaked in cetrimide. Then remove the protective gauze swab and proceed to intestinal anastomosis. In an attempt to limit contamination, some surgeons divide the intestine between two pairs of light crushing clamps (i.e. six clamps in all) and insert the posterior seromuscular layer of sutures, before removing the outer clamps and excising the narrow rim of crushed tissue (Fig. 6.16).

6. Perform a two-layer, end-to-end anastomosis, as described in the previous section.

Partial resection

1. A diverticulum on the antimesenteric border may be locally excised. Clamp and cut it off at the neck, then close the defect in two layers as a transverse linear slit. Try to avoid narrowing the intestinal lumen during this procedure.

2. A diamond-shaped area of the antimesenteric border may be included in the resection of a localised tumour or wide-mouthed Meckel's diverticulum. Apply two light crushing clamps (Lang Stevenson's or Pringle's) across the antimesenteric border meeting in a V (Fig. 6.17). Incise the bowel flush with the outer aspect of each clamp, and close the wall in two layers, leaving a transverse suture line.

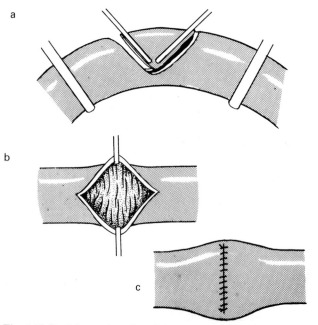

a

b

c

Fig. 6.17 Partial resection of small bowel. (a) A wedge of antimesenteric bowel is removed; (b) The defect is opened out transversely; (c) Closure across the long axis of the bowel prevents narrowing.

3. A similar defect results if the antimesenteric lesion is excised through a longitudinal ellipse. Approximate the ends of the ellipse, pull apart the sides and close transversely as before.

Difficulty?

1. The bowel is obstructed. Decompress obstructed jejunum by milking its contents upwards until they can be aspirated through the nasogastric tube. Decompress obstructed ileum by inserting a sucker tube either into the end of the proximal bowel after releasing the clamps or via a separate enterotomy (see p. 117). Do this without allowing bowel contents to spill.

2. In the presence of obstruction there may be marked disparity between the diameters of the bowel ends. In practice moderate incongruities can be overcome by adjusting the size of bite, while suturing proximal to distal bowel. The diameter of the distal bowel can be increased by transecting it more obliquely (sparing the mesenteric border) and by opening it along the antimesenteric border. If there is gross disparity, consider oblique or side-to-side anastomosis (see preceding section).

3. Resection and anastomosis can usually be completed outside the abdomen. Sometimes this is not possible, in which case you may not be able to apply all the clamps described above (either four or six). Try and retain the non-crushing clamps placed at a distance from the anastomosis, if possible. If difficult circumstances, concentrate on completing the all-coats suture without defect, if necessary using interrupted sutures. You may subsequently be able to insert seromuscular sutures around all or most of the circumference.

4. A haematoma develops in the mesentery or in the submucosa at the point of intestinal transection. Compression of the area with a swab will usually stop the bleeding. Alternatively, gently close swab-holding forceps or non-crushing clamps across the bleeding point and wait for a few minutes. If the bleeding is not fully controlled, incise the peritoneum, find the bleeding point, pick it up with fine artery forceps and ligate it. Check the colour of the bowel to confirm that the blood supply is not prejudiced.

5. One or other intestinal end becomes dusky during the anastomosis. Time will usually declare the issue. Nonviable bowel will not heal, so if you are in any doubt it is better to excise a few more centimetres of bowel and make a fresh start. Leave the mesentery attached to the bowel as close as possible to the point of transection, and check for visible pulsations in the edge of the mesentery.

Check list

1. Take a last look at the anastomosis. Check that the bowel is pink, that haemostasis is secure and that all mesenteric defects are closed.

2. It is easy to lose a swab among the coils of small intestine. Check the entire abdominal cavity and make sure that the swab count is correct. Remove any ends of suture material that might provoke subsequent adhesions. Replace the intestine and the greater omentum in their normal anatomical position.

3. Suck out the peritoneal cavity. Place a fine-bore suction drain to the region of the anastomosis.

Aftercare

1. Anticipate a period of postoperative ileus, during which the patient is maintained on intravenous fluids. The nasogastric tube should be left on open drainage and aspirated regularly for the first 24–48 hours. Allow 30 ml of water per hour by mouth. The tube can usually be removed when bowel sounds return, the volume of aspirate drops below the volume of fluid taken by mouth and there is passage of flatus. Peristalsis returns to the small bowel before the stomach and colon regain their motility.

2. Remove the drain when the fluid loss diminishes, generally at 2–3 days.

3. A leaking anastomosis will often present with pain, fever, tachycardia and erythaema of the wound or drain site before intestinal contents begin to discharge. The management of an established small-bowel fistula is described at the end of this chapter.

4. It is occasionally necessary to undertake massive resection of the small bowel, e.g. for volvulus complicating an obstruction. Repeated enterectomies in Crohn's disease can similarly remove a substantial percentage of the small intestine. Increased frequency of bowel actions may follow loss of a third to a half of the small bowel. During the initial phase of recovery and adaptation, anticipate and replace losses of fluid and electrolytes, notably potassium. Give codeine or loperamide to control diarrhoea. The body compensates better for proximal than distal enterectomy. After an extensive ileal resection regular injections of vitamin B_{12} may be needed indefinitely; cholestyramine may diminish the irritative diarrhoea that results from bile-acid malabsorption. Consider nutritional support by the enteral or parenteral routes in severe short bowel syndrome. Cimetidine or, rarely, vagotomy may be needed for gastric acid hypersecretion.

Further reading

Pennington L, Hamilton S R, Bayless T M, Cameron J L 1980 Surgical management of Crohn's disease. Influence of disease at margin of resection. Annals of Surgery 192: 311–318

Williamson R C N 1978 Intestinal adaptation. New England Journal of Medicine 298: 1393–1402, 1444–1450

Williamson R C N, Malt R A, Welch C E 1983 Adenocarcinoma and lymphoma of the small intestine: distribution and etiologic associations. Annals of Surgery 197: 172–178

ENTERIC BYPASS

Appraise

1. Small-bowel loops may become obstructed as a result of carcinomatosis peritonei or a particularly dense set of adhesions, sometimes deep in the pelvis. Irradiated small bowel may fistulate into other organs, such as the bladder or vagina. In these unfavourable circumstances it is often better just to bypass the affected segment of intestine (Fig. 6.18) rather than embark on a difficult and hazardous

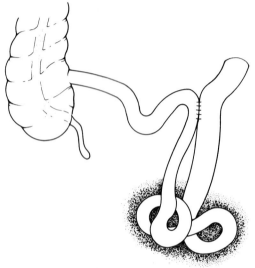

Fig. 6.18 Bypass procedure for small-bowel obstruction resulting from irresectable pelvic cancer. A side-to-side anastomosisis is fashioned between a (proximal) distended loop of bowel and a (distal) collapsed loop.

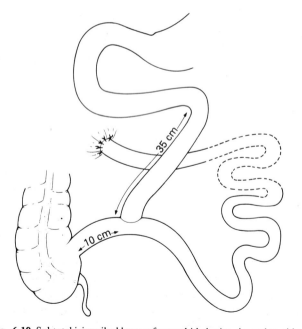

Fig. 6.19 Subtotal jejunoileal bypass for morbid obesity. An end-to-side anastomosis is fashioned between 35 cm of functioning jejunum and 10 cm of functioning ileum. The top end of the blind loop is closed and invaginated and tacked to the posterior abdominal wall to prevent intussusception.

disentanglement. In radiation enteritis choose overtly normal bowel for the anastomosis, since healing is likely to be impaired.

2. Resection is almost always a better option than simple defunction in Crohn's disease of the small bowel (see p. 111). For irresectable carcinoma of the caecum, however, side-to-side bypass is indicated between the terminal ileum and the transverse colon (ileotransversostomy).

3. Subtotal jejunoileal bypass has been recommended for intractable morbid obesity (Fig. 6.19). Patients lose weight because of malabsorption, diarrhoea and impaired appetite. The operation provides a metabolic insult to the body, and there are many potential long-term complications. The alternative procedures of subtotal gastric bypass and gastric partitioning cause fewer metabolic upsets but offer a formidable technical challenge and have a higher reoperation rate.

4. Bypass of the distal one-third of the small intestine is rarely indicated for certain types of hyperlipidaemia. The ileum is divided, the distal end is closed and the proximal end is reimplanted into the caecum. The operation reduces the levels of cholesterol and triglyceride in the blood.

Action

Bypass of an irresectable lesion

1. A midline incision is usually appropriate. Aim to anastomose healthy bowel on either side of the diseased segment. Side-to-side anastomosis avoids the risk of closed loop obstruction developing in a sequestered loop of bowel.

2. Occasionally if there are multiple sites of actual or imminent obstruction, two or more side-to-side anastomoses between adjacent loops may cause less of a short circuit than one enormous bypass.

3. Approximate a distended loop of proximal intestine to a collapsed loop of distal small bowel (Fig. 6.18) or transverse colon. Pack off the remaining viscera. Consider decompression of the obstructed loops.

4. Carry out a two-layer, side-to-side anastomosis, as previously described (p. 110). Take care with the anastomosis and subsequent wound closure, since healing may be impaired, but do not prolong the operation unnecessarily if the patient has advanced disease.

Bypass for morbid obesity

1. I prefer a right transverse incision just above the umbilicus, if possible cutting only one rectus abdominis muscle. The subcutaneous fat should be 'fractured', i.e. torn apart by the surgeon's fingers; this procedure limits bleeding. Enlist plenty of assistance when tackling an obese patient.

2. End-to-side bypass is both simple and satisfactory. Although the precise lengths of residual functioning intes-

tine may not be crucial to success of failure, I leave 35 cm of jejunum in continuity with 10 cm of ileum (Fig. 6.19). Measure the segments of jejunum and ileum to be left in circuit immediately after the initial abdominal exploration. Using a string or chain of the correct length, take the mean of three measurements along the antimesenteric border of the bowel from the ligament of Treitz and the ileocaecal valve; mark the points for enterotomy with a silk suture.

3. Transect the jejunum, close and invaginate the distal cut end and tack it to the posterior abdominal wall to prevent intussusception. Incise the ileum to accommodate the diameter of the jejunum and construct an end-to-side anastomosis, as previously described (p. 110).

4. Close the abdominal wall with care, leaving fine-bore suction tubes to drain the deeper layers.

Aftercare

The principles of management are as for enterectomy (see previous section). Short bowel syndrome is inevitable after subtotal (about 90%) jejunoileal bypass, although adaptation can still be anticipated. Fluid and electrolyte losses may need intravenous replacement at first, but diarrhoea usually subsides. Protein malnutrition and bacterial colonisation of the long blind loop may be responsible for liver damage, which occasionally necessitates restoration of intestinal continuity. Fat-soluble vitamins should be given, together with measures to combat excessive oxalate absorption.

Further reading

Galland R B, Spencer J 1979 Surgical aspects of radiation injury to the intestine. British Journal of Surgery 66: 135–138

Halverson J D 1980 Obesity surgery in perspective. Surgery 87: 119–127

Mason E E 1981 Surgical Treatment of Obesity. W B Saunders, Philadelphia

THE ROUX LOOP

Appraise

1. A defunctioned segment of jejunum provides a convenient conduit for connecting various upper abdominal organs to the remaining small bowel. Originally described by César Roux in 1907 for oesophageal bypass, the technique has proved invaluable in gastric, biliary and pancreatic surgery. Its uses in these circumstances are considered in the relevant chapters. Creation of the fundamental loop is described below.

2. Roux-en-Y anastomosis has two advantages over the use of an intact loop: it can stretch further and it is empty of intestinal contents, thus preventing contamination of the organ to be drained (e.g. bile duct). Active peristalsis down the loop encourages this drainage.

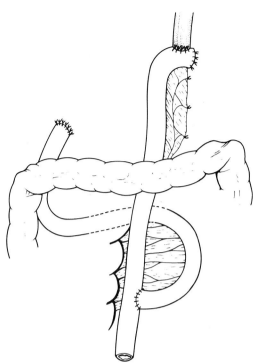

Fig. 6.20 One indication for a Roux loop: Roux-en-Y anastomosis between the oesophagus and jejunum after total gastrectomy.

3. Probably the commonest indications for Roux-en-Y anastomosis are biliary drainage in irresectable carcinoma of the pancreatic head and reconstruction after total gastrectomy (Fig. 6.20) or oesophagogastrectomy. Conversion to a Roux loop may cure duodenogastric reflux after partial gastrectomy, provided the loop is 40–50 cm long. Allison has shown that with meticulous attention to technique it is possible to bring a Roux loop up to the neck to replace the oesophagus.

4. Although Roux-en-Y anastomosis is the most versatile technique, other types of jejunal loop are sometimes indicated (Fig. 6.21). Intact loops are used for cholecystoenterostomy, gastroenterostomy and Polya (Billroth II) reconstruction after partial gastrectomy. Isolated loops may be interposed between the stomach and duodenum in an isoperistaltic or antiperistaltic direction for different facets of the postgastrectomy syndrome. A reversed loop can be used further downstream in certain cases of intractable diarrhoea. These alternatives are further discussed in Chapter 5.

Action

1. Select a loop of proximal small bowel, beginning 10–15 cm distal to the ligament of Treitz. Hold up the jejunum and transilluminate its mesentery to display the precise blood supply, which varies from patient to patient. The number of vessels requiring division depends on the length of conduit required.

2. Starting at the point chosen for intestinal transection, incise the peritoneal leaves of the mesentery in a vertical

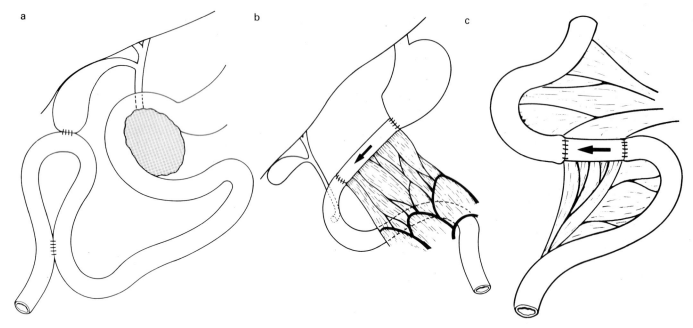

Fig. 6.21 Other types of enteric loop. (a) Intact loop used to drain the distended gallbladder in a case of irresectable pancreatic cancer; side-to-side anastomosis below the cholecystjejunostomy may divert food away from the biliary tree; (b) Isoperistaltic 20 cm jejunal loop interposed between the stomach remnant and the duodenum to treat reflux alkaline gastritis after partial gastrectomy; (c) Reversed 10 cm loop inserted 1 m distal to the ligament of Treitz to treat severe postoperative diarrhoea.

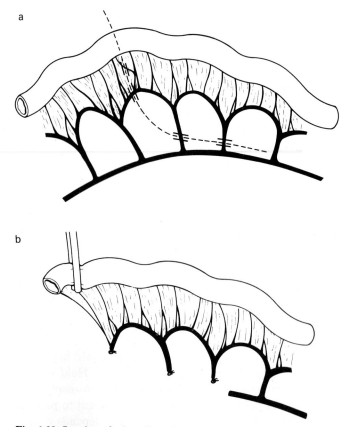

Fig. 6.22 Creation of a long Roux loop. (a) Three arcade vessels have been divided; (b) The bowel is transected at a point previously selected and the loop is mobilised.

direction (Fig. 6.22). Divide at least one vascular arcade and the smaller branches that lie between the arcade vessels and the bowel. Ligate these vessels neatly in continuity and avoid using artery forceps, which can bunch up the tissues and prevent mobilisation of the loop. Now divide the bowel between clamps.

3. If a longer loop is required sacrifice two or three main jejunal vessels, preserving an intact blood supply to the extremity of the bowel via the arcades (Fig. 6.22). The peritoneum may require further incision to facilitate elongation of the loop without tension. Individual ligation of the arteries and veins is recommended, using fine silk sutures. Check the viability of the bowel at the tip of the loop, and sacrifice the end if it is dusky.

4. Straighten out the efferent limb and take it up by the shortest route for anastomosis to the oesophagus, stomach, bile duct, common hepatic duct or pancreatic duct. It is often easier to close the end of the limb and fashion a new subterminal opening of the correct diameter. Make a window in the base of the transverse mesocolon, to the right of the duodenojejunal flexure, for passage of the Roux loop. At the end of the operation suture the margins of this defect to the Roux loop to prevent internal herniation.

5. Restore intestinal continuity by uniting the short afferent limb to the base of the long efferent limb, using an end-to-side anastomosis (p. 110). Ensure that the efferent limb is at least 30 cm long and that the afferent loop is joined to its left-hand side.

Further reading

Allison P R, da Silva L T 1953 The Roux loop. British Journal of
    Surgery 41: 173–180

ENTEROTOMY

Appraise

1. Probably the commonest reason for making an incision into the lumen of the small bowel is to decompress the intestine proximal to the site of an obstruction. The enterotomy should be made halfway between the ligament of Treitz and the site of obstruction, so that the sucker can be inserted both proximally and distally to reach all the distended loops. It is sometimes possible to avoid enterotomy in a high obstruction by advancing the nasogastric tube through the duodenum and squeezing luminal contents upwards until they can be aspirated. In other circumstances the decompressing sucker can be inserted through the proximal cut end of bowel, if enterectomy is planned, or through the caecum and ileocaecal valve after appendicectomy.

2. Sometimes enterotomy is needed to extract a foreign body, for example in gallstone ileus or bolus obstruction. After partial gastrectomy, the absence of the antropyloric mill means that orange pith is inadequately broken up and may impact further down the gut. Benign mucosal or submucosal tumours may be explored and removed through an enterotomy incision.

3. Traumatic enterotomy can result from blunt or penetrating abdominal injuries. After a closed injury there is typically a rosette of exposed mucosa on the antimesenteric border of the upper jejunum. After knife or gunshot injuries, look for entry and exit wounds; holes in the small bowel nearly always come in multiples of two.

4. Very occasionally operative enteroscopy may be indicated for unexplained bleeding localised to the small bowel. A flexible colonoscope can be introduced through a mid enterotomy and threaded up and down the gut.

Action

Decompression enterotomy

1. The objective is to empty the small bowel without contaminating the peritoneal cavity. Pack off the area and apply non-crushing clamps on either side of the site chosen for enterotomy. Insert a catgut purse-string stitch, make a small nick through the wall of the bowel and introduce a Savage decompressor, which consists of a long trocar and cannula connected to the sucker tubing (Fig. 6.23).

2. Pass the sucker up and down the bowel, removing first one clamp and then the other. The assistant feeds the distended loops of gut over the end of the sucker, while the surgeon controls the force of suction by placing a finger

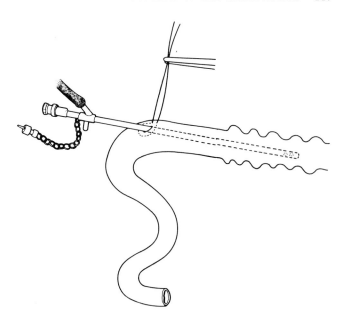

Fig. 6.23 Decompression enterotomy. After insertion of the Savage decompressor, the trocar is withdrawn and the cannula is gently passed along the distended loops of bowel in either direction. Suction tubing is attached to the side-arm of the decompressor.

over a side-port on the decompressing cannula. Sometimes the bowel appears to be only partly deflated, because of interstitial oedema.

3. After emptying the bowel, remove the sucker, tighten and tie the purse-string and discard the contaminated packs. Place a second purse-string suture or Lembert sutures to bury the wound.

Extraction enterotomy

1. It may be possible to knead a foreign body, especially a bolus of food, onwards into the caecum. If so, it will pass spontaneously per rectum. Do not persist with this manoeuvre if it is difficult.

2. Before opening the bowel, pack off the area carefully. Try and manipulate an impacted foreign body upwards for a few centimetres, away from the inflamed segment in which it was lodged.

3. Apply soft clamps across the intestine on either side of the enterotomy site. Open the bowel longitudinally over the foreign body or tumour and gently extract or resect the lesion. Close the bowel transversely in two layers to prevent stenosis.

4. In gallstone ileus examine the right upper quadrant of the abdomen. Consider whether it is appropriate to proceed to cholecystectomy, choledochotomy and possible closure of the biliary-enteric fistula. Since the patient is often elderly and unfit, relief of the intestinal obstruction must be the dominant consideration. Examine the rest of the small bowel to exclude a second gallstone.

Traumatic enterotomy

1. Excise devitalised tissue and close the intestinal wound(s) in two layers. An associated haematoma in the mesentery should be explored, with ligation of any bleeding points. Check the viability of the bowel thereafter, and if in doubt resect the damaged segment with end-to-end anastomosis.

2. Examine the other abdominal viscera for concomitant injuries (see p. 52).

Further reading

Celestin L R 1981 Small intestine. In: Keen G (ed) Operative Surgery and Management. Wright P S G, Bristol p 128–144
Robbs J V, Moore S W, Pillay G P 1980 Blunt abdominal trauma with jejunal injury: a review. Journal of Trauma 20: 308–311

ENTEROSTOMY

Appraise

1. A feeding jejunostomy permits enteral nutrition in patients who are unable to take sufficient food by mouth. The development of parenteral nutrition has limited its use to certain circumstances, for example the preoperative hyperalimentation of malnourished patients with cancer of the stomach or oesophagus. Better still, it may be possible to pass a fine transnasal feeding tube through the malignant stricture under endoscopic control.

2. A feeding tube should always be placed as high as possible in the jejunum. Nevertheless it can be difficult to introduce enough calories and nitrogen by this route without causing troublesome diarrhoea. Some surgeons use feeding jejunostomy routinely after major oesophagogastric resections. Others reserve it for post-operative complications (fistula etc.) or serious upper gastrointestinal conditions, such as corrosive oesophagogastritis or pancreatic abscess.

3. The ideal feeding jejunostomy is easily inserted, if necessary under local anaesthesia, and seals off immediately it is removed. It neither obstructs the bowel nor permits the escape of intestinal contents. I favour the use of a T-tube for this purpose.

4. A terminal ileostomy replaces the anus after total colectomy for multiple neoplasia, ulcerative proctocolitis or Crohn's colitis. The ileostomy may be temporary, if subsequent ileorectal anastomosis is planned, or permanent after panproctocolectomy. Improvements in stoma care make ileostomy less of a burden to patients, many of whom are young. It is desirable and usually possible to select and mark the site for ileostomy preoperatively. Choose a point just below waist level and 5 cm to the right of the midline, unless there is a previous scar in this region. It is important to create a spout that will discharge its irritative contents well clear of the skin.

5. Other types of ileostomy are sometimes fashioned. A loop ileostomy can be used for temporary protection of a precarious anastomosis in the right colon. Split ileostomy (separated stomas) will completely defunction the distal bowel and has been advocated in selected cases of colitis; the distal cut end is exteriorised as a mucous fistula. Kock's continent ileostomy consists of an ileal reservoir discharging by a short conduit to a flush stoma; a nipple valve is created to preserve continence, and the patient empties the reservoir regularly with a soft catheter. Lastly, a 'wet' ileostomy together with an ileal conduit provides one of the commoner methods for achieving urinary diversion (see p. 232).

Action

Feeding jejunostomy

1. Expose the upper jejunum through a small left upper paramedian or transverse incision. Trace the bowel proximally to the duodenojejunal flexure. Select a loop a few centimetres distal to this point, so that it will easily reach the anterior abdominal wall.

2. Insert a catgut purse-string suture on the antimesenteric border of the bowel. Make a tiny enterotomy in the centre of the purse-string and introduce a T-tube (14 FG) into the lumen of the bowel (Fig. 6.24). Tighten the purse-string snugly around the tube.

3. An alternative method employs a Foley catheter subsequently inflated with 5–10 ml of water. After tightening the purse string, the catheter and its point of entry into the

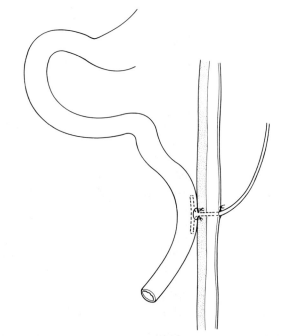

Fig. 6.24 Feeding jejunostomy. The T-tube is brought out through the abdominal wall, and the jejunum is stitched to the peritoneum around the margins of the stab incision.

bowel are buried with Lembert sutures (Witzel jejunostomy).

4. Whichever tube is used, it should be introduced first through a stab incision in the abdominal wall and then into the jejunum. Traction on the tube will approximate the bowel to the underside of the abdominal wall, where the intestine should be sutured to the peritoneum.

Terminal ileostomy

1. Excise a circular disc of skin and subcutaneous fat, 3 cm in diameter, at the site marked preoperatively. Make a cruciate incision in the exposed anterior rectus sheath, split the fibres of the rectus muscle and open the posterior sheath and peritoneum. The defect should comfortably accommodate two fingers.

2. The terminal ileum will previously have been clamped and transected. Now exteriorize 6–8 cm of bowel (with its mesentery intact) through the circular opening in the abdominal wall, leaving its end securely clamped. Make sure that the mesentery is neither twisted nor tight and that the tip of the ileum remains pink.

3. Some surgeons close the lateral space between the ileostomy and the abdominal wall, using a running catgut suture (Fig. 6.25). Others tunnel the ileum extraperitoneally. I prefer transperitoneal ileostomy, leaving the lateral space widely open. In this case, however, it is important to suture the seromuscular layer of the bowel to

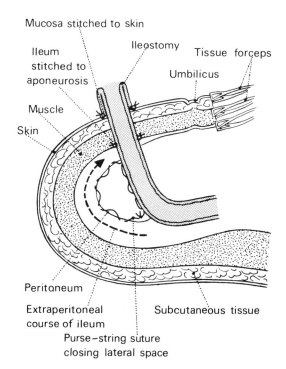

Mucosa stitched to skin

Ileostomy

Tissue forceps

Umbilicus

Ileum stitched to aponeurosis

Muscle

Skin

Peritoneum

Extraperitoneal course of ileum

Subcutaneous tissue

Purse–string suture closing lateral space

Fig. 6.25 Terminal ileostomy. Two methods of closing the lateral space are shown: a purse-string suture or taking the ileum along an extraperitoneal track. Alternatively, the lateral space can be left widely open. Tissue forceps on each layer of the wound edge prevent retraction of the layers while the ileostomy is being fashioned.

the margins of the defect at peritoneal level. Take great care not to enter the lumen of the ileum when inserting these stitches.

4. After closing the main abdominal incision, remove the clamp and trim the crushed portion of ileum. Now suture the edge of the ileum directly to the skin, using catgut mounted on an atraumatic taper-pointed needle. After inserting three or four evenly-spaced sutures, the bowel will begin to evert spontaneously; if not, use Babcock's forceps to encourage eversion. Complete the circumferential sutures, producing a spout which should project about 3 cm from the abdominal wall.

5. Carefully clean and dry the skin around the ileostomy and apply an ileostomy bag at once.

Aftercare

1. Feeding jejunostomy. Keep the tube patent by introducing 5–10 ml of sterile water hourly. When bowel sounds return, increase the amount of water before switching to half-strength and then full-strength liquid feed. Consult the dietitian about the patient's individual nutritional needs. Give codeine or loperamide to control diarrhoea. When oral feeding is resumed, spigot the tube for 24–48 hours before removal.

2. Ileostomy. Increase oral fluids when the stoma commences to discharge. The effluent will be very loose at first but will gradually thicken as the ileum adapts. Give bulking agents or anti-diarrhoeal drugs as needed. Consult the stomatherapist directly, if she has not already seen the patient before operation. Make sure that the patient is competent and confident at managing the stoma before he leaves hospital.

Further reading

Goligher J C. 1980 Surgical treatment of ulcerative colitis. In: Surgery of the anus, rectum and colon, 4th edn. Bailliere Tindall, London p 733–826
Todd I P 1980 A critical review of stomas, stomatherapy and newer operative techniques. In: Taylor S (ed) Recent advances in surgery 10. Churchill Livingstone, Edinburgh P 281–292

MISCELLANEOUS CONDITIONS

MECKEL'S DIVERTICULUM

1. Potential complications include bleeding, infection, peptic ulceration, perforation, intestinal obstruction or fistulation to the umbilicus. Usually this remnant of the allantois gives no trouble at all, however, throughout the patient's life. Meckel's diverticulum should be left alone if encountered at laparotomy, unless it is thought to be the cause of symptoms.

2. The first step in Meckelian diverticulectomy is to divide the small vessel that crosses the ileum to supply it.

Depending on the size of the mouth of the diverticulum, it can simply be transected across the neck or excised with a portion of the antimesenteric border of the bowel (see p. 112). Local resection of the ileum with end-to-end anastomosis may be preferable in a complicated case.

INTUSSUSCEPTION

In infants

1. Ileocolic intussusception usually presents in a child of a few months old with abdominal colic and rectal passage of blood and mucus. Besides confirming the diagnosis, barium enema may reduce the intussusception totally or subtotally. On examination under anaesthetic, if not before, a mass can be felt in the central or upper abdomen with an 'empty' right iliac fossa.

2. Open the abdomen through a right Lanz incision and find the sausage-shaped mass. Starting at the apex, squeeze the intussusceptum back along the intussuscipiens as though extracting toothpaste from the bottom of the tube. Do not remove the bowel from the abdominal cavity during this manoeuvre.

3. The final portion of the intussusception is the most difficult to reduce. Deliver the affected segment from the abdomen and gently compress it with a moist swab, before resuming the squeeze. Make certain that reduction is complete before replacing the bowel. No fixation is required, except in the rare event of a recurrent intussusception.

4. If the bowel is clearly gangrenous or the intussusception cannot be reduced, proceed to resection. Usually an end-to-end ileoileostomy can be performed.

In adults

1. Intussusception is rare and is nearly always associated with an underlying lesion in the bowel wall, e.g. benign tumour or Meckel's diverticulum.

2. Reduce the intussusception as far as possible, then proceed to local resection of the affected segment of bowel with end-to-end anastomosis.

INTESTINAL ISCHAEMIA

1. The small intestine is supplied by the superior mesenteric (midgut) vessels. Thrombosis may occur on arteriosclerotic plaques at the origin of the superior mesenteric artery, especially if the patient is shocked. The superior mesenteric artery is an uncommon site for peripheral embolism in patients with cardiac arrhythmia or a recent myocardial infarction. Venous gangrene may result if the superior mesenteric or portal veins suddenly thrombose, for example in extreme dehydration or disseminated intra-

vascular coagulation. Lastly, patchy ischaemia can result from damage to the microcirculation in vasculitic conditions or septicaemia.

2. Patients with severe mesenteric vascular insufficiency are extremely ill with evidence of peritonitis and shock. Early operation is needed to prevent death. At laparotomy, the bowel appears ischaemic or frankly infarcted without evidence of strangulation.

3. Examine the whole intestinal tract and feel for pulsation in all accessible gut arteries. Examine the aorta and its main divisions to determine the extent of atherosclerosis. If the main intestinal vessels and their arcades are patent, the circulation is probably occluded at capillary level.

4. Obviously-necrotic bowel must be resected. Recovery is unlikely if the entire midgut is infarcted following occlusion of the main superior mesenteric vessels. If an extensive segment is affected, be as conservative as possible to avoid severe short bowel syndrome (see p. 113). Multiple patches of ischaemia can be oversewn or locally resected.

5. Early cases of arterial embolus or acute in-situ thrombosis may be amenable to revascularization. It is much easier to mobilise the caecum and identify the ileocolic artery than to expose the origin of the superior mesenteric artery itself. Control the vessel with tapes and perform a longitudinal arteriotomy. Pass a Fogarty catheter proximally into the superior mesenteric artery and aorta to dislodge the clot, and try to establish free flow. Rapid injection of heparin saline up the vessel may achieve the same effect. If the bowel regains its normal colour, close the arteriotomy with a venous patch. Otherwise consider side-to-side anastomosis between the ileocolic and right common iliac arteries.

6. Following direct arterial surgery or in any case in which bowel of doubtful viability has been left in the abdomen, plan to repeat the laparotomy after 24 hours. Further resection of bowel may be clearly indicated at this time.

SMALL-BOWEL FISTULA

1. The spontaneous discharge of bowel contents onto the abdominal wall is a rare event. The vast majority of external fistulas arise from either a leaking anastomosis or operative injury to the intestine. Besides impaired healing, radiation enteritis, multiple adhesions, diffuse carcinoma and Crohn's disease predispose to fistula formation.

2. Do not rush to reoperate once there is an established small-bowel fistula. Correct fluid and electrolyte depletion. Switch to total parenteral nutrition both to maintain health and to reduce the amount of intestinal contents discharged. Consult a stomatherapist on how best to protect the wound and abdominal wall from the effluent, using adhesive seals and collecting bags as appropriate. Consider

constant suction through a catheter placed in the fistula if the discharge is particularly profuse.

3. Obtain an early fistulogram to delineate the leak. A side-hole may well close if there is no distal obstruction, but a complete anastomotic dehiscence is almost certain to require reoperation once the patient's general condition allows.

4. If the patient is toxic, early drainage of an associated abscess may improve his general health and sometimes allow the fistula to heal. If a complete dehiscence is encountered at this time, it is probably better to exteriorise the bowel ends rather than attempt a repeat anastomosis under unpromising circumstances. This counsel may not be appropriate for a high jejunal fistula, however.

5. Definitive operation to close a small-bowel fistula should not ordinarily be undertaken by an inexperienced surgeon. Resection of the damaged portion of bowel is generally indicated. Take care to divide any adhesions that could partially obstruct the distal gut and lead to recurrence of the fistula. Continue nutritional support during the postoperative healing phase.

INTESTINAL OBSTRUCTION

See Chapter 4.

Further reading

Alexander-Williams J, Irving M H 1982 Intestinal fistulas. Wrights, Bristol
Marston J A P 1977 Intestinal ischaemia. Arnold, London
Moore T, Johnston A O 1976 Complications of Meckel's diverticulum. British Journal of Surgery 63: 453–454
Pollet J E 1980 Intussusception: a study of its surgical management. British Journal of Surgery 67: 213–215

Surgery of the appendix and abdominal abscess

Appendicectomy
Appendix abscess
Subphrenic and subhepatic abscess

APPENDICECTOMY

Appraise

1. Appendicitis is still the commonest single reason for laparotomy. At any age, tenderness and guarding in the right iliac fossa raise the possibility of acute appendicitis, but consider alternative diagnoses particularly in two groups of patients:

a) Girls between the menarche and the age of 25 are the commonest group to undergo a needless appendicectomy. Be prepared to repeat clinical examination at regular intervals if the physical signs are equivocal. Consider laparoscopy (see Ch. 17) to exclude lesions of the uterine tube and ovary.

b) The elderly are by no means immune from appendicitis, but they are more likely than the young to have other causes of peritonitis, such as perforating carcinoma of the caecum and diverticulitis. Keep an open mind, therefore, and give thought to the best incision (see below).

2. A good case can be made for delaying appendicectomy if the patient has an obvious mass in the right iliac fossa by the time of admission. Be prepared to intervene surgically if there is any evidence of clinical deterioration. Operation for an appendix abscess is described later in this chapter. If an appendix mass has been treated conservatively, proceed to interval appendicectomy within 1–2 months. Over the age of 40–50 consider having a barium enema examination performed, when the acute condition has settled, to exclude caecal carcinoma.

3. Beware of removing a normal appendix casually during other operations. If laparotomy for suspected appendicitis (either acute or recurrent) proves negative, you should look for another cause for symptoms and or-

dinarily proceed to appendicectomy. Problems can arise, however, if you struggle to remove the appendix through an inadequate incision, for example during cholecystectomy or vagotomy.

4. Do not forget to examine the abdomen once the patient has been anaesthetized for operation. The finding of a mass at this stage should never deter you from proceeding to laparotomy, but it may well help you to site the incision correctly.

5. Consider antibiotic prophylaxis. It is a safe principle to insert one metronidazole suppository (1 g) when you make the original decision to operate. Start parenteral antibiotics preoperatively in the presence of generalised peritonitis.

Access

The skin incision

1. The neatest incision for appendicectomy is undoubtedly the horizontal (Lanz) modification of the oblique gridiron incision. I use this incision routinely in young and middle-aged patients, unless they are very obese or the diagnosis is in serious doubt. The incision starts about 2 cm below and medial to the right anterior superior iliac spine and extends medially for 5–7 cm, either transversely or with a slight downward obliquity. The exact level of the incision may be modified by the examination under anaesthetic, but in a girl it is worth trying to place it close to the bikini line.

2. The classical gridiron incision (Fig. 7.1) can be extended in either direction a little more readily than the Lanz incision. I favour this approach in elderly or fat patients or if the diagnosis of appendicitis is tenous. The incision is 7–10 cm long in the adult. It starts 2 cm above the iliac crest and should cross McBurney's point, which lies at the junction of the middle and outer thirds of a line joining the umbilicus to the right anterior superior iliac spine; the incision ends medial to the linea semilunaris.

3. The excellence of a gridiron incision (with or without

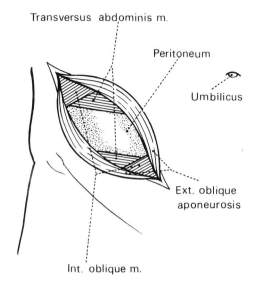

Transversus abdominis m.

Peritoneum

Umbilicus

Ext. oblique aponeurosis

Int. oblique m.

Fig. 7.1 Gridiron incision for appendicectomy. In the Lanz modification the skin incision is transverse, but the abdominal muscles are similarly split in the line of their fibres

the Lanz modification) is such that it should be preferred to a vertical incision if appendicitis seems at all likely. If there are no localizing signs whatsoever to explain peritonitis, then proceed as described in Chapter 4 (p. 53).

Opening the abdomen

1. Make a clean incision through the skin with the belly of the knife. Divide the subcutaneous fat, Scarpa's fascia and subjacent areolar tissue to expose the glistening fibres of the external oblique aponeurosis. In the classical gridiron approach these fibres run parallel to the skin incision.

2. Stop the bleeding. Incise the external oblique aponeurosis in the line of its fibres. Start the cut with a scalpel, then use the partly-closed blades of the scissors to complete the split while your assistant retracts the skin edges (Fig. 7.2).

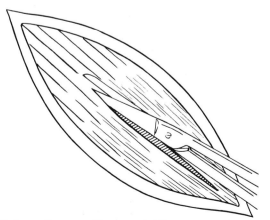

Fig. 7.2 Appendicectomy. The external oblique anastomosis is split by pushing partly closed scissors in the line of the fibres

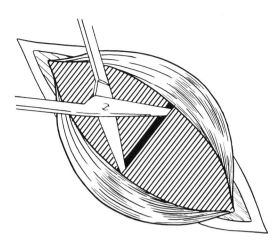

Fig. 7.3 Appendicectomy. The internal oblique muscle is split by opening Mayo's straight scissors in the line of the fibres

3. Retract the external oblique aponeurosis to display the fibres of the internal oblique muscle, which run at right angles. Split the fibres of the internal oblique and transversus abdominis muscles, using Mayo's straight scissors (Fig. 7.3). Open the blades in the line of the fibres and use both index fingers to widen the split. Provided the scissors are not thrust in violently, the transversalis fascia and peritoneum are pushed away unopened.

4. Stop the bleeding. Have the muscles retracted firmly to display the fused transversalis fascia and peritoneum.

5. Pick up a fold of peritoneum with toothed dissecting forceps and grasp the tented portion with artery forceps. Release the dissecting forceps and take a fresh grasp to ensure that only peritoneum is held. Make a small incision through the peritoneum using a knife. Allow air to enter the peritoneal cavity, so that the viscera fall away. Use scissors to enlarge the hole in the line of the skin incision. Now protect the wound edges with swabs or skin towels.

Assess

1. Aspirate any free fluid or pus, preserving a specimen for laboratory examination and culture for organisms.

2. Find the caecum and identify its taeniae. If it does not present immediately in the wound, insert a finger into the peritoneal cavity, pass it to the right under the anterior abdominal wall, laterally into the iliac fossa and then medially until the caecum is reached. Gently deliver the caecum into the wound, more by pushing from within than by pulling from without.

3. Follow the anterior taenia of the caecum downwards to the base of the appendix. Trace the appendix right to its tip and if it is free, gently deliver it by pushing from within.

4. Confirm the diagnosis by observing swelling, vascular congestion, fibrin deposition, inflammatory adhesions, necrosis, turbid free fluid or frank pus.

5. If the appendix is not obviously inflamed, examine the caecum and terminal 1.5 m ileum together with its mesentery to exclude other local causes of inflammation. Insert two fingers into the abdomen and palpate the posterior abdominal wall, ascending colon, lower pole of right kidney, liver edge and fundus of gallbladder, pelvic brim, right iliac vessels, fundus of bladder and right inguinal region. In the female examine the right ovary and uterine tube and try to reach the uterus, left ovary and tube.

6. If there is obvious appendicitis, the examination of other organs can be less detailed, but it is sensible to exclude Meckel's diverticulum, Crohn's disease or obvious pelvic pathology. In the presence of severe local sepsis the laparotomy should be curtailed for fear of disseminating the infection.

7. Exclude carcinoid tumour of the appendix, usually a localised yellowish tumour at the tip, for which appendicectomy will nearly always be curative. Exclude also the rare adenocarcinoma of the appendix, which requires right hemicolectomy. Remember that carcinoma of the caecum or ascending colon occasionally presents with obstructive appendicitis.

Action

1. Mobilize the appendix from base to tip, gently freeing it with an index finger. Remember that the appendix may be adherent to the caecum in a paracaecal or retrocaecal position. The blood supply to the appendix reaches its medial aspect, so that it is usually safe to break down any adhesions laterally with blunt finger dissection. If the tip of the appendix is adherent in a pelvic or retrocaecal position, have the assistant retract one or other end of the wound to display the anatomy and allow you to separate the adhesions under direct vision. Never pull hard on the base of the appendix and never use scissors to cut blindly.

2. Apply Babcock's tissue forceps to enclose the organ without crushing it, so that it can be lifted vertically (Fig. 7.4). View the vessels in the mesoappendix against the light. Make a hole through a window near the base of the appendix.

3. Pass one blade of an artery forceps through the hole and clamp the appendicular vessels. If the mesoappendix is wide or thick, it may be safer to clamp it in two separate bites. Often there is a small vessel near the caecal wall, which may be ligated separately. Cut through the mesoappendix close to the appendix, leaving a generous fringe of tissue projecting from the forceps. Gently but firmly ligate the mesoappendix as the forceps are opened and withdrawn; use 0 or 2/0 chromic catgut or silk.

4. Do not worry about the small amount of back bleeding from the appendiceal side of the mesoappendix. Proceed to crush the base of the appendix with a haemostat. Release and reapply the haemostat 0.5 cm distally. Ligate the crushed portion of the appendix with 0 chromic catgut. Apply a forceps close to the knot and cut off the ends of suture material (Fig. 7.5).

5. Using a knife, cut off the appendix immediately proximal to the haemostat. Briefly cauterise the exposed mucosa of the stump, using the knife to transmit the diathermy current. Stop! You have now entered the bowel; the knife, appendix, artery forceps and tissue forceps must immediately be placed in a dish reserved for contaminated articles.

6. Insert a seromuscular purse-string or Z stitch into the caecum, using 2/0 catgut mounted on a round-bodied needle. Place each bite at least 10–15 mm from the base of the appendix stump, or you will have difficulty invaginating it.

7. Use the forceps applied to the stump ligature to invaginate the stump while tightening the purse-string or Z stitch. Remove the forceps. Tie the purse-string.

8. Always send the appendix for histological examin-

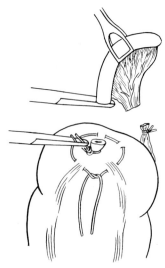

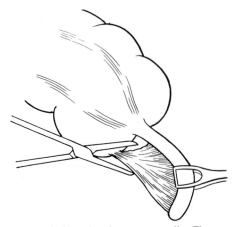

Fig. 7.4 Appendicectomy. Clamping the mesoappendix. The appendix is held up with tissue forceps

Fig. 7.5 Appendicectomy. The resected appendix, together with the haemostat at its base and the tissue forceps, is placed in a separate dish. The ligated stump of the appendix is invaginated while tying the purse-string suture.

ation. Besides confirming the clinical diagnosis, it may reveal unsuspected conditions such as threadworm, actinomycosis, carcinoid or carcinoma, which may require further treatment.

Difficulty?

1. You cannot carry out any of the preceding steps with ease and safety, usually because of inadequate exposure. The incision was planned for the minimum difficulty, so there is no shame in enlarging it. Indeed, infection resulting from excessive retraction and trauma to the wound edges is much more likely to spoil the cosmetic appearance of the incision. As a first step cut all the muscles in the line of the skin incision in one or other direction. Do not hesitate to enlarge the whole incision; carry it into the loin to reach a high retrocaecal appendix or medially to reach an adherent pelvic appendix. If you extend the incision medially, curve it downwards at the edge of the rectum sheath. If necessary, enter the sheath, ligate and divide the inferior epigastric vessels and displace or transect the rectus muscle. Stop all the fresh bleeding.

2. You cannot find the caecum. If small bowel keeps prolapsing through the wound, explore further laterally with your finger. Sometimes large bowel presents, but further exploration reveals that it is the sigmoid or even the transverse colon. Replace it and start again. Remember that the caecum is sometimes high and tucked up under the liver. Preoperative examination should alert you to this possibility.

3. Having found the caecum, you cannot identify the appendix. This problem is usually encountered with a retrocaecal appendix. Incise the parietal peritoneum in the right paracolic gutter and elevate the caecum to inspect its posterior surface. If you draw a blank, remember that the appendix can lie in a pre-ileal or post-ileal position and try to display the ileocaecal junction.

4. You cannot deliver the tip of the appendix. Do not just pull blindly or the organ may rupture, especially if it is turgid and inflamed. Improve the view by carefully placing retractors, adjusting the light, extending the incision.

5. Retrograde appendicectomy is sometimes useful for a high retrocaecal organ, but it still requires adequate exposure. First clamp, ligate and divide the base, leaving a forceps on the transected organ as before. Then pulling very gently on this forceps, open up the space between the adherent appendix and the caecum, clamping and dividing the mesoappendix as you go. In this way you can gradually free the organ towards its tip.

6. The appendix bursts as you deliver it. Try and anticipate this problem and avoid it by gentle manipulation, but have suction ready if the organ is obviously friable. If perforation has occurred before or during appendicectomy, look for faecaliths and consider saline lavage and postoperative drainage.

7. The base of the appendix is grossly oedematous, necrotic or perforated. Do not crush it as usual, but ligate it and cut off the appendix 5 mm distally. If the ligature cuts through, one or two all-coats sutures may close the hole. Infold the area with sutures applied to a portion of healthy caecal wall. Sometimes it is better not to attempt to invaginate the stump but to ligate it securely and cauterise the exposed mucosa. Try and find a nearby piece of omentum or an appendix epiploica to tie over the area.

8. Rarely gangrene extends onto the caecal wall. Apply a non-crushing clamp to healthy caecum, making sure not to include any of the ileocaecal junction. Resect the apex of the caecum together with the appendix and close the caecal wall in two layers, as for an intestinal anastomosis. If all else fails, place a large tube drain in the hole, bring the area to the surface and stitch the surrounding caecum to the skin. The caecostomy will probably close spontaneously after the tube is removed.

9. You find Crohn's disease. If the appendix is not inflamed, do not remove it. If there is Crohn's terminal ileitis and coincident acute appendicitis, it is safe to remove the appendix provided the caecal apex is healthy. In the rare situation in which acute appendicitis coexists with Crohn's disease of the caecum or right colon, proceed to ileocaecal resection or right hemicolectomy.

10. If the appendix cannot be found within a localized abscess cavity, do not hesitate to drain the abscess and leave the appendix.

11. If there is generalised purulent peritonitis, first deal with the appendix, making sure that you have adequate exposure. Now gently remove with sucker and swabs all the pus and debris, remembering that it may have percolated along the paracolic gutter and down into the pelvis. Drain the wound (at least) post-operatively (see below).

Check list

1. If the appendix was not grossly inflamed, is there another cause for the clinical picture?
(a) Examine the caecum, ascending and sigmoid colon for signs of inflammation, ulcer, diverticula or growth.
(b) If the terminal ileum is red and oedematous with thickening of the mesentery, the patient has terminal ileitis, probably Crohn's disease but possibly yersinial or even tuberculous. Remove a lymph node both for bacteriological culture and histological examination. Soft, oedematous glands and a normal ileum probably represent mesenteric adenitis, a benign self-limiting disease.
(c) Exclude Meckelian diverticulitis by examining the last 1–1.5 m of ileum
(d) Is the bowel healthy, with a good blood supply?
(e) If you feel gross pathology in the liver, gallbladder, duodenum, or right kidney, consider whether it would be best to enlarge the incision and deal with the lesion

(if acute) or close the abdomen and investigate the patient thereafter. Similar principles should guide your management of pelvic lesions, for example of the female reproductive organs.

2. If free fluid was found, has its presence been explained? If there was also free gas, you must locate the site of visceral perforation; it will usually be necessary to close the Lanz or gridiron incision and proceed to midline laparotomy.

3. Re-examine the operation site. Is the appendix stump safely closed? Are the ligatures on the mesoappendix secure?

4. Is a wound drain required? I use these more readily than peritoneal drains in appendicitis. If contamination has been modest, systemic antibiotics (e.g. metronidazole suppositories) or a local antiseptic spray (e.g. povidone iodine) will usually suffice. If the wound has been more severely contaminated, insertion of a fine corrugated drain down to the site of peritoneal closure is probably a sensible precaution.

5. Suture the split edges of the internal oblique and transversus abdominis muscles (together), using 1 or 2 interrupted sutures of 0 chromic catgut. Tie the stitch(es) just tightly enough to appose the muscle edges. Consider leaving this layer open if you have inserted a wound drain.

6. Close the external oblique aponeurosis, using a running stitch of 0 or 2/0 chromic catgut.

7. Ensure complete haemostasis. Close the skin using either interrupted sutures or (in a 'clean' case) a running subcuticular stitch. Apply a small dressing to the wound.

Aftercare

1. In the absence of general peritonitis, free oral fluids can usually be tolerated within 24 hours of operation.

2. In gangrenous appendicitis, it is reasonable to continue antibiotic prophylaxis, e.g. in the form of metronidazole suppositories, for 24 hours postoperatively. In perforated appendicitis parenteral antibiotics should be given for a minimum of 3 days.

3. Wound drains can usually be removed within 2–3 days.

4. If postoperative pyrexia develops, exclude chest and urinary infection. Examine the wound carefully for signs of local sepsis. Perform rectal examination; high, anterior tenderness and a boggy swelling suggest the development of a pelvic abscess. Repeated pelvic examinations will indicate when the abscess is beginning to point. At this stage, thorough digital examination may allow the pus to burst into the rectum. Alternatively, carry out rectal (or vaginal) examination under general anaesthetic. Try and aspirate pus with a needle inserted through the rectal or vaginal wall, and then thrust a pair of artery forceps through the wall to drain the abscess.

Further reading

Keddie N 1975 Appendicectomy. British Journal of Hospital Medicine 14: 175–188

Lewis F R, Holcroft J W, Boey J, Dunphy J E 1975 Appendicitis: a critical review of diagnosis and treatment in 1000 cases. Archives of Surgery 110: 677–684

Mosegaard A, Nielsen O S 1979 Interval appendicectomy: a retrospective study. Acta Chirurgica Scandinavica 145: 109–111

Pinto D J, Sanderson P J 1980 Rational use of antibiotic therapy after appendicectomy. British Medical Journal 280: 275–277

Silen W 1979 Cope's early diagnosis of the acute abdomen, 15th edn. Oxford University Press, London

APPENDIX ABSCESS

Appraise

1. An appendix mass results when perforation of the appendix is walled off by omentum and adherent viscera. This condition may settle with conservative treatment, but increasing pyrexia and leucocytosis indicate suppuration. Prompt drainage of the abscess is now required, with or without appendicectomy.

2. Modern antibiotics have made it less hazardous to operate at the appendix mass stage and thus avoid the delay inherent in conservative management. It is usually possible to identify and remove the appendix without risking injury to the caecum or small bowel, but if in doubt forego appendicectomy and leave a drain in situ.

Access

Define the limits of the mass by careful examination under anaesthetic. Proceed to make a standard gridiron or Lanz incision. You may encounter oedema in the deeper layers of the abdominal wall.

Action

1. You may enter directly into the abscess cavity on incising the peritoneum. Do not rush to open the wound any further. Gently and thoroughly aspirate all pus and debris, saving a specimen of pus for bacteriological culture. Explore the cavity carefully with your finger to see if it is safe to enlarge the opening without damaging viscera or breaking down the cavity walls.

2. If the abscess cavity can safely be opened up, you may see the appendix and be able to remove it, sometimes piecemeal. Make sure that the whole appendix is removed, not just the healthy proximal stump of a completely disintegrated organ.

3. If you cannot find the appendix or if it is unsafe to open up the abscess cavity, insert a tube or corrugated drain and close the wound in layers loosely around the drain.

4. You may open into the peritoneal cavity and find the mass lying posteriorly. Once again decide whether simply to drain the mass or to separate the adherent omentum and viscera and search for the appendix. If you decide to proceed, pack off the rest of the peritoneal cavity and gently explore the mass, looking for a line of cleavage, before committing yourself. Remember that inflamed tissues are extremely friable, and retreat if the going becomes difficult.

5. The mass or abscess may be retrocaecal, retroileal or pelvic in position. Be prepared to mobilise the caecum and terminal ileum and explore gently below the pelvic brim. As before try and pack off the healthy viscera before breaking down adhesions to find the appendix.

6. Whether or not you remove the appendix, it is sensible to leave a drain in the peritoneal cavity at the end of the operation.

Further reading

Bradley E L III, Isaacs J 1978 Appendiceal abscess revisited. Archives of Surgery 113: 130–132

Foran B, Berne T V, Rosoff L 1978 Management of the appendiceal mass. Archives of Surgery 113: 1144–1145

SUBPHRENIC AND SUBHEPATIC ABSCESS

Appraise

1. Following major abdominal operations, abscesses may develop above the liver (subphrenic), below the liver (subhepatic), along either paracolic gutter, between loops of bowel in the mid abdomen or in the pelvis (see above). Causes include retained foreign bodies or necrotic tissue, inadequate drainage of blood or contaminated fluid and subclinical anastomotic leakage.

2. The diagnosis is suggested by continuing fever, toxicity and leucocytosis. Paralysis of the hemi-diaphragm and 'sympathetic' pleural effusion often accompany a true subphrenic collection. Modern methods of scanning (ultrasound, CT, isotope) are invaluable for localising the abscess. Besides confirming the site, needle aspiration can provide pus for culture and sometimes avoid the need for formal operative drainage of the abscess.

3. Strictly, the term 'subphrenic' should be reserved for an abscess lying immediately below the diaphragm, confined on the right by the liver and on the left by the liver, spleen or stomach (Fig. 7.6). Right subhepatic collections can be anterior (paraduodenal) or posterior (above the right kidney) (Fig. 7.7). Similarly, left subhepatic collections lie anterior to the stomach and transverse colon or posteriorly in the lesser sac.

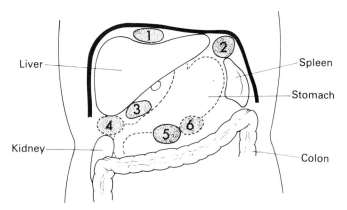

Fig. 7.6 Common sites of abscess above and below the liver. 1. right subphrenic; 2. left subphrenic; 3. right anterior subhepatic; 4. right posterior subhepatic (hepatorenal); 5. left anterior subhepatic; 6. left posterior subhepatic (lesser sac).

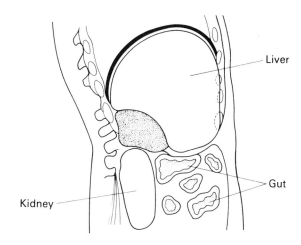

Fig. 7.7 Abscess in the hepatorenal pouch (right posterior subhepatic). This type of posterior collection may be drained by an extraperitoneal approach from behind, through the bed of the 12th rib, or from an anterolateral direction.

Action

Choice of approach

1. Drainage of the abscess by an extrapleural, extraperitoneal route is ideal, but in practice it is only appropriate for a loculated posterior collection, usually on the right. Such an abscess can be entered posteriorly through the bed of the twelfth rib or anterolaterally without opening the peritoneal cavity.

2. Abscesses that are multiple, poorly localised or anteriorly placed are best approached transperitoneally by formal laparotomy.

Posterior approach

1. Place the patient in the full lateral position with the side of the abscess uppermost. Identify the twelfth rib, and

make a transverse incision 10 cm long crossing its midpoint.

2. Cut down to the rib, incise the periosteum and resect the rib, as for the approach to the kidney (p. 222). Incise the bed of the rib transversely, taking care to avoid entering the pleural cavity. Divide the attachment of the diaphragm. Displace the kidney forwards.

3. Feel for the lower edge of the liver, and explore with syringe and needle to locate a right posterior subhepatic abscess. If pus is found, open into the cavity and suck out the pus and debris. Insert a tube drain into the cavity.

4. Separate peritoneum from the undersurface of the diaphragm to reach a right or left subphrenic abscess.

Anterolateral approach

1. Place the patient supine with a sandbag to elevate the flank on the affected side.

2. Make a lateral subcostal incision 1 cm below the costal margin and cut through all layers down to but not including the peritoneum.

3. Strip the peritoneum from the undersurface of the diaphragm until the abscess is reached; open it and drain it.

4. If no pus is found, consider if the peritoneum should be opened to allow exploration of the abdomen.

Transperitoneal approach

1. Choose a midline or subcostal incision according to the likely site of the abscess.

2. Carry out a formal laparotomy. Explore the right and left subphrenic spaces. Examine the area beneath the right lobe of the liver and the hepatorenal pouch. Enter the lesser sac through the greater omentum.

3. If you encounter an abscess, pack off the rest of the peritoneal cavity before opening it. Suck out the pus and drain the cavity through a separate stab wound.

Further reading

Dunphy J E 1983 Peritoneal cavity. In: Way L W (ed) Current surgical diagnosis and treatment, 6th edn. Lange Medical Publications, Los Altos, p 422–436

Norton L, Eule J, Burdick D 1978 Accuracy of techniques to detect intraperitoneal abscesses. Surgery 84: 370–378

Colonic surgery

EXAMINATION OF THE LARGE BOWEL

Pre-operative assessment

Obtain a full history and carry out a complete examination before any surgical procedure. Examine the abdomen and anus and rectum in every patient before undertaking surgery of the large bowel. This implies a thorough digital examination of the rectum and the passage of a rigid sigmoidoscope which is an out-patient or bedside procedure. Carry out further investigations as necessary.

1. *Fibreoptic sigmoidoscopy.* A simple out-patient procedure undertaken after clearing out the left colon with one or two hypophosphate enemas. This will immediately reveal the diagnosis of polyps or a carcinoma in the proximal sigmoid or descending colon.

2. *Barium enema.* Carry out a barium enema on patients with suspected pathology above the reach of a sigmoidoscope. This should routinely be a double contrast (Malmo) enema as this records much more pathology such as polyps and fine degrees of ulceration than the single contrast technique.

3. *Instant barium enema.* Barium is instilled into the rectum without any preparation. This is very useful in inflammatory bowel disease when the upper limit of disease can be obtained during the out-patient visit.

4. *Colonoscopy.* This has not taken the place of air contrast barium enema but compliments it. Carry out this investigation to evaluate equivocal findings on a barium enema. Pedunculated polyps will be removed by colonoscopic snaring. Biopsies of tumours and inflammatory bowel disease can be obtained from the proximal colon. Carry out colonscopy in the evaluation of gastro-intestinal bleeding suspected from the colon.

5. *Other examinations.* Other examinations which may be of value in the assessment of large bowel disease include mucosal biopsy in inflammatory bowel disease to help in the differentiation of ulcerative colitis, Crohn's disease and infective colitis. Stool microscopy and culture to differentiate bacterial and parasitic infection from inflammatory bowel disease. Straight X-ray of the abdomen in suspected large bowel obstruction or perforation. Serial abdominal films are important in evaluating the progress of acute colitis and the onset of toxic megacolon. Scans are of value in elucidating abdominal masses, abscesses and possible metastases. Ultrasonography is more readily available than computerised tomography but the accuracy of diagnosis is much more user dependant. Angiography must be carried out to evaluate severe gastrointestinal haemorrhage and will localise haemagniomatas malformations.

No elective operation on the colon or rectum should be undertaken without every step being undertaken to establish a firm diagnosis. There is now virtually no place for diagnostic laparotomy to exclude a filling deffect in the right colon on barium enema or be uncertain if an area of sigmoid diverticular disease hides a carcinoma. Skilled endoscopy will provide the answer.

ELECTIVE OPERATIONS

CARCINOMA

1. Examine the whole abdomen. Examine the whole of the colon from the appendix to the rectum. Small adenomatous polyps cannot be felt. Synchronous carcinomas occur in 4% of patients. Avoid handling the carcinoma and cover with a swab soaked in 1 : 500 mercury perchloride solution. Feel for enlarged lymph nodes in the mesentery and in the para-aortic regions. Look for peritoneal metastases.

2. Estimate the resectability and curability of the tumour. Palpate and visualize the liver to exclude metastases. If present biopsy to confirm. If up to five small metastases are present on the surface of the liver excise with diathermy. If a large solitary metastasis is present within the substance of the liver carefully note its position as this may be suitable for partial hepatectomy in from 3–6 months time. Tumours which are locally resectable but fixed to other organs such as bladder, uterus, another piece of large or small intestine, the duodenum, stomach, gall-bladder, liver or kidney may still be curable so resect it with part or all of the adjacent organ. If the carcinoma is resectable but metastases are present modify surgical treatment. Resection of the tumour gives better palliation than a bypass procedure.

3. Treat potentially curable carcinoma of the right colon by one stage right hemicolectomy taking the ileocolic vessels at their origin on the superior mesenteric vessels. If metastases are present a less extensive resection without wide mesenteric clearance can be carried out.

4. Treat carcinoma of the transverse colon by transverse colectomy taking the hepatic or splenic flexure if the lesion is situated proximally or distally in the transverse colon. Ligate the middle colic vessels at their origin from the superior mesenteric vessels.

5. Treat carcinoma of the descending and sigmoid colon by left hemicolectomy or sigmoid colectomy taking the inferior mesenteric artery at its origin from the aorta and the inferior mesenteric vein at the same level.

6. Treat carcinoma of the rectum as a rule by anterior resection using either a sutured, stapled or peranal anastomosis. Some tumours of the lower third of the rectum, of a high grade of malignancy and bulky fixed tumours are treated by abdomino-perineal excision of the rectum because it may be technically impossible to remove them by anterior resection if the patient is obese and has a narrow pelvis or to obtain a 5 cm distal clearance of the tumour if it is of a high grade of malignancy.

For metastatic rectal carcinoma carry out anterior resection if this can be safely done without a defunctioning colostomy, as many of these patients will deteriorate and never have the colostomy closed. If the rectal carcinoma is low, or there is local extension to the side walls of the pelvis or internal iliac nodes are involved, select a palliative abdomino-perineal excision of the rectum or a Hartmann's operation.

DIVERTICULAR DISEASE

1. Diverticular disease is very common and most elderly patients having surgery for other abdominal conditions have some diverticula, mainly in the sigmoid colon. Although diverticular disease may be widespread in the colon, symptomatic disease is usually produced by the muscle hypertrophy, thickening and shortening of the sigmoid colon.

2. Even in elective resection, the disease may be associated with marked pericolic inflammation and oedema with pericolic abscess formation in the mesentery.

3. Indications for elective resection are not always definite, and with the introduction of high roughage diets and the addition of bran fewer operations are undertaken. However, patients with severe attacks of lower left-sided and suprapubic pain with marked diverticular disease on a barium enema with muscle hypertrophy and narrowing of the colonic lumen which is unresponsive to dietary change and antispasmodic drugs should be offered resection provided their general health is good. The barium enema findings and pathology do not always correlate and patients often wait too long before being offered surgical treatment.

Definite indications for surgical treatment include male patients under the age 50 years with symptomatic disease as statistically over 80% will eventually come to surgery many with complications; patients with urinary infection associated with their attacks indicating adhesion to the bladder or ureter and an impending fistula and indeed those with an established colovesical fistula; patients with two or more attacks of acute diverticular disease within a short period of time associated with a fever, mass and radiological signs of a pericolic abscess.

Avoid operation in patients with the irritable bowel syndrome and a few diverticula, their symptoms will persist.

4. It is unnecessary to remove all the proximal diverticula but resect the whole of the sigmoid colon and perform an anastomosis between the middle or upper descending colon and the upper third of the rectum below the sacral promontory.

5. Operative treatment is always by resection and anastomosis, and myotomy either longitudinally or transversely is no longer advocated.

ULCERATIVE COLITIS

1. Elective operation is indicated in patients with persistent or recurrent attacks of diarrhoea with the passage

of blood, anaemia, weight loss and general ill health which is unresponsive to treatment with corticosteroids and salazopyrine. The majority of these patients will have total or extensive colitis and it is rare to have to operate on patients with purely distal (sigmoid or left-sided) disease. Patients with several severe attacks of acute colitis should be operated upon during remission if possible.

Total colitis of 10–15 years duration or longer may result in dysplastic epithelial changes and eventual carcinoma even in the absence of any symptoms. These patients must be carefully followed up by colonoscopy and mucosal biopsy. Those who eventually develop persistent severe dysplasia require surgical treatment. Patients with total colitis and strictures or filling defects on barium enema also require surgery.

Steroid therapy is no contraindication to surgery as it makes no difference to the outcome, but these patients must have steroid cover during and after the operation.

2. In quiescent total colitis, the colon is slightly thickened, shortened and greyish white in colour. Even at elective operation, part of the colon may appear much more actively inflamed with thickening, oedema and marked hyperaemia. The paracolic and mesenteric nodes may be considerably enlarged.

3. The most straightforward operation is to carry out a proctocolectomy with a conventional Brooke ileostomy.

4. Alternative procedures must be considered. If the patient comes to surgery early in the course of the disease when the rectum is still distensible and there is no dysplasia in rectal biopsies, consider a colectomy and ileorectal anastomosis. If proctocolectomy is undertaken the patient may wish to avoid a permanent conventional ileostomy. This is possible with a Kock reservoir ileostomy or a conservative proctocolectomy leaving the anal sphincters and constructing a J ileo-anal pouch. If you are inexperienced in these newer methods of treatment, carry out a colectomy and ileostomy, and retain the rectum.

CROHN'S DISEASE

1. Appraise. Because the disease can occur throughout the gastrointestinal tract primary treatment is always medical. Undertake surgical treatment if medical treatment fails to control the disease, or for complications such as stenosis causing obstructive symptoms, abscesses or internal or external fistula formation.

2. The whole or part of the colon may be involved with Crohn's disease. Carefully examine the stomach and duodenum and the whole of the small bowel to exclude other sites. Measure the length of the small bowel and record the situation and extent of Crohn's disease.

3. When the disease affects the terminal ileum and/or caecum and ascending colon, carry out a right hemicolectomy. In a primary operation remove 5–10 cm

of macroscopically normal ileum proximal to the lesion. If there is a chronic abscess cavity in the right iliac fossa, extend the right hemicolectomy so that the anastomosis lies in the upper abdomen away from the abscess cavity.

4. If the whole colon is severely involved and requires resection, perform a colectomy and ileorectal anastomosis or a total proctocolectomy and convenitonal ileostomy. Distal disease involving only the rectum may require an abdomino-perineal excision with an end colostomy. Segmental colonic resection is rarely required.

POLYPS AND POLYPOSIS

1. Appraise. Polyps in the rectum are often discovered on routine sigmoidoscopy when patients present with minor anal conditions. Remove one or more for histology and if an adenoma carry out an air-contrast barium enema. Sessile villous adenomas usually occur in the rectum and can be removed by endoanal local excision. Pedunculated adenomas are removed endoscopically thrugh a sigmoidoscope or colonoscope. Colotomy and operative removal of pedunculated adenomas is no longer necessary.

2. Colonic and rectal polyps may be neoplastic in origin — adenomas or hamartomas — Peutz Jeghers polyps, juvenile polyps or metaplastic polyps. Adenomatous polyps are common and potentially malignant.

3. If several large polyps are present in a patient with carcinoma extend the resection to include these. In a patient with one or more carcinomas and several large polyps, colectomy and ileorectal anastomosis may be required.

4. Circumferential villous tumours extending above 10 cm from the anal verge require anterior resection or a modified Soave procedure.

5. Familial polyposis (adenomatosis) coli requires a colectomy and ileorectal anastomosis. Plan to perform follow-up sigmoidoscopy every 6 months. Fulgerate rectal polyps or polyps which subsequently develop, if they are over 5 mm in diameter. Exceptionally a proctocolectomy with ileostomy or ileoanal pouch may be indicated when there are confluent polyps or a carcinoma in the rectum.

URGENT OPERATIONS

Urgent operations on the colon or rectum are carried out for obstruction, perforation, abscess formation, acute fulminating inflammatory bowel disease and acute haemorrhage. Ensure the patient is in the best possible condition before undertaking surgery. Replace blood, fluid and electrolyte loss and in major septic conditions commence antibiotic therapy with gentamicin or a cephalosporin together with metronidazole.

Decide on the best time for operation. If the patient has severe bleeding or major abdominal sepsis or perforation, it should be undertaken as soon as the patient's condition allows but operations for large bowel obtruction and inflammatory bowel disease do not require operation in the middle of the night and can almost always be done the next morning. Many of these patients will require major operation and difficult decisions and the best results will be obtained when theatre staff, surgeon and anaesthetist are fresh.

OBSTRUCTION

1. Define the level of obstruction with sigmoidoscopy or an urgent barium enema.

2. If an urgent resection is carried out, it must be as radical a procedure as for an elective operation at the same site, provided cure is possible. If there are metastases carry out palliative resection. It is rare to find a proximal tumour which is not resectable but if you find yourself in this situation, carry out a bypass procedure. Remember this will relieve the obstruction but not stop bleeding from the tumour and the consequent anaemia or pain and complications from the mass invading other strictures. In an unresectable left-sided tumour carry out a proximal defunctioning colostomy.

3. Obstructing carcinoma of the right colon causing acute intestinal obstruction is treated by right hemicolectomy. Treat left-sided obstruction by stages, carrying out a defunctioning transverse colostomy, an interim resection and finally closure of the colostomy. An alternative procedure for a carcinoma of the upper sigmoid or descending colon is to carry out a one-stage, subtotal colectomy with ileosigmoid or ileorectal anastomosis. A carcinoma of the lower sigmoid or rectosigmoid junction can be treated by an immediate resection with a Hartmann's procedure or peroperative irrigation of the colon and anastomosis with a defunctioning transverse colostomy.

4. Acute obstructive diverticular disease is often complicated by paracolic abscess formation. Immediate resection with a Hartmann's procedure is the operation of choice. It may be safe to carry out a resection and anastomosis with a defunctioning transverse colostomy, if the infection is localised and completely removed by the resection and peroperative irrigation of the colon is carried out.

PERFORATION

Perforation of a carcinoma or diverticular disease requires resection and anastomosis with a covering colostomy or, in the presence of abscess formation, a Hartmann's procedure. Drainage of the abscess and defunctioning colostomy in a severely ill, debilitated patient may be necessary but is usually the less satisfactory alternative.

ACUTE INFLAMMATORY BOWEL DISEASE

Acute fulminating colitis with or without toxic megacolon is treated by colectomy and ileostomy with a mucous fistula. The rectum should not be excised and it is much safer to make a mucous fistula than close the rectal stump.

Acute ischaemic colitis requiring urgent surgery should be treated by excision and proximal and distal colostomy. Again the rectum and sigmoid colon should always be left as this usually recovers sufficiently for anastomosis to be carried out later.

ACUTE MASSIVE HAEMORRHAGE

Determine if possible the site of bleeding by sigmoidoscopy and colonoscopy. Carry out a single contrast barium enema. This will show the site of diverticular disease and occasionally be therapeutic and stop the bleeding. Remember that 50% of patients with episodes of haemorrhage and diverticular disease will have another cause for the bleeding. If the site can be accurately determined, carry out a limited resection but if laparotomy has to be carried out with the site of bleeding unknown, it is wise to carry out a colectomy and ileorectal anastomosis.

SURGERY OF THE LARGE BOWEL

Prepare

1. In elective operation, the diagnosis will have been reached preoperatively by barium enema and/or colonoscopy. Ensure that barium enema films are available at operation.

2. The colon should always be empty when elective operation is undertaken. A variety of methods have been used to mechanically clean the colon; castor oil, magnesium sulphate, sodium picosulphate, mannitol and irrigation from above with a nasogastric tube and enemas from below. We favour giving fluids only by mouth for 48 hours preoperatively together with two doses of 30 ml of castor oil. Enemas are not usually required.

3. Pre-operative oral antibiotics are of little value. Give peroperative prophylactic gentamycin 80–120 mg intramuscularly with the premedication or on induction of anaesthesia, together with 500 mg of metranidazole intravenously during the operation. Continue gentamycin 80 mg together with metranidazole 8 hourly for 24–48 hours or longer if there is established infection.

4. Catheterize the patient after induction of anaesthetic and monitor urinary output during and after surgery.

Action

1. The morbidity and mortality following colonic surgery is higher than resections of the small bowel. The blood supply is more tenuous and easily damaged. Perfusion postoperatively is often decreased resulting in a degree of ischaemic colitis. Infection is more common resulting in abscess formation with the potentiation of collagenase activity, collagen lyses and anastomotic dehiscence.

2. Clamp the bowel to be resected with Parker-Kerr clamps. If the patient has been well prepared and the colon is empty place no clamps on the ends to be sutured.

3. Clean the ends of the bowel to be sutured with moistened swabs wetted in 1:2000 aqueous chlorhexidine solution in the absence of malignancy or 1 : 500 mercuric perchloride solution when carcinoma is being resected.

4. Divide the colon at right-angles to the mesentery. If there is a disparity in size, particularly when carrying out a right hemicolectomy or an ileorectal anastomosis, slit up the anti-mesenteric border of the ileum or narrower colon until the two ends approximate in size. Do not cut off the edges of the slit bowel as this only narrows the bowel again. When a long length of mobilised colon is to be anastomosed to the rectum make certain there is not a 360° twist in the colon.

5. Carry out anastomosis of the colon end-to-end with the proximal bowel rotated 90° to the right, so that the mesenteric borders are not opposite each other, particularly when making a rectal anastomosis.

6. Suture the bowel in the Mayo method with an all-coat continuous 2/0 chromic catgut and interrupted 3/0 seromuscular silk, in one or two layers of interrupted 3/0 polyglycolic acid (Dexon) or polyglactin 910 (Vicryl) sutures, or one layer of synthetic non-absoluble sutures such as 4/0 polypropylene. Invert the edges but not so much as to produce a cuff which will cause an obstructive anastomosis. When anastomosis is sutured mark it with haemostatic clips for future radiological identification. Rectal anastomosis may be undertaken using a stapling device such as the EEA stapler using 28 or 31 mm cartridges or the disposable gun.

7. Take care to avoid contamination during the operation. If the colon is loaded, place a non-crushing clamp across the bowel 10 cm from the end before this is swabed out and cleared. If possible, screen the anastomosis from the peritoneal cavity and contents while it is being constructed. When it is complete discard and replace the towels, gloves and instruments, before the closing the abdomen.

8. It is traditional for British surgeons to drain any colonic anastomosis. This is unnecessary. Drain an intraperitoneal abscess. Drain an extraperitoneal low anterior resection through the peritoneal cavity into the pelvis.

TRANSVERSE COLOSTOMY

Appraise

1. Carry out a transverse colostomy in cases of distal obstruction in patients unfit to have an urgent resection carried out or you are too inexperienced to do this. It may be necessary as a preliminary operation in patients with severe distal sepsis with abscesses and fistular formation, for example, in Crohn's disease or diverticular disease or in vesico-colic fistula and severe urinary tract infection.

2. Site the stoma in right upper quadrant midway between the umbilicus and the costal margin.

3. Place the colostomy well to the right of the transverse colon. The next stage of the operation may require taking down the splenic flexure and mobilising the distal transverse colon.

Access

1. Make a transverse incision 8–10 cm long centred on the upper right rectus muscle between the umbilicus and the costal margin so that an appliance can be fitted without encroaching upon either. Divide the anterior and posterior rectus sheath and the rectus muscle transversely in the line of the incision. Through this locate the bowel, explore the abdomen, and feel the liver.

2. The abdomen may be already open when a decision is made to perform a colostomy. When a midline or left paramedian incision was used, make a transverse incision as described above but only 6 cm or 7 cm long. If a right upper paramedian incision was used, bring the colostomy through the upper end of the incision, provided it is clear of the costal margin.

Assess

1. If the operation is undertaken to relieve a distal obstruction, examine the relevant structures and feel the obstructing mass in the distal colon. It may be impossible to determine if this is due to carcinoma or diverticular disease.

2. Feel the liver for metastases.

3. Feel the rest of the colon and the peritoneal cavity to determine if there are other metastases.

Action (Fig. 8.1)

1. Draw the right side of the transverse colon and omentum out of the wound. Manipulate it so a loop of proximal transverse colon lies in the wound without tension.

2. Separate the omentum from the colon and turn it upwards to expose the mesentery.

3. Pull the loop upwards through the incision and make

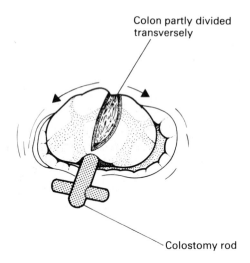

Colon partly divided transversely

Colostomy rod

Fig. 8.1 Transverse colostomy. Bring a loop of colon through the wound and keep it in place with a colostomy device or simple glass rod. Open the colostomy by a transverse incision.

a hole through the mesentery close to the bowel wall at the apex of the loop with a pair of long artery forceps, taking care not to damage the blood supply.

4. Pass a piece of narrow rubber tubing or a Jaques catheter under the mesentery. Pull the loop right out through the incision with the rubber tubing making certain that the loop is not twisted and the proximal opening will be to the right and the distal opening to the left.

5. Pass a plastic colostomy device (e.g. Squibb System 2) through the mesentery to form a bridge for the colostomy. Open the end of the colostomy device to stop it slipping out. Alternatively, use a small glass rod if no colostomy device is available.

6. No internal sutures are required.

7. Open the colostomy transversely for half the circumference at the apex of the loop. If a colostomy is made to relieve obstruction, open it immediately. Clean the contents away, with mounted swabs wetted with 1 : 500 mercuric perchloride if the condition is thought to be carcinoma.

8. Turn back the edges of the opened colon and suture the whole thickness of the colon wall to the edge of the skin incision with interrupted 2/0 catgut sutures on a cutting needle.

9. Insert a finger into each loop of the colostomy to make sure it is not too narrow and that the finger passes straight into the underlying colon.

10. Fix a suitable disposable appliance (e.g. Squibb System 2) over the loop colostomy rod.

Aftercare

1. A transverse colostomy is a temporary defunctioning stoma, made with a view to closure. Closure should be as

easy as possible and not require excision of the colon and re-anastomosis.

2. Remove the colostomy device forming the bridge in 7–10 days depending on the obesity of the patient and the difficulty in bringing up the loop of colon.

CLOSURE

Appraise

1. Do not close the colostomy until at least 1 month after it has been formed. This allows the oedema to settle down and makes the operation safer and easier.

2. Before closure ensure that the distal anastomosis is satisfactory as shown on sigmoidoscopy and/or gastrografin enema, and prepare the proximal bowel as for colonic resection and anastomosis (see p. 132).

Action (Fig. 8.2)

1. Make an incision in the skin close to the mucocutaneous junction.

2. Insert six 2/0 silk stay sutures into the mucocutaneous junction, each held in an artery forceps so that traction may be applied while dissecting.

3. Deepen the incision to reveal the colon and the external rectus sheath. Dissect the colonic loops from the abdominal wall until the whole of the loop is freed and can easily be drawn out from the abdominal cavity.

4. Excise the mucocutaneous junction and clean the edges of the colon with 1 : 2000 aqueous chlorhexidine solution prior to re-anastomosis.

5. Close the colostomy transversely using one layer of 4/0 interrupted vertical mattress sutures of polypropyline or alternatively use an all-coat stitch of continuous 2/0

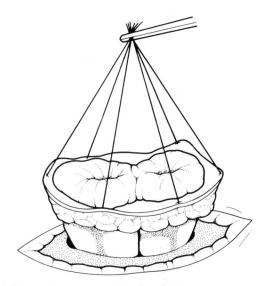

Fig. 8.2 Closure of transverse colostomy. Insert stay sutures to help mobilisation.

chromic catgut, and a second layer of interrupted sero-muscular silk.

6. Replace the resutured colostomy into the peritoneal cavity, place the omentum over it, and manipulate it so that it lies away from the abdominal incision.

7. Close the abdominal wound in one layer with a continuous or interrupted nylon suture. If the patient is fat, drain the subcutaneous space with a slip of corrugated latex sheet brought out through the end of the wound, or through a separate stab wound. Close the skin.

SIGMOID DEFUNCTIONING COLOSTOMY

Appraise

1. Employ this in inoperable carcinoma of the rectum if obstruction is present or insipient.

2. It may be necessary when there is anal incontinence due to sphincter damage.

3. Use it to defunction a rectovaginal fistula requiring repair.

Action

1. Make an oblique incision 8 cm long, halfway between the anterior superior iliac spine and the umbilicus, on the left side of the abdomen. Divide the anterior rectus sheath and external oblique aponeurosis in the line of the incision.

2. Separate the internal oblique fibres and open the peritoneum.

3. Deliver a loop of sigmoid colon through the wound and keep it in place using a colostomy device.

4. Open the colon and suture it as for a transverse colostomy.

5. If the colostomy is to be permanent make a skin bridge by constructing a flap of skin and suturing it under the loop.

CAECOSTOMY

Appraise

1. This is a bad defunctioning operation in cases of obstruction.

2. It is occasionally useful to decompress a distal anastomosis in a prepared colon. As such it is always made as an accessory procedure when the abdomen is open.

3. An open caecostomy is never indicated. If the caecum is grossly dilated with patchy gangrene in distal obstruction, it is rarely sufficient to exteriorize it as the ischaemic changes are extensive, involving much of the proximal colon. Carry out excision with proximal ileostomy and distal colostomy or perform ileocolic or ileorectal anastomosis.

Action

1. Carry out appendicectomy.

2. Place a purse-string suture of 2/0 chromic catgut in the caecum around the anterior tenia coli.

3. Make an incision in the anterior tenia through the purse-string suture and open the caecum. Insert a 30f Foley catheter through a stab wound in the abdominal wall and into the caecum. Partially inflate the balloon and tie the purse-string suture.

4. Insert a second purse-string to 'inkwell' the catheter, then fix the caecum to the anterior abdominal wall with 3 interrupted 2/0 catgut around the abdominal opening.

COLOTOMY

This is now rarely indicated, as all polyps and most foreign bodies suitable for removal by simple colotomy can be removed via a colonoscope.

RIGHT HEMICOLECTOMY

Appraise

1. Undertake this operation for carcinoma of the caecum and ascending colon and for the occasional benign tumour of the right colon. Also undertake this operation for a perforated caecal diverticulum, the so-called solitary ulcer of the caecum. Carcinoma of the appendix or a carcinoid tumour at the base of the appendix is also treated by a limited right hemicolectomy.

Never carry out an ileocolic by-pass for an extensive carcinoma even if the operation is palliative. Try and carry out a right hemicolectomy.

2. Benign disease of the terminal ileum, particularly Crohn's disease, is treated by resection of an appropriate amount of ileum together with part of the right colon. When this is associated with abscess formation in the right iliac fossa extend the operation so that the anastomosis lies in the upper abdomen away from the abscess. This will prevent fistula formation postoperatively.

3. Never make a small bowel anastomosis close to the ileocaecal valve. It is preferable to remove the caecum and a small part of the ascending colon and to carry out an ileo-colonic anastomosis.

4. In obstruction usually due to carcinoma of the ileo-caecal region or the right colon carry out an urgent right hemicolectomy extending the operation distally as appropriate.

Action (Fig. 8.3)

Resect

1. Handle the tumour as little as possible. If the serosa and surrounding fat are infiltrated by carcinoma, cover it

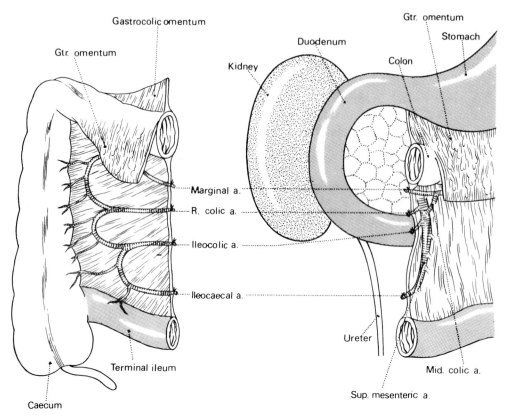

Fig. 8.3 Radical right hemicolectomy. The resected specimen is on the left and comprises the right half of the colon, the terminal ileum and the mesentery with vessels and nodes. Also included are the right halves of the gastrocolic and greater omentum. The ileocolic artery and vein are divided in their origin from the superior mesenteric vessels. The right branch of the middle colonic artery is divided. The duodenum, pancreas and right kidney and ureter have been identified and protected from damage.

with a pack soaked in 1 : 500 mercuric perchloride solution.

2. Leave the omentum adherent to the right colon.

3. Draw the caecum and ascending colon medially. Cut through the parietal peritoneum lateral to the colon from the caecum to the hepatic flexure. If the carcinoma infiltrates the lateral abdominal wall, cut out a large disc of peritoneum and underlying muscle with the specimen.

4. Dissect the right colon from the posterior abdominal wall. Identify and preserve the right ureter, gonadal vessels and duodenum.

5. Mobilise the hepatic flexure and divide any ileal bands so that the whole of the right colon can be lifted from the abdomen.

6. Transilluminate the mesentery to show the vessels, identify, clamp and divide the ileocolic artery and vein, close to the superior mesenteric vessels. Divide the right colic vessels and the right branch of the middle colic vessels close to their origin.

7. The extent of the resection depends to some extent on the size and site of the tumour but normally will include approximately 30 cm of terminal ileum to the middle third of the transverse colon.

8. Remove the right half of the greater omentum with the specimen. If the tumour is situated near the hepatic

flexure remove the right side of the gastroepiploeic arch of vessels to obtain a wider clearance.

9. Place a Parker-Kerr clamp across the ileum and transverse colon at the site of division. Unless the patient is obstructed and the colon unprepared do not clamp the ends to be anastomosed.

10. Divide the bowel and remove the specimen.

11. Hold the ends of the ileum and colon to be anastomosed in Babcock forceps and clean them with mounted swabs wetted with 1 : 500 mercuric perchloride solution.

Unite

1. Anastomose the terminal ileum end-to-end to the transverse colon, widening the ileum with an anti-mesenteric slit if necessary. Mark the anastomosis with haemostatic clips.

2. Suture the cut edges of the mesentery with a continuous 2/0 chromic catgut suture.

3. Cover the anastomosis with the remaining omentum.

Technical points

1. If the resection is for a benign condition such as Crohn's disease, or a caecal diverticulum, it need not be so

extensive and the vessels can be divided in the middle of the mesentery rather than at their origin.

2. If the carcinoma is locally extensive but can be excised radically, widen the scope of the operation to include abdominal wall or part of other organs involved.

3. If the carcinoma is situated at the hepatic flexure or in the right side of the transverse colon, mobilise the splenic flexure as well. Divide the middle colic vessels close to their origin and anastomose the terminal ileum to the descending or sigmoid colon. If there are multiple metastases carry out a limited segmental resection rather than a bypass procedure.

Check list

1. Make sure the bowel each side of the anastomosis is viable and check that the anastomosis is lying easily without kinking.

2. Examine the raw surfaces particularly in the right flank and stop any bleeding. Remove any blood collected above the right lobe of the liver and in the pelvis.

LEFT HEMICOLECTOMY

Appraise

1. Undertake left hemicolectomy for carcinoma of the left and sigmoid colon. Carry out this operation for diverticular disease.

2. If the operation is carried out for an obstructed neoplasm, either carry out a staged procedure, a Hartmann's operation, or if the patient is in good condition, a colectomy and an ileosigmoid or ileorectal anastomosis or a resection with irrigation of the obstructive proximal colon and an anastomosis protected by a defunctioning colostomy.

3. In diverticular disease, resect the sigmoid colon and as much of the ascending colon as is necessary to remove severe diverticular disease. Isolated diverticula in the upper descending and transverse colon can be left providing the bowel wall is not thickened. It is important to anastamose the proximal bowel to the upper third of the rectum below the sacral promontory and not to the sigmoid colon.

4. In any left hemicolectomy the splenic flexure and the left half of the transverse colon must be mobilised.

Prepare (Fig. 8.4)

For any left sided colonic or rectal resection place the patient in the lithotomy Trendelenberg (Lloyd-Davies) position. Catheterize the patient to ensure an empty bladder and to monitor the urine flow during and after the operation.

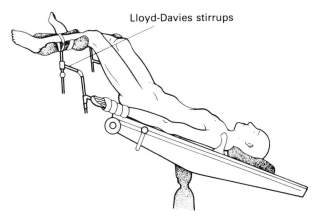

Fig. 8.4 Place the patient in the lithotomy Trendelenburg position of Lloyd-Davies for any operation on or involving the left side of the colon or rectum. This allows simultaneous approach to the perineum or rectum and the abdomen without altering the patient's position.

Access

1. Stand on the patient's left side.

2. Make a long midline incision. Remember you will be working up around the spleen when the splenic flexure is mobilised, and in the pelvis when the anastomosis is constructed. Access must be adequate without a struggle.

Assess

1. If the operation is performed for a carcinoma, palpate the liver, examine the colon and the whole of the small bowel, palpate the mesenteric and para-aortic nodes, and the whole of the peritoneal cavity and pelvis.

2. Palpate the carcinoma and assess mobility. Touch the carcinoma as little as possible and if the serosal surface is involved, cover it with a swab soaked in 1 : 500 mercuric perchloride solution.

3. If the partial colectomy is performed for a benign condition, assess the diseased colon and decide the extent of resection and then explore the abdomen completely as in a case of carcinoma.

How radical is a resection?

1. If a carcinoma is confined within the limits of a radical operation, carry this out if the patient is fit. Tie the inferior mesenteric artery at its origin from the aorta and the inferior mesenteric vein at a similar level.

2. If the patient is very elderly and clearly unfit, and the blood supply to the colon is tenuous due to severe atheroma, undertake a less radical procedure retaining the inferior mesenteric artery, and ligating the left colon and sigmoid branches as appropriate.

3. If the resection is for a benign condition, or a palliative resection for carcinoma, then the bowel resection need not be so wide and the vessels may be ligated and divided close to the bowel wall.

RADICAL RESECTION OF THE LEFT COLON

Action (Fig. 8.5)

1. Place damp packs over the wound edges. Suture the peritoneum overlying the bladder to the lower part of the skin wound and packs.

2. Lift the whole of the small bowel to the right side, out of the wound, and cover it with moist pack. Never pack the small bowel into the wound as it severely restricts access.

3. Divide the congenital adhesions which bind the sigmoid colon to the abdominal wall in the left iliac fossa and then divide the adhesions between the descending colon and the lateral peritoneum.

4. Move to the right side of the patient. Rotate the patient to the right side and then mobilise the splenic flexure by dividing the phrenicocolic ligament. Ligate the few vessels in it. Avoid damaging the spleen and the tail of the pancreas. If the carcinoma is distal the greater omentum may be preserved by dividing the adhesions between the omentum and the colon as far proximally as the middle of the transverse colon and dividing the peritoneum along the end of the lesser sac. If the tumour is situated near the flexure excise the left half of the greater omentum with the tumour by dividing the left side of the

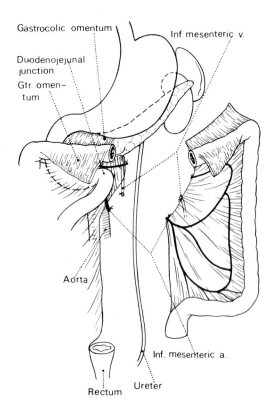

Gastrocolic omentum

Duodenojejunal junction

Gtr. omen-tum

Inf. mesenteric v.

Aorta

Inf. mesenteric a.

Rectum   Ureter

Fig. 8.5 Radical left hemicolectomy. The resected specimen is on the right and comprises the left half of the colon, the mesocolon and the left halves of the gastrocolic and greater omentum. The left division of the middle colic artery and the origin of the inferior mesenteric artery have been ligated and divided. The duodenojejunal junction, left ureter and kidney, pancreas and spleen have been protected from damage.

gastroepiploic arch and removing the lesser and greater omentum with the specimen.

5. Elevate the left colon on its mesentery and dissect free from the duodeno-jejunal flexure, the left ureter and gonadal vessels.

6. Incise the peritoneum overlying the aorta and mobilise the interior mesenteric artery to its origin. Ligate and divide the artery and then identify the inferior mesenteric vein lying well laterally and clamp, ligate and divide it a little be low the lower border of the pancreas.

7. Mobilise the sigmoid colon if the anastomosis is to be made to the upper third of the rectum. Do not divide the sigmoid higher than about 10 cm above the rectum or its blood supply may be endangered.

8. Divide the mesentery and marginal vessels to the edge of the colon at the site chosen for resection in the transverse colon and rectum or sigmoid colon.

9. Place a Lloyd-Davies right-angle clamp across the rectum at the site of resection. Then irrigate the rectum by means of a catheter passed through the anus, with 1:500 mercuric perchloride solution if the resection is for carcinoma, or a 1 : 2000 aqueous chlorhexidine solution if the condition is benign, until it is perfectly clean. Then swab the rectum dry.

10. While the rectal irrigation is being carried out prepare the proximal colon for division. Place a Parker-Kerr clamp across the bowel. If the colon is well prepared do not clamp the proximal bowel to be used in the anastomosis. Divide the colon, hold the proximal end in Babcock forceps and swab the bowel out with 1 : 500 mercuric perchloride or 1 : 2000 aqueous chlorhexidine solution.

11. Divide the rectum or sigmoid colon below the right angle clamp and remove the specimen consisting of the left half of the colon, the inferior mesenteric artery and vein, and the whole of the mesentery.

12. If it is necessary to mobilise the transverse colon or hepatic flexure to ensure a tension free anastomosis do this before dividing the colon.

Unite

1. Unite the bowel ends with one or two layers of sutures according to the preferred technique. Make the anastomosis end-to-end with the proximal colon rotated 90° to the left so that the proximal mesentery lies opposite the cut edge of the peritoneum overlying the aorta.

2. Suture the cut edge of the transverse mesocolon to the cut edge of the peritoneum overlying the aorta.

Technical points

1. If the abdominal wall is involved with carcinoma excise part of the wall with the tumour and repair the defect later. If small bowel is involved be prepared to resect

one loop or more as necessary and anastomose the cut ends of the bowel. A portion of the bladder fundus may be removed. If the left ureter is obstructed by carcinoma, excise a portion with the mass and either reimplant the upper end of the ureter into the bladder or excise the whole of the ureter and kidney. Remove the uterus, ovaries and tubes or the spleen or kidney invaded by direct extension of the tumour.

2. If the tumour is situated in the left half of the transverse colon or at the splenic flexure excise most of the transverse colon and unite the hepatic flexure or ascending colon to the lower descending or sigmoid colon.

CARCINOMA OF THE RECTUM

Appraise

1. All patients are assessed before operation by a sigmoidoscopy and rectal biopsy and in the majority of cases by a barium enema to evaluate the proximal colon.

2. Two-thirds of patients with a rectal carcinoma are suitable for a conservative anterior resection with the anastomosis carried out in a number of different ways.

3. One third of patients still require an abdominoperineal excision of the rectum.

4. A few patients with small early carcinomas are suitable for a peranal local excision.

ANTERIOR RESECTION OF THE RECTUM

Prepare

1. Place the anaesthetised patient in the lithotomy Trendelenberg (Lloyd-Davies) position.

2. Insert an indwelling Foley catheter.

Access

Make a long midline incision, as the splenic flexure will require mobilisation and the rectal anastomosis may be deep within the pelvis.

Assess

1. Palpate and visualise the liver to establish if there are metastases. Biopsy metastases. If one or two small superficial metastases are present completely excise them with diathermy. If there is a large intrahepatic secondary in the substance of one or other lobe assess it for possible hemi-hepatectomy in 3–6 months time if the procedure is otherwise radical.

2. Palpate the gall bladder and note any calculi. Examine the whole of the gastrointestinal tract from the stomach to the rectum.

3. Note any local or distant peritoneal metastases. Examine the omentum.

4. Palpate any nodes in the mesentery and note any paraortic nodes.

5. Finally palpate the tumour, note its size and position above or below the peritoneal reflexion and decide whether it is mobile or adherent to other organs, or fixed within the pelvis.

Action (Fig. 8.6)

1. Mobilise the left side of the peritoneum from the congenital adhesions to the sigmoid to the splenic flexure.

2. Stand on the patient's right side and fully mobilise the splenic flexure and the left half of the transverse colon,

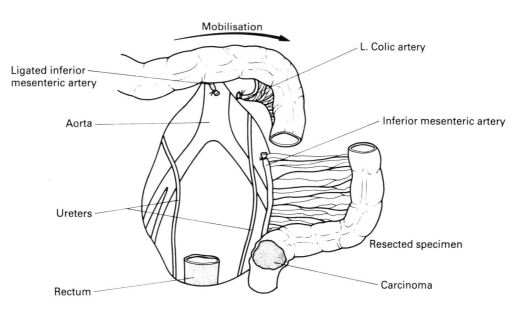

Fig. 8.6 Anterior resection of the rectum. The resected specimen is on the right and consists of the upper rectum, the sigmoid and part of the descending colon, together with the mesentery. The inferior mesenteric artery has been ligated and divided on the aorta and the inferior mesenteric vein at the upper border of the pancreas. The splenic flexure has been mobilised. Both ureters have been identified and preserved.

preserving the omentum unless there are metastases present. Avoid damage to the spleen.

3. Mobilise the left colon, pull it to the right on its mesentery and separate and preserve the left ureter and gonadal vessels. Take care not to damage the duodeno-jejunal flexure or the tail of the pancreas.

4. Incise the peritoneum overlying the aorta and look for and preserve the right ureter. Separate the inferior mesenteric artery and vein from the posterior abdominal wall and clamp, divide and ligate the inferior mesenteric artery at its origin from the aorta unless the patient is old and arteriosclerotic, when it may be wise to preserve the left colic artery. Divide the inferior mesenteric vein at a slightly higher level, close to the lower border of the pancreas. Select a suitable area in the descending colon for division of the colon and divide the mesentery up to this point.

5. Divide the peritoneum over each side of the pelvis close to the lateral wall and join the incisions in the midline at the most dependent part of the peritoneal floor.

6. The extent of mobilisation of the rectum depends upon the level of the tumour. If it is retroperitoneal, complete mobilisation of the rectum is necessary.

7. Pull the rectum forwards and dissect anteriorly to the sacral promontory and presacral fascia as far down as the tip of the coccyx and the pelvic floor muscles. Take care to visualise and preserve the presacral sympathetic nerves.

8. Hold the seminal vesicles forwards with a St. Mark's lipped anterior retractor and dissect between the vesicles and the rectum to uncover Denonvilliers' fascia. Incise this transversely across and dissect down between this and the rectum as far distally as necessary, even behind the prostate and down to the pelvic floor. In a female dissect distally between the rectum and vagina as far down as necessary even to the pelvic floor.

9. By traction on the rectum to one side and then the other side of the pelvis, identify and divide the lateral ligaments close to the lateral pelvic wall. Identify the cut ends of the middle rectal vessels, clamp and ligate.

10. Straighten out the rectum and draw the tumour upwards. Choose a suitable site for division of the rectum. If possible allow 5 cm clearance below the lower edge of the carcinoma. If the tumour is low down this degree of clearance may be impossible to achieve if a restorative procedure is to be undertaken so be willing to compromise without jeopardising any possibility of performing a curative procedure. Obtain at least a 2 cm Clearance. If the mesorectum is present at the site selected for division of the rectum divide this between long forceps and ligate the distal end of the superior rectal artery and veinvein. Place a Lloyd-Davies right-angled clamp across the rectum at the site of division.

11. Irrigate the rectum through the anus with 1 : 500 mercuric perchloride solution If only a small cuff of sphincter and rectum remains, simply swab it out with mercuric perchloride solution.

12. At the site selected for division of the descending colon, place a Parker-Kerr clamp at right angles across the bowel and divide above it, holding the upper end of the colon with Babcock forceps so that it can be swabbed out with mercuric perchloride solution.

13. Divide the rectum below the clamp. Remove the specimen containing the rectal carcinoma, the complete mesentery and nodes up to the origin of the inferior mesenteric artery.

Unite

The anastomosis may be carried out in one of three ways, depending upon the level of anastomosis, the ease of access to the pelvis and the obesity of the patient.

Sutured anastomosis (Fig. 8.7)

A high anastomosis may be sutured in one or two layers depending upon your choice. A low anterior resection is best sutured using a one-layer technique to produce an end-to-end inverted anastomosis. Insert vertical mattress sutures into the posterior layer and hold each suture in artery forceps until they have all been inserted. Now 'railroad' the descending colon down to the rectum. This means the sutures are all held taught while the descending colon is pushed down until its posterior edge is in contact with the rectum. Tie the sutures with the knots in the lumen. Hold the two most lateral sutures and cut the others. Suture the anterior layer using interrupted all coat vertical mattress stitches inserting them all before they are tied. Place a haemostatic clip on each side of the anastomosis to mark it radiologically.

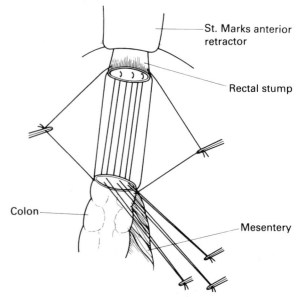

Fig. 8.7 Anterior resection of the rectum. Sutured anastomosis. One layer anastomosis showing insertion of sutures in preparation for the descending colon to be railroaded down to the rectum.

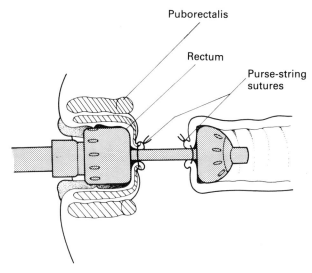

Fig. 8.8 Anterior resection of the rectum. Stapled anastomosis showing insertion of the circular stapling device through the anus with the rectum and descending colon tied over the cartridge and anvil.

Stapled anastomosis (Fig. 8.8)

1. If the anastomosis is too low to suture conventionally or if you prefer the technique, unite the bowel with the EEA circular stapling device. Carry out the operation exactly as described until the ends of the bowel have been prepared for anastomosis. Now insert the sizing heads into the rectum and colon to see if the cartridge of staples or the disposable gun should be of 25, 28 or 31 mm in diameter. For the colon it is best to select a 28 or 31 mm cartridge. Remember the stapler removes an extra 8 mm of rectum and this can be taken into account when estimating the distal clearance below the tumour. Insert a purse-string suture of 1 prolene around the rectum and colon, using a simple over-and-over stitch with the knot on the outside.

2. Introduce the EEA gun through the anus and open the cartridge. Tie the lower purse-string suture as tightly as possible around the shaft of the instrument above the cartridge. Manipulate the end of the descending colon over the top of the anvil and tie the purse-string suture as tightly as possible below the anwil.

3. Have the assistant operating the gun approximate the anvil to the cartridge while you make sure that the gun is pushed firmly upwards and that the descending colon is pulled up tightly over the anvil. Ensure that no appendices epliploica fall between the ends of the bowel to be stapled. Rotate the descending colon 90° to the left so that the mesentery lies to the right side. Fire the staple gun to construct the anastomosis. Open the gun to separate the anvil from the cartridge, twist it to make sure the anastomosis is lying free, and then gently rock it and pull it free from the anus.

Check the integrity of the stapled anastomosis

1. Examine the 'doughnuts' of colon and rectum removed from the cartridge. They should be complete. Identify the proximal and distal doughnuts and send them for histological examination.

2. Feel the anastomosis digitally with a finger through the rectum.

3. Pass a 1 cm sigmoidoscope to examine the anastomosis.

4. Fill the pelvis with 1 : 2000 aqueous chlorhexidine solution and gently blow air into the colon through the sigmoidoscope. If no bubbles appear and the doughnuts are complete, the anastomosis is satisfactory.

Peranal anastomosis (Fig. 8.9)

1. If the rectum has been divided across at the level of the puborectalis muscle, or just above, it is difficult to carry out a satisfactory stapled anastomosis since part of the sphincter is removed in the distal 'doughnut'. It may also be be impossible to insert the purse-string suture into the rectum from above and it may be difficult to insert it satisfactorily by the peranal route. In these circumstances choose to make a peranal anastomosis.

2. Insert an anal retractor of the Parks or Eisenhammer type through the anus and bring the descending colon down to the anal canal with stay sutures. Make the anastomosis either end-to-end at the upper anal canal, or excise the 1.5 cm of rectal mucosa from the dentate line to the upper anal canal, draw down the colon and suture it to the dentate line. In either method use interrupted polyglycolic-

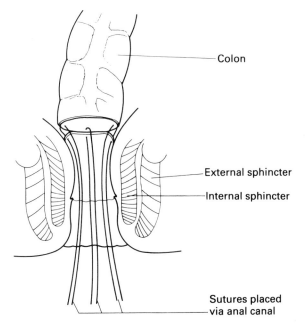

Fig. 8.9 Anterior resection of the rectum. Peranal anastomosis. The descending colon has been drawn down to the upper anal canal. A self-retaining retractor in the anus allows access for interrupted sutures to be inserted.

acid (Dexon) or polyglactin 910 (Vicryl) inserted through the anal canal to suture the whole thickness of the colon wall to the anal canal and underlying internal sphincter muscle.

3. Palpate after completion to make sure the anastomosis is complete. A peranal anastomosis demands the protection of a transverse colostomy. A low stapled or sutured anastomosis can be carried out without a defunctioning colostomy but perform one if the anastomosis is incomplete, technically difficult, if viability is questionable at the end of the operation, if soiling occurred during the procedure, or if the colon was badly prepared in an obstructed patient.

Check list

1. Make certain there is no bleeding, particularly in region of the splenic flexure and spleen.

2. Check that the anastomosis is under no tension and that the descending colon lies in the sacral hollow.

3. Ensure that the descending colon is viable.

4. In a low anastomosis do not close the mesentery.

5. Drain the pelvis, preferably using a sump suction drain, through a stab wound in the left iliac fossa.

6. Arrange the small bowel and cover it with omentum before closing abdomen.

HARTMANN'S OPERATION

Appraise

After carrying out an anterior resection of the rectum or rectosigmoid it may be inadvisable to proceed with an anastomosis in the following circumstances:

1. If the procedure is palliative and the anastomosis would demand the addition of a defunctioning colostomy.

2. If there is residual carcinoma in the lateral pelvic wall or internal iliac nodes.

Action

1. Close the distal rectum. If the rectum is cut off low down and the end is difficult to suture, leave it open and insert a drain through the anus into the pelvis.

2. Close the peritoneum over the rectal stump if possible. Bring out an end colostomy as described following abdomino-perineal excision of the rectum.

ABDOMINOPERINEAL EXCISION OF THE RECTUM

Prepare

1. Before operation mark on the skin of the left iliac fossa the site of the colostomy.

2. This operation may be carried out by one surgical team carrying out the abdominal and then the perineal part of the operation, or by a synchronous combined approach with two teams.

3. Place the patient in the lithotomy Trendelenberg position of Lloyd-Davies.

4. Rest the sacrum on a pad to allow the coccyx to overhang the end of the table.

5. Insert a self retaining catheter into the bladder, connected to a plastic bag of closed continuous drainage.

6. Suture or strap up the scrotum clear of the perineal operation field.

7. Assess the carcinoma digitally to ascertain that the tumour is technically operable. If the tumour is too low for anastomosis to be constructed after excising it, excision of the rectum is the preferred procedure.

8. The anus is closed with a strong silk purse string suture.

ABDOMINAL OPERATOR

Access

1. Stand on the patient's left side.

2. Construct a trephine in the left iliac fossa at the previously marked site for the colostomy. Remove a disc of skin 2 cm in diameter together with the subcutaneous fat and aponeurosis. Separate the underlying muscle fibres rather than cut across them. Make a cruciate incision in the peritoneum.

3. Suture the aponeurosis to the subcutaneous fascia with four interrupted chromic catgut sutures.

4. Open the abdomen through a lower midline incision extending above the umbilicus.

Assess

1. Palpate the liver for metastases.

2. Palpate the gallbladder for calculi.

3. Examine the whole of the colon and then the small intestine.

4. Examine the mesentery and para-aortic region for enlarged lymph nodes.

5. Examine the peritoneal cavity, particularly in the rectovesical pouch for peritoneal metastases.

6. Finally palpate the tumour which will be retroperitoneal.

Action (Fig. 8.10)

1. Cover the wound edges with damp packs and suture the lower cut edge of the peritoneum to the skin.

2. Place the small bowel to the right side of the incision so that it is lying outside the wound if possible, and cover it with a pack.

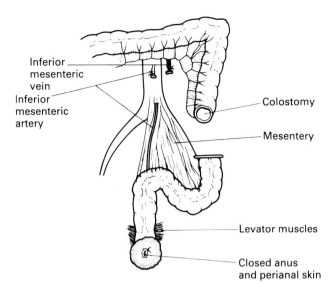

Inferior mesenteric vein

Inferior mesenteric artery

Colostomy

Mesentery

Levator muscles

Closed anus and perianal skin

Fig. 8.10 Abdominoperineal excision of the rectum. The excised specimen consists of the rectum, anus, perianal skin and sigmoid colon and mesentery. The inferior mesenteric artery is divided at its origin from the aorta and the inferior mesenteric vein at a similar level.

3. Cut the lateral adhesions from the sigmoid colon and along the lateral aspect of the descending colon.

4. Lift the colon upwards and to the right and find the left ureter and gonadal vessels, which are swept away from the vascular pedicle.

5. Retract the sigmoid colon to the left and incise the peritoneum over the aorta up as far as the duodenum. Mobilise the vascular pedicle and ligate and divide the inferior mesenteric artery at its origin from the aorta, and the inferior mesenteric vein at the same level or a little higher.

6. Select a suitable site in the sigmoid colon for division of the bowel. Pull the colon down until it easily reaches the symphysis pubis and this will be found to leave approximately the correct length of colon for construction of the colostomy. Cut the mesocolon, ligating and dividing the marginal vessels to this point.

7. Commence the pelvic dissection by incising the peritoneum down on each side of the rectum to the level of the vesicles.

8. Lift the rectosigmoid mesentery forwards from the promontory of the sacrum and insert a pair of blunt-ended scissors in the midline downwards and backwards in front of the first piece of the sacrum and behind the mesorectum. The plane of clearance is anterior to the presacral fascia. Take care to see and preserve the presacral sympathetic nerves. Continue the separation downwards by blunt-ended scissor dissection as far as the coccyx. At this stage the abdominal and perineal operators meet behind the mesorectum. Define the course of both ureter in the pelvis and carefully preserve them.

9. Continue the dissection anteriorly. Joint the peritoneal incisions anteriorly 1 cm in front of the lowest part of the peritoneal pouch. Expose the base of the bladder and

both vesicles, or the vaginal wall in the female. Place a lipped St Mark's retractor behind the vesicles and draw them upwards exposing the fascia of Denonvilliers on the anorectal wall. Incise this transversely to enter a distinct line of cleavage posterior to it, extending down as far as the apex of the prostate. Define the anterior border of the lateral ligaments.

10. Divide the lateral ligaments laterally by retracting the rectum to one side and then the other. Pick up and ligate the middle haemorrhoidal vessels after dividing the lateral ligaments.

11. Divide the colon between Zachary Cope clamps. When the perineal dissection is completed have the excised colon and rectum withdrawn through the perineum.

12. Irrigate the pelvic cavity with 500 ml of 1:500 mercuric perchloride solution.

13. Pass a long artery forceps through the colostomy trephine hole and use this to elevate the left side of the abdominal wall and expose the paracolic gutter. Insert a non-absorbable purse string suture between the lateral edge of the peritoneum and the colostomy site, including some muscle fibres, continuing under the peritoneum of the paracolic gutter to the cut edge of the peritoneum lying along the antimesenteric border of the colon. Tie this purse string suture and obliterate the lateral space.

14. Pass the Zachary Cope clamp on the proximal end of the colon through the colostomy trephine hole.

15. Before closure of the pelvic peritoneal floor, both the pelvic and abdominal operators must make certain that complete haemostasis has been achieved.

16. Mobilise the peritoneum from the lateral walls of the pelvis and the iliac fossae gently with the fingers and suture the edges together over the empty pelvis with a continuous 2/0 chromic catgut suture.

17. Close the abdominal wound.

18. Remove the Zachary Cope clamps from the colon then trim it to leave 1 cm projecting above the skin. Suture the edge of the colon to the edge of the skin wound with a 2/0 chromic catgut suture on a cutting needle.

PERINEAL OPERATOR

Start the perineal operation when the abdominal operator has opened the abdomen, carried out a full laparotomy and has ligated and divided the inferior mesenteric artery and vein.

In the male (Fig. 8.11)

1. Make an elliptical incision around the closed anal canal from a point midway between the anus and the bulb of the urethra anteriorly, and extending backwards to the sacrococcygeal articulation. Deepen the incision to expose the lobulated fat of the ischiorectal fossae and the coccyx.

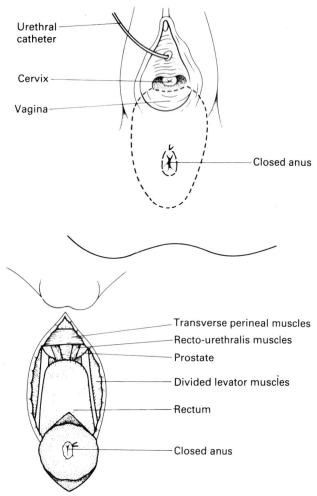

Fig. 8.11 Perineal approach of abdominperineal excision of the rectum. The female pelvis on the left and male on the right. The broken lines indicate the extent of the excision. In the female the posterior vaginal wall is removed up to the posterior fornix. In the male the initial plane is posterior to the transverse perineal muscles.

Pick up the skin edges and the anal skin with tissue forceps.

2. In the male with a small pelvis and a patient with a large posterior tumour low in the rectum, remove the coccyx. Flex the coccyx to open a coccygeal joint and divide across with a scalpel to separate the distal portion of the coccyx. Coagulate the middle sacral vessels.

3. Make small incisions on either side of the coccyx through the fibrous attachment at the coccygeal raphe and with a finger separate the levator muscles from the underlying rectal fascia of Waldeyer.

4. Divide the levator muscles well out on the lateral wall of the pelvis and ligate or coagulate the inferior haemorrhoidal vessels.

5. Insert a St Mark's pattern self-retaining perineal retractor. Clearly identify Waldeyer's fascia and cut it across just in front of the divided coccyx. Extend the incision laterally to expose the mesorectum.

6. Separate the mesorectum from the anterior aspect of the presacral fascia and join up with the abdominal operator.

7. Retract the rectum posteriorly and make a transverse incision anteriorly to expose the superficial and the deep transverse perineal muscles. The plane of dissection must be behind these muscles to avoid injury to the urethra.

8. Divide the broad strap-like pubococcygeus muscle on either side of the rectum. Then divide the underlying fascia, which is the lateral continuation of the fascia of Denonvilliers and Waldeyer, to expose the rectal wall. Palpate the prostate anteriorly and define the plane between the rectum and prostate.

9. Insert an artery forceps anteriorly between the rectum and the prostate to separate the rectourethralis muscle fibres. Divide these fibres to expose the prostatic capsule. Cut the visceral pelvic fascia which is condensed anteriorly to the lateral aspect of the prostate, to expose the whole of the prostate and the vesicles above. Anteriorly your dissection now meets that of the abdominal operator.

10. Divide the lower parts of the lateral ligaments and then draw the rectum and sigmoid colon through the perineal incision.

11. Flatten the operating table and secure pelvic haemostasis.

12. If haemostasis can be secured and there is no significant sepsis place a sump suction drain, such as the Shirley drain, into the pelvis through a lateral stab wound, and secure it to the skin.

13. Close the incision with subcutaneous and skin sutures of 3/0 interrupted polyglycolic acid (Dexon) or polyglactin 910 (Vicryl). If the wound is unsuitable for primary closure leave the centre open to take three fingers, and insert a corrugated drain into the pelvis.

In the female

1. Unless the tumour is small and situated in the midline posteriorly always remove the posterior vaginal wall. Make an incision from the posterior lateral aspects of the labia around the anus to the coccyx.

2. The posterior part of the dissection is as in the male until the anterior part of the dissection is reached. Carry the anterior incision upwards through the lateral aspect of the vagina as far as the posterior fornix. Make a transverse incision to join the two lateral incisions and deepen it to expose the rectal wall, to meet the abdominal operator.

3. Make no attempt to reconstruct the vagina. Obtain haemostasis by oversewing the cut edge of the vagina with a continuous 2/0 chromic catgut suture.

4. Close the subcutaneous tissue and skin with interrupted mattress sutures of 3/0 polyglycolic acid (Dexon) or polyglactin 910 (Vicryl).

5. Drain the pelvis by placing a currugated drain through the re-formed vaginal orifice.

Difficulty

1. In the male or female, it may be impossible to close the peritoneal floor to prevent small bowel herniation to the skin incision or out through the vagina. In these circumstances place a plastic (Aldon) bag into the pelvis, fill it with gauze from rolls, to pack the bag and keep the small intestine in the abdominal cavity. Loosely close the skin of the perineal wound to keep the bag in place. Remove the gauze and bag after 3–5 days.

2. If the pelvic haemorrhage cannot be controlled, pack the pelvis with gauze directly. Leave the packs for 72 hours and gently remove them under an anaesthetic so that the pelvis can be inspected.

OTHER OPERATIONS FOR CARCINOMA OF THE LARGE BOWEL

PAUL-MIKULICZ OPERATION

Appraise

This is largely superseded, but can occasionally be valuable in an emergency. Exteriorize the colon loop and remove the lesion, leaving a double-barrelled colostomy which can be closed later. It can be used only if both ends of the colon can be brought out onto the surface of the abdomen. It could be used in cases of obstructive carcinoma, colonic trauma or perforation, sigmoid volvulus, ischaemic colitis, when the patient is very sick with intercurrent disease, there is severe contamination with peritonitis or the perfusion of the ends of the colon is doubtful and would not support an anastomosis.

PULL-THROUGH ANASTOMOSIS

This is largely historical and has been replaced by anterior resection with anastomosis. Before low anterior resection became established this method was used. The operation is carried out as for an anterior resection of the rectum. Instead of carrying out an anastomosis the proximal colon is pulled through the sphincters and approximately 10 cm left projecting beyond the anus. When good union has taken place between the cut end of the rectum and the pulled through colon, the excess colon is removed on the 7–10th day. An alternative procedure is to evert the cuff of the rectum and carry out an end-to-end anastomosis between this and the end of the pulled-through colon. The anastomosis is then replaced in the pelvis.

COLECTOMY FOR INFLAMMATORY BOWEL DISEASE

COLECTOMY AND ILEOSTOMY FOR ACUTE COLITIS

Appraise

1. Acute fulminating colitis, with or without toxic megacolon, usually occurs in idiopathic ulcerative colitis but may occur in Crohn's colitis.

2. The operation of choice is to carry out a colectomy and ileostomy. It is incorrect to carry out an emergency proctocolectomy as the mortality and morbidity are increased and there is no opportunity to carry out a secondary ileorectal anastomosis.

3. Treat acute colitis medically with steroids. Correct anaemia with blood transfusion. Replace fluid and electrolyte loss.

4. If the patient does not improve in 24 hours and still has over six bowel actions containing blood each day, there is a fever of over 38°C and a tachycardia over 100, surgical treatment is likely.

5. Carry out daily plain X-ray of abdomen to see if toxic dilatation develops.

6. If there is toxic dilatation or evidence of perforation carry out emergency surgery.

7. If the patient's condition does not improve within 72 hours, carry out surgery.

8. Beware of being lulled into a false sent of security as the patient's condition is more critical than apparent.

Prepare

1. Continue steroid therapy with 100 mg of hydrocortisone 6 hourly. Commence full antibiotic cover with gentomicin and metronidazole.

2. Mark site of ileostomy if patient is fit enough.

3. Place the patient in the Lloyd-Davies position. If there is any degree of toxic dilatation gently insert a sigmoidoscope and suck gas from the rectum and colon.

4. Catheterize the patient.

Access

1. Make an ileostomy trephine 2 cm in diameter at the previously marked site. If the patient is very sick and this has not been done, make it in the right iliac fossa over the infraumbilical fat pad. The trephine is made in the same way as in the construction of a colostomy (see p. 142).

2. Open the abdomen through a long midline incision.

Assess

1. The colon is hyperaemic, thickened and oedematous. Do not handle it excessively and do not pull away adherent

omentum or lateral pelvic wall adhesions as these may be the site of sealed perforations.

2. Note any free fluid and obtain a swab for culture and antibiotic sensitivity. Note any free gas denoting that perforation has occurred. If there is a perforation, try and close it with a purse-string suture and placing omentum over it before proceeding.

3. Examine the liver to note the presence of cirrhosis, and the small bowel to see if the diagnosis could be Crohn's disease. Examine the mesentery for enlarged lymph nodes.

Action (Fig. 8.12)

1. Gently dissect the omentum from the lateral walls starting at the caecum and mobilise the colon completely down to the rectum taking care not to apply too much traction and there is good access. In any severe case, remove the omentum with the colon as any attempt to dissect it away may lead to a perforation. If the colon is fixed to the lateral wall remove a disc of peritoneum with the colon rather than risk opening a sealed perforation.

2. Transilluminate the mesentery and divide the vessels at a suitable place in the centre of the mesentery.

3. Mobilize the terminal ileum and divide it between Zachary Cope clamps 1–2 cm proximal to the ileocaecal valve.

4. Divide the colon between Parker-Kerr clamps through the sigmoid colon so that a distal mucous fistula can be brought out through the abdominal wall without tension. Do not divide the colon close to the sacral promonotory in the mistaken belief that all the colon must be resected.

5. Bring the ileum through the ileostomy trephine hole and close the lateral space with a continuous purse-string suture (see p. 119). Alternatively, suture the cut edge of the small bowel mesentery to the anterior abdominal wall,

placing interrupted non-absorbable sutures between the cut edges of the mesentery and the anterior abdominal wall, from the falciform ligament down to the edge of the trephine hole.

6. Secure haemostasis and close the abdomen with the sigmoid colon brought out through the lower end of the wound.

7. Construct the ileostomy (p. 119).

8. Place suitable instrument, for example a Lloyd-Davies enterotome, on the distal colon under the Parker-Kerr clamp, which is then removed. The enterotome is convenient for preventing the colon retracting and is tightened over successive days and usually separates in 7–10 days when the colon is firmly adherent to the abdominal wall.

Technical

1. If colectomy and ileostomy are carried out electively, the sigmoid colon can be oversewn and replaced in the peritoneal cavity.

2. In any operation for inflammatory bowel disease or polyposis coli, never carry out a proctocolectomy without considering whether a sphincter-saving operation would eventually be more appropriate. If there is any doubt in your mind, leave the rectum intact.

ELECTIVE COLECTOMY AND ILEORECTAL ANASTOMOSIS

Appraise

1. In elective surgery for ulcerative colitis or Crohn's disease or in polyposis coli, a colectomy and ileorectal anastomosis may be the appropriate operation.

2. In ulcerative colitis there must be no carcinoma or severe dysplasia associated with colitis. The rectum must be distensible to act as a reservoir and the anal sphincter function normal.

3. In Crohn's disease the rectum must be relatively free of disease and the sphincter function normal with no evidence of severe perianal disease such as fistulas.

4. In polyposis coli there must be no carcinoma in the rectum. If the rectum contains confluent polyps, it is not suitable for ileorectal anastomosis and proctocolectomy possibly with an ileoanal pouch is appropriate.

5. Never assume a patient with multiple polyps has familial adenomatosis coli until several have been biopsied and proved to be adenomas. 20% of patients will give no family history and arise as a genetic mutation.

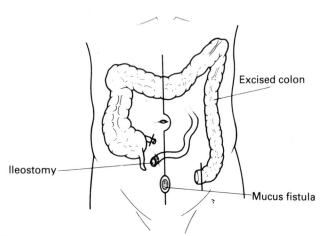

Fig. 8.12 Colectomy for acute colitis. The colon is resected to the mide-sigmoid colon which is brought out as a mucus fistula through the lower part of the midline incision. An end ileostomy is constructed in the right iliac fossa.

Access

1. The patient is placed in the lithotomy-Trendelenburg position with the legs supported on Lloyd-Davies Stirrups.

Insert a Foley catheter into the bladder for continuous drainage.

2. Open the abdomen through a long mid-line incision.

Assess

1. Palpate and visualise the liver. Examine the gallbladder to exclude calculi.

2. Examine the whole of the gastrointestinal tract, the stomach, the duodenum, the whole of the small bowel and the colon.

3. In a patient with familial polyposis coli examine the duodenum carefully for possible adenomas. If any abnormality is felt make certain the patient has upper gastrointestinal endoscopy. Examine the colon and rectum carefully to make certain no carcinoma is present. If it is, carry out a radical operation as for carcinoma. An ileorectal anastomosis is still possible provided the carcinoma is not in the rectum. In Crohn's disease examine particularly the small bowel and make certain that this is not diseased.

Action

1. Mobilise the colon completely as previously described, starting at the caecum. Work around to the rectosigmoid junction. Preserve the omentum by separating the congenital adhesions from the transverse colon.

2. Divide the mesenteric vessels at a suitable place in the mid part of the mesocolon. Preserve the superior rectal artery and vein and avoid damaging the presacral nerves. In ulcerative colitis or Crohn's disease, ligate the superior rectal artery in continuity to decrease the vascularity of the rectum. This is claimed to decrease the chances of exacerbation of inflammation in the rectum.

3. Place a Lloyd-Davies right-angle clamp across the rectosigmoid junction and irrigate the rectum through the anus with 1:2000 aqueous chlorhexadine solution.

4. Divide the terminal ileum. Place a Parker Kerr clamp at right-angles across the terminal ileum close to the ileocaecal valve. Wrap a gauze swab soaked in 1:2000 aqueous chlorhexidine around the ileum at the site of division and hold it between forefinger and thumb of the left hand. After protecting the abdominal contents with packs, divide the ileum close to the proximal side of the clamp.

5. Pick up the divided ileum with Babcock forceps, which also grasps the surrounding swab, holding it in place. Swab out the lumen with chlorhexadine solution.

6. Divide the rectum below the Lloyd-Davies' clamp with scissors and remove the specimen. Hold up the rectum with Babcock forceps.

7. The ileal lumen is usually narrower than that of the rectum. Widen the ileum with a longitudinal cut along the anti-mesenteric border. This matches the ileum and colon for size ready for anastomosis.

8. Construct an anastomosis with a single layer of inter-rupted 4/0 polypropylene sutures. Rotate the ileum to the left side through 90°. Alternatively construct the anastomosis in two layers with continuous 2/0 chromic catgut and interrupted seromusular silk.

9. Place a haemostatic clip at the lateral margins of the anastomosis.

10. Suture the rotated mesentery of the ileum to the cut edge of the peritoneum on the right side with 2/0 continuous chromic catgut. Arrange the terminal ileum so that the terminal loop lies in the left iliac fossa. This prevents acute kinking of the anastomosis. Arrange the remaining loops of bowel anatomically and cover with the omentum. Do not drain the anastomosis.

11. Close the abdomen.

Technical

If the colectomy and ileorectal anastomosis is carried out for polyposis, excise or destroy with diathermy any polyps which are going to impinge on the anastomosis, through the cut end of the rectum, before constructing the anastomosis.

ELECTIVE TOTAL PROCTOCOLECTOMY

Appraise

1. Whenever a proctocolectomy or excision of the rectum is undertaken in inflammatory bowel disease or polyposis, excise the rectum conservatively to conserve the pelvic floor and protect the pelvic autonomic nerves.

2. Excise the rectum as part of the proctocolectomy or following previous colectomy and ileostomy with a mucous fistula.

3. Mark the ileostomy preoperatively. Place it in the right iliac fossa in the infraumbilical fat pad through the right rectus muscle.

Access

1. Place the patient in the lithotomy-Trendelenburg position of Lloyd-Davies.
2. Ensure an indwelling bladder catheter is in place.
3. Open the abdomen through a long mid-line incisiion.

Action (Fig. 8.13)

1. Carry out the colectomy and ileostomy as previously described (p. 145). If a patient has previously had a colectomy and a mucous fistula, mobilize the mucous fistula when the wound is reopened, and oversew the sigmoid colon.

2. Mobilize the rectum with peritoneal incisions on both sides of the rectum close to the rectal wall, joined anteriorly just above the lowest part of the peritoneal pouch. Preserve

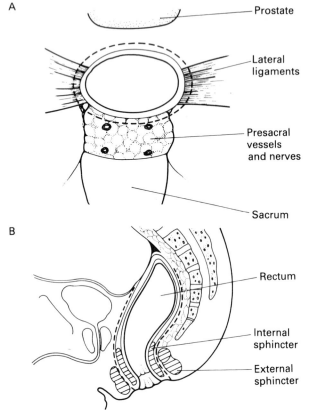

A
— Prostate
— Lateral ligaments
— Presacral vessels and nerves
— Sacrum

B
— Rectum
— Internal sphincter
— External sphincter

Fig. 8.13 Proctocolectomy for inflammatory bowel disease. The rectal excision is not the same as for malignant disease. The abdominal operator on the left preserves the superior rectal vessels, presacral fat and nerves. The perineal excision below is in the plane between the internal and external sphincter.

the superior rectal artery, together with the presacral fat and nerves. Clamp, divide and ligate the individual sigmoid and rectal arteries close to the rectal wall with fine ligatures.

3. Dissect posteriorly as far as the coccyx to meet the upward dissection of the surgeon operating in the perineum.

4. Dissect anteriorly between the rectum and the vagina in the female. In the male, hold up the seminal vesicles with a St Mark's lip retractor. Divide the fascia of Denonvilliers transversely and dissect downwards between the rectum and the prostate.

5. Divide the lateral ligaments close to the rectal wall.

6. If the operation is being carried out as a synchronous combined excision the perineal surgeon will have completed the rectal excision and the specimen can be removed through the perineal wound.

7. Close the pelvic peritoneum with a continuous 2/0 chromic catgut suture.

Perineal operation

1. Place a strong purse-string suture around the anus close to the anal margin since a minimum of skin will be removed.

2. Make a circumferential incision over the intersphincteric groove and deepen it to expose the intersphincteric plane between the pale fibres of the internal sphincter and the dark red fibres of the voluntary muscle of the external sphincter.

3. Divide the longitudinal fibres crossing the internal sphincter of fix the mucosa at the dentate line. Separate the internal sphincter from the puborectalis and levator muscles, easily establishing a plane into the pelvis. Carry out a similar dissection on the other side of the anus and then dissect the posterior part of the external sphincter from the puborectalis muscle.

4. Deepen the anterioir part of the dissection behind the superficial and deep transverse perineal muscles and then continue the dissection upwards between the vagina and the rectal wall. The wound is small and a self-retaining retractor cannot be inserted. Improve the exposure using a Langenbeck retractor, or a pelvic lateral wall retractor of the Lockhart-Mummery type. In the male, the external sphincter decussates in the midline and becomes attached to the fibres of the rectourethralis muscle. Cut the strip-like parts of the rectourethralis muscle to expose the posterior aspect of the prostate. Divide the visceral pelvic fascia laterally on each side where it is condensed onto the lateral lobes of the prostate. The seminal vesicles are then apparent in the upper part of the wound.

5. Divide Waldeyer's fascia posteriorly and meet the abdominal surgeon. Divide the lower parts of the lateral ligament and then remove the specimen through the perineal wound. This excision leaves a small wound with the external sphincter and the whole of the levator muscles intact.

Closure

1. Drain the pelvis with a sump suction catheter inserted through a lateral stab wound and placed above the levator muscles.

2. Approximate the puborectalis and levator muscles with 3/0 polyglycolic acid (Dexon) or polyglactin 910 (Vicryl) sutures. Approximate the subcutaneous fat and close the skin with interrupted mattress sutures also of polyglycolic acid or polyglactin 910.

3. Start continuous suction drainage immediately.

Technical

In patients with ulcerative colitis or polyposis coli who wish to avoid a permanent conventional ileostomy but are not suitable for an ileorectal anastomosis two alternative procedures can be carried out:

1. A Koch reservoir ileostomy. This consists of a reservoir constructed from 45 cm of terminal ileum with an intussuscepted nipple valve in the efferent ileum. The

reservoir is continent and emptied by catheterisation so that no external appliance is necessary.

2. A restorative proctocolectomy. The rectum is divided across at the level of the puborectalis and the internal and external sphincter muscles are preserved. Through the anus the mucosa between the dentate line and the puborectalis is removed from the underlying internal sphincter muscle. A pelvic reservoir, preferably of the J type can then be constructed and anastomosed to the anal canal. Such a procedure must be covered by a defunctioning ileostomy.

DUHAMEL OPERATION

Appraise

1. This is the most satisfactory procedure for treating adult Hirschsprung's disease. A variety of operations are carried out for this condition in children but will not be considered (see Ch. 32).

2. Confirm the diagnosis of Hirschsprung's disease by anorectal manometry to show the absence of the rectosphincteric reflex. Remove a full thickness biopsy to show the absence of ganglia and abnormal autonomic nerve plexuses within the bowel wall.

3. Adults with Hirschsprung's disease do not always have short segment disease.

Prepare

1. It is unnecessary to carry out a preliminary colostomy in these patients.
2. Place the patient in the lithotomy-Trendelenburg position of Lloyd-Davies.
3. Insert an indwelling catheter.
4. Open the abdomen through a long midline incision.

Assess

1. After carrying out a general laparotomy examine the colon carefully. The narrow segment may be quite short.

2. The bowel proximal to the narrow segment is dilated and thickened and then gradually becomes of normal diameter.

3. Plan to excise the thickened dilated bowel.

Action (Fig. 8.14)

Abdominal operation

1. Mobilise the colon. The splenic flexure will probably need to be taken down so mobilise it initially as previously described (see p. 138).

2. Mobilize the rectum to its upper third.

3. Place a right-angle clamp across the middle third of the rectum at the site of division, to leave a rectal stump of approximately 10 cm Have the rectum below the clamp carefully washed out through the anus with 1:2000 aqueous chlorhexadine solution.

4. Dissect behind the rectum down to the tip of the coccyx.

5. Divide the rectum across below the clamp and close the divided rectum in two layers with a continuous catgut suture and inverting seromuscular sutures.

6. Divide the colon at an appropriate place above the dilated hypertrophied segment in the descending or sigmoid colon.

7. Remove the specimen. Arrange for frozen sections to be carried out on the upper end of the specimen to make sure ganglia are present. Swab out the colon with 1:2000 aqueous chlorhexadine solution.

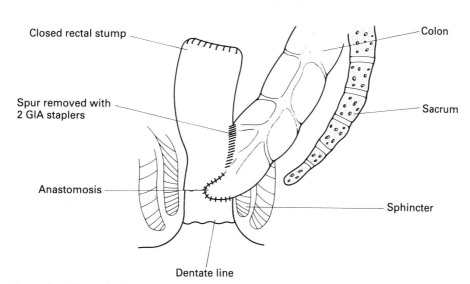

Closed rectal stump

Spur removed with 2 GIA staplers

Anastomosis

Dentate line

Colon

Sacrum

Sphincter

Fig. 8.14 Duhamel operation. The retained rectum with the colon anastomosed to the posterior wall at the level of the puborectalis. The septum between the rectum and colon is removed with the GIA stapler.

Peranal operation

1. Insert a self-retaining anal retractor and make a transverse incision through the posterior half of the rectal wall at the level of the puborectalis.

2. Deepen the wound until the space which has been dissected behind the rectum is entered.

3. Bring down the mobilised colon to the upper anal canal with stay sutures.

4. Suture the lower edge of the anal incision of the posterior edge of the colon with interrupted sutures of polyglycolic acid (Dexon) or polyglactin 910 (Vicryl). Similarly suture the anterior wall of the rectum to the upper end of the anal incision.

5. Apply a modified Duhamel clamp or Parker Kerr clamps to crush the spur between the rectum and the colon which has been brought down posteriorly. Leave the clamps in place until the rectal and colonic wall between the jaws becomes necrotic and separates. Alternatively, immediately resect this spur by placing two GIA staple lines from the lateral aspects of the anastomosis to meet at the top of the rectal stump. The intervening piece of the rectal and colonic wall will be removed. It is usually necessary to suture the top end of the rectum and colon between the lines of staples.

6. Close the abdominal wound with drainage.

Technical

A colectomy and ileorectal anastomosis is the operation of choice in patients who are constipated due to slow transit or ideopathic megarectum and megacolon.

SOAVE OPERATION

Appraise

1. This operation was described initially to treat Hirschsprung's disease, but is rarely used for this in adults.

2. A modified Soave operation is very useful to treat large villous tumours, irradiation proctitis, rectovaginal and rectoprostatic fistulas and haemangeomas of the rectum.

Access

1. Place the patient in the lithotomy-Trendelenburg position. Drain the bladder with an indwelling catheter.

2. Open the abdomen through a long mid-line incision.

3. Assess the nature and extent of the pelvic disease. Carry out a general exploration of the abdomen.

Action (Fig. 8.15)

1. Mobilize the sigmoid colon, descending colon and splenic flexure. Divide the rectum across to leave 10 cm or 12 cm.

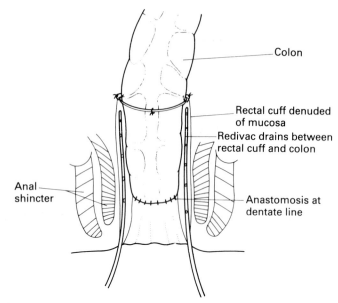

Fig. 8.15 Soave operation. The mobilized left colon is drawn through the retained rectum denuded of mucosa and sutures to the dentate line. Fine suction drainage tubes are inserted through the perianal skin to drain the potential space between the rectum and colon.

2. Resect any diseased bowel above this.

3. Working from above and through the anus with a self-retaining retractor inject a solution of 1:300 000 adrenaline in saline under the mucosa to lift it off the underlying circular muscle.

4. Remove the mucosa from the whole of the rectum down to the dentate line.

5. Bring down normal colon through this muscular tube and suture with polyglycolic acid (Dexon) or polyglactin 910 (Vicryl) sutures to the dentate line, making certain that the anal sutures include part of the internal sphincter muscle. Three or four sutures approximate the upper end of the rectal cuff of the descending colon.

6. Close abdomen without drainage.

7. Place Redivac drains close to the anus, led up through the intersphincteric plane to drain the space between the colon and the rectal cuff.

Further reading

Dudley H A F 1983 Operative surgery: alimentary tract and abdominal wall. 4th edn. Butterworths, London
Goligher J C 1984 Surgery of the anus, rectum and colon, 5th edn. Bailliere Tindall, London
Schwartz S I, Ellis H 1985 Maingot's abdominal operations. 8th edn. Vol 2. Butterworth, London.
1978 Surgical techniques illustrated Vol 3, No. 2 Little Brown, Boston

Anorectal surgery

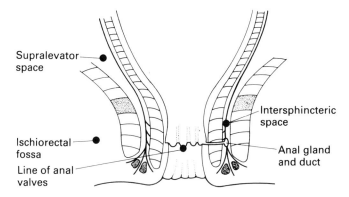

Fig. 9.1 A diagram to show the essential anatomy of the anal canal.

INTRODUCTION

Operations on the anal canal and peri-anal area are relatively simple but there is a need for finesse, meticulous attention to detail and carefully supervised postoperative care. Thus, a sound understanding of the anatomy of the area and precision in diagnosis is essential for effective treatment. Therefore always perform a full rectal examination including inspection, palpation, sigmoidoscopy and proctoscopy, before carrying out any procedure. If indicated, exclude serious diseases, such as neoplastic or inflammatory bowel disease with barium enema X-ray and colonoscopy.

ANATOMY

The anal canal extends from the anorectal junction superiorly to the anus below and is approximately 3–4 cm long. The lining epithelium is characterised by the anal valves midway along the anal canal. This line of the anal valves is often loosely referred to as the 'dentate line' (Fig. 9.1). It does not represent the point of fusion between the embryonic hind-gut and the proctoderm which occurs at a higher level, between the anal valves and the anorectal junction. In this zone, sometimes called the transitional

zone, there is a mixture of columnar and squamous epithelium.

SPHINCTERS

The anal canal is surrounded by two sphincter muscles. The internal sphincter is the expanded distal portion of the circular muscle of the large intestine. It is composed of smooth muscle and is white in colour. The external sphincter lies outside the internal sphincter. It is composed of striated muscle and is brown in colour. Superiorly it is contiguous with the puborectalis and levator ani muscles, forming one continuous striated muscle sheet (Fig. 9.1). The external sphincter is supplied by the pudendal nerve entering the muscle from its outer aspect posterolaterally, and the levator ani from branches of the fourth sacral nerve on its superior aspect. The levator ani and puborectalis muscles are responsible for holding the anal canal at its correct position in relationship to the bony pelvis; this is with the top of the anal canal on the line joining the tip of the coccyx to the inferior aspect of the symphysis pubis. They also maintain the correct angle between the rectum and anal canal at less than 90° (Fig. 9.2).

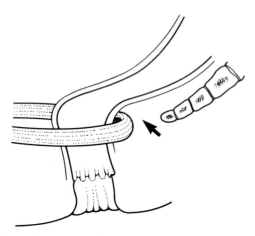

Fig. 9.2 A sagittal diagram to show the relationship of the distal rectum to the anal canal. The anorectal angle is just less than a right angle in normal people.

SPACES

There are three important spaces around the anal canal — the intersphincteric space, the ischiorectal fossa and the supralevator space (Fig. 9.1). These spaces are important in the spread of sepsis and in certain operations.

1. *The intersphincteric space* lies between the two sphincters and contains the terminal fibres of the longitudinal muscle of the large intestine. It also contains the anal intermuscular glands, approximately 12 in number, arranged around the anal canal. The ducts of these glands pass through the internal sphincter and open into the anal crypts.

2. *The ischiorectal fossa* lies lateral to the external sphincter and contains fat. Abscesses may occur in this site as the result of horizontal spread of infection across the external sphincter.

3. *The supralevator space* lies between the levator ani and the rectum. It is important in the spread of infection.

Prepare

1. Familiarize yourself with the small range of essential instruments for examination of the patient, such as the proctoscope and the rigid sigmoidoscope. In patients with anal sphincter spasm, use a small paediatric sigmoidoscope.

2. Operating proctoscopes of the Eisenhammer, Parks and Sims type are essential for operations on and within the anal canal.

3. Use a pair of fine scissors, fine forceps (toothed and non-toothed), a light needle holder, Emetts forceps and a small No. 15 scalpel blade for inter-anal work.

4. For fistula surgery have a set of Lockhart-Mummery fistula probes (Fig. 9.3), **together** with a set of Anel's lacrimal probes.

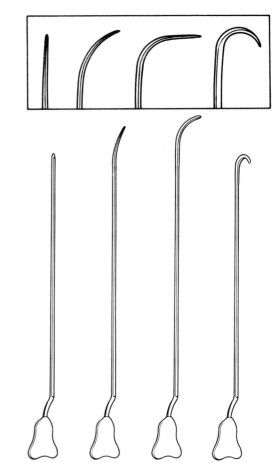

Fig. 9.3 A set of four Lockhart-Mummery fistula probes.

5. Most patients require no preparation, or two glycerine suppositories to ensure an empty rectum before anal surgery. If for any reason the bowels need to be confined post-operatively, then carry out a full bowel preparation to empty the whole large intestine.

6. Take a blood sample from all patients. In addition to a routine haemoglobin estimation, take blood for blood group determination. Request that serum be held in the laboratory. Primary, reactionary and secondary haemorrhage may occur in any anal operation. For complex fistula operations, request cross matched blood for the operation.

7. Minor operations can be performed under local infiltration anaesthesia, larger procedures demand regional or general anaesthesia.

8. Position of the patient. For outpatient procedures use the left lateral position, or alternatively the knee-elbow position. For anal operations most United Kingdom surgeons favour the lithotomy position, although the jack-knife position (Fig. 9.4) has its advocates.

9. Shave the whole area before starting any anal operation, best done in the operating theatre yourself where there is good illumination. This is much easier for the patient and more efficient than a shave in the ward before operation.

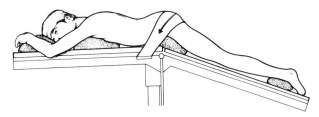

Fig. 9.4 The jack-knife position.

HAEMORRHOIDS

Appraise

1. Exclude pelvic tumours, large bowel carcinoma and inflammatory bowel disease.

2. Haemorrhoids do not always need treatment if the symptoms are minimal.

3. We treat small internal haemorrhoids by injection sclerotherapy, prolapsing haemorrhoids by elastic band ligation and large prolapsing haemorrhoids, which are usually accompanied by a significant external component, by haemorrhoidectomy.

4. All procedures are contra-indicated if the patient also has Crohn's disease.

INJECTION SCLEROTHERAPY

Although injection sclerotherapy is an outpatient procedure and does not require any anaesthesia, we shall describe it for completeness. It is most conveniently done after full rectal examination if no further investigation is required. The patient is usually in the left lateral position.

Action

1. Pass full length proctoscope and withdraw slowly to identify the anorectal junction — the area where the anal canal begins to close around the instrument.

2. Place a ball of cotton wool into the lower rectum with Emetts forceps to keep the walls apart (the patients, as it is not usually removed, should be told they will pass the cotton wool with the next motion).

3. Identify the position of the right anterior, left lateral and right posterior haemorrhoids.

4. Fill a 10 ml (Gabriel pattern) syringe with 5% phenol in arachis oil with 0.5% menthol (oily phenol BP).

5. Through the full length proctoscope, insert the needle into the submucosa at the anorectal junction at the identified positions of the haemorrhoids in turn. Inject 3–5 ml of 5% phenol in arachis oil into the submucosa at each site, to produce a swelling with a pearly appearance of the mucosa in which the vessels are clearly seen. Move the needle slightly during injection to avoid giving an intravascular injection.

6. After injecting, delay removal of the needle for a few seconds to lessen the escape of the solution. If necessary, press on the injection site with cotton wool to minimize leakage.

7. Warn the patient to avoid attempts at defaecation for 24 hours.

Care

1. Avoid injecting the solution too superficially. This produces a watery bleb which may ulcerate and subsequently cause haemorrhage

2. Avoid injecting the solution too deep. This produces an oleogranuloma with subsequent features of an extrarectal swelling. Too deep anterior injection in male patients causes perineal pain and even haematuria from prostatitis.

3. If the patient complains of sudden right subcostal pain, stop the injection. Phenol solution may have entered a portal vein radical.

ELASTIC BAND LIGATION

Elastic band ligation is also an outpatient procedure and does not need anaesthesia. There are several different designs of band applicators and the simplest is illustrated (Fig. 9.5). Have a pair of grasping forceps such as Patterson's biopsy forceps.

Action

1. Load two elastic bands on to the band applicator.

2. Pass the full length proctoscope and withdraw it slowly to identify the anorectal junction. Position the end of proctoscope midway between the anorectal junction and the dentate line.

3. Pass the tips of the grasping forceps through the ring of the band applicator, through the proctoscope and take hold of the selected haemorrhoid.

4. Pull the haemorrhoid through the ring of band applicator whilst pushing the band applicator upwards. Establish whether or not the patient experiences any additional discomfort. If he does *not*, 'fire' the band on to the haemorrhoid. If he does, reposition the grip on the haemorrhoid slightly higher and retest before applying the band.

5. We band only one or two haemorrhoids on each occasion. Others are applied at intervals of 4 weeks.

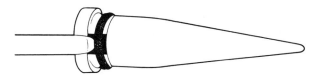

Fig. 9.5 A simple instrument with which to perform elastic band ligation of haemorrhoids.

Aftercare

1. Warn the patient to avoid attempts at defaecation for 24 hours.

2. Warn the patient that there may be discomfort, but no pain if band is in correct site, and that mild analgesics may be needed. If the patient experiences severe pain the band has been applied too low on to sensitive epithelium. If analgesics do not control the pain, remove the bands in the operating theatre under general anaesthesia, using an operating proctoscope.

3. Pain developing slowly in 1–2 days may be from ischaemia. Analgesics relieve the pain and metronidazole tablets 200 mg thrice daily reduce inflammation.

4. Warn the patient that the haemorrhoid and the band should drop off after 5–10 days. There may be a small amount of bleeding at this time.

5. Warn the patient of the risk of secondary haemorrhage — approximately 2% — and that it may occur any time up to 3 weeks after application. He should report to hospital if this is severe since he may require transfusion and operative control of the bleeding.

6. Stenosis of the upper anal canal presents with difficulty in defaecation and the passage of very narrow stools. It is usually avoided if no more than two band applications are made at any one time.

HAEMORRHOIDECTOMY

There are different methods of performing a haemorrhoidectomy, but we shall describe the ligation and excision technique of Milligan and Morgan. Haemorrhoidectomy should be a curative procedure and must be done very carefully and thoroughly. The anaesthetized patient is in the lithotomy position with some head-down tilt.

Action

1. Place small curved haemostats on the skin at the anal margin in the patient's left lateral, right posterior and right anterior positions. Draw them outwards to expose the internal components of the haemorrhoids.

2. Place similar curved haemostats on the internal components. Traction applied to all pairs of haemostats produces the 'triangle of exposure' (Fig. 9.6).

3. Infiltrate approximately 5 ml of 1 : 200 000 adrenaline in 1% lignocaine hydrochloride solution into each haemorrhoid to aid dissection and haemostasis.

4. Cut through the skin with straight scissors starting at the periphery of each haemorrhoid to free it towards the anal canal, starting with the left lateral haemorrhoid. Preserve a complete muco-cutaneous bridge between each hae-

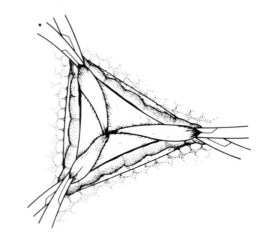

Fig. 9.6 Haemorrhoidectomy: the triangle of exposure.

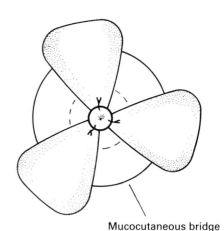

Mucocutaneous bridge

Fig. 9.7 Haemorrhoidectomy: it is essential to preserve three mucocutaneous bridges.

morrhoid dissection (Fig. 9.7). Take care to identify and avoid damage to the brown fibres of the external sphincter muscle, and the white fibres of the internal sphincter muscle. Both of them must be carefully dissected away from the haemorrhoid.

5. When the base of the haemorrhoid is reached, just below the anorectal junction, ligate it with strong silk with the knot on the lumen side (Fig. 9.8). Some surgeons prefer a transfixion suture with catgut. Excise the haemorrhoid distal to the ligature. Deal in turn with the right anterior and right posterior haemorrhoids.

6. Now examine the three mucocutaneous bridges which are the sites of the secondary haemorrhoids. Excise any vascular tissue under the skin or mucosa using fine scissors and fine toothed forceps (Fig. 9.9).

7. Suture the mucocutaneous bridges on to the internal sphincter muscle using 000 chromic catgut, at the mid point of the anal canal (Fig. 9.10). Simply ligate any redundant mucosa above this point.

8. Insert a full length proctoscope to exclude narrowing and ensure that the three pedicles are secure.

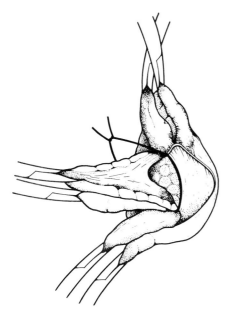

Fig. 9.8 Haemorrhoidectomy: ligation of the haemorrhoid just below the anorectal junction.

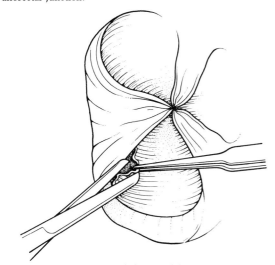

Fig. 9.9 Haemorrhoidectomy: it is essential to remove secondary haemorrhoidal tissue from beneath the mucocutaneous bridges.

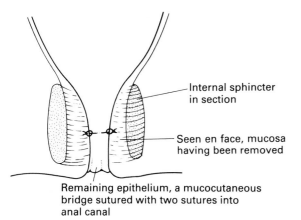

Internal sphincter in section

Seen en face, mucosa having been removed

Remaining epithelium, a mucocutaneous bridge sutured with two sutures into anal canal

Fig. 9.10 Haemorrhoidectomy: suturing the bridges to the internal sphincter to prevent redundant skin tags.

9. Make certain that the external wounds are of adequate size. Skin heals faster than mucosa. An inadequate skin wound may result in a persistent unhealed internal wound.

10. Insert a small soft rubber drain into the anal canal to prevent the wounds adhering to each other. Place a gauze swab soaked in 1:40 sodium hypochlorite solution on the external wounds or alternatively, gauze soaked in topical adrenaline (1:1000). Some surgeons still prefer to insert gauze dressings into the anal canal to ensure that the mucocutaneous bridges are held flat against the internal sphincter.

11. Apply a perineal pad and apply pressure with a firmly tied T-bandage.

Aftercare

1. Make sure the patient does not develop urinary retention. Pass a catheter to relieve it.

2. It is important that the first bowel movement occurs at the latest by the third day. Give laxatives such as Milk of Magnesia and ispaghula. Order an intramuscular injection of 50 mg pethidine 30 minutes before the first defaecation to lessen the patient's discomfort. A normal diet should be taken as soon as the patient feels able.

3. Remove the dressings after giving an intramuscular injection of pethidine 100 mg or papaveretum 20 mg on the third postoperative day if they have not previously been dislodged by a bowel movement. The wounds are managed by a routine of twice-daily baths, irrigation and the application of a flat dressing soaked in hypochlorite solution.

4. Perform a gentle digital examination on the fifth to seventh day, to exclude tightness, spasm, or faecal retention. Treat tightness or spasm with twice daily passage of an anal dilator lubricated with lignocaine gel. Try giving glycerine suppositories or an enema to relieve faecal retention. If these fail, consider manual evacuation under general anaesthesia.

5. Warn the patient that there may be haemorrhage around the tenth postoperative day, and that wound healing may not be complete until 4–6 weeks postoperatively.

6. Impaired healing may produce narrowing, skin tags, fistula or fissure. Cauterise exuberant granulation tissue with silver nitrate stick.

Other procedures

1. *Maximal dilatation of the anus.* The principle of maximal dilatation of the anus is the destruction by stretching of the constriction in the distal and canal. This is done gently under general anaesthesia, avoiding strain on the midline anteriorly and posteriorly so that six or eight of the surgeon's fingers may be inserted at the end of the procedure. A sponge is inserted for 1½ hours post-operatively

and there follows a regimen of bulk laxatives and the passage of an anal dilator for 6 months.

Complications include haematoma formation and damage to the sphincter leading to incontinence or prolapse. Because of the risk of incontinence, it is a procedure of which, although widely used, we have no personal experience.

2. Partial internal sphincterotomy. Surgical division of the distal internal sphincter has been advocated by some as a more controlled form of maximal dilatation of the anus. The technique is used for the management of fissure (see below) but has not been widely adopted in the treatment of haemorrhoids.

3. Cryotherapy. The freezing of haemorrhoids again has its advocates. A liquid nitrogen probe (−180°C) or a nitrous oxide probe (−75°C) can be used. There is postoperative discomfort and discharge. The external component and skin tags are not effectively treated.

4. Infrared coagulation is a new alternative to injection sclerotherapy. The controlled burn produced at the base of the haemorrhoid is less invasive than injection. There is an increased risk of postoperative haemorrhage. These newer techniques still require full evaluation.

CLOTTED VENOUS SACCULE EVACUATION (PERI-ANAL HAEMATOMA)

If the patient is seen within 24 hours of onset and the pain is very severe, evacuate the clot.

Action

1. Place the patient in the left lateral position and inject 5–10 ml 1% lignocaine hydrochloride with 1 : 200 000 adrenaline into and around the base of the swelling.

2. With scissors excise the top of the lesion and express the clot.

3. Close the wound with 000 chromic catgut, apply a pressure pad. Alternatively, pack it with Surgicel. Postoperative haemorrhage may be severe if these measures are not adopted.

FISSURE

Appraise

1. Most ulcers at the anal margin are simple fissures-in-ano, possibly associated with a sentinel skin tag and/or hypertrophied anal papilla or anal polyp.

2. Exclude excoriation in association with pruritus ani, Crohn's disease, primary chancre of syphilis, herpes simplex, leukaemia and tumours.

3. Treat superficial fissures with topical local anaesthesia

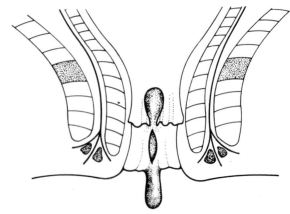

Fig. 9.11 A fissure with a sentinal skin tag, an anal polyp and undermining of the edges of the ulcer.

(2% lignocaine hydrochloride gel applied before and after defaecation). Advise the patient to take a high fibre diet.

4. The value of an anal dilator has been questioned but it is often tried. Tell the patient to lie on his left side, insert the dilator lubricated with local anaesthetic gel (2% lignocaine hydrochloride) and hold it in the anal canal for 5 minutes by the clock. This is repeated 2–3 times a day. It is a good idea for the patient to bathe after the passage of the dilator to remove excess gel to which the patient might become hypersensitive.

5. In the long term only approximately 20% remain cured. Most patients therefore require operative treatment especially if there is a sentinel tag, an anal polyp, exposure of the internal sphincter or undermining of the edges (Fig. 9.11).

The standard procedure used is a lateral (partial internal) sphincterotomy.

LATERAL SPHINCTEROTOMY

Appraise

1. This is very successful, curing 95% of patients. Anal dilatation, stretching the internal and external sphincters and lower rectum increases the risk of incontinence and we do not use it.

2. Because of pain, preparation is usually avoided. The operation can be carried out as a 'day case' procedure.

Action

1. Have the patient in the lithotomy position, under general or regional anaesthesia.

2. Pass an Eisenhammer bivalve operating proctoscope. Examine the fissure to make certain there is no induration suggesting an underlying intersphincteric abscess. If there is, proceed to dorsal sphincterotomy.

3. Transfix and excise hypertrophied anal papillae or fi-

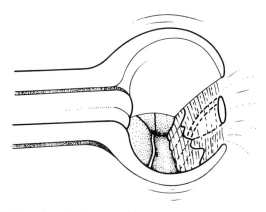

Fig. 9.12 Lateral partial internal sphincterotomy.

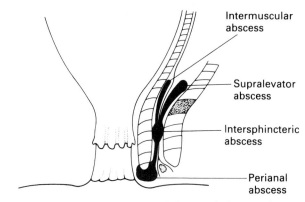

Fig. 9.13 Vertical spread upwards and downwards from a primary intersphincteric abscess.

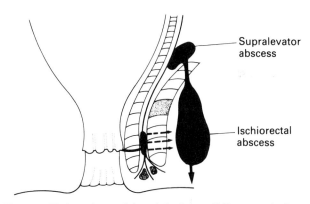

Fig. 9.14 Horizontal spread from infection medially across the internal sphincter into the anal canal and laterally into the ischiorectal fossa.

brous anal polyp and send for histopathological examination. Also remove a sentinel skin tag.

4. Rotate the operating proctoscope to demonstrate the left lateral aspect of the anal canal. Palpate the lower border of the internal sphincter muscle.

5. Make small incision 1 cm long in line with the lower border of internal sphincter. Insert scissors into the submucosa to gently separate the epithelial lining of the anal canal from the internal sphincter, and into the intersphincteric space to separate the internal and external sphincters.

6. If you make a hole in the mucosa open it completely to avoid the risk of sepsis.

7. With one blade of the scissors on each side of it, divide the internal sphincter muscle up to the level of the dentate line (Fig. 9.12). Do not extend the division of the internal sphincter above the upper limit of the fissure and never above the line of the anal valves.

8. Press on the area for 2–3 minutes then close the small wound with two 000 chromic catgut sutures.

9. Insert a small dressing into the anal canal.

10. Apply a perineal pad and apply pressure with a firmly tied T-bandage.

Aftercare

1. Remove the dressing next morning.

2. Prescribe a bulk laxative such as sterculia (Normacol) 10 ml once or twice a day.

3. Detect a haematoma by bruising under the perianal skin. It requires no treatment.

4. Minor transient degrees of incontinence of flatus occur after this procedure in a few patients.

ANAL ABSCESS AND FISTULA

Appraise

1. Most abscesses and fistulas in the anal region arise from a primary infection in the anal intersphincteric

glands. Furthermore, they represent different phases of the same disease process. An abscess, the acute phase, occurs when free drainage of the pus is prevented by closure of either the internal or external opening (or both) of the fistula which is the chronic phase.

2. Other causes of sepsis in the perianal region include pilonidal infection, hidradenitis suppurativa, Crohn's disease, tuberculosis, and intrapelvic sepsis draining downwards across the levator ani.

3. Once established an intersphincteric absecss may spread vertically downwards to form a perianal abscess, or upwards to form either an intermuscular abscess or supralevator abscess, depending upon which side of the longitudinal muscle spread occurs (Fig. 9.13). Horizontal spread medially across the internal sphincter may result in drainage into the anal canal, but spread laterally across the external sphincter may result in an ischiorectal abscess (Fig. 9.14). Finally, circumferential spread of infection may occur from one intersphincteric space to the other, from one ischiorectal fossa to the other and from one supralevator space to the other (Fig. 9.15).

4. Once an abscess has formed surgical drainage must be instituted — antibiotics have no part to play in the primary management. As the tissues are inflamed and oede-

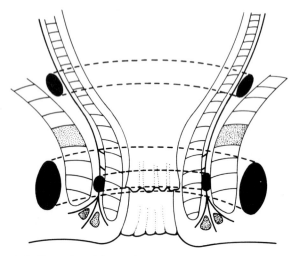

Fig. 9.15 Circumferential spread.

matous, it is best to do the minimum to ensure resolution of the infection. More tissue can be divided later to totally resolve the problem. Send a specimen of pus to the laboratory for culture. (The presence of intestinal organisms suggests that a fistula is present).

5. Pre-operative preparation of the bowel is best avoided as it causes unnecessary pain.

6. Have the anaesthetized patient in the lithotomy position and shave the patient on the table.

PERI-ANAL ABSCESS

1. Recognise the abscess as a swelling at the anal margin.

2. Make a radial incision and excise overhanging edges. Allow pus to drain and send a sample to the laboratory.

3. Gently examine the wound to see if there is a fistula.

4. Insert gauze dressing soaked in 1:40 sodium hypochlorite solution. Do not pack the wound tightly. Do not use oily dressing since there is a risk of producing an oleogranuloma.

INTERMUSCULAR ABSCESS

1. Recognise the abscess as an indurated swelling, sometimes mobile within the lower rectal wall.

2. As this is an upward extension of an intersphincteric abscess, the steps are similar, but the upper limit of division of the internal sphincter and/or circular muscle of the rectum is higher.

3. If the divided edges of the rectal wall bleed, insert a running 000 catgut suture to establish haemostasis.

4. Insert gauze dressing soaked in 1 : 40 sodium hypochlorite solution to the upper limit of the wound. Do not

pack the wound tightly. Do not use oily dressing since there is a risk of producing an oleogranuloma.

SUPRALEVATOR ABSCESS

1. Recognise as a fixed indurated swelling palpable above the anorectal junction.

2. Drainage of a supralevator abscess extends upwards to a similar level as an intermuscular abscess, except that the whole rectal wall needs to be divided.

3. Insert a gauze dressing soaked in 1:40 sodium hypochlorite into the anal canal to the upper limit of the wound. Do not pack the wound tightly. Do not use oily dressing since there is a risk of producing an oleogranuloma.

ISCHIORECTAL ABSCESS

1. Recognise as a brawny inflamed swelling in the ischiorectal fossa.

2. As an ischiorectal abscess often spreads circumferentially from one side to the other, carefully examine the patient under anaesthesia to determine if this has occurred. Recognise the abscess by induration inferior to the levator ani muscle.

3. For the same reason, employ a circumanal incision to establish drainage. Excise the skin edges to create an adequate opening and send a specimen of pus to the laboratory.

4. Be very careful when exploring the cavity with the finger. You may spread infection or damage the levator ani or even the rectum itself. Never use a probe.

5. Insert a gauze dressing soaked in 1 : 40 sodium hypochlorite solution gently to the upper limit of the wound. Do not pack the wound tightly. Do not use oily dressing.

Aftercare

1. Remove the dressing on the second postoperative day while the patient lies in the bath after having an intramuscular injection of pethidine 100 mg or omnopon 20 mg.

2. Initiate a routine of twice daily baths, irrigation of the wound, and the insertion of a tuck-in gauze dressing soaked in 1:40 sodium hypochlorite solution.

3. If the patient has evidence of persistent local or systemic sepsis, administer antibiotics guided by the culture report. Metronidazole is valuable against anaerobic organisms.

4. Assess the patient for the possible presence of a fistula detected at time of abscess drainage, a history of recurrent abscesses, palpable induration of the perianal area, anal canal and lower rectum or the presence of gut organisms

in the pus. If so, plan to re-examine the patient under anaesthesia and carry out the appropriate treatment.

FISTULA

Appraise

1. A fistula is an abnormal communication between two epithelial lined surfaces. Therefore in the context of fistula-in-ano, there should be an external opening on the perianal skin, an internal opening into the anal canal and a track between the two.

2. There may be no external opening, or it may be healed over. Likewise there may be no internal opening as the sepsis arises in the area of the intersphincteric gland which is the primary site of infection. It may not drain across the internal sphincter into the anal canal. Finally, the track may follow a very complicated path.

3. The presence of infection is characterised by the physical sign of induration, detected by palpation with a lubricated, covered finger.

SUPERFICIAL FISTULA

Assess

1. Have the anaesthetised patient in the lithotomy position. Sigmoidoscopy should be done in all cases, especially looking for inflammatory bowel disease.

2. Palpate the perianal skin, anal canal and lower rectum thoroughly for induration. This will be confined to the distal anal canal and localised to one area as superficial fistulas are really fissures covered with skin and lower anal canal epithelium (Fig. 9.16).

Action

1. Insert bivalve operating proctoscope and pass a fine probe along the track.

2. Lay open the fistula using a No. 15 bladed knife.

3. Curette the granulation tissue and send a specimen for histopathology.

4. If there is no induration deep to the internal sphincter, fashion the external skin wound so that it becomes pear-shaped and perform a lateral sphincterotomy (p. 156).

5. Insert gauze dressing soaked in hypochlorite solution to the upper limit of the wound.

INTERSPHINCTERIC FISTULA

An intersphincteric fistula results when the sepsis is inside the striated muscle of the pelvic floor and the anal canal (Fig. 9.17)

Assess

1. Have the anaesthetized patient in the lithotomy position. Sigmoidoscopy should be done in all cases, especially looking for inflammatory bowel disease.

2. Palpate carefully for induration. There is often a long subcutaneous perianal track leading to the external opening. Induration will be present in the wall of the anal canal — readily felt between a finger in the anal canal and the thumb externally. With an upward extension, induration will be felt in the rectal wall. Although the internal opening into the rectum may be above the anorectal ring, laying open is not difficult as the striated muscle will not be divided. Remember there may not be an internal opening.

Action

1. Insert a bivalve operating proctoscope and pass a fistula probe, Lockhart-Mummery or Anel's lacrimal probe, along the track. This will run parallel to the long axis of the anal canal. Never force a probe as false passages may be made.

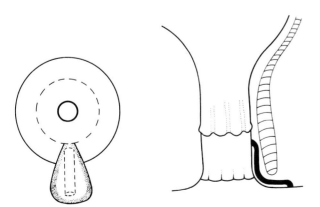

Fig. 9.16 A diagram to show a superficial fistula and the pear-shaped wound required to treat it.

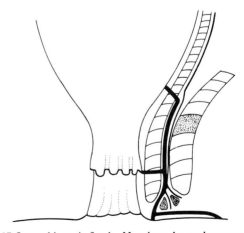

Fig. 9.17 Intersphincteric fistula. Note how the track may extend upwards into the rectum above the level of puborectalis and subcutaneously some distance from the anus.

2. If there is a long subcutaneous track, the probe will be directed from the external opening towards the anus. Lay it open and remove the granulation tissue with a curette. The upward extension between the sphincters becomes apparent as granulation tissue exudes from the opening.

3. Divide the internal sphincter as high as the tip of the probe. Again remove granulation tissue by curettage. If no granulation tissue is seen to protrude from a residual part of the track, and palpation reveals no more induration do no more.

4. If necessary, totally divide the internal sphincter and the muscle of the lower rectum, to completely lay open the fistula.

5. Create an adequate external wound to allow drainage.

6. Insert a gauze dressing soaked in 1 : 40 sodium hypochlorite solution. Do not pack wound tightly. Do not use an oily dressing.

7. Apply tight perineal pad with a T-bandage.

TRANS-SPHINCTERIC FISTULA

In a trans-sphincteric fistula, the primary track passes across the external sphincter from the intersphincteric space to the ischiorectal fossa. The infection may also have drained across the internal sphincter into the anal canal — the internal opening of the fistula which is usually at the level of the anal valves (Fig. 9.18). It is always important to remember that:

1. There may be no internal opening — the infection has not crossed the internal sphincter.

2. If there is an internal opening at the level of the anal valves, the level at which the primary track crosses the external sphincter may not be the same — it may be lower or higher (Fig. 9.19).

3. Infection can spread vertically in the intersphincteric space and open into the rectum in addition to spreading across the external sphincter.

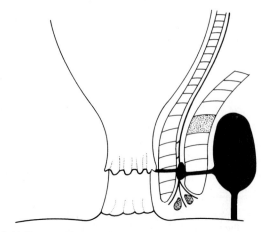

Fig. 9.18 Trans-sphincteric fistula.

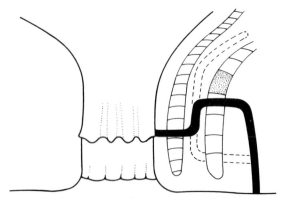

Fig. 9.19 The level at which the primary track crosses the external sphincter is not necessarily at the same level as the internal opening into the anal canal. It may be higher or lower, furthermore, there may be an upward intersphincteric extension.

4. Circumferential spread of infection and other secondary tracks may also occur.

Assess

1. Have the patient anaesthetised in the lithotomy position with the buttocks well down over the end of the table. Sigmoidoscopy should be done in all cases especially looking for inflammatory bowel disease. Ensure that 2 units of blood are crossmatched if this is a large or complex fistula, a significant blood loss can occur during operation.

2. Palpate carefully for induration. The external opening(s) are usually laterally placed and indurated, but there is not usually any induration extending towards the anus subcutaneously in a trans-sphincteric fistula. Palpation may reveal induration within the wall of the anal canal, the site of the primary anal gland infection. Induration will also be detected under the levator ani muscles and is often circumferential; palpation between a finger (in the lower rectum) and thumb (on the perianal skin) will reveal a large area of induration. This is especially obvious if circumferential spread has not occurred and the contralateral side is normal.

Action

1. Pass a bivalve operating proctoscope. Use a curved Lockhart-Mummery fistula probe to attempt to identify the internal opening.

2. Pass a probe into the external opening. It may extend several centimetres and be felt very close to a finger in the rectum. Do not force the probe, and do not pass it into the rectum, as this is never the site of the internal opening.

3. If there is spread of infection towards the midline posteriorly direct the probe previously inserted into the external opening posteriorly towards the coccyx. With a scalpel (No. 10 blade) in the groove of the probe divide the

tissue between the skin and the probe (skin and fat only — no muscle should be divided). Tissue-holding forceps are then applied to the skin edges and any major bleeding points secured. Avoid excessive use of the diathermy.

4. Curette away granulation tissue (send some for histopathological examination) and look for a forward extension from the site of the external opening. Lay it open.

5. Seek any extension of the sepsis to the opposite side by palpation, probing and looking for granulation tissue pouting from an opening in the previously curetted track. Use a No. 10 bladed knife to divide skin and fat to lay open any further tracks.

6. Insert the bivalve proctoscope again and re-identify the internal opening. It may or may not be possible to pass a probe either through the internal opening into the previously opened tracks, or from the previously opened tracks into the anal canal.

7. Divide the anal canal epithelium and the internal sphincter to the level of the internal opening (if present) with a No. 15 bladed knife, thus opening up the intersphincteric space. If there is no internal opening, open the intersphincteric space in a similar way to the level of the anal valves. Curette any granulation tissue.

8. The primary track across the external sphincter should now be identifiable. If it is at or below the line of the anal valves, divide the muscle. If it is higher, as it often is, do not divide the muscle but drain the track by insertion of a length of fine silicone tubing (1 mm diameter) or monofilament nylon (1). Such a piece of material is called a seton.

9. In summary, the phases of the procedure are:
(a) Drainage of the secondary tracks
(b) Drainage of intersphincteric abscess of origin
(c) Drainage of primary track — either by dividing the muscle or inserting a seton.

10. Once all the septic areas have been drained fashion the wound so that drainage will continue to take place and the wound heal from its depth. Skin and fat will almost certainly need to be trimmed.

11. Insert gauze dressings soaked in 1:40 sodium hypochlorite into the wounds and the anal canal. Do not pack the dressings tightly. Do not use oily dressings.

12. Apply a perineal pad and pressure to assist haemostasis with a T-bandage.

SUPRASPHINCTERIC FISTULA

In a suprasphincteric fistula, the primary track crosses the striated muscle above all the muscles of continence (Fig. 9.20). As this is a variant of a 'high' trans-sphincteric fistula, manage it on similar principles.

This is a very rare form of fistula. When possible refer the patient to a surgeon specialising in this field.

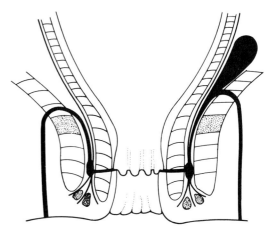

Fig. 9.20 Suprasphincteric fistula. There may be an associated supralevator abscess.

EXTRASPHINCTERIC FISTULA

1. An extrasphincteric fistula arising from an upward extension of infection from the ischiorectal fossa is again an unusual occurrence, possibly due to the injudicious use of a probe during operation.

2. Create a defunctioning loop colostomy as a preliminary to closing the opening in the rectum and treat the fistula along the lines indicated above.

3. A fistula arising from pelvic sepsis from, for example, acute appendicitis, Crohn's disease or diverticular disease (not therefore of anal gland origin) needs to be managed by treating the primary disease (see Chapters 7 and 8).

Aftercare

1. Remove the dressing on the second or third postoperative day after giving an intramuscular injection of pethidine 100 mg or omnopon 20 mg. Carry out the first dressing in the operating theatre under general anaesthesia if the wound is very extensive.

2. Initiate a routine of twice-daily baths, irrigation of the wound, and insertion of gauze soaked in 1:40 sodium hypochlorite solution.

3. Inspect the wound at regular intervals until healing is complete.

4. Encourage the bowel movements to coincide with these dressing times by giving laxatives. If they do not coincide, arrange bath-irrigation-dressing routines as necessary.

5. If voluminous pus discharges, review the wound in theatre under general anaesthesia after 10–14 days. In patients with large wounds, this may need to be repeated. Lay open any residual tracks and curette away the granulation tissue.

6. Administer antimicrobial agents such as erythromycin 250 mg 8-hourly and metronidazole 200 mg 8-hourly for up to 28 days, to assist in the elimination of the sepsis.

7. A seton does not complicate the postoperative routine. Allow the wound to heal around it; this may take 3 months. Then under general anaesthesia, remove the seton and curette its track free of granulation tissue. Spontaneous healing occurs in approximately 40% of patients. If healing does not occur, lay open the residual track. The advantage of this staged division of the external sphincter is that healing occurs around the 'scaffolding' of the external sphincter. When it is subsequently divided, and this is not always necessary, its ends separate only slightly. This gives a better functional result than if it were divided at the outset.

Complications

1. Failure to heal may be from inadequate or inappropriate drainage of intersphincteric abscess of origin, of secondary tracks, or of the primary track. Inadequate postoperative dressings allow bridging of the wound edges and pocketing of pus. Do not fail to instruct the nurses adequately. If there is excessive granulation tissue growth, cauterise it with silver nitrate, or curette it away (general anaesthetic required). Healing may be slow if the patient is malnourished or suffers from zinc deficiency. If hairs grow into the wound, shave the area. Has a specific cause for the fistula, such as Crohn's disease been missed?

2. Secondary haemorrhage may occur from any potentially septic open wound, healing by second intention.

3. Anal incontinence of varying degrees may follow division of the sphincter muscles. If all the sphincter complex has inadvertently been divided, consider repairing it once the sepsis has been eradicated and healing has occurred.

4. Successful fistula surgery depends upon accurate definition of the pathoanatomy, drainage of the intersphincteric abscess of origin, the primary and secondary tracks, and excellent post-operative wound care.

PILONIDAL DISEASE

A simple pilonidal sinus, detected as a chance finding during routine examination, probably does not require treatment. Operate only if it is painful or infected, producing a pilonidal abscess.

Position

Place the anaesthetised patient in the left lateral position with the right buttock strapped to hold it up. Elastic adhesive strapping is adequate and adheres better if the skin has been sprayed with compound tincture of benzoin. Carefully shave the area.

Action

1. Determine the extent of sepsis by palpation for induration, and the use of probes.

2. Completely excise the skin of the septic area.

3. Curette away the granulation tissue and embedded hairs.

4. Check the base of wound for any side tracks with a probe, and look for any residual granulation tissue which may be pouting from a side track.

5. Fashion the wound so that there are no overhanging edges. Obtain haemostasis by pressure only, avoiding the use of diathermy which might delay wound healing.

6. Dress the wound with haemostatic gauze if haemostasis is not complete. Otherwise use gauze soaked in 1 : 40 sodium hypochloride solution and apply pressure.

Aftercare

1. Remove the dressing on the second postoperative day, if necessary after an injection of intramuscular analgesic such as pethidine 100 mg or omnopon 200 mg.

2. Initiate a twice-daily routine of bath, irrigation and dressing.

3. Keep the wound edges shaved. You may need bright light and a magnifying glass to ensure that this is adequate. Continue frequent shaving for at least 6 months after healing to allow scar to mature.

4. Cauterize any excess granulation tissue with silver nitrate.

5. Complications include haemorrhage, delayed healing and recurrence, nearly always due to lack of satisfactory postoperative wound care and shaving. The operative procedure may need to be repeated to get healing.

HIDRADENITIS SUPPURATIVA

Appraise

1. Hidradenitis suppurativa is a septic process which involves the apocrine sweat glands. It occurs in the perineum as well as the axillae.

2. Recurrent abscess formation often results from inadequate drainage. There is no communication with the anal canal and the infection is superficial. Occasionally, hidradenitis occurs in association with Crohn's disease.

Action

1. Drain the pus from each abscess. They are often multiple and may intercommunicate.

2. Curette away all the granulation tissue.

3. Remove all overhanging skin.

4. Allow the defect to heal by second intention.

ANAL MANIFESTATIONS OF CROHN'S DISEASE

Appraise

1. Anal manifestations of Crohn's disease occur in approximately 50% of patients.

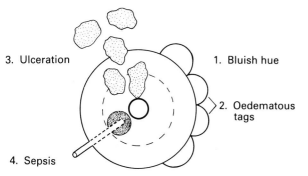

3. Ulceration

1. Bluish hue

2. Oedematous tags

4. Sepsis

Fig. 9.21 A diagram to show the anal manifestations of Crohn's disease.

2. The perianal area has a bluish discolouration, there may be oedematous skin tags. Ulceration, which may be extensive, may involve the perianal skin, anal margin and anal canal. Sepsis may occur in the form of either an abscess or a fistula (Fig. 9.21).

Action

1. Always think of the possibility of anal Crohn's disease. It may be the first manifestation.
2. Take a small biopsy of a skin tag, or granulation tissue together with a rectal mucosal biopsy for histopathological examination.
3. Drain any abscess in the usual way taking care not to divide any muscle.
4. Fully investigate the patient.

CONDYLOMATA ACUMINATA

Appraise

1. Condylomata acuminata (warts) are the result of a virus infection of the squamous epithelium. Papilliferous lesions are produced which may occur on the perianal skin, within the anal canal and on the genitalia. Exclude other forms of sexually transmitted disease and attempt to trace contacts.
2. Treat scattered lesions by applying 25% podophyllin in compound benzoin tincture. Treat more extensive lesions by operation — a technique of scissor excision.

Action

1. Have the anaesthetized patient placed in the lithotomy position.
2. Infiltrate a solution of 1:300 000 adrenaline in normal saline under the epithelium bearing the perianal lesions to reduce bleeding when the warts are removed and to separate the individual lesions so that the maximum amount of normal skin may be preserved.
3. Remove the warts with fine pointed scissors, holding them with fine toothed forceps.

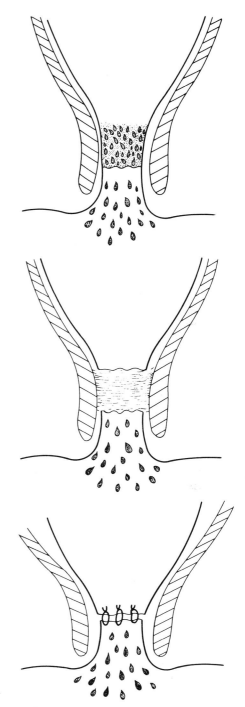

a

b

c

Fig. 9.22 (a) Confluent intra-anal canal warts above the dentate line.
(b) The warts, together with all the mucosa, are removed leaving a section of muscle denuded of mucosa.
(c) The lower rectal mucosa is attached to the dentate line by means of a series of catgut sutures.

4. Remove intra-anal canal warts in the same way after inserting a bivalve operating proctoscope. There is often a confluent ring of lesions in the upper anal canal. Remove these in toto and then join the mucosa of the lower rectum to that of the anal canal at the dentate line with sutures of 000 chromic catgut (Fig. 9.22). In addition to achieving mucosal apposition, this mucosal anastomosis is haemostatic.

5. Send the excised lesions, particularly the intra-anal ones, for histopathological examination.

Aftercare

1. No special measures need be adopted.

2. Carry out regular examinations to detect further wart formation, which usually occurs in the first three months. Treat scattered lesions with podophyllin. More extensive recurrences require further inpatient treatment.

3. 5-fluorouracil ointment (Efudix) may be of value in the resistant case, but its precise place is as yet undetermined. Apply it sparingly twice daily for several weeks.

ANAL TUMOURS

Tumours in this region may be divided into two groups. Anal canal tumours arise from the dentate line and above. Anal margin tumours arise below the dentate line.

ANAL CANAL TUMOURS

Appraise

1. These are almost always malignant and include squamous cell carcinoma, basaloid carcinoma, adenocarcinoma and malignant melanoma.

2. Examine the tumour under anaesthesia and remove a biopsy specimen.

3. If the tumour is operable, excise the rectum (see Ch. 8) and anal canal, widely excising the perianal skin, ischiorectal fossa fat and the levator ani muscles near the lateral pelvic wall. Create a terminal left iliac fossa colostomy.

4. Excise inguinal lymph nodes if they are enlarged. Consider radiotherapy if histologically they contain carcinoma.

ANAL MARGIN TUMOURS

Appraise

1. These may be benign or malignant. Condylomata acuminata (see p. 163), keratoacanthoma, apocrine gland tumours and the premalignant Bowen's disease and Paget's disease are benign.

2. Excise condylomata acuminata with scissors.

3. Totally excise other tumours. If the defect is not too large, allow the wound to heal by second intention. Close large defects with split skin grafts.

4. Histopathological information is essential in deciding whether or not any further treatment is required.

5. Malignant tumours of the anal margin are mainly squamous cell carcinomas, although basal cell carcinoma

can occur. Induration is the physical sign which suggests malignancy. If the tumour is less than 3 cm in diameter, widely excise it. Treat larger squamous cell carcinomas by excision of the rectum and construction of an end colostomy. Enlarged inguinal nodes are excised. Consider radiotherapy if they contain carcinoma.

RECTAL ADENOMAS

Appraise

1. Adenomas of the rectum may be classified on a histopathological basis into tubular, tubovillous and villous. From the clinical viewpoint these three types of adenoma are similar in their behaviour as there is no invasion of neoplastic cells across the muscularis mucosae. A more useful classification is according to their clinical appearance, that is, are they pedunculated or sessile?

2. Are there any other neoplastic lesions in the large intestine — benign or malignant? In patients with lesions >2 cm in diameter, there is an incidence of further tumours of 25%: benign 18%, malignant 7%. The patient will need a barium enema examination and/or a colonoscopy.

N.B. Multiple small adenomatous polyps in the rectum suggest the diagnosis of familial adenomatous polyposis.

3. Is the lesion totally benign, or does it have malignant areas? There is a 50% chance of malignant areas in patients with lesions >2 cm in diameter.

4. Be sure to remove the whole lesion, a *total excision biopsy*, which will be diagnostic as well as therapeutic if the lesion proves to be totally benign.

EXCISE

1. Totally remove by twisting with a pair of Patterson biopsy forceps, lesions less than 5 mm across.

2. Employ diathermy snare excision for those which are pedunculated.

3. Excise submucosally those which are sessile, non-circumferential and confined to the lower two-thirds of the rectum (see below).

4. Use a modified Soave operation for those in the lower third of the rectum which are circumferential (see p. 165)

5. Employ anterior resection for sessile non-circumferential tumours with the lower border in the upper third, and circumferential tumours with the lower border in the upper two-thirds of the rectum

SUBMUCOSAL EXCISION OF SESSILE ADENOMA

Appraise

1. Undertake this technique only if there are no malignant lesions at a higher level. Resect a carcinoma of the sigmoid colon first.

2. Undertake this technique provided the tumour does not feel indurated on palpation with the finger or the end of the sigmoidoscope, suggesting malignant change.

3. Order full bowel preparation. Conduct the operation in the lithotomy position or the jack knife position, which is especially suitable for anterior lesions.

Action

1. Insert a bivalve operating proctoscope and ensure that illumination is adequate. You may prefer to wear a headlamp.

2. Inject 1:300 000 adrenaline in normal saline into the sub-mucosa under the tumour. Remember if it is benign it is entirely mucosal, therefore difficulty in creating artificial oedema in the submucosa suggests malignant invasion (Fig. 9.23).

3. With sharp scissors incise the mucosa approximately 1 cm from the edge of the tumour and then dissect it free of the circular muscle of the rectum (white fibres) in the distended submucosal layer (Fig. 9.24).

4. Seal bleeding points with diathermy.

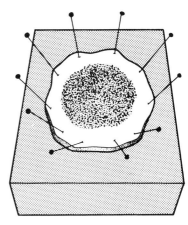

Fig. 9.25 The specimen with a margin of normal mucosa is pinned to a cork board prior to fixing to assist the histopathologist.

5. Allow the wound to heal spontaneously without suturing it. Close any defect inadvertently created in the muscle with 00 catgut sutures.

6. Pin the specimen to a cork board before fixing so that the pathologist can determine whether or not there is any malignant invasion, by taking serial sections (Fig. 9.25).

Aftercare

1. No special measures need be adopted other than to ensure that constipation does not occur.

2. Acquaint yourself with the result of the histopathological examination. If there are malignant foci, decide whether or not to proceed to a more radical procedure.

3. Follow up the patient to detect any recurrence and metachronous lesions.

4. Haemorrhage is very rarely a problem.

5. Stenosis of the rectum may develop if excision was performed for too large a lesion.

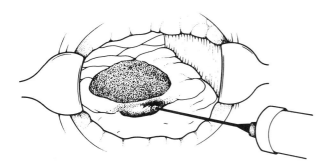

Fig. 9.23 1 : 300 000 adrenaline in normal saline is injected into the submucosa to elevate the mucosa and the tumour within it.

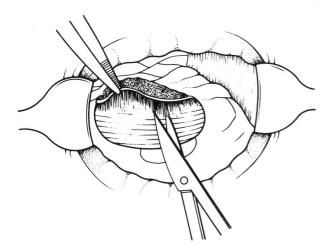

Fig. 9.24 The mucosa is dissected from the underlying circular muscle (white fibres)

MODIFIED SOAVE OPERATION

Reserve this operation for large circumferential lesions with their lower border in the lower third of the rectum and extending into the upper third. All the tumour is excised submucosally by a combined abdominal and peranal approach. The rectal muscular tube is relined with descending colon anastomosed through the anus to the level of the dentate line (Fig. 9.26). This is an unusual operation and should be done only in a specialist centre. Circumferential lesions extending over only a few centimetres can be treated by submucosal excision, with plication of the muscle tube to allow mucosal anastomosis.

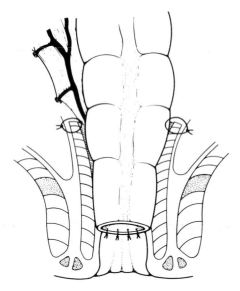

Fig. 9.26 Modified Soave operation. The mucosa has been removed from the distal rectum both by the abdominal and perineal surgeon. The descending colon is now passed into the muscle tube and sutured at the dentate line.

COMPLETE RECTAL PROLAPSE

Appraise

1. The symptom of prolapse, tissue slipping through the anus, may be due to causes other than complete rectal prolapse. Distinguish haemorrhoids, anal polyps, mucosal prolapse and rectal adenomas.

2. Treatment consists of control of the prolapse, re-education of the bowel habit, and improvement, if necessary, of sphincter function.

3. First control the prolapse. While an internally intus-susscepted rectum lies in the lower third of the rectum (the first phase of prolapse) sphincter function is inhibited as it will be as a complete prolapse passes through the anal sphincter and keeps it open. Many operations have been described to achieve control. The one which is justifiably popular in the United Kingdom is the polyvinyl alcohol sponge abdominal rectopexy.

4. Bowel habit re-education requires advice on dietary and fluid intake, and the use of laxatives, suppositories, and enemas to reduce or stop straining at defaecation.

5. After rectopexy only a few patients have sphincter dysfunction severe enough to produce significant incontinence. Pelvic floor physiotherapy, faradism and electrical stimulators give little longterm benefit. The problem is anatomically the result of pelvic floor neurogenic myopathy producing a shortened anal canal with widening of the anorectal angle. Postanal pelvic floor repair reduces the anorectal angle and lengthens the anal canal, restoring satisfactory continence in 80% of patients.

ABDOMINAL RECTOPEXY

Prepare

1. Order full bowel preparation (see Ch. 8). Warn the nurses that as these patients have defective sphincter function they may be incontinent during preparation.

2. Place the anaesthetized patient in the Lloyd-Davies (lithotomy Trendelenberg) position.

3. Order metronidazole 500 mg i.v. and gentamicin 80 mg i.v. at induction of anaesthesia and at 6 and 12 hours later.

4. The patient should be catheterised.

Action

1. Make a long left paramedian or midline incision. Elderly females may have shortening between the costal margin and symphysis pubis from vertebral collapse and a transverse abdominal or extended Pfannensteil incision affords better access.

2. Carry out full exploration.

3. Mobilise the sigmoid colon by dividing the congenital adhesions.

4. Starting at the level of the sacral promontory, incise the peritoneum beside (but not damaging) the superior haemorrhoidal artery. The ureters lie laterally on both sides, but check their position at all times. Extend the peritoneal incision to the bottom of the pre-rectal pouch, then across the midline between the rectum and vagina or bladder, so that the rectum may be separated from them.

5. Enter the post-rectal space and open it up by scissor dissection, holding the rectum forward with your left hand or a tipped anterior St. Mark's retractor. Adequate tension on the rectum displays the areolar tissue. Seal any vessels with diathermy.

6. Now that the anterior and posterior dissection of the rectum is complete its only attachments are the two lateral ligaments. It is usually necessary to divide only the upper half of these between ligatures.

7. Achieve perfect haemostasis.

8. Suture. Polyvinyl alcohol sponge to the presacral fascia. Use four full lengths of 00 linen, passing it first through the sponge then the fascia and finally through the sponge again. Remove the needle and clip the two ends. Place the first suture at the level of the tip of the coccyx, and the last just below the sacral promontory. The other two are spaced equally between them. When all sutures are inserted ease the sponge into place and tie the sutures loosely (Fig. 9.27). Control bleeding from a damaged presacral vein by leaving the suture in place, applying local pressure with a 'swab on a stick' for 5 minutes. The bleeding always stops!

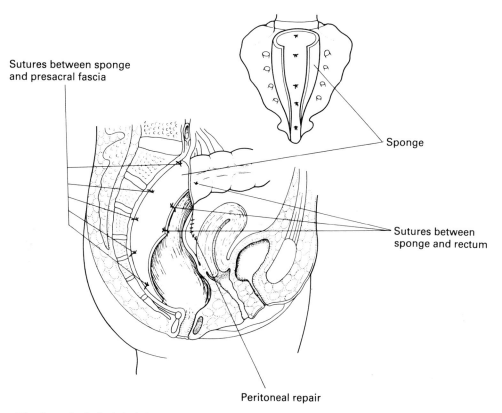

Sutures between sponge and presacral fascia

Sponge

Sutures between sponge and rectum

Peritoneal repair

Fig. 9.27 Abdominal rectopexy. The sheet of polyvinyl alcohol sponge is inserted behind the rectum, and after it has been completely mobilised to the tip of the coccyx. The Ivalon is anchored to the presacral fascia by non-absorbable sutures, it is then anchored to the rectum by similar sutures. The rectum is not completely encircled to allow expansion.

9. Pull the rectum so that there is slight traction on the anus. Suture the sponge to the rectum with interrupted 000 silk sutures, leaving a gap anteriorly.

10. Close the peritoneum of the pelvic floor and repair the sigmoid mesocolon. Cover all the sponge to prevent small bowel adhesion, and to ensure that the site of pelvic peritoneum closure does not narrow the rectum.

11. A drain is not usually necessary, but if there is a persistent collection of blood and fluid in the pelvis, insert a suction drain for 24 hours.

12. Close the abdominal wound.

Aftercare

1. Maintain the patient on intravenous fluids. Allow drinking when there are good bowel sounds and flatus has been passed.

2. Remove the catheter on the fifth post-operative day after sending a sample of urine for culture.

3. Avoid constipation. Give a mild osmotic laxative such as Milk of Magnesia to initiate bowel movement. Subsequently use suppositories such as glycerine and Dulcolax.

4. Inject or excise any residual mucosal prolapse.

Complications

1. Haemorrhage may lead to a pelvic haematoma.

2. An abscess may develop around the implanted foreign material after an interval of up to 2–3 years. If necessary, remove the polyvinyl alcohol sponge through a small incision in the back of the rectum.

3. If any polyvinyl alcohol sponge remains exposed small intestinal obstruction may develop.

POST-ANAL PELVIC FLOOR REPAIR

Post-anal pelvic floor repair is valuable in patients who have residual incontinence after rectopexy and in patients who have so-called idiopathic incontinence. It should be done only by those with a special interest in anorectal surgery.

Prepare

1. Order a full bowel preparation.

2. The patient is given general or regional anaesthesia and lies in the lithotomy position.

Action

1. Make a curved 180° posterior circumanal incision 3 cm from the anus from the left to the right lateral position (Fig. 9.28).

2. Dissect the skin contained within the incision forwards and medially, exposing the external sphincter.

3. Open up the intersphincteric space all round with the striated muscle of the external sphincter, puborectalis and levator ani outside, and the rectum and anal canal with the internal sphincter and longitudinal muscle fibres inside (Fig. 9.29).

4. Dissect the rectum forwards and medially to develop the supralevator space. If necessary divide Waldeyer's fascia.

5. Insert monofilament nylon or prolene sutures from one levator ani muscle to the other and tie them loosely; tension further damages the muscle. Place these sutures in four or five layers with approximately three sutures in each layer (Fig. 9.30). As the suturing becomes more superficial the fibres of the external sphincter approximate without tension. These sutures effectively elevate the anorectal junction and place it nearer the symphysis pubis. Furthermore the anal canal is lengthened and the anorectal angle narrowed (made more acute).

6. Close the wound partially, perhaps creating a V-Y plasty (Fig. 9.31). Because of the lengthening of the anal canal, some of the epithelium is carried into the anal canal anteriorly. Allow the defect to heal by second intention.

7. Insert a suction drain into the supralevator space.

Aftercare.

1. Dress the wound regularly.

2. Avoid constipation. Give an osmotic laxative to en-

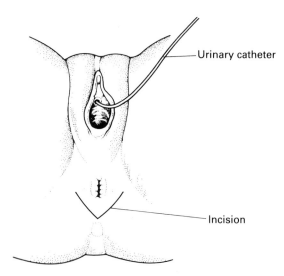

Fig. 9.28 Postanal pelvic floor repair: the incision.

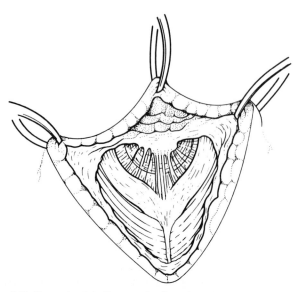

Fig. 9.29 Postanal pelvic floor repair: dissection of the intersphincteric space. The terminal fibres of the longitudinal muscle guide one to this.

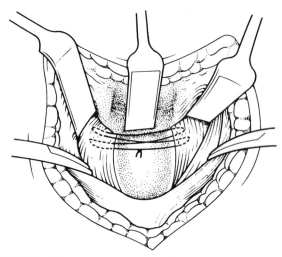

Fig. 9.30 Monofilament nylon sutures are inserted and loosely tied so as not to damage muscle tissue, they will form a hammock on which the distal rectum rests.

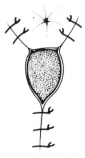

Fig. 9.31 A V-Y plasty to close the wound. As the result of lengthening of the anal canal, the skin is drawn into it. As the apex of the V frequently becomes ischaemic, it is best excised and the central part of the wound allowed to heal by second intention.

sure diarrhoea in the early post-operative period. The patient may not be able to control this.

3. Before discharging the patient, teach him to initiate defaecation with glycerine or bisacodyl suppositories to eliminate the risk of repeated straining which might break down the repair.

FAECAL INCONTINENCE

Appraise

1. Determine the cause of faecal incontinence. If the anal sphincter is normal consider faecal impaction and urgent diarrhoea as the cause.

If the anal sphincter is abnormal consider a congenital abnormality, complete rectal prolapse (see above), a lower motor neurone lesion, disruption of the sphincter ring due to trauma (often surgical) and so-called idiopathic incontinence, which is probably due to a pelvic floor neurogenic myopathy.

2. Operative treatment may be employed for the correction of some congenital abnormalities, complete rectal prolapse (abdominal rectopexy) disruption of the sphincter ring (sphincter repair) and idiopathic incontinence (postanal pelvic floor repair).

3. Disruption of the sphincter ring may be suggested by a history of trauma — accidental, obstetric or surgical — and diagnosed by detecting a defect in the sphincter ring. Such a defect may be confirmed by electromyography.

4. Idiopathic incontinence is associated with descent of the perineum on straining (valsalva manoeuvre) and a lax gaping anus. On palpation there is little or no tone in the puborectalis and as a result the tip of the coccyx is readily palpable. Again on straining, the anal canal shortens and the angle between the anal canal and the rectum posteriorly widens. The operation of postanal pelvic floor repair (described above) restores the anorectal angle (approximately 90°) and lengthens the anal canal.

SPHINCTER REPAIR

It is accepted practice that while the sphincter repair is healing, a temporary loop colostomy should be employed to divert faecal stream.

Prepare

1. Order a full bowel preparation.
2. The patient is given a general anaesthetic and lies in the supine position for construction of the loop sigmoid colostomy (see Ch. 8) The patient is then placed in the lithotomy position for the sphincter repair.
3. A urinary catheter is passed.

Action

1. A generous circumanal incision extending either side of the pre-existing scar is made approximately 1–2 cm away from the anus (Fig. 9.32)
2. Dissect towards the anus under the skin to identify the brown fibres of the external sphincter on either side of the scar and then remove the ischiorectal fat by dissecting superiorly (Fig. 9.33)

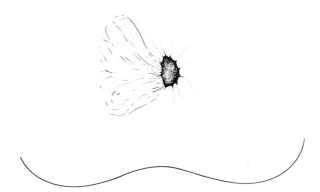

Fig. 9.32 Sphincter repair: the incision extends approximately 180° around the circumference of the anal canal, the scarred skin is excised.

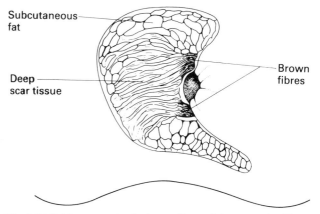

Fig. 9.33 Sphincter repair: the brown fibres of the external sphincter are identified.

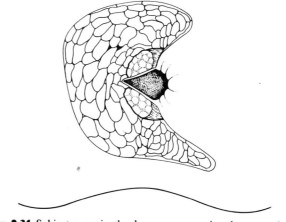

Fig. 9.34 Sphincter repair: the deep scar connecting the two ends of striated muscle, together with the mucosa, are excised.

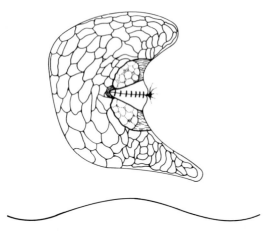

Fig. 9.35 Sphincter repair: the mucosa is repaired using a continuous 2/0 chromic catgut suture. It should be possible to insert the surgeon's index finger into the contained tube.

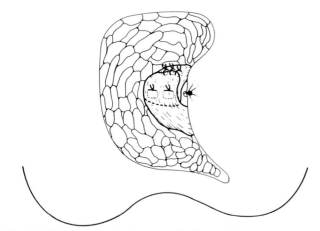

Fig. 9.36 Sphincter repair: the two ends of the sphincter muscle are approximated by overlapping their ends (rather than performing a direct suture).

3. Insert a bivalve operating proctoscope and infiltrate the submucosa with a solution of 1:300 000 adrenaline in normal saline. The mucosa will not lift where there is scar tissue. Incise the mucosa and dissect it from the internal sphincter for a short distance.

4. Cut away the scar tissue in the form of a wedge (Fig. 9.34)

5. Reconstitute the mucosa and submucosa with a continuous 00 chromic catgut suture, making sure that the anus and anal canal will admit the surgeon's index finger (Fig. 9.35)

6. Insert three 0 prolene or monofilament nylon sutures into the combined internal and external sphincter so that when they are tied (not too tight so that ischaemia results) one side of the sphincter complex overlaps the other (Fig. 9.36)

7. The wound is left open to granulate.

8. When healing is complete the defunctioning colostomy is closed (usually 6–8 weeks).

Further reading

Goldberg S M, Gordon P H, Nivatvongs S 1980 Essentials of anorectal surgery. J B Lippincott, Philadelphia

Goligher J C 1984 Surgery of the anus, rectum and colon, 5th edn. Bailliere Tindall, London

Sir Alan Parks Symposium Proceedings 1983 Annals of the Royal College of Surgeons of England (Supplement)

Thomson J P S, Nicholls R J, Williams C B 1981 Colorectal disease. Heinemann Medical Books, London

Todd I P, Fielding L P 1983 Rob and Smith's operative surgery: alimentary tract and abdominal — 3. Colon rectum and anus. 4th edn. Butterworths, London

Surgery of the biliary tract and pancreas

GENERAL NOTES

1. This chapter will concentrate on operations for gallstones and palliative procedures for pancreatic cancer. Other pancreatobiliary operations are much less commonly performed and should not ordinarily be undertaken by the inexperienced.

2. When operating on the biliary tract or pancreas, always ensure that the patient is positioned on the operating table so that the upper abdomen overlies a radiolucent tunnel. Alert the radiographer in advance that an operative cholangiogram or pancreatogram may be required.

3. Routine antibiotic prophylaxis is a wise precaution in pancreatobiliary surgery. Choose a broad-spectrum agent excreted in bile such as one of the cephalosporins. A single parenteral dose given shortly before operation may suffice, unless the bile is obviously infected.

CHOLECYSTECTOMY

Appraise

1. Whether symptomatic or symptomfree, gallstones are the overwhelming indication for cholecystectomy. Their prevalence makes cholecystectomy the second commonest intra-abdominal operation in Western countries (after appendicectomy). Cholecystectomy is occasionally indicated for acalculous cholecystitis or cholecystoses (cholesterosis, adenomyosis) or during the course of partial hepatectomy or pancreatoduodenectomy. A diseased gallbladder encountered incidentally at operation should usually be removed, provided there is adequate access and an additional procedure would not be inappropriate.

2. Dissolution therapy with cheno- or urso-deoxycholic acid is a reasonable alternative to cholecystectomy in very elderly or infirm patients with a functioning gallbladder and a limited number of small, radiolucent calculi. Treatment is often prolonged, and recurrence commonly follows its cessation.

3. The timing of operation after an acute attack of cholecystitis or biliary colic is disputatious. My preference is to confirm the diagnosis at an early stage by ultrasonography and contrast radiology and to put the patient on the next 'cold' operating list. This policy of early cholecystectomy avoids recurrent attacks or complications, such as acute pancreatitis, but occasionally results in a more difficult operation. Often, however, the inflammatory oedema assists dissection of the gallbladder from the liver bed.

4. Transient jaundice is compatible with stones confined to the gallbladder. Continuing jaundice suggests obstruction of the bile duct and requires further investigation, including an 'invasive' cholangiogram (either percutaneous transhepatic or endoscopic retrograde). Perioperative precautions in obstructive jaundice are outlined on page 191.

5. Half the population have some variation from 'normal' in the arterial supply of the gallbladder or the disposition of the bile ducts. Therefore, do not embark upon cholecystectomy without learning the common anatomical variations.

Access

1. Choose between a right upper paramedian, oblique (or transverse) subcostal or vertical midline incision. Try

each of them on different occasions, and decide which you prefer.

2. In a paramedian incision it is simpler to split the fibres of rectus abdominis than to mobilise and retract the muscle belly. In practice, no harm ensues from denervation of the medial portion of the rectus. The incision starts at the costal margin 5 cm from the midline and runs down to just below the umbilicus.

3. Some surgeons prefer Kocher's oblique subcostal incision which extends parallel to the costal margin for about 15 cm. If the incision is taken further to the right, isolate and preserve the ninth thoracic nerve. The muscles are divided by diathermy in the line of the skin incision. A transverse incision provides a better cosmetic scar at the expense of slightly limited access.

4. Though quick to perform, a midline incision provides less satisfactory access to the gallbladder region, except in a thin subject.

Assess

1. Examine the gallbladder to see if it is inflamed, thickened or contains stones. With the patient supine, stones sink to the neck of the gallbladder. If the organ is hard and adherent to the liver, consider the possibility of carcinoma.

2. Gallstone symptoms can mimic those of other diseases. Explore the rest of the abdomen, looking in particular for hiatus hernia, peptic ulcer, diverticular disease of the colon and diseases of the liver, pancreas and appendix.

3. Examine the (common) bile duct. It should not exceed 6–8 mm in diameter. Insert the left index finger through the epiploic foramen (of Winslow) and feel the duct between finger and thumb. Is it thickened, does it contain stones? The lower duct may be felt after splitting the peritoneum in the floor of the foramen with the edge of the finger.

4. Examine the head of pancreas between finger and thumb, again with the left index finger passed through the epiploic foramen and down behind the gland. Normal pancreas has a nodular feel, but with experience you will learn to detect the induration that denotes chronic inflammation or neoplasia.

Action

1. Place your hand over the liver and gently manipulate the right lobe downwards into the wound.

2. Ask the anaesthetist to empty the stomach by aspirating the nasogastric tube. Divide any omental adhesions to the under surface of the gallbladder.

3. Place one pack in the subhepatic space to retract the intestines and another just covering the duodenal bulb.

4. Decide whether to commence gallbladder dissection at the fundus or in the region of the cystic duct. I prefer to display the structures in Calot's triangle (Fig. 10.1) and

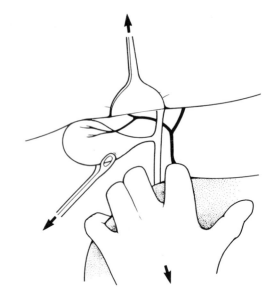

Fig. 10.1 Cholecystectomy. Traction in three directions displays Calot's triangle, which is bounded by the cystic duct, common hepatic duct and inferior border of the liver. The triangle has been extended by mobilisation of the neck of the gallbladder. The cystic artery normally arises from the right hepatic artery within Calot's triangle.

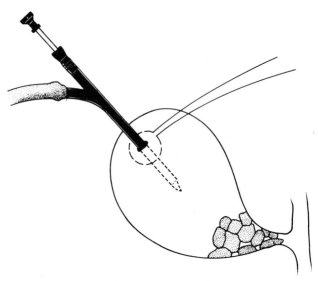

Fig. 10.2 Decompression of an obstructed gallbladder before cholecystectomy (or cholecystostomy). The side-arm of the Ochsner trocar is connected to the sucker tubing.

to ligate and divide the cystic artery before proceeding to the fundus and working back towards the cystic duct. If chronic inflammation is severe, it is safer to start at the fundus; some surgeons advocate this approach routinely.

5. Cholecystectomy may be performed with the surgeon standing on the right or left hand side of the operating table. Try both positions on different occasions and see which you find more comfortable.

6. If the gallbladder is very distended, it should be aspirated before proceeding (Fig. 10.2). Pack off the fun-

dus and insert an Ochsner trocar, which is connected to the sucker tubing. Alternatively, use a syringe and wide-bore needle. Afterwards, seal the defect by grasping it with tissue-holding forceps.

'Duct-first' technique

1. The first assistant's left hand draws the duodenal bulb downwards, while a retractor draws the liver upwards. Grasp the neck of the gallbladder with sponge-holding forceps and draw it to the patient's right. This three-way traction provides good exposure (Fig. 10.1).

2. Incise the peritoneum over the neck of the gallbladder and continue for a short distance along its superior border. With blunt dissection gently open the space between the gallbladder and the liver at this point and expose the cystic artery. Follow the vessel onto the gallbladder wall and confirm that it is the cystic artery and not the right hepatic artery. Ligate the vessel twice in continuity and divide it between the ligatures.

3. Prior division of the cystic artery helps to straighten out the cystic duct. The duct is now exposed by a combination of sharp and blunt dissection and traced to its junction with the common hepatic duct to form the bile duct. It is vital to display this three-way junction before dividing the cystic duct.

4. Perform an operative cholangiogram via the cystic duct (see next section). Take a swab of the bile for bacteriological culture on opening the duct.

5. While awaiting the X-ray films, proceed to dissect the gallbladder from its liver bed. Leave the cholangiogram catheter in situ but complete the division of the cystic duct, grasping its gallbladder end with Moynihan's cholecystectomy forceps. Incise the peritoneum along the anterior and

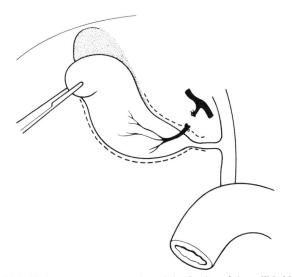

Fig. 10.3 Cholecystectomy: separation of the fundus of the gallbladder from the liver. The lines of peritoneal division are shown. The fundal dissection may be carried out after ligation and division of the cystic artery (as shown) or as the first stage of cholecystectomy.

posterior aspects of the gallbladder, proceeding either towards or away from the fundus. Traction on the fundus assists the dissection (Fig. 10.3). Numerous small vessels and occasionally accessory bile ducts traverse the areolar tissue between the liver and the gallbladder. Diathermy can be used to secure these vessels, but it may be simpler to ligate leashes of tissue on the hepatic side and then divide with scissors. Remove the gallbladder, preserving it for subsequent gross and histological examination.

6. If the cholangiogram pictures are technically satisfactory, withdraw the catheter and ligate the cystic duct close to the origin of the bile duct. Try and avoid leaving too long a cystic duct stump, but do not struggle to place the ligature exactly flush with the bile duct. Avoid tenting or narrowing the bile duct while tying the ligature. I use a 2/0 catgut tie reinforced by a 2/0 silk tie away from the bile duct. If the cystic duct is large, use a transfixion suture.

7. Use diathermy to stop any residual oozing from the liver bed. If you observe a leak of bile from a small cholecyst-hepatic duct, close the duct with a catgut stitch. Do not attempt to close the raw area of liver with sutures.

8. Remove the packs and aspirate any blood.

'Fundus-first' technique

1. Grasp the fundus of the gallbladder with tissue-holding forceps. Incise the peritoneum between the fundus and the liver, using frequent diathermy to secure the many fine vessels. Larger vessels can be ligated on the hepatic side and divided.

2. Extend the peritoneal incision along the anterior and posterior aspects of the gallbladder (Fig. 10.3). Open up the plane between the liver and the gallbladder, and proceed towards the neck of the organ. Identify the cystic artery. Ligate and divide the artery close to the gallbladder wall.

3. The advantage of the 'fundus-first' technique is that it brings you directly onto the cystic duct from the safe side and lessens the risk of bile-duct injury. Trace the cystic duct to its junction with the common hepatic duct. Perform a cholangiogram. Ligate and divide the cystic duct and remove the gallbladder.

4. Secure haemostasis in the liver bed. Remove the packs.

Difficulty?

1. The gallbladder is stuck to the duodenum or transverse colon and obscured by inflammatory adhesions. The organ can usually be freed by gentle digital dissection, but remember that calculi may have fistulated into the adherent viscus.

2. You cannot identify the cystic artery or the three-way union of ducts. Perhaps the tissues are fibrotic or bleed too easily. The liver may be enlarged and stiff, the gallbladder

may be inaccessible because the costal margin is low or the patient obese. Do not proceed until you have improved the view. Enlarge the incision if necessary. Have the light adjusted. Use the sucker. Make sure the assistants are usefully employed or summon further assistance.

3. You still cannot safely progress. Adopt the 'fundus-first' technique. Seek senior help. If all else fails, content yourself with cholecystostomy (see p. 180).

4. You are proceeding with the dissection, but the anatomy is anomalous or confusing. In these circumstances do not divide any structure until the anatomy of the area is fully displayed and understood. Remember the common variations, summon a textbook of surgical anatomy or seek assistance from the consultant. If the cystic duct can be identified with confidence, cholangiography may clarify the remaining ductal anatomy.

5. You suspect damage to the common hepatic duct or the bile duct. If the possibility exists, you must declare the issue and not just hope for the best. Enlist the help of the most experienced surgeon available. Cholangiography may be helpful. Partial or complete division of the main duct should be repaired immediately, using fine catgut sutures and placing a T-tube across the anastomosis through a separate stab incision. If a length of the duct has been resected, dissect out the upper end and bring up a Roux loop of jejunum to drain the bile. Resolve to make accurate notes, with drawings to display the exact situation.

6. Severe bleeding is encountered. Do not panic or apply haemostats blindly; the situation is almost certainly recoverable. Control the bleeding by local pressure. Arrange for blood to be available, for arterial sutures, tapes and bulldog clamps. Summon further advice and assistance if necessary.

(a) If the bleeding is *arterial*, compress the free edge of the lesser omentum between finger and thumb or apply a non-crushing intestinal clamp just tightly enough to control bleeding (Pringle's manoeuvre (Fig. 10.4)). Dissect out and control the hepatic artery, which normally lies on the left-hand side of the bile duct. Remember that accessory hepatic arteries arising from the left gastric or superior mesenteric arteries will not be controlled by occluding the main hepatic artery. Expose the damaged vessel. If large, repair it with arterial sutures; if small, ligate each end. You may find that you have pulled the cystic artery off the right hepatic artery. If so, suture the defect in the parent vessel. In the absence of jaundice or hypotension, ligature of the right hepatic or common hepatic artery (though best avoided) will not lead to infarction of the liver.

(b) If the bleeding is *venous*, control it by compression for 5 minutes timed by the clock, then explore, evaluate and repair the damage as necessary.

7. The gallbladder cannot be separated from the liver. Suspect carcinoma, and consider frozen-section examination if the diagnosis is equivocal. Carcinoma of the gall-

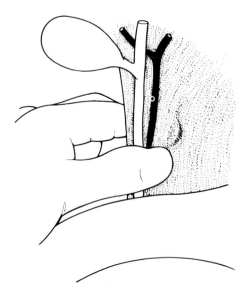

Fig. 10.4 Pringle's manoeuvre. Digital compression of the hepatic artery within the free edge of the lesser omentum controls haemorrhage from branches of the vessel beyond that point.

bladder should be removed together with a segment of subjacent liver and the nodes at the porta hepatis. Alternatively, some surgeons favour partial hepatectomy, but operative treatment is invariably unsuccessful once carcinoma has spread into the adjacent liver. If severe (benign) fibrosis makes it extremely difficult to develop a safe plane of dissection, it is permissible to leave the back wall of the gallbladder attached to the liver and diathermy the exposed mucosa.

Check list

1. Review the clinical and radiological criteria for continuing to exploration of the bile duct (see below).

2. Examine the gallbladder bed, the common duct and the ligatures on the cystic duct and cystic artery.

3. Place a fine-bore suction drain to the subhepatic pouch.

Aftercare

1. The nasogastric tube can usually be removed at 12–24 hours and the drain at 48 hours. In straightforward cases a light diet can be reintroduced at 24–36 hours, and patients are ready for discharge at 5–8 days.

2. Copious bile drainage through the wound or drain site suggests unrecognised injury to the bile duct or a slipped ligature on the cystic duct. Damage to the main duct may be accompanied by jaundice. The diagnosis is confirmed by cholangiography, obtained either by transhepatic needling or by retrograde cannulation of the ampulla. Reoperation will be needed.

3. Wound infection is uncommon unless the bile duct is explored. Subphrenic abscess and septicaemia are rare.

4. The mortality rate of cholecystectomy is well under 1%. Most post-cholecystectomy symptoms result from unrecognised intercurrent disease.

Further reading

Dawson J L 1981 Cholecystectomy. In: Lord Smith of Marlow, Sherlock Dame S Surgery of the gall bladder and bile ducts, 2nd edn. Butterworths, London. p 313–328

Linden W van der, Edlund G 1981 Early versus delayed cholecystectomy: the effect of a change in management. British Journal of Surgery 68: 743–757

Espiner H J 1982 Emergency cholecystectomy: towards guaranteed safety. In: Wilson D H, Marsden A K (eds) Care of the acutely ill and injured. Wiley, London. p 385–387

OPERATIVE CHOLANGIOGRAPHY

Appraise

1. Cholangiography is an integral part of cholecystectomy and should always be carried out at some stage of the operation, unless preoperative visualisation of the ducts (e.g. by retrograde cholangiography) has been excellent and they are normal.

2. Warn the X-ray Department pre-operatively. Ensure that the patient is correctly place on the operating table, with the upper abdomen overlying a radiolucent tunnel.

3. Cholangiograms should normally be obtained via the cystic duct. Alternatively, contrast material can be injected directly into the common hepatic or bile ducts. If ductal stones are obviously present at operation, it may still help to discover their number and size and the state of the duct before proceeding to exploration.

4. After choledocholithotomy, it is always sensible to check that all stones have been removed by repeating the cholangiogram.

Action

1. Fill a 20 ml syringe and attached fine plastic cannula with saline, making sure no air bubbles remain in the syringe or tubing. Prepare a second syringe filled with 25% sodium diatrizoate (Hypaque) and clearly marked.

2. Isolate 2 cm of cystic duct and ligate on the gallbladder side. Pass a second ligature around the duct, but do not tie. Partly divide the cystic duct between these ligatures about 2 cm from its entry into the main duct (Fig. 10.5).

3. Pass the cannula down the cystic duct for about 2 cm and ligate in situ. If difficulty is encountered from spiralling of the ductal mucosa (Heister's valve), withdraw the cannula, gently pass a probe and try again.

4. Check the patency of the cannula when it is tied in place. Inject a small quantity of saline, or detach the syringe and observe bile pass back up the tubing.

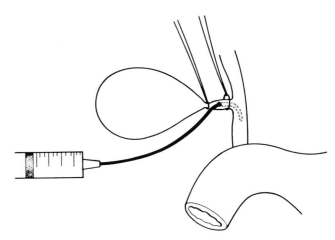

Fig. 10.5 Operative cholangiography. Through a small opening in the cystic duct, a fine polythene cannula is passed into the bile duct and secured in position by tightening a ligature around the cystic duct.

5. Remove instruments and swabs from the field. Cover the wound with a sterile towel and allow the radiographer to position the X-ray machine. Spectators, assistants and nursing personnel should now leave the theatre or take their place behind a lead screen. The anaesthetist remains for the moment to control the patient's respiration.

6. Inject 3–4 ml of contrast medium and have an X-ray film exposed. Insert a further 5–10 ml and obtain a second film.

7. Other techniques are convenient in particular circumstances. The contrast material can be injected directly into the main duct through a fine 'butterfly' needle. Alternatively, the neck of the gallbladder may be clamped and contrast is injected immediately beyond this point. When duodenotomy has been performed, a retrograde cholangiogram may be obtained by cannulation of the papilla.

8. Post-exploratory films are obtained via a T-tube inserted into the bile duct. Care must be taken to clear the tube and the ductal tree of air. The T-tube is repeatedly irrigated during closure of the choledochotomy incision, the last stitch being inserted and tied under water. One or two films are obtained after injection of 10–20 cc of 25% Hypaque.

9. If the films are technically unsatisfactory, do not hesitate to repeat them.

Interpretation

1. Inspect the films carefully. Make sure that the right and left hepatic ducts are displayed together with their tributaries. The bile duct usually overlies the spine, and occasionally this can obscure certain features. If necessary, obtain further films with the operating table rotated 15° to the right to throw the bile duct clear of the spine (some surgeons adopt this precaution routinely).

2. On the pre-exploratory films, exclude the following features: filling defects, obstruction of a major hepatic radicle, dilatation of the bile duct (>10 mm), failure of contrast to enter the duodenum. Remember that the bile duct normally tapers before smoothly entering the duodenum. If you suspect spasm rather than organic obstruction of the papilla, consider obtaining a further X-ray after an intravenous injection of hyoscine hydrobromide (Buscopan) 40 mg.

3. On the post-exploratory films the most important feature is the presence or absence of a filling defect, consistent with a residual calculus. It is quite common for contrast not to enter the duodenum at this stage, especially after instrumentation of the papilla.

Further reading

Cranley B, Logan H 1980 Exploration of the common bile duct; the relevance of the clinical picture and the importance of peroperative cholangiography. British Journal of Surgery 67: 869–872

EXPLORATION OF THE BILE DUCT

Appraise

1. Absolute indications for choledochotomy are stones unequivocally shown on a pre-operative or operative cholangiogram, stones that can be palpated within the bile duct and stones causing obstructive jaundice.

2. Relative indications for exploration are any abnormalities shown on operative cholangiography apart from obvious stones. If the radiological criteria are doubtful the following clinical factors would tend to favour exploration of the duct: a history of jaundice or acute pancreatitis, dilatation and opacification of the wall of the bile duct, multiple small calculi in the gallbladder and a short wide cystic duct.

3. If narrowing of the terminal bile duct is the only abnormality, it is sometimes possible to rule out appreciable stenosis by passing a soft Jacques catheter (No. 8 FG) through the cystic duct stump and into the duodenum.

4. If doubt remains, explore the duct. Negative exploration is safer than ignoring disease (usually stones but conceivably tumour).

5. Remember that a jaundiced patient needs proper perioperative precautions taken (see p. 191).

Access

1. If continuing on from cholecystectomy, make sure the existing incision is adequate; otherwise, extend it.

2. If starting from scratch, choose a right upper paramedian incision, unless there is a convenient scar to reopen from a previous operation.

3. At re-operation there may be dense adhesions. Find the liver at the upper end of the wound and trace its undersurface, where stomach, small bowel or transverse colon may be adherent. Identify the stomach, follow it distally to the duodenum and draw this downwards to display the region of the common duct.

Assess

1. During abdominal exploration pay particular attention to the extrahepatic biliary tree, liver and pancreas. Decide if a liver biopsy should be taken.

2. Expose the supraduodenal portion of the bile duct by careful dissection within the free edge of the lesser omentum. Examine the duct carefully. Split the peritoneum in the floor of the epiploic foramen to feel its lower end.

3. If previous cholecystectomy has been performed, it may or may not be necessary to obtain operative cholangiograms, depending upon the adequacy of pre-operative investigation. Otherwise proceed to cholecystectomy and operative cholangiography, as described above.

Action

1. Place two catgut stay sutures in the wall of the bile duct. Incise the duct vertically between the sutures (Fig. 10.6) and take a culture swab of the bile. Extend the choledochotomy for 15–20 mm. Obtain haemostasis from the cut edges of the duct.

2. Remove any obvious stones with forceps. Palpate the duct and try to milk stones towards the choledochotomy. Gently explore the biliary tree upwards and downwards, using Desjardin's or Randall's forceps with the appropriate degrees of angulation. Reconcile the calculi extracted with the cholangiographic appearances.

3. Pass a soft polyethylene catheter (Jaques No. 8 FG)

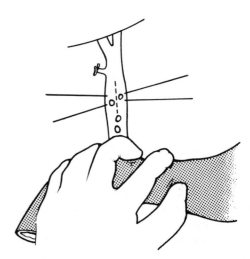

Fig. 10.6 Exploration of the bile duct. Stay sutures are placed, and a vertical choledochotomy is performed.

connected to a 50 ml syringe upwards into the hepatic ducts. Irrigate briskly with saline and repeat until the returning fluid is entirely clear. Now pass the catheter downwards and irrigate the bile duct. If there are multiple stones and gravel, it is sensible to occlude the common hepatic duct with a bulldog clip or tape during this procedure.

4. Pass the catheter through the papilla and into the duodenum, where it can be felt by rolling the bowel between finger and thumb. Failure to pass the catheter suggests either a calculus impacted at the ampulla or some other obstruction, e.g. papillary fibrosis. Mobilise the duodenum, using Kocher's technique. It may be possible to disimpact the calculus or crush it with forceps (if it is soft) and wash out the fragments. Passage of graded Bakes' metal dilators may overcome papillary stenosis, but this manoeuvre should be performed with great care.

5. After all apparent stones have been removed, use a choledochoscope (if available) to check that the ducts are clear. Both rigid and flexible endoscopes require a free flow of irrigant to distend the ductal tree for adequate inspection. The choledochotomy is temporarily occluded by crossing the stay sutures.

6. Insert the T-piece of a latex T-tube into the bile duct and close the duct with a running 2/0 catgut suture, so that the tube emerges from the lower end of the suture line (Fig. 10.7). The T-tube will normally be between sizes 10–16 FG, depending on the size of the duct.

7. Whether or not choledochoscopy has been performed it is sensible to obtain a post-exploratory T-tube cholangiogram (see previous section), unless no stones have been found in the duct and the original grounds for exploration were equivocal.

8. Bring the T-tube directly to the surface of the abdominal wall, to exit through a separate stab incision. Suture the tube to the skin and connect it to a drainage bag.

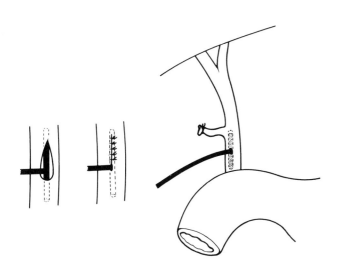

Fig. 10.7 T-tube drainage of the bile duct. The tube is brought out through the lower end of the sutured choledochotomy.

Difficulty?

1. Adhesions from previous biliary surgery make the bile duct difficult to find. Explore the area with a syringe and fine needle, aspirating to see if bile is obtained.

2. Multiple stones are present with or without biliary mud and gravel. It will obviously be difficult to ensure complete clearance of the dilated ductal tree. Perform a permanent drainage operation, either choledochoduodenostomy or transduodenal sphincteroplasty (see below). Greater readiness to take this step would undoubtedly reduce the incidence of retained calculi (about 10%).

3. There is a problem at the lower end of the bile duct. You cannot remove an impacted calculus or manage to pass an instrument through the papilla. The patient may be jaundiced. Proceed to transduodenal sphincteroplasty.

Aftercare

1. Leave the T-tube on free dependent drainage for 3 days, then lift the bag level with the wound for 2–3 days and elevate to the shoulder thereafter. Output of bile will decrease, provided there is no residual obstruction in the duct. If pain develops after elevating the bag, return to dependent drainage.

2. Obtain a T-tube cholangiogram 7–10 days after operation. Check the films to ensure that there is free drainage of contrast into the duodenum and there are no filling defects. Repeat the X-ray if appearances are equivocal.

3. If the X-rays are satisfactory, spigot the T-tube and remove it on the 10th post-operative day. A firm pull is usually required. Observe the patient overnight before discharge from hospital.

4. If it is clear that you have left a stone behind, do not remove the T-tube. Small stones can sometimes be cleared by flushing the duct with normal saline. Give an antispasmodic to relax the sphincter of Oddi and infuse 1 litre of saline from a bag suspended 1 m above the wound. If this technique fails, leave the T-tube in situ for 6 weeks to obtain a mature fibrous track and repeat the X-ray. It may now be possible to pass a steerable catheter down the T-tube track and remove residual calculi under X-ray control (Burhenne technique). Other treatment options for retained stone include endoscopic papillotomy and reoperation, but prevention is very much better than cure.

Further reading

Motson R W, Wood A J, de Jode L R 1980 Operative choledochoscopy: experience with a rigid choledochoscope. British Journal of Surgery 67: 406–409

INTERNAL DRAINAGE FOR DUCTAL STONES

Appraise

1. Some form of permanent drainage operation is indicated during exploration of the bile duct when multiple

stones and biliary mud are encountered, or when papillary stenosis impedes the onward passage of contrast or instruments. Such patients are likely to have a history of jaundice and dilatation of the extrahepatic biliary tree.

2. A calculus that is impacted in the ampulla and cannot be extracted is a clear indication for transduodenal sphincteroplasty. The intention is to create a passage into the duodenum equal in size to the diameter of the bile duct, so that any remaining stones can enter the duodenum. Correctly performed, this is probably the procedure of choice for establishing long-term drainage of the duct. Indeed, a few surgeons use the transduodenal approach for routine exploration of the bile duct. There is no indication for operative sphincterotomy alone, since healing by fibrosis is likely to cause renewed stenosis of the papilla.

3. Choledochoduodenostomy is a satisfactory alternative, especially in the elderly. An ample side-to-side anastomosis is created, bypassing the lower part of the bile duct. Occasionally stasis in the bypassed duct leads to recurrent cholangitis ('sump' syndrome). This operation is technically simpler to perform in most cases than sphincteroplasty.

4. Endoscopic papillotomy can provide ductal drainage without the need for a major surgical operation and is therefore particularly useful in the elderly or infirm. The diathermy incision usually abolishes the pressure gradient between the duodenum and the bile duct and is therefore a form of sphincterotomy. Calculi can often be extracted by retrograde instrumentation or will pass spontaneously. Of proven value in the management of ductal stones left behind at operation, the technique has also been advocated in the primary treatment of choledocholithiasis, especially in the presence of jaundice or severe cholangitis. Subsequent cholecystectomy would ordinarily be indicated in such patients, however.

Action

Choledochoduodenostomy (Fig. 10.8)

1. First mobilize the duodenal loop, using Kocher's manoeuvre.

2. If the operation has been considered before exploration of the bile duct, make a vertical incision low down in the supraduodenal portion of the duct to avoid subsequent tension on the anastomosis.

3. Incise the duodenum either vertically or transversely (as appropriate) at the junction of its first and second parts. Pass a finger downwards to examine the ampulla and exclude a lesion at this site.

4. Roll the duodenum upwards and effect a side-to-side anastomosis with the bile duct, using one layer of fine catgut sutures, either continuous or interrupted. It is important to create a stoma that is at least 2.5 cm in diameter.

5. Place a suction drain into the subhepatic pouch.

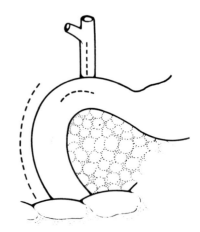

Fig. 10.8 Choledochoduodenostomy. The bile duct and duodenum are opened as shown and then approximated. Kocherisation of the duodenum reduces tension on the anastomosis.

Transduodenal sphincteroplasty (Fig. 10.9)

1. Mobilize the duodenal loop and make an oblique or vertical duodenotomy incision, about 4 cm long, opposite the papilla. The papilla can usually be palpated in the descending duodenum, especially if diseased. Otherwise it can be localized by passing a catheter or bougie down the bile duct via a supraduodenal choledochotomy.

2. Once the duodenum has been opened, grasp the mucosa with Babcock's forceps and search for the papilla on the posteromedial wall. Again an instrument passed from above may be of assistance.

3. Pass a blunt-nosed polyethylene cannula (No. 8 FG) through the papilla from above. If necessary, first make a short relieving incision to allow extraction of an impacted

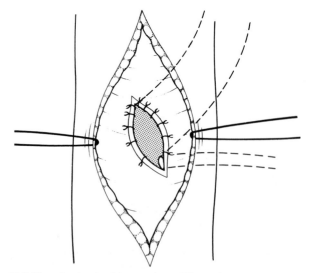

Fig. 10.9 Transduodenal sphincteroplasty. The papilla is approached via a longitudinal duodenotomy and is incised. Interrupted sutures coapt the mucosae of the terminal bile duct and duodenum. The orifice of the major pancreatic duct can be seen at the lower end of the sphincteroplasty.

calculus or dilate a stenosed papilla forcibly under direct vision. Cut off the end of the cannula, insert a grooved hernia director into its lumen and withdraw the cannula so that the director enters the lower bile duct with its groove towards the liver.

4. Use the groove to insert two 3/0 catgut sutures into the papilla at about 10 o'clock and 12 o'clock. Tie these sutures and divide the papilla for a short distance between them, using sharp scissors. Now place and tie two further stay sutures towards the apex of the cut and proceed methodically in this manner until a wide stoma has been created, which will usually accept the tip of the little finger. Each suture unites the lax pink intestinal mucosa to the paler and tighter mucosa of the terminal bile duct. Insert the final stitch into the apex of the V.

5. Search for the orifice of the major pancreatic duct. The orifice can nearly always be found on the lower lip of the papilla at about 5 o'clock. Clear juice can usually be seen emerging from the duct. Ensure that the opening is in no way obstructed by the sutures. If appropriate, gently pass a fine polythene cannnula (No. 4 or 5 FG) to check the patency of the duct and consider if retrograde pancreatography is indicated.

6. Close the duodenotomy in the line that it was created, using a running catgut suture. Place the second (seromuscular) layer of sutures with care to avoid excessive narrowing of the duodenum.

7. Though T-tube drainage of the supraduodenal duct is not essential after an adequate sphincteroplasty has been carried out, it does provide a safety-valve if the stoma is narrowed by postoperative oedema and it permits subsequent cholangiography. I always insert a T-tube, therefore.

8. Drain the subhepatic pouch as before.

Endoscopic papillotomy

1. Treat this procedure like a surgical operation. Admit the patient to hospital, check the coagulation status and exclude hepatitis B antigen. Group and save serum, in case emergency blood transfusion becomes necessary. Starve the patient for 6 hours beforehand. Obtain a preliminary X-ray of the upper abdomen. Sedate the patient with a combination of pentazocine (or pethidine) and diazepam. Give intravenous hyoscine hydrobromide (Buscopan: 40 mg) or glucagon (2 mg) to inhibit duodenal peristalsis.

2. Pass a long insulated side-viewing duodenoscope through the pylorus and into the descending duodenum. Turn the patient prone. Rotate the instrument to bring the lens 'face-on' to the papilla, which can be identified as a pink nipple partly covered by a proximal transverse fold of mucosa.

3. Cannulate the bile duct by inserting a diathermy catheter into the papilla along the axis of the duct, i.e. in a retrograde fashion. Insert a small quantity of water-sol-

uble contrast (e.g. Conray 420) under fluoroscopic control to check that the correct duct has been cannulated.

4. Partly withdraw the cannula and exert traction, so that its contained wire arches against the roof of the ampulla at about 11 o'clock. Using alternative bursts of cutting and coagulation current, make a 10–15 mm incision and secure haemostasis.

5. Small stones (<10 mm diameter) can be removed by atraumatic balloon catheters or be left to pass spontaneously. Sometimes repeated endoscopic examinations or instrumentation can be avoided by leaving a catheter in the bile duct after sphincterotomy and bringing it out through the patient's nose. Lavage with saline and check cholangiograms are facilitated.

Difficulty?

1. In the presence of suppurative cholangitis any form of internal surgical drainage is probably inadvisable. Content yourself with removing obstructing calculi from the duct, irrigation and insertion of a T-tube. If necessary, further procedures may be attempted when the emergency has passed.

2. If the duodenum and/or the bile duct are grossly adherent to surrounding structures and cannot be approximated without tension, choledochoduodenostomy is inadvisable. Thorough mobilisation of the duodenum assists both types of operative drainage procedure, however.

3. Do not hesitate to pass an instrument from above, if the papilla cannot be found after opening the duodenum. Retractors placed inside the duodenum may help to display an inaccessible papilla. The 'stitch-and-cut' technique described controls haemorrhage and allows a precise incision to be created and sutured. The worrying complication of acute pancreatitis can be avoided by ensuring that the orifice of the major pancreatic duct is not occluded by sutures.

4. Do not attempt endoscopic papillotomy until you are fully proficient both at gastroduodenoscopy and at retrograde cholangiopancreatography. Remember that attempts at cannulation are doomed to failure unless the papilla is seen 'face-on'. A slick technique is needed to achieve successful papillotomy before the patient and the endoscopist become fatigued. Bleeding or suspected perforation require emergency operative intervention in about 3% of cases.

Further reading

Cotton P B, Williams C B 1982 Practical Gastrointestinal Endoscopy, 2nd edn. Blackwell, Oxford

Lygidakis N J 1981 Choledochoduodenostomy in calculous biliary tract disease. British Journal of Surgery 68: 762–765

Vogt D P, Hermann R E 1981 Choledochoduodenostomy, choledochojejunostomy or sphincteroplasty for biliary and pancreatic disease. Annals of Surgery 193: 161–168

CHOLECYSTOSTOMY

Appraise

1. Cholecystostomy is a temporary expedient for draining an obstructed or infected gallbladder to the exterior. Nowadays it is seldom indicated.

2. Cholecystostomy should be considered where gross disease of the gallbladder or intercurrent illness make cholecystectomy unsafe. In the very elderly or infirm with empyema of the gallbladder or necrotising cholecystitis, cholecystostomy under local anaesthetic can be life-saving. If cholecystectomy is planned, but obesity and/or severe inflammation cause serious technical difficulties, cholecystostomy is a reasonable option, especially for an inexperienced surgeon. A second operation may well be needed at a later date, however, and subtotal cholecystectomy is an alternative.

3. Cholecystostomy is sometimes performed to relieve obstructive jaundice before proceeding to resection of a periampullary cancer (see p. 191).

4. If gallstones are encountered during laparotomy for severe acute pancreatitis, cholecystostomy may permit drainage of an obstructed biliary tree (see p. 186).

Access

1. Planned cholecystostomy should be carried out through a short transverse incision in the right upper quadrant. The incision is placed over the fundus of the gallbladder, when this is palpable.

Action

1. Protect the margins of the wound and pack off the area of the gallbladder to prevent contamination by infected bile. Free adhesions sufficiently to expose the fundus of the gallbladder.

2. Aspirate the fluid contents of the gallbladder by suction through an Ochsner trocar and cannula or syringe and wide-bore needle.

3. Grasp the partly-collapsed fundus with tissue-holding forceps to control the organ and prevent its retraction. Make a short incision in the fundus and obtain a culture of the bile. Suck out residual bile.

4. Explore the lumen of the gallbladder with a finger and extract all the stones. Saline irrigation may help or insertion of a gauze swab to trap small calculi. If the patient's condition allows, try and determine the presence or absence of gangrene, perforation and obvious calculi in the cystic duct or Hartmann's pouch, which could be gently disimpacted and milked towards the fundal incision.

5. After the gallbladder has been cleared of stones, insert a large Foley or Malecot catheter into the lumen and secure it with catgut sutures to effect a watertight closure (Fig. 10.10). Bring the tube to the exterior through a stab

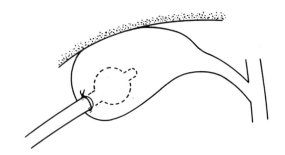

Fig. 10.10 Cholecystostomy. A large Foley catheter is sutured into the gallbladder, taking care not to puncture the balloon when inserting the stitches.

wound immediately over the gallbladder, and suture it to the skin of the abdominal wall. A corrugated drain should be inserted to the subhepatic space if there has been quite an extensive dissection.

Difficulty?

1. The gallbladder is friable or necrotic and tears during the dissection. Excise devitalised segments and close the remnant around the tube. If the cystic duct is cleared of stones and bile flow is re-established, subtotal cholecystectomy without external tube drainage is a reasonable alternative in unfavourable circumstances.

2. Calculi cannot easily be disimpacted from the depths of the gallbladder. The options are to remove as much debris as possible and insert a tube as before or proceed to subtotal or complete cholecystectomy despite the patient's poor condition.

Aftercare

1. Record the amount of cholecystostomy drainage and replace electrolytes as needed. Obtain a tube cholecystogram at 7–10 days. If there are no residual stones and contrast enters the bile duct, clamp and then remove the tube. Consider elective cholecystectomy at a later date.

2. Residual stones are a clear indication for re-operation when the patient's condition allows.

Further reading

Dawson J L 1981 Cholecystostomy. In: Lord Smith of Marlow, Sherlock Dame S (eds) Surgery of the gall bladder and bile ducts, 2nd edn. Butterworths, London. p 329–336

INTERNAL DRAINAGE FOR BILE-DUCT STRICTURES

Appraise

1. Inadvertent injury during cholecystectomy is the commonest cause of a benign stricture of the bile duct or

common hepatic duct. Immediate recognition and careful repair of the injured duct at the original operation reduces but does not abolish the risk of subsequent stenosis. The postoperative development of obstructive jaundice, with or without fever and an external biliary fistula, suggests a traumatic stricture.

2. In the absence of previous surgery ductal strictures are likely to be malignant, either primary carcinoma of the bile-duct epithelium (cholangiocarcinoma) or, more commonly, compression and invasion of the duct by secondary carcinoma. Carcinoma of the pancreas can obstruct the bile duct either in its supraduodenal portion or close to the ampulla. The presentation and management of primary carcinoma of the ampulla are similar to those of pancreatic cancer (see p. 191), but the results of resection are superior. Both resection and palliative bypass for malignant stricture generally require some type of biliary-enteric anastomosis.

3. Sclerosing cholangitis and certain types of congenital biliary atresia are occasional indications for a ductal drainage procedure. It may be necessary to perform a high hepaticojejunostomy to re-route the bile. Choledochal cyst can be drained into a Roux loop of jejunum; primary excision of the cyst is more difficult but probably gives better results.

4. A cholangiogram should be obtained before operating on a patient with stricture of the bile duct. Impaired liver function usually ensures that the percutaneous transhepatic or endoscopic retrograde routes must be chosen. Perioperative precautions to be taken in obstructive jaundice are described later in the chapter (p. 191).

5. The simplest type of biliary-enteric bypass is a cholecystenterostomy, but this should be reserved for short-term relief of jaundice in irresectable cancer of the pancreas (see p. 191). Anastomosis of a defunctioned (Roux) loop of jejunum to the bile duct (choledochojejunostomy) or common hepatic duct (hepaticojejunostomy) provides the best permanent biliary drainage. Anastomosis can be performed with or without resection of a benign or malignant stricture. The closer the lesion to the hilus of the liver, the greater the technical difficulty. When tackling a high cholangiocarcinoma or a repeat operation for traumatic stricture, it will be necessary to dissect within the hilus or even split the liver (hepatotomy) to obtain access. These operations are among the most taxing in abdominal surgery, and some alternative options are discussed below.

Access

1. Choose an incision that will provide generous access to the structures at the porta hepatis, e.g. long midline or bilateral Kocher. Dissection within the hilus of the liver occasionally requires extension of the incision into the right chest.

2. If this is a re-operation for traumatic stricture, there may be extensive adhesions in the right upper quadrant. Try and locate the right lobe of the liver and separate attached stomach, duodenum or transverse colon from its lower border. Identify and mobilise the duodenal loop, and explore gently above this point to find the bile duct. Be prepared to aspirate any potential tube with syringe and needle, looking for bile.

3. During a high dissection within the hilus of the liver keep close to the common hepatic duct and remember that its bifurcation usually lies in front of those of the hepatic artery and portal vein. In the case of a malignant obstruction, removal of a distended gallbladder may improve access to the dilated common hepatic duct.

Assess

1. With a traumatic stricture the objective is to fashion an accurate and watertight anastomosis between supple proximal bile duct and a Roux loop of jejunum, with the complete avoidance of tension. Resection of the strictured duct and reunion of the cut ends is unlikely to succeed at this stage (unlike primary repair at the time of injury). Resection of the stricture with ligation of the lower end may assist hepaticojejunostomy, however.

2. For primary cholangiocarcinoma, including carcinoma of the ampulla, resection is the preferred treatment, where feasible. For cancer of the supraduodenal duct, local resection of the tumour and adjacent nodes should be followed by anastomosis of the proximal duct to a Roux loop of jejunum. For cancer of the terminal bile duct or ampulla, partial pancreatoduodenectomy should be undertaken (see p. 194).

3. If a bile-duct tumour is irresectable or has widely metastasized, the surgeon should still make every effort to relieve obstructive jaundice. Possible methods include transection of the main duct above the tumour plus hepaticojejunostomy, opening of the bile duct and insertion of a stent or transhepatic drainage tube, or a Longmire operation (see below).

4. Consider whether operative cholangiography might help to display the anatomy, if you are in difficulty.

Action

Cholecystjejunostomy (Fig. 10.11)

1. Lift up the greater omentum and transverse colon to identify the duodenojejunal flexure. Draw the first loop of jejunum in front of the transverse colon and ensure that it will reach the gallbladder without tension.

2. Pack off the gallbladder area. Partly aspirate the contents of the distended gallbladder with an Ochsner trocar and cannula connected to the sucker. Now grasp the puncture site with tissue-holding forceps to seal it.

3. Milk the loop of jejunum free of contents and apply a non-crushing clamp to occude the lumen.

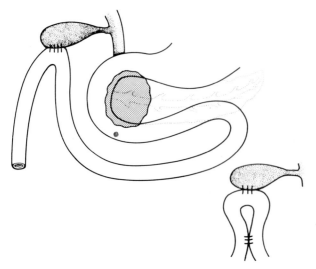

Fig. 10.11 Cholecystjejunostomy. A jejunojejunostomy may be added (inset) to divert food from the biliary-enteric anastomosis.

4. Run a catgut seromuscular stitch between the posterior surface of the gallbladder and the loop of jejunum. It may be easier to leave the structures slightly apart while completing the suture line, then tighten the loops individually to draw the surfaces together. Do not insert the gallbladder stitches too deeply or they will pierce the whole wall and allow bile leakage.

5. Incise both the fundus of the gallbladder and the apex of the jejunal loop for about 3 cm. Suck out the rest of the bile and obtain a culture.

6. Insert an all-coats running 2/0 catgut stitch to create the anastomosis. Complete the encircling seromuscular stitch.

7. Some surgeons perform a side-to-side enteroenterostomy at a convenient point below the biliary-enteric anastomosis to prevent food entering the gallbladder.

8. Close the abdomen after removing the packs, aspirating any bile spillage and inserting a separate stab drain to the anastomosis.

Choledochojejunostomy and hepaticojejunostomy

1. Dissect out the supraduodenal portion of the bile duct and/or the common hepatic duct. Encircle them with soft rubber slings, taking great care not to injure the portal vein lying posteriorly.

2. The point of transection of the main duct depends upon the underlying lesion. During resection or bypass for benign disease (e.g. traumatic stricture, chronic pancreatitis), divide the duct as low as possible. It will ordinarily be the bile duct that you have divided, unless there is a very low entry of the cystic duct. During resection or bypass for malignant disease (e.g. cholangiocarcinoma, carcinoma of pancreas), divide the duct at a higher level, at least 1 cm above the tumour. This may involve transection of the common hepatic duct, in which case cholecystectomy should be carried out. A bulldog clamp on the proximal duct will control bile spillage.

3. After ductal division culture the bile. Ligate or oversew the lower end of the duct, depending on its size.

4. Select a length of upper jejunum for conversion into a Roux loop (see Ch. 6). Transilluminate the mesentery, ligate and divide 2–3 arterial arcades, transect the bowel and close the distal cut end with a double layer of catgut sutures. Create a mesocolic window and bring the Roux loop up behind the transverse colon, so that it reaches the transected bile duct or common hepatic duct without any tension.

5. Make a small enterotomy some 3 cm from the closed end of the Roux loop. The incision should be slightly shorter than the diameter of the bile duct, bearing in mind that an enterotomy will stretch.

6. The choledochojejunostomy or hepaticojejunostomy is fashioned using a single layer of interruped 3/0 catgut sutures. Insert the corner stitches followed by the back row. Clip each stitch and do not tie until the entire back row has been placed.

7. If the bile duct is of normal size (<1 cm diameter) it is wise to splint the anastomosis with a fine T-tube (Fig. 10.12). With a dilated duct this step is optional. After tying the back row of sutures pass a right-angled Lahey forceps up the duct, and incise the duct wall over the tip of the forceps. Grasp the T-piece of the tube and pull it into the duct. Place the T-tube so that its long lower limb

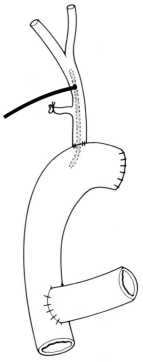

Fig. 10.12 Hepaticojejunostomy Roux-en-Y. The anastomosis is splinted by the long descending limb of a T-tube. Cholecystectomy has been performed.

traverses the anastomosis. Insert 1–2 catgut sutures to tighten the point of entry of the T-tube into the proximal duct.

8. Now complete the anterior row of interrupted catgut sutures to create a watertight anastomosis.

9. Intestinal continuity is restored by end-to-side jejunojejunostomy (two-layer catgut anastomosis).

10. Close the abdomen with drainage as before.

Operations for high bile-duct stricture

1. *Hepatojejunostomy.* It may be possible to excise a malignant stricture at the hilus of the liver, taking care to preserve the divisions of the hepatic artery and portal vein. It may be necessary to split the liver partly between the right and left lobes to approach the origin of the common hepatic duct. The gallbladder must first be mobilised or resected, and the liver substance in its bed is then divided as for hemihepatectomy (see Ch. 11). After resection of the tumour the right and left hepatic ducts or their major divisions must be sutured to a Roux loop of jejunum. Each anastomosis should be splinted by a transhepatic tube (a Redivac® suction tube is convenient). The top end of the tube is brought to the exterior, and the lower end is placed within the jejunal loop. There should be several holes in the tube on either side of the anastomosis.

2. *Smith's 'mucosal graft' operation* (Fig. 10.13). During re-operation for traumatic stricture, the mass of scar tissue at the porta hepatis may prevent accurate coaptation of the biliary and jejunal epithelia. A seromuscular disc of jejunum is removed to expose the mucosa. A transhepatic tube is sutured to the mucosal graft and used to draw a sleeve of jejunal mucosa through the scar tissue and into the intrahepatic duct system. No sutures are used except to anchor the Roux loop to the liver capsule.

3. *Central hepatic resection.* This operation has also been advocated for benign or malignant stricture at the hepatic bifurcation. It is an extension of hepatojejunostomy involving excision of a core of hepatic substance together with the affected bile ducts. Continuity is again restored by suturing the transected ducts separately to a Roux loop of jejunum, with transhepatic splinting tubes.

4. *Intubation.* This procedure may be appropriate for an irresectable malignant stricture. The collapsed bile duct is exposed and opened below the stricture between stay sutures. Dilators are passed upwards to gauge the length of the stricture and to try and enter an obstructed proximal duct. An attempt should be made to biopsy the tumour. The ducts are washed out through a fine catheter and cholangiograms may be obtained. A length of stiff polyethylene tubing is passed through the stricture and is left as an internal stent before closing the bile duct. Alternatively, a transhepatic U-tube is placed across the stricture and both ends are brought to the surface of the abdominal wall. If preoperative assessment shows that the tumour is clearly irresectable, the need for laparotomy may be avoided by percutaneous transhepatic placement of a biliary stent.

5. *Longmire's operation* (Fig. 10.14). As an alternative to draining the ducts at the hilus of the liver, they may be drained to the surface of the liver following a limited hepatic resection. Usually both sides of the liver have to be drained for successful relief of jaundice. The left and/or right hepatic lobe is mobilised, and its tip is amputated beyond a non-crushing intestinal clamp. A cholangiogram may be obtained. A Roux loop of jejunum is brought up for anastomosis preferably to individual large duct(s) or if necessary to the liver capsule around several smaller ducts. Again, the anastomosis may be splinted by transhepatic tube(s).

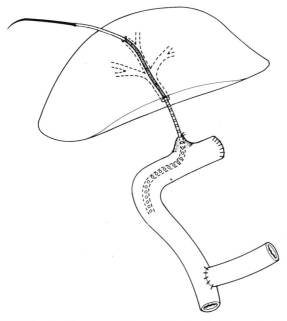

Fig. 10.13 Hepaticojejunostomy Roux-en-Y, using the 'mucosal graft' procedure of Lord Smith. A sleeve of jejunal mucosa is sutured to the transhepatic tube and drawn up into the intrahepatic biliary tree.

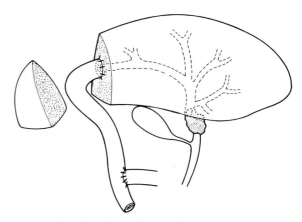

Fig. 10.14 Longmire's operation for irresectable tumour at the hilus of the liver. After resection of the lateral pole of the right (and/or left) hepatic lobe, a Roux loop of jejunum is sutured around the exposed dilated bile ducts.

6. *Kasai's hepatic portoenterostomy.* This procedure may permit surgical correction of otherwise non-correctable congenital biliary atresia. The atretic ducts are followed into the porta hepatis, and a small disc of liver tissue is excised at this point, revealing small bile ducts. The end of a Roux loop is then sewn to the surrounding liver capsule, using 5/0 catgut sutures.

Aftercare

1. Many of the above operations involve placement of a splinting tube across the anastomosis. The tube permits postoperative sampling of bile and repeat cholangiography. Where rapid healing is anticipated (e.g. after choledochojejunostomy Roux-en-Y), the tube can usually be removed at about 10 days. In less favourable cases (e.g. hepatojejunostomy for high traumatic stricture), the tube should be left for several weeks to assist healing. The advantage of a transhepatic U-tube is that is can be flushed through at each end and even be replaced if it becomes blocked.

2. The peritoneal drain can be removed after 3–4 days, provided there is no overt bile leak.

Further reading

Rickham P P, Hersig J 1981 Congenital biliary atresia. In: Lord Smith of Marlow, Sherlock, Dame S (eds) Surgery of the gall bladder and bile ducts, 2nd edn. Butterworths, London. p 117–152
Hart M J, White T T 1980 Central hepatic resection and anastomosis for stricture or carcinoma at the hepatic bifurcation. Annals of Surgery 192: 299–305
Terblanche J, Saunders S J, Louw J H 1972 Prolonged palliation in carcinoma of the main hepatic duct junction. Surgery 72: 720–731
Lord Smith of Marlow 1979 Obstructions of the bile duct. British Journal of Surgery 66: 69–79
Harrington D P, Barth K H, Maddrey W C, Kaufman S L, Cameron J L 1979 Percutaneously placed biliary stents in the management of malignant biliary obstruction. Digestive Diseases and Sciences 24: 849–857
Blumgart L H, Drury J K, Wood C B 1979 Hepatic resection for trauma, tumour and biliary obstruction. British Journal of Surgery 66: 762–769

EXPLORATION AND BIOPSY OF THE PANCREAS

Access

1. Examination of the pancreas is usually performed as part of a general abdominal exploration.

2. If examination of the whole pancreas is the major purpose of the operation, select either an upper midline incision or a curved transverse incision midway between umbilicus and xiphoid and convex upwards.

Assess

1. Before approaching the pancreas, pay particular attention to the duodenum, liver, spleen and bile duct.

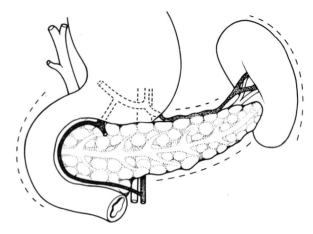

Fig. 10.15 Exposure of the pancreas. The lines of peritoneal incision are shown. The head and neck of pancreas and uncinate lobe are nourished by the superior and inferior pancreaticoduodenal arteries, and the body and tail by the splenic artery.

2. Mobilise the duodenal loop and pancreatic head by Kocher's manoeuvre (Fig. 10.15). Gently clear the omentum from the anterior aspect of the head of pancreas, which can now be directly inspected and palpated between finger and thumb.

3. Expose the body and tail of the pancreas through the lesser sac, which can be entered through the greater (or lesser) omentum. Separate the congenital adhesions between the stomach and the pancreas. If necessary, the peritoneum may be divided along the superior border of the pancreas, so that a finger can be insinuated beneath the gland.

4. The inferior border of the pancreas can also be mobilised by dividing the overlying peritoneum, taking care not to wound the superior or inferior mesenteric vein. Trace the middle colic vein downwards to find the superior mesenteric vein.

5. Lying at the splenic hilum, the tail of pancreas is the least accessible part of the gland. It can usually be approached by dividing the greater omentum and retracting the stomach upwards. Occasionally it may be necessary to divide the peritoneum lateral to the spleen and lift the spleen and tail of pancreas forwards into the wound.

6. Learn to recognise the firm, nodular consistency of normal pancreas by palpating the gland during all upper abdominal operations. You should then be able to differentiate the hard sclerotic gland of chronic pancreatitis or a localised tumour, which may be hard (carcinoma) or soft (cyst). The pancreatic duct is not palpable unless it is dilated.

7. If a mass can be felt in the region of the ampulla, it may assist diagnosis to open the duodenum and directly visualise the pancreatic papilla. Suspected carcinoma at this site should be confirmed by immediate frozen-section examination of a suitable biopsy (if endoscopic biopsy has not already provided the diagnosis).

PANCREATIC BIOPSY

1. No method of biopsying the pancreas is devoid of risk, yet a positive tissue diagnosis may be important for the proper management of suspected malignant disease in particular. Select the safest method appropriate. The following biopsy techniques are listed in order of increasing hazard.

2. To confirm metastatic carcinoma, it is better to biopsy the site of possible metastasis (liver nodule, adjacent lymph node) than the pancreatic primary itself.

3. Using a fine (No. 1) needle and a 20 ml syringe, aspirate the site of the lesion. Apply strong suction while advancing and withdrawing the needle within the lesion, then release the suction and remove the needle and syringe. Eject the material in the needle track onto a glass slide, and make a smear for cytological examination.

4. If the surface of the pancreas is diseased, perform a 'shave' biopsy with a scalpel. Remember the possibility that an inflammatory 'halo' may surround the actual neoplastic tissue.

5. A core of tissue for histological examination can be obtained using a Trucut or Menghini needle. If the lesion is in the head of pancreas it may be safer to approach it through the duodenum.

6. If the above techniques are inadequate and a biopsy is essential, incise the gland directly over the lesion and obtain a small piece of tissue. However, it may be better to carry out a formal partial pancreatectomy under these circumstances.

7. The complications of biopsy include acute pancreatitis and pancreatic fistula. If pancreatic juice escapes from the site of incision or the needle puncture, consider pancreatectomy or Roux-en-Y drainage of this area (see below).

Further reading

Lightwood R, Reber H A, Way L W 1976 The risk and accuracy of pancreatic biopsy. American Journal of Surgery 132: 189–194

OPERATIVE PANCREATOGRAPHY

Appraise

1. On-table X-rays are of greatest help in choosing between resection or drainage in chronic pancreatitis and in determining the proper extent of either procedure. Preoperative endoscopic pancreatograms may be inadequate for this assessment. Ductography may also be useful during operations for carcinoma or pancreatic trauma.

2. The choice of route depends upon the operation being performed. During operations on the biliary tract, a retrograde pancreatogram may be obtained by transduodenal cannulation of the papilla. If ductal disease is suspected in the head of pancreas after resection of the distal gland, the duct can be cannulated at the site of amputation. In chronic pancreatitis or carcinoma, a dilated duct may be palpable as a soft cord in a sclerotic gland. Pancreatograms are obtainable either by needle puncture of the duct or by incision and intubation in the body of the pancreas.

3. Operative cystography may be useful to delineate pancreatic pseudocysts and their ductal communication.

4. Use a dense water-soluble contrast medium, such as Conray 420 or 40% Hypaque. Be careful not to overdistend the ductal tree, especially during retrograde pancreatography, since there is a risk of inducing acute pancreatitis.

Action

1. *Retrograde pancreatography* (Fig. 10.16a). Sphincterotomy is helpful but may not be essential. The major pancreatic duct enters the duodenum horizontally, and its orifice is located at about 5 o'clock on the lower lip of the papilla. Usually a No. 5 FG umbilical catheter can be passed for 2–3 cm, but it is necessary to occlude the orifice around the catheter to prevent spillage of contrast (I use Babcock's forceps). Obtain the first picture after introducing 1–2 ml of contrast.

2. *Prograde pancreatography* (Fig. 10.16b). The pancreas has been divided across the body or neck. Search carefully for the transected duct. Pass a fine catheter down it for 1–2 cm and suture the duct around the catheter to effect a watertight seal.

3. *Ambigrade pancreatography* (Fig. 10.16c). Mobilise the body of the pancreas and feel carefully for the softer sensation of a dilated duct. Insert a butterfly needle into the duct and observe the colourless pancreatic fluid flow back into the tubing. Several millilitres of contrast medium may be needed to fill a dilated ductal system, but do not continue injecting if pressure builds up. If needle puncture is unsuccessful and pancreatography is necessary, make a short vertical incision in the body of pancreas and deepen it until the duct is entered. Insert a fine T-tube into the duct and close the gland about the tube. Afterwards, it is important either to resect the gland distal to the point of incision or to drain the duct into a Roux loop of jejunum.

4. *Pancreatic cystography* (Fig. 10.16d). Intrapancreatic cysts will also feel softer than the surrounding gland. Parapancreatic (pseudo-) cysts are collections of fluid within the lesser sac or loculated against the anterior aspect of the gland. To obtain a cystogram, partly aspirate the cyst contents and introduce a similar quantity of contrast material.

Interpretation

1. The normal pancreatic duct tapers from a diameter of 3–4 mm in the head to <2 mm in the tail. Ductal anomalies in the Wirsung and Santorini systems and their communication and drainage are common. Look for sites

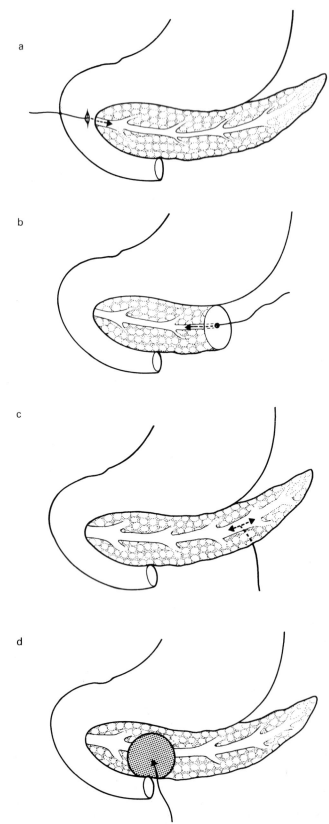

Fig. 10.16 Various methods of operative pancreatography. (a) transduodenal (retrograde) cannulation. (b) prograde cannulation following distal pancreatectomy. (c) ambigrade pancreatogram obtained by cannulation of a distended duct in the body of the gland. (d) pancreatic cystogram.

of stricture and dilatation both in the main duct and its side-branches. Contrast injected by the prograde route should enter the duodenum.

2. Determine the size of a cyst and the number of loculi, its relation to the gland and the presence or absence of any communication with the main duct.

Further reading

White T T, Silverstein F E 1976 Operative and endoscopic pancreatography in the diagnosis of pancreatic cancer. Cancer 37: 449–461
Cooper M J, Williamson R C N 1983 The value of operative pancreatography. British Journal of Surgery 70: 577–580

LAPAROTOMY FOR ACUTE PANCREATITIS

Appraise

1. Diagnostic laparotomy is usually undertaken to determine the cause of generalised or upper abdominal peritonitis. Perhaps acute pancreatitis has not been suspected, or the elevation of serum amylase is not enough to be pathognomonic.

2. Sometimes laparotomy is required within the first 2–3 days of an established attack of acute pancreatitis, when deterioration of the patient's condition raises the possibility of a complication such as ascending cholangitis. Subtotal or total pancreatectomy at this stage carries a formidable mortality.

3. In gallstone pancreatitis, it has been suggested that urgent removal of a calculus impacted at the ampulla of Vater might prevent progression of the disease; both surgical and endoscopic sphincterotomy have been advocated. In most series, however, at least one-third of patients do not appear to have gallstones as the underlying cause of acute pancreatitis, and this aggressive approach has not yet become standard practice.

4. Besides these early diagnostic and therapeutic indications, laparotomy may be needed after the first week of the disease for complications such as pseudocyst and pancreatic abscess.

5. If gallstones are identified, early cholecystectomy is indicated to prevent the risk of a subsequent attack of acute pancreatitis.

Access

1. The patient is likely to have had a midline or right paramedian incision performed for abdominal exploration. If necessary, extend the incision upwards to permit examination of the biliary apparatus and pancreas.

2. When operating for established pancreatitis use an upper midline incision, which may skirt the umbilicus if extra length is required.

Assess

1. Blood-stained free fluid is usually present in the abdominal cavity. Whitish plaques of fat necrosis are visible on serosal surfaces, especially in the region of the pancreas.

2. Lift up the greater omentum and transverse colon. There is oedema and blackish discolouration of the retroperitoneal tissues. The pancreas itself is swollen and may be haemorrhagic or even necrotic.

3. Examine the gall bladder and, if possible, the bile duct to determine if these organs are diseased. A more thorough examination is required if the patient has obstructive jaundice.

Action

1. Once the diagnosis has been made, do nothing unless there is a definite indication. Attempts at debridement of the pancreas at this stage can be disastrous. Formal exploration of the pancreas is usually unnecessary to obtain a diagnosis and may be meddlesome.

2. The management of coincidental gallstones is controversial, so be prepared to seek senior advice. In oedematous (mild) pancreatitis it is probably safe to carry out cholecystectomy with operative cholangiography and proceed to exploration of the duct and even transduodenal sphincteroplasty, if necessary. In haemorrhagic (severe) pancreatitis these manouvres are probably best avoided, but consider T-tube drainage for an obstructed bile duct.

3. It is unusual to encounter loculated fluid or pus during the first week of an attack of acute pancreatitis, but any such collection should be drained to the exterior.

4. Consider placing a peritoneal dialysis catheter through a stab incision into the pelvis for postoperative peritoneal lavage.

5. Wound dehiscence is common after laparotomy for acute pancreatitis. Take extra care in closing the linea alba or rectus sheath, and consider the use of tension sutures.

Aftercare

1. Continue standard supportive measures for acute pancreatitis. If lavage is employed, continue for 2–3 days or until the return fluid is clear. Most patients tolerate hourly cycles with 2 l of isotonic dialysate.

2. After recovery from an acute attack keep the patient in hospital for ultrasound and contrast radiological studies of the biliary tree. If gallstones are confirmed, proceed to *cholecystectomy* during the same hospital admission. Have a high index of suspicion regarding ductal stones.

3. An epigastric mass with or without recurrence of pain suggests the development of a *pseudocyst*, which can be confirmed by ultrasound scan. Unless the mass subsides spontaneously, it should be drained (see below).

4. Toxaemia developing during the second or third week of an attack heralds the development of a *pancreatic abscess*, which carries a substantial mortality rate (>30%). Do not delay laparotomy. Open the retroperitoneal tissues widely, drain all collections of pus and enucleate the peripancreatic slough, which resembles a retained gauze swab. Remember that the slough will digest the root of the mesentery and the transverse mesocolon, though the vascular pedicles are usually preserved. Examine the pancreas gently; sometimes it is completely necrotic and can be removed with a sponge-holding forceps. Carry out vigorous saline lavage and insert several wide-bore tube drains to the retroperitoneal tissues and the pelvis. Take particular care to obtain good wound closure.

Further reading

Osborne D H, Imrie C W, Carter D C 1981 Biliary surgery in the same admission for gallstone-associated acute pancreatitis. British Journal of Surgery 68: 758–761

Saxon A, Reynolds J T, Doolas A 1981 Management of pancreatic abscesses. Annals of Surgery 194: 545–552

Cooper M J, Williamson R C N, Pollock A V 1982 The role of peritoneal lavage in the prediction and treatment of severe acute pancreatitis. Annals of the Royal College of Surgeons of England 64: 422–427

Williamson R C N 1984 Early assessment of severity in acute pancreatitis Gut 25: 1331–1339

DRAINAGE OF PANCREATIC CYSTS

Appraise

1. True cysts are congenital or neoplastic and are rare. Cysts complicating acute or chronic pancreatitis and pancreatic trauma are 'false' (pseudocysts) in that they have no epithelial lining. Both types are best diagnosed by ultrasound and CT scanning of the upper abdomen.

2. A collection of fluid around the pancreas is probably quite a common event during an attack of acute pancreatitis, but many of these resolve spontaneously. Drainage is required for an expanding mass, which often causes pain, or for vomiting and jaundice, or for a mass that fails to resolve or becomes infected. Within 3–4 weeks of the acute attack, the cyst wall is unlikely to be sufficiently mature to take sutures, and external drainage is required. Thereafter, internal drainage becomes feasible, either cystgastrostomy or cystjejunostomy Roux-en-Y.

3. Percutaneous aspiration of pancreatic pseudocysts is becoming increasingly popular. The procedure is carried out under ultrasound control, and a pigtail catheter can also be inserted to effect external drainage. Percutaneous needling and drainage may be suitable for small cysts discovered in the early weeks after an attack of acute pancreatitis. Surgical drainage seems a more appropriate technique for large, mature or recurrent cysts.

4. Sometimes an encysted collection of blood and/or pancreatic fluid may follow blunt abdominal trauma. Traumatic cysts are prone to complications and require early drainage, usually to the exterior.

5. Destructive cysts developing in association with chronic pancreatitis are often multiple, are contained within the pancreas and frequently communicate with the main ductal system. Endoscopic retrograde pancreatography therefore runs the risk of introducing infection into the cyst cavity. Small cysts can be resected together with diseased pancreas or drained into the duct and thence to a Roux loop of jejunum. Large cysts should be treated by cystenterostomy, unless a pre-operative angiogram shows pseudoaneurysms in the wall, in which case resection may be safer.

Assess

1. After an acute attack of pancreatitis or pancreatic trauma an encysted collection of fluid may be entered on approaching the pancreas. This type of collection is usually best drained to the exterior. The resultant pancreatic fistula does not cause skin excoriation, since the pancreatic enzymes are not activated, and it will nearly always close spontaneously. If a large cyst is palpable within the lesser sac, try and determine whether the posterior wall of the stomach is adherent to the front of the cyst, in which case cystgastrostomy may be appropriate. If not, internal drainage into a Roux loop of jejunum is a satisfactory method of dealing with a mature cyst.

2. During laparotomy for chronic pancreatitis, plan your attack according to the operative findings in the underlying pancreas, supplemented by ductography (see 5 above). A cyst in the head of the pancreas can sometimes be marsupialised into the duodenum. Elsewhere in the gland cystjejunostomy Roux-en-Y is the best option.

3. Operative cystography (see p. 185) is a useful adjunct to the findings at exploration. It will outline any communication with the pancreatic ducts and will show whether the type of procedure planned is likely to achieve dependent drainage.

4. Try and create a good-sized stoma between the cyst and the viscus chosen for internal drainage, so that tube drains are not needed.

Action

Cystgastrostomy (Fig. 10.17)

1. This is only indicated for effusions into the lesser sac that have been present long enough to have developed a fibrous wall. The stoma will probably close once the cavity has filled in after drainage.

2. After packing off the stomach, make a longitudinal incision through the anterior gastric wall fairly close to the greater curvature and opposite the incisura angularis. Suck out the gastric contents.

3. Now incise the posterior gastric wall for a short distance opposite the anterior gastrotomy. Deepen the inci-

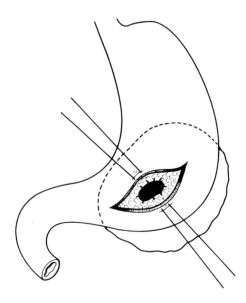

Fig. 10.17 Pancreatic cystgastrostomy. The anterior wall of the stomach is held open by stay sutures. A collection of pancreatic fluid in the lesser sac ('pseudocyst') is drained into the stomach through a posterior gastrostomy.

sion and enter the cyst, obtaining samples of the fluid for culture and chemical analysis. Evacuate the contents of the cyst and gently break down any loculi with your finger.

4. Insert a running Dexon suture round the margins of the posterior gastrotomy, ensuring a stoma of at least 4 cm diameter. Close the anterior gastrotomy in two layers and close the abdomen with drainage.

Cystduodenostomy

1. Reserve this procedure for a small cyst in the head of pancreas close to the duodenal loop.

2. Make a longitudinal duodenotomy opposite the cyst. Insert a needle into the cyst. Aspiration of bile warns you that the bile duct is nearby and you should not proceed.

3. If the aspirate is clear, leave the needle in place and incise the duodenal wall to enter the cyst. Suture the margins of the opening as above. Close the duodenum in two layers, taking care not to narrow its lumen. Close the abdomen with drainage.

Cystjejunostomy

1. This technique is applicable to all types of cyst with walls thick enough for suturing. It is the most likely method to obtain dependent drainage.

2. Mobilise the pancreas and obtain an operative cystogram. Now incise the anterior wall of the cyst, sample and drain its contents and explore its recesses for any obvious ductal communication.

3. Create a Roux loop of jejunum (p. 115) and close its end. Approximate the upper end of the Roux loop to the

front of the cyst without tension. Create a generous side-to-side anastomosis between the opening into the cyst and a longitudinal jejunotomy. Use one or two layers of suture according to the thickness of the cyst wall, but use Dexon or Vicryl for the inner layer.

4. Restore intestinal continuity by jejunojejunostomy at the base of the Roux loop. Drain the abdomen through a stab incision as above.

Further reading

Frey C F 1978 Pancreatic pseudocyst-operative strategy. Annals of Surgery 188: 652–662
Williamson R C N 1981 The pancreas. In: Keen G (ed) Operative Surgery and Management. Wright P S G, Bristol. p 105–127

DRAINAGE OF THE PANCREATIC DUCT

Appraise

1. Ductal drainage is preferable to resection for the relief of pain in chronic pancreatitis, since it preserves the remaining functioning tissue. However, only an anastomosis between the pancreatic duct and adjacent viscus that is several millimetres in diameter is likely to remain patent. Therefore do not ordinarily undertake a drainage operation unless the duct is 2–3 times its normal diameter.

2. The operation of choice is longitudinal pancreaticojejunostomy, which creates a long side-to-side anastomosis between the incised duct and a Roux loop of jejunum. A lateral anastomosis between the amputated body of pancreas and a Roux loop is less likely to stay open unless the duct is grossly dilated at the site of transection, in which case it should probably be opened up in the proximal gland. Sometimes it is reasonable to combine conservative distal resection with lateral pancreaticojejunostomy.

3. Formerly popular for the treatment of chronic pancreatitis, sphincteroplasty has in fact little to offer. It is reasonable to carry out sphincteroplasty (p. 178) followed by a similar procedure to widen the orifice of the pancreatic duct (Wirsungoplasty), when there is moderate dilatation of the whole duct tapering to a stricture at its orifice.

4. Drainage of an obstructed distended duct into the back of the stomach (pancreaticogastrostomy) is quite a simple technique that may bring dramatic relief of pain from irresectable carcinoma of the head of pancreas.

5. Techniques for draining normal-calibre and dilated pancreatic ducts after proximal pancreatectomy (Whipple resection) are considered at the end of this chapter.

Access

Operations for chronic pancreatitis require generous access to the upper abdomen. Excellent exposure is afforded by a transverse subcostal incision that divides both recti and is gently curved with an upward convexity ('low gable'). Alternatively, choose a long midline incision.

Assess

1. Expose the pancreas carefully at each end and examine it thoroughly. Is the gland indurated throughout, or is the disease partly localized? Can you feel the pancreatic duct as a soft dilated tube in the body of the gland? Are there any associated cysts? If there is serious suspicion of carcinoma, obtain a biopsy (p. 185).

2. Look for evidence of gallstones, which are quite commonly associated with chronic pancreatitis. The bile duct may be slightly dilated with a thickened opaque wall. Examine the stomach and duodenum for peptic ulcer disease. Exclude cirrhosis of the liver, portal hypertension and splenomegaly. Consider liver biopsy if the patient is an alcoholic.

3. Do not hesitate to obtain an operative pancreatogram (p. 185) if you are in any doubt about the best procedure for chronic pancreatitis. If the disease is not very severe, amputation of the tail of pancreas (for histological examination) and prograde pancreatography may provide useful information for subsequent clinical management.

Action

Longitudinal pancreaticojejunostomy (Fig. 10.18)

1. Expose the body, neck and part of the head of pancreas through the lesser sac. It is usually not necessary to mobilise the gland completely. If needle pancreatography has been performed, leave the needle in position as a guide to the duct.

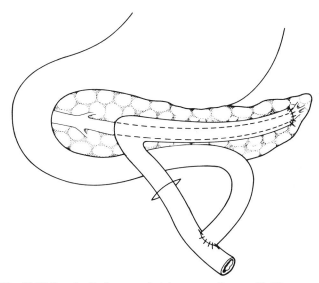

Fig. 10.18 Longitudinal pancreaticojejunostomy Roux-en-Y. The dilated duct is opened widely, and a long side-to-side anastomosis is created.

2. Incise the front of the pancreas between stay sutures at a convenient place in the body of the gland. If the duct is clearly dilated, make the incision in the long axis of the gland. If not, make a small exploratory incision across the axis.

3. On entering a dilated ductal system aspirate the pale greyish pancreatic juice. Extend the incision in each direction, using scalpel or pointed scissors, and underrun any major bleeding vessel. Open the duct widely from head to tail. Remove any calculi and try to open any cysts into the main duct.

4. Select a Roux loop of jejunum and close its end. Bring the loop through a mesocolic window so that it lies comfortably along the entire pancreas. Insert interrupted silk sutures to approximate the fibrotic 'capsule' of the pancreas and the seromuscular layers of the jejunum. Now make a long jejunotomy to match the incision in the pancreatic duct and place a running all-coats suture between the two, using 2/0 Dexon or 3/0 Prolene. The ductal lining is tough and takes sutures quite well. Finish with an anterior seromuscular layer of silk.

5. Restore intestinal continuity by end-to-side jejunojejunostomy. Close the abdomen with a drain to the region of the pancreas.

Lateral pancreaticojejunostomy (Fig. 10.19)

1. Reserve this procedure for draining a dilated duct in the neck or proximal body after conservative distal resection. It may be sensible to open up the duct at the site of transection by a short incision through its anterior wall and the overlying pancreas.

2. Fashion a retrocolic Roux loop of jejunum as above and close its end. Make a small subterminal jejunotomy to

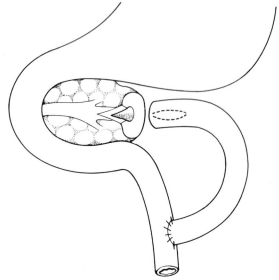

Fig. 10.19 Lateral pancreaticojejunostomy Roux-en-Y. Following distal pancreatectomy a dilated pancreatic duct is opened for a short distance and sutured to the Roux loop.

match the diameter of the duct and insert an all-coats suture, using fine non-absorbable stitches. Tack the peripheral pancreatic substance to the seromuscular layer of jejunum with a second layer of similar sutures. Consider splinting the anastomosis with a fine polythene tube brought out through the Roux loop and a stab incision to the exterior.

3. Restore intestinal continuity as usual.

Intubated pancreaticogastrostomy (Fig. 10.20)

1. Examine the body of pancreas for the tell-tale sensation of a dilated duct. Needling the duct with or without pancreatography may help to confirm your finding.

2. Make a short vertical incision across the body of pancreas and deepen this until you enter the duct. Insert a T-tube into the duct; suture the gland around the entry of the tube. Make tiny posterior and anterior gastrotomies several centimetres apart. Bring the tube through each wall of the stomach and thence by a stab incision to the exterior. Make sure there are two or three holes in the tube within its intragastric course, and tighten a purse-string suture around the anterior gastrotomy. By traction on the tube, draw the stomach down onto the front of the pancreas, and approximate the two organs with a few tacking sutures.

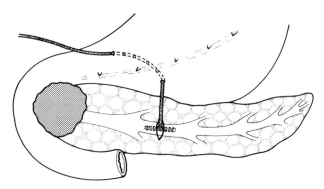

Fig. 10.20 Intubated pancreaticogastrostomy. In an attempt to relieve back pain from an irresectable carcinoma of the head of pancreas, the obstructed pancreatic duct is decompressed into the stomach. The small incisions in the back of the stomach and the front of the pancreas are approximated, and the T-tube is brought to the exterior.

Aftercare

1. The peritoneal drain can usually be removed after 3–4 days.

2. If the pancreatic ductal anastomosis has been splinted with a tube that emerges through the abdominal wall, consider postoperative pancreatography at about 7 days. Ordinarily the tube can be clamped at or before this time and can be removed at about 10 days. After pancreaticogastrostomy the T-tube may drain the stomach in preference to the nasogastric tube, but it can usually be clamped with safety after flatus has been passed per rectum.

Further reading

Proctor H J, Mendes D C, Thomas C G Jr, Herbst C A 1979 Surgery for chronic pancreatitis. Drainage versus resection. Annals of Surgery 189: 664–671

Prinz R A, Greenlee H B 1981 Pancreatic duct drainage in 100 patients with chronic pancreatitis. Annals of Surgery 194: 313–320

Coopen M J, Williamson R C N 1984 Drainage operations in chronic pancreatitis. British Journal of Surgery 71: 761–766

LAPAROTOMY FOR PANCREATIC CANCER

Appraise

1. Carcinoma of the head of pancreas is often irresectable; moreover, resection usually fails to prevent recurrence. Carcinoma of the body of pancreas is almost incurable. Nevertheless, most patients with pancreatic cancer require laparotomy to confirm the diagnosis and achieve palliation. Resection of the head of pancreas is inadvisable over the age of 70–75.

2. Other carcinomas of the periampullary region (terminal bile duct, ampulla, duodenum) are less invasive and carry a better prognosis than carcinoma of the pancreatic head. Differentiating one tumour from another at operation is sometimes very difficult.

3. Pre-operative investigations help to localise the tumour and depict the extent of spread. Percutaneous transhepatic cholangiography (PTC) or endoscopic retrograde cholangiopancreatography (ERCP) will show the level of obstruction in a jaundiced patient. Liver scans (ultrasound, CT) may demonstrate dilated bile ducts and/or metastases. Selective visceral angiography provides an arterial 'road-map' for operation and may reveal portal vein invasion or occlusion, indicating irresectability.

4. Whether benign or malignant, endocrine tumours of the pancreas are more amenable to surgical cure than adenocarcinoma of the exocrine gland. The diagnosis is suspected because of clinical syndromes resulting from excessive hormonal secretion: hypoglycaemia (insulin), intractable peptic ulceration (gastrin) and rarely profuse diarrhoea (vasoactive intestinal polypeptide). Angiography or transhepatic portal venous sampling may localise the tumour.

PERI-OPERATIVE MANAGEMENT OF OBSTRUCTIVE JAUNDICE

1. Patients with prolonged obstruction of the extrahepatic biliary tree tolerate major resectional procedures very poorly. The following specific problems should be anticipated and countered:
(a) *Coagulopathy*. If hypoprothrombinaemia is present, give sufficient parenteral vitamin K to restore the prothrombin time of the blood to normal. Routine pre-operative administration of vitamin K is a sensible precaution in any jaundiced patient.
(b) *Hepatorenal syndrome*. Renal failure may be precipitated by intra-operative hypotension, and this should be avoided as far as possible. Catheterise the patient after induction of anaesthesia, ensure adequate hydration and administer intravenous mannitol (40 g) to achieve an osmotic diuresis during the operation.
(c) *Sepsis*. Though infected bile is more likely with gallstones than a malignant stricture, 'invasive' cholangiography or operation may provoke infection in any obstructed biliary tree. Both procedures should be covered by prophylactic antibiotics.
(d) *Malnutrition*. Decreased hepatic synthesis of albumin will inevitably follow obstructive jaundice and may not improve until the obstruction has been relieved. Consider parenteral nutrition postoperatively if convalescence is prolonged.
(e) *Wound failure*. The healing of wounds is impaired in jaundiced patients. Take particular care with abdominal closure.

2. Pre-operative decompression of the obstructed biliary tree is controversial. External transhepatic drainage may improve general health at the risk of various complications, e.g. infection, bile leakage, electrolyte loss. Internal decompression by transhepatic or endoscopic retrograde intubation of the stricture may be safer but requires considerable technical expertise.

3. Staged resection is a reasonable alternative for patients with unrelenting obstructive jaundice for more than 2–3 weeks. At the first operation, determine that the tumour in the region of the pancreatic head is mobile and potentially resectable. Do not prolong the dissection but carry out cholecystjejunostomy. Re-operate at 3–4 weeks when serum bilirubin levels have fallen and serum albumin has risen.

Access

A near-transverse muscle-cutting incision in the right upper quadrant will suffice for cholecystjejunostomy alone. If (as usual) further bypass procedures or pancreatectomy are indicated, extend the incision across the midline, dividing both recti to complete a 'low gable' incision.

Assess

1. The gallbladder is distended and there is such diffuse metastatic spread that the patient is unlikely to live very long. Relieve obstructive jaundice by the simple expedient of cholecystjejunostomy (see p. 181). If you are in doubt about the patency of the cystic duct, consider obtaining an operative cholecystogram via a Foley catheter inserted into the fundus.

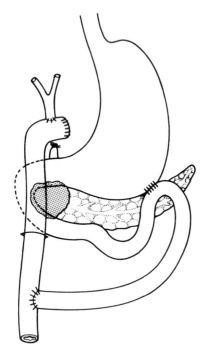

Fig. 10.21 Bypass procedures for an irresectable carcinoma of the head of pancreas. The bile duct is transected above the growth, cholecystectomy is performed and biliary drainage is achieved by hepaticojejunostomy Roux-en-Y. An antecolic gastroenterostomy is included.

Further reading

McPherson G A D, Benjamin I S, Habib N A, Bowley N B, Blumgart L H 1982 Percutaneous transhepatic drainage in obstructive jaundice: advantages and problems. British Journal of Surgery 69: 261–264

Moossa A R, Lewis M H, Mackie C R 1979 Surgical treatment of pancreatic cancer. Mayo Clinic Proceedings 54: 468–474

Sarr M G, Cameron J L 1982 Surgical management of unresectable carcinoma of the pancreas. Surgery 91: 123–133

PANCREATECTOMY

Appraise

1. Distal pancreatectomy may be undertaken for chronic inflammation, trauma or tumour in the body and tail of the gland or as part of a radical gastrectomy for carcinoma of the stomach. Splenectomy is nearly always performed in addition, though it is technically feasible to dissect healthy distal pancreas from the splenic vessels and thus preserve the spleen.

2. Distal pancreatectomy is usually completed by dividing the gland in front of the portal vein, but the resection may be extended to include the neck and part of the head of pancreas. Occasionally performed for diffuse pancreatitis, a subtotal pancreatectomy removes upwards of 80% of the gland. Care must be taken to preserve the bile duct and at least one of the pancreaticoduodenal arteries. Varying degrees of pancreatic insufficiency (diabetes, steatorrhoea) can be anticipated, depending on the functional status of the residual pancreas.

3. The intimate relation to the duodenal loop means that resection of the pancreatic head must also remove the duodenum and terminal bile duct. Distal hemigastrectomy is nearly always added to widen the lymph-node clearance and reduce the risk of stress ulceration in the stomach. Carcinoma of the head of pancreas or carcinoma of the ampulla are the usual indications for this major resection procedure (Whipple's operation). Consider a pylorus-preserving pancreatoduodenectomy for chronic pancreatitis or ampullary cancer.

4. Combined distal and proximal excision results in total pancreatectomy, again including the antrum and duodenum. This operation is occasionally needed for severe and generalised chronic pancreatitis. Unless already present, diabetes and steatorrhoea are inevitable sequelae. In carcinoma of the pancreas it is debatable whether the possibility of improving the very poor prognosis after Whipple's operation by completing a total pancreatectomy is balanced by the disadvantage of making the survivors diabetic.

2. The tumour is clearly irresectable but not as advanced as the above; alternatively, the gallbladder is collapsed or contains calculi. Better medium-term biliary diversion is achieved by choledochojejunostomy Roux-en-Y (see p. 182), dividing the bile duct above the 'leading edge' of tumour to limit upward spread (Fig. 10.21). Cholecystectomy generally facilitates the operation and is certainly advisable if there is a low entry of the cystic duct.

3. The tumour could be resectable and there is no overt metastasis. Embark upon a trial dissection. If the superior mesenteric and portal veins can be separated from the neck of pancreas, proceed to pancreatoduodenectomy (see next section).

4. You have decided against resection. Try and obtain a positive tissue diagnosis by appropriate biopsy (see p. 185). Palliative procedures should be considered to relieve jaundice, vomiting and pain. Carry out biliary diversion as described in 1 and 2 above. Unless the prognosis is extremely limited, create an antecolic gastroenterostomy (see Ch. 5) to bypass present or future duodenal obstruction (Fig. 10.21). Options for pain relief include intubated pancreaticogastrostomy, if the pancreatic duct is clearly dilated (see previous section), or coeliac plexus block. An intraoperative nerve block involves injection of 15–20 ml of 50% alcohol on each side at the level of the diaphragmatic crura. Aspirate the syringe each time to ensure that the needle has not entered the aorta or vena cava.

Access

Good exposure of the upper abdominal cavity is essential for any type of pancreatectomy. Probably the best access is provided by the long transverse or 'low gable' incision.

Assess

1. In operations for chronic pancreatitis the likelihood and extent of resection will have been indicated by pre-operative investigations, including endoscopic pancreatography and pancreatic function tests. At laparotomy, however, the entire gland should be examined (see p. 184), and operative pancreatography should be performed (see p. 185) if there is any chance of a dilated ductal system, since drainage might be more appropriate than resection in such a case (see p. 189).

2. When operating for upper abdominal trauma, first inspect the liver, spleen and mesentery and deal with any site of bleeding. Pancreatic or duodenal injury should be suspected if there is a retroperitoneal haematoma. Mobilise the duodenum and inspect both surfaces. Enter the lesser sac and examine the pancreas thoroughly. Major contusion or fracture of the pancreatic neck should be treated by distal pancreatectomy.

3. Resection of carcinoma of the body of pancreas is nearly always precluded by direct involvement of the superior mesenteric vessels and/or metastatic spread. Follow the middle colic vein back to find the superior mesenteric vein, and establish the relation of this vessel to the tumour.

4. Do not forget that endocrine tumours of the pancreas can be multiple or malignant. Examine the entire pancreas and look for secondaries in adjacent lymph nodes; these can sometimes be removed together with the primary.

5. In the absence of overt metastases or fixity you may need to embark upon a lengthy trial dissection to determine whether a periampullary tumour is resectable. Mobilise the duodenal loop and head of pancreas by Kocher's manoeuvre. The key to successful resection is the ability to free the neck of pancreas from the subjacent superior mesenteric and portal veins. Identify the superior mesenteric vein at the lower border of the gland. Dissect carefully within the free edge of the lesser omentum to find the portal vein between the bile duct and hepatic artery but at a deeper level. Sling the duct and the artery to facilitate the approach to the portal vein. Keeping close to the vein, place one index finger below the pancreas and one above. If the two fingers can be gently insinuated to meet behind the neck of the gland, resection will be feasible. If malignant induration prevents this manoeuvre, proceed to bypass as described in the previous section.

Action

Distal pancreatectomy (Fig. 10.22)

1. Mobilize the spleen upwards by dividing its posterior peritoneal attachment (posterior layer of the lienorenal ligament). Ligate and divide the short gastric vessels. If the spleen is torn during the dissection, ligate its vascular pedicle and complete the splenectomy at this stage.

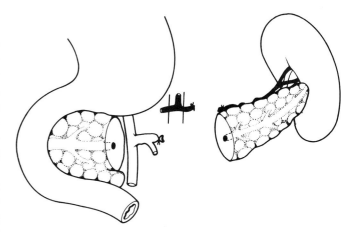

Fig. 10.22 Distal pancreatectomy (including splenectomy). Transection just to the right of the portal vein removes 50–60% of the gland.

2. The pancreatic tail lies at the splenic hilum and will therefore have been mobilised already. Divide the peritoneum along the upper and lower borders of the distal pancreas. Several small vessels need to be ligated or coagulated by diathermy. Continue the dissection towards the midline, lifting the body and tail of pancreas forwards and to the right.

3. The splenic vein can be seen running along the posterior surface of the body of pancreas. As it approaches its right-angled junction with the superior mesenteric vein, it is usually joined by the inferior mesenteric vein. Carefully insert a pair of Lahey forceps between the pancreas and the splenic vein. Ligate and divide the splenic vein, if possible preserving the entry of the inferior mesenteric vein.

4. Identify, ligate and divide the splenic artery as it reaches the upper border of the pancreas from the coeliac plexus. The pancreas can now be lifted gently off the portal vein. Great care must be taken in the presence of chronic inflammation, since it is easy to tear the great veins.

5. Decide where to transect the pancreas. Division in front of the portal vein is usually considered to represent hemi-pancreatectomy. Insert 2/0 silk stay sutures at the upper and lower border of the pancreas at this point, and place a soft intestinal clamp across the neck. Divide the pancreas to the left of the clamp and stay sutures and remove the specimen. Be careful not to injure the underlying vein during transection of the gland.

6. Remove the clamp and secure haemostasis. Look for the amputated main pancreatic duct, which should measure about 3 mm across at this point. Consider operative pancreatography (and a drainage procedure) if the duct is dilated. Otherwise, underrun the duct and close over the pancreatic stump, using 2/0 or 3/0 silk sutures.

7. Check that the splenic bed and pancreas are dry. Insert a suction drain and close the abdomen.

Proximal pancreatoduodenectomy

1. Mobilisation of the head of pancreas and separation of the neck from the portal vein have already been described. Identify and ligate the gastroduodenal artery immediately above the pancreas.

2. Four major structures must now be divided, but the order of division may be varied according to the progress of the dissection. Transect the body of the stomach to include distal hemigastrectomy. Divide the bile duct well above the tumour. Divide the neck of pancreas in front of the portal vein. Mobilise the ligament of Treitz and transect the jejunum just beyond this point.

3. The most tedious part of the resection is the separation of the head and uncinate process from the portal and superior mesenteric veins. Several short thin-walled vessels require ligation, and the pancreas must be separated from the connective tissue overlying the aorta and vena cava. Finally, division of the inferior pancreaticoduodenal artery and veins and the vessels supplying the duodeno-jejunal flexure allows the specimen to be removed (Fig. 10.23).

4. Advance the upper jejunum through the transverse mesocolon and commence reconstruction. The type of pancreaticojejunostomy chosen should depend on the size of the pancreatic duct. If the duct is dilated, close the end of the jejunum and construct an end-to-side pancreatico-intestinal anastomosis, using fine interrupted silk sutures (Fig. 10.24). Splint the anastomosis with a fine polythene cannula brought to the exterior through the jejunum and abdominal wall and sutured with catgut to the bowel mucosa close to the anastomosis. If the duct is of normal

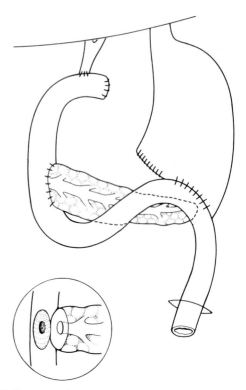

Fig. 10.24 Reconstruction after pancreatoduodectomy when the pancreatic duct is dilated. To create the pancreaticojejunostomy (inset), the pancreatic duct is sutured directly to the jejunal mucosa; the anastomosis is splinted by a fine polythene tube.

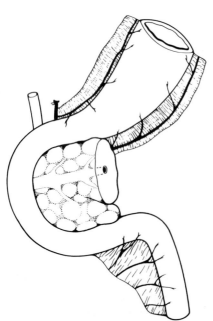

Fig. 10.23 Pancreatoduodenectomy (Whipple's operation). The resection specimen is shown and includes the distal half of the stomach, the duodenal loop and duodenojejunal flexure, the terminal bile duct and the head and uncinate process of the pancreas.

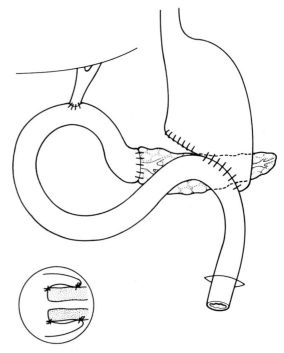

Fig. 10.25 Reconstruction after pancreatoduodenectomy when the pancreatic duct is of normal calibre. To create the pancreatojejunostomy (inset), the amputated neck of pancreas is sutured to the end of the jejunum; a second layer of stitches is placed to invaginate the bowel.

calibre, suture the end of jejunum directly to the amputated pancreas, using circumferential 3/0 silk sutures (Fig. 10.25). Bury this suture line with a second row of silk sutures that invaginate the jejunum.

5. Biliary continuity is restored by end-to-side choledochojejunostomy (see p. 182). A splinting T-tube is usually unnecessary, since dilatation of the duct makes for an easy anastomosis. Complete the reconstruction by performing a valved gastroenterostomy (Ch. 5).

6. Check haemostasis and insert at least two drains to the region of the pancreaticojejunostomy.

Total pancreatectomy

1. This operation combines the above two procedures. When operating for chronic pancreatitis, proceed from left to right. When operating for cancer, ensure that the portal vein is free before mobilising the spleen.

2. Reconstruction after total pancreatectomy is simpler than after Whipple's operation, since the difficult pancreatico-intestinal anastomosis is avoided. Close the end of the jejunum and insert first the bile duct and then the stomach.

3. In benign disease it may be possible to preserve the antrum, pylorus and duodenal cap, ligating the superior pancreaticoduodenal artery distal to its origin from the gastroduodenal artery or the parent vessel itself. Intestinal continuity is restored by end-to-side duodenojejunostomy.

Aftercare

1. After resection of the pancreatic head it is sensible to give intravenous cimetidine for a few days to prevent erosive gastritis.

2. Remove drains after 3–4 days, provided they have ceased to function. Leakage of bile or pancreatic juice are less likely to occur if splinting tubes are used for awkward anastomoses. Minor leaks may dry up spontaneously, but a major leak requires reoperation. Consider parenteral nutrition if convalescence is prolonged.

3. Diabetes and steatorrhoea are inevitable after total pancreatectomy and may be precipitated by partial resection of a diseased gland. Adjust insulin dosage according to blood (or urine) sugar estimations. If permanent diabetes is anticipated, teach the patient to recognise the warning symptoms of hypoglycaemia and instruct him to have sugar to hand at all times. For exocrine insufficiency institute a low fat diet and give enzyme supplements by mouth as required.

Further reading

Braasch J W, Vito L, Nugent F W 1978 Total pancreatectomy for end-stage chronic pancreatitis. Annals of Surgery 188: 317–322

Traverso L W, Longmire W P Jr 1978 Preservation of the pylorus in pancreaticoduodenectomy. Surgery Gynecology and Obstetrics 146: 959–962

White T T, Slavotinek A H 1979 Results of surgical treatment of chronic pancreatitis. Annals of Surgery 189: 217–224

Cohen J R, Kuchta N, Geller N, Shires T, Dineen P 1982 Pancreaticoduodenectomy: a 40-year experience. Annals of Surgery 1982; 195: 608–617

Cooper M J, Williamson R C N Conservative pancreatectomy. British Journal of Surgery 1985; 72: 801–803

Surgery of the liver and portal venous system

INTRODUCTION

The liver is considered by many surgeons to be a hallowed organ and one which presents them with insurmountable problems. They fear massive haemorrhage after any violation of the capsule and dread the thought of attempting any elective procedure. These are unfounded myths and the liver is as amenable to surgery as any other organ, providing certain principles are respected.

TRAUMA

The most frequent procedure the emergency surgeon is called upon to perform on the liver is to arrest haemorrhage following trauma or spontaneous rupture of a tumour.

Injuries to the liver can be contusions from crush injuries, penetrating lacerations from stab wounds, or a mixture of the two from gun shots. Contusion carries a very high mortality rate.

Appraise

1. A patient will present in a shocked state with an obvious history. Remember to assess the general condition of the whole patient to exclude other lesions. Examine the head, chest and limbs as well as the abdomen. If his external injuries cannot explain his degree of shock you must assume he is bleeding internally. Management of this must take priority over the other problems. However, stop external haemorrhage by direct pressure, splint any broken limbs, protect a fractured spine, treat a crushed chest by mechanical ventilation and assess any head injury.

2. If you are still in doubt about a possible intra-abdominal lesion in a severely shocked patient, you can try inserting gently a number one needle (21G) attached to a 20 ml syringe into each of the four quadrants of the abdomen (four quadrant tap). If aspiration reveals the presence of blood or heavily blood-stained fluid you can be confident of the diagnosis. However, if you are still in doubt and the patient fails to respond to normal resuscitation, carry out an emergency laparotomy.

3. Patients with occult liver tumours which rupture spontaneously frequently present with an 'acute abdomen' of unknown cause which requires urgent laparotomy. A four quadrant tap before laparotomy may reveal intra-peritoneal blood. A young woman who presents with this clinical picture may be thought to have a ruptured ectopic pregnancy; a gynaecolgist then opens the lower abdomen only to discover the bleeding lesion in the liver and calls you.

EXPLORATION OF A DAMAGED LIVER

Prepare

1. Ensure you have the collaboration of an experienced anaesthetist, for you are about to embark on a major surgical procedure which carries a high mortality rate.

2. Pass a bladder catheter to measure urine output. To avoid the complication of hepatorenal failure it is important to ensure urine flow continues during major liver surgery.

3. Pass a central venous catheter to measure central venous pressure and if facilities permit, insert an arterial catheter to allow constant measurement of arterial pressure.

4. Ensure there is plenty of blood available (at least 12 units) together with fresh frozen plasma and platelets to replace lost clotting products in the event of an exchange transfusion being necessary.

Access

1. If the diagnosis is suspected pre-operatively, then use a right subcostal incision 3 cm below the costal margin. Cut through all tissues in the line of the incision and use diathermy coagulation to obtain haemostasis. If necessary the incision can be extended across the mid line 3 cm below the left costal margin as an inverted 'V' or vertically upwards as a low sternal split. If you need to gain access above the liver, make another incision in the 10th rib bed from the anterior axillary line to the original subcostal incision, joining it at right angles. This will allow you to open the chest, divide the costal margin and so gain control of the inferior vena cava above the diaphragm.

2. If the rupture is discovered at diagnostic laparotomy through a paramedian incision, extend this to the costal margin to gain access and assess the need for further extensions.

3. If the rupture is discovered by a gynaecologist through a totally inappropriate lower abdominal incision then close it and re-explore through a more appropriate incision.

Assess

1. There will be a lot of blood clot in the peritoneal cavity and probably some fresh bleeding. Do not panic. Remove clot with your hands and with the help of a sucker.

2. Look for damage to the liver, the gut from oesophagus to rectum, the spleen, the pancreas, the anterior and posterior abdominal wall and the diaphragm.

Action

1. If there is obvious damage and haemorrhage from other intra-abdominal viscera, pack the bleeding area of the liver with large sterile packs and have an assistant apply gentle pressure to control the bleeding. Attend to the lesions in the other organs first.

2. Try and identify bleeding points in any damaged organs and clip them with haemostats. Then ligate them with fine silk ligatures. Use vascular clamps to control haemorrhage from major vessels. Repair damage in major vessels using vascular sutures.

3. Identify any torn gut or other peritoneal organs and cover them with packs when you have controlled the haemorrhage.

4. Remove blood and blood clot to gain adequate exposure of the bleeding area of the liver. Do not panic but attempt quietly to gain control of the haemorrhage. Most patients do not require major surgical procedures.

5. Attempt only the minimum surgery necessary to control haemorrhage. Avoid exploration and rough handling of injuries which are not bleeding at the time of exploration despite a normal blood pressure.

6. Explore locally the tear of the liver and remove any avascular tissue. If the laceration is still bleeding and extends deeply into the liver parenchyma it is important to explore the depth of the wound. This procedure is very important in contusion injuries, for major branches of the liver vessels may be ruptured producing large areas of devascularized tissue.

7. Identify bleeding points and apply fine haemostats. Ligate with fine silk.

8. If there is vascular oozing from a large raw area of liver, cover this with one layer of absorbable haemostatic gauze ('Surgicel', Johnson and Johnson Ltd.) and apply a pack. Avoid using deep mattress sutures to control such bleeding, for they may produce areas of devascularized tissue which will predispose to subsequent infection.

Difficulty?

1. Uncontrolled haemorrhage from torn liver — if haemorrhage is massive, attempt to obtain control by inserting a finger through the aditus to the lesser sac behind the hepatic hilum and apply a Satinsky or other vascular clamp across the hilar structures. If vascular clamps are not available in a real emergency, use a noncrushing intestinal clamp with great care. Try to identify any large vessels crossing the tear and ligate them or suture any tears in their walls. Injuries which involve the inferior vena cava are very difficult to treat and even very experienced liver surgeons find these are associated with a high mortality rate. Bleeding from such injuries may not be controlled by clamping the liver hilum. In these patients, attempt to mobilise the inferior vena cava above and below the liver, identify the caval tear and attempt to suture it. Unless you are very experienced, do not attempt total vascular isolation of the liver by using intra-caval shunts. They are rarely necessary, and even when used by the most experienced surgeons, are accompanied by a 60–70% mortality rate. Remember total hepatic devascularization should not be maintained for single periods longer than 10 minutes. Before releasing any vascular clamps, have the anaesthetist infuse calcium and bicarbonate solutions to protect against the effects of massive acidosis and potassium release which can cause cardiac arrest.

2. If you cannot achieve control using these techniques, do not attempt a major resection as an emergency procedure without the assistance of an experienced hepatic surgeon. Such operations are rarely necessary in an emergency and are accompanied by an unacceptably high mortality rate. In these circumstances it is better to obtain

control of the bleeding by packing the liver with gauze rolls and closing the abdomen. This will give you time to assess the next move.

3. Damage to the biliary tree — if the extrahepatic biliary tree is damaged you should attempt reconstruction by anastomosing cut ends of the biliary tract end-to-end over a T-tube splint inserted through healthy bile duct. Use interrupted absorbable sutures. If the damage to the duct is excessive, identify the most distal section of normal duct and anastomose this to a loop of jejunum (see Ch. 10.)

Check

1. When you have gained control of the bleeding from the liver carry out a full, careful and gentle exploration for other intraperiotoneal injuries. Explore the entire gut from the oesophagus to rectum and pay special attention to the retroperitoneal duodenum. Explore the pancreas and the spleen carefully.

2. When you are certain haemorrhage is controlled and other lesions have been attended to in the appropriate manner, unless you have had to pack the liver to control haemorrhage, inspect it again. Ensure there are no devascularized areas, which must be removed to prevent infection, and no bile leaking from damaged intrahepatic bile ducts, which must be ligated or sutured.

Closure

Close the abdomen in a standard fashion. The insertion of a peritoneal drain is controversial. If you have operated on any part of the biliary tract then a drain, and preferably a closed system drain, will be needed. If there is only liver parenchymal damage then probably a drain is unneccessary.

Aftercare

1. Give the patient a broad spectrum antibiotic mixture such as netilmicin and metronidazole if there has been damage to the biliary tract or any part of the gut. Correct any remaining electrolyte imbalance and blood and clotting factor loss. Assess the patient's general condition and if further surgery is needed because you have had to employ packing to control haemorrhage, arrange for his transfer to a unit experienced in handling major liver trauma if possible. If such transfer is impossible then the abdomen and liver will require re-exploration after 48 or 72 hours.

2. Nurse the patient in an intensive care area.

3. Mechanically ventilate the patient electively and maintain his blood gases within normal range until he is haemodynamically stable, other injuries have been treated and his core temperature has returned to normal.

4. Maintain intravascular volume and normal clotting, electrolyte and colloid balance. Measure blood sugar hourly

and albumin levels 4-hourly and treat any abnormality immediately. Estimate biochemical liver function tests daily.

5. Maintain urine flow. If it falls below 30 ml per hour, first check that the circulating blood volume is adequate (normal blood pressure and central venous pressure). If you are in any doubt about this, give a 'fluid challenge' of 200 ml of colloid-containing fluid intravenously. If this fails to stimulate urine flow, despite an adequate blood pressure and normal central venous pressure, give an intravenous injection of a diuretic such as frusemide 40 mg.

6. If gastrointestinal activity does not return within 2 or 3 days, start intravenous nutrition.

7. Sudden collapse suggests the patient has developed further internal bleeding or septicaemia. Measure the patient's girth and attempt four quadrant aspiration of the abdomen. If blood is aspirated, it must be assumed there is internal bleeding. Carry out another exploratory laparotomy and attempt to control it as before.

8. If you are in any doubt, re-exploration is safer than waiting.

9. If you suspect septicaemia then start full investigations to determine the source. Culture blood, urine and any leaking body fluid, X-ray the chest and carry out an ultrasound of the abdomen to look for an abscess.

10. Give the patient an adequate dose of appropriate broad spectrum antibiotics and correct any hypovolaemia. An intraperitoneal abscess must be drained either by a further laparotomy or by ultrasound-guided needle aspiration. If the patient is very shocked and the diagnosis is uncertain, it is safer to re-explore the abdomen than to wait. Sepsis is very common following liver trauma and if you fail to recognise and treat it, the patient may die.

RE-EXPLORATION

Prepare

Ensure the patient is stable and biochemical and haematological abnormalities have been corrected. Order 12 units of blood and at least 4 units each of platelets and fresh frozen plasma.

Access

1. Open the previous incision.
2. Remove the packs gently and send them immediately to the microbiological laboratory for culture.

Assess

Usually everything is dry. Avoid any major exploration of the liver.

Action

1. If bleeding recurs apply haemostats to any obvious bleeding vessels and ligate them.

2. Aspirate any bile collections and attempt to ligate or suture any leaking bile ducts.

3. If major bleeding starts again then attempt to identify the main vessel and suture it. On rare occasions, carry out lobectomy (see below) if the injury is confined to one lobe.

4. Occasionally, following a severe blunt crushing injury, the damage is so great that no surgical procedure can save the patient's life.

Closure

If you are sure there are no more local problems, close the abdomen without drainage and continue antibiotic therapy, adjusted in due course when the results of the culture of the removed packs is available.

Aftercare

As before.

PRINCIPLES OF ELECTIVE SURGERY

Appraise

1. Do not undertake an elective operation on the liver without complete pre-operative investigation and a fairly certain working diagnosis. Modern investigative techniques permit this goal. If you have any doubt about the nature of a liver problem, refer the patient to a centre with experience in this type of complex surgery if possible.

2. Take a history — this may give you a lead since the patient may complain of past or recent jaundice, of a lump in the right upper quadrant of the abdomen, of pain or discomfort in that region, of rigors suggesting septicaemia or of upper gastrointestinal bleeding from endoscopically-proven oesophageal varices. There may be a history of the patient having lived in an area where *Taenia echinococcus* or amoebic dysentery are endemic, of taking high oestrogen-containing contraceptive pills or of excessive alcohol intake.

3. Carry out a clinical examination — there may be jaundice or other systemic signs of liver disease or a mass or tenderness in the right upper quadrant of the abdomen. Of course, the only sign may be a chance finding of a liver abnormality at a laparotomy carried out for another reason.

4. Carry out biochemical liver function tests. These may indicate the type of liver disease. Measure the alpha feto-protein since a raised level suggests the presence of a malignant liver tumour. Check the hepatitis antigen status (HBsAg).

5. Arrange for ultrasound (US) or computerized tomography (CT) scans of the upper abdomen. These can demonstrate the size of the liver and the biliary ducts within and outside it and may show gallstones. Patency of major vessels and the nature of any space-occupying lesions in the liver can be assessed. A picture characteristic of cirrhosis may be seen.

6. If an hepatic lesion is identified or if the patient has oesophageal varices then carry out vascular angiography. Selective coeliac and superior mesenteric angiography will demonstrate the arterial anatomy outside and within the liver and the vascularization of any intrahepatic lesion. These X-rays may be diagnostic. Furthermore, the venous phase of angiograms will demonstrate patency or distortion of the portal vein. It will demonstrate the position and nature of any abnormal portasystemic shunts in portal hypertension. In proven portal hypertension, percutaneous splenic portography can be done and this technique will demonstrate the venous anatomy and any shunts too. However, there is always the risk of splenic damage and subsequent haemorrhage as a result of this procedure. It should never be carried out unless the blood clotting is normal and it is dangerous if the platelet count is low.

7. Always obtain histological confirmation of the nature of any liver disease. Once any clotting or platelet abnormalities have been corrected biopsy can be carried out either blind by percutaneous stab or percutaneously with CT or US direction or at peritoneouscopy. Use either a Tru-cut or a Menghini needle. It is also possible to take a biopsy during laparotomy.

8. Consider portal pressure measurement. Measurement of portal pressure alone will identify portal hypertension if it is above 15 cm water. However, the actual pressure does not help you to decide the best treatment or indicate the prognosis. It may be of relative value during procedures designed to produce portal decompression when a fall in pressure will indicate a successful operation. Portal pressure can be measured by inserting a needle connected to a manometer into the spleen, a dilated umbilical vein or at laporatomy into any portal venous branch. In specialist centres, wedged hepatic venous pressure measurements are made and these may reflect the portal pressure.

6. Before undertaking any operative procedure on a patient with liver disease, check the blood film, platelet count and clotting profile. Correct these if possible by giving blood and blood products. Rarely are platelet infusions necessary but all patients undergoing liver surgery, especially if jaundiced or with severe biochemical dysfunction, benefit from injections of Vitamin K_1. If the clotting profile is badly deranged, the patient may need an infusion of fresh frozen plasma.

OPERATIVE LIVER BIOPSY

Prepare

Check the patient's blood group. Cross-match an adequate quantity of blood and platelets and have available some frozen plasma for replacement therapy during surgery if you anticipate a more major procedure.

Access

Use a right upper paramedian or right subcostal incision 3 cm below the costal margin.

Action

1. Always take the liver biopsy at an early stage during any laparotomy. Prolonged trauma to the liver during laparotomy can produce changes which make histological interpretation of the specimen difficult.

2. Select an area of diseased liver or an edge which presents easily through the incision.

3. Place two mattress stitches using 3–0 catgut on an atraumatic round bodied needle to form a V, the apex of this pointing towards the hilum of the liver (Fig. 11.1a).

4. Gently but firmly tie these stitches (Fig. 11.1b) and remove the wedge of tissue between them with a sharp

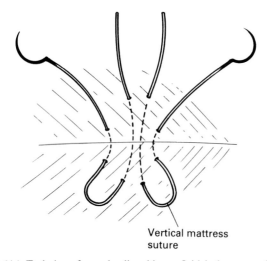

Vertical mattress suture

Fig. 11.1(a) Technique for wedge liver biopsy. Initial placement of two mattress stitches

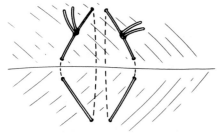

Fig. 11.1(b) Tie each firmly

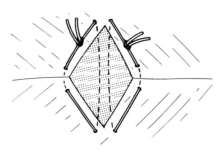

Fig. 11.1(c) Remove wedge of tissue between them

knife (Fig. 11.1c). The cut edges of the liver should be dry. Insert another suture of similar material if haemostasis is not complete.

5. Complete your examination of all abdominal structures.

6. Close the incision in the standard way.

INFECTIVE LESIONS

BACTERIAL LIVER ABSCESS

Appraise

1. This condition is still associated with a high mortality rate. However, recently this has been reduced by aspirating the pus under ultrasound or CT direction and giving antibiotics. Inititially these should be netilmicin and metronidazole until the exact nature and antibiotic sensitivities of the causative organism is known.

2. Localize the abscess with US or CT scanning. Aspirate pus using a percutaneous needle guided by US or CT, culture organisms and determine antibiotic sensitivity.

3. Avoid surgical exploration if possible because the operation may be complicated by local and systemic sepsis.

4. You may have to aspirate the abscess several times but if it fails to respond to repeated aspirations and antibiotics or the percutaneous insertion of a drain, then you may be forced to operate. Localise the abscess first with US or CT.

Access

Use a right subcostal incision 3 cm below the costal margin or right upper paramedian incision for an anterior abscess. Approach a posterior abscess through the bed of the right posterior 12th rib.

Action

1. Isolate the peritoneal contents from the area of the abscess by packs.

2. Insert a needle into the abscess to confirm the diagnosis. Aspirate some of the contents and send to the microbiology laboratory for immediate examination and culture including anaerobic culture.

3. Incise the abscess and suck out the contents. Insert gently a finger to ensure that all loculi are broken.

4. Wash out the cavity with physiological saline.

5. Insert a tube drain. Ideally use a 'closed system' such as a Robinson drain. Pass the distal end of the drain through the abdominal wall at a suitable site, not the incision.

6. Ensure haemostasis at the edge of the liver incision by using 3/0 catgut mattress sutures on an atraumatic needle.

7. If it is practicable, place the omentum such that some of it enters the abscess cavity.

8. Close the abdomen.

9. Leave the drain until drainage ceases and the cavity can be shown to have collapsed by radiological sinogram techniques.

10. Continue treatment with appropriate antibiotics until the cavity has obliterated on ultrasound screening or by radiological sinogram.

AMOEBIC ABSCESS

Appraise

1. This condition rarely requires surgical treatment.

2. Diagnosis is confirmed by positive identification of trophozoites in the abscess aspirate or a positive serological test. It is not necessary to identify amoebae in stools or on rectal biopsy since an amoebic abscess can occur many years after the initial infection.

3. Treatment is with metronidazole until the abscess has been shown to have resolved on ultrasound screening. Occasionally chloroquine is valuable if metronidazole fails to cure the lesion.

4. If it becomes secondarily infected or is discovered at laparotomy then it should be treated as any other liver abscess.

CYSTS

HYDATID CYST

Appraise

1. Suspect a hydatid cyst in patients who present with a liver mass and live in an endemic area. Confirm it by the presence of an eosinophilia, positive hydatid complement fixation tests and classical US and CT appearances.

2. Do **NOT** aspirate by needle a hydatid or suspected hydatid cyst. This would expose the patient to the great dangers of the rupture of the cysts with dissemination of the disease, or anaphylactic shock.

3. There is no proven medical treatment for this condition although high dose metronidazole and a new drug, albendazole, are currently under investigation.

4. Treatment therefore remains surgical.

Prepare

1. Have available fluid with which to wash out the cyst to kill any remaining scolices. This can be absolute alcohol, 1% cetrimide, 10% formalin, 0.5% silver nitrate solution or the safest, which his sterile satured saline.

2. Have available sterile black towels with which to pack off the surrounding tissues. Some clinicians like to soak these in formalin solution.

3. Have available a refrigerated funnel ('cryo-funnel') if possible. (Fig. 11.2a)

4. Warn the anaesthetist to be prepared for sudden anaphylactic shock in the event of spillage of cyst contents into the peritoneal cavity.

Access

Use an extended right subcostal incision 3 cm below the costal margin or if the abscess is very posterior, a 10th rib thoraco-abdominal incision.

Action

1. When the cyst is seen, take care in handling it for it can rupture very easily.

2. Isolate the cyst from the rest of the peritoneal or chest contents by packs. Traditionally, these should be covered by black towels which are said to make any spilt daughter cysts or scolices visible.

3. If it is available use a metal 'cryo-funnel' with a narrow-end 5 cm diameter fused to which is a circular metal tube with an inlet and outlet connection through which liquid nitrogen can be passed (Fig. 11.2a). Connect the inlet tube via an insulated plastic tube to a Dewar flask of liquid nitrogen. The outlet tube should be connected to another insulated plastic tube and allowed to go to waste on the floor. Place the narrow cooled end on the exposed cyst

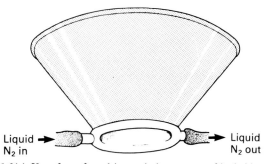

Fig. 11.2(a) Use of cryofunnel in surgical treatment of hydatid cyst of the liver. Stainless steel cryofunnel

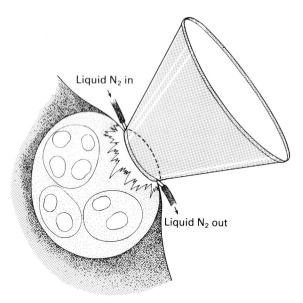

Fig. 11.2(b) Diagrammatic representation of cryofunnel frozen to presenting surface of cyst

and turn on the liquid nitrogen (Fig. 11.2b). The freezing produces perfect adhesion between cyst wall and lower end of the funnel and prevents any split contents from contaminating surrounding structures. You can carry out all the operative procedures through the funnel.

4. Insert a wide bore needle into the cyst and aspirate carefully as much of the fluid contained therein as possible.

5. Incise the wall of the cyst and gently remove the yellow grey cyst membrane together with any free daughter cysts. At all stages take great care not to spill any of the cyst fluid or any of the daughter cysts or membranes in such a way that they can infest any other part of the abdomen.

6. When the cyst is empty fill it with a fluid ideally saturated brine which will destroy any remaining scolices. Leave the fluid in the cyst for at least 10 minutes, then aspirate it and repeat the procedure.

7. Finally aspirate the fluid and if a 'cryo-funnel' has been used, turn off the liquid nitrogen and allow the frozen contact between funnel and liver to thaw. Remove the funnel. Remove the packs carefully to prevent any contamination.

8. Insert a closed suction drain into the cyst and pack into it any available omentum if this is possible.

9. Ensure haemostasis is complete and close the wound.

Technical points

1. Some surgeons advocate excision of the cyst intact. In some circumstances this is possible, but it is a bloody operation.

2. Communication between the cyst and the biliary tree is usually obvious pre-operatively, since the patient will have suffered jaundice and cholangitis. Cholangiography, especially by the endoscopic retrograde route (ERCP), will demonstrate the communication. In these patients the biliary tract will require exploration, lavage and T-tube drainage. Since the bile salts in the bile are probably adequate to kill the scolices, it is unnecessary and possibly dangerous to flush the cyst with the usual scolicidal fluids.

OTHER CYSTS

Appraise

1. The majority of liver cysts are totally asymptomatic and only discovered at autopsy or during a routine laparotomy. When symptoms develop, they include right upper quadrant abdominal swelling, discomfort or acute pain associated with haemorrhage into the cyst or rupture of the cyst. Occasionally cysts become infected or the patient may have recurrent cholanitis due to biliary tract narrowing from pressure. A very rare liver cyst is caused by a biliary cystadenoma and this needs excising.

2. Symptomatic cysts will be diagnosed before surgery is undertaken from the results of tests carried out to investigate the symptoms.

3. Do **not** attempt percutaneous aspiration of a cyst as a diagnostic test until you are certain it is not hydatid.

4. In 50% of patients with polycystic liver disease, there is associated polycystic renal disease. The renal lesions are more serious and life-threatening than the liver lesions. Some patients have associated pancreatic cysts also.

Access

Use an extended right subcostal incision 3 cm below the costal margin.

Action

1. Carry out a thorough exploratory laparotomy, paying particular attention to palpation of the kidneys and pancreas.

2. If you cannot exclude hydatid disease as the cause of the lesion then proceed cautiously and manage the cyst as if it were a hydatid cyst.

3. If you are certain the cyst is not hydatid, firstly carry out needle aspiration and send the fluid for cytological, microbiological and chemical analysis.

4. If you have found the cystic lesion during a laparotomy for something else, and the lesion is totally asymptomatic and smaller than 8 cm in diameter, no further action is needed.

5. If the cyst is symptomatic or large then carefully unroof it and allow it to drain freely into the peritoneal cavity. You can insert some omentum into it loosely. A cyst treated in this way may recur but can then be treated by percutaneous aspiration or formal resection.

6. If the cyst is superficial you can carry out simple wedge excision if you have had experience of this surgical technique.

7. If the lesion is large, multilocular or appears to be vascular then it is probably better to attempt no further action at this stage but rather to close the abdomen to await the results of the tests on the cyst fluid. Later on you can treat the lesion as you would a liver tumour after full and appropriate investigations.

NEOPLASMS

Appraise

1. Neoplastic lesions in the liver can be solid or cystic, benign or malignant. The latter can be primary or secondary and all can be single or multiple.

2. Pre-operative assessment as outlined on page 199 is essential to determine the need for surgical treatment. Of particular diagnostic value are alpha fetoprotein levels, US and CT scans, vascular angiograms and biopsy.

3. Not every neoplasm requires excision once it can be proved that it is benign. However, no patient with malignant or suspected malignant disease should be denied a laparotomy to confirm the diagnosis and assess operability.

Prepare

1. If you think a major liver resection will be necessary advise your anaesthetist accordingly and order 12 units of blood, 4 units of platelets and 4 units of fresh frozen plasma. Warn the blood bank you may need more.

2. Correct any clotting abnormality before surgery. Give the jaundiced patient vitamim K. However if the tumour has caused so much liver damage that the patient is jaundiced, resection is unlikely to be successful.

3. Inform the theatre team of the nature of the operation and ask them to have available chest retractors, vascular clamps and sutures in addition to your usual laparotomy instruments.

4. After the patient has been anaesthetised, ask the anaesthetist to insert a central venous catheter and an arterial cannula for pressure measurements. Pass a bladder catheter to allow urine flow to be measured.

WEDGE EXCISION OF SOLITARY LIVER LESION

Access

1. Use a right subcostal incision 3 cm below the costal margin to explore the lesion first. This can be extended across the mid-line below the left costal margin as an inverted 'V' to gain greater exposure. Split the lower sternum or right costal margin in the 10th rib bed to gain access to the upper part of the liver. This is rarely necessary.

Assess

1. Carry out a general exploration to exclude other intra-abdominal pathology.

2. Identify the site of the liver tumour and ensure your incision is adequate to allow you to resect it. If it is too small, enlarge it.

3. Explore the liver hilum and identify the hepatic artery and portal vein and their right and left branches. This will allow a vascular clamp to be applied to them in the event of severe haemorrhage.

Action

1. Incise through the liver capsule a short distance away from the tumour.

2. Use a finger-and-thumb pinch technique and divide the liver substance identifying any major ductal or vascular structures crossing the line of incision. Clip these with fine haemostats and divide them.

3. Remove the tumour and ligate the ducts and vessels held in the haemostats with fine silk. Diathermy coagulate any remaining small bleeding points.

4. If the cut surfaces of the liver are not dry, cover them with absorbable haemostatic gauze ('Surgicel', Johnson and Johnson Ltd) and apply a pack. After 10 minutes remove the pack gently. The area should be dry. Coagulate any remaining bleeding points.

Check

1. Inspect carefully the liver hilum to ensure that no major structures have been damaged.

2. Carry out cholangiography if there is any question of biliary tract damage.

Closure

1. Once the cut surface of the liver is dry, apply the omentum to the outer surface of the absorbable haemostatic gauze and close the wound without drainage.

HEPATIC LOBECTOMY

Anatomy

1. The liver is divided into two anatomical lobes, each being supplied by its own branch of the hepatic artery, portal vein and hepatic duct. The junction of the two lobes is about 4 cm lateral to the attachment of the falciform ligament and in the line of the gallbladder bed (Fig. 11.3). By ligating the vessels to either lobe, it is possible to see the junction between them as a fairly sharp colour change. The lobes can then by separated by dividing the small vessels and ducts which cross this junctional area.

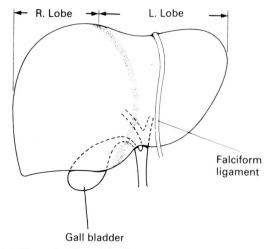

Fig. 11.3 The main lobes of the liver

2. It is also possible to remove all the liver tissue to the right of the falciform ligament by ligating the vessels supplying the right part of the left lobe together with all the vessels supplying the right lobe. Such a resection is called an extended right hepatic lobectomy or trisegmentectomy. This resection is difficult and should not be undertaken by an inexperienced surgeon.

3. Removal of the left lateral lobe, that is removal of the part of the liver to the left of the falciform ligament, is also possible and is a comparatively straight-forward surgical procedure.

Appraise

Left lateral, left, right or extended right (trisegmentectomy) hepatic lobectomy can be carried out in order to excise a solitary tumour affecting one part of the liver.

Access

As for wedge excision (see p. 203). However, it will be necessary to extend the incision for this more radical operation.

Action

1. After full exploration of all abdominal viscera, dissect the hepatic hilum and identify the branches of the hepatic artery, portal vein and bile duct supplying the affected lobe.

2. If the right lobe is to be removed, identify and dissect the cystic duct and artery too.

3. Doubly ligate with silk and divide the structures supplying the lobe to be removed (Fig. 11.4a).

4. Divide the peritoneal reflections between the back of the liver lobe and the diaphragm and retract the lobe from the diaphragm and posterior abdominal wall until the inferior vena cava is seen.

5. Identify veins from the lobe entering the inferior vena cava, dissect, doubly ligate with silk and divide them (Fig. 11.4b).

6. Return to the anterior surface of the liver. A demarcation line should be obvious between the devascularized lobe to be removed, and the normal vascularized liver.

7. Make an incision through the capsule just on the vascularized side of this demarcation line.

8. Use a finger-and-thumb pinching technique and divide the liver substance between this incision and the inferior vena cava.

9. Doubly clip with fine haemostats any vascular or biliary tract structures crossing the line of transection as they are encountered.

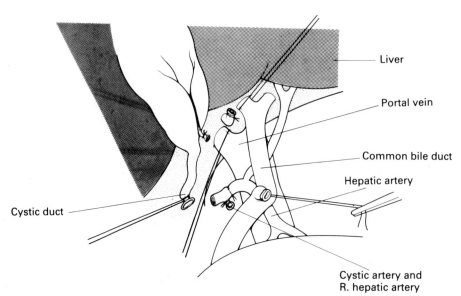

Fig. 11.4(a) Hepatic lobectomy. The vessels supplying the lobe to be removed are ligated

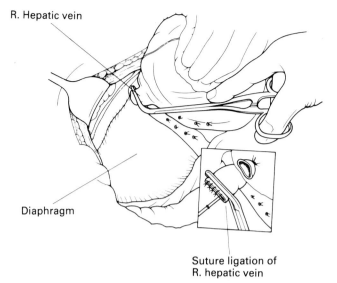

R. Hepatic vein

Diaphragm

Suture ligation of
R. hepatic vein

Fig. 11.4(b) The hepatic veins from the lobe to be removed are ligated

10. Remove the diseased lobe and ligate with fine silk the structures in the haemostats on the remaining liver.

11. Control any smaller bleeding points by diathermy coagulation.

12. Cover the raw area of the liver with absorbable haemostatic gauze ('Surgicel') and apply a pack for 10 minutes.

Check

1. When haemostasis is complete, explore the hilar structures to ensure no major damage has occurred.

2. Carry out cholangiography if there is any doubt about damage to the biliary system.

Closure

Cover the transected area of liver with omentum and close the abdomen without drainage.

Technical point

Some surgeons advocate T-tube drainage of the biliary tract but in normal circumstances this is unnecessary unless some distal obstruction is suspected or there has been any damage.

Aftercare

1. Post-operative management of these patient is critical.

2. Maintain careful fluid and electrolyte balance. Maintain urine flow at about 40 ml per hour. If this falls, suspect either hypovolaemia due to blood loss or septicaemia. Treat this initially with a 'fluid challenge' of 200 ml of colloid-containing fluid. If urine flow increases immediately then this is an indication that the fall in urine output was due to hypovolaemia and the patient may require more blood or other intravenous, colloid-containing fluid.

3. Regularly monitor blood glucose and protein levels. Treat any fall actively.

4. Carefully watch for signs of infection which should be treated early and fully.

SURGICAL MANAGEMENT OF HAEMORRHAGE FROM OESOPHAGEAL VARICES

The most life-threatening complication of portal hypertension which requires surgical treatment is that of bleeding from oesophageal varices. Management of these patients is extremely complex and should ideally be undertaken by a surgeon in consultation with a medical hepatologist, specialist radiologists and pathologists.

Management

1. Resuscitate the patient.
2. Find the cause of the bleeding.
3. Stop the bleeding.

These three processes must be carried out simultaneously. The prognosis of the condition is directly related to the severity of any underlying liver disease. Minimal damage should carry a good prognosis whereas, if there is severe liver disease, the prognosis is poor. However, as there is no way of telling in advance which patients will fare badly or well, all should be actively treated initially.

Appraise

1. Endoscope a patient admitted to hospital with massive upper gastrointestinal haemorrhage. This is the most certain way of discovering if bleeding is from ruptured oesophageal varices. Although a previous history and clinical examination may suggest such a diagnosis, direct visualization of the bleeding area is mandatory before undertaking treatment since some patients, especially alcoholics with known varices, bleed from other gastrointestinal lesions. In the presence of active bleeding, it may be difficult to see the actual bleeding point due to the presence of a lot of blood. Be prepared to wash out the oesophagus and stomach and repeat the endoscopy (see p. 58).

2. Resuscitate by infusing compatible blood, platelets and clotting products given as fresh frozen plasma. If intravenous fluid is needed while the blood is being crossmatched, maintain the circulating volume with 5% dextrose. If bleeding persists then attempt to stop it by giving an intravenous injection of a vasoactive drug such as Pitressin. If this fails, you can control bleeding usually by oesophagogastric tamponade using an orogastric balloon

tube. This is unlikely to be curative but 'buys time' prior to more definitive measures.

3. Collect as much information as possible regarding liver pathology, liver function and the anatomicial arrangement of the liver blood supply.

4. After resuscitation and full assessment, decide if more definitive procedures are required. These can be summarized as 'veno-occlusive', designed to stop the venous haemorrhage or 'portal decompression', by which the portal pressure is reduced. The exact choice of technique depends on local expertise and facilities. In general it is better to attempt to stop the bleeding by a vaso-occlusive technique. These techniques are less hazardous for acute bleeding than portal decompression, which is associated with a 50% mortality rate and a 40% chance of portasystemic encephalopathy in the survivors.

VENO-OCCLUSIVE PROCEDURES

Appraise

1. The most important need is to stop the bleeding. Different centres produce figures to justify their own preferred technique.

2. There are three approaches to the problem. Firstly, induction of thrombosis and sclerosis in the oesophageal varices by injecting a sclerosing agent through a catheter inserted into the vessels using a percutaneous transhepatic technique. Secondly, the varices can be injected with sclerosant directly through an oesophagoscope. Thirdly, the portal feeding vessels or the varices themselves can be ligated by a variety of thoracic or abdominal surgical approaches. The most satisfactory way of doing this at present is oesophagogastric transection and reanastomosis using a circular stapling device.

PERCUTANEOUS TRANSHEPATIC SCLEROTHERAPY

This can be undertaken only in a major centre possessing appropriate radiological equipment and expertise. In expert hands this procedure controls acute haemorrhage but rebleeding is common a few weeks later. Thus it must be regarded as a holding procedure, giving time for full assessment prior to more definitive treatment.

Action

1. Using fluoroscopic control, sedation, and local anaesthesia, insert a needle percutaneously into an intrahepatic branch of the portal vein.

2. Thread a catheter through this with the aid of a guide wire until the tip comes to lie in the lumen of a branch of the portal vien, usually the coronary vein, which is feeding the oesophageal varices.

3. Inject sclerosant material such as thrombin, absorbable gelatin sponge ('Gel-Foam'), cyanoacrylate or alcohol with the object of causing thrombosis in the bleeding varices.

4. Block the catheter pathway through the liver by injecting 'Gel-Foam' as it is withdrawn.

ENDOSCOPIC SCLEROTHERAPY

Attempt this only if you are experienced in endoscopy. It can be carried out with either a flexible endoscope or a rigid Negus type oesophagoscope and the technique chosen should be governed by personal experience and preference.

Prepare

1. Consider the type of anaesthetic to be used. If you are going to use a rigid oesophagoscope then the patient will need a general anaesthetic given by an experienced anaesthetist. If you are going to use a flexible endoscope then sedation alone may be adequate. However, some clinicians still prefer to use a general anaesthetic for this technique also.

2. If you are going to use a rigid oesophagoscope, use the Bailey and Dawson modified instrument (Fig. 11.5).

3. A similar shaped semi-flexible, but fairly rigid sheath can be passed over the flexible instrument and some clinicians find this helpful.

Action

1. Pass the oesophagoscope.
2. When you can see the oesophageal varices in the

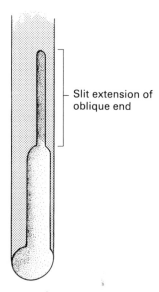

Slit extension of oblique end

Fig. 11.5 Bailey and Dawson modification of the rigid Negus oesophagoscope

lower third of the oesophagus, inject sclerosant (e.g. ethanolamine oleate 5%) either directly into the lumen of the veins or into the submucosa adjacent to them. Do not inject more than 5 ml intravenously or 2 ml submucosally.

3. After each injection rotate the oesophagoscope or the sheath over the flexible instrument in order to compress the injection site.

4. Visualise another varix and repeat the procedure. Do not inject a total or more than 25 ml of 5% ethanolamine oleate at any one time.

5. It is often difficult to see within the oesophagus during an acute bleeding episode. Attempt to control haemorrhage temporarily, using balloon tamponade tube before attempting the injections.

6. Repeat endoscopic sclerotherapy at intervals during the following weeks until the varices disappear, to prevent further bleeding episodes. Occasionally, a second or third injection will be needed in the acute phase to control bleeding. Once this is controlled, allow periods of about 2 weeks between further injections. Local ulceration contraindicates further injections and if you find this on endoscopy, wait until it has healed. When the varices have disappeared, repeat endoscopy every 3 months and inject recurrent veins to prevent further bleeding.

OESOPHAGOGASTRIC DISCONNECTION

This procedure which is designed to occlude all veins filling the oesophageal plexus from below, is now safely and rapidly carried out using a mechanical circular stapling instrument.

Prepare

1. Have available disposable circular stapling instruments (EEA 25, 28 and 31, or similar) and the accompanying measuring bougies.

2. Ask the anaesthetist to give a single prophylactic intravenous injection of 2 g cefotaxime and 500 mg matranidazole at the start of the operation.

Access

Use a left subcostal incision 3 cm below the costal margin.

Assess

1. Aspirate ascitic fluid from the peritoneal cavity and measure the volume carefully. This helps you to calculate subsequent fluid replacement.

2. Carry out a general exploration and perform a liver biopsy if histological diagnosis of the liver disease has not been obtained.

Action

1. Identify the oesophagogastric junction after the anaesthetist has passed a nasogastric tube.

2. Gently retract the left lobe of the liver from this region using a Deaver retractor.

3. Incise the peritoneum adjacent to the lower end of the oesophagus and gently pass a finger behind the oesophagus and immediate perioesophageal tissues. Encircle these structures with a tape.

4. Extend the dissection proximally and distally until two fingers can be passed easily around the whole of the lower oesophagus. It is not necessary to identify separately the vagi, however if they prevent adequate mobilisation they can be excluded from the mobilised tissues.

5. Make a vertical gastrotomy in the anterior stomach wall 10–15 cm from the oesophagogastric junction and insert through this one of the measuring bougies. Start with the 31 mm diameter bougie and introduce it into the lower oesophagus to ensure that the lumen is large enough to accommodate it and thus the 31 mm staple instrument. If it will not pass easily do not force it but try one of the smaller ones. Usually the 31 mm instrument passes easily.

6. Unpack and remove the staple gun of the same size.

7. Remove the tape from the lower oesophagus and replace it with a stout thread ligature.

8. Pass a finger through the gastrotomy and into the lumen of the lower oesophagus. Have the anaesthetist slowly withdraw the nasogastric tube until the tip just disappears proximally up the oesophagus.

9. Pass the well-lubricated head of the selected staple gun into the lower oesophagus and separate the anvil from the staple cartridge by adjusting the screw on the handle. Have an assistant steady the instrument and palpate the groove between the separated parts of the head of the instrument through the wall of the oesophagus.

10. Tie the thread ligature firmly in this groove and cut the ends (Fig. 11.6a).

11. While protecting the lower end of the oesophagus with a hand placed around it, tighten the screw to bring the staple cartridge and anvil together. Check the mobility of the lower oesophagus and 'fire' the gun.

12. Unscrew the nut in the handle of the instrument two turns to separate anvil from staple cartridge. Firmly hold the lower oesophagus and, with a gentle twisting motion, remove the instrument.

Check

1. Put a large pack into the upper peritoneal cavity in the region of the transection and inspect the instrument. Separate the anvil and staple cartridge, remove the anvil and the plastic ring. Within the circular knife blade you will find the resected portion of oesophagus. Remove this and ensure that a complete 'doughnut' of oesophageal wall

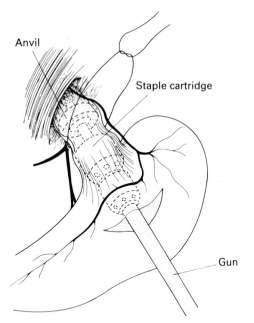

Fig. 11.6(a) Use of EEA staple instrument to carry out oesophagogastric transection. Instrument passed into lower oesophagus, staple cartridge and anvil separated and ligature tied around the entire oesophagus in the groove between the two

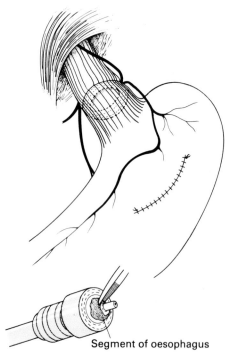

Fig 11.6(b) After firing the gun the instrument is removed

has been obtained. (Fig. 11.6b). If it is incomplete, it means that there is a portion of the oesophageal wall that has not been adequately stapled, and patent varices may be present still.

2. Remove the pack from the upper abdomen and check that haemostasis is complete. If it is not or if the transec-

tion was incomplete, inspect the anastomosis. Insert some additional mattress catgut sutures through the entire thickness of the oesphageal wall to control bleeding from any remaining vessels. If the transection has been complete the area will be dry.

3. Check that there is no bleeding from gastric fundal varices. If there is, it may be necessary to carry out gastric devascularization coupled with splenectomy. Mobilise the spleen as for splenectomy (p. 214). Ligate and divide the vessels in the splenic pedicle. Identify, dissect, ligate and divide all the short gastric vessels between the greater curvature of the stomach and the spleen. Remove the spleen. Check the rest of the greater curvature of the stomach and dissect, ligate and divide any remaining vessels between it and the diaphragm. Turn your attention to the lesser curve of the stomach. Dissect this and identify, ligate and divide any vessels passing to it from the lesser omentum. Continue this dissection to the region of the antrum. The entire stomach should now be separated from any feeding vessels along its greater and lesser curves. Fortunately the internal vascularisation of the stomach is almost always adequate to prevent any avascular necrosis.

Closure

1. Pass a finger through the gastrotomy into the lower oesophagus across the line of transection, have the anaesthetist slowly repass the nasogastric tube, and with your finger, guide it back into the lumen of the stomach.

2. Close the gastrotomy in two layers with absorbable sutures.

3. Close the abdominal incision in layers in the usual way without drainage.

Protect

Since a viscus infected by gut organisms has been opened and the contents have flooded the peritoneal cavity, continue the prophylactic antibiotic regimen used at the start of the operation for 3 days after operation.

Aftercare

Arrange initial management in an intensive care unit with the help of medical hepatologists since accurate water, electrolyte, colloid and blood balance is essential.

PORTAL DECOMPRESSION

Appraise

1. Portal decompression can be total end-to-side (portacaval shunt); semi-total side-to-side (splenorenal or mesocaval shunt) or selective (Warren proximal splenorenal shunt). There is no evidence to suggest that any one op-

eration is in the long term any better than any of the others so choose the one with which you have had most experience.

2. The incidence of the major complication, portasystemic encephalopathy, is similar after any of these operations although it may be less in the early days following Warren splenorenal shunt.

3. Do not attempt portal decompression without full preoperative consultation with an experienced medical hepatologist. You must discuss liver function, identification of the nature of the liver pathology and the vascular anatomy. This means that it is rarely a procedure that can be entertained in an emergency. Patients who tolerate this operation well with minimal encephalopathy are those with good liver function. These include patients with portal venous occlusion, primary biliary cirrhosis or hepatic fibrosis. The decision to carry out a shunt operation should not be undertaken lightly if the patient has a job which would bd threatened if he suffered any intellectual impairment.

PORTACAVAL SHUNT

Prepare

1. You will need to correct any electrolyte or blood clotting imbalance pre-operatively. Order 6 units of blood and 4 units each of fresh frozen plasma and platelets and warn the blood bank you may need more.

2. Advise your anaesthetist that you will be carrying out major surgery on a very sick patient.

3. Advise your operating department assistant that you will require vascular instruments and sutures.

Access

1. Place the patient supine on the operating table with sand bags under right shoulder and pelvis to rotate the patient slightly towards the left.

2. Use a right subcostal incision 4 cm below the costal margin and extending from the left costal margin to the right mid-axillary line.

Assess

1. Aspirate and measure the volume of any ascitic fluid. This helps in calculating the postoperative fluid requirements.

2. Carry out a thorough exploration to exclude any other intra-abdominal pathology which may make you review the wisdom of a porta caval shunt.

3. If histological assessment of the liver pathology has not been made, take a liver biopsy.

Action

1. Mobilise and retract distally the hepatic flexure of the colon. Mobilise the duodenum using Kocher's manouevre by dividing the peritoneal reflection between it and the posterior abdominal wall which allows you to identify and expose the inferior vena cava below the liver.

2. Incise the right hand edge of the lesser omentum between liver and duodenum and identify the portal vein behind the common bile duct.

3. Dissect the portal vein free of attachments from its origin up to its bifurcation. Ligate and divide any branches. You can gain extra length by gently dissecting off the vessel the tissue of the pancreas, again doubly ligating and dividing any small pancreatic vessels entering the portal vein. During this dissection retract the common bile duct anteriorly and to the left, taking care not to damage the blood supply to its wall.

4. Pass a tape around the portal vein.

5. Dissect the anterior surface of the inferior vena cava from the suprarenal vein to the lower edge of the liver.

6. Clamp the portal vein as close to its origin as possible with a Satinsky or DeBakey clamp.

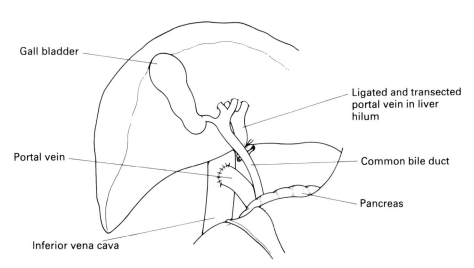

Fig. 11.7 Portacaval shunt

7. Encircle the hepatic end of the portal vein with a stout ligature and tie it firmly. Transect the portal vein cleanly immediately proximal to this ligature. Flush the now collapsed segment of portal vein distal to the clamp with a heparin, 1 : 500 000 in physiological saline solution.

8. Draw the vein to the inferior vena cava. Apply a Satinsky clamp to the anterior surface of the inferior vena cava without totally occluding the lumen.

9. Trim the end of the portal vein obliquely so that it will join the anterior wall of the inferior vena cava without kinking.

10. Remove an oval segment of the anterior wall of the inferior vena cava the same size as the oblique cut end of the portal vein.

11. Using standard vascular anastomotic techniques, suture the end of the portal vein to the side of the inferior veno cava with 4/0 Ethiflex or similar vascular suture material. Just before completing the anastomosis flush the lumen of the portal vein and the occluded segment of the inferior vena cava with heparinised saline.

12. Complete the anastomosis. Remove the clamp on the inferior vena cava followed by the clamp on the portal vein (Fig. 11.7).

Check

Ensure a good flow through the shunt by palpation of a venous thrill or observation of a measured fall in portal pressure when the clamps are removed. Ensure that haemostasis is complete.

Closure

Close the abdominal wall in a standard way, without drainage.

Aftercare

1. Manage the patient initially in the intensive care unit together with an expert medical hepatologist.

2. Water, electrolyte and colloid balance must be accurate.

3. Take steps to prevent or control portosystemic encephalopathy. In consultation with your hepatologist colleague prescribe twice daily magnesium sulphate enemata to keep the colon empty, oral lactulose when gastrointestinal activity returns at a dose producing one to two soft motions a day, and restriction of protein intake. Start at 20 gm a day and increase by 10 gm every second day if the electro-encephalogram (EEG) remains normal. In some severe cases of portosystemic encephalopathy the patient needs oral nonabsorbed antibiotics such as neomycin in addition.

SPLENORENAL SHUNT

Appraise

This operation was once considered to be superior to the portacaval shunt because it was claimed there was a lower incidence of postoperative portosystemic encephalopathy. This has not been confirmed. The incidence of thrombosis is commoner and this of course, leads to recurrence of portal hypertension and rebleeding from the oesophageal varices. It may be indicated for patients with portal vein thrombosis.

Access

1. Have the patient lying on his right side and support the pelvis and shoulder with straps.

2. Use either an extended left subcostal incision or preferably a left ninth rib thoraco-abdominal incision. This makes the operation simpler but involves subjecting the patient to the additional problems of a thoracotomy.

Assess

After opening the abdomen, as for portacaval shunt.

Action

1. Mobilise the spleen, doubly ligating and dividing all adhesions which are usually vascularised in portal hypertension. Doubly ligate and divide the short gastric vessels. The spleen will now be attached only by its main artery and vein.

2. Doubly ligate and divide the splenic artery.

3. Ligate the splenic vein close to the splenic hilum and apply a small DeBakey vascular clamp to it before its first attachment to the pancreas. Divide the vein cleanly between the vascular clamp and the ligature close to the ligature and remove the spleen.

4. Use the vascular clamp as a gentle handle and retract the splenic vein from the pancreas. Pairs of pancreatic veins will be seen entering the splenic vein. Doubly ligate and divide these individually. This is a tedious surgical procedure: carry it out slowly and meticulously. If any of these vessels is not ligated it will retract into the body of the pancreas and cause haemorrhage which may be very difficult to control.

5. Continue mobilizing the splenic vein from the upper posterior border of the pancreas towards its junction with the superior mesenteric vein until a sufficient, usually 5 cm length of vein is available to permit a curved, non-kinked anastomosis with the renal vein. Apply a second DeBakey vascular clamp close to the still attached end of the splenic

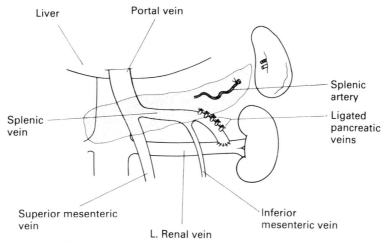

Fig. 11.8 'Linton' splenorenal shunt

vein and remove the first clamp. Flush the collapsed segment of vein with heparinized saline.

6. Identify the left kidney by palpation. Gently dissect down towards the hilum and in the region of the renal hilum identify and expose the left renal artery and vein. Be very careful not to damage any branches of the vein. Encircle the artery and vein with tapes.

7. Dissect the renal vein until sufficient vessel is exposed to permit an anastomosis with the mobilized splenic vein. If necessary adrenal, testicular or ovarian veins entering the renal vein can be doubly ligated and divided.

8. Apply a Satinsky clamp to the superior surface of the renal vein and remove an oval segment of the wall in the right place and of the right size to permit the splenorenal anastomosis. If the Satinsky clamp on the renal vein totally occludes the lumen then apply a vascular clamp to the renal artery to prevent renal engorgement. Note the time since the left kidney should not remain avascular for more than 30 minutes.

9. Anastomose the end of the splenic vein to the side of the renal vein with 5/0 Ethiflex using a conventional vascular technique (Fig. 11.8). Before completing the anastomosis flush the occluded vessels with heparinised saline.

10. Remove the renal vein clamp followed by the clamp on the splenic vein and finally the renal artery clamp.

Check

1. Confirm flow through the shunt by feeling for a local thrill or by measuring a reduction of portal pressure. There should be no kinking of the vessel after the anastomosis is complete for if there is it will thrombose.

2. Check the colour of the kidney to ensure it has revascularized.

3. Check for haemostasis.

Closure

1. Close the wound in the conventional way with no peritoneal drainage.

2. If the chest has been opened then insert an under water sealed chest drain.

Aftercare

The patient should be nursed postoperatively as a patient having a portacaval shunt.

MESOCAVAL SHUNT

Appraise

This is an easy, fast operation but since it usually employs foreign material for the shunt there is a high incidence of later thrombosis and for that reason has been largely abandoned.

Action

1. Use a transverse upper abdominal incision.

2. Identify the superior mesenteric vein and dissect it in the base of the transverse mesocolon.

3. Identify the inferior vena cava by extending the dissection in the base of the mesocolon to the right and deeply, and expose the anterior surface. The inferior part of the junction of the second and third parts of the duodenum lies between these two vessels. Mobilise this and retract it upwards.

4. Anastomose an 18 mm diameter prosthetic graft (e.g. Dacron) to the side of the superior mesenteric vein and the side of the inferior vena cava (Fig. 11.9). Some surgeons prefer to use autogenous jugular vein for this.

5. Close the wound without drainage.

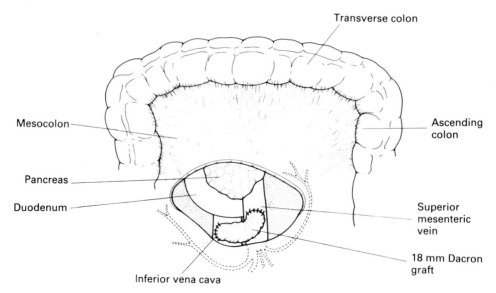

Fig. 11.9 'Drapanas' H mesocaval shunt

WARREN DISTAL SPLENORENAL SHUNT

Appraise

1. Theoretically this operation allows decompression of oesophageal varices while maintaining high pressure portal venous inflow to the liver.

2. It was designed to prevent the high incidence of encephalopathy postoperatively. However, during the early months following surgery, the incidence of encephalopathy is lower than following the other shunts. Only as the years pass the incidence comes to equal that of the other shunts. The operation is much more difficult than the alternatives and should only be undertaken by an experienced surgeon who has been taught the technique.

Action

1. Use an upper transverse abdominal incision.

2. Open the lesser sac, mobilize the lower edge of the pancreas and identify the splenic vein on its posterior superior surface. Dissect this away from the pancreas by carefully doubly ligating the paired pancreatic veins which drain into the vein. Mobilize about 5 cm of vein from its junction with the superior mesenteric vein.

3. Identify and dissect the renal vein as for a conventional splenorenal shunt.

4. Ligate the splenic vein close to its junction with the superior mesenteric vein. Place a vascular clamp on the vein, divide it and approximate the splenic end to the left renal vein.

5. Fashion an end-to-side anastomosis avoiding any kinking (Fig. 11.10).

6. Close the wound without drainage.

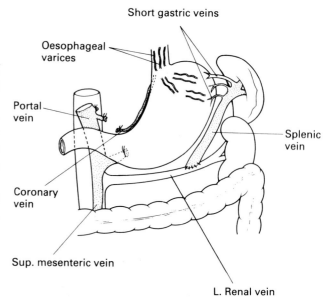

Fig. 11.10 Warren distal splenorenal shunt

Technical points

1. Additional procedures advocated by some surgeons include splenic artery ligation or ligation of the coronary vein or other large veins connecting the portal vein with the now decompressed left upper quadrant venous circulation (Fig. 11.10). These additional procedures are probably unnecessary since they do not seem to affect the long term outcome.

2. Some surgeons advocate a posterior approach to make this operation easier.

Further reading

Dudley H, Pries W, Carter D 1983 Robb and Smith's Operative surgery: Alimentary Tract and Abdominal Wall vol 2, 4th edn. Butterworth, London

Editorial 1982 Percutaneous drainage of the abdominal abscess. Lancet 1: 889–890

Mottaghian H, Saidi F 1978 Postoperative recurrence of hydatid disease. British Journal of Surgery 65: 237–242

Walt A J 1978 The mythology of hepatic trauma — or Babel revisited. Americal Journal of Surgery 135: 12–18

Wright R, Alberti KGMM, Karran S, Milward-Sadler G H 1985 Liver and Biliary Disease. 2nd edn W B Saunders, London

Surgery of the spleen

Splenectomy
Splenic conservation
Staging laparotomy

SPLENECTOMY

Appraise

1. Elective splenectomy may be indicated for certain lymphomas and leukaemias, for splenomegaly with hypersplenism and occasionally for conditions such as cyst, abscess or haemangioma. Hypersplenism can complicate primary splenomegaly (e.g. spherocytosis, idiopathic thrombocytopenic purpura) or secondary splenomegaly (e.g. malaria, portal hypertension); anaemia, other cytopenias and coagulopathies may require preoperative correction.

2. Splenectomy is routinely carried out as a part of other operations, such as total gastrectomy, radical proximal gastrectomy, distal pancreatectomy and 'conventional' splenorenal shunt.

3. Emergency splenectomy may be indicated for traumatic rupture or accidental splenic injury sustained during operations such as vagotomy or left hemicolectomy. Enlarged spleens are at increased risk of rupture, which can even occur spontaneously. Most cases of ruptured spleen follow road traffic accidents. Classically patients are shocked, with pain in the left hypochondrium and shoulder-tip and evidence of left lower rib fractures. Diagnostic paracentesis may confirm a haemoperitoneum, and urgent laparotomy is normally required after initial resuscitation. Occasionally minor splenic injuries can be managed conservatively with vigilant clinical observation and blood transfusion.

ELECTIVE SPLENECTOMY

Access

1. An upper midline or left upper paramedian incision is usually appropriate.

2. Occasionally a left thoracoabdominal approach facilitates the removal of a very large spleen.

Assess

1. Explore the whole abdomen, particularly noting the liver and any enlarged lymph nodes.

2. Make a careful search for accessory spleens (splenunculi). These are usually to be found near the splenic hilum, in the gastrosplenic ligament or greater omentum. Remove all splenunculi if splenectomy is being undertaken for a blood dyscrasia.

Action

1. If the spleen is enormous, first tie the splenic artery in continuity (Fig. 12.1). Enter the lesser sac by dividing 8–10 cm of greater omentum between ligatures, keeping to the colic side of the gastroepiploic vessels. Divide the adhesions between the back of the stomach and the front of the pancreas. Palpate along the superior border of the body of pancreas for arterial pulsation. Incise the peritoneum at this point, mobilise the vessel with right-angled forceps and ligate it with 0 or 1 silk.

2. Pass the left hand over the top of the spleen to draw it medially, and retract the left side of the abdominal wall. Coagulate and divide any adhesions between the convex surface of the spleen and the parietal peritoneum.

3. Swab any blood out of the groove behind the spleen, then cut through the peritoneum just lateral to the spleen (left leaf of the lienorenal ligament) slitting it upwards and downwards (Fig. 12.2).

4. Gently mobilise the spleen forwards and medially, using the fingers of the left hand. Identify the left colic flexure and free it from the spleen. Identify the tail of pan-

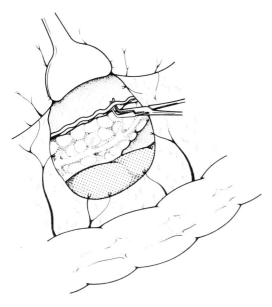

Fig. 12.1 Ligation of the splenic artery at the superior border of the body of pancreas. Part of the greater omentum has been divided allowing access to the lesser sac.

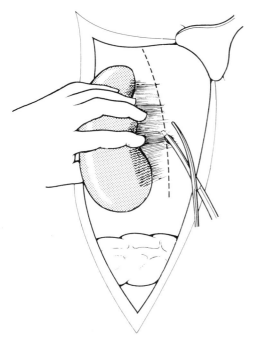

Fig. 12.2 Division of the left peritoneal leaf of the lienorenal ligament as a preliminary to mobilisation of the spleen.

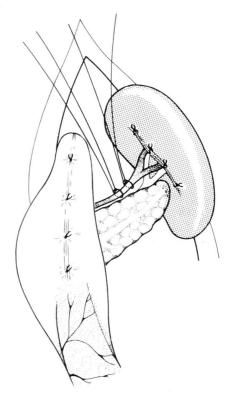

Fig. 12.3 Exposure of the splenic artery and vein after prior division of the gastrosplenic ligament. Two ligatures have been passed around the splenic artery.

creas as it turns forwards into the splenic hilum, and dissect it gently free. Place a pack in the splenic bed while completing the splenectomy.

5. Proceed to free the spleen from its attachments to the diaphragm (avascular) and greater curvature of the stomach (containing the vasa brevia). Carefully incise the anterior peritoneal leaf of the gastrosplenic ligament. Identify, ligate and divide the short gastric vessels, taking care not to include any of the stomach wall in the ligatures. Sometimes

it is easier to delay this manoeuvre until you have dealt with the splenic artery and vein.

6. Control the vascular pedicle of the spleen between fingers and thumb and dissect away the fatty tissue to expose the splenic artery and vein (Fig. 12.3). Doubly clamp, ligate and divide each vessel. Be careful not to injure the tail of pancreas at this point. After dividing the remaining peritoneal attachments (right leaf of the lienorenal ligament) the spleen can be removed.

EMERGENCY SPLENECTOMY

Access

Use a midline upper abdominal incision. Do not hesitate to make a T-shaped extension towards the left costal margin, if access is difficult and the patient is exsanguinating.

Assess

1. First check that a ruptured spleen is the source of bleeding. It is often easier to feel than to see whether the spleen is intact.

2. Remove or repair a ruptured spleen without further ado, postponing exploration of the rest of the abdomen until later.

3. Particularly in young children try to avoid total splenectomy if at all possible, for reasons explained in the next section of this chapter. If the spleen is shattered or bleeding profusely, however, you will probably have no alternative but to remove it promptly to save life.

Action

1. Quickly but carefully mobilise the spleen and bring it forwards into the abdominal wound. In ruptured spleen it is often possible to break down the left peritoneal leaf of the lienorenal ligament using your fingers. If splenic repair is at all likely, however, try to avoid further injury to the spleen during this manoeuvre.

2. Once the spleen has been brought up into the wound, compress its vascular pedicle between finger and thumb to control the bleeding. Inspect the organ thoroughly and assess the extent of damage.

3. If total splenectomy is inevitable proceed as for an elective operation, securing the splenic artery and vein at an early stage. Consider scattering a handful of splenic pulp into the splenic bed at the end of the operation to encourage splenosis. Conservative splenic operations are described later in this chapter.

Difficulty?

1. The patient is bleeding to death from the spleen, but you cannot identify the precise source of haemorrhage. There may not be time to summon senior help. Consider extending the incision as described above. Place your hand over the top of the spleen, break down its posterior attachments and deliver it into the wound as quickly as possible. Now compress or clamp the pedicle, and you will bring the situation under control.

2. You have inadvertently injured the stomach or pancreas during splenectomy, usually because of inadequate mobilisation of the spleen. Remove the spleen and place a pack in the splenic bed. Inspect the damage carefully. Repair a gastric defect in two layers. Repair or resect the tail of pancreas, using non-absorbable sutures. Ask the anaesthetist to insert a nasogastric tube and drain the splenic bed.

Closure

1. Remove the pack, inspect the splenic bed and coagulate any oozing vessels.

2. Examine the ligatures on the main vascular pedicles. Make sure that the adjacent viscera are undamaged.

3. Placed a suction drain to the splenic bed. If there is an enormous cavity or if the stomach or pancreas have been wounded, a wide-bore tube drain may be preferable.

4. Consider nasogastric intubation for 24–48 hours.

Aftercare

1. Remove the nasogastric tube when gastric aspirates diminish.

2. Check the haemoglobin, white cell and platelet counts postoperatively. Leucocytosis and thrombocythaemia nearly always ensue, with peaks at 7–14 days. Persistent leucocytosis and pyrexia may suggest a subphrenic abscess. Consider some form of prophylactic anticoagulation if the platelet count exceeds 1000×10^9/l.

3. Consider prophylactic immunisation and/or antibiotics. Young patients undergoing splenectomy for haematological diseases are at particular risk of post-splenectomy sepsis (see below).

Further reading

Cochrane J P S 1980 Ruptured spleen. British Journal of Hospital Medicine 24: 398–404
Irving M 1978 Splenectomy. British Journal of Hospital Medicine 19: 623–629
Schwartz S I 1981 Splenectomy for hematologic disease. Surgical Clinics of North America 61: 117–125

SPLENIC CONSERVATION

Appraise

1. It is now recognised that the spleen is not a superfluous organ. Its immunological function of producing opsonins (tuftsin, properdin) seems more important than its haematological function of clearing effete and abnormal erythrocytes from the circulation. Following splenectomy there is a 1.0–2.5% risk of developing overwhelming septicaemia from encapsulated bacteria (especially the pneumococcus), usually within 2 years of operation. The mortality of post-splenectomy sepsis is at least 50%. The risk is higher in young children and after splenectomy for haematological disease, but fatal cases have been reported in adults after removal of a ruptured spleen.

2. Non-operative management may be appropriate for lesser degrees of splenic injury, especially in children; repeated scintiscanning of the spleen helps to monitor progress. Embolization therapy has been attempted in hypersplenism. With these exceptions, alternatives to total splenectomy can only be assessed at laparotomy.

Assess

1. At operation for abdominal trauma a spleen that is either fragmented or avulsed from its vascular pedicle should be removed forthwith. Under these circumstances consider autotransplantation of some splenic pulp into the peritoneal cavity (see above). If the extent of damage (and bleeding) is less severe, gently mobilise the spleen into the wound after dividing its peritoneal attachments. Examine

the organ thoroughly. Decide whether topical haemostatic agents, partial splenectomy or some form of splenic repair (splenorrhaphy) might be feasible, with or without ligation of the splenic artery.

2. Capsular tears and other minor injuries to the spleen inadvertently sustained at operation seldom necessitate splenectomy. Retract or extend the incision adequately to inspect the spleen without mobilising it. Application of a haemostatic agent will usually suffice.

3. The spleen is removed along with adjacent viscera either to widen the extent of lymph-node clearance (as in gastrectomy for cancer) or for technical reasons (as in distal pancreatectomy or 'conventional' splenorenal shunt). Make sure that these indications are relevant in each individual case explored.

4. Removal of the entire organ can sometimes be avoided in certain elective operations on the spleen. Thus marsupialisation may be adequate for congenital splenic cysts and segmental splenectomy for tropical splenomegaly.

Action

1. Haemostatic applications should avoid the need for splenectomy in superficial lacerations of the capsule or splenic pulp. Full mobilisation of the spleen is unnecessary if the damaged area is accessible, but use suction to obtain a clear view. Apply an appropriate disc of gelatin sponge to the laceration and maintain light pressure until the sponge soaks up the blood and becomes adherent. Alternatively, sprinkle some microfibrillar collagen powder over the site of injury. Gently pack off the area and leave it for 5–10 minutes before checking that haemostasis has been achieved.

2. Deeper or more extensive lacerations may still be suitable for repair. Mobilise the spleen at least in part. As in operations on the liver, use catgut sutures swaged onto a long blunt needle. Take deep bites of splenic tissue on either side of the tear, and tie the sutures snugly. Use omentum or teflon buttresses to prevent the stitches cutting

through (Fig. 12.4), together with a topical haemostatic agent to control surface bleeding. Consider ligating the splenic artery along the superior border of the pancreas (see p. 214).

3. For partial splenectomy, fully mobilise the organ and carefully dissect in the splenic hilum to identify and ligate the segmental arteries and veins. Then incise the capsule at the point chosen for transection of the organ, and use a finger-fracture technique to resect the upper or lower pole (Fig. 12.4). Secure haemostasis by means of catgut sutures.

Difficulty?

If bleeding continues despite these endeavours, you should probably proceed to total splenectomy. Be sure to leave a drain to the area of the spleen following conservative operations.

Aftercare

1. Monitor the haemoglobin level and remove the drain when it ceases to function. Splenic size and function can be checked by serial scintiscans and haematological investigations.

2. Consider giving all splenectomised patients a poly-valent vaccine, which covers several types of pneumococci plus some other potential pathogens. Children, especially those under the age of 2 years, should also receive pro-phylactic penicillin for 2–3 years.

Further reading

Buntain W L, Lynn H B 1979 Splenorrhaphy: changing concepts for the traumatized spleen. Surgery 86: 748–760

Cooper M J, Williamson R C N 1983 Splenectomy: indications, hazards and alternatives. British Journal of Surgery 71: 173–180

Francke E L, New H C 1981 Postsplenectomy infection. Surgical Clinics of North America 61: 135–155

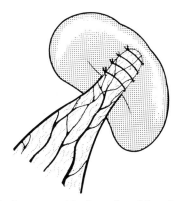 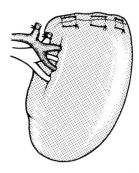

Fig. 12.4 Alternatives to total splenectomy: (a) a laceration of the splenic pulp has been sutured over a tongue of greater omentum; (b) resection of the upper pole of the spleen with ligation of its feeding vessels.

STAGING LAPAROTOMY

Appraise

1. The indications for this operation are declining as more patients with early Hodgkin's disease receive chemotherapy. Staging laparotomy still has a role in detecting occult abdominal disease in patients who might otherwise receive radiotherapy alone.

2. The operation involves splenectomy, liver biopsy and sampling of any palpable lymph nodes, especially in the upper abdomen. Bipedal lymphography can be sufficiently accurate to obviate the need for sampling nodes in the iliac or lower para-aortic chains. Bone marrow biopsy is less often required nowadays.

Action

Laparotomy

1. Through a long midline incision carry out a thorough exploration of the abdomen.

2. Remove the spleen and biopsy any nodes in the splenic hilum.

3. Remove a representative wedge of liver for histological examination (see p. 200). Obtain two needle biopsies from each lobe of the liver in addition. Examine the porta hepatis and biopsy any suspicious nodes.

4. Remove specimen lymph nodes from the coeliac, mesenteric and upper para-aortic regions and from any other groups that appear to be enlarged. Mark the site of any suspicious node with a silver clip. Put each gland in a separate container, labelled with the site of origin.

5. Consider routine appendicectomy and (in younger women) transposition of the ovaries to the midline, with suture to the uterine fundus.

6. Before closing the abdomen, remember that this operation is of no direct therapeutic benefit to the patient. Avoid the temptation to be casual, and check each area to ensure that there is no bleeding and no undue disturbance of structures.

Marrow biopsy

1. Make a 5 cm incision over the anterior part of the iliac crest. Deepen it to bone, incising the gluteal fascia just below the crest and stripping the underlying muscle to expose a small area of bone.

2. Using a gouge remove a portion of the crest (including bone marrow), tapping the gouge lightly with a mallet. Alternatively use a trephine held in a handchuck, making sure not to thrust it too powerfully into the bone.

3. Stop all bleeding, using bone wax if necessary.

4. Resuture the fascia and skin.

Further reading

Glees J P, Barr L C, McElwain T J, Peckham M J, Gazet J C 1982 The changing role of staging laparotomy in Hodgkin's disease: a personal series of 310 patients. British Journal of Surgery 69: 181–187
Miller D, Gillett R, Irving M H 1980 Is multiple lymph node biopsy essential during staging laparotomy for Hodgkin's disease? Clinical Oncology 6: 49–53

Surgery of the adrenal gland

Adrenalectomy

ADRENALECTOMY

Appraise

1. Adrenalectomy is indicated for tumours of the adrenal cortex and medulla and for some cases of bilateral cortical hyperplasia and metastatic breast (or prostatic) carcinoma. It is usually hormonal oversecretion that draws attention to an adrenal tumour, but neuroblastoma in children and a nonfunctioning adrenocortical cancer in adults can present with a mass or evidence of metastases.

2. Detailed preoperative investigation is mandatory to establish the diagnosis with certainty. Adrenal lesions can often be localised by computed tomography scans, ^{131}I-cholesterol scintiscans, intravenous urograms and arteriograms.

3. Features of Cushing's syndrome include hypertension, osteoporosis, glycosuria, hirsutism and an altered distribution of body fat. Much commoner in women, the syndrome results **either** from excess adrenocorticotropin (ACTH) secreted by the pituitary (adenoma, hyperplasia) or an ectopic site (e.g. bronchial carcinoma) **or** from an autonomous adrenocortical tumour (benign or malignant). Cushing's syndrome is confirmed by finding raised plasma and urinary levels of cortisol, which are not suppressed by dexamethasone. The plasma concentration of ACTH helps to distinguish the underlying lesion. Pituitary tumours are best treated by irradiation or surgical excision, but total bilateral adrenalectomy is sometimes required. Adrenocortical tumours require adrenalectomy, which can usually be unilateral.

4. Primary hyperaldosteronism (Conn's syndrome) causes hypokalaemia and moderate hypertension. About 80% of patients have a small, solitary adrenal adenoma, the rest having multiple adenomas, carcinoma or bilateral cortical hyperplasia. Unlike in secondary hyperaldosteronism, plasma renin values are low. Hypokalaemic alkalosis must be corrected preoperatively. Adenomas should be removed, but hyperplasia can often be controlled by spironolactone. Unilateral exploration is indicated for a tumour that can be localised. Otherwise bilateral exploration is needed, with total (or subtotal) removal of adrenal tissue in hyperplasia.

5. Phaeochromocytoma causes episodic or sustained hypertension with features of sympathetic overactivity (headache, sweating, palpitations). A benign tumour of the adrenal medulla is usually responsible, but multiple, malignant and extra-adrenal tumours also occur, especially in children. Elevated levels of catecholamines or their derivates are found in the blood and urine. Phenoxybenzamine should be given, followed by propranolol, to produce full alpha- and beta-adrenergic blockade. Then, but only then, both adrenals should be explored. At operation, arterial pressure and cardiac function should be closely monitored, and the surgeon should avoid manipulating the tumour more than is essential until the major draining veins have been ligated.

6. Rarely virilisation or feminisation result from adrenal tumours, many of which are malignant; excision is required. Congenital adrenal hyperplasia can cause virilisation and Cushing's syndrome in young girls and may be controlled by hormonal manipulation.

Access

Choice of approach

1. Select an anterior transperitoneal approach to obtain good exposure of both adrenal glands through the same incision. Use this route for bilateral adrenal disease, for large tumours such as many phaeochromocytomas, and if you plan concomitant oophorectomy for advanced breast cancer. Some degree of postoperative ileus is inevitable, however.

2. A lateral approach through the 12th rib bed is ideal for a unilateral adrenocortical adenoma that has been localised preoperatively. The retroperitoneal subpleural route causes little or no interference with intestinal motility

and is particularly useful in the obese or where poor healing is anticipated, e.g. in Cushing's syndrome. If necessary, turn the patient after completing unilateral adrenalectomy, and explore the opposite side through a symmetrical incision.

3. A lateral thoracoabdominal approach is occasionally indicated for a very large adrenal tumour. Place the patient in the anterolateral position. Expose the right adrenal through the bed of the 9th or 10th rib, incising the diaphragm and displacing the liver upwards into the chest. Expose the left adrenal by an extrapleural approach through the bed of the 11th rib. You may need to excise en bloc contiguous organs such as the kidney, spleen or tail of pancreas for invasive carcinoma of the adrenal.

4. Separate posterior incisions with the patient lying prone offer an alternative approach for bilateral adrenalectomy in thin patients. Expose each gland through the bed of the 11th or 12th rib, but remember that access is likely to be restricted.

5. Only the anterior and lateral approaches are described further, since these are generally most suitable for surgeons with limited experience of adrenalectomy. For either incision use a pelvic strap to secure the patient to the operating table.

Anterior approach

1. Use a long transverse supraumbilical incision with a gentle upwards convexity (the 'low gable' incision). It may help to break the table slightly so as to stretch the retroperitoneal tissues.

2. After completing a thorough laparotomy and removing the ovaries (if indicated), direct your attention to each adrenal gland in turn. Stand on the side of the table opposite the gland to be removed, and tilt the table towards yourself by 20°. Pack off the small intestine and colon, and get your assistant to retract the costal margin.

3. Approach the **left** adrenal gland as follows. Enter the lesser sac by ligating and dividing 10–15 cm of greater omentum. Retract the stomach upwards and incise the peritoneum along the lower border of the body and tail of pancreas. Using blunt dissection, gently mobilise the pancreas and splenic vein upwards to display the upper pole of the kidney.

4. Alternatively, approach the **left** adrenal gland as follows. Place a hand over the spleen and incise the left peritoneal leaf of the lienorenal ligament. Now carefully mobilise the spleen and tail of pancreas and displace them downwards to reach the upper pole of the kidney.

5. Approach the **right** adrenal gland as follows. Mobilise the right colic flexure. Displace the colon downwards and the liver upwards, and identify the inferior vena cava deep to the duodenum. Steady the right kidney with your left hand and incise the posterior parietal peritoneum immediately above its upper pole, i.e. directly over the adrenal.

Lateral approach

1. Place the patient in the full lateral position with the lower ribs sited over the break in the table. Jack-knife the table to open up the gap between the 12th rib and the iliac crest. Remember that the ribs can be fragile in Cushing's syndrome.

2. Make an incision over the 12th rib, starting posteriorly at the edge of the erector spinae muscles and continuing obliquely forwards onto the abdominal wall. Deepen the incision down to the rib and identify its free anterior end. Free the rib from its muscular attachments and elevate the periosteum; try to avoid injuring the subcostal vessels and nerve.

3. Resect the rib. Incise its bed and divide the origin of the diaphragm. Take care not to damage the pleura, which should be reflected gently upwards. An audible hiss indicates that the pleura has been opened. Ask the anaesthetist to inflate the lung, and close the defect with 2/0 catgut sutures before proceeding.

4. Extend the incision forwards through the muscles of the anterior abdominal wall. Insert a self-retaining retractor to open the wound widely. Incise the renal fascia to expose the upper pole of the kidney.

5. Alternatively, use an approach through the bed of the 11th rib. The procedure is essentially the same, except that even greater care is needed to avoid entering the pleura.

Action

Identifying the adrenals

1. Each adrenal gland lies on the relevant diphragmatic crus, separated from the kidney by perinephric fat and fascia. Whereas the right adrenal caps the upper pole of the kidney, the left adrenal is related to its upper medial border (Fig. 13.1).

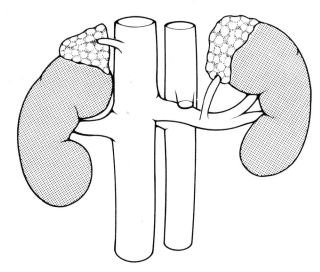

Fig. 13.1 Position and venous drainage of the adrenal glands.

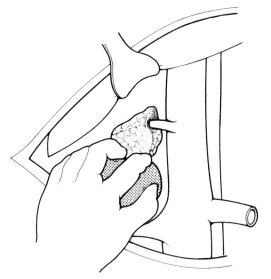

Fig. 13.2 Exposure of the right adrenal vein, which enters the inferior vena cava directly after a short extraglandular course.

2. The adrenal has a characteristic firm consistency on palpation and a yellow-ochre colour on inspection.

Right adrenalectomy

1. The gland is attached to the lateral border of the inferior vena cava by a short (5 mm) and relatively wide adrenal vein. Use pledgets to dissect gently between the cava and the gland to identify this vein, which should then be ligated and divided (Fig. 13.2). The adrenal arteries are small and variable and can usually be cauterised with diathermy.

2. Mobilise the lateral border of the gland, using blunt dissection. Divide any residual, tenuous attachments and remove the adrenal.

Left adrenalectomy

1. Again the vein is usually solitary, but it is longer (2–3 cm) than on the right and it enters the left renal vein. Secure it at its point of entry into the renal vein.

2. Mobilise the gland laterally and cauterise its fine, medial arterial attachments before removal.

Difficulty?

Brisk venous haemorrhage ensues if the right adrenal vein is avulsed from the cava. Pack the wound and ensure that you have adequate exposure. Consider proceeding to left adrenalectomy before removing the pack. When ready, use the sucker to identify the damage. If the cava has already been mobilised, it may be possible to apply a vascular clamp tangentially to control the bleeding. If not, a pair of Allis forceps may be applied directly to the vein to occlude the defect. Once you have controlled the bleeding, suture the defect in the cava with 5/0 Prolene.

Closure

1. Search for any ectopic adrenal tissue. Check that haemostasis is secure. Place a fine suction drain to the adrenal bed on either side if you have removed a sizeable gland or encountered troublesome bleeding.

2. Straighten the table. Close the wound in layers.

Aftercare

1. Unilateral adrenalectomy does not require perioperative corticosteroid therapy. Removal of an aldosteronoma occasionally causes temporary aldosterone deficiency (hypotension, hyperkalaemia), because the tumour has suppressed function of the normal gland. Give fludrocortisone (0.1 mg/day orally) until endogenous secretion of mineralocorticoids is restored.

2. Bilateral adrenalectomy demands adequate steroid replacement therapy for the rest of the patient's life. Start hydrocortisone hemisuccinate (100 mg 8-hourly i.v.) immediately after operation, and halve the dose after 24–48 hours. Convert the patient to oral hydrocortisone when free fluids can be taken by mouth, and gradually reduce the dose towards a maintenance level of about 30 mg/day. Add fludrocortisone (0.1 mg/day) when the dose of hydrocortisone drops below 50 mg/day. Increase the dose of steroids if postoperative complications develop. Before the patient leaves hospital, explain the crucial importance of this replacement therapy, including the need to increase the dose in the presence of systemic infection.

Further reading

Delaney J P 1978 Surgical management of Cushing's syndrome. Surgery 84: 465–475
Kerwig K R 1979 Primary aldosteronism: experience with 38 patients. Surgery 86: 470–474
Modlin I M 1979 Phaeochromocytomas in 72 patients: clinical and diagnostic features, treatment and long term results. British Journal of Surgery 66: 456–465
Hunt T K, Biglieri E G, Roizen M F, Tyrrell J B 1983 Adrenals. In: Way L W (ed) Current Surgical Diagnosis and Treatment, 6th edn. Lange, Los Altos, p. 683–695

Surgery of the upper urinary tract

INTRODUCTION: UROLOGICAL OPERATIONS

The practice of urology has grown out of the field of general surgery. There are several branches in which specialization occurs from within the scope of general urology, for instance paediatric urology, urological oncology, dialysis, and transplantation.

For the surgeon training in general surgery it is essential to have a knowledge of urology. Likewise, a urologist cannot escape a wide training first in general surgery. To practise urology in its fullest extent a knowledge of bowel, vascular, plastic and paediatric surgery is essential, as well as a knowledge of the management of renal failure. The urologist must be a very versatile man.

The general surgeon working away from a urological unit must be able to manage urinary retentions, simple strictures, stones, and trauma to the urinary tract. When faced with urinary tract tumours the general surgeon must be in a position to know which cases he can deal with, for instance simple papillary tumours, and which cases must be referred. The outcome in the majority will usually depend on the initial treatment.

Thus, the general surgeon practising urology has to be constantly aware of his limitations and be prepared to refer those cases which require specialist care. A knowledge of the possible outcome in difficult cases is a strong indicator when considering referral.

PAEDIATRIC AND CONGENITAL PROBLEMS

These procedures should be undertaken only by a specialist urologist in this field. To acquaint yourself with these procedures, other texts must be referred to, such as 'Paediatric Urology' (D Innes Williams (ed) 1968 Butterworth London).

SIMPLE NEPHRECTOMY

Appraise

This is indicated especially for gross hydronephrosis, pyonephrosis, severe calculous disease, chronic pyelonephritis.

Access

1. Position the patient so that the side to be operated on is not only uppermost but right up to the edge of the operating table. Have the break in the table under the lowermost ribs. It is pointless to have the break at the patient's waist, as this will not open up the flank. Break the table so that the shoulder and buttock are just resting on the surface. Maintain the position with suitable restrainers and an arm rest. Do not allow the patient to roll forward as this makes access difficult. Make sure the lower arm is not compressed by the patient's weight. Be sure that you are fully satisfied with the position before you scrub up.

2. The approach to the kidney: there are various incisions which may be used. In children, a lumbar incision

below the 12th rib is usually all that is necessary. This divides successively the external oblique, internal oblique and transversus abdominis. Beneath this will be the lumbar fascia and once you have incised this, the perirenal fat will be exposed. Divide all these below and in line with the 12th rib. In the adult this incision is usually insufficient, unless there is a very small 12th rib, as you will find yourself approaching the kidney from below. In this case it is better to cut down on to the 12th rib, denude it of periosteum and remove it with bone cutters. It is important to get as far back and as high as possible in approaching the kidney. The anterior part of the incision is often made unnecessarily long. The best incision if you are experienced in the technique is a supra-12th rib incision, leaving the rib and stripping the pleura and diaphragm away from the inner surface until the tubercle can be felt. Now incise with a diathermy point along the upper border of the rib until you can feel the superior costotransverse ligament as a sharp band running upward from the back end of the rib. Once you have divided this with scissors, the whole rib will fall down and afford great exposure.

3. Whichever technique you choose, once you have either excised or dislocated the 12th rib, carry the incision forward for about 8 cm dividing all the muscles as described. A large self-retaining retractor is very helpful.

Action

1. Using fingers as dissectors, widen the incision in the lumbar fascia and separate the perirenal fat from the kidney.

2. Grasp the kidney with the left hand and gently strip the fat off in all directions, using large blunt dissecting forceps. In cases of gross calculous disease many adhesions will be found, particularly round the pelvis of the kidney. Identify the vascular pedicle, clamp and divide the artery and the vein. The kidney will now be free and the ureter identified. Clamp the ureter and remove the kidney.

3. Close the wound with through-and-through interrupted 1 chromic catgut, or else close each muscle layer in turn with a continuous suture. Unbreak the table during this procedure. If there is any oozing or infection, leave in a tube drain attached to a drainage bag.

Difficulty?

1. Always beware of the pleura. Should you make a hole in it, the easiest manoeuvre to re-expand the lung is to place a simple catheter into the pleural cavity and completely close the wound including the skin. Now dip the catheter into a jug of sterile water and get the anaesthetist to forcibly inflate the lungs; when the bubbles cease to flow on full inflation, remove the catheter. The hole will automatically seal itself.

2. With a gross hydronephrosis always aspirate first.

This will shrink the kidney down to a manageable size and make nephrectomy easier.

3. Look out for polar vessels and double vascular pedicles.

4. Try to avoid a mass ligature round the pedicle. However, with a pyonephrosis it may be impossible to adequately define the artery and vein, and a mass ligature is the only way out.

5. If you should damage one of the great vessels, simply pack firmly around to stop the bleeding. Wait a few minutes and then gently remove the packs. The bleeding vessel will usually be evident and can be picked up with a large curved artery forceps.

PARTIAL NEPHRECTOMY

Appraise

1. A hemi- or partial nephrectomy is rarely practised these days. The commonest indication is where the lower pole of the kidney is removed along with a dilated lower group of calyces containing stones. Less common indications are for residual calyceal dilatation or cavities after adequate antituberculous chemotherapy and rarely in the removal of a hypernephroma in a solitary kidney.

2. A partial nephrectomy is an integral part of a heminephro-ureterectomy in cases of ectopic duplex systems causing problems.

Prepare

1. An aortogram may give very useful information about the arterial distribution to the kidney.

2. Local renal hypothermia or the intravenous injection of Inosine and arterial clamping may be essential adjuncts, especially in solitary kidneys.

3. In really hazardous cases, refer the patient to a centre with dialysis facilities.

Action

1. Obtain adequate exposure and identify the vessels.

2. In duplex systems where one half is to be ablated, the problem is easier, as clamping the artery to the half to be removed will demonstrate the line of demarcation.

3. Try to identify the vessels to the pole to be removed so that these can be ligated.

4. Strip the capsule off the affected part if feasible.

5. The amount of renal tissue to be removed will depend on the condition and extent of the disease. If possible, amputate the pole in a wedge-shaped fashion to facilitate repair (Fig. 14.1).

6. Secure individual bleeding points by underrunning with fine catgut.

7. Repair the pelvicalyceal system.

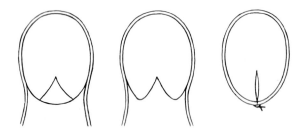

Fig. 14.1 Partial nephrectomy

8. Approximate the stripped capsule if possible; this will bring the surfaces of the wedge together.

9. Always drain.

RADICAL NEPHRECTOMY

Appraise

1. Radical nephrectomy is undertaken for renal cell carcinoma. It entails removing not only the kidney but also its complete envelope of surrounding fat; this will include the suprarenal gland. It is sometimes necessary to remove part of the diaphragm, back muscles, peritoneum, the spleen and even bowel. This is in order not to disturb the tumour should it have penetrated the capsule into the perinephric tissues. A para-aortic node dissection is also carried out.

2. In this procedure one must also anticipate intentionally opening the inferior vena cava, particularly with tumours on the right. Pre-operative assessment is often of great help in deciding which approach is the most appropriate. There is, unfortunately, considerable controversy as to which is the best exposure as each approach has its own merits.

3. In the very large, and presumably very vascular tumours, considerable advantage can be obtained by arterial vascular occlusion as a preliminary to the operation. This can be achieved by passing a trans-femoral catheter selectively into the renal artery and embolising the artery completely using a combination of gel-foam or autologous clot and/or combining this with small metal springs. In order to reduce the vascularity of the tumour, this can be done immediately pre-operatively. There is speculation that this may have an additional immunological benefit to patients, in that 'dead' embolised kidney and tumour tissue is left in-situ for 4–7 days. However, leaving the patient for these number of days following embolisation may well render the operation much more difficult and also lead to considerable pain and discomfort. The validity of the claim for better results in these cases is very doubtful, and the author has, himself, abandoned all such techniques.

ABDOMINAL APPROACH

1. A long midline, paramedian or transverse incision may be used. Carry out a preliminary laparotomy. Even in the presence of secondary deposits, unless they are very widespread, perform a nephrectomy if possible.

2. Isolate the vascular pedicle and divide the vein and artery separately. This necessitates mobilization of the bowel.

3. The kidney with its envelope of tissue is now dissected free and removed.

4. The merit of this approach is with left-sided tumours when it is suspected that the inferior vena cava may have to be opened.

LOIN APPROACHES

There are two ways of reaching the kidney from the loin.

Supra-12th or 11th rib incision

1. This really gives an excellent exposure, and it can be easily extended anteriorly if necessary. Approach the kidney from behind, mobilizing the whole fatty envelope posteriorly until the vessels are reached and ligated. At this stage the dissection is carried out superiorly and inferiorly, and finally the whole mass is dissected free from in front.

2. Difficulty is often experienced with large aberrant veins which have to be divided separately in order to dissect the mass free. From this approach the peritoneum can be opened for a laparotomy and part of the diaphragm and other structures excised if necessary. It gives an excellent view for node dissection. However, on the left side the inferior vena cava is inaccessible.

Nagamatsu incision.

1. Here the 12th rib is removed as far back as possible and a 2–3 cm segment of the midportion of the 11th and 10th ribs is excised.

2. The skin incision for this approach is 'hockey-stick' shaped, along the line of the 12th rib and then extending upward for an appropriate distance to expose the 11th and 10th ribs. The incision is then carried forward into the loin.

3. The diaphragm is separated from its lateral attachments and a very wide exposure is afforded. It is highly suitable for upper pole tumours, but again there is the problem of the inferior vena cava on the left side.

THORACOLUMBAR APPROACH

This approach gives the widest exposure of all; it is especially useful in very large upper pole lesions. If the incision is carried across the abdomen far enough and the patient suitably positioned, the inferior vena cava is accessible from both sides.

Difficulty?

1. In all cases of hypernephroma, one of the main operative problems is controlling the bleeding which may occur from the often very large thin-walled aberrant veins.

2. It is always said that the renal vein should be exposed and ligated first. This may be difficult or even impossible and is probably not important. In fact, by ligating the renal artery first, the vascularity of the kidney is considerably reduced and this may be preferable.

3. With very large tumours it is wise to have a bowel preparation as occasionally it is necessary to remove a segment of bowel with the tumour mass.

4. In polycythaemic patients preoperative control of the polycythaemia is essential and time should be taken to allow the vascular tone to recover.

NEPHROURETERECTOMY
A. FOR TRANSITIONAL CELL TUMOURS OF THE RENAL PELVIS AND/OR URETER

Appraise

It has for a long time been taught that transitional cell tumours in the upper tracts should be treated by a total clearance on that side, unless it was a solitary system. Considerable doubt has been thrown on to the validity of this approach, and where possible a conservative 'renal preserving' operation is used. The author has practised this conservative ideal for over a decade, with no untoward problems. Such cases, however, must be dealt with in specialised centres.

Action

1. Perform a preliminary cystoscopy to establish that the bladder is clear; remember this is potentially a panurothelial disease. If necessary perform a bulb ureterogram.

2. Position the patient for a nephrectomy from the loin.

3. Complete the nephrectomy and node dissection and free the ureter as far down as is possible, but do not divide it. Tuck the kidney down into the space formed by the exploration. Close the wound.

4. Reposition the patient for a lower abdominal exploration.

5. Through an extended Pfannenstiel or long lower muscle cutting incision, expose the lower ureter and place a sling around it. Retrieve the kidney and ureter from above and continue freeing the ureter down to the bladder. bladder.

6. Mobilize the side of the bladder and perform a partial cystectomy so as to remove the intramural part of the ureter.

7. Wash with distilled water and close the bladder with an indwelling urethral catheter.

Difficulty?

1. With a renal pelvic tumour, always explore the kidney first to establish its local operability. The reverse applies to a lower ureteric tumour.

2. If the kidney is too large to tuck down into the loin, it may be enclosed in a sterile glove and left hanging outside the incision, closing the wound around it.

3. To get good histology, always distend the specimen with formal saline and tie off the lower end.

4. As this is a panurothelial disease, more conservative procedures such as local removal of tumours from the renal pelvis, partial ureterectomies and partial nephrectomies may have to be considered. This is particularly pertinent when the opposite kidney has previously been removed. Each case must be treated on its own merits.

B. FOR TUBERCULOSIS

This operation is essentially the same procedure as for transitional cell tumours. There is no need to perform a node dissection. The ureter should only be taken down as far as the bladder wall, obviating the necessity of opening the bladder.

URETEROLITHOTOMY

Appraise

1. Single stones can obstruct the ureter or become arrested in their descent.

2. Arrest occurs commonly at three sites:
(a) The pelviureteric junction or upper third of the ureter.
(b) The junction of the middle and lower third of the ureter where it crosses the ala of the sacrum.
(c) The lower end of the ureter.

3. Each of these requires a different approach. It is a mistake to compromise on the incision.

4. In all cases have a plain X-ray taken immediately prior to operation to make sure the stone has not moved. If you cannot locate the stone at operation, do not hesitate to X-ray at the time.

STONES IN THE UPPER END OF THE URETER.

Action

1. Expose as for a simple nephrectomy. The whole kidney need not be mobilized. Search for the ureter and pass two small tapes round it above and below the stone.

2. Incise on to the stone longitudinally with a small knife. Having removed the stone, it is traditional to pass a small plastic bougie up into the kidney and down into the bladder. This manoeuvre has no merit if there is a single stone and may indeed do damage. If there is more than one stone, it can help to locate the level of a lower one.

3. Leave the ureteric incision wide open with a tube drain down to the site of removal.

STONES OVER THE ALA OF THE SACRUM

Action

1. Make a classical gridiron incision down to the peritoneum. Do not incise the peritoneum, but sweep it aside so that your fingers can be inserted between the peritoneum and the transversus and internal oblique muscles.

2. Cut these muscles in the line of the external oblique both upward and downward. This will give a wide exposure.

3. Sweep the peritoneum medially so exposing the retroperitoneal structures. Search for the ureter and place a tape round it above the stone. It is unusual for the stone to escape downward.

4. Incise over the stone as before.

5. Close the wound round a tube drain.

Difficulty?

1. In the first instance with a stone in the upper part of the ureter it can be a nuisance if the stone slips back into the pelvis. By using a renal exposure, a simple pyelolithotomy will overcome this hazard should it occur.

2. Should there be difficulty locating the ureter in its lower third, remember it usually strips forward with the peritoneum. Another landmark is the bifurcation of the common iliac artery at which point the ureter will cross.

3. Do not be tempted to remove stones in 'in-between' positions with an inadequate incision. A reasonable compromise incision for stones midway between these two sites is that for a lumbar sympathectomy.

STONES IMPACTED AT THE LOWER END OF THE URETER

This is a difficult operation and should you have any doubt, refer the case to a urologist.

Action

1. An extended Pfannenstiel incision will expose the bladder extra-peritoneally.

2. If the bladder is full, empty it with a wide-bore aspiration needle attached to the sucker.

3. Mobilize the bladder toward the midline on the appropriate side and seek the ureter, taping it.

4. Divide the superior vesical pedicle, and in the male mobilize the vas. This enables the bladder to be retracted medially.

5. Trace the ureter down, taking care not to apply too much traction, as it can be avulsed from the bladder.

6. Locate the stone by palpation and cut down on to it from behind.

7. Close the wound with a tube drain.

Difficulty?

1. If the stone is exceedingly low, it is preferable after locating it to incise the ureter 1–2 cm above where it can be visualized. Pass a long pair of stone extracting forceps, of the Turner-Warwick variety, down the ureter and remove the stone from above. When this manoeuvre is adopted, it is necessary to pass a bougie downward as small fragments may break off which can obstruct the intramural ureter. The bougie will push them into the bladder.

2. This procedure requires considerable manipulation and the stone may be dislodged upward. A tape or small arterial bulldog clip round the ureter well above the stone is essential.

3. Adequate exposure and good retraction make this procedure easier.

Closure

1. Never close the ureter.
2. Always drain

ENDOSCOPIC STONE EXTRACTION

For stones which get impacted in the lower 2–3 cm of intramural ureter, various endoscopic techniques can be used.

INTRAMURAL STONES

Here the stone is seen to bulge the intramural ureter or may even be seen emerging from the orifice. In these cases the ureteric orifice may be slit up with a diathermy knife, so releasing the stone into the bladder. An alternative technique is gently to use the resectoscope to resect the lower part of the orifice, again releasing the stone. If the latter procedure has been used, it is usually possible to extricate the stone completely with the loop. Otherwise it will have to be washed out with an evacuator.

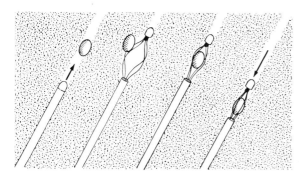

Fig. 14.2 Dormia basket extraction of ureteric stone

STONES IN THE LOWER 2–3 CM OF THE URETER

For these stones a ureteric stone extractor is used, usually the Dormia basket and preferably under image intensifier control. Pass the extractor up just beyond the stone, open the basket and under visual control attempt to engage the stone in the opened basket. Once this has happened, gently close the basket and retrieve the extractor and stone from the orifice (Fig. 14.2).

Difficulty?

1. Do not use the basket for stones bigger than 0.5 cm in diameter.

2. Do not attempt this for a stone higher than 2–3 cm, or at most 4 cm above the orifice. Severe ureteric damage may occur if the basket is used in cases of high stone.

3. If there is difficulty in getting the extractor and stone out of the orifice, do not pull fiercely but apply gentle but continuous traction over several minutes.

4. If the extractor and stone cannot be released from the orifice, detach the extractor from the cystoscope and leave it in situ. It will usually be found lying free in the bladder the following day.

5. If several attempts to engage the stone have failed, then abandon the procedure. The stone may well have been dislodged and will often pass spontaneously over the next few days.

EXTRACTION OF STONES USING THE RIGID URETEROSCOPE

In well equipped departments, since the introduction of the ureteroscope, the visual retrieval of stones from the ureter has become possible. Even stones high up in the ureter can be extracted. The handling of this instrument must be left to the expert, as great damage can be inflicted.

SIMPLE PYELOLITHOTOMY

Appraise

1. This operation is indicated for the removal of simple stones from the renal pelvis or a stone impacted at the pelviureteric junction.

2. The removal of staghorn calculi and multiple stones in the pelvis and calyces should be referred to someone with specialist training.

Action

1. Expose and mobilize the kidney as for a simple nephrectomy.

2. Hold the kidney forward and expose the pelvis from behind. The plane between the sinus of the kidney and pelvis should be entered; it is usually free of adhesions.

3. Clean all the fatty tissue off the pelvis, and identify the pelvi-ureteric junction.

4. Incise the pelvis longitudinally over a sufficient length to remove the stone(s).

5. If the incision is extensive it should be approximated with one or two fine chromic catgut sutures. Never close the incision tightly. If the incision is short then leave it open.

6. Close the wound with a wide-bore tube drain down to the renal bed, attached to a drainage bag.

Difficulty?

1. The pyelographic appearances will indicate if there is any degree of idiopathic hydronephrosis associated with the stone. If this is the case, then some form of pyeloplasty must be undertaken. This type of case should be referred to a urologist.

2. There may be very dense adhesions surrounding the pelvis. The posterior approach avoids endangering the major vessels.

3. With a large but simple stone, i.e. not a staghorn calculus, it may be difficult to deliver the stone out of the pelvis without carrying the incision across the pelviureteric junction. The incision over this junction should not be sewn up.

4. If the stone is small it may disappear into one of the calyces; if there is any difficulty in locating it, do not hesitate to X-ray the kidney with special renal plates.

5. A stone which is entirely within a calyx is best left to a specialist. If, however, having exposed the kidney you find the stone to be a calyceal one, it is best to make a small radial incision over the stone of sufficient size to remove it. Do not attempt to dilate the calyceal neck and drag the stone out that way. Close the small nephrotomy incision with fine chromic catgut through the cortex and capsule of the kidney.

APPROACHES FOR STAGHORN OR RECURRENT RENAL CALCULI

Appraise

1. These operations are difficult, so adequate operating time should be allowed. Meticulous care must be taken to mobilize the kidney. There are two reasonably standard methods in use. One is to isolate and clamp the renal arterial supply with small bulldog artery clips and then to employ local renal hypothermia, dropping the kidney temperature to the region of 15–20°C monitored by thermocouple probes. There are various cooling coils on the market. This procedure allows for ample operating time in a bloodless field to search for and remove all the calculi, both from the pelvis and through separate nephrotomy incisions where necessary. Alternatively, the anti-metabolite 'Inosine' can be injected into a peripheral vein, and the renal artery subsequently clamped. This again gives a reasonable margin of safety, with warm ischaemia.

2. The second approach is to use the Gil-Vernet method. The Gil-Vernet plane is in the renal sinus, between the kidney and the pelvis along with its attached fat and fibrous tissue. By dissecting into this plane one can usually establish an excellent view of the pelvis and often the calyceal necks.

3. The actual removal of the stones must depend on their size and shape and the configuration of the renal collecting system. It may well be necessary to cut through the necks of the staghorns, and remove the horns through separate radial nephrotomy incisions. This is far preferable to dilating the calyceal necks and dragging the stones through. It is mandatory to perform these difficult stone-removing operations using X-ray control. It is surprising how easy it is to miss quite large fragments. Flushing out each individual major calyx after operation is necessary to remove any remaining dust. Some urologists employ the daily instillation of Renacidin for about a week through a nephrostomy tube in an effort to dissolve these particles; should the patient experience renal pain during this technique it should be stopped immediately.

NON-OPERATIVE REMOVAL OR RENAL CALCULI

PERCUTANEOUS EXTRACTION

Appraise

1. Since endoscopic instruments have become so sophisticated, this has led to the development of the nephroscope. In expert hands and in suitable cases this instrument renders removal of renal calculi, even quite large ones, a very short procedure.

2. By performing a preliminary percutaneous nephrostomy, a standard procedure in most urological departments, a nephroscope can be introduced into the kidney.

This may need successive dilatations of the nephrostomy opening over a period of 4 or 5 days in order to allow sufficient size for the instrument to be introduced. Small stones can be extracted with forceps or loops, using this technique. Bigger stones can be tackled in exactly the same way, but first they have to be broken up, utilising an ultrasonic disintegrator and subsequently extracting and washing out the fragments and dust.

3. Such techniques are in their infancy, and of necessity are confined to a few specialised units.

EXTRA-CORPOREAL SHOCK WAVE LITHOTRIPSY (ESWL)

This of necessity is exceedingly specialised and also exceptionally expensive. The anaesthetised patient is placed in a special water bath. The stone is accurately pinpointed, using two X-ray probes, and then shock-waves are directed at the stone, which will disintegrate. The fragments are subsequently passed by the patient. Again, this technique is in its infancy.

NEPHROSTOMY AND PYELOSTOMY

Appraise

1. Nephrostomy is indicated as a drainage procedure after a formal operation on the kidney or pelvis, such as the repair of a hydronephrosis.

2. It may be used in an emergency to decompress an acutely obstructed kidney.

3. Refer to a urologist urgently a patient with a grossly obstructed upper tract, to establish preliminary drainage before operative relief of the obstruction. This is often bilateral and will mainly apply to children.

NEPHROSTOMY AS PART OF A FORMAL RENAL OPERATION

Action

1. Through the pelvic incision insert a curved artery forceps into the middle group of calyces (Fig. 14.3.).

2. Once the forceps have reached the renal substance, force it through to the outer surface.

3. Grasp the tip of a small Malecot catheter and by pulling on the Malecot flatten the wings (Fig. 14.4).

4. Pull the forceps back into the kidney and relax the traction on the catheter. Release the forceps and withdraw them. The Malecot will now be situated in the pelvis (Fig. 14.5).

5. Anchor the catheter with a small catgut suture in the capsule.

6. Complete the original procedure.

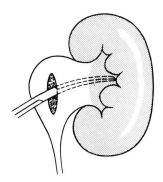

Fig. 14.3 Nephrostomy

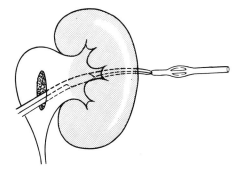

Fig. 14.4 Nephrostomy

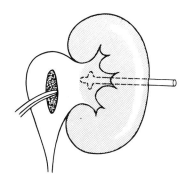

Fig. 14.5 Nephrostomy

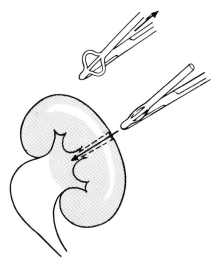

Fig. 14.6 Nephrostomy

You will find the perirenal tissues oedematous and the kidney swollen.

2. Make a 0.5 cm incision into the capsule over the convex border and thrust a large pair of straight artery forceps directly into the renal parenchyma and so into the pelvis. This will form a pathway for the catheter.

3. Take a small pair of artery forceps and grasp the tip of a small Malecot catheter. Stretch the Malecot catheter backward along the length of the forceps so flattening the wings (Fig. 14.6).

4. Thrust the fine forceps and the flattened catheter down the track into the pelvis, relax the tension on the catheter and release the forceps.

5. Anchor with a fine catgut suture to the capsule.

NEPHROSTOMY AS A PLANNED DRAINAGE PROCEDURE

This may be bilateral and is usually done for severe obstructive disease before reconstructive surgery is undertaken. It is often necessary in childhood obstructive uropathy and should be left to a urologist.

The technique is similar to the previous two, care being taken to preserve as much renal tissue as possible.

PYELOSTOMY

This is a similar drainage procedure to a nephrostomy, but the catheter is brought out from the renal pelvis. It has the advantage that no renal tissue is damaged. The disadvantages are that it needs greater renal mobilization than for a simple nephrostomy, there is not such direct urinary drainage and catheter kinking can occur.

NEPHROSTOMY AS AN EMERGENCY PROCEDURE FOR AN ACUTELY OBSTRUCTED KIDNEY.

1. In the majority of instances, with a good uro-radiologist, there is no need for an emergency operation to drain an acutely obstructed kidney.

2. Percutaneous nephrostomy under X-ray control is now virtually routine. Where such expertise is not available, the following standard procedure must be employed.

Action

1. Make a loin incision below the 12th rib. Allow sufficient length to expose the convex border of the kidney.

DRAINAGE OF PERINEPHRIC ABSCESS

Appraise

Perinephric abscess is becoming a rarity. It is usually the result of a pyonephrosis, and in this instance the safest procedure is a preliminary drainage followed by a nephrectomy.

Action

1. Position the patient as for a nephrectomy.
2. Make a short incision below the 12th rib.
3. The tissues will often be oedematous and rather wooden.
4. Expose down to the perinephric space. Pus will usually gush out once this has been reached.
5. Pass the forefinger through the incision and into the abscess cavity. This will usually lead straight into the kidney in cases resulting from pyonephrosis. Sweep the finger around to make sure the whole cavity is exposed.
6. Pass a wide-bore tube into this cavity and secure to the skin.
7. Do not close the wound.
8. When the patient's general state and the local condition permits, proceed to a simple nephrectomy if the kidney is irreparably damaged.

Difficulty?

1. Waiting for too long a period will result in extensive fibrosis and make the definitive procedure more difficult.
2. Do not be tempted to do a nephrectomy straight away unless you have great experience and the patient's condition warrants it.

EXCISION OF A SOLITARY RENAL CYST

Appraise

1. Excise a cyst which is of such a size that it causes pain, discomfort or an unsightly swelling.
2. The diagnosis is confirmed by pyelography, arteriography, ultrasound and cyst puncture. When the cyst refills after puncture and causes the above symptoms, it may be an indication for its removal. Some authorities advocate the removal of all cysts because of the occasional finding of malignant elements in the cyst wall.

Action

1. Expose the kidney as for a simple nephrectomy.
2. Aspirate the cyst, so outlining its boundaries.
3. Excise the cyst round this boundary, leaving that part of the wall embedded in the renal substance.
4. Obtain haemostasis round this margin.

5. Send the cyst wall for histology.
6. If you suspect that the cyst may in fact be malignant, i.e. all investigations are normal but there are areas of calcification in the wall, then it is safer to perform a nephrectomy. The alternative is to excise the cyst, await the histology report and then face the problem of deciding whether to reoperate to perform a nephrectomy or to follow the patient carefully. If in doubt in such cases, it is preferable to refer the patient to a specialist in this field.

PYELOPLASTY FOR HYDRONEPHROSIS

Appraise

There are three well-recognized techniques for repairing a hydronephrosis. The type of operation will depend on the case in question and the experience and personal choice of the surgeon.

HYNES-ANDERSON PYELOPLASTY

This is the most widely practised operation and has a particular merit with a large renal pelvis.

Action

1. Position the patient as for a nephrectomy.
2. Expose the kidney and completely clean the pelvis and pelviureteric junction of fatty tissue.
3. Clean and isolate the vessels so that they will not interfere with the procedure. Look for any aberrant vessels; it is unusual for these in fact to cause a hydronephrosis, but they may accentuate the appearances of one.
4. Place a small 3/0 stay suture at the level you wish to transect the ureter and again at the lowermost part of the pelvis to be preserved.
5. Make your incisions as shown in Figure 14.7; beware in a large hydronephrosis of cutting too close to the kidney or you may divide into the calyces.
6. Run a continuous 4/0 chromic catgut suture from point A to B and anchor it at the latter (Fig. 14.8).
7. Next slit down the upper end of the ureter on its renal side so as to approximate it to the opening in the pelvis (Fig. 14.9).
8. With continuous or interrupted 4/0 sutures, join the ureter back on to the pelvis as shown. Size will largely determine which method of suturing should be used.
9. Close with drainage to the renal bed.
10. To splint or not to splint? To drain the kidney or not? These are always two difficult questions. To do both of these things causes no regrets, but to do neither will often lead to problems. It is therefore safer to do both. A convenient method is to use a small Malecot catheter for the nephrostomy which has either a solid (Williams' cath-

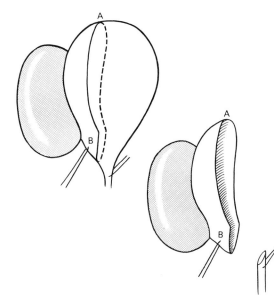

Fig. 14.7 Hynes-Anderson pyeloplasty

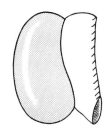

Fig. 14.8 Hynes-Anderson pyeloplasty

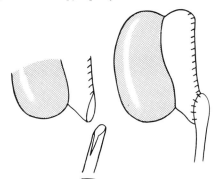

Fig. 14.9 Hynes-Anderson pyeloplasty

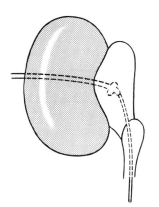

Fig. 14.10 Hynes-Anderson pyeloplasty with nephrostomy and splint in situ

eter) or hollow tail (Cummings' catheter) attached to it to act as a splint. These come in various sizes suitable for all age groups. Leave the splint and nephrostomy tube for ten days (Fig. 14.10).

CULP PYELOPLASTY

This is suitable for a hydronephrosis with a moderate pelvis, where you do not wish to dismember the pelvis from the ureter.

Action

1. Proceed as for a Hynes-Anderson pyeloplasty.
2. Approach the pelvis and ureter from behind so as to avoid the vessels.
3. Incise across the pelviureteric junction for about 2–3 cm. down the ureter and a similar distance into the pelvis. (Fig. 14.11).
4. Carry the pelvic incision laterally for 0.50–0.75 cm and then downward to the bottom of the renal pelvis (Fig. 14.12).
5. Turn the flap downward so that point A reaches point B without tension.
6. Sew this flap into the opened ureter and close the pelvic defect above (Fig. 14.13).
7. It is again wise to drain the kidney and to splint the anastomosis.

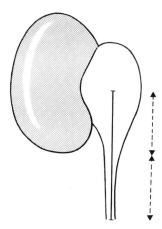

Fig. 14.11 Culp pyeloplasty

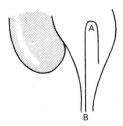

Fig. 14.12 Culp pyeloplasty

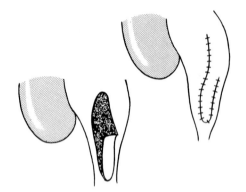

Fig. 14.13 Culp pyeloplasty

FOLEY PYELOPLASTY

This is for a hydronephrosis with a small pelvis.

Action

1. Proceed as before.
2. Incise down from just above the pelviureteric junction along the ureter for a distance of 1–2 cm.
3. From the upper end of this incision fashion a broad-based V, so turning the incision into a Y (Fig. 14.14).
4. Approximate points A and B, so converting the incision into a V and thus widening considerably the pelviureteric junction (Fig. 14.15).
5. Splint and drain as before.

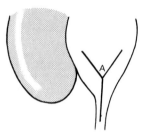

Fig. 14.14 Foley pyeloplasty

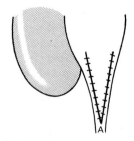

Fig. 14.15 Foley pyeloplasty

Difficulty?

In all pyeloplasties the big problem is prolonged leakage. This tends to occur more often in cases where the kidney has not been drained or the anastomosis splinted.

If you do encounter prolonged leakage, i.e. over many weeks, it is essential to be patient. By far the majority heal spontaneously. Only rarely is it necessary to re-explore, when the safest procedure is to perform a nephrostomy and wait for healing.

STANDARD URINARY DIVERSIONS

Appraise

1. These procedures are an integral part of cystectomy, but they are also performed in a variety of other conditions, as for instance in extrophy and neurogenic bladders.
2. Refer to a standard text for the more diverse indications.

ILEAL LOOP DIVERSION (WALLACE TYPE)

Action

1. Isolate a segment of lower ileum approximately 20 cm in length. The length will obviously vary with the size of the patient and should be about 25 cm from the ileocaecal junction.
2. Anastomose the two remaining ends of ileum in the standard fashion.
3. Mark the proximal end of this loop.
4. With finger dissection fashion a tunnel beneath the peritoneum so that the free left ureter can be brought across the midline to join its fellow on the right. Make sure the left ureter does not kink as it passes across.
5. The two divided ureters now lie in the right iliac fossa. Slit up the ureters on their anterior surfaces for about 1.5–2 cm.
6. According to the natural lie of these two ureters, join their adjacent borders with fine catgut to form a single opening (Fig. 14.16).
7. Pass a splint up each ureter into the renal pelvis, the size varying with the amount of ureteric dilatation. Soft nasogastric tubes are excellent for this purpose.
8. Pass a long straight artery clamp down the isolated loop from its distal end and grasp the splints, so withdrawing them through the loop.
9. Anastomose the proximal end of the loop either with fine continuous or interrupted catgut sutures on to the conjoined ureters.
10. Attach the adjacent free peritoneum to the proximal end of the loop.
11. Bring the distal free end out as a classical ileostomy spout.

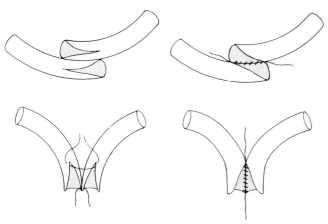

Fig. 14.16 Wallace type of ileal loop diversion. Methods of joining lower ends of ureters

12. Anchor the splints to the tip of the spout. They will usually detach themselves and fall out; otherwise remove them after about 7–10 days.

ILEAL LOOP DIVERSION (BRICKER TYPE)

Action

1. In this diversion the proximal end of the loop is closed and the two ureters anastomosed separately into the loop either with a direct mucosa-to-mucosa suture and a small muscle tunnel, or with a collar-and-cuff technique. It is wise to splint each ureter. Alternatively, one ureter may be anastomosed to the proximal free and the other into the side.

2. Either the whole loop can be extraperitonealized by reflecting the caecum medially and bringing the loop out lateral to this, or it should be left entirely free within the peritoneal cavity.

3. If the patient has had radiotherapy, either a planned small pre-operative course or a radical course, care must be taken with fashioning the loop. Should the bowel look thickened or whitish then use a loop of jejunum. Special care should be taken in rejoining the bowel because a breakdown in the anastomosis can occur in these cases.

4. If the diversion is a separate procedure, always drain the operative site.

COLONIC LOOP DIVERSION

Action

1. Sometimes it may be an advantage to utilise a short segment of colon to perform the diversion; the spout is not quite so satisfactory, but good bags give an excellent result. The ureters are usually implanted into the side of the loop, either directly, or with a Leadbetter technique, (see below).

2. An essential part of skin diversions is the stoma care. A cooperative patient with help and encouragement from a stomatherapist copes well with modern bags.

URETEROCOLIC ANASTOMOSIS (URETEROSIGMOIDOSTOMY)

Appraise

1. The indications for this particular type of diversion are varied. There are a few basic guidelines which can be followed. Ileal loop diversion should not be seriously considered if the patient cannot be independent, i.e. in the presence of severe rheumatoid arthritis. Ureterocolic anastomosis should not be considered if there is anal incontinence, obstructed and dilated ureters, severe diverticular disease or after extensive radiotherapy to the pelvis. If there is any doubt as to the advisability of a bowel diversion, a good general rule is that a loop should be used.

2. The most important preoperative preparation is to make sure that the bowel is completely empty. Sterilization is important but is probably not so imperative as the mechanical clearance of faeces.

3. This procedure has gone through various phases, most of which are historical, and the commonly practised method of anastomosis is the Leadbetter technique which is outlined here.

Action

1. Bring the lower sigmoid colon into the operative field and select the site in the anterior longitudinal muscle band (taenia coli) for anastomosis. Place two small tissue forceps on this taenia about 6 cm apart.

2. Incise through the muscle coats of the bowel rather in the fashion of a Ramstedt operation until the mucosa pouts out.

3. Incise through the mucosa at its distal end.

4. Slit up the ureter on its posterior surface for about 1 cm and anastomose this, end-to-mucosa, to the bowel.

5. Close the muscle layers of the bowel over the ureter so making a tunnel of muscle for it. Slit the muscle laterally where the ureter enters this tunnel.

6. Anchor the ureter 1 cm above the tunnel to avoid any traction (Fig. 14.17). The left ureter usually lies comfortably at the higher level so that the right one does not kink too severely as it comes across.

7. Anchor the bowel so that the ureters are under no tension.

Drainage and splinting

1. Drainage is essential; a large Depezzar catheter with window holes added to its tubing must be inserted high into the rectum.

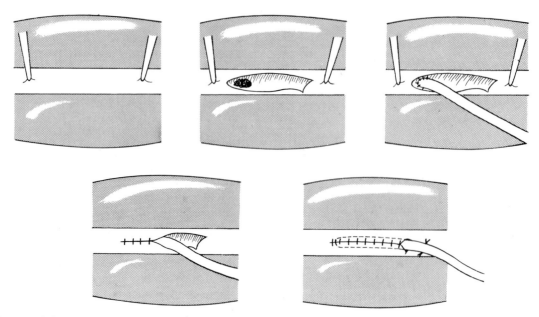

Fig. 14.17 Leadbetter technique of ureterocolic anastomosis

2. A good method of splinting the ureters is to have the patient's thighs well cleaned and draped and insert the large Depezzar catheter with its top cut off before the operation.

3. At the time of the ureterocolic anastomosis, the Depezzar head can be manipulated high up into the sigmoid colon and the two ureteric splints can be passed down the catheter and one up into each of the ureters. This enables free urinary drainage through the splints, and a suitable fitting can be made so that the urine will drain into a Uribag. Firmly suture the Depezzar catheter to the buttocks.

URETEROSTOMY

Appraise

Ureterostomy is rarely needed, and the special circumstances for which this operation is undertaken must be sought in texts of advanced urology. It may be unilateral or bilateral, temporary or permanent.

URETEROSTOMY IN SITU

This is usually an emergency temporary measure.

Action

1. Perform a gridiron incision on the appropriate side. Do not open the peritoneum but reflect it medially to expose the ureter.

2. Make a small incision into the ureter without mobilizing it unduly. Thread a plastic nasogastric tube of appropriate size up into the renal pelvis.

3. Close the wound round this ureterostomy catheter. Firmly anchor the catheter to the skin and attach to a Uribag.

4. The catheter may be left in situ for several weeks and can be changed by slipping it out and immediately replacing it with another one.

LOOP URETEROSTOMY

Appraise

This procedure is virtually confined to gross obstructive uropathy in infants and children and is often needed bilaterally. It is an alternative to bilateral nephrostomy and is a temporary measure.

Action

At an appropriate site, either in the loin or iliac fossa, cut down on to the dilated and tortuous ureter, mobilize it and bring it to the surface. Close the wound round the ureter in such a way that it is unobstructed. Incise the ureter so that it drains freely and attach a suitable urostomy bag over the site. A ureteric drainage splint may be temporarily employed.

END URETEROSTOMY

Appraise

This operation is nearly always a definitive method of urinary diversion. It may be employed as a long-term temporary measure before establishing an ileal loop diversion.

In childhood, the two dilated ureters may be brought together, bivalved and brought to the surface as a single spout. Bringing a single ureter of normal calibre to the surface is quick and easy; however, the long-term results are often poor due to stenosis of the spout. Various techniques for overcoming this problem, such as establishing a skin nipple, have been tried but usually without success. The end result in this instance is often the use of a permanent tube inserted into the ureterostomy which is changed at appropriate intervals.

REPAIR OF THE DAMAGED URETER

Appraise

1. The ureter may be damaged during pelvic operations. Undertake immediate repair if the injury is noticed at the time. Usually, however, it is not until a week or more has gone by that the injury manifests itself. These two situations present different problems.

2. The usual site for injury is low down in the pelvis; for this reason direct repair of the injury is rarely possible unless it is immediate, and reimplantation into the bladder is the usual procedure. If the pelvic surgery has been extensive and the injury re-explored later on, direct reimplantation may be difficult. Here a transuretero-ureterostomy may be the best manoeuvre.

3. Occasionally both ureters may be damaged, and then some compromise procedure will have to be employed. These latter instances should be referred to a urologist.

4. Reflux. In all cases of ureteric reconstruction remember that reflux is better than no flux! Do not jeopardize free urinary drainage in the hope of preventing reflux, only to finish up with an obstructed kidney.

SIMPLE DIVISION OF THE URETER RECOGNIZED AT THE TIME OF SURGERY

Action

1. Make sure that both ends of the divided ureter are accessible for anastomosis.

2. Pass a plastic tube of suitable calibre upward through the divided upper end of the ureter until it reaches the renal pelvis. Pass the lower end of this tube down through the distal divided ureter into the bladder. Use a double pigtail stent if one is available.

3. Approximate the two cut ends, fashioned obliquely, with four 4/0 chromic catgut sutures.

4. At the completion of the original operation, leave a large tube drain to the site of the ureteric anastomosis.

5. Make no attempt to anchor the plastic tube either to the ureter or bladder.

6. Leave the tube splint in situ for 10 days and then with a small lithotrite passed into the bladder, grip the tube and

remove it. The injury usually occurs in women, and this technique of removing the tube is relatively simple.

LATE REPAIR OF A LOW URETERIC INJURY

Appraise

1. These repairs should be undertaken by a surgeon with specialized training. The ureter should be repaired as soon as the injury becomes manifest. Waiting will only add to the fibrosis and difficulty of the operation; it should be avoided unless the patient's condition contraindicates early surgery. With prompt exploration the planes of the previous pelvic surgery are readily reopened.

2. There are various techniques for re-implantation of the ureter into the bladder and these will be outlined; the decision as to which to use must depend on the operative findings.

Action

1. Identify the ureter well above the operative field and trace it down as far as possible. It will usually come away into your dissecting fingers at its lowest point.

2. The decision now has to be made as to whether the ureter can be re-implanted direct into the bladder, whether the bladder will need mobilizing and bringing up to the ureter, or whether a flap of bladder should be turned up, rolled into a tube, and then anastomosed to the ureter.

3. For direct reimplantation, the collar-and-cuff technique is preferable as it has an antireflux action. If the ureter is very dilated it should be possible to turn it back on itself for a distance of approximately 1 cm. If it is not dilated then it will be necessary to slit it up for about 1 cm in order to turn it back on itself (Fig. 14.18). This will only fold back for a half to three-quarters of its circumference, but the defect will epithelialize.

4. Anchor the turned-back cuff with two or three 4/0 chromic catgut sutures, so forming a ureteric spout.

5. Make a central incision into the bladder, and hooking a forefinger into it, tent up a suitable site for ureteric anastomosis.

6. Incise the bladder over the forefinger, making a small opening. By passing a curved artery forceps through this opening it will be possible to draw the ureteric spout into

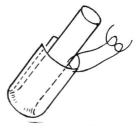

Fig. 14.18 Lower end of ureter fashioned into collar and cuff

the bladder. Anchor the ureter firmly both inside the bladder, with mucosa-to-mucosa sutures muscle sutures on the outside. Make sure there is no tension.

7. Splint with a suitable plastic tube which can conveniently be brought out suprapubically.

8. Close the bladder with a urethral catheter.

PSOAS HITCH OPERATION

Appraise

1. Where there is insufficient ureter remaining so that direct re-implantation into the bladder is impossible, then either the bladder must be mobilized and brought up to the ureteric stump (the psoas hitch operation) or a tube of bladder can be turned upward to bridge the gap (the Boari flap procedure).

2. For a psoas hitch it will be necessary to mobilize and divide both superior vesical pedicles and usually the inferior pedicle on the contralateral side, so that the bladder can be swung upward to meet the ureter.

Action

1. Having mobilized the bladder as fully as is necessary, open it in the midline.

2. Hitch the bladder up to the necessary height to overcome the ureteric defect and maintain it in this position with two or three 2/0 chromic sutures, taking good muscle bites and anchoring them to the psoas minor tendon.

3. Anastomose the ureter into the mobilized and lengthened bladder, as previously described for direct anastomosis, and splint.

BOARI FLAP PROCEDURE

Action

1. Distend the bladder and mobilize the sides and dome.

2. Fashion a broad-based flap which should consist of the whole anterior surface of the bladder. The flap should be at least 3–4 cm. across; it will shrink considerably in size when cut (Fig. 14.19).

3. Turn this flap upward and fashion it into a tube using a continuous two-layer fine chromic catgut suture. Continue this suture so as to close the bladder defect. The bladder will now effectively be a long tube (Fig. 14.20).

4. Anastomose this tube end-to-end with the ureter over a splint, or else fashion a collar and cuff with the ureter and anastomose this to the Boari flap. It is a curious feature that these bladder tubes usually do not lead to reflux if an end-to-end anastomosis is made.

Difficulty

1. Never anastomose if there is any tension; always mobilize the bladder or form a tube.

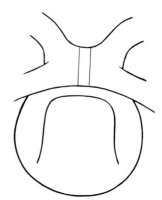

Fig. 14.19 Boari flap. bladder incision

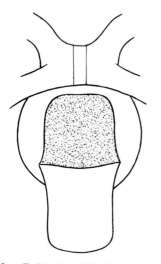 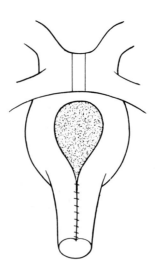 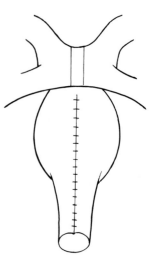

Fig. 14.20 Boari flap. Fashioning of 'bladder flap' tube

2. Always splint the anastomosis.
3. Soft nasogastric tubes make suitable splints.
4. Always drain the site of anastomosis.

TRANSURETERO-URETEROSTOMY

This procedure is useful for bridging a long lower ureteric defect. This may occur after conservative surgery for a lower ureteric tumour, or after extensive damage to a ureter where it may be impossible to re-implant into the bladder.

Action

1. Free the damaged ureter sufficiently to bring it across to the opposite side retroperitoneally, making a retroperitoneal tunnel with your fingers.
2. Mobilize the midpart of the normal ureter so that an anastomosis end-to-side can be made between the two ureters.
3. Make a small incision into the normal ureter, about 0.75–1.00 cm in length, and intubate with a plastic splint.
4. Anastomose the damaged ureter on to this opening with fine interrupted sutures, removing the splint before the final sutures are inserted (Figs. 14.21, 14.22).

It may be necessary to slit up the damaged ureter in order to get a satisfactory anastomosis.

ILEAL REPLACEMENT OF THE URETER

This procedure is rarely practised today, but the occasion may arise when it is necessary.

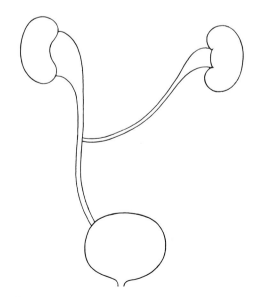

Fig. 14.21 Transuretero-ureterostomy

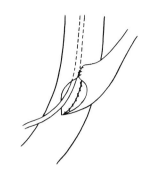

Fig. 14.22 Transuretero-ureterostomy

Action

1. Ileal replacement should encompass the full length of the ureter, i.e. pelvis to bladder.
2. Having isolated the segment, the appropriate left or right colon should be mobilized medially, thus exposing the kidneys. Pass the loop through the colonic mesentery and anastomose the upper (i.e. isoperistaltic) end, as this will usually usually become clogged with mucus.
3. Drain both upper and lower anastomoses and the bladder with a urethral catheter. Do not attempt any fancy reflux-preventing operations on the lower end, as these may interfere with the working of the loop.

SYNTHETIC URETERIC REPLACEMENTS

There are reports in the literature of inert valved synthetic ureters. Again, they are usually full-length prostheses. Their use is probably very limited and their need and effectiveness require much further evaluation.

RENAL TRANSPLANTATION

Appraise

1. This whole field is highly specialised, and the reader wishing knowledge on this apect of urology must seek information from advanced texts on the subject.
2. Following advances in immunosuppression and tissue typing, renal transplantation is now a necessary and satisfactory adjunct to the management of renal failure. The standard technique of immunosuppression is with azathioprine (Imuran) or cyclosporin and steroids.
3. Tissue typing and other histocompatibility testing have now made the selection of donor kidneys, both live and cadaver, more accurate. By far the best results are obtained in transplanting a kidney from one identical twin into the other. This ideal situation is obviously very rare.
4. The next most satisfactory technique is with live related donors. Transplantation with cadaver kidneys is the method most widely practised but gives less good results.

COLLECTION OF LIVE DONOR KIDNEYS

There is no doubt that closely matching, live related donor kidneys give better results than cadaver kidneys. Particularly is this so with identical twins, where the results are excellent. Full pre-operative assessment of the donor, including the vascular pattern of the kidney, is essential.

The procedure is best carried out in twin operating theatres; one surgeon prepares the recipient, and not until the recipient field is ready is the donor kidney removed and transferred to the recipient by the second operator.

RETRIEVAL OF CADAVER KIDNEYS

Once the decision has been made to remove the kidneys from the cadaver you must move swiftly. Use a normal operative aseptic technique.

Action

1. Make a full-length cruciate incision to expose the whole abdominal content.
2. Reflect the caecum, ascending colon, and the small bowel and their mesenteries medially. Reflect also the duodenum and pancreas, so that both kidneys are exposed along with the aorta and inferior vena cava.
3. Cross-clamp the aorta and vena cava well above and below the renal vessels. Remove the whole block of tissue containing both kidneys, pelvis, ureters and all vessels, including the segments of aorta and inferior vena cava intact. Leave plenty of perirenal and periureteric tissue.
4. Flush the vessels with a suitable solution cooled at 4°C.
5. Place this block of tissue in a sterile plastic bag and seal.
6. Place this bag within another sterile one and again seal.

7. Immerse in a large Thermos container of ice and water and transport to the recipient hospital(s) immediately. Do not forget to close the abdomen neatly.

RENAL TRANSPLANT PROCEDURE

1. The recipient site is usually the right iliac fossa. Where there has been a previous transplant on this side, then the left may be used.
2. Use an extraperitoneal approach through an oblique muscle-cutting incision above the inguinal ligament. This incision can easily be extended upward so that the diseased kidney on that side may be removed.
3. Isolate and divide the internal iliac artery before its branches commence. The common iliac vein is fully cleaned and isolated but not divided.
4. The left donor kidney is utilized for anastomosis into the right iliac fossa so that the renal pelvis lies anteriorly. The reverse applies with the right kidney into the left iliac fossa. The renal artery is anastomosed end-to-end with the divided proximal end of the internal iliac artery. The renal vein is joined end-to-side to the common iliac vein.
5. Open the bladder and anastomose the ureter to it with a reflux-preventing procedure, usually employing a submucous tunnel. Some transplant surgeons utilize the patient's own ureter, but this of course must be a normal one.
6. Where there are renal anomalies, for instance a double renal artery, modifications of the above basic technique must be used, such as the utilization of a cuff of aorta.

Further reading

Blandy J P 1978 Transurethral Resection, 2nd ed. Pitman, London.
Glenn J P, Boyce W H 1975 Urologic Surgery, 2nd edn. Harper & Row, Hagerstown
Innes-Williams D 1968 Paediatric Urology. Butterworths, London.
Mitchell J P 1972 Transurethral Resection and Haemostasis. Wright, Bristol

Surgery of the lower urinary tract

URETHRAL DILATATION AND URETHROTOMY

Appraise

1. Over the last decade, the general management of urethral stricture in the male has completely changed. There is still place for stricture dilatation in the time-honoured tradition, but this is severely limited; and it is mainly employed in elderly patients who have been dilated over many years and are totally resistant to any treatment change.

2. The visual urethrotome, as described by Sachse, with the 0° end-viewing telescope, has revolutionised the closed management of virtually all strictures. Its use must of course be confined to skilled operators, usually in departments of urology, since in unskilled hands it is a dangerous instrument.

URETHROTOMY
Action

Not only is there direct visualisation of the stricture, but also of the urethrotome knife and what it is dividing. By gently manipulating the whole instrument, the stricture is divided dorsally until it springs open. Even very long strictures can be divided. Should it be difficult to visualise the stricture easily due to multiple false passages, a guide can be passed down under vision to probe these until the correct channel is found. The impenetrable strictures can in this way be negotiated with the optical urethrotome.

Aftercare

1. After urethrotomy small strictures can be left without a catheter. Indeed these can be dealt with on an outpatient basis, and some advocate the use of local anaesthesia. Longer and more difficult strictures are probably best left with a nonirritating Foley catheter, 16–18 French gauge. It does not appear to make much difference if these are left in for 24 hours or 6 weeks.

2. Some cases dealt with using the optical urethrotome will stay patent for months or years; the majority, however, close down and have to be divided again. The time interval is usually much longer in these cases, when compared to the previous blind dilatations.

STANDARD URETHRAL DILATATION

Assess

1. This can be done under local or general anaesthesia. For strictures being dilated for the first time, or where difficulty has been encountered before, always use general anaesthesia.

2. Instruments. There are various dilators available. The most commonly used are the Clutton metal dilators, plastic and filiform bougies. These latter have 'female' screw ends, on to which graduated plastic bougies with 'male' ends are fitted. All dilators are in graduated sizes.

Action

1. Clean and drape the penis.

2. Local anaesthesia will be described. Squeeze into the urethra a tube of 2% lignocaine gel, preferably containing an antiseptic. Apply a penile clamp to the end of the penis and massage the gel back into the posterior urethra. Cover with a sterile drape and leave for 5 minutes.

3. Choose a medium-sized metal dilator, and firmly elevating the penis with the left hand, insert the dilator into the urethra, maintaining the beak of the dilator against the dorsal surface of the urethra.

4. Advance the dilator until the stricture is encountered. Now with gentle manipulation, still holding the penis stretched with the left hand, try to negotiate the stricture. Always maintain the back in an upward direction.

5. Should it be impossible to pass the stricture then use the next smaller sized dilator and so on until the stricture is negotiated. For posterior strictures as you pass the dilator through the bulbous urethra and into the membranous urethra, it will be necessary to depress the handle of the dilator down between the patient's legs. It will then easily slip into the bladder. This you can confirm by rotating the sound.

Difficulty?

1. Never force the dilators or else you may make a false passage.

2. If you encounter difficulty, stop and try again under general anaesthesia.

3. Avoid overdilatation, which is indicated by excessive bleeding.

4. It is best to stretch the stricture with the same range of dilators as was used previously.

5. For anterior urethral strictures, the plastic bougies are usually sufficient.

Impassable stricture

1. If it is impossible to pass the metal dilators or plastic bougies, then gently insert four or five filiform bougies. Hold the penis taut as before and gently tease each of these bougies in. Eventually one will find its way through the tight stricture and you will feel it give. Holding this in place, remove the others and in turn attach increasing sizes of followers until the stricture has been dilated.

2. If all these manoeuvres fail and the patient is in acute retention, some form of suprapubic drainage must be performed.

3. After dilating a very difficult stricture, leave a small catheter in situ for 48 hours.

4. With infected urine, the appropriate antibiotic cover must be used.

5. Should the patient spike a high temperature either following the dilatation or when he next passes urine, then treat immediately as for a Gram-negative bacteraemia.

SUPRAPUBIC CYSTOTOMY DRAINAGE

Appraise

1. This is indicated in cases of acute retention when it is impossible to enter the bladder in any other way.

2. Use also, when it is necessary to divert the urine temporarily in such instances as urinary extravasation or after closing a urethroplasty. In the former emergency cases, it is quite satisfactory to perform the cystotomy under local anaesthesia.

3. In cases of acute retention the bladder will be distended well above the symphysis.

Action

1. After fully preparing and draping the patient, select a point 3–4 cm above the midpoint of the symphysis. Infiltrate with local anaesthetic down to the bladder, so that the infiltrating needle enters the bladder and clean urine can be aspirated.

2. You may now select one of two differing techniques, according to the length of time you anticipate using the temporary diversion. For short duration of drainage, it is perfectly acceptable to use one of the disposable Supracaths now on the market. These are threaded through a sharp stab needle. Take care to thread sufficient length into the bladder so that when the bladder collapses, the catheter is not left high and dry outside.

3. For more prolonged drainage or when the suprapubic area is scarred, it is better formally to expose the bladder and sew in a larger catheter

(a) Make a 3–4 cm transverse incision 3 cm above the symphysis. Expose the rectus sheath and separate the muscles in the midline. Hold the muscles apart with retractors and pick up the bladder with two tissue forceps. With considerable scarring it may be difficult to identify the bladder; however, it is safe to continue in a downward and backward direction provided the bladder is distended.

(b) Divide between the forceps and enter the bladder. Pass in a selected catheter, a large Foley usually being satisfactory. Bring the bladder together with one or two all-coats 2/0 chromic catgut sutures.

(c) Appose the recti and sew the catheter to the skin wound.

(d) Do not forget to inflate the Foley Balloon. Anchor the catheter with skin sutures.

SUPRAPUBIC CYSTOTOMY DRAINAGE WHERE THE URETHRA IS PATENT

This is performed as a formal operation and is often part of other procedures.

Action

1. Pass a small catheter so that you can distend the bladder.

2. Pass a medium-sized metal dilator into the bladder so that its tip can easily be felt suprapubically. It is best to use a special sound with a small hole drilled across its tip (Fig. 15.1).

3. Incise down on to the tip of the sound and force it out of the suprapubic wound so formed.

4. Thread a long piece of no. 1 monofilament nylon through the hole and tie it through the eye of a large Foley catheter.

5. Now withdraw the sound and so pull the catheter into the bladder. Leave sufficient length of nylon so that it can be cut outside the urethra and removed (Fig. 15.2).

6. Inflate the Foley balloon and secure the catheter with a skin stitch.

Difficulty?

1. Do not attempt this manoeuvere where there is a scarred suprapubic area. It is better to cut down in these cases.

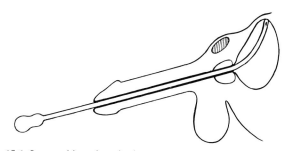

Fig. 15.1 Suprapubic catheterisation

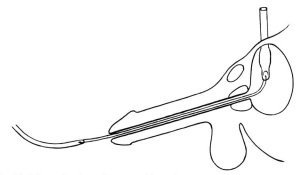

Fig. 15.2 Introduction of suprapubic catheter.

2. Fill the bladder sufficiently so that the sound is pushed against the anterior abdominal wall extraperitoneally.

3. Leave the nylon long enough to be able to release and cut it.

CYSTOSCOPY

Appraise

1. For the urologist, this is a fundamental technique. Always it is accompanied by a preliminary urethroscopy, using a 30° or 0° telescope. One can thus view the whole length of the urethra, and should one encounter a stricture, it is seen before it is damaged! The panurothelial nature of bladder tumours makes it mandatory to view the urethra as well as the bladder. The sphincter area, prostate and bladder neck, in cases of outflow obstruction, taken in conjunction with urodynamic studies, will complete the investigation in such cases.

2. The fibre-optic lighting systems and the rod-lens telescope, both invented by Hopkins, have made endoscopic assessment of the lower urinary tract a sophisticated and delightful procedure.

3. For the general surgeon, cystoscopic examination should be confined to the bladder and only the simplest manoeuvres attempted.

4. Good light, a good lens system and irrigation are essential.

Action

1. Place the patient in the lithotomy position. Avoid cystoscoping flat unless the patient has severe osteoarthritis of the hips.

2. Use general anaesthesia where at all possible.

3. Clean and appropriately drape the patient.

4. Check the cystoscope for lighting and irrigation.

5. Pass the sheath with its obturator as described for the passage of a metal sound. Difficulty may be found in patients with large prostates; most cystoscopes are beaked to overcome this difficulty.

6. Empty the bladder. If the urine is dirty or bloody you will need to irrigate several times. If there are large blood clots, these will need breaking up and forcibly washing out with a large bladder syringe.

7. When you are satisfied that you will have a clear view, pass the telescope, connect the light, and view with the fluid running in. You will be able to watch the bladder distend.

8. Have a set plan of inspection so that all areas of the bladder are viewed.

9. It is possible with the irrigating cystoscope to bring it down, under vision and with the fluid running, into the

prostatic urethra. This will enable you to assess the prostatic size before deciding on enucleation prostatectomy.

10. Always empty the bladder after cystoscopy, unless you wish to proceed to a transvesical operation.

MANIPULATION OF DIATHERMY ELECTRODES AND RETROGRADE CATHETERS

1. If you are a general surgeon confine yourself to the treatment of the simplest of tumours.

2. Obtain a biopsy first. Unless you have modern biopsy forceps, it may be difficult to obtain an adequate specimen; in this circumstance refer the case to a specialist centre.

3. Electrodes and retrograde catheters once passed down the operating channel are manipulated into position, using the platform wheel in combination with manoeuvring the cystoscope sheath. By varying the fullness of the bladder with the irrigating mechanism, it is possible to get to most parts of the bladder. For lesions on the dome, suprapubic pressure with the fingers is exceedingly helpful.

4. For retrograde catheterization, once the tip of the catheter is well in view, it is best to advance the whole cystoscope and catheter so that the catheter tip engages in the orifice. Then advance the catheter up the ureter, removing the stilette once you are progressing easily. Each catheter is marked in centimetres and has double, treble and quadruple rings for each increment of 5 cm.

5. If there is difficulty in negotiating the orifice then try a bulb catheter; impinge the bulb into the lower end and inject contrast up the ureter.

ENDOSCOPIC RESECTION OF BLADDER TUMOURS

A comprehensive biopsy specimen of large superficial or infiltrating bladder tumours can be obtained using the resectoscope. It is also a very satisfactory method for totally removing superficial tumours. It should, however, be left in the hands of the expert, as it is considerably more hazardous than the routine resection of the prostate.

EXCISION OF BLADDER STONES

Appraise

1. Do not undertake simple open excision of bladder stones unless the stone or stones cannot be dealt with by litholapaxy, or there is some other bladder pathology such as an enlarged prostate or diverticulum to be dealt with at the same time.

2. It is essential to overcome outflow obstruction, i.e. prostatic disease, before or at the same time as removing the stones.

Action

1. Pass a cystoscope so that not only can you visualize and assess the stones and any other pathology, but also fill the bladder with water.

2. Use a Pfannenstiel incision. Make a slightly convex, downward transverse incision 7–9 cm long, so that its lowest part crosses the upper margin of the symphysis pubis.

3. Expose the rectus sheath.

4. Incise the rectus sheath over each rectus muscle from one lateral margin to the other, so exposing each muscle belly.

5. Use curved dissecting scissors to enlarge each end of his incision laterally to include the external oblique aponeurosis.

6. Grasp the midline of the upper and lower borders of the rectus sheath with long artery forceps, and with finger dissection free the rectus sheath from both muscles. Use scissors for the linea alba. Carry this downward to the symphysis and upward for about 6 cm. The recti will now be exposed with or without the pyramidalis muscles (Fig. 15.3).

7. Thrust blunt scissors between the recti, opening them longitudinally.

8. Hook two index fingers into the space so formed and forcibly retract the two recti apart. This will expose the bladder with its overlying fat and areolar tissue.

9. Use a short-bladed Millin or other suitable self-retaining retractor to hold the recti apart. Clean the fatty tissue off the bladder. Pick up the bladder with two transverse stay sutures and enter the bladder between these with scissors (Fig. 15.4).

10. Place the left forefinger into the bladder and, hooking it posteriorly, lift it upward. Clean away the fat anteriorly and posteriorly sufficiently to enlarge the bladder opening to obtain easy access.

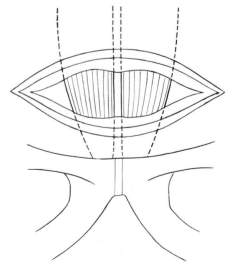

Fig. 15.3 Exposure of recti muscles

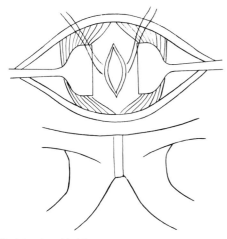

Fig. 15.4 Incision into bladder

11. Remove the stones, making sure there is no other pathology to deal with.

12. Grasp the anterior and posterior ends of the incision with tissue forceps, so tenting the incised bladder out of the wound.

Closure

1. Close the bladder with a 2/0 chromic catgut, continuous, two-layer suture. The first stitch at the anterior end of the wound is tied and takes all-coats. Clip the end. The first half of the second stitch is all-coats, the second half being mucosa only. Continue with the mucosal stitch posteriorly until the mucosa is completely closed (Fig. 15.5).

2. Leave a small suprapubic Malecot catheter in the upper end of the bladder incision, or else use a urethral catheter for drainage.

3. At the upper end of the incision, secure the catgut and return the continuous suture to the lower end, this

time taking the muscle only; secure the suture to the original clipped end.

4. Approximate the recti with a few No. 1 catgut sutures. Close the external oblique aponeurosis and rectus sheath with a continuous No. 1 catgut suture. Close the skin without drainage.

5. If you have used a urethral catheter for drainage, leave it for 10 days. If however, you have used a suprapubic catheter, change to a urethral catheter as soon as the urine is clean and again leave for 10 days.

LITHOLAPAXY

Appraise

1. This means the crushing of bladder stones and the subsequent washing out of the fragments. Lithotrites come in varying sizes and may be blind or viewing. The advantage of the latter is that one can see what one is doing, but it has the disadvantage of being a large and rather clumsy instrument which may inflict urethral damage.

2. As this procedure should in the main be performed by urologists, the less damaging blind lithotrite is usually employed.

Action

1. Assess the stones cystoscopically.

2. Fill the bladder with water and pass the lithotrite.

3. Point the jaws upward and open them.

4. Depress the end of the lithotrite downward towards the rectum; the stone or stones will usually engage in the jaws which can then be closed, so crushing the stone (Fig. 15.6).

5. Repeat this process many times until the stones have been pulverized, and then wash the fragments out. Make sure that all pieces have gone.

6. There are various types of instruments for washing

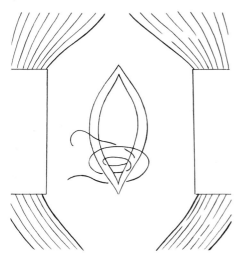

Fig. 15.5 Closure of bladder incision

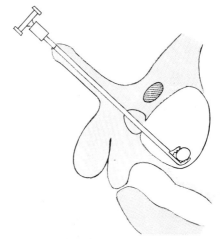

Fig. 15.6 Lithotrite grasping stone

out the fragments. A wide-bore resectoscope sheath is probably the best, as a 70° viewing telescope can be used in conjunction with this to assess the situation periodically. The sheath is attached to an evacuator; there are a variety of these, for instance the Bigelow, Freyer or Ellick types.

7. For minute, dusty fragments which attach themselves to the bladder mucosa, daily washouts with Renacidin for 5 days are recommended.

8. The viewing lithotrite is used in the opposite way, the jaws facing downward. They are opened under vision so that the stone can be accuately grasped and crushed. This may seem to be advantageous, but in order to crush large or hard stones the instrument is so big that it may cause severe urethral damage. It is therefore only suitable for small and soft stones.

BIOPSY OF THE PROSTATE

TRANSURETHRAL BIOPSY

1. This is in essence a modified resection of the prostate. This technique helps to improve the obstructed outflow symptoms and signs of the patient and at the same time obtains excellent biopsy material.

2. It is not possible to obtain biopsy specimens from the posterior capsule and indeed it would be dangerous to do so. If this is necessary then a perineal biopsy should be combined with the resection.

PERINEAL BIOPSY

1. It is usual to perform this biopsy under general anaesthesia, as it is often combined with endoscopic assessment and bimanual examination. One good biopsy needle on the market is the Travenol Tru-Cut disposable biopsy needle. This is guided through the perineum into the suspicious area with the forefinger in the rectum. The instructions for its manipulation are clearly given with each needle.

TRANSRECTAL BIOPSY

1. Some urologists advocate the use of the Travenol needle transrectally, but the hazards of doing this are entirely unjustified.

2. Aspiration biopsy using the thin-bore Franzen needle is a satisfactory transrectal approach. The needle is guided with the forefinger in the rectum as for perineal biopsy, but the needle carrier is attached to the forefinger so the needle can be directed into the appropriate area of the prostate. The aspirated material must immediately be spread and fixed on a clean microscope slide.

3. The fine-needle technique has the advantage that it can be used in the outpatient department with little upset to the patient and also that multiple areas can be biopsied. Its disadvantage is that its accuracy is not great.

PROSTATECTOMY

Appraise

1. Patients with acute retention due to prostatic hypertrophy select themselves. It is not often that surgery is withheld in this circumstance. Beware of senile patients and those with severe Parkinsonism, as they may become incontinent. The alternative is a permanent indwelling catheter, and the problems of each of these situations must be considered.

2. Patients with chronic retention and overflow, or chronic retention with back pressure on their upper urinary tracts, again select themselves for surgery. If renal impairment is considerable, preliminarily decompress them, watching in this instance for the occasional massive diuresis or bladder haemorrhage which may occur. Such patients often require preliminary blood transfusion.

3. Symptomatic patients are considered for surgery according to their degree of disability. Beware of patients with urgency, frequency, and often urge incontinence; such men often have primary bladder instability and do not benefit from surgery. If, however, they have accompanying outflow obstructive symptoms of hesitancy, poor stream and dribbling, then offer them surgery. In case of doubt, assess them with urodynamic studies.

4. Preliminary assessment with urography is helpful, but not mandatory. Ultrasound examination of the upper tracts can be every bit as informative. Urine and blood analysis are essential. Flow studies and, if necessary, urodynamic studies, will often be helpful in deciding on surgery in doubtful cases.

5. Panendoscopy prior to surgery is essential to exclude associated lesions.

Select

1. Prostatectomy for benign hyperplasia is the commonest operation performed by urologists. It also forms a large part of surgical work for general surgeons who have to practise without a urological colleague.

2. The trained urologist selects transurethral resection (T.U.R) almost exclusively, reserving the open procedures either for the large gland, weighing upwards from 100 g, or where concomitant conditions have to be dealt with, such as a large, hard stone. Even under these latter circumstances, the author personally prefers to perform a T.U.R., followed by suprapubic removal of the offending stone.

3. For the general surgeon working without urological assistance, the author would strongly advise the selection

of the retropubic or transvesical route, the latter probably leading to less problems. Unless you have been specifically orientated to transurethral work, the use of this instrument cannot be condoned. There are so many hazards, some of which may prove fatal, in inexpert hands. Extravasation due to capsular perforation is high on the list, as is the undermining of the trigone. There is a high incidence of incontinence and stricture formation, and of course, inadequate resection which can at times lead to formidable blood loss.

4. Do not approach clinically malignant prostates through the open route. Unless you have resection experience, try to refer them to a specialist unit.

5. Very small prostates, often only amounting to a tight unrelaxing bladder neck, are far better approached transurethrally.

6. The author recommends that when in doubt, it is far better for the patient to travel to the nearest centre for his surgery, if this is at all possible.

Aftercare

1. This is aimed at preventing blood loss and clot retention. I always employ a fast irrigation system with a three-way catheter, and I use a suprapubic irrigation for transvesical procedures.

2. Another major problem is bacteraemia, which may lead to septicaemia. Carefully watch the temperature chart.

3. Be aware of fluid absorption during long transurethral resections, and of the subsequent hyponatraemia.

4. Keep the irrigation going until there is no further fear of clot retention. Remove the catheter on the third or fourth day, provided there is no further bleeding.

5. For transvesical procedures, leave the urethral catheter for 10 days; the suprapubic catheter will have been removed when the fear of bleeding and clot retention has passed.

RETROPUBIC PROSTATECTOMY

Action

1. Perform a preliminary cystoscopy to establish that the gland is suitable for enucleation and that there is no bladder pathology.

2. Position yourself on the left side of the patient; clean the lower abdomen, genitalia and upper thighs. Drape so that the genitalia can be easily reached.

3. Perform a preliminary simple vasectomy. This will not only give the anaesthetist and theatre staff plenty of time to have everything ready, but will also go a long way to prevent acute epididymitis post-operatively.

4. Have the patient in the Trendelenburg position.

5. Make a Pfannenstiel incision exactly as described for simple removal of stones.

6. Once the recti have been parted, sweep the right index finger beneath the symphysis and so clean the retropubic space. Position a long-bladed Millin self-retaining retractor.

7. With diathermy forceps coagulate all the veins coursing across the prostatic capsule. After this clean the capsule of fatty tissue.

8. Define the anterior capsule stretched over the prostate and therefore its upper border.

9. Get your assistant to use a sponge-holder and sponge to depress the bladder downward and backward, thus throwing into relief the upper border of the prostate (Fig. 15.7).

10. Make a 2 cm long transverse incision through the capsule of the prostate just below the upper border with a cutting diathermy point (Fig. 15.8). The capsule may be up to 0.5 cm thick, and vessels in it will need coagulating. The two lobes of the prostate will be seen bulging together.

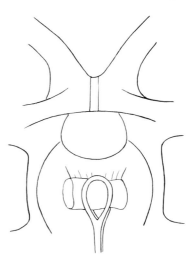

Fig. 15.7 Exposure of prostatic capsule

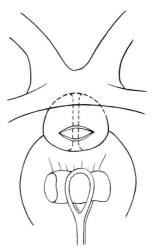

Fig. 15.8 Incision into prostatic capsule

11. Insert long dissecting scissors between the two lobes, i.e. into the prostatic urethra, and open them longitudinally. Remove the retractor and other instruments.

12. Insert the right index finger into the prostatic urethra. You will feel it gripped between the two lobes. Now push the finger downward until it reaches the back of the prostatic urethra and then curl it toward yourself. You will be able to break into a plane between the urethra and the left lobe of the 'adenomatous' gland. Extend this plane to the apex of the prostate and backward to the bladder neck (Fig. 15.9).

13. Next come back to the apex of the prostate. With the index finger under the lobe and the thumb on the outside of the capsule, you will be able to nip through the apex and so free it. Now carry the index finger round the front and lateral border, so freeing the lobe completely except for that part attached to the bladder neck.

14. Repeat the process on the opposite lobe. It is often convenient to start this lobe using the left index finger and complete it with the right one.

15. Dislocate the two lobes out of the capsule and nip them off at the bladder neck, using thumb and forefinger as pincers.

16. Insert a bladder neck spreader into the bladder. The Badenoch spreader is one of the most satisfactory available.

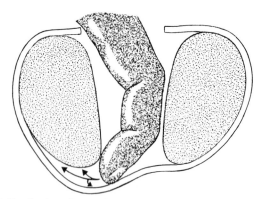

Fig. 15.9 Enucleation of prostatic 'adenomas'

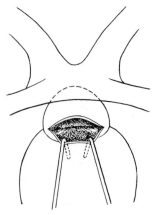

Fig. 15.10 Bladder neck retractor in position

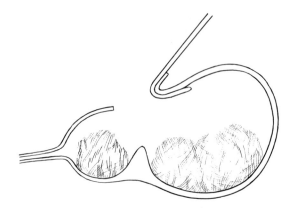

Fig. 15.11 Swabs in prostatic cavity and bladder, exposing the bladder neck to be excised

Get your assistant to hold it in position (Fig. 15.10). This will throw into relief the bladder neck and middle lobe if present, both of which must be totally excised. It is often a good idea to pack a swab into the prostatic cavity to stop the field being obscured by blood, and likewise into the bladder to stop the bladder mucosa folding upward (Fig. 15.11). The bladder neck can then be grasped with long-toothed forceps and excised with a diathermy point. The shaded area in the illustration must be removed. Do not be tempted just to take a small 'V'. Arrest all bleeding points with diathermy.

17. Insert the appropriate catheter, and secure with a nylon stitch or with its self-retaining balloon (see below).

18. Close the prostatic capsule using a No. 1 chromic catgut continuous suture. Make sure both lateral angles are firmly secured. A boomerang needle or needle and holder may be used.

19. Wash the bladder to make sure your suture line is watertight.

20. Bring the catheter suture, if present, through the rectus sheath and skin.

21. Close the recti, rectus sheath and skin as before but in this case always use a drain down to the retropubic space, either a Redivac or wide-bore perforated tube attached to a drainage bag.

22. Finally wash the bladder out, ascertaining that the water will flow freely, and then secure the catheter stitch with an Emessay button or bar. Attach the catheter to a Uribag.

What catheter and whether to irrigate

1. There is no doubt that with the advent of good irrigating non-collapsing catheters, the problems of bleeding and clot retention have been almost banished from the postoperative scene.

2. If you have decided to irrigate, there is no doubt that this must be started as soon as the capsule is closed and continued at a high rate until the effluent is just pink, and then it can be slowed down. It is far better to do this rather

than wait until bleeding troubles ensue. It is much easier not to get clot retention in the bladder than it is to get rid of it.

3. Clot in the bladder and prostatic cavity prevents proper drainage and will lead to increasing problems, until the patient is thoroughly 'washed out.' This may mean returning the patient to the theatre and washing the bladder out thoroughly under a general anaesthetic.

Difficulty?

If there is a very large middle lobe, it is often easier to cut this off the bladder neck, again with a diathermy cutter. This will leave the bladder neck behind, which can then be excised under direct vision. Sometimes with a very large, trilobed gland the neck becomes insignificant.

TRANSVESICAL PROSTATECTOMY

Appraise

1. Use when it is necessary to have good access to the bladder at the same time as performing a prostatectomy: for instance in removing very large stones, a diverticulum or very rarely a superficial bladder neoplasm.

2. After an abdominoperineal resection of the rectum a transvesical prostatectomy is often easier than a retropubic one.

Action

1. Proceed as described for a retropubic prostatectomy up to and including stage 5. However, in this instance leave the bladder distended.

2. Part the two recti; the bladder will be immediately identifiable. Free the fat off the bladder, coagulating any veins coursing over its surface.

3. Pick up the bladder with two stay sutures and open between these longitudinally. Hook the bladder out of the wound with the left forefinger and free it sufficiently to enlarge the opening to about 7 cm.

4. Insert a suitable self-retaining bladder retractor. In this instance the third blade, particularly with a swab tucked under it, will expose the base of the bladder. Examine the bladder carefully and deal with the pathology which necessitated a transvesical approach.

5. Remove the retractor and all other instruments, and insert the right index finger in through the internal meatus and so into the prostatic urethra.

6. In exactly the same way as for a retropubic prostatectomy, enucleate the 'adenomas'. In this approach it is more difficult to free the apex, particularly if it is a large gland. Again it is not easy to obtain haemostasis or clear the bladder neck as in a retropubic approach. This is mainly because you are working away from yourself instead of down on to the prostate.

7. Close the bladder and wound as described for simple removal of stones. It is wise to insert not only a suprapubic catheter but also a urethral whistle-tip as in the retropubic approach.

8. Irrigate postoperatively through either the urethral or suprapubic catheter. Once the urine is clear, remove the suprapubic catheter and maintain closed drainage through the urethral one, which is left for 10 days.

Aftercare

In a transvesical approach the bladder must be allowed to heal before the catheter is removed. This usually takes 10 days; should any suprapubic leakage occur, then replace the urethral catheter. For the same reason, post-operative clot retention is a problem because the bladder cannot be washed out forcibly without endangering the suture line; this is the reason for irrigating in the immediate postoperative period.

TRANSURETHRAL PROSTATECTOMY

Appraise

1. In this procedure, instead of enucleating the prostatic 'adenomas', they are cut up and the chippings are washed out. It is highly suitable for small prostates and for patients who are otherwise unfit for general anaesthesia and open surgery. In the hands of the expert urologist, it has virtually replaced the operation of open prostatectomy.

2. The instrument consists of a rigid sheath down which are passed the viewing telescope (in this case a 30° telescope which gives a more direct view) and the movable cutting loop, which is therefore under vision. Irrigating fluid (isotonic) flushes down the sheath and keeps the end of the telescope clear of blood.

3. The resectoscope sheath comes in various sizes. Select the one which will slide easily within the urethra. If the meatus is too tight, divide it with the Otis urethrotome. Do not dilate it to accommodate the sheath.

Action

1. Assess the prostatic size bimanually and endoscopically to see if it is suitable for resection. Examine the bladder to ascertain that there are no lesions which would make a different approach more appropriate. All this can be done either with a conventional viewing irrigating cystoscope or else with the appropriately sized resectoscope sheath, down which is passed a 70° viewing telescope.

2. Visualize the landmarks; these are basically the bladder neck and the verumontanum.

3. With a cutting current or a blended cutting and coagulating current, resect the bladder neck completely. Each resection cut is made by visualizing the area to be

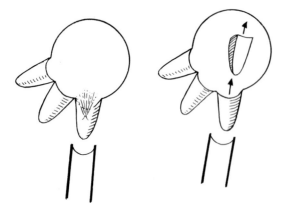

Fig. 15.12 Transurethral resection of the prostate

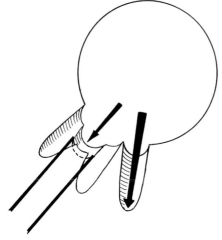

Fig. 15.13 Transurethral resection of the prostate. Resection of the ridges left behind, between previous cuts

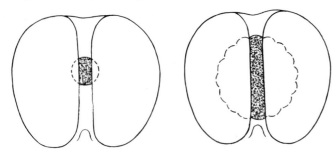

Fig. 15.14 Transurethral resection of the prostate. Preliminary resection of the bladder neck

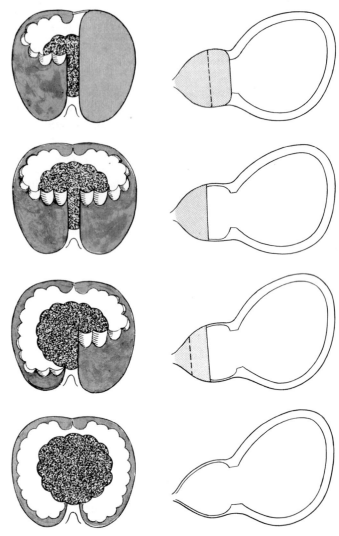

Fig. 15.15 Transurethral resection of the prostatic 'adenomas'

resected, passing the loop beyond this and then, while pressing the foot on the diathermy pedal, bringing the loop under vision backward into the sheath (Fig. 15.12).

The resected piece of bladder neck or prostate will be flushed into the bladder. Do not attempt to resect the lateral lobes until the neck is completed. This will avoid the hazard of going back again and again to the neck, which sometimes results in the resection being carried up under the trigone. Always resect under vision and coagulate the bleeding points as they show themselves. (Fig. 15.13).

4. Having satisfied yourself that the neck is completely resected, start on the lateral lobes (Fig. 15.14). Work on each lobe resecting toward yourself, keeping the resection of each in step. Avoid completing one lobe before starting on the other. Figure 15.15 demonstrates the progressive reduction in lobe size until the resection is complete.

5. When the 'cotton wool' appearance of the prostate gives way to transverse pinkish fibres, the capsule has been reached. Do not resect deeper than this.

6. At the level of the verumontanum the lobes often protrude just distal to it. Unless you have expert knowledge in this procedure it is wiser to leave these little areas behind.

Difficulty?

1. This operation must be left to the expert.

2. Always make sure the verumontanum is not obscured and never resect distal to it.

3. Coagulate bleeding points as they occur.

4. If the bleeding becomes so severe that vision is lost, then abandon the procedure. It is safer in these circumstances to wait a few days and start again or else proceed to an open enucleation if the amount resected at this time has been small.

5. The introduction of the 'Iglasis' continual irrigating resectoscope enables this procedure to be carried out continually, with constant pressure within the bladder. This not only speeds up the procedure but also probably renders it more safe, as high intra-prostatic cavity pressures are not reached and the absorption of the irrigating fluid may not be so great.

DIVERTICULECTOMY OF THE BLADDER

Appraise

1. It is not always necessary to remove inert diverticula. They often come to light in association with outflow problems, and if it is judged necessary to remove the diverticulum, it is often done immediately after a prostatic resection or as a planned procedure sometime later.

2. The approach to this operation, which is a difficult one, is a combination of extravesical and intravesical dissection.

Action

1. Cystoscope the patient. This will give you information about other bladder lesions, such as stones or tumours, and also the relationship of the diverticulum to the ureteric orifices. Leave a moderate amount of water in the bladder.

2. Expose the bladder widely, and without opening it, dissect the diverticulum as free as possible from surrounding fat and areolar tissue.

3. Trace the diverticulum as far down toward its neck as possible; it will often arise from behind the bladder, near the ureteric orifice.

4. Open the bladder in the midline, and by placing the forefinger within the diverticulum, complete your dissection down to the bladder.

5. Excise the diverticulum close to the bladder wall. For this excision it is often wise to pass a stiff probe or ureteric catheter within the adjacent ureter so that it can be identified.

6. Close the defect in the bladder muscle and mucosa separately with 2/0 chromic catgut. It is often easier to do this from within the bladder. By moving the ureteric probe you will make sure that you have not picked up the ureter with one of the closure sutures.

7. Drain the extravesical tissues with a tube drain and the bladder with a urethral catheter.

Difficulty?

1. The big problems in this procedure are the access — a wide Pfannenstiel incision should be used — and the proximity of some diverticula to the ureter. It may be necessary to expose the ureter fully as well as passing a ureteric catheter.

2. If it is necessary to divide the ureter then it will need reimplantation. For details of this procedure see page 235.

PARTIAL CYSTECTOMY

Appraise

1. There are two broad indications for partial cystectomy. The first is for primary bladder pathology; this is rarely required and is almost entirely confined to solitary superficial bladder tumours situated in or near the dome of the bladder, or for a urachal tumour.

2. The second is where the bladder is locally invaded by a primary carcinoma of the sigmoid colon or occasionally of the caecum, or where the colon is extensively involved in diverticular disease or more rarely Crohn's disease.

PARTIAL CYSTECTOMY FOR PRIMARY BLADDER PATHOLOGY

Action

1. The pathology and extent of the disease will have been previously assessed, so preliminary cystoscopy is unnecessary. Pass a small catheter, empty the bladder and distend it with distilled water. This has the advantage of possibly breaking down any free malignant cells.

2. Expose the bladder and mobilize fully. This may necessitate dividing the superior vesical pedicles, where present.

3. Open the bladder well clear of the growth and completely excise the growth with a margin of at least 3–4 cm. It may mean leaving a small bladder capacity; this however, readily distends.

4. Wash the bladder remnant and perivesical space several times with distilled water.

5. Close the bladder in two layers with a urethral catheter for 10 days. Drain the perivesical space.

Difficulty?

1. Never be tempted to do a partial cystectomy for more than one lesion. This will mean that the mucosa is unstable, and your incision will therefore incoporate unstable mucosa.

2. Do not perform partial cystectomy after radiotherapy.

3. In a case where the growth is near the ureter, refer to a specialist as it may well need re-implantation.

4. Consider postoperative radiotherapy should the definitive pathology show muscle invasion.

PARTIAL CYSTECTOMY IN CONJUNCTION WITH A PRIMARY BOWEL RESECTION

This is basically an extension of anterior resection of the rectosigmoid, where the growth or diverticular disease involves the bladder, often with a fistula.

Action

1. When you have decided that a partial cystectomy is necessary, distend the bladder. Mobilize it as necessary and perform the partial cystectomy first. This you will find frees the bowel and so facilitates resection.

2. Close the bladder with a urethral catheter and proceed with the bowel resection.

Difficulty?

1. If the growth is near the ureter, then refer to a specialist as a re-implantation or transureteroureterostomy will be necessary.

2. If you are sure that the disease is diverticular disease, then all that may be necessary is to nip the bowel off the bladder and drain the bladder urethrally for 10 days.

OPEN EXCISION OF BLADDER TUMOUR

Appraise

1. This is a rare procedure, and the decision is made entirely on the cystoscopic appearance, biopsy and bimanual examination. It should be reserved for a solitary tumour that is not invading the bladder muscle.

2. The main reason for open excision is that the lesion is too big for endoscopic resection.

3. Never be tempted to do this procedure for multiple lesions or where the bladder mucosa appears unstable.

Action

1. Distend the bladder with distilled water.

2. Expose the bladder and open it well away from the tumour.

3. Excised the tumour well down to the bladder muscle with a diathermy loop and coagulate the base.

4. Radioactive gold grains may now, if thought necessary, be inserted round the base of the lesion. This is done by the radiotherapist, who estimates the dosage and distribution of the grains.

5. Wash the bladder and wound several times with distilled water.

6. Close with a urethral catheter, never a suprapubic catheter.

Difficulty?

For a lesion situated round or near one ureteric orifice, ignore the orifice, for although there is often reflux afterwards, very little harm comes to the ureter or kidney.

SIMPLE CYSTECTOMY

Appraise

Use when the urinary stream has to be diverted for non-malignant conditions of the bladder, i.e. neurogenic bladder. Leaving the bladder in these instances is usually safe, but occasionally a pyocystis develops necessitating its removal.

Action

1. If the urine has previously been diverted, an extra-peritoneal approach through an extended Pfannenstiel or lower left paramedian incision can be used.

2. Keeping close to the bladder, expose, ligate and divide the superior and inferior pedicles.

3. In men, in an endeavour to maintain potency, the bladder may be excised leaving the prostate. Usually it is very difficult to retain the vesicles and vas. Doing this may lead to collections of seminal fluid in the retropubic space which periodically infect and discharge. This leads to unnecessary morbidity. As these patients are usually impotent anyway, this precaution may be unnecessary.

4. Should you decide to remove the prostate and the vesicles, expose the prostate anteriorly and laterally with blunt and sharp dissection. With finger dissection, break through behind the urethra so that the forefinger can be hooked round the urethra. Clamp the urethra proximally with a suitable curved clamp and divide distal to this.

5. Turn the prostate upwards, and with blunt and scissor dissection free the prostate, vesicles and bladder from the rectum.

6. Protecting the rectum with your assistant's fingers, divide through the lateral fascial attachments on each side and so remove the bladder.

7. There is usually considerable venous oozing from under the pubic arch. If possible arrest this with coagulation.

8. Pass a Foley catheter with a large balloon and inflate the balloon to its maximum. Attaching a Uribag containing 100 ml water to this catheter, and hang it over the foot of the bed to stop all the retropubic oozing by direct pressure; it also acts as a pelvic drain.

9. Close the wound with a large tube drain attached to a drainage bag.

10. If a urinary diversion has not previously been carried out, perform this now.

RADICAL CYSTECTOMY

RADICAL CYSTECTOMY IN THE MALE

Action

1. Place the patient in a steep Trendelenburg position.

2. Perform a preliminary laparotomy through a lower left paramedian incision, not only to access local operability but also to look for any evidence of liver or peritoneal secondaries.

3. Increase the length of the incision so that the lower end is down to the symphysis pubis, the upper end being either level with or above the umbilicus according to the size of the patient.

4. Expose each ureter as it crosses the bifurcation of the common iliac artery.

5. Divide the ureters at this level if an ileal loop diversion is to be fashioned, or lower down for a ureterocolic anastomosis. Ligate the lower ends only, to act as markers, leaving the ureters to drain freely.

6. Ligate each internal iliac artery in continuity, unless arterially contraindicated.

7. With finger dissection sweep the retropubic space clean in front and as far laterally as is possible. Keeping well away from the bladder, divide the peritoneum, vas and vesical pedicles as close to the pelvic wall as possible.

8. Once both sides have been cleared using scissor dissection, cut down retropubically until the forefinger can be insinuated between the urethra and rectum. The prostate will serve as a guide.

9. Hooking the forefinger round the urethra and retracting it backward on the prostate, place a long curved clamp on the urethra and divide distally. There is usually venous oozing at this point.

10. Turn the clamp and urethra upwards and, with a combination of finger and scissor dissection, peel the prostate and vesicles off the rectum.

11. There will now remain the lateral attachments of the bladder; divide these with scissors, taking care to guard the rectum which is in very close proximity.

12. Pack the pelvic space firmly and proceed with the urinary diversion.

13. Remove the packs; a lot of the oozing will have ceased. Secure any bleeding points that are evident.

14. Carry out a node dissection up to the aortic bifurcation.

15. Insert a large Foley urethral catheter and inflate the balloon to maximum, i.e. 30 ml. Attach this catheter to a Uribag with about 100 ml water; hang the bag over the foot of the operating table, and ultimately over the foot of the patient's bed. This amount of traction will usually arrest any tiresome venous oozing from the retropubic and periurethral areas.

16. Close the wound with a wide-bore soft tube drain attached to a drainage bag.

RADICAL CYSTOURETHRECTOMY IN THE MALE

Action

1. Place the patient in a steep Trendelenburg position and employ Lloyd-Davies leg rests.

2. Proceed as for a radical cystectomy up to and including stage 8.

3. Pass a Foley catheter and inflate the balloon.

4. Make a vertical incision on the ventral surface of the penis over its proximal two-thirds.

5. With sharp dissection establish the plane between the urethra and corpora.

6. Dissect the urethra free, tying it distally around the catheter.

7. Split the glans ventrally and completely free the urethra distally.

8. Using traction on the catheter, free the urethra and spongy tissue on all sides until the plane is established with the pelvic exploration. Pass the catheter end with the freed urethra back into the retropubic space.

9. Reflect the whole urethra upwards, and with it the prostate and vesicles, and proceed with the radical cystectomy.

RADICAL CYSTECTOMY IN THE FEMALE

Action

1. As well as preparing the abdomen and thighs, prepare the vulva and vagina.

2. Proceed as for a radical cystectomy in the male up to and including stage 6.

3. Divide each ovarian pedicle and so free both fallopian tubes and ovaries.

4. With finger dissection sweep the retropubic space clean and divide the peritoneum, superior vesical, inferior vesical and uterine pedicles.

5. Clean and dissect down anteriorly immediately beneath the pubic arch until the urethra is reached. Retract firmly on the bladder and divide the urethra as far distally as possible. One is usually able to remove the entire urethra.

6. Continue dividing downwards until the vagina is entered. Hook the forefinger into the vagina and retract the bladder and anterior vaginal wall upwards and backwards.

7. With scissors divide along each lateral wall of the

vagina, eventually meeting these two incisions just below the cervix.

8. Divide the lateral vesical and uterine attachments and so remove the whole bladder, anterior half of the vagina, the uterus, fallopian tubes and ovaries. The posterior strip of vagina is left in situ and of course protects the rectum from any damage.

9. Carry out a pelvic node dissection.

10. Proceed with the urinary diversion and close the wound with vaginal and suprapubic drains.

Difficulty?

Radical cystectomies and cystourethrectomies should not be undertaken unless the surgeon has special training in such procedures. Difficulty may be encountered where there has been previous, often ill-advised, open bladder surgery, after radiotherapy and after extensive transurethral resections of bladder tumours.

The two big hazards are haemorrhage and damage to the rectum. In the former by retracting the bladder medially in order to display the pedicles, the common iliac vein can be tented and damaged. Rectal damage can lead to very serious problems particularly after radiotherapy; it is usually apparent at the time of surgery and the defect must be carefully repaired and, if necessary, a defunctioning colostomy performed.

MANAGEMENT OF URINARY EXTRAVASATION

Appraise

1. These remarks do not apply to the management of a ruptured bladder or posterior urethra, where there may be intraperitoneal and perivesical extravasation. They refer to superficial extravasation due to a urethral injury following dilatation, or more commonly, as a result of an anterior urethral stricture, abscess formation and so extravasation of urine into the superficial tissues.

2. In these cases the extravasation of urine is very toxic and causes extensive necrosis of subcutaneous tissues and eventually the skin. It is limited posteriorly by the attachment of Colles fascia, which also limits its spread down the thighs, being attached just below the inguinal ligament. It will spread subcutaneously throughout the scrotum and the shaft of the penis and will ascend up the anterior abdominal wall.

3. If the urine is not already infected, the necrotic tissues will certainly become so.

Action

1. Perform a suprapubic drainage of the bladder.

2. Make as many incisions as are necessary in the perineum, scrotum, penile shaft and anterior abdominal wall to let out the infected urine and necrotic tissue. Never be afraid to widely open up the spaces.

3. Use the appropriate antibiotic where known, or else a broad-spectrum one.

4. Deal with the stricture when all has settled down.

EMERGENCY TREATMENT OF RUPTURE OF THE URETHRA

Appraise

1. There are essentially two varieties of ruptured urethra. One is the direct perineal injury which may partially or completely damage the bulbous or even penile urethra. The second is either a partial or complete tear of the posterior urethra. This latter injury is often associated with severe multiple injuries and is always associated with fracture of the pelvic ring, which results in a shearing force disrupting the prostatic urethra from the membranous urethra. For full clinical details of these injuries, refer to standard texts.

2. In all these cases, life-saving is imperative. The safest, easiest and most informative investigation that can be performed to evaluate the urethral injury is a gentle urethrogram with an aqueous solution. Should the dye enter the bladder then the rupture is either insignificant or incomplete, and in this instance a simple suprapubic drainage procedure is all that is necessary should the patient be unable to void.

RUPTURED BULBOUS URETHRA

With 'falling astride' injuries, the patient's general condition is usually good and exploration should be undertaken as soon as feasible. Avoid attempts at catheterization.

Action

1. Place the patient in the lithotomy position.

2. Make a midline incision over the bruised area. The tissues will be difficult to recognize.

3. Identify the bulbar muscles and separate each laterally from the midline.

4. Pass a metal sound gently down to the site of the injury and open the urethra in the midline immediately distal to the injured area. For this manoeuvre Riddle's grooved sound is very useful. Run a fine mattress catgut suture along each side of the opened urethra to stop the bulbar tissues bleeding profusely.

5. Continue your incision to open up the urethra right through the injury. This will show the completeness of the rupture.

6. Now that the injured area is opened up, approximate the dorsal surface of the urethra only with two or three interrupted fine catgut sutures.

7. Pass a small urethral plastic Foley catheter down the penis, across the repaired urethra and into the bladder.

8. Gently pack the wound with paraffin gauze and leave it well open to drain.

9. Encourage frequent baths and dressing changes.

10. Allow the whole area to heal spontaneously.

11. Any residual stricturing can be dealt with in later years by intermittent dilatations or urethroplasty.

Difficulty?

1. If the patient's general condition does not allow exploration within 48 hours, leave a suprapubic catheter in situ for 3–4 months and then refer for a formal urethroplasty. In these cases the fibrosis can be exceedingly severe.

2. After the whole area has healed, do not be tempted to pass sounds or a urethroscope just to see how things are getting on. Rather, perform regular urethrograms which are so much more informative.

RUPTURE OF THE POSTERIOR URETHRA

Appraise

1. There are two very definite approaches to the management of this condition. One postulates that this injury is practically never a complete severance of the urethra and all that is necessary is to drain with a suprapubic catheter for 2–3 weeks, by which time the urethra will have re-epithelialized and a small panendoscope can be passed into the bladder. Certainly if in doubt as to the management of a particular case, or if the other injuries are too severe, a suprapubic drainage procedure is very safe.

2. It is however, difficult to believe that with severe dislocation of the prostate and rupture of the urethra that there is not complete severance, and in this instance operative reduction and realignment of the two ends of the urethra is essential. This line of thought is the one most commonly adopted. Certainly this management will afford ample drainage of the peri-prostatic and vesical spaces, so minimizing the resultant fibrosis.

3. Only when the general condition of the patient permits is operative repair possible. The technique of railroading is still the most satisfactory for realigning the torn urethra; the method of holding the urethral ends together is questioned.

Action

1. Position the patient with Lloyd-Davies leg supports and drape the whole area.

2. Use a generous Pfannenstiel incision if there is no need to explore the abdomen. If in doubt, a long left lower paramedian incision will afford ample exposure for the urethral injury as well as for a laparotomy. Do not hesitate to use two incisions if you suspect an upper abdominal injury as well.

2. Explore the retropubic space. It will be very oedematous and haemorrhagic. Feel for the prostate; in young boys identifying the urethra will be difficult.

3. Open the bladder and identify the internal meatus.

4. Pass one metal sound up the urethra and another down through the internal meatus. You will feel the two ends meet. By advancing the lower sound in contact with the upper one, guide it into the bladder.

5. Attach a suitable piece of rubber tubing to the tip of the lower sound. Again, a sound with a small hole drilled in its tip is useful. Pull the tubing out through the urethra and attach to its distal end a Foley catheter. Now pull the catheter back through the penile urethra, across the rupture and into the bladder.

6. By inflating the balloon and applying traction to the catheter the two ends can certainly be held together.

At this stage there are various problems. In young boys prolonged traction on the bladder neck may render them incontinent. It is probable that this is because the balloon is not inflated enough and the traction is too strong, so that a sausage of balloon is forcing the bladder neck and posterior urethra open. Another problem is that of a penoscrotal urethral fistula due to pressure necrosis. This is usually because the traction is applied over the end of the bed; it should be at 45° upwards. The third disadvantage is that if the catheter should fall out, it may be exceedingly difficult, if not impossible to replace it, and indeed the patient may have to be re-explored. All these disadvantages can be overcome by taking appropriate precautions. Inflate the balloon fully so that the pressure is not concentrated on the bladder neck. Use only the minimum of traction, i.e. 100 g or a Uribag with 100 ml water in it; use even less in children. Apply the traction in an upward direction to about 45° to the horizontal. Use a nylon suture and Emessay button to hold the tip of the catheter in situ. Finally drain the bladder suprapubically.

7. Leave the urethral catheter for 14 days, gradually reducing the traction over this time. The tissues should be reasonably firm after about 1 week.

8. Maintain the suprapubic catheter until either the patient can void spontaneously or a urethrogram has shown an intact passage.

9. With multiple orthopaedic injuries where the patient may be immobilized for a considerable time, the suprapubic catheter may be left as a matter of expedience.

Technical points

1. Because of the problems associated with catheter traction, other techniques have been evolved. These are difficult and should be left to the realm of a urologist. They consist of either direct suture of the torn ends or else

holding them together by sutures passed through the prostate and held on the perineum by buttons or bars.

2. Always work in close co-operation with the orthopaedic surgeons.

3. The two essentials are to get as good an alignment as possible and to ensure free bladder drainage.

4. Use a minimum of traction.

5. Avoid instrumentation.

6. Refer residual stricture problems to a urologist.

INTRAPERITONEAL RUPTURE OF THE BLADDER

Appraise

1. This is an unusual injury to occur by itself, and other injuries must therefore be dealt with accordingly.

2. Gently perform a urethrogram using an aqueous solution to ascertain the damage to the bladder and also to give the vital information as to whether it is associated with a urethral injury.

Action

1. Expose the bladder intra- and extraperitoneally. This enables you to perform an exploratory laparotomy at the same time.

2. Clean the peritoneal cavity.

3. Open the bladder so that other injuries can be seen which may have escaped notice.

4. Close the bladder incision and injuries in two layers if possible. Drain either urethrally if there is no urethral injury or suprapubically if there is any doubt.

CYSTOPLASTIES

Appraise

1. These operations are used to increase the capacity of chronically contracted bladders. The commonest indications are quiescent tuberculosis or severe Hunner's ulcer.

2. There are three methods used: ileocystoplasty, colocystoplasty and caecocystoplasty. Use of the caecum is probably the most satisfactory as it acts as a good reservoir and is anatomically adjacent to the area.

3. Just to make a hole in the bladder or to remove a small segment of bladder wall and attach the bowel to it is incorrect. This merely creates a diverticulum. It is necessary to remove virtually the whole bladder just leaving the internal meatus and a fringe around the trigone of sufficient size to enable attachment of the bowel. It is essentially a bowel replacement of the bladder on to the trigone.

4. The advantage of employing the caecum is in being able to utilize the terminal ileum as part of the new bladder. This ileal segment can be used for ureteric implantation should this prove necessary. If the procedure fails then it is not difficult to convert this ileal segment into a conduit.

5. In all cystoplasties it may be necessary to lower the outflow resistance in order to obtain satisfactory emptying of the new bladder. This is particularly so in the male.

REPAIR OF VESICOVAGINAL FISTULA

1. The surgical approach in this condition depends on the size and position of the fistula, whether or not there has been previous radiotherapy, and the particular preference of the surgeon.

2. The gynaecologist usually approaches the fistula through the vagina, the urologist through the bladder or else by a combined intra- and extravesical approach.

3. The principle of the operation is to establish the two layers, i.e. bladder and vagina, and close them separately. The interposition of omentum when done from above is a useful adjunct, especially so after radiotherapy. Carefully avoid the ureters.

4. Where radiotherapy has been extensive and repeated attempts have failed to close the fistula, there are two ways open for treatment. One is to close the vaginal introitus, colpocleisis, so that the vagina merely becomes a diverticulum to the bladder. The second procedure is to perform a urinary diversion, usually with an ileal conduit.

OPERATIONS FOR INCONTINENCE AND URETHRAL STRICTURE

STRESS INCONTINENCE

Operations for stress incontinence in women are well described in advanced texts of urology and gynaecology, as are the modern techniques for postprostatectomy incontinence. The reader interested in this particular topic should also read the appropriate literature on the use of electronic stimulators in the control of incontinence. The description of their use is beyond the scope of this book.

URETHROPLASTIES FOR STRICTURE

There are four basic techniques for the plastic repair of urethral strictures. These should only be undertaken by experts in this particular field.

1. For short strictures with little or no adjacent scarring, mobilisation, excision, and end-to-end anastomosis in a one-stage procedure is highly satisfactory.

2. Strictures of limited length, but which may have adjacent scarring, can be treated by laying them open sufficiently to include all strictured and scarred tissue. The next step is to suture in place a pedicled full-thickness skin-graft from the adjacent scrotal skin, so forming a one-stage patch urethroplasty. A free full-thickness graft, using foreskin skin or a split-skin graft, can also be employed in selected cases.

3. Staged urethroplasties. The basic concept of these operations is to open widely the stricture, continuing the incision distal and proximal to it so that the largest sound or the index finger can be introduced into the bladder. Scrotal skin is sutured to the opened-out edges of this area and the hole is left to heal. The patient is reviewed at regular intervals.When all has healed and no further stricturing has occurred, which may take many months, a circumferential incision is made to include the urethral roof and immediate surrounding skin. This is closed over as a tube and the scrotum is then reconstructed. Epilation of the scrotal skin to be used as the inlay is carried out during review examinations (refer to the works of Turner-Warwick and Blandy for operative details).

4. Transpubic urethroplasty. This is performed for totally disrupted urethras, combined with severe pelvic fractures. Usually the injuries are several months or even years old, and are often associated with a suprapubic urinary diversion. This procedure is highly specialised. A combined suprapubic and perineal approach is used. Urethra and bladder neck are identified, and the whole scarred area is excised, including all encroaching bone. The ends are then anastomosed over a catheter. Continence, although not 100%, can often be quite pleasing in these cases.

DRAINAGE OF PERIURETHRAL ABSCESS

Appraise

This condition is usually the result of a urethral stricture. It may therefore be necessary before drainage of the abscess to establish adequate urinary drainage with a suprapubic catheter. Forcibly dilating the stricture under these conditions is hazardous.

Action

1. Incise over the most prominent part of the abscess and lay it completely open.

2. Break down any loculi and pack the cavity with a Eusol or similar dressing.

3. Once healing is proceeding well, it is safe to pass a dilator and establish urethral drainage if necessary.

4. When all has healed over, perform a urethrogram to establish the extent of the stricture; use this information to decide on future management.

16

Surgery of the penis, scrotum and regional glands

CIRCUMCISION

Appraise

The only medical indication for circumcision is phimosis, which falls into three categories:

1. Infantile.
2. Phimosis in the middle years of life, almost invariably balanitis xerotica obliterans.
3. Senile.

In hot, unhygienic countries, circumcision has developed into a religious cult, and carcinoma of the penis and balanitis are virtually non-existent. However, with good education and hygiene the need for wholesale circumcision, with its inevitable morbidity and mortality (however small these may be) is questioned. Some of the tribal circumcision rites in certain African states are barbaric and cannot be condoned.

From a surgical point of view, an unnecessary operation is an unnecessary operation and, in particular, infants should not be exposed to unnecessary hazards. Each surgeon must, however, make up his own mind when confronted with a request for infant circumscision.

Action

1. Grasp the tip of the dorsal surface of the foreskin in the midline with a small artery forceps and gently pull downward until it is held on the stretch.

2. If the phimosis is particularly severe, use a second pair of artery forceps as a dilator to enlarge the opening.

3. Gently, using a silver probe in the infant or artery forceps in the adult, free the foreskin from the glans so that it can be completely retracted, leaving no adhesions or inspissated smegma behind. Wash with non-spirituous solution.

4. Pull the foreskin down over the glans and apply two straight artery forceps side by side in the midline on the dorsal surface of the foreskin. Divide between these two (Fig. 16.1).

5. Continue the incision in the same direction with straight scissors about 3–6 mm short of the corona according to the size (Fig. 16.2).

6. From the apex of this incision, cut laterally until the incision reaches the lateral border of the glans (Fig. 16.3).

7. Now carry the incision towards the fraenum, making sure that both surfaces of the foreskin are cut together.

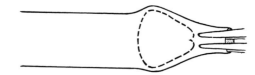

Fig. 16.1 Circumcision

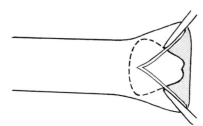

Fig. 16.2 Circumcision

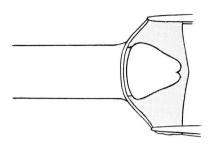

Fig. 16.3 Circumcision

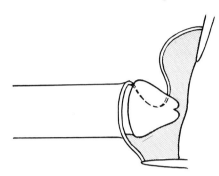

Fig. 16.4 Circumcision

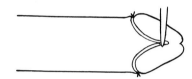

Fig. 16.5 Circumcision

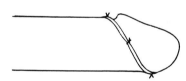

Fig. 16.6 Circumcision

This ensures that the undersurface of the glans is not denuded of skin (Fig. 16.4).

8. Place a small artery forceps across the fraenum, so catching the inverted-V extension of skin and fraenum together, and excise the foreskin from this (Fig. 16.5).

9. Transfix the fraenum and apex of shaft skin with a fine chromic catgut stitch and tie firmly, releasing the artery forceps.

10. Search for and pick up all the bleeding vessels and tie with fine catgut. There is usually one artery, on each side of the shaft of the penis, which tends to retract.

11. Bring the two layers of the foreskin together with three sutures, two lateral ones and one dorsal. Always avoid excess suturing (Fig. 16.6).

Difficulty?

1. Do not pull downward on the foreskin once the initial two artery forceps have been applied, thus avoiding the removal of too much skin.

2. Never, ever, use diathermy.

3. An adherent foreskin may be very difficult to separate from the glans and may even require sharp dissection. This is particularly so with long-standing phimosis in adults after repeated infections or in balanitis xerotica obliterans.

4. Always make sure all bleeding is arrested. Infants cannot tolerate blood loss.

5. Never sew on dressings. Do not use dressings unless absolutely necessary and then very loosely.

SURGERY FOR PARAPHIMOSIS

Operation is indicated when it is not possible to reduce the paraphimosis under general anaesthesia.

Action

1. Hold the penis on the fingers of one hand, placing the thumb uppermost on the glans.

2. Depress the glans downwards so exposing the constricting band. After many hours of paraphimosis, it may be exceedingly difficult to identify this ring clearly due to the gross oedema.

3. Incise the ring longitudinally with a small knife. This incision should be of sufficient length and depth to release the constriction and so enable the paraphimosis to be reduced.

4. Leave the incision wide open and cover with loose dressings.

5. Proceed to formal circumcision when all inflammation and oedema has settled.

MEATOTOMY

Appraise

1. The indications for this operation are meatal stenosis or insufficient meatal size to allow free passage of endoscopic instruments.

2. In a urological department, the 'Otis' urethrotome is the standard method of meatotomy. Make the incision dorsally, having introduced the urethrotome into the distal urethra, and open it to a 20–30 F gauge. This dorsal incision heals perfectly and leaves no resulting stenosis.

3. For the virtually occluded distal urethra, a meatoplasty utilizing a skin-flap to widen the urethra goes a long way to avoiding the misdirected stream or spraying seen following this standard meatotomy.

4. However, the operation probably most commonly performed in general departments, will be the standard meatotomy. Any resultant spraying can later on be helped by referral to a specialist unit for meatoplasty.

Action

1. Gently dilate the meatus until one blade of a straight artery forceps can be introduced into the orifice.

2. Direct the forceps just to one side of the midline and introduce one blade until its tip lies in the fossa naviculare. Firmly clamp the forceps and leave for 5 minutes (Fig. 16.7).

3. Remove the forceps and divide the crushed area with straight scissors. If there is any bleeding, use a fine catgut suture to under-run the bleeding point.

4. Instruct the patient how to keep the cut edges apart. He should do this each time he passes urine and when he has a bath, until the wound is well healed. The use of a small spigot as a meatal dilator is often advantageous in the healing stage.

Check list

1. Have you opened far enough back into the urethra?

2. Failure to keep the incision wide open until it has healed results in restenosis.

3. Loss of the directional effect of the meatus may occur, with resultant spraying of the stream.

OPERATIONS FOR HYDROCOELE IN THE ADULT

EXCISION OF HYDROCOELE

This procedure is suitable for very large or thick-walled hydrocoeles.

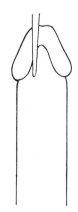

Fig. 16.7 Meatotomy

Action

1. Grasp the scrotum firmly with one hand and stretch the skin over the hydrocoele.

2. Choose an appropriate area between the vessels in the skin to make a transverse incision. The vessels usually run transversely. Carry the incision through all layers of the scrotum. Make the incision long enough to allow the whole scrotal contents to be delivered. The scrotal skin stretches easily, so this incision need not be of great length. Secure all bleeding points.

3. Use dissecting scissors and clean all the coverings off the hydrocoele sac until it is completely free.

4. Incise the sac and allow the fluid to escape. Continue the incision until the testicle can be freely delivered.

5. Excise the sac only, keeping close to the testicle.

6. Run a fine continuous haemostatic catgut suture along the cut edge of the sac.

7. Secure all small bleeding points with fine catgut.

8. Return the testicle to the scrotum.

9. Grasp the dartos muscle at each end of the incision with tissue forceps. Elevating these will bring the muscle into view.

10. Approximate the dartos with a continuous catgut suture. This will gather the muscle together and with it the skin, obviating the need for skin sutures.

11. Apply a firm 'Litesome' or similar scrotal support or use a 10 cm crepe bandage to wind round the scrotum to minimize any subsequent swelling.

12. With a very adherent sac which needs scissor dissection to free it from the scrotum, it may be difficult to stop all oozing. Do not hesitate to use a drain in these circumstances.

13. An alternative technique is Jaboulay's operation. Instead of running a haemostatic suture along the cut edge of the sac, the edge is sutured together behind the epididymis.

RIDDLE'S PROCEDURE FOR HYDROCOELE

Action

1. Incise the scrotum as before. The incision should be long enough to deliver the testicle only.

2. Carry the incision, over its full length, down into the hydrocoele sac. Allow all fluid to escape.

3. Deliver the testicle from the sac and out through the scrotal incision.

4. Apply gentle traction on the testicle and counter-traction on the scrotum. This will evert the hydrocoele sac behind the testicle.

5. Plicate together the two walls of the sac, which will now lie behind the testicle, with fine catgut. Make sure you avoid the epididymis and cord structures.

6. Return the testicle into the scrotum and close the incision as before.

Difficulty?

The bulk of tissue to be returned to the scrotum may be too big. Lift up the skin edges with tissue forceps and with blunt scissor dissection free beneath the dartos until the cavity is sufficiently enlarged.

LORD'S PROCEDURE FOR HYDROCOELE

Action

1. Incise the scrotum down to and including the hydrocoele sac, securing all bleeding points in this incision.

2. Widen the incision so that visual and instrumental access is obtained into the hydrocoele.

3. Using six interrupted sutures, three on each side of the testis, pick up the edge of the sac and gather up the sac wall with a series of bites according to the sac size, finally taking a bite of the tunica.

4. When all these sutures are in place, tie them, so bunching up and obliterating the hydrocoele around the testis (Figs. 16.8 to 16.12).

5. Finally close the scrotal incision.

6. Apply a scrotal support.

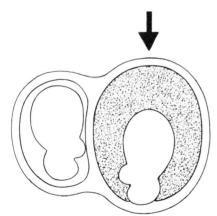

Fig. 16.8 Lord's hydrocoele operation

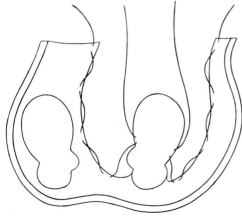

Fig. 16.9 Lord's hydrocoele operation

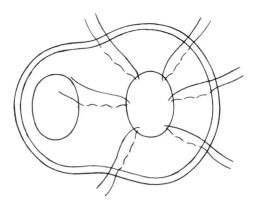

Fig. 16.10 Lord's hydrocoele operation

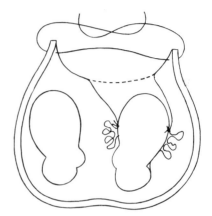

Fig. 16.11 Lord's hydrocoele operation

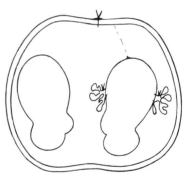

Fig. 16.12 Lord's hydrocoele operation

HYDROCOELE IN THE INFANT

These hydrocoeles are essentially hernias and should be treated as such, no attempt being made to excise the sac.

TORSION OF THE TESTICLE

Never delay operation: every minute counts. Never be tempted to leave the good side for another time; the child may leave the district and never return to hospital.

Action

1. Incise the scrotum transversely as described for hydrocoele operations. Continue the incision in depth until the testicle and cord can be delivered.

2. Untwist the torsion and wrap the testicle in a warm pack.

3. Make a similar incision in the other side of the scrotum and deliver the non-twisted testicle, noting any abnormal anatomy that may be present.

4. With a fine nylon stitch take a firm bite of the tunica of the testicle and anchor it to the side wall of the scrotum. Do this at both upper and lower poles.

5. Close the scrotal incision on the non-twisted side.

6. Remove the pack from the twisted testicle and examine it carefully for viability. If it is obviously dead and remains black it must be removed. Place a strong artery forceps across the cord and then remove the testicle and tie the cord with strong catgut.

7. If there is any hope of viability, return the testicle to the scrotum, fixing it with fine nylon sutures as described for the other side.

ORCHIECTOMY

SIMPLE ORCHIECTOMY

Remember to get the patient's consent before operation.

Indications

1. Severe or recurrent attacks of acute epididymitis.

2. Chronic epididymitis, including tuberculous epididymitis.

3. Severe testicular trauma. Only if the testicle is not salvageable should it be removed. Provided the appendages are intact, the majority of disrupted testes can be safely left, once the haematoma has been evacuated.

4. Testicular infarction from a neglected torsion.

Action

1. If the condition is inflammatory and involves the skin, then make the incision in the scrotum so as to excise the overlying attached infected skin. The incision will therefore vary in shape and size according to the condition.

2. The involved skin should be left attached to the underlying structures. Enter the scrotal sac away from the inflamed area.

3. Deliver the testicle with the overlying attached area of skin. Do not hesitate to remove all the involved surrounding skin.

4. Apply gentle traction to the testicle and clean the cord structures so that 4–6 cm of cord are freed.

5. Cross-clamp the cord at this level with two strong artery forceps, and divide between these. Do not pull on

the testicle or else the divided upper end may retract from view.

6. Tie the clamped upper end with strong catgut, but do not release the forceps until a second tie has been applied. If the cord is very thick, tease it into two structures and cross-clamp each, so avoiding a bulky tie.

7. Use finger dissection and traction on the lower divided cord to remove the testicle.

8. Leave the scrotal wound unsutured to drain freely. Never be tempted to close the wound.

9. Apply loose dressings only.

Difficulty?

Do not apply traction when clamping and dividing the cord. A divided, untied cord which retracts up into the inguinal canal will mean a higher exploration and can be dangerous.

BILATERAL SIMPLE ORCHIECTOMY

This operation is indicated for advanced carcinoma of the prostate.

Action

1. Make two small skin incisions immediately over each external ring. They may be placed obliquely or transversely.
2. Identify the cords by rolling them over the pubic tubercles.
3. Free the cords and pull each testicle out of the scrotum into the groin
4. Cross-clamp and divide the cords as before.
5. Close the skin wounds. Testicular prostheses may be inserted before wound closure.

Alternatively a single scrotal incision can be used and both testes excised, as described for unilateral orchiectomy.

SUBCAPSULAR ORCHIECTOMY

After exposure of the testes, the tunica is incised and the testicular contents are scooped out. It has the advantage that some men may feel slightly less inclined to refuse this procedure, but it has the theoretical disadvantage that the epididymis may well secrete androgen. This is not borne out clinically, however.

RADICAL ORCHIECTOMY

The radical orchiectomy is the biopsy in cases of suspected tumour; never be tempted to biopsy first. Remember to get the patient's permission.

Action

1. Clean the whole of the inguinal region, scrotum, penis and upper thighs.

2. Drape to expose the inguinal region on the affected side. The drapes should be arranged so that easy access is available to the scrotum.

3. Make an incision parallel to but 2 cm above the medial two-thirds of the inguinal ligament. The medial end of this incision should be centred on the pubic tubercle. Carry this incision down to the external oblique aponeurosis. Secure all bleeding points.

4. Clean the external oblique aponeurosis and identify the external ring. Open the external oblique over the length of the wound along the line of its fibres, dividing into the external ring.

5. Identify the cord by rolling it under the forefinger as it crosses the pubic tubercle.

6. Free the cord with forefinger and thumb at this point and cradle it in the crooked forefinger.

7. Apply traction on the cord with this forefinger, and with a blunt pair of dissecting forceps, completely free the cord from the inguinal canal.

8. Cross-clamp the cord with two large artery forceps at the internal ring and divide between them. Tie as described before.

9. Apply gentle traction to the divided lower cord, and by pushing the testicle from below through the scrotum manipulate the testicle up into the groin. You will usually invert the scrotum by doing this. Free the testicle from the scrotum by blunt dissection.

10. Close the external oblique aponeurosis with continuous 1 chromic catgut.

11. Close the skin with or without subcutaneous fat sutures.

12. After applying the dressing fit a firm Litesome or similar scrotal support, or use a 10 cm crepe bandage to bind the scrotum and so minimize subsequent swelling.

If a tumour is suspected, but doubt still exists, then proceed up to No. 7. Instead of artery forceps, an occluding bowel clamp is now applied. The testicle can be safely delivered and examined with the naked eye, before proceeding to excision.

TESTICULAR BIOPSY

Always ask your pathologist which fixative will be required before you start.

Action

1. Grasp the testicle firmly with the hand so that the skin is stretched over it.

2. Make a small 1 cm skin incision carried down through the layers of the scrotum until you reach the tunica albuginea.

3. Make a small incision through the tunica albuginea so that it just gapes open and a minute amount of testicular tissue protudes.

4. With a clean sharp knife remove the protruding testicular tissue and place it in the fixative.

5. Close the scrotal incision with one or two fine catgut sutures.

EXCISION OF EPIDIDYMAL CYSTS

Epididymal cysts should be excised when they become uncomfortably large. Removal of epididymal cysts is contraindicated in the young or unmarried, as it often renders that side sterile.

Action

1. Incise the scrotum as described for excision of a hydrocoele sac.

2. Deliver the testicle along with its appendages, including the cysts. Remember that cysts are often multiple and commonly occur in the upper pole of the epididymis.

3. With blunt and scissor dissection, holding the testicle yourself with one hand or using an assistant to hold it, clean off all the adventitial tissue surrounding the cyst.

4. Using the same scissor dissection, completely excise the cyst or else marsupialize it by cutting off the whole protruding surface.

5. If there are very many cysts it is best to excise that part of the epididymis bearing them. Oversew the raw area left after this manoeuvre with find chromic catgut.

6. Return the testicle to the scrotum and continue as described for hydrocoeles.

A Lord's type of procedure as described for hydrocoele is often practical for large simple epididymal cysts. One has to be sure, however, that further cysts are not present.

EXCISION OF VARICOCOELE

Action

1. Make an incision in the inguinal region as for a hernia.

2. Expose the external oblique aponeurosis and open it in the line of its fibres into the external ring.

3. Free the cord from the canal and deliver the testicle out of the scrotum.

4. With dissection and and fine catgut ties, remove all the enlarged and tortuous veins which make up the pampiniform plexus. Do this over the whole length of the cord. Do not be afraid to remove all the enlarged veins; leaving a few will spoil the result.

5. Make sure that all bleeding points are secure and return the testicle to the scrotum.

6. Close the external oblique aponeurosis with continuous 1 chromic catgut and close the skin.

7. Fit a Litesome or similar scrotal support.

VASECTOMY FOR STERILIZATION

There are various methods for vasectomy; two safe techniques are described. Always use general anaesthesia if possible. The first technique can be used under local if necessary.

For all vasectomies make sure the appropriate consent and instructions are signed and understood.

METHOD 1

Action

1. Grasp the scrotum between the first two fingers and the thumb so as to be able to roll the scrotal skin between them.

2. Doing this in the upper part of the scrotum, feel the hard round structure of the vas apart from the cord (Fig. 16.13).

3. Grip the vas between the middle finger, which invaginates the scrotum, and the thumb on the outside. Move the index finger nearer to the thumb. Now spread the index finger and thumb apart, so holding the vas firmly across the invaginated middle finger. This will hold the vas in relief.

4. Make a 1 cm transverse cut into the scrotal skin, down to but not including the vas.

5. Still firmly holding the vas, grasp it with secure tissue forceps.

6. Release the finger and thumb. The vas will now protrude from the incision held by the forceps.

7. Force an artery forceps under the vas so that it cannot escape back into the scrotum, and release the tissue forceps. Next incise the tissues over the vas with a fine scalpel in the line of the vas. This will release the vas from its adventitial coverings and expose it as a shiny white structure.

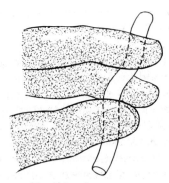

Fig. 16.13 Vasectomy: identifying the vas

8. Regrasp the vas with tissue forceps, but this time without its adventitial coverings. Use traction on this forceps and with blunt dissection strip the vas clean of all its surroundings over a distance of 6–7 cm. This will expose the convoluted lower part of the vas.

9. Apply artery forceps to the upper and lower ends of this 6–7 cm segment and completely excise it. Tie both ends firmly with catgut. Secure any bleeding points and suture the skin with 2/0 chromic catgut.

10. Repeat the process on the other side.

11. Send the excised segments for histology to confirm that you have in fact performed a bilateral vasectomy.

Difficulty?

1. Do not attempt this operation under local anaesthesia unless the patient and his scrotum are relaxed.

2. If you lose the vas in the scrotum, it is best to start again. Never be tempted to blindly grope for structures in the scrotum.

3. Under local anaesthesia, it is difficult to remove a satisfactory length of vas. Do not be satisfied with a simple division.

RIDDLE'S METHOD

In this technique only a small portion of each vas is removed and it has the advantage of being potentially reversible. Another advantage is that it is impossible for recanalization to occur with this technique.

Action

1. Proceed under general anaesthesia as described in the previous method up to stage 8. Riddle's method cannot be performed under local anaesthesia.

2. Before dividing the first vas, free the second vas completely.

3. High up the vas on one side, place a curved artery forceps.

4. Through the opposite skin incision, thrust a straight artery forceps through the median raphe and grasp the same vas just distal to the curved forceps (Fig. 16.14).

5. Divide between these two and pull the straight forceps with the lower end of the vas into the opposite side of the scrotum (Fig. 16.15).

6. Next thrust a curved artery forceps through the first skin incision, crossing the median raphe, and grasp the second vas in its lower part. Apply a straight forceps below this and divide between the two.

7. Pull the curved artery forceps back through the median raphe and out through the first incision.

8. Now tie both upper ends together with chromic 1 catgut on one side of the raphe and the two lower ends on

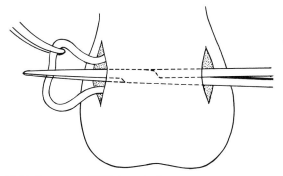

Fig. 16.14 Vasectomy: Riddle's method

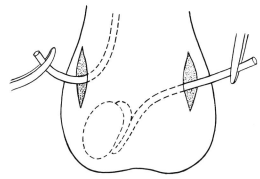

Fig. 16.15 Vasectomy: Riddle's method

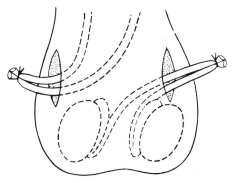

Fig. 16.16 Vasectomy: Riddle's method

the opposite side (Fig. 16.16). Take a small segment of each for histology.

9. Close each wound as before.

REVERSAL OF VASECTOMY AND EPIDIDYMO-VASOSTOMY

Appraise

1. Since the advent of vasectomy as a commonly accepted method of family planning, there is an increasing number of men coming forward wishing for the procedure to be reversed. It is perhaps an indication of poor counselling of the couple in the first instance that has led to this problem.

2. The overall figures suggest that at best there is a 50% chance of further pregnancies.

Action

The operative technique is to expose both ends of the vas and anastomose them with 5/0 or 6/0 unabsorbable sutures, with or without a fine nylon splint. There are various modifications beyond the scope of this book.

EPIDIDYMO-VASOSTOMY AND SPERM POUCHES

These are techniques, usually doomed to failure, to overcome a normal but blocked testicle. The techniques, some involving micro-surgery, are beyond the scope of this work.

ORCHIDOPEXY

Appraise

Employ for ectopic or undescended testicles.

Action

1. Make a small inguinal incision centred over the external ring. In young and fat boys Scarpa's fascia may be very thick and can be confused with the external oblique.

2. Expose the external oblique over its medial third. In cases of ectopic testes, where the testis will be lying outside the external oblique, care must be taken not to damage either the testicle or cord while exposing the external oblique.

3. If the testis is found lying in the superficial inguinal pouch, then free it and the cord until the latter can be traced passing backwards into the external ring.

4. The testis and cord should now be lying free, but there will not be enough cord length to bring the testicle down into the scrotum. Open the external oblique in the line of its fibres into the external ring.

5. Free the cord from within the canal right up to the internal ring. This will add more length.

6. Gently insert the little finger under the cord and in through the internal ring, sweeping it gently from side to side. This will free the cord, vas and vessels from any posterior adhesions, again adding length.

7. Hold the testis with one hand and apply gentle traction to the cord so that it is held taut. Now with fine non-toothed forceps gently separate the vas and vascular pedicle. Free all the adventitia from these structures over their full lengths. You may need to use sharp dissection for this. Take care not to damage either the vas or vessels. This will obtain the maximum length of cord available.

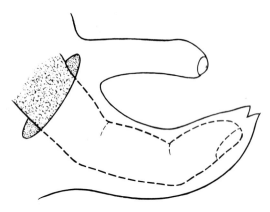

Fig. 16.17 Orchidopexy: skin incision for dartos pouch

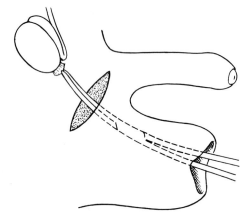

Fig. 16.18 Orchidopexy: manipulating testis into dartos pouch

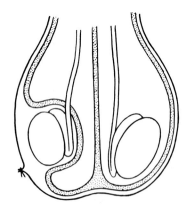

Fig. 16.19 Orchidopexy: testis in dartos pouch

8. Insert the forefinger into the scrotum, so widening the neck into this structure. There will then be easy access for the testis to be brought down. Now hold the scrotum stretched over the forefinger and make a small 1 cm long transverse cut in the scrotal skin over its most dependent part (Fig. 16.17). Just incise the skin, leaving the dartos muscle intact. Now with fine curved dissecting scissors, free a subcutaneous pouch between skin and dartos muslce for a distance of about 1 cm all round the incision.

9. Thrust a fine artery forceps through the exposed dartos and out through the groin incision, and grasp the remains of the gubernaculum (Fig. 16.18).

10. Bring the testicle down through the scrotum and tease it out through the small hole in the dartos made by the forceps. Make sure the cord structures are not twisted. Place the testicle in the subcutaneous pouch and close the skin of the scrotum with fine catgut (Fig. 16.19).

11. Close the inguinal incision.

Using this technique of anchoring the testicle will avoid any tension on the cord, which might endanger the vascular supply to the testicle.

Difficulty?

1. For undescended testis, which may lie within the canal or just within the internal ring, exactly the same technique is used. However, for these the cord length is often shorter and great care should be taken to obtain as much length as possible without either damaging the vessels or applying traction.

2. When there is not enough cord to bring the testicle into the scrotum, it is best to leave it as low as you can and try again when the child is older.

3. If the testicle is of miserable size with little cord length and the contralateral one is normal, then remove it.

4. If you cannot find the testicle and cord structures at all, then close the wound and refer the case to a specialist.

5. Should the condition be bilateral, then do both sides at the same operation. It is unkind to submit the child to two procedures.

6. Always bring the testes down before the age of 5 years. After this time spermatogenesis decreases.

SURGICAL TREATMENT OF PRIAPISM

Appraise

1. Whatever the cause, treatment must be instituted as soon as possible.

2. Should delay occur, then the resulting sludging of the blood in the corpora and eventual fibrosis will lead to impotence. Even with early treatment, impotence is an all too common event.

IRRIGATION

1. Pass a catheter as these patients have difficulty in voiding.

2. Either under local anaesthesia, i.e. spinal or epidural, or preferably general anaesthesia, insert a wide-bore aspiration needle into the distal end of one corpus

cavernosum and another into the proximal end of the opposite one.

3. Irrigate with 100–200 ml physiological saline or heparin/saline into the proximal needle.

4. After a while the fluid will come out reasonably clear from the opposite needle. Each injection of fluid will cause a considerable hardening of the priapism, but by massage, the fluid will escape and the corpora become flaccid. It may be necessary to have four needles in situ.

5. Apply a firm bandage and return the patient to the ward.

6. It may be necessary to repeat this process three or four times over the ensuing 48 hours before the corpora remain flaccid.

SAPHENOCORPORAL SHUNT

The irrigation technique is not very successful and it is usually necessary to establish some form of venous drainage to the corpora. The two corpora communicate and therefore only one shunt need be established.

Action

1. Expose the saphenous vein and dissect it free. Carefully ligate its tributaries.

2. Clean the saphenofemoral junction so that the vein can be swung medially without kinking.

3. Obtain about 8 cm of vein, less of course in children.

4. Make a longitudinal incision at the base of the penis and expose the tough fibrous covering of the corpus cavernosum.

5. Irrigate the penis as described before so that it is flaccid.

6. Make a window in the fibrous covering of sufficient size to anastomose it to the slit-up end of the saphenous vein with fine arterial sutures.

7. The patency of the shunt will be obvious as the anastomosed vein will fill out.

8. Close the skin incisions.

Difficulty?

1. Always irrigate the saphenous vein intermittently during the procedure with heparin/saline so that it does not thrombose.

2. If it appears unsuccessful then repeat the process on the opposite side.

3. If the process is successful for 24–48 hours and then the priapism returns, it is necessary to perform a shunt on the other side.

4. Systemic anticoagulants and fibrinolysins appear to have no effect in the management of this condition.

CORPUS CAVERNOSUM-SPONGIOSUM ANASTOMOSIS

The saphenocorporal shunt has the best chance of success. Should it fail, an anastomosis between the corpus cavernosum and spongiosum may be tried.

AMPUTATION OF THE PENIS
PARTIAL AMPUTATION

1. Use a rubber band type of tourniquet round the base of the penis.

2. Choose the level of amputation and make a circular incision round the penis through the skin.

3. Carry this incision through the two corpora cavernosa, but stop short of the spongiosum and urethra.

4. Dissect the urethra free distally for about 2 cm and amputate the end of the penis at this level (Fig. 16.20).

5. Slit up the ventral surface of the urethra so turning it into a flat surface.

6. Secure any bleeding points on releasing the tourniquet. The best method to stop the corpora bleeding is to firmly oppose their fibrous walls (Fig. 16.21).

7. Turn the urethra upwards and suture it to the skin circumferentially. (Fig. 16.22).

8. Leave in a small catheter for a few days.

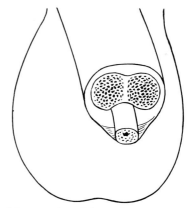
Fig. 16.20 Partial amputation of the penis

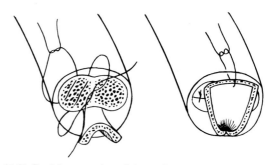
Fig. 16.21 Partial amputation of the penis

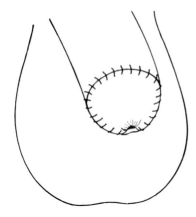

Fig. 16.22 Partial amputation of the penis

TOTAL AMPUTATION

Avoid the temptation of leaving the testes in this procedure. It makes the operation difficult and the end result of the urethrostomy poor.

1. Once the skin has been incised round the dorsum of the base of the penis and the scrotum entered, remove both testes.

2. Dissect both corpora completely off the pubic rami and detach them as far back as possible. This will leave the urethra and bulb attached.

3. Divide this at a ·covenient level to bring the urethra out through a perineal opening in the scrotum.

4. Excise any excess scrotal skin and reconstitute the bare area with the scrotum.

5. Suture the slit-up urethra to the window in the remaining scrotal skin.

BLOCK DISSECTION OF ILIOINGUNAL NODES

A radical block dissection of the ilioinguinal nodes may be incorporated into either of the foregoing procedures. The dissection itself has a high morbidity in that the wounds rarely heal by primary intention and a 12–14 week convalescent period is often necessary.

OTHER OPERATIONS ON THE PENIS AND SCROTUM

SURGICAL CORRECTION OF PEYRONIE'S DISEASE

1. If the resulting deformity from burnt-out Peyronie's disease is too great to allow intercourse to take place, then surgical correction is warranted.

2. The procedure most commonly adopted is Nesbit's operation. The principle of this is to artifically induce an erection on the operating table, and having established the degree and direction of the bend, to correct it by excising an appropriate ellipse of tunica from the opposite corpus to the bend, and closing the ensuing corporal defect. This will effectively counteract the bending force by preventing corporal expansion on the opposite side.

3. The author finds it much easier to take in a tuck on the opposite side with a series of unabsorbable sutures; these can be altered until the desired straightening is obtained, and then tied.

OPERATIONS FOR IMPOTENCE

The only satisfactory procedure to date is the surgical introduction of splints into the corpora; these are either rigid or preferably of the malleable variety, so that the penis can be bent down when not in use.

SCROTAL CARCINOMA EXCISIONS

The extent of the excision will depend entirely on the size of the growth. The scrotal skin has great powers of healing, so that the scrotum can usually be reconstructed. There are times, however, when one or both testicles may have to be removed. Occasionally when the growth encroaches on the shaft of the penis with possible infiltration, the whole of the genitalia will need to be ablated with the establishment of a perineal urethrostomy. The need for an ilioinguinal node dissection must be judged clinically.

BLOCK DISSECTION OF GROIN LYMPH GLANDS

Appraise

1. Radical groin dissection is usually carried out for resection of proven or suspected malignant lymph nodes.

2. In general surgery the operation is employed most frequently to excise metastatic melanoma deposits from primary sites in the leg, perineum and gluteal regions.

3. The inguinal glands may be involved by epidermoid carcinoma of the external male or female genitalia, or of the anal skin. In these cases the nodal dissection is usually accomplished in continuity with the primary lesion.

INGUINAL NODES

Access

1. Make a linear incision, 2.5 cm below and parallel to the inguinal ligament.

2. Alternatively make the incision elliptical, so that skin overlying involved glands can be excised en bloc.

Action

1. Raise the upper skin flap so that the superficial and deep fascia can be incised 2–3 cm above and parallel to the inguinal ligament to display the lower fibres of the external oblique aponeurosis. Sweep the connective tissues downwards to leave the lower portion of external oblique stripped clean.

2. Dissect the lower flap to reach the fascia lata over the lateral edge of sartorius muscle and incise it here, preparing to sweep it medially with the superficial fascia. Look for, and preserve if possible, the lateral and intermediate cutaneous nerves of the thigh.

3. At the medial border of sartorius muscle, the dissection reaches into the femoral triangle as the femoral nerve, femoral artery and femoral vein are displayed in turn. At the groin, the superficial circumflex iliac, superficial epigastric and superficial external pudendal vessels should be identified, doubly ligated and divided, to avoid tearing them or their junctions with the main vessels.

4. Ligate and divide the saphenous vein at the lower extremity of the clearance and again as it joins the femoral vein, so that the segment within the femoral triangle is removed with the specimen.

5. Sweep the superficial tissues and lymph nodes medially as far as possible, then incise the fascia lata vertically over the adductor magnus muscle.

6. The specimen is still attached by the fat and lymphatic tissue entering the femoral canal. Gently draw down the lymph node lying within the canal and remove it with the specimen.

Closure

1. Insert one or two tubular drains attached to suction apparatus either at the ends of the incision or through separate stab wounds.
2. Close the skin.

ILIAC NODES

This dissection may be made in continuity with the inguinal node dissection, before or after the groin clearance (Fig. 16.23).

Access

1. For a combined approach, a vertical incision may be made, starting superiorly at the midpoint of a line joining the umbilicus and anterior superior iliac spine and finishing inferiorly at the apex of the femoral triangle. The incision should not be straight, or future contracture will restrict hip movements. A sinusoidal path should therefore be followed.

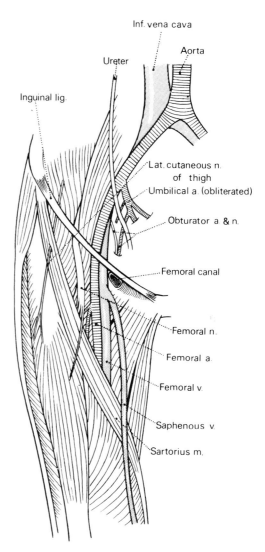

Fig. 16.23 Ilioguinal block dissection of lymph nodes

2. In a very thin person it may be possible to excise the iliac glands through the intact femoral canal following inguinal gland clearance.

Action

1. Enter the iliac region through the inguinal ligament, by dividing the ligament over the femoral canal, subsequently repairing it. Alternatively, dissect the medial insertion from the pubic tubercle, re-attaching it when the dissection is complete.

2. Incise the external oblique, internal oblique and transversus abdominis muscles 1–2 cm above and parallel to the inguinal ligament, so that the whole or part of the inguinal ligament can be swung laterally.

3. Doubly ligate and divide the inferior epigastric vessels.

4. Sweep up the intact peritoneum from the iliac vessels, making sure that the ureter remains attached to the peri-

toneum and is thus preserved from damage. The obliterated umbilical artery must be divided.

5. Starting in the hollow of the sacrum, sweep out the connective tissue and lymph nodes from the iliac vessels and their branches, including the obturator vessels and nerve. Remove glands at the obturator foramen.

6. Strip out the loose tissue and lymph nodes from the femoral canal.

Closure

1. Reattach or repair the inguinal ligament and abdominal muscles.

2. Insert one or more tubular drains attached to suction apparatus.

3. Close the skin.

Aftercare

1. Oedema may develop in the leg. Try to keep this to a minimum by elevating the leg. When the patient becomes mobile, support the leg using carefully applied bandages and subsequently a full length elastic stocking.

2. Keep the drains on suction until the lymphatic drainage has ceased or become slight.

17

Gynaecological surgery

GENERAL CONSIDERATIONS

INTRODUCTION

1. General surgeons may be called upon to perform gynaecological or even obstetric operations in certain circumstances. There may be an unexpected finding at an emergency operation, or there may be an incidental gynaecological lesion, or in an emergency there may be no gynaecologist available. Try and become familiar with the gynaecological pathology that you are likely to encounter therefore, and learn how to deal with it. But remember that most elective gynaecological operations are of a specialised nature and should not be tried on an occasional basis.

2. When operating on women in the reproductive phase of life, be particularly careful and gentle in handling the pelvic organs. Careless surgery in the female pelvis will result in pelvic adhesions, which may drastically disturb a woman's fertility and affect the rest of her life and happiness.

3. Gynaecologists use the Pfannenstiel incision for many operations, but in emergencies dealt with by the general surgeon a midline or paramedian incision will often have been chosen because of the uncertain nature of the diagnosis.

PRE-OPERATIVE CARE

1. Nowhere is informed consent more important than in gynaecological surgery. Give a full explanation of the probable operative procedure and its consequences, particularly if future fertility is likely to be affected; whenever possible, obtain the husband's consent as well.

2. Before most abdominal procedures an enema should be given. Shaving of pubic and vulval hair should be kept to a minimum; it is particularly uncomfortable when it is re-growing.

3. Patients should stop the oral contraceptive pill 6 weeks before elective gynaecological surgery. Menstruation is not a contraindication to gynaecological surgery nor indeed to thorough examination.

PREPARATION IN THEATRE

1. *Positioning of patient.* Vaginal operations are carried out in the lithotomy position. Laparoscopy is best carried out with the patient in Lloyd-Davies stirrups with steep head-down tilt. Abdominal operations are carried out with the patient supine and 5–10° of head-down tilt.

2. *Catheterisation.* Empty the bladder by catheterisation before all abdominal procedures, laparoscopy included. Separate the labia and swab the urethral meatus with antiseptic solution. Without allowing the labia to close again, pass a silver or plastic catheter well into the bladder. Now let the labia approximate and press firmly and continuously suprapubically. When the urine flow ceases, gradually withdraw the catheter, taking care not to allow air to be sucked into the bladder.

MINOR GYNAECOLOGICAL OPERATIONS

DILATATION AND CURETTAGE

Appraise

The general surgeon may need to perform a diagnostic dilatation and curettage on a patient with abnormal vaginal bleeding, or a therapeutic dilatation and curettage for bleeding associated with retained products of conception. In the presence of bleeding give an intravenous injection of ergometrine 0.5 mg or syntocinon 10 units immediately before the operation.

Action

1. Perform a bimanual examination to determine the size and axis of the uterus and to detect any adnexal swellings.

2. Insert a Sim's or Auvard's speculum into the vagina and grasp the cervix with two Volsellum forceps.

3. Gently pass a uterine sound to determine the length and direction of the uterus, but omit this step if you think there has been a recent pregnancy. The soft pregnant uterus is easily perforated by a sound.

4. Dilate the cervix progressively by passing Hegar's dilators, increasing by 1 mm at a time. Some pressure may be needed to pass through the internal cervical os, but be careful to reduce the pressure as soon as the resistance has been passed. If there is difficulty, go back to the previous dilator. An 8 mm diameter dilator is adequate for a diagnostic D & C, 10 mm for a therapeutic one.

5. Pass a pair of polyp forceps, open them, twist through 90°, close them and withdraw any tissue present. Repeat two or three times in different planes or more frequently if there are retained products of conception.

6. Pass a curette, small and sharp in the non-pregnant, large and blunt in the patient who has been pregnant, until the fundus of the uterus is reached. With firm pressure on the uterine wall, withdraw the curette and collect the specimen on a swab. Repeat the manoeuvre going round the whole surface of the uterine cavity. In the pregnant patient, make sure that the cavity is completely empty. Send the curettings for histology.

BARTHOLIN'S CYST OR ABSCESS

Appraise

Bartholin's abscess is an acutely painful condition and should be dealt with as an emergency. A cyst may be dealt with electively. The operation of marsupialisation is the procedure of choice, as recurrence is very likely following simple incision and drainage.

Action

1. Make a vertical incision 1 cm long just inside the hymenal ring.

2. Remove a semicircle of skin and cyst wall from each side of the incision.

3. Insert half a dozen or so fine catgut sutures circumferentially to bring the cyst wall and skin into apposition, so leaving a wide ostium to the gland. A gauze ribbon drain may be left in the cavity for 1–2 days.

LAPAROSCOPY

Appraise

1. This is a very useful and important diagnostic procedure in the diagnosis of pelvic pain, both acute and chronic. It is particularly valuable in cases of suspected ectopic pregnancy.

2. The general surgeon may find laparoscopy useful in the diagnosis of ascites, for direct liver biopsy and for peritoneal biopsy.

3. Laparoscopy must only be carried out by those trained in the technique and should never be done in the presence of generalised peritonitis, intestinal obstruction or ileus, or when extensive adhesions are suspected. Pre-existing cardiovascular and respiratory disease may also be a contraindication.

Position

The semi-lithotomy position is used with the legs in Lloyd-Davies stirrups and with steep head-down tilt.

Action

1. Empty the bladder and perform bimanual examination. Apply Volsellum forceps and a Spackman cannula to the cervix.

2. Make a horizontal incision 0.75 cm long just below the umbilicus.

3. Introduce a Verres needle for a few centimetres beneath the skin. Then alter its direction towards the pelvic cavity until the parietal peritoneum is entered, when a characteristic loss of resistance is felt.

4. Aspirate the needle with a syringe to check that neither a blood vessel nor a viscus has been entered.

5. Connect the needle to the carbon dioxide insufflator and introduce the gas at low flow. Provided the pressure is less than 40 mm Hg, the gas may be turned up to 'high flow' until approximately 3 litres have been instilled.

6. Remove the Verres needle, and pass the large trocar and cannula into the peritoneal cavity, using the same direction as used for the Verres needle. It is helpful to hold up the abdominal wall between fingers and thumb to provide counter-pressure.

7. Remove the trocar and insert the telescope through the cannula; attach the fibrelight cable.

8. The uterus can be moved by an assistant grasping the Spackman cannula to facilitate visualisation of all parts of the pelvis. If necessary, a second instrument may be inserted suprapubically to use as a probe and manipulator.

9. After thorough inspection of the pelvic organs, the telescope in its cannula may be rotated to inspect the upper abdomen and peritoneum. Any necessary biopsies can then be taken, using Palmer forceps with diathermy coagulation to obtain haemostasis.

10. When the procedure is completed, let out as much of the carbon dioxide as possible, remove the trocar and insert one skin suture in each incision.

OVARIAN OPERATIONS

Appraise

1. It is of great importance for the general surgeon to recognise the features of tumours which are likely to be benign and of those which are likely to be malignant. In a woman of reproductive age it is better to err on the side of conservatism, even if a further laparotomy is needed, rather than risk sacrificing healthy ovaries. In general, a smooth surface and the absence of ascites, peritoneal, omental or nodular metastases are features of benign tumours; bilaterality is no guide to the likelihood of malignancy.

2. It is equally important to distinguish a mature Graafian follicle or a corpus luteum cyst from a neoplastic cyst. Luteal cyst may occur in early pregnancy, and unnecessary removal can result in abortion.

3. Do not remove any ovarian cyst under 5 cm in diameter without good evidence either that it is neoplastic or that it has undergone haemorrhage or rupture, giving rise to acute abdominal pain.

4. The operation of ovarian cystectomy is the preferred treatment for benign ovarian cysts. Salpingo-oophorectomy is carried out
a) If there is evidence of malignancy.
b   If the cyst has undergone torsion and is gangrenous
c) If the tumour is very large and little normal ovarian tissue could be conserved.

5. In suspected malignancy explore the whole abdomen, including the diaphragmatic surface of the liver. Palpate the para-aortic nodes, and send off ascitic fluid or peritoneal washings for cytology. Further treatment will depend upon accurate staging. If there are no metastases and the contralateral ovary is grossly normal, split it open and send a slice for histology (frozen section if available), before closing the ovary with plain catgut or fine non-absorbable sutures.

6. If the ovarian tumour is obviously malignant, remove the uterus, both ovaries and tubes, the omentum and as much metastatic tumour bulk as possible. The only exception to such radical surgery would be in a young woman with disease confined to one ovary and no sign of abdominal metastases.

Action

Ovarian cystectomy

1. Separate the tumour from adhesions and draw it out of the wound.

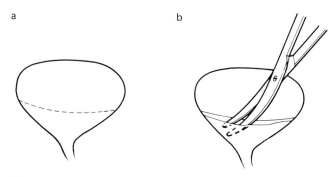

Fig. 17.1 Ovarian cystectomy (a) Circumcision (b) Separation of cyst from ovary

2. Surround the operation site with large gauze packs, and have a sucker ready in case the cyst is accidentally ruptured.

3. Make an incision in the ovarian cortex around the base of the tumour (Fig. 17.1a).

4. Find the plane of cleavage and shell the tumour out, using scissors and gauze swab dissection (Fig. 17.1b). If the cyst ruptures, it is important to remove all the cyst lining.

5. Repair the residual ovarian tissue, using 2/0 plain catgut sutures or fine monofilament nylon; good haemostasis is important to prevent future adhesion formation.

Salpingo-oophorectomy

1. If you decide to remove the whole ovary, place one clamp across the ovarian pedicle (infundibulopelvic fold) and a second across the ovarian ligament and fallopian tube, adjacent to the uterus. Resect the ovary together with the tube and the broad ligament between the clamps.

2. Doubly ligate each pedicle with 0 or 1 chromic catgut. Use a transfixion suture or gently release and reapply the clamp while tying the ligature. At the end of the operation check the pedicles before closing the abdomen.

SURGERY OF ECTOPIC PREGNANCY

Appraise

1. A classical ruptured ectopic pregnancy is easily diagnosed, but a tubal abortion or slowly leaking ectopic is much more likely to be misdiagnosed pre-operatively. Laparoscopy can be helpful, but often the first suspicion is the finding of blood in the peritoneal cavity at laparotomy.

2. Once the diagnosis of ruptured ectopic has been made the patient should be taken to theatre as soon as possible. It is no good waiting for blood to be cross-matched or hoping that the patient's condition will improve. She will improve only when the fallopian tube is clamped.

Action

1. Make a generous incision, either midline or Pfannenstiel (if you are used to this incision).

2. Have the sucker ready to aspirate blood and plenty of large abdominal packs.

3. Pass a hand into the pelvis and bring the uterus with appendages up into the wound. Identify the ruptured tube. Place one or more clamps across the mesosalpinx and another clamp across the cornual end of the tube, then excise the damaged tube. In most cases it is neither necessary nor desirable to remove the ovary. Doubly ligate the pedicles beneath the clamps, using 0 or 1 chromic catgut.

4. Inspect the contralateral tube and ovary. The other tube may have a hydrosalpinx or haematosalpinx, but do not be tempted to tamper with it. Bilateral tubal pregnancy is excessively rare. Record the state of the pelvis carefully.

5. Before closing the abdomen, aspirate and swab out as much blood as possible, and make an estimate of the blood loss. Washing the peritoneal cavity with Hartmann's solution may help to reduce adhesion formation.

TUBAL LIGATION

Appraise

1. General surgeons may be asked to carry out a sterilisation procedure, either in the course of a Caesarean section operation (see below), or as an additional procedure during the course of an abdominal operation. Obtain prior consent of the patient and her husband. Avoid sterilisation in women under the age of 30, unless there is a good medical reason to perform it.

2. Sterilisation may be carried out by one of the modifications of Pomeroy's method (as described below) or by the application of a Hulka clip.

Action

1. Pick up a loop of fallopian tube with a Spencer Wells forceps 2–3 cm from the uterus (Fig. 17.2a).

2. Tie a catgut ligature tightly round the base of the loop, and excise the end of the loop. Each end of the tube may be sealed with the diathermy needle as an additional precaution (Fig. 17.2b).

HYSTERECTOMY

Appraise

1. The general surgeon may be called upon to perform a hysterectomy under various circumstances, for example as part of a larger surgical procedure such as the removal of a rectal cancer, because of fibromyomata or other benign

a

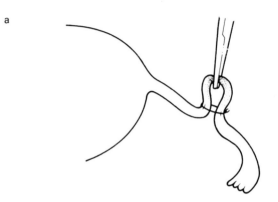

b

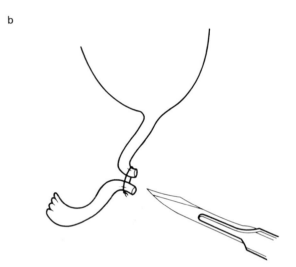

Fig. 17.2 Pomeroy sterilisation (a) Ligature round loop of tube (b) Excision of loop of tube

uterine disease causing severe menorrhagia, or for ovarian carcinoma which has not been diagnosed pre-operatively. Do not be tempted to carry out a hysterectomy during the course of another operation because of the incidental finding of large uterine fibroids, unless you have discussed the possibility with the patient pre-operatively.

2. Unless there is gynaecological malignancy, conserve at least one ovary whenever possible in pre-menopausal women.

Access

1. Empty the bladder by catheterisation and cleanse the vagina with an antiseptic. Bonney's Blue has the advantage of staining the vaginal skin, making it more easily recognised at operation.

2. A Pfannenstiel incision is suitable for many hysterectomies, but should be avoided if either malignancy is suspected, the uterus is larger than the size of a 16-week pregnancy or the diagnosis is in doubt. In these cases use a vertical incision.

3. Carefully pack off the intestines, both large and small, to render the operation easier and safer. It is well worth spending a few minutes displacing all the intestines from the pelvis, and packing them above the pelvic brim.

4. Insert a self-retaining retractor of the Gosset type, preferably one with a third blade.

Action

1. Place a strong straight clamp of the Kocher's or Howkins' type as close to the uterus as possible across the fallopian tube, round ligament, ovarian ligament, and upper part of the broad ligament. If these structures are held on the stretch, an avascular window will be seen at a depth of about 3 cm into the broad ligament. Aim to put the tip of the clamp into this avascular window.

2. Place a second straight clamp just lateral to the first clamp, again with the tip in the avascular window (Fig. 17.3).

3. Divide the tissue between the clamps down to their tips, and ligate the lateral pedicle with 1 chromic catgut, doubly tied.

4. Repeat this procedure on the opposite side.

5. Open the layers of the broad ligament below the sutured pedicle by inserting closed scissors and gently opening them. Incise the anterior leaf of the broad ligament and gradually continue opening the broad ligament, until you reach the loose fold of utero-vesical peritoneum.

6. Now pass the closed scissors in a medial direction, open them and cut the loose utero-vesical peritoneum. Carry out the same manoeuvre on the other side until the bladder peritoneum is completely incised in front of the cervix.

7. Pick up the bladder flap with dissecting forceps and apply tension. This manoeuvre will display the loose connective tissue between bladder and cervix, and this can be cut with one or two judicious snips, keeping the point of the scissors towards the cervix.

8. The bladder may now be pushed off the cervix, either with a swab on the sponge-holder or with the swab wrapped around the thumb, the pressure being applied onto the cervix rather than the bladder. Once the longitudinal fibres of the vagina are visible, no further displace-

ment of the bladder is necessary. Adequate displacement of the bladder may also be checked by gripping the cervix between thumb and forefinger until you can feel that you are below the level of the cervix.

9. Using the two clamps which are still applied to the uterine cornu, pull the uterus up with as much tension as possible, so accentuating the fold of the utero-sacral ligaments. These can now be divided with a scalpel, and the uterus will lift even higher out of the pelvis. If the utero-sacral ligaments look thick and vascular, a Spencer Wells forceps may be applied to them before incision.

10. The uterine vessels are now clamped. Apply a strong straight or curved clamp at right angles to the uterus just above the level at which the utero-sacral ligaments have been divided. Make sure that the tips of the clamp are as close as possible to the uterus. Divide the uterine vessels by cutting with a knife close to the clamp, and continue cutting until you are just into the uterine wall.

11. Next clamp the para-cervical tissue by applying another straight clamp at right angles to the uterine vessel clamp. The depth to which this clamp is applied will depend upon the length of the cervix, but it is rarely necessary to apply it to a depth of greater than 1 cm. Using the scalpel again, cut the pedicle, keeping the direction of incision somewhat medial and towards the cervix.

12. Now open the vagina by inserting a scalpel in the midline through the vaginal fascia and then into the vagina itself. Pick up the anterior vaginal edge with Littlewood's forceps, and extend the vaginal incision circumferentially. Pick up each vaginal angle with another Littlewood's forceps, and a fourth one should be placed posteriorly in the midline.

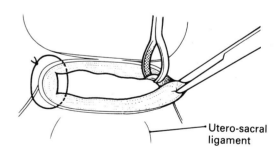

Fig. 17.4 Closure of vault; tying of vaginal angle

Utero-sacral ligament

Closure

1. The most important sutures are at the vaginal angle. Place an interrupted suture just below the tip of the para-cervical clamp so as to include the vaginal angle. Having tied the suture, apply a Spencer Wells forceps to the end of the suture to use as a holder (Fig. 17.4).

2. Close the vaginal vault with a series of interrupted catgut sutures. Alternatively, leave it open, and arrest oozing by inserting a running suture around the vault (Fig. 17.5).

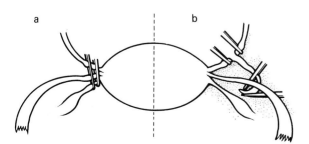

Fig. 17.3 Hysterectomy: incision of broad ligament (a) Conservation of adnexa (b) With adnexa removed

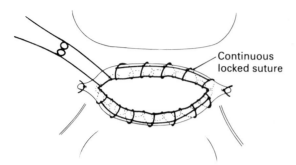

Fig. 17.5 Vaginal vault circumsuture, leaving vagina open for drainage

3. Doubly ligate the uterine vessels with 1 chromic catgut.

4. Check that there is no bleeding from the vaginal vault or uterine vessels, and close the pelvic peritoneum with a continuous suture starting at one ovarian pedicle and concluding at the other.

Difficulty?

Occasionally, if there are very dense pelvic adhesions and the uterus remains fixed in a deep pelvis, or if there is an extensive ovarian malignancy, it may be difficult to remove the cervix. It may then be safer to perform subtotal hysterectomy. Proceed exactly as described above, but there is no need to apply a clamp to the para-cervical tissue (step 11). At this stage, cut across the stump to close the cervical canal. Cover the stump with the pelvic peritoneum.

MYOMECTOMY

Assess

1. In a young patient with fibromyomata it may be preferable to remove the myomata, conserving the uterus. If the fibroids are multiple, the operation can be a good deal more time-consuming and hazardous than hysterectomy. A solitary pedunculated subserous fibroid (which may have undergone torsion) is easily removed.

2. Remove as many fibroids as possible through one uterine incision. Try to avoid incisions in the posterior wall of the uterus, since these often give rise to small-intestinal adhesions. You can often make an anterior incision and go through the cavity of the uterus to remove a posterior fibroid.

3. If you have to remove multiple fibroids, it is worth applying a Bonney's myomectomy clamp or tying a rubber sling around the cervix to reduce haemorrhage.

Action

1. Make an incision in the uterus, usually over the largest fibroid.

2. Grasp the fibroid with tissue-holding forceps. It is easy to identify a plane of cleavage and to shell out the tumour either with a finger or the handle of a scalpel.

3. Trim off any excess uterine muscle and insert deep catgut sutures to obliterate the cavity left after removal of the fibroid. Several layers of sutures may be needed to achieve hamostasis.

4. Close the serous surface of the uterus with 0 or 00 chromic catgut sutures.

5. If the uterus falls back into retroversion, plicate the round ligaments with linen thread or silk in order to antevert the uterus. This manoeuvre prevents adhesion formation.

INCIDENTAL GYNAECOLOGICAL CONDITIONS

PELVIC INFLAMMATORY DISEASE

1. Not uncommonly a patient explored for suspected appendicitis is found to have acute salpingitis. The condition is almost always bilateral, although one tube may be more affected than the other. The tubes are oedematous and reddened, and pus is often seen dripping from the fimbrial end. Take a swab for bacteriological culture and close the abdomen.

2. Sometimes tubal infection may have progressed to the development of a tubo-ovarian abscess or a pyosalpinx. Alternatively, a pelvic abscess may have developed. Adhere to the usual surgical principle of drainage of pus, preferably inserting a drain through a separate abdominal incision. Send swabs for culture, and give appropriate antibiotics.

FIMBRIAL CYST AND PAROVARIAN CYST

Small cysts may be seen in relation to the distal end of the fallopian tube or broad ligament. They arise in remnants of the mesonephric (Wolffian) duct and occasionally undergo torsion to produce acute abdominal pain. Remove them only if they have undergone torsion. Tie the pedicle before excision.

ENDOMETRIOSIS

1. This condition may involve the ovaries, forming chocolate cysts, or the pelvic peritoneum, when it is seen as small purple or dark brown nodules. Occasionally it involves the intestine, where the appearance may mimic a carcinoma. In the large intestine it may produce subacute obstruction and can be extremely difficult to differentiate from carcinoma. It is important to try and do so, because excision of an endometrioma can be more limited than for

a carcinoma. Rarely, endometriomas may be seen in an abdominal scar.

2. Many patients with endometriosis are now treated medically with hormones, so do not be radical if you find pelvic endometriosis unexpectedly.

CAESAREAN SECTION

Appraise

1. The general surgeon may be asked to perform a Caesarean section if he works in a hospital where there is no specialist obstetrician. It is likely that the patient will have been in labour for some hours, although occasionally it is necessary to perform the operation on a patient who is bleeding heavily from a placenta praevia.

2 The lower segment operation is almost universally employed nowadays, being associated with less bleeding and fewer post-operative complications than 'classical' section.

3. Crossmatch at least 2 units of blood preoperatively.

Access

1. The operating table should have about 15° of lateral tilt to avoid compression of the inferior vena cava during the operation. Either tilt the operating table or place a rubber wedge under the patient's buttocks.

2. Empty the bladder by catheterisation and leave the catheter in place during the operation.

3. A Pfannenstiel incision is suitable, but if you are inexperienced, you may find a vertical midline incision easier.

4. When the peritoneal cavity is opened, place a large Doyen retractor into the lower edge of the wound.

Action

1. Identify the loose fold of utero-vesical peritoneum. Pick it up with dissecting forceps and incise it with scissors in the midline. Extend the incision laterally almost to the broad ligament on each side.

2. Push the bladder downwards with a swab, and replace the Doyen retractor over the bladder to retract it well away from the lower uterine segment.

3. Incise the lower segment transversely, beginning in the midline. The lower segment may be very thin, especially if the patient has been in labour for long, so care must be taken not to cut too deeply. Once the incision is large enough to admit two fingers insert the index finger of each hand and extend the incision laterally by stretching until the incision is approximately 11 cm in length (Fig. 17.6).

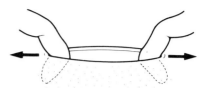

Fig. 17.6 Caesarean section. Digital enlargement of incision

4. Rupture the exposed membranes with scissors, while the assistant removes liquor and blood with a sucker.

5. Insert the right hand into the uterus below the presenting part, easing it out of the pelvis. If it is deeply wedged in the pelvis, ask for head-down tilt of the table.

6. Deliver the foetal head into the wound. Once the face is exposed, the infant's nose and throat may be aspirated. Now ask the assistant to apply fundal pressure, and gently withdraw the baby from the uterus. Once the head is delivered, the anaesthetist should give an intravenous injection of ergometrine 0.5 mg or syntocinon 10 units.

7. Lay the baby on the mother's thighs, and apply two clamps to the umbilical cord. Divide the cord and hand the baby to the midwife.

8. Grasp the lateral ends of the uterine incision with Green-Armytage forceps, and also place two of these forceps on the upper and lower flap of the uterine incision. This will control most of the bleeding from the uterus.

9. Deliver the placenta by applying gentle cord traction and light fundal compression.

Closure

1. Replace the Doyen's retractor.

2. Using an atraumatic 0 or 1 chromic catgut suture, insert a stitch in one angle of the uterine incision and close the incision with a continuous running suture. If there is sufficient thickness of the uterine muscle, do not include the full thickness in this first layer of sutures. Insert a second continuous running suture to invaginate the first, so closing the uterus in two layers.

3. Apply a swab firmly over the uterine incision for 2 minutes. When it is removed there may be one or two small bleeding vessels, which need to be dealt with by individual stitches.

4. Close the utero-vesical peritoneum using 0 chromic catgut.

5. Swab out any blood or liquor from the paracolic gutters on each side.

6. Close the abdominal incision.

Difficulty?

In exceptional circumstances it may be necessary to carry out a 'classical' upper segment Caesarian section. This might be necessary if there is an anterior placenta praevia, a fibroid over the lower segment, or if the operation is being done at an early stage of pregnancy. In this case use a vertical skin incision, and make a large midline incision in the upper segment of the uterus. The uterine wall is much thicker in the upper segment and three layers of sutures will be needed to close it.

PREGNANCY AND EMERGENCY SURGERY

The presence of a pregnancy may cause considerable confusion in the diagnosis of an acute abdomen and may make access more difficult at laparotomy. It should not, however, deter the surgeon from performing emergency abdominal operations when necessary.

APPENDICITIS

The appendix is pushed upwards and outwards during pregnancy, so that the physical signs of appendicitis may be considerably altered. Because the large pregnant uterus may prevent the normal walling-off of acute appendicitis, generalised peritonitis occurs more readily. Make a gridiron incision above and lateral to the normal site, or consider a right paramedian incision if there is doubt about diagnosis.

CHOLECYSTITIS

Acute cholecystitis and biliary colic are not uncommon in pregnancy, but the symptoms may be atypical, simulating hyperemesis or indigestion of pregnancy. If the diagnosis of gallbladder disease is made in pregnancy, prefer to wait until after delivery before carrying out cholecystectomy. If there is a need to perform the operation during pregnancy, it is best carried out in the mid-trimester.

RED DEGENERATION OF A FIBROID

Pregnancy and fibroids often co-exist, and a fibroid growing rapidly during pregnancy may undergo red degeneration. This is an extremely painful condition; sometimes the pain is so severe that exploratory laparotomy is carried out. Once the diagnosis of fibroids is confirmed, **do not attempt to remove the fibroids,** as myomectomy in pregnancy is attended with catastrophic haemorrhage and loss of the foetus. The only exception to this rule is if a pedunculated fibroid has undergone torsion and is gangrenous.

PLACENTAL ABRUPTION

The condition of abruptio placentae results in severe abdominal pain and uterine tenderness, which may or may not be accompanied by vaginal bleeding. A major degree of abruption will cause profound shock and usually result in foetal death, but lesser degrees may cause diagnostic difficulty. Tenderness is localised over the uterus, and in the severe form the uterus acquires a characteristic woody-hard feel to it. Induction of labour is usually appropriate.

RECTUS SHEATH HAEMATOMA

Occasionally a spontaneous haematoma occurs in the rectus sheath as a result of spontaneous haemorrhage from the inferior epigastric vessels in pregnancy. A tender mass appears in the abdominal wall. The condition is best treated conservatively.

Further reading

Howkins J, Hudson C N 1977 Shaw's textbook of operative gynaecology, 4th edn. Churchill Livingstone, Edinburgh
Howkins J, Stallworthy J 1974 Bonney's gynaecological surgery. Balliere & Tindall, London
Lees D, Singer A 1978 Clinics in obstetrics and gynaecology, vol. 5, no. 3, Saunders, London
Lees D, Singer A 1981 A colour atlas of gynaecological surgery. Wolfe Medical, London
Roberts D W T 1977 Operative surgery, gynaecology and obstetrics. Butterworths, London
Steptoe P C 1967 Laparoscopy in gynaecology. Churchill Livingstone, Edinburgh

Oesophageal surgery

OESOPHAGOSCOPY

Appraise

1. Endoscope every patient with dysphagia except when this is fully explained by the presence of neurological or neuromuscular disease.

2. Endoscope patients with suspected disease in the oesophagus producing pain on swallowing (odynophagia), heartburn, bleeding, or if accidental and iatrogenic damage are suspected.

3. Flexible instruments are versatile and can be passed with minimal sedation and pharyngeal anaesthesia in most patients. They are safe, relatively comfortable for the patient, and allow examination of the stomach and duodenum beyond. Use the end-viewing instrument routinely since it is versatile and modern endoscopes have remarkably flexible tips. Through it can be passed biopsy forceps, cystology brushes, snares, guide wires for dilators and needles for injection. Newer instruments promise to overcome the disadvantages of a small biopsy channel and inadequate suction facilities.

4. Rigid oesophagoscopy is best performed under general anaesthesia. Skill and experience are required and the combination of small mouth, large teeth, receding and stiff jaw, osteoarthritic neck and kyphotic spine may make it impossible to carry out. The major advantage of the rigid instrument is that generous biopsy specimens may be removed and dilatation and even intubation can be performed under direct vision.

5. Whenever the rigid instrument is used, also have the flexible instrument available.

6. Whenever oesophageal carcinoma is suspected have a bronchoscope available.

Prepare

1. Obtain signed informed consent from the patient.

2. Remove dentures from the patient.

3. Except in an emergency have the patient starved of food and fluids for at least 5 hours.

4. Obtain a preliminary barium swallow X-ray if you are inexperienced, if there is suspected pharyngeal pouch, a stricture, or an anatomic anomaly.

5. If the flexible instrument is used, give the patient a lozenge of amethocaine to suck 1 hour, and half an hour before endoscopy. Alternatively, spray the pharynx with lignocaine solution just before passing the endoscope. Insert a 'butterfly' needle into a peripheral vein and through it inject slowly 10–20 mg of diazepam until the patient's speech is slurred and he becomes sleepy. If it becomes necessary to cause discomfort by dilating a stricture or other manoeuvre, inject up to 50 mg pethidine (meperidine, Demerol) slowly intravenously.

6. For rigid oesophagoscopy arrange for normal premedication and general anaesthesia with endotracheal intubation. The anaesthetist usually stands with his trolley to the left of the patient and alongside him.

FIBRE-OPTIC ENDOSCOPY

1. Lay the patient on his left side with hips and knees flexed. Endoscopy can be safely performed with the patient lying supine and when passing the modern thin inspecting instrument with minimum or no sedation, the patient may sit upright in a chair. Place a plastic hollow gag between

the teeth. Ensure that the patient's head is in the midline and that the chin is lowered onto the chest.

2. Lubricate the previously checked end-viewing instrument with water-soluble jelly.

3. Pass the endoscope tip through the plastic gag, over the tongue to the posterior pharyngeal wall. Depress the tip control slightly so that the instrument tip passes down towards the cricopharyngeal sphincter. If necessary insert a finger alongside the gag to direct the tip in the midline over the epiglottis.

4. Ask the patient to swallow. Do not resist the slight extrusion of the endoscope as the larynx rises but maintain gentle pressure so that it will advance as the larynx descends and the cricopharyngeal sphincter relaxes. Advance the endoscope under vision, insufflating air gently to open up the passage. Aspirate any fluid. Spray water across the lens if it becomes obscured. If no hold up is encountered pass the tip through the stomach into the duodenum then withdraw it slowly, noting the features. Remove biopsy specimens and take cytology brushings from any ulcers, tumours or other lesions.

5. If a stricture is encountered note its distance from the incisior teeth. Sometimes the instrument will pass through, allowing the length of the stricture to be determined. Always remove biopsy specimens and cytology brushings from within the stricture.

Decide if the stricture should be dilated now because it is benign and requires no further treatment, or because it is malignant and the patient will benefit from improved oral feeding prior to surgical treatment, or because it is unsuitable for surgical treatment and palliative dilatation is indicated, possibly with intubation. Pass a well-lubricated Eder-Puestow guide wire through the biopsy channel, through the stricture and for at least 10 cm beyond it. If the tip of the Eder-Puestow wire impacts in the stricture, slightly withdraw and rotate it before trying again. Use no force or the wire will damage the gullet, kink, jam, or all of these. Gently withdraw the endoscope, feeding through more wire so that the tip remains well beyond the stricture after the instrument has been taken out.

RIGID OESOPHAGOSCOPY (Fig. 18.1)

1. As a rule use a wide-bore instrument since vision is very restricted through a narrow tube. Occasionally it is impossible to pass the widest oesophagoscope. Lubricate the shaft with water-soluble jelly. Check the light source, suction apparatus beforehand and ensure that bougies and biopsy forceps are available.

2. Check that the anaesthetized patient lies supine with his head in the midline, supported on the hinged section of the table or by a seated assistant.

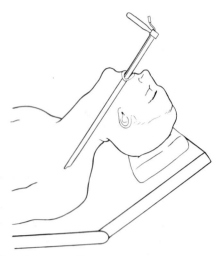

Fig. 18.1 Oesophagoscopy. When the instrument is first introduced, the neck is not extended. Notice how far posteriorly the instrument points as it enters the upper thoracic oesophagus.

3. Sit at the head of the table. Have the patient's neck fully flexed. Pass the end of the instrument into the patient's mouth with the extended tip against the tongue. As the oesophagoscope enters further, angle it vertically and as it enters the pharynx continue to move the eyepiece in the sagittal plane to keep the tip centred in the pharynx. Look through the instrument to guide the tip behind the epiglottis and along the posterior pharyngeal wall, aspirating any fluid through the sucker. Do not yet extend the neck but allow the head to extend on the occipito-axial joints so that the oesophagoscope does not press heavily on the upper incisor teeth or gums.

4. Identify the cricopharyngeal sphincter. If you cannot, gently press with the sucker tip or a flexible bougie, checking that the oesophagoscope and the patient's head and neck are all strictly in the midline. If much angling pressure is required because of the backward pressure of the inflated endotracheal tube cuff, ask for it to be temporarily deflated while the tip of the instrument is gently insinuated through the sphincter. Do not use force. The oesophagoscope now enters the upper thoracic oesophagus, curving posteriorly, then gradually running forwards. Only now should the neck be extended completely so that the lumen is constantly centred in the field of view.

5. Note any abnormalities and their distance from the incisor teeth during the advancement. Remove biopsy specimens from suspicious areas with side-biting forceps, taking a bite from each quadrant of circumferential lesions. Remove biopsy specimens from within a stricture, if necessary first dilating it with graded gum elastic bougies. Following such dilatation the instrument may sometimes be advanced through the stricture or a slim fibre-optic instrument can be passed through the rigid instrument and on through the stricture to view the structures beyond.

Assess

1. Note the level of each feature. The cricopharyngeal sphincter is approximately 16 cm from the incisor teeth. The deviation around the aortic arch is 28–30 cm, the cardia lies at 40 cm and here the lining changes abruptly from the pale bluish stratified oesophageal to the florid, pinker, gastric columnar-cell epithelium.

2. Oesophagitis is usually from gastro-oesophageal reflux but is not necessarily associated with hiatal hernia. Classically it appears red with erosions and white adherent exudate, bleeding easily on contact with the tip of the instrument. It may appear relatively normal and only the increased vascularity seen on biopsy specimens suggests its presence. Oesophagitis also develops above a stricture or in achalasia of the cardia from contact with stagnant food. Thick white plaques indicate monilial infection, usually in association with oral involvement. Confirm the diagnosis by taking mucosal scrapings.

3. Sliding hiatal hernia produces a loculus of stomach above the constriction of the crura with a raised gastro-oesophageal mucosal junction. Reflux and oesophagitis may be visible. A rolling hernia is visible only from within the stomach by inverting the tip of a flexible instrument to view the apparent fundic diverticulum.

4. Ulcers may be superficial erosions in oesophagitis. Peptic ulcer may also develop in the presence of acid reflux. In Barrett's oesophagus the lower gullet is lined with modified gastric mucosa and an ulcer may develop at the junction of squamous and columnar-cell epithelia. Ulcerating carcinomas may develop at any level and are usually squamous cell in type but in the lower third the majority are adenocarcinomas usually invading from the gastric cardia. Take multiple biopsies and cytological brushings from a number of areas of all ulcers.

5. Strictures from peptic oesophagitis or ulceration develop at any time from birth onwards but more frequently occur in middle or old age. Usually but not always, there is a sliding or fixed hiatal hernia. Do not assume they are always benign: in my experience half of the strictures seen above hiatal hernias are malignant although it is controversial which is cause and effect. Take multiple biopsies and brushings for cytology. Caustic strictures develop at the sites of hold-up of swallowed liquids at the cricopharyngeus, aortic arch crossing, and at the cardia. The pharyngeal web in the Patterson-Brown-Plummer-Vinson syndrome is in the upper oesophagus. This may also become malignant, so remove biopsy specimens. Stricture may arise from external pressure: in the neck the thyroid and enlarged lymph nodes, in the mediastinum from aortic aneurysm, aberrant left subclavian artery, enlarged glands and invasion from bronchial carcinoma.

6. Mega-oesophagus is seen in achalasia of the cardia, scleroderma and in the South American Chagas' disease.

7. Pulsion diverticula are seen at the cricopharyngeus muscle (Zenker's diverticulum or pharyngeal pouch), and above segments of presumed spasm. Traction diverticula develop as a result of chronic inflammation of mediastinal glands, especially from tuberculosis.

8. Oesophageal varices are usually recognised just above the cardia as convoluted varicose veins which may extend into the upper stomach.

DILATATION OF STRICTURES (Fig. 18.2)

1. Fragile strictures, including constriction following overtightening of the crura at hiatal hernia repair or early recurrence of inflammatory strictures from gastro-oesophageal reflux, or spasm from trauma complicating a mild chronic stricture do not always require endoscopic dilatation if the diagnosis is not in doubt or has been confirmed by endoscopy. The safest oesophageal dilator is soft solid food provided that each bolus contains only aggregated small particles.

2. Hurst's mercury-filled hollow rubber or plastic bougies are safe and often effective in such strictures. Give the patient, after starving him of food and fluid for 5 hours, an amethocaine lozenge to suck. After half an hour, sit the patient upright and have him swallow the well lubricated smoothly rounded end of the bougie. Support the other end above the patient so that it is almost vertical but has

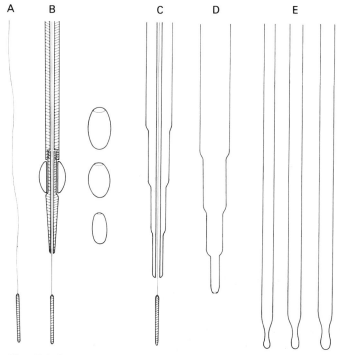

Fig. 18.2 Oesophageal dilators. A is the Eder-Puestow guide wire. B is the Eder-Puestow dilator shaft, with, to the right, three graded metal olive dilators. C is the Celestin stepped-shaft dilator with the large sized shaft to the right. D shows three standard gum-elastic bougies with olivary tips.

a little slack, and maintain this for 1 hour. The weight of the mercury should exert gentle pressure to carry the tip through the stricture. Check the position of the tip by a plain erect abdominal X-ray film before assuming it has passed through. Larger sizes can be passed subsequently. Patients with recurring strictures from caustic burns, oesophagitis and achalasia can be trained to swallow Hurst's bougies regularly to maintain an adequate passage if more permanent treatment cannot be contemplated or is refused.

3. Dilatation through the rigid oesophagoscope under direct vision is best carried out using gum elastic or plastic olivary-tipped bougies. As the stricture is negotiated the neck behind the olive tip lies loosely within the stricture, giving an estimate of its length. Do not use too fine a bougie initially since the 'feel' of the stricture is reduced. Try passing the closed tips of alligator forceps through the stricture, gently open them slightly and withdraw them. This allows the length and consistency of the stricture to be assessed. Dilate the stricture further with graded bougies not forcibly overstretching it, leaving the final one in position until the patient awakens.

4. The Eder-Puestow dilators can be used with the rigid oesophagoscope under general anaesthesia but are usually passed using the endviewing fibre-optic instrument under local anaesthesia giving increments of pethidine (meperidine, Demerol) of 10 mg intravenously as necessary up to 50 mg. Record the distance of the stricture from the incisor teeth. Ensure that the guide wire is unkinked. Pass it through the endoscope, through the stricture, and beyond for 30 cm or so — the wire will loop within the stomach. Withdraw the flexible endoscope, meanwhile feeding the wire through it so that it is not inadvertently withdrawn. The rigid oesophagoscope can be left in place provided the largest dilator can be passed through its lumen. Mount a suitable olive on the introducing shaft, lubricate the wire and dilator with water-soluble jelly. Slide the flexible hollow introducer over the guide wire until it engages the stricture, making sure that the guide wire is kept straight without being withdrawn. Gently push the olive through the stricture, judging success by feeling the grip of the stricture freed, and by measuring the length of introducer that has passed beyond the incisor teeth against an externally placed shaft. Withdraw the olive and replace it with one of the next size until the stricture is sufficiently dilated without the use of force. Each time the olive is changed, take care not to withdraw or kink the guide wire. Do not use force or overstretch the stricture at a single session. Rather, repeat the manoeuvre after an interval of 1–2 weeks.

Celestin has designed two hollow, stepped, plastic dilators that are complimentary to each other, that can be used instead of the individual Eder-Puestow dilators. These are safe, convenient and simplify the procedure. First make sure that a sufficient length of guide wire is past the stricture to accommodate the full length of steps on the slim dilator. Now thread the well lubricated smaller dilator over the guide wire and passed down through the stricture. Each successive step can be felt to engage the stricture until it is fully inserted. Withdraw the dilator but not the guide wire and pass the well lubricated thicker dilator over the guide wire and through the stricture. Withdraw the dilator and wire.

Preferably pass a flexible end-viewing endoscope through the stricture and beyond, to confirm the intact passage and exclude disease beyond the stricture and damage at the site of the stricture. X-ray the chest without delay.

5. Dilatation from below is safer than dilatation from above. If laparotomy and gastrotomy are necessary to draw the tail of a Mousseau-Barbin or Celestin tube to splint the stricture, pass gum elastic bougies or a finger to dilate the stricture from below. Now advance a bougie up to the pharynx where the anaesthetist can grasp it, and tie the leader of an appropriate sized tube to it. Draw the leader and tube down to impact the tube in the stricture, cut off the excess tube below the stricture, close the gastrotomy wound and the abdomen.

REMOVAL OF FOREIGN BODIES

Appraise

1. Swallowed articles impact at the sites of narrowing. Objects at the cricopharyngeus muscle are regurgitated but those that pass this point may impact at the crossing of the aortic arch or at the cardia. However, the normal oesophagus is extremely distensible and smooth objects usually pass into the stomach. The most frequent causes of impaction are pre-existing stricture or sharp foreign body which penetrates the oesophageal wall.

2. Remember that many impacted foreign bodies are radiolucent. Sometimes they are demonstrable on X-rays by giving the patient a drink of water-soluble contrast medium.

3. Do not embark on foreign body removal if you are inexperienced if there is a skilled endoscopist available.

4. Foreign bodies may be removed using ingenious methods in conjunction with fibre-optic endoscopes and local anaesthesia with sedation. Impacted foreign bodies that cannot be easily grasped with the instrument available with fibre-optic instruments will require full anaesthesia and the passage of a rigid endoscope. Deeply and firmly impacted foreign bodies may require thoracotomy and oesophagotomy to remove them.

5. A smooth foreign body may be gently pushed into the stomach. As a rule it will pass through the gut but if it remains in the stomach removal is easier than from the oesophagus.

Action

1. The technique of removal through the rigid oesophagoscope with the patient anaesthetized is well developed. The grasping forceps are strong and versatile and special varieties are made that aid the removal of open safety pins and coins. Do not attempt to remove a foreign body before assessing how this can best be achieved with minimum damage. A sharp foreign body may be withdrawn into the lumen of the instrument but large foreign bodies may need to be removed together with the oesophagoscope, with any sharp edges pulled within the protection of the distal lip of the endoscope.

2. Ingenious methods have been used to remove foreign bodies using the end viewing fibre-optic endoscope. The foreign body may be grasped with forceps or caught with a snare and withdrawn together with the instrument. An external flexible sheath may be pushed over the end of the endoscope tip into which a sharp foreign body can be drawn to protect the mucosa from injury.

INJECTION OF VARICES

Appraise (See p. 206)

1. Recognise these as soft, collapsible projecting columns in the lower oesophagus sometimes continuing into the gastric cardia.

2. In patients with upper gastrointestinal bleeding who are found to have varices, do not assume that the bleeding is from the varices. A high proportion of such patients have another cause such as peptic ulcer, so always carry out a complete examination.

3. The varices thrombose when injected with ethanolamine oleate warmed to reduce its viscosity. The rigid or flexible oesophagoscope may be used and 2–5 ml are injected into each varix. The injections are repeated at intervals of 3–4 weeks until the varices are obliterated.

INTUBATION OF STRICTURES

Appraise

1. It is not necessary to intubate all strictures that cannot be resected or do not respond to dilatation. Malignant strictures that will be submitted to radiotherapy may deteriorate temporarily and later expand, so it is worthwhile deferring intubation. Benign strictures that respond to dilatation at intervals of 3–6 months should not be intubated. Intubation produces a rigid channel through which food must fall by gravity and which can easily block so reserve its use for patients with real need.

2. There are two methods of introducing tubes through strictures (Fig. 18.3). The one in vogue at present is pulsion intubation in which the tube is pushed through

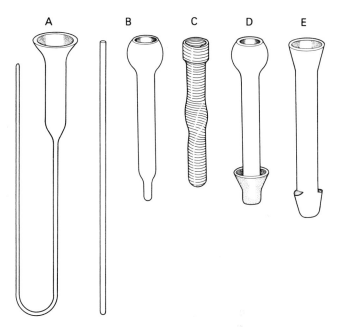

Fig. 18.3 A is the Mousseau-Barbin tube. B is the Celestin tube with plastic leader on the left. A and B are pulled through oesophageal strictures from below. C is Souttar's brass wire tube. D is Celestin's tube with latex frill to prevent the tube from slipping upwards. E is the Atkinson tube with projections to prevent the tube from slipping upwards. C, D and E can be pushed through strictures from above.

from above. No incision is made and if necessary the procedure can be accomplished with sedation and analgesia. In the second method performed under anaesthesia, the tube is attached to a leader which is drawn through the stricture by traction from below, through a gastrotomy incision: the excess tube and leader are then cut off and the gastrotomy is closed. This method is useful when dilatation from above proves impossible because the dilators and the guide wire impact against the wall and cannot be passed through the stricture. When it is intended to use oesophageal dilatation and traction intubation, leave a Celestin semiflexible leader in place through the stricture with the lower end in the stomach. Whenever it is likely that intubation from above will be difficult, obtain consent for intubation from below and make preparations to carry it out immediately.

3. Intubation of oesophageal strictures is dangerous and should be performed only by experienced operators. The tube may split a rigid, friable stricture. This is not necessarily disastrous provided a tube can be impacted across the split.

PULSION INTUBATION WITH FLEXIBLE ENDOSCOPE (Fig. 18.4)

1. Introduce the endoscope in the sedated or anaesthetized patient and pass an Eder-Puestow guide wire through the biopsy channel, the stricture, and beyond into the

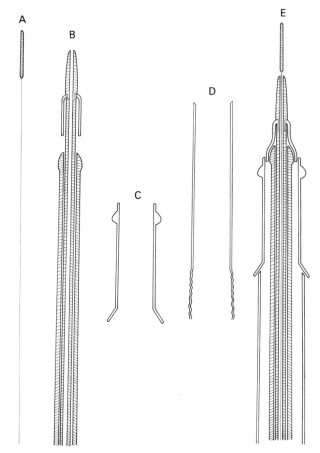

Fig. 18.4 Pulsion intubation using the Nottingham introducer. A is the Eder-Puestow guide wire, B is the carrier that grips the tube from within by means of an expanding segment. C is the tube and D the pusher. At E, the whole assembly is shown.

stomach. Withdraw the endoscope, retaining the guide wire in place. Pass graded Eder-Puestow or Celestin dilators over the guide wire and through the stricture until it is maximally dilated.

2. Withdraw the dilators, leaving the guide wire in place.

3. Assemble the selected tube on the Nottingham introducer shaft. The tube size and length must be estimated from the measured length of the stricture and the size to which it has been dilated. The distal end of the tube is gripped by an expanding rubber section of the shaft. A flexible pusher tube fits into the expanded proximal end of the tube.

4. If the tube is to be introduced under sedation, give an intravenous bolus of analgesic such as 25 mg pethidine (meperidine, Demerol). Thread the introducer assembly onto the guide wire and gently push it through the mouth and pharynx into the oesophagus. The flexible tip of the carrier shaft guides the distal end of the tube through the stricture. Push the tube home until the resistance is felt as the expanded proximal end of the tube impacts just above the stricture. This part of the procedure is facilitated using

a radiographic image intensifier but the distance of the pusher length beyond the incisor teeth can be measured as a guide.

5. Unlock the expanding shaft of the introducer and withdraw it, holding the tube in place with the pusher tube. Now remove the pusher tube. It is valuable to re-pass the small flexible endoscope through the tube and beyond, checking that the tube is correctly sited, that there is no damage and that the passage is clear.

6. Withhold oral feeding overnight and next morning be sure that the patient is free of chest pain, of air emphysema in the neck, and that a chest X-ray shows no abnormality before allowing oral fluid feeding.

PULSION INTUBATION USING RIGID OESOPHAGOSCOPE

1. Pass the oesophagoscope in the anaesthetized patient and dilate the stricture to its maximum without splitting it. Select a suitable Souttar-type wire or plastic tube, a trimmed Mousseau-Barbin or Celestin tube, or an Atkinson tube. Insert a gum-elastic bougie through the stricture of a size that the lubricated tube will slide easily over it.

2. Withdraw the oesophagoscope, slide the tube over the bougie and guide its tip through the mouth and pharynx. Now insert the tip of the oesophagoscope into the expanded end of the tube to act as a pusher and carefully slide the tube down until the expanded neck impacts at the upper end of the stricture. This can be checked by noting the depth of insertion of the oesophagoscope.

3. Withdraw the oesophagoscope and the bougie.

4. Determine to have a plain X-ray of the patient's chest and neck to exclude mediastinal air emphysema that would suggest rupture of the oesophagus. Check the patient's neck clinically after operation to exclude air emphysema. If there is no chest pain or other sign of rupture, cautiously start oral fluids the following day.

TRACTION INTUBATION

1. If dilatation or intubation from above proves impossible because the angulated or distorted lumen prevents onward progress of the dilators or guide wire, dilatation from below is often possible and safe, and a tube can then be drawn through. Sometimes the dilators will pass but the tube cannot be satisfactorily inserted through it, perhaps because the stricture is irregular, elastic, has a lip which catches the end of the tube, or if the guide wire cannot be passed sufficiently far beyond it to allow full introduction of the tube carrier.

2. The prepared patient is anaesthetized, intubated and lies supine on the operating table. If oesophagoscopy has

been performed, leave a bougie or Eder-Puestow guide wire in place with its lower end in the stomach.

3. Prepare the skin, make a vertical incision 5–7 cm long through all layers of the abdominal wall from the left costal margin through the middle of the left rectus muscle, splitting the fibres. Insert the right hand to feel the liver, left gastric and coeliac nodes, stomach, cardia and lower oesophagus. Feel for the end of a bougie, leader, guide wire or nasogastric tube.

4. Draw the stomach down to bring the upper anterior wall into the wound and make a 2 cm gastrotomy midway between the greater and lesser curves. Aspirate the contents with a sucker.

5. Grasp and draw out the lower end of a nasogastric tube, leader, guide wire or bougie. If it was not possible to pass one, insert a medium sized bougie from below, guide it through the cardia into the lower oesophagus and up to the pharynx where the anaesthetist can recover the tip and draw it out of the mouth. Sometimes it is safer to insert a finger through the gastrotomy and cardia, to feel and dilate a lower oesophageal stricture before passing up the bougie.

6. Ask the anaesthetist to attach the Celestin tube to its leader, or attach the tail of a Mousseau-Barbin type of tube to the upper end of the nasogastric tube or olive of a bougie passed from below. If a bougie or Eder-Puestow guide wire has been passed from above, attach a strong thread to the lower end, ask the anaesthetist to draw out the instrument and thread, detach the thread and tie it securely to the leader of a tube. Now gently draw the leader of the tube into the stomach as the anaesthetist guides the lubricated tube through the mouth and pharynx. Draw the lower end of the tube through the stricture into the stomach until the expanded proximal end of the tube is felt to impact at the upper end of the stricture.

7. Cut off the excess tube high in the stomach, making sure there are no sharp edges. Some surgeons fix the tube with a stitch to the stomach wall to prevent it from being regurgitated into the oesophagus above the stricture. I have rarely had problems with tubes slipping upwards, so do not attempt this.

8. Close the gastrotomy in two layers and close the abdomen routinely.

Aftercare

1. Make sure the patient does not have chest pain, air emphysema in the neck, or a raised temperature and have a plain chest radiograph.

2. If there is evidence of leak, confirm it and identify the site with X-rays using a water-soluble contrast medium and plan to explore the chest immediately in a suitable patient. Intubation of low strictures are likely to damage the oesophagus on the left side, possibly with rupture into the left pleural cavity. At left thoracotomy, repair and

drain the leak. If the rupture is low it may be preferable to impact a large Mousseau-Barbin type tube through the split by traction from below and then insert a chest drain. Minor injury in the neck usually responds to conservative management with parenteral feeding but it is usually wise to insert a drain.

3. If the patient is satisfactory, start oral fluid feeding next day and progress rapidly to solids. Warn the patient against swallowing unchewed food, particularly lumps of meat, fruit skins and stones and to wash down the food with sips of water. Aerated drinks such as sodium bicarbonate solution (half of teaspoonful in half a glass of water half an hour before meals) helps to wash away adherent mucus that may block the tube.

4. Very occasionally the oesophagus cannot be intubated from above or below. Suitable patients withstand operative bypass but some already have severe aspiration pneumonia. Many surgeons deprecate the use of gastrostomy in such patients and think that sedatives and analgesics alone should be given. This is a philosophical decision. Personally I never withhold gastrostomy after discussing the problem with the patient.

OESOPHAGEAL EXPOSURE

NECK (Fig. 18.5)

1. The cervical oesophagus may be approached from either side. Operations for the removal of pharyngeal pouch or cricopharyngeal myotomy are usually carried out from the left side. Approach to the lower cervical oesophagus on the left endangers the thoracic duct, therefore whenever possible approach it from the right side.

2. The anaesthetised intubated patient lies supine on the operating table with the head turned to the opposite side from which the exploration will be made and resting on a ring. After preparing the skin, wrap the head, endotracheal tube and hair within a sterile towel.

3. Incise along the anterior border of sternomastoid muscle, through platysma muscle, cervical fascia, omo-hyoid muscle, ligating and dividing the middle thyroid vein to enter the space between the oesophagus, trachea and thyroid gland medially and the sternomastoid muscle and carotid sheath laterally, The inferior thyroid artery crosses the space: ligate and divide it only if it inteferes with the dissection, preferring to retain it if the oesophagus is to be mobilized for subsequent anastomosis.

4. Rotate the whole oesophageal-tracheal-thyroid column towards the opposite side bringing into view the tracheo-oesophageal groove and display the posterior surface of the oesophagus and lower pharynx.

5. If the oesophagus is to be separated from the trachea, carefully identify the recurrent laryngeal nerve to preserve it. Gently insinuate blunt forceps between the trachea and oesophagus, taking care not to damage either the oesoph-

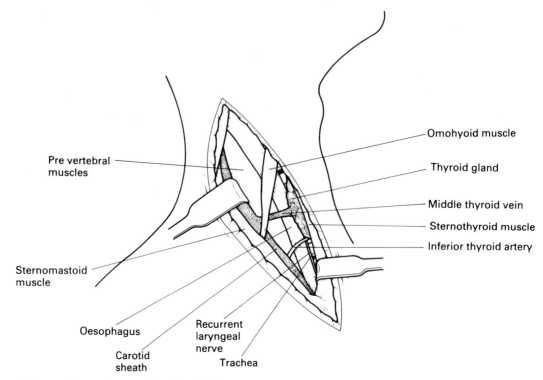

Fig. 18.5 Exposure of the cervical oesophagus on the right side. Sternomastoid muscle and the carotid sheath are drawn laterally. The space between these structures and the midline column of the pharynx and oesophagus, trachea and thyroid gland, is crossed by omohyoid muscle, middle thyroid vein and inferior thyroid artery.

agus or the membranous posterior wall of the trachea. The recurrent laryngeal nerve on the opposite side cannot be seen and is endangered. Insert a curved Moynihan's or Lahey's forceps between the tubes, turn the point posteriorly to make contact with the anterior vertebral muscles on the opposite side. Insert a finger behind the oesophagus to reach the forceps point and guide it through so that a tape can be fed into its jaws. Now withdraw the forceps leaving the tape encircling the oesophagus. This can be the starting point for further dissection.

6. If a gastric, jejunal or colonic conduit is to be united to the oesophagus and is short, continue the skin incision down to the manubriosternal joint in the midline. Insert a finger behind the sternum to separate the posterior aspect of the sternum from the innominate vein. Split the sternum down its centre using a sternal splitter. Carefully separate the medial end of the clavicle and first rib from the underlying vessels. Cut through the clavicle 3 cm from its medial end and the rib 2 cm from the manubrium. Remove the freed bone. Access is markedly improved.

THORACIC

Right thoracotomy (Fig. 18.6)

1. The anaesthetised patient, intubated with a double-lumen tube to allow exclusion of the right lung, lies on his

left side. Carry out right thoracotomy at the level of the fifth or sixth rib (see Ch. 19).

2. Ask the anaesthetist to collapse the right lung. Draw it downwards and forwards to reveal the mediastinal pleura. The oesophagus cannot be seen but the azygos vein can be seen arching over the lung root. Incise the mediastinal pleura, mobilize, doubly ligate and divide the azygos vein. This reveals the oesophagus running posterior to the trachea and lung root. The lower oesophagus is not visible between the left atrium and the vertebral column as it veers to the left. The upper stomach can be approached after dilating or incising the diaphragmatic crus to enlarge the hiatus.

Right anterior thoracotomy

An alternative but less adequate approach can be made through a right anterior thoracotomy with the patient supine. This allows the oesophagus to be reached as part of the resection in the manner described by McKeown (see p. 303) without the need to turn the patient onto his left side. Make a 15–20 cm incision over the right anterior fifth rib deepening it until the pectoralis major muscle is reached. Dissect the intact pectoralis muscle from the rib. Enter the chest through the bed of the resected right fifth rib.

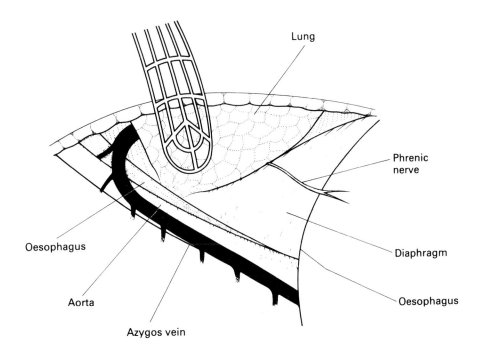

Fig. 18.6 Diagram of approach to the oesophagus through the right pleural space. The right lung is retracted anteriorly.

Left thoracotomy

1. The lower thoracic oesophagus may be approached by left thoracotomy at the level of the seventh or eighth rib (see Ch. 19).

2. The left dome of diaphragm or the diaphragmatic crus may be incised to enter the upper abdomen.

Left thoracoabdominal approach (Fig. 18.7)

1. The lower thoracic oesophagus and upper stomach are best approached using a combined thoracoabdominal approach.

2. Lay the anaesthetized intubated patient on his right side, left leg extended, right leg flexed at hip and knee,

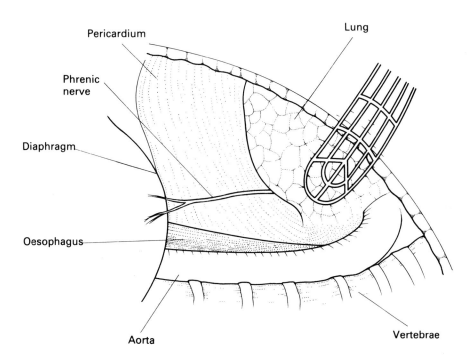

Fig. 18.7 Diagram of approach to lower oesophagus through the left pleural space. The left lung is retracted anteriorly.

both arms flexed with forearms before the face as though performing the hornpipe dance. Allow the patient to lay back with the shoulders at 30° from the vertical. Fix the patient's hips with an encircling band, support the left upper scapula against a padded post.

3. Prepare the skin and drape the area with sterile towels.

4. Start the incision just above the umbilicus, carry it obliquely upwards and to the left to cross the costal margin along the line of the seventh or eighth rib, extending to the posterior angle of the chosen rib. Deepen the incision to enter the thorax along the line of the rib, cutting the costal margin and incising the diaphragm radially towards the oesophageal hiatus.

5. In case of doubt make the abdominal or thoracic part of the incision first: assess the condition and now, if indicated, extend it fully.

6. After completing the procedure, close the diaphragm using strong non-absorbable thread. Suture the abdomen in the usual manner. Close the chest after inserting an underwater-sealed drain.

ABDOMINAL (Fig. 18.8)

1. The lower oesophagus is approachable through the abdomen and oesophageal hiatus.

2. Make an upper midline incision extending to the costal margin, opening the peritoneum just to the left of the falciform ligament. Ligate the ligamentum teres. Divide it and the falciform ligament.

3. Draw down the stomach while an assistant elevates the left lobe of the liver with a flat-bladed retractor. The lower oesophagus can be felt at the hiatus.

4. If necessary cut the left triangular ligament and fold the left lobe of the liver to the right. To improve the view of the oesophagus remove the xiphoid process and if necessary split the lower sternum subcutaneously (p. 63).

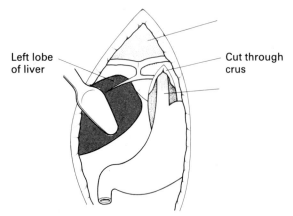

Left lobe of liver

Cut through crus

Fig. 18.8 Transabdominal approach to the lower oesophagus. The left lobe of liver is folded to the right. If necessary the diaphragmatic crus can be incised anteriorly.

5. To display the lower thoracic oesophagus, transversely incise the peritoneum and fascia over the abdominal oesophagus for 5 cm, preserving the anterior vagal trunk. If greater exposure is necessary insert a finger into the posterior mediastinum. Turn it forwards to separate the pericardium from the upper surface and incise the crus and diaphragm anteriorily for 5–7 cms.

6. In patients of suitable build the oesophagus can be viewed almost up to the carina of the trachea if the heart is gently elevated with a flat retractor. It is usually unnecessary to close the incision in the crus and diaphragm.

OPERATIVE CONSIDERATIONS

Appraise

1. Most other parts of the bowel are covered with serosa that rapidly forms fibrinous adhesions, sealing small defects and preventing leaks. The oesophagus has no serous coat except on the anterior wall of the abdominal segment.

2. A considerable part of the oesophageal wall is composed of longitudinal muscle. Longitudinally placed sutures thus have a marked tendency to cut out. The powerful longitudinal muscle produces remarkable shortening of the oesophagus when it contracts, reducing it to half its original length. Unless this is allowed for, the most carefully placed sutures may be torn out.

3. When the oesophagus is relaxed the circular muscle makes the diameter appear to be small. However it can be stretched to a remarkable extent. Closely spaced sutures into the relaxed oesophagus become widely separated on stretching and leakage can easily occur between them.

4. The blood supply to the oesophagus is tenuous when it is mobilised.

5. The healthy oesophagus is easily damaged but disease makes it exceptionally fragile.

6. Although oral feeding may be stopped temporarily following oesophageal surgery, swallowed saliva must still pass through.

7. Intrathoracic oesophageal leakage produces posterior mediastinitis and if the pleura is damaged a pleural collection develops. The best hope for the patient's survival is rapid clinical recognition with early re-operative repair and drainage.

Safeguards

1. Never intubate the oesophagus unnecessarily. Never pass a rigid tube when a flexible one will suffice.

2. Never carry out extensive oesophageal mobilization before forming an anastomosis.

3. Never leave the oesophagus sutured under tension. When joining it to another viscus make sure there will be no traction, even when the oesophagus fully contracts.

4. Whenever possible aim to fashion an oesophageal anastomosis where leakage would be a nuisance, such as in the neck or subcutaneously, rather than where leakage would be disastrous as in the mediastinum.

5. Never attempt an oesophageal anastomosis when access is poor. Improve the view or change tactics.

ANASTOMOSIS

1. The tenuous blood supply of the oesophagus makes it rarely possible to excise a segment, mobilize the cut ends and carry out an end to end union except in neonates. Anastomosis is therefore usually to stomach, jejunum or colon.

2. Sutured anastomoses have been described using many different methods and materials, with up to three layers of interrupted sutures. This only demonstrates again that it is the meticulous care with which an anastomosis is performed rather than the technique used that determines the outcome. I shall describe a two-layer anastomosis using continuous sutures of chromic catgut on eyeless needles that has worked well in my hands

3. Mechanical circular stapling devices are now available. Do not assume that perfection automatically follows their use. As with sutures, staplers give results commensurate with the care with which they are used. Which to choose? The stapling device saves a little time. It may allow an anastomosis to be accomplished where suturing is difficult high in the abdomen, under the aortic arch, or high in the thorax — but if it fails, suturing is usually impossible and a higher resection is necessary. The stapling gun has an inevitable crushing effect on the tissues. If a dilated and thickened oesophagus is to be joined to the cut end of bowel, the resulting tissue bulk cannot be accommodated in the staple gun. It is safer to use a sutured anastomosis. Hand suturing is sometimes preferable in the neck since

there may be insufficient bowel accessible below the anastomosis for insertion of the gun.

Sutured anastomosis

1. Have you made sure that the oesophagus and bowel can be joined without tension, are not twisted and both have a good blood supply?

2. Place the posterior surfaces together.

3. Insert traction stitches at each end of the flattened oesophagus through all coats, including the stoma of the viscus to be united, if this is already prepared. These stitches allow the stoma to be stretched (Fig. 18.9).

4. Run a 2/0 chromic catgut Lembert stitch on an eyeless needle between the posterior walls of the parts to be joined about 0.5 cm from the cut edges. This picks up the seromuscularis of the stomach or bowel, but catches the muscularis and submucosa of the oesophagus.

5. If the stoma of the viscus has not yet been prepared, cut through it so that the hole matches the size of the cut end of the oesophagus. Insert traction stitches at each end so that it can be stretched to match the oesophageal opening.

6. Insert the 2/0 chromic catgut all-coats suture, mounted on an eyeless needle as a running over-and-over stitch. Place the stitches every 2–3 mm along the gently stretched bowel edges. Do not pull them too tight.

7. If you intend to pass an aspiration tube through the anastomosis ask the anaesthetist to advance it now and guide the tip into the distal bowel. A tube passed well beyond the anastomosis can be used not only to decompress the bowel but also for enteral feeding after operation.

8. Continue the all-coats over and over stitch to invert and unite the anterior edges. Tie off the stitch.

9. Remove the traction sutures.

10. Continue the Lembert stitch along the anterior wall. Pick up the viscus to be joined to the oesophagus about

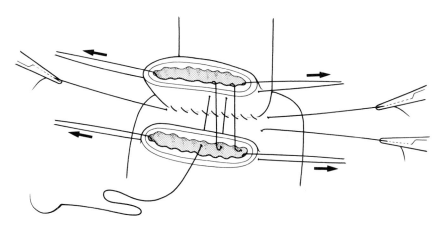

Fig. 18.9 Oesophageal anastomosis. The traction stitches are used to stretch the anastomosis (arrows). The posterior seromuscular stitch is inserted and the all coats stitch is started.

1 cm from the anastomosis, pick up the oesophageal wall 0.5 cm from the anastomosis. This produces an ink-well effect, drawing the viscus over the anastomosis.

11. If possible suture omentum, or pleura, to cover and seal the anastomosis.

12. This two-layered anastomosis, using continuous chromic catgut stitches, works satisfactorily in my hands. Alternatively, a single layer of interrupted sutures of fine monofilament nylon, prolene, or stainless steel wire may be used. As always, it is not the material, or the details of the method that are important, but the meticulous care with which each stitch is inserted.

Stapled anastomosis

1. Make sure that the oesophagus and bowel can be joined together without tension, are not twisted, and that both ends have a good blood supply.

2. If the oesophagus has not yet been transected, this may be accomplished using the special clamp that allows for the insertion of a purse-string suture (Fig. 18.10). The clamp may be applied to the cut end of the transected oesophagus. Take a fine monofilament nylon or prolene suture on a straight eyeless needle. Insert the needle through the channel on one jaw of the clamp and return it through the other jaw. Transect the oesophagus just below the clamp if it has not yet been cut. Remove the clamp. Check that the purse-string suture is perfectly inserted.

Alternatively insert the purse-string suture into the cut end of the oesophagus without the clamp, using a running all-coats over and over stitch around the cut edge.

3. Assess the size of the oesophageal lumen by gently opening the jaws of an empty swab-holding forceps within it to allow the insertion of a test sizing head, lubricated with sterile water-soluble jelly. Select a suitable sized stapling head.

4. Assemble the circular stapling device after applying the safety catch. Follow the maker's instructions step by step. The device may have a single or a double row of staples.

5. The well-lubricated stapler must first be introduced into the viscus that will be joined to the oesophagus. If the stomach is used, create a temporary anterior gastrotomy,

insert the stapler without the anvil head, so that the stem bulges the fundus at least 2 cm from any suture line. Make a small incision and allow the stem to protrude (Fig. 18.11). If the jejunum or colon are joined end-to-side, insert the stapler without the anvil head through the cut end, which will be closed later. Protrude the stem through the antimesenteric wall at a suitable point. If jejunum or colon are joined end to end, insert the fully assembled instrument through a temporary antimesenteric enterotomy 5–7 cm distal to the cut end. Protrude the head past the bowel end and open the anvil from the staple head. Insert an all-coats, purse-string suture around the cut end, tighten

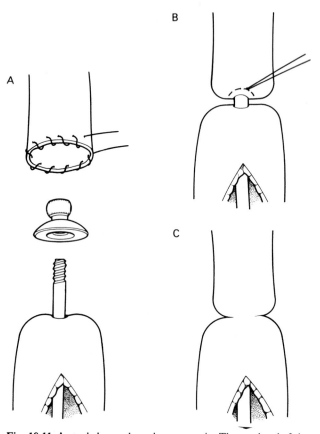

Fig. 18.11 A stapled oesophageal anastomosis. The stapler shaft has been pushed through a hole in the stomach. The anvil is attached so that it can be introduced into the oesophagus. The purse-string is tightened, the device closed and actuated, producing an anastomosis.

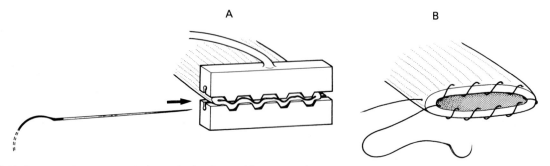

Fig. 18.10 A purse-string suture can be inserted using the special clamp or directly without a clamp.

and tie it to draw the end of the bowel over the staple head, snugly on the stem. Ensure that the bulk of the purse-stringed bowel end is as small as possible.

6. If the anvil has been removed, replace it and unscrew the jaws to separate the anvil from the staple head.

7. Insert the well-lubricated anvil into the cut end of the oesophagus, tighten and tie the purse-string to draw the end of the oesophagus over the anvil onto the stem.

8. Check that both oesophagus and viscus to be joined are not twisted but are correctly positioned, as the instrument is closed to bring them together. Make sure that nothing else becomes trapped within the jaws, and that the closure is complete without crushing the bowel.

9. Release the safety catch.

10. Compress the handle fully and firmly, slightly release them and recompress them. The gun has now been 'fired'.

11. Reapply the safety catch.

12. Unscrew the nut to separate the jaws. Gently rotate the device and draw it clear of the stapled anastomosis. Completely withdraw the instrument.

13. Remove the anvil head and check the toroidal ('doughnut-shaped') oesophageal and viscus cuffs trimmed from the inside of the anastomosis. Make sure they are complete and then place them in fixative solution prior to histological examination.

14. Insert a finger through the anastomosis to check it. If an aspiration tube is to be passed, ask the anaesthetist to pass it now and guide it through the anastomosis with a finger.

15. Close the opening through which the instrument and finger were passed.

16. Carefully check that the anastomosis is complete all the way round and lies without tension.

Difficulty?

1. A thick walled viscus and thick walled oesophagus joined end to end may produce too great a bulk of tissue between the jaws of the stapling device. Is it possible to convert the anastomosis to end-to-side, so that the stem merely requires to be pushed through a small hole in the distal viscus wall?

2. A fragile oesophagus compressed normally within the jaws of the stapling machine may be damaged. The tenuous blood supply may be crushed between the staple carrier and the anvil, or between the staples. The longitudinal muscular wall may be traumatized. Either abandon the anastomotic technique or first dissect back the thick muscle wall and engage only the mucosa and submucosa of the oesophagus in the purse string suture to be trapped in the stapling device. Subsequently insert an external layer of sutures uniting the muscular and submucous layers of the oesophagus to the viscus.

3. If the anastomosis is imperfect, be prepared to reinforce the staple line with an encircling suture. Alternatively, abandon attempts to staple the viscera and rely on a carefully sutured anastomosis. Hoping for the best is a recipe for disaster in oesophageal surgery.

TRAUMA, SPONTANEOUS AND POST-OPERATIVE LEAKS

Appraise

1. Swallowed foreign body, stab or missile wounds may immediately rupture the oesophagus but crush injuries such as those sustained in road traffic accidents may cause necrosis with late rupture. Inco-ordinated retching may tear the lower oesophagus usually just above the hiatus, to the left side: this is Boerhaave's syndrome of spontaneous rupture.

2. Iatrogenic rupture may follow endoscopy, dilatation of stricture or achalasia, removal of a foreign body, or follow an operation on the oesophagus including cardiomyotomy, vagotomy and resection or bypass.

3. The history of events, complaint of pain, collapse after injury or operation, presence of air emphysema in the neck and on plain radiographs demand radiological study with contrast media and endoscopy to determine the site, extent, and localization of leakage in case of doubt. Tracheo-oesophageal fistula, producing respiratory symptoms and signs is localized by contrast radiology, oesophagoscopy and bronchoscopy.

4. Late presentation may show signs of cellulitis including mediastinitis and peritonitis, abscess formation and fistula.

5. Following accidental or violent injury, assess the possibility of other injuries which must be dealt with.

6. Small cervical leaks following instrumental damage usually seal·if the patient is fed parenterally for a few days. Except for minor leaks, insert a drain.

7. Intrathoracic leaks are almost uniformly fatal if not sealed or drained without delay.

8. If the oesophagus is split during dilatation of a carcinoma, which it was intended to intubate, always proceed with intubation. The plastic tube will help to seal the leak.

Prepare

1. Resuscitate the patient with intravenous fluids and if necessary cross match blood.

2. Start treatment with a versatile antibiotic.

Access

1. Approach the oesophagus by the most direct route.

2. If abdominal injuries are suspected use a left thoraco-abdominal incision or be prepared to explore the abdomen subsequently.

3. If this is a post-operative leak, resolve whether the underlying disease process allows direct correction of the complication. Possibly the disease will need to be eradicated by resection. It may be defunctioned by bypass or the creation of proximal and distal stomata.

4. Expose the oesophagus adequately to allow full assessment of the damage to the oesophagus and related structures.

5. Rupture of the lower thoracic oesophagus following endoscopy, dilatation or attempted intubation of a neoplastic stricture may be best approached through an upper abdominal incision with exposure through the enlarged hiatus.

Assess

1. Is there but a single site of damage? Can you identify healthy mucosa around the whole circumference? If not extend the hole in the wall until you can.

2. Are the tissues healthy or ischaemic? Closing defects with unhealthy margins is doomed to failure.

3. Can the defect be repaired? Is there enough tissue for closure without tension?

4. Is there any foreign material. If so, remove it.

5. What is the condition of adjacent structures? Ensure that only healthy tissues remain.

6. If this is a postoperative leak is the cause evident? What can be learned for future incorporation in your technique?

7. Take a swab for culture of organisms and tests for antibiotic sensitivity.

Action

1. Remove any foreign material and excise dead or doubtful tissue.

2. Small tears of the cervical oesophagus need no sutures but it is wise to drain the area.

3. If the defect can be repaired with simple sutures, close it in a single layer using non-absorbable sutures in one or two layers. Reinforce this if possible with pleura, pericardium or lung sutured over it. Lower oesophageal holes may be reinforced by wrapping with gastric fundus.

4. A leaking or ruptured neoplasm may not be sealed by conventional methods. Impact in it a Mousseau-Barbin type of tube to act as an obturator plugging the leak.

5. If the defect cannot be repaird, if may be sufficient to drain it. Arrange also to keep the oesophagus empty and facilitate enteral feeding below the leak. Achieve this by arranging a double gastrostomy or jejunostomy: one tube passes up the point of leakage, and is joined to a gentle sucker apparatus, the other passes down into the jejunum for feeding.

6. Seal an unclosable leak in the lower oesophagus by mobilizing the gastric fundus and suturing the seromuscularis around the margins of the defect (Thal, 1968).

7. Isolate a severe leak by disconnecting the oesophagus above and below it, either as a temporary or permanent measure. Transect the oesophagus in the neck after closing the lower cut end with a ligature and bring out the proximal end to the skin as a temporary cervical oesophagostomy or unite it to stomach, jejunum or colon brought up as a bypass conduit. Transect the oesophagus below the leak (see p. 305). The isolated segment of oesophagus will produce only a little mucus.

8. Dissect a tracheo-oesophageal or broncho-oesophageal fistula, close the two holes and interpose pleura, pericardium or even lung.

Closure

1. Insert underwater sealed drains to apex and base of the pleural cavity after thoracotomy.

2. Insert closed suction drains into the neck or mediastinum and upper abdomen if the leak or site of trauma has been approached through the abdomen and hiatus.

Aftercare

1. Continue parenteral feeding, and antibiotics.

2. Remove chest drains after 48 hours or when they cease to drain and swing.

3. Monitor the patient's recovery clinically by progress charts and plain radiographs.

4. Check the repair and healing with a screened radio-opaque swallow on the fifth postoperative day. If there is no leak, or if there is a small leak well loculated, or a small leak well drained, oral feeding may be started, initially with clear fluids.

5. As drains cease to discharge, shorten or remove them. If fresh collections develop, drain them.

PHARYNGEAL POUCH

Appraise

1. This pulsion diverticulum of Zenker is a mucosal herniation between the transverse and oblique fibres of the inferior pharyngeal constrictor muscle, thought to result from incoordination or achalasia of the cricopharyngeal sphincter.

2. Recommend operation if the patient has dysphagia or regurgitation with the likelihood of aspiration pneumonia.

Access (Fig. 18.12)

1. The anaesthetized patient, with a cuffed endotracheal tube in place lies supine with the head on a ring, turned to the right and neck extended. Some surgeons pass an oesophageal speculum, identify the pouch and pack it with ribbon gauze to help identify it but I do not.

2. After preparing the skin and towelling off the left side

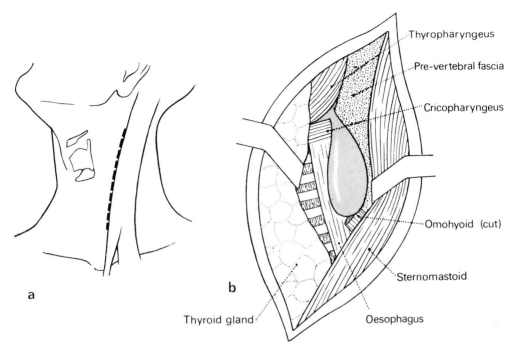

Fig. 18.12 Excision of pharyngeal pouch (a) Incision. Head rotated to right and neck extended. (b) Pouch and its relations.

of the neck make an incision along the anterior border of the left sternomastoid muscle from the greater horn of the hyoid bone to 5 cm above the sternoclavicular joint. Deepen the incision through the platysma muscle, ligating and dividing the external jugular vein if necessary, and then incise the deep fascia.

3. Identify the carotid sheath and retract it and the sternomastoid muscle posteriorly to view the groove between the carotid sheath laterally and the tracheo-oesophageal column medially.

4. Three structures cross the groove. Identify the belly of omohyoid muscle and divide it. The middle thyroid vein may require double ligation and division but is usually lower. The inferior thyroid artery is lower and deeper than this dissection.

5. Rotate the thyroid gland, larynx, trachea and oesophagus to the right and gently separate the loose tissue in the groove to reach the prevertebral fascia. View the back of the lower pharynx and upper oesophagus to identify the pouch which lies collapsed against the oesophagus unless it has been previously packed. The neck of the sack lies at the level of the cricoid cartilage.

Action

1. Gently separate the sac from the oesophagus and elevate it from below until it is attached only by the neck. Avoid dissecting away from the sac and in particular keep away from the tracheo-oesophageal groove where lies the recurrent laryngeal nerve.

2. While the sac is still attached, identify the transverse fibres of cricopharyngeus passing just distal to the neck.

Carefully insinuate the tips of non-toothed forceps between the neck and the fibres and direct the forceps longitudinally towards the upper oesophagus. Incise the fibres with a scalpel or with the tips of nearly closed scissors for about 1 cm. The lower end of the sphincter is obvious because the fibres of the upper oesophagus appear to be predominantly longitudinal. It is usually convenient to make the incision on the left of the neck of the sac rather than in the midline posteriorly. Make absolutely sure that no horizontal muscle fibres remain.

3. The most important part of the operation is now completed.

4. Conventionally the sac may now be incised at its neck. Do not remove too much tissue or you may encroach on the pharynx. It is wise to cut a little distal to the neck, closing the defect as the cut is extended transversely, using a continuous invaginating stitch of catgut. When the sac is completely excised there should be a horizontal suture line. Reinforce this with a second layer of continuous sutures.

5. Alternatively, especially in old people and especially if the sac is small, invert the sac instead of excising it. Stitch the fundus to the prevertebral fascia with one or two non-absorbable sutures so that it is upside down. This prevents the sac from filling and removes it from directly beneath the pharynx.

Closure

1. If the sac has been excised, insert a closed drainage system of the Redivac type.

2. Repair the deep fascia, platysma, and close the skin.

Aftercare

1. If the sac has been inverted it is safe to start the patient feeding immediately.

2. If the sac has been excised, feed the patient parenterally for 24–48 hours to allow the defect to seal. Remove the drain after 2–3 days.

HIATAL HERNIA AND GASTRO-OESOPHAGEAL REFLUX

Appraise

1. Incontrovertible symptoms of gastro-oesophageal reflux may be present when reflux cannot be demonstrated radiologically. Certainly reflux may exist without hiatal hernia, and hiatal hernia occurs without reflux.

2. Rolling hernia infrequently results in reflux but combined forms of hernia occur. Rolling hernia may be complicated by obstructive symptoms or by ulceration and bleeding and ordinarily requires reduction and repair.

3. Uncomplicated reflux rarely requires operative treatment. Weight loss and the observance of a few simple rules usually control the symptoms. The patient should avoid wearing tight abdominal clothing, smoking, stooping and bending and should sleep propped up at night and allow a simple antacid tablet to dissolve in the vestibule between the teeth and cheek between meals and last thing at night. Some patients respond to a course of H_2 receptor blocking drugs or carbenoxolone. Offer operation only if the patient remains incapacitated, despite obeying these rules.

4. Reflux may complicate dilatation of strictures, vagotomy, cardiomyotomy and surgical damage to the hiatal mechanism. It may be particularly severe if the cardia has been injured or resected. In suitable patients, reflux can be prevented by interposing a 15–20 cm isoperistaltic jejunal segment or isoperistaltic segment of left colon between oesophagus and stomach or by uniting the oesophagus to a Roux-en-Y jejunal loop.

5. Gastro-oesophageal reflux is not directly indicated in oesophageal carcinoma. Nevertheless, reflux oesophagitis and carcinoma may co-exist. Therefore do not neglect endoscopic biopsy and brush cytology.

6. An anti-reflux operation should be carried out for oesophagitis in Barrett's oesophagus. There is usually no hiatal hernia but incompetence at the cardia is the likely mechanism. Such patients should thereafter have an annual endoscopic biopsy and cytology examination to detect any early neoplastic change, which is a risk in this condition.

7. Offer operation for complications that cannot be managed conservatively such as chronic bleeding, oesophageal ulcer, stricture or persistent aspiration and pneumonia with the possibility of pulmonary fibrosis.

8. Do not blame indeterminate dyspepsia upon an incidentally-discovered hiatal hernia. Properly investigate the patient before offering surgical repair.

9. Depending upon your training and philosophy, you may repair a hiatal hernia through the abdominal or thoracic route. The abdominal route offers the opportunity to search for and treat other intra-abdominal disease that may be contributing to symptoms. If the oesophagus is shortened or if the patient is obese, access if often better by the transthoracic route. The Belsey technique was devised as a transthoracic method and cannot be easily performed through the abdominal route. Satisfactory operations can be accomplished through either approach so select the one with which you are most familiar.

10. Anti-reflux procedures: Not all patients with gastro-oesophageal reflux have hiatal hernias. The margins of some hiatal hernias are so poor and stretched that successful repair is impossible. Fixed hiatal hernias cannot be reduced so that repair is not possible. Anti-reflux operations have become increasingly popular as adjunctive operations to hiatal hernia repair or to replace attempts at repair when this is difficult or ineffectual. They are designed to augment the natural mechanisms that prevent reflux. The method of Nissen can be carried out through the chest or abdomen. The Belsey Mark IV repair is accomplished through the chest. The Nissen gastropexy and Hill techniques are performed through the abdomen. Read the original descriptions. The procedures will be described in outline. I have personal experience with the Nissen and Belsey's techniques only. Because I believe that a thorough abdominal exploration is vital, I favour the abdominal approach and have only passing knowledge of transthoracic anti-reflux operations.

TRANSABDOMINAL REPAIR

Prepare

1. Do not operate upon an overweight patient until he has lost as much weight as possible.

2. Never operate before performing endoscopy to confirm the presence of a hernia and oesophagitis. Exclude a stricture, peptic ulcer, neoplasm and pyloric stenosis in particular.

Access (Fig. 18.13)

1. Use an upper midline abdominal incision, opening the peritoneum to the left of the ligamentum teres and falciform ligament.

2. Mobilize the left lobe of the liver and fold it to the right.

3. If necessary, excise the xiphoid process.

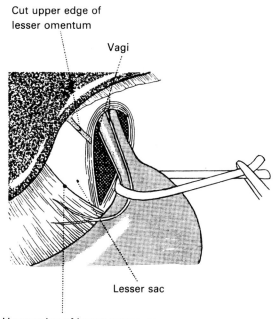

Cut upper edge of lesser omentum

Vagi

Lesser sac

Upper edge of lesser omentum

Fig. 18.13 Abdominal approach for the repair of hiatal hernia. The hernial sac has been excised to define the margins of the hiatus, and the upper edge of the lesser omentum has been detached from the diaphragm. Either an anterior or posterior repair may now be performed.

Assess

1. Explore the abdomen.

2. Confirm the presence of a sliding hiatal hernia. The hiatus will usually be patulous, so that one or more fingers can be inserted alongside the abdominal oesophagus between the diaphragmatic crura. If the gastric cardia is grasped between finger and thumb it can be slid upwards through the hiatus; this manoeuvre confirms sliding hiatal hernia.

3. In rolling hernia the gastric fundus herniates alongside the gullet into the chest. The cardia may remain in the abdomen or slide into the chest.

4. Anterior or posterior repair? Successes are gained by competent surgeons using either repair. The higher the hiatus, the greater the chance that the lower oesophagus will remain in the abdomen. Following the posterior repair, the anterior and highest part of the crus becomes the new hiatus. The anterior repair lowers the point at which the gullet enters the abdomen. It has the practical advantage, however, that the anterior part of the hiatus can be formed into a tunnel rather than a sheet with a hole in it.

Action

1. While the first assistant pulls down the stomach with his left hand, identify the gullet by feeling the nasogastric

tube in its lumen. Avoiding the subphrenic veins, incise the thinned-out peritoneum and the phreno-oesophageal ligament transversely for 3–4 cm in front of the gullet. Identify and preserve the anterior vagus nerve.

2. Try to make the right thumb and index finger meet behind the gullet. They are separated by a 'mesentery' in which lies the posterior trunk of the vagus nerve. Taking care to avoid damaging the nerve, break through the tissue behind the nerve. Pass a 30 cm length of soft rubber tubing round the gullet. Catch the ends of the tube in strong artery forceps so that traction may be applied to the gullet.

3. Working from the front around to each side, cut away the sac and loose tissue from the palpably firm margins of the hiatus until they are well defined. On the right side, deliberately divide the upper portion of the gastrohepatic omentum, to display the right margin of the hiatus.

Anterior repair

1. Draw the anterior lip of the hiatus forwards by means of a traction stitch. Displace the gullet posteriorly. The defect now becomes an anteroposterior slit.

2. Insert three or four horizontal mattress stitches of 00 silk or monofilament nylon, preferably mounted on eyeless needles. Each stitch picks up good muscular tissue on either side, while avoiding damage to the pericardium. When the stitches are tied, the repaired hiatal margins bulge into the abdomen as a keel, forming a tunnel for the gullet.

3. Insert stitches of the same material to form a loose darn over the anterior surface of the repair, picking up the diaphragm 3–4 cm on each side of the hiatus.

POSTERIOR REPAIR

1. Displace the gullet forwards and stitch the margins of the hiatus together behind it using 3–4 horizontal mattress sutures. Continue the repair upwards until the gullet is snugly grasped at the anterior part of the hiatus.

2. A darn may be applied over the suture line in the same manner as described for an anterior repair.

FUNDOPLICATION (Nissen) (Fig. 18.14)

1. Ask the anaesthetist to pass a peroral 38F tube into the stomach. It will be removed at the end of the operation.

2. Carry out the mobilization and preparation for transabdominal hiatal hernia repair if this is feasible. Place the sutures for an anterior or posterior hiatal repair. Tie them after completing the fundoplication.

3. Separate the lower 5–8 cm of the oesophagus from

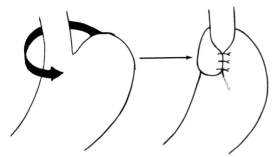

Fig. 18.14 Nissen's fundoplication. The gastric fundus is wrapped posteriorly around the upper stomach.

the hiatal margin and pass a tape around it to include the anterior and posterior vagal trunks so that they are preserved from damage.

4. Mobilize the gastric fundus, dividing the gastrophrenic ligament. Doubly ligate and divide the upper three or four short gastric arteries while avoiding damage to the spleen. Place the ligatures using aneurysm needles, tie them and cut between them. Alternatively, use carefully placed haemostatic clips.

5. Clear the upper 3–4 cm of gastric lesser curve, preserving the nerves of Latarjet, but ligating and dividing the ascending branch of the left gastric artery if necessary.

6. Draw the freed fundus posteriorly around the cardia.

7. Place a series of interrupted nonabsorbable sutures picking up the gastric fundus, the oesophagus and anterior gastric wall, one below the other. As these are tied the lower 4 cm of oesophagus and the cardia are wrapped with a cuff of gastric fundus, to augment the lower oesophageal sphincter.

8. If this operation fails, it does so because the oesophagus and cardia are drawn up through the fundic cuff which now forms a constriction around the upper stomach, allowing free gastro-oesophageal reflux from the upper loculus. Avoid this by ensuring that the cuff is sutured correctly to the oesophagus. I try to place a row of sutures attaching the posterior gastric wall to the fundic wrapping as well as those joining the fold to the anterior wall.

9. Tie the sutures to narrow the hiatus so that the crura fit snugly around the oesophagus above the cuff.

10. Ask the anaesthetist to withdraw the orogastric tube.

ANGELCHIK PROSTHESIS

Appraise

1. This is a silicone, incomplete 'doughnut' with tapes that can be tied to produce a complete circle.

2. Although such prostheses were initially considered to be inert they may generate fibrosis. Early models tended to become displaced.

3. The cushionlike ring is placed around the lower oesophagus and appears to exert gentle compression simulating the action of a sphincter. Good results are reported

in a number of series but longterm controlled trials have not yet been reported.

Action

1. Open the abdomen through a vertical upper abdominal midline incision and elevate the left lobe of the liver with a broad bladed retractor. Do not use metal haemostatic clips or staples, since they may rupture the envelope of the silicone prosthesis if they come into contact with it.

2. Identify the abdominal oesophagus. Incise the peritoneum and transversalis fascia to reach the oesophagus.

3. Gently encircle the oesophagus with a finger just above the gastro-oesophageal junction. Include the anterior vagal trunk but pass between the posterior trunk and the gullet. Pass a curved forceps behind the oesophagus and grasp one tape end of the prosthesis to draw it round the back of the oesophagus and out at the other side.

4. Remove all metal instruments from the area for fear of rupturing the capsule of the prosthesis. Gently ease the prosthesis round so that it encircles the oesophagus.

5. Tie the tapes just tightly enough to appose the ends of the prosthesis and cut off the excess tape.

6. Close the abdomen.

ANTERIOR GASTROPEXY

1. This is an especially useful procedure to carry out on a poor-risk patient or one having an abdominal operation for another condition, who has a troublesome sliding hiatal hernia, when formal repair is difficult.

2. Decide to which edge of the wound the lesser curvature of the stomach will most easily be sutured. This is usually the left side. Place a line of long Spencer Wells forceps along the peritoneum to evert the edge.

3. Draw down the stomach so that the lesser curvature continues the line of the lower oesophagus.

4. Stitch the taut lesser curvature to the undersurface of the everted wound edge, using non-absorbable material such as silk or linen. Pick up the submucous coat of the bowel and the fascial layer of the posterior rectus sheath.

5. Make sure the stitches in the abdominal wall are placed at least 2 cm from the edge. When closing the abdominal wall take care to avoid damaging the stomach that has been drawn close to the suture line.

POSTERIOR GASTROPEXY (HILL)

1. Divide the left triangular ligament, mobilize the left lobe of liver and fold it to the right.

2. Hill now measures the lower oesophageal sphincter pressure using a calibrated manometric tube attached to a nasogastric tube. The surgeon monitors the site of the tube.

3. Divide the peritoneum and phreno-oesophageal ligament to expose the pre-aortic fascia and free the oesophagus in the hiatus.

4. Doubly ligate and divide the upper two short gastric vessels, preserving the spleen.

5. Divide the upper part of the lesser omentum and have the stomach drawn to the left.

6. Identify the aorta, coeliac axis and overlying coeliac plexus. Draw the coeliac plexus caudally to expose the median arcuate ligament crossing the front of the aorta.

7. Identify and preserve the inferior phrenic arteries on each side while elevating the median arcuate ligament from below, keeping strictly in the midline from the aorta.

8. Loosely oppose the crura behind the oesophagus using three or four nonabsorbable horizontal mattress sutures picking up crus, peritoneum and fascia.

9. Place four to six nonabsorbable sutures one above the other, each of which picks up in turn the oesophageal anterior and posterior phreno-oesophageal ligaments, while avoiding vagal trunks, and the median arcuate ligament and preaortic fascia while they are lifted forwards clear of the aorta.

10. Hill now ties the highest stitch with a slip knot, so that it can be adjusted. He measures the lower oesophageal sphincter pressure, progressiely tightening the stitch until the pressure is 50–55 mm Hg. He then applies further ties to fix the stitch.

11. Tie the remaining lower ties.

ROLLING HERNIA

1. Access is as for sliding hernia.

2. The gastric fundus can be seen disappearing through the oesophageal hiatus alongside the oesophagus. In the combined hernia, the whole upper stomach appears to have passed through the hiatus into the mediastinum.

3. Mobilize and reduce the herniating gastric fundus from within the chest by inserting an index finger between the margins of the defect and the stomach. This is usually very easy since the fundus does not readily adhere to the sac.

4. Define the emptied sac of peritoneum, draw it down into the abdomen and excise it, leaving the cleared hiatal margins.

5. Close the defect using horizontal mattress sutures of nonabsorbable material, if necessary augmented with a darn.

TRANSTHORACIC REPAIR

Access

1. With the patient lying on his right side carry out a left thoracotomy at the level of the seventh or eighth rib (see Ch. 19).

2. Free the lower lobe of the left lung by dividing the pulmonary ligament as far as the inferior pulmonary vein. Display the oesophagus through an incision in the mediastinal pleura just anterior to the thoracic aorta.

Action

1. Gently encircle the lower oesophagus together with the anterior and posterior vagal trunks, taking care not to breach the right mediastinal pleura. Pass a tape around the oesophagus and vagi.

2. Identify the loose, stretched phreno-oesophageal ligament and carefully incise the sac which it has formed, to gain access to the abdomen.

3. Excise the sac until the oesophagus is cleared of everything but the intact vagal trunks, and the right crus of the diaphragm can be seen as an intact muscular loop.

4. Decide whether the repair can be carried out most easily in front of the oesophagus or behind it. The intention will be to close the hiatus to form a small, firm anteroposterior slit.

5. Suture together the limbs of the right crus, using sutures of nonabsorbable material such as 2/0 monofilament nylon, 2/0 silk or 6/0 linen thread. Insert each stitch before tying any of them, so that the hiatus remains open to allow the needle tip emerging in the abdomen to be safely directed and recovered. Then tie the sutures to trap the oesophagus snugly.

6. If the dissection or repair cannot be accomplished safely and effectively through the chest, carefully make an incision radically in the diaphragmatic aponeurosis, stopping short of the right crural muscle fibres, allowing you to approach the hernia both through the chest and also abdominally through the hole in the diaphragm. After repairing the hernia, suture the diaphragm using nonabsorbable material.

Closure

1. Close the chest in a routine manner, leaving in an underwater seal drain for 24–48 hours.

2. If the right pleural cavity was inadvertently opened, repair the mediastinal pleura with stitches and subsequently insert a right underwater seal drain.

BELSEY MARK IV REPIAR

This is the fourth modification by Mr Belsey of Bristol, of the transthoracic repair originated by Philip Allison of Leeds

Access

Perform a left posterolateral thoracotomy through the sixth intercostal space.

Action (Fig. 18.15)

1. Mobilize the lower oesophagus with intact vagi from the lung root to the hiatus.

2. Free the gastric cardia by dividing its attachments and gently draw it into the chest. Ligate and divide the upper one or two short gastric arteries to free the fundus.

3. Carefully avoiding damage to the vagal nerves, clear the cardia of adherent fat.

4. Insert linen thread sutures between the limbs of the diaphragmatic crus posteriorly, while drawing the oesophagus anteriorly. Clip the ends. They will be tied later, to reduce the size of the haitus.

5. Wrap the gastric fundus round the anterior two-thirds of the lower oesophagus, holding it in place by means of three linen mattress sutures picking up the seromuscularis of the stomach and the submucosa, but not the mucosa, of the oesophagus, 1.5 cm above the cardia.

6. Insert a second set of three sutures 1.5 cm higher than the first set. Each of these first passes down through the central tendon of the diaphragm where it meets the muscular crus, sutures the gastric fundus to the oesophagus, and then passes back through the diaphragm. After replacing the cardia in the abdomen, tie the sutures above the diaphragm just tightly enough to maintain apposition.

7. Tie the sutures previously placed posteriorly in the crus, barely tightly enough to appose the edges.

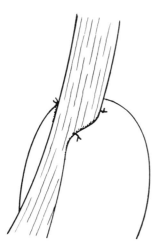

Fig. 18.15 Belsey Mark IV repair. The fundus is wrapped around the anterior two thirds of the oesophagus with a row of linen mattress sutures. A second row of sutures draws the fundal wrap higher and also picks up the anterior crural fibres of the diaphragmatic hiatus.

GASTROPLASTY

This allows a segment of upper stomach to be formed into a tube to lengthen a shortened oesophagus. In effect, it creates a 'Barrett's oesophagus'. I am therefore reluctant to perform this technique.

Action

1. Use a left thoraco-abdominal approach to excise the hernial sac, preserving the right crus of the diaphragm.

2. Apply two parallel, thin, crushing clamps across the fundic portion of the stomach, from the neck of the herniated portion, with blades parallel to the lesser curve (Fig. 18.16).

3. Cut between the clamps.

4. Close the separated portions of the stomach, so creating a tube of lesser curve upper stomach.

5. Close the right crus of the diaphragm around the new 'cardia'.

6. Close the diaphragm, abdomen and chest.

BENIGN STRICTURE

PEPTIC STRICTURE

Appraise

1. This results from gastro-oesophageal reflux and oesophagitis.

2. Make sure by endoscopy, biopsy and cytology that the stricture is truly benign.

3. Take account of the age and fitness of the patient. Some procedures carry a high risk. Be prepared on behalf of frail patients to accept less than perfect results. Carry them along with per-oral dilatations as necessary but remember the safest dilator is a solid well-chewed bolus of food. Institute medical therapy as for reflux oesophagitis (p. 292).

4. If stricturing recurs rapidly and severely, say within 3 months after adequate dilatation, in spite of a full regime of conservative management, a few patients can still be managed by training them to swallow mercury-filled Hurst's bougies by themselves at regular intervals. Initially dilate the stricture after endoscopy. The next day sit the patient upright. Ask him to swallow a well-lubricated bougie, if necessary using an anaesthetic throat spray and an intravenous injection of diazepam 5–10 mg. Hold the bougie vertical while the patient swallows it, so that the

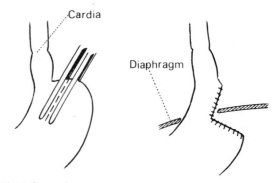

Fig. 18.16 Gastroplasty.

mercury runs downwards and by its weight carries the bougie through the stricture. Confirm that the lower end is in the stomach with a plain radiograph. By trial and error, select a suitable size of bougie, to keep the patient comfortable. He will learn to dispense with medication. Autobouginage is performed daily at first, but the period between dilatations may be gradually increased in most patients.

5. Most peptic strictures can be controlled by surgical measures to prevent gastro-oesophageal reflux, reduce gastric acid secretion, and prevent delayed gastric emptying, especially if the patient can keep his weight low. The combination of hiatal hernia repair and Polya partial gastrectomy reduces gastric acidity, ensures rapid gastric emptying, prevents reflux and helps keep the patient's weight low. Partial gastrectomy with Roux-en-Y gastroenterostomy has been recommended to prevent alkaline reflux. Hiatal hernia repair may also be combined with proximal gastric vagotomy or with truncal vagotomy and an adjunctive drainage procedure.

In recent years anti-reflux operations such as Nissen's fundoplication or the Belsey Mark IV have increased in popularity on their own, or more usually combined with a procedure to reduce gastric acid output. My current routine is to combine fundoplication with truncal vagotomy and gastroenterostomy, repairing a sliding hiatal hernia at the same time.

At the time of operation the stricture can be safely dilated from below through a gastrotomy.

6. Thal describes a technique I have not used. Through a left thoraco-abdominal incision, he cuts longitudinally through the stricture. After opening out the oesophagus, he then uses the mobilized gastric fundus to patch the defect. The fundic seromuscularis thus forms part of the oesophageal circumference, but in some cases he covers this with a split skin graft taken from the thigh. A flap valve is constructed and the hiatus is repaired.

7. A few strictures cannot be safely dilated or require frequent hazardous instrumentation. Resection and replacement offer the only satisfactory solution. The strictured oesophageal segment is resected, usually through a left thoraco-abdominal incision. The mobilized, vagotomised stomach may be drawn up and anastomosed to the oesophagus above the stricture. Alternatively an isoperistaltic segment of jejunum or colon is taken out of circuit and used to bridge the gap from oesophagus to stomach, acting as a one-way valve to prevent reflux. The oesophagus may be disconnected in the neck and abdomen, and drained into a Roux loop of jejunum below. Mobilised stomach, jejunum or colon is then taken subcutaneously or substernally to the neck as a conduit. The techniques for these are described on page 305.

8. Barrett's oesophagus may produce a severe peptic stricture. It can sometimes be managed conservatively. There is a risk of adenocarcinoma developing locally, so these patients should have regular endoscopy with biopsy and cytological examination. Operation to prevent gastro-oesophageal reflux may improve the symptoms, but it is not known whether this reduces the incidence of malignant transformation.

NON-PEPTIC STRICTURES

Appraise

1. Caustic ingestion classically causes ulceration with probable future stenosis which may be extensive. Avoid instrumentation in the early phase if possible. If a stricture develops be prepared to use regular dilatation or autobouginage, hoping that the periodicity of restenosis will lengthen. Severe stenosis that will not respond to dilatation demands gastrostomy (p. 68). Excision and replacement is occasionally necessary.

2. Anastomotic stricture usually responds to gentle dilatation. Since most anastomoses follow resection or bypass of carcinoma, do not lightly reoperate on the patient, but confirm by endoscopic biopsy and cytology that there is no anastomotic recurrence. Occasionally, resection and re-anastomosis or the interposition of a jejunal or colonic loop, is worthwhile.

3. Lower oesophageal ring of Schatzki responds to simple dilatation.

4. Cricopharyngeal web of sideropaenic anaemia, described by Patterson and Brown Kelly and by Plummer and Vinson, requires dilatation and biopsy, since there is a risk of squamous carcinoma developing. Always fully assess and treat the anaemia.

CARDIOMYOTOMY

Appraise

1. Achalasia, in which the lower segment of the oesophagus fails to relax as peristalsis reaches it, is probably part of a generalized condition of neuromuscular origin associated with myenteric ganglionic degeneration. Thus the failure to relax may be associated with a failure of propulsion above.

2. Achalasia can be treated using forceful dilatation of the lower oesophagus using an improved form of Plummer bag. Increasing sizes of bags may be used on successive days. The bag may be passed under endoscopic control and may indeed be fitted onto the shaft of a fibre-optic endoscope, or it may be passed under radiological control until it sits at the correct level. This method requires great judgement and experise and should never be used without preliminary training and without full facilities for surgical intervention if the oesophagus is inadvertently ruptured.

3. The usual surgical method of dealing with achalasia is to perform a modification of Heller's cardiomyotomy.

The circular muscle of the lower oesophagus is divided down to the mucosa. There is no argument about how high the incision is carried — it should extend well onto the dilated segment. There is some disagreement about how low the incision is carried onto the stomach. In the past the myotomy was carried down for about 5 cm onto the stomach but it is suggested that this produces gastro-oesophageal reflux.

4. The surgical approach may be through the abdomen or through the left chest.

5. Rarely severe achalasia fails to respond to Heller's operation and oesophagectomy or oesophageal bypass is necessary to allow the patient to maintain normal nutritional intake.

6. Diffuse spasm of the oesophagus may be so severe that it can be relieved only by long myotomy. Since it is usually more severe distally, this can be accomplished through the left chest.

Access

1. The abdominal approach, which I prefer, is through an upper midline incision. When necessary, remove the xiphoid process and fold the left lobe of the liver down to the right.

2. Thoracic surgeons approach the lower oesophagus through the left chest (see p. 285), incising the left mediastinal pleura over the lower oesophagus. Gently mobilize the oesophagus, freeing it without damaging the right mediastinal pleura, sufficiently to be able to place a tape around it to exert gentle traction.

Assess

1. Before disturbing the anatomy determine how easily the cardia slides into the chest. Some patients develop severe gastro-oesophageal reflux following this operation and it may be from surgical destruction of the lower oesophageal sphincter, or it may be from incipient or actual hiatal hernia. If the oesophageal hiatus is lax, plan to repair it at the end of the operation.

2. If the abdominal approach is used, explore the abdomen.

Action

1. Place the lower oesophagus under slight tension. Have the stomach drawn down if this is an abdominal approach (Fig. 18.17), have the oesophagus drawn upwards if this is a thoracic approach.

2. Identify the anterior vagal trunk, its division into hepatic and gastric branches, and its continuation as the anterior nerve of Latarjet. Safeguard the trunk and its branches by gently freeing them and moving them to the

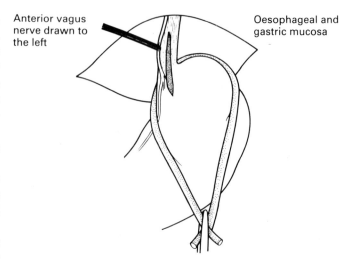

Anterior vagus nerve drawn to the left

Oesophageal and gastric mucosa

Fig. 18.17 Heller's operation for achalasia of the cardia.

right, although one or two fine branches to the gastric fundus may be sacrificed.

3. Starting just on the gastric side of the cardia, incise the muscle longitudinally on the middle of the anterior surface, until the mucosa bulges through. The reason for starting here is that if the mucosa is inadvertently perforated, it can easily be repaired and reperitonealised.

4. Insinuate fine dissecting or haemostatic forceps under the muscle of the anterior wall of the lower oesophagus, allow the blades to separate and cut through the muscle allowing the mucosa to bulge through. Continue in this fashion until the intact mucosa bulges along a longitudinal muscle split extending well on to the dilated part of the oesophagus.

5. In the rarely performed operation for diffuse spasm the myotomy is continued upwards to the aortic arch.

Check

1. If possible gather some air into the segment of lower oesophagus to distend the mucosa and exclude leaks. If there is a leak carefully repair it with fine catgut sutures, reinforced if possible by peritoneum or pleura.

2. Check the lowest extent of the split. It should definitely encroach about 1–2 cm onto the stomach. If it does not, part of the lower oesophageal physiological sphincter may still be intact.

3. Decide whether to repair the hiatus if it is lax. This may be carried out equally well from above or below.

Closure

1. If this was an abdominal approach, repair the phreno-oesophageal and peritoneal incision and close the abdomen routinely.

2. If this was a thoracic approach, insert a left basal chest drain connected to an underwater seal before closing the thorax.

CARCINOMA

Appraise

1. Pursue the diagnosis assiduously. The prognosis of early carcinoma is very good. Determine the extent of the growth by endoscopy, by radiology including tomography, and by scanning techniques. Ultrasonic imaging detects hepatic secondaries. Computerized tomography displays local infiltration, glandular spread within the thorax, abdomen and neck, and liver involvement. Bronchoscopy reveals infiltration and possible fistula formation.

2. All the operations on the oesophagus are complex and best learned from experienced masters and original descriptions. Therefore they are outlined here. There are many choices, so a selection of sound techniques is given.

3. Post-cricoid carcinoma is usually treated by radiotherapy initially but selected larger tumours and radiotherapy failures are sometimes treated by pharyngo-laryngectomy, which is outside the scope of this book.

4. The intrathoracic oesophagus is usually divided into thirds. Upper third squamous tumours are usually treated by radiotherapy and some surgeons also prefer this method for middle and lower third tumours. However, surgery is more usually attempted for middle third tumours. Lower third carcinomas are usually treated by surgery when possible. Some of these are gastric adenocarcinomas extending upward, which are insensitive to irradiation.

5. Carefully assess the age and fitness of the patient, the extent of the disease and your own capabilities. Oesophagectomy carries a high mortality and the risks are increased if the surgeon's skill, or his support facilities, are imperfect.

6. Adequate resection of gastric adenocarcinoma and especially oesophageal squamous carcinoma demands an apparent tumour-free margin of up to 12 cm on either side to avoid the possibility of the patient developing recurrent malignant dysphagia. This is not always possible but try to protect the patient by leaving a minimum of 6 cm of tumour-free margins above and below. Do not submit the patient to a lesser 'palliative' resection at risk of leaving tumour at the anastomosis. Rather use other methods such as wide bypass, irradiation, dilatation and intubation.

Prepare

1. Discuss the possibilities with the patient. His co-operation is essential to the success of major procedures.

2. Restore the dysphagic patient to a good nutritional state with soft oral foods, elemental fluid diet, if necessary dilating the oesophagus first, or introduce a fine nasogastric drip-feed tube into the stomach. If the patient is very undernourished create a jejunostomy for pre-operative and postoperative feeding. This is more effective than parenteral intravenous alimentation.

3. Enteral feeding of any kind is precluded for 4–5 days after operation. Set up a central venous line before operation if necessary, to augment the nutritional intake. Otherwise ask the anaesthetist to set up a line during the operation which can be used in the post-operative period for parenteral feeding.

4. Make sure that the best possible cardio-respiratory state is achieved with physiotherapy, blood replacement, correction of serum protein and electrolytes. Order 4 units of cross matched blood.

5. Ensure the oesophagus, stomach and colon are empty. Allow oral fluids only for 48 hours before operation. Have a nasogastric tube passed before the patient leaves the ward or when anaesthesia is induced. If colon may be used, have it cleaned with enemata daily or twice daily for 3–4 days.

6. Arrange prophylactic antibiotic cover to be started intravenously as the operation begins. Gentamycin and metronidazole have been used routinely but a cephalosporin may be more versatile than gentamycin.

7. Arrange for prophylaxis against deep venous thrombosis, usually with subcutaneous heparin, 5000 units at the start of the operation and subsequently twice daily until the patient is mobile.

8. Arrange for urethral catheter drainage so that urinary output can be monitored during and after operation.

RESECTION FOR CARCINOMA OF LOWER OESOPHAGUS

Appraise

The orthodox operation is resection of the lower half of the thoracic oesophagus together with a cuff of cardiac stomach, followed by intrathoracic oesophago-gastrostomy. Unless the tumour is short, it is difficult to allow an adequate tumour-free margin above and below the visible tumour.

Access

1. Lie the anaesthetized, intubated patient on his right side, left shoulder rotated back against a support attached to the operating table (Fig. 18.18).

2. Open the left upper abdomen obliquely in the line of the seventh or eighth left rib, starting in the midline, half way between the umbilicus and the tip of the xiphisternum, extending to the left costal margin. Feel the liver and the pelvis to detect distant spread. Determine the

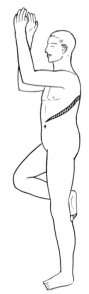

Fig. 18.18 Left thoracoabdominal approach to the lower oesophagus. The shaded section shows the extent of the incision.

fixity of the cardia and feel for extensive lymph node involvement that would make resection useless.

3. If resection seems feasible, cut across the costal margin and along the seventh or eight left rib to its neck. Open the chest close to the upper border of the rib. In elderly patients with fixed ribs, be prepared to excise the rib, or to excise a 3–5 cm portion near its neck to allow adequate access.

4. Cut radially through the diaphragm towards the right crus. Leave the crus intact so that a portion can be included with the oesophageal resection if necessary.

5. Insert Finochietto's self-retaining rib retractor and gently open it in stages.

6. Stop all bleeding. This is an extensive incision. Continuous slight oozing results in considerable blood loss.

7. Gently free the lower lobe of the left lung, dividing the pulmonary ligament, taking care not to injure the pulmonary veins.

8. Locate the thoracic aorta and incise the mediastinal pleura just anterior to it. Have the lower lobe of the lung elevated forwards to display the posterior mediastinum up to the aortic arch.

9. Gently display the lower oesophagus, taking care not to accidentally open the right pleural cavity.

10. Incise the avascular portion of the gastric lesser omentum and the avascular portion of the gastrocolic omentum to obtain a good view of the lesser sac.

Assess

1. Determine the extent of spread to the gastric cardia and glands along the left gastric vessels and around the coeliac axis.

2. If the infradiaphragmatic oesophagus, stomach and associated glands are quite free, plan to retain the fundic

stomach for oesophagogastrostomy. If the cardia or upper stomach are involved, total gastrectomy is preferable to upper partial gastrectomy since there is a temptation to facilitate oesophagogastrostomy by carrying out inadequate longitudinal excision.

3. If the growth is fixed, extends for more than 6–8 cm longitudinally, if there are multiple hepatic or intraperitoneal metastases, resection is inappropriate. Be willing to carry out an adequate longitudinal resection in a fit vigorous patient with resectable growth but with not too extensive metastatic lymph node or liver metastases. Treat unresectable growths by bypass, taking stomach, jejunum or colon well above the tumour to unite it to the oesophagus in the chest or the neck (see p. 305). For extensive obstructing growths in poor risk patients, insert a Mousseau-Barbin or Celestin type tube and close the chest and abdominal wounds.

Resect (Fig. 18.19)

1. Lift the oesophagus free of the aorta, ligating and dividing the oesophageal arteries. If sharp dissection is necessary, free aorta from growth, not oesophagus from aorta. Remove all possible adventitia and glands around the oesophagus, near the inferior pulmonary veins, and from the right mediastinal pleura. If necessary, excise the posterior pericardium and a portion of right pleura after warning the anaesthetist that the right chest is open.

2. Free the oesophagus and glands downwards, if necessary excising a cuff of right diaphragmatic crus.

3. Ligate and divide the left gastric vessels flush with the coeliac axis so any involved glands will be removed. Transect the cardia, aiming to excise a cuff of lesser curvature with its associated glands and the left main gastric vessels. This is conveniently achieved using the TA90 straight stapling device. Otherwise temporarily occlude the gastric defect with a large, curved, non-crushing bowel clamp.

4. Transect the oesophagus at least 6–8 cm above the growth after applying a non-crushing occlusive clamp across the oesophagus to prevent it from retracting. Remove the specimen for histological examination.

Unite

1. Bury the line of staples with a seromuscular stitch, or close the defect in the gastric lesser curve with two layers of sutures.

2. Mobilize the stomach. Incise the gastrocolic omentum in an avascular portion outside the gastroepiploic arch and incise it proximally outside the arcade, doubly ligating any divided vessels. Divide the left gastroepiploic and short gastric vessels to free the fundus of the stomach, retaining any anastomotic links to the gastric fundus. Remove the spleen only if this is convenient or if it is accidentally damaged. Incise the gastrocolic omentum distally, but

juxtapyloric isoperistaltic gastroenterostomy may be preferable.

5. Gently draw the upper stomach into the chest. After ensuring that the blood supply is satisfactory, cut a hole in the fundus to match the oesophageal lumen, and carry out an oesophagofundic anastomosis. First insert an all-coats stitch of 00 chromic catgut mounted on an eyeless needle. If a nasogastric tube is used, pass it into the stomach before completing this layer. Insert a second layer of 00 catgut to draw the fundus of the stomach up over the anastomotic line.

6. Alternatively, use the circular stapling device (see Fig. 18.11 p. 288). Remove the anvil head. Create a 3 cm long temporary anterior gastrotomy. Insert the device through the gastrotomy and push the spindle to tent the gastric fundus. Make a small incision over the spindle so that it projects. Screw on the anvil. Insert a purse-string nylon suture through all coats around the cut lower end of the oesophagus. Manoeuvre the anvil head into the oesophageal lumen and tighten the purse-string suture, cutting off the excess thread. Close the gun, release the safety catch, 'fire' the gun, remove it and close the gastrotomy. Check that the 'doughnut' oesophageal and gastric trimmings are intact, send them for histology, and check the anastomosis. A nasogastric tube can now be passed through the anastomosis, if desired.

7. Make sure there is no tension on the anastomosis, no twisting of the stomach and no kinking of the right gastric and right gastroepiploic vessels.

Difficulty?

1. Does the oesophageal growth extend down to the cardia or involve the stomach? If radical resection seems possible, carry out total gastrectomy, close the duodenal stump, and fashion a Roux-en-Y loop (p. 115). Perform oesophagojejunostomy.

Sometimes the upper half of the stomach can be excised but still oesophagogastrostomy is possible. If this brings the transection line close to tumour, prefer to close the lower portion of the stomach and complete the anastomosis with a Roux-en-Y loop of jejunum.

It is most important to make sure the anastomosis remains free from recurrence. Therefore never skimp the resection of growth to facilitate the anastomosis.

2. Does the oesophageal growth extend higher than expected? If so, the proximal cut end retracts behind the aorta. It is usually possible to free the oesophagus gently and draw it out above the aortic arch, allowing the anastomosis to be fashioned lateral to the arch. A high anastomosis is facilitated by carrying out a second thoracotomy above the fourth rib. It is usually safer, however, to free the upper thoracic oesophagus, and draw it out in the neck. The gastric fundus can then be drawn into the neck, for cervical oesophagogastrostomy. If the stomach passes through the posterior mediastinum it may be

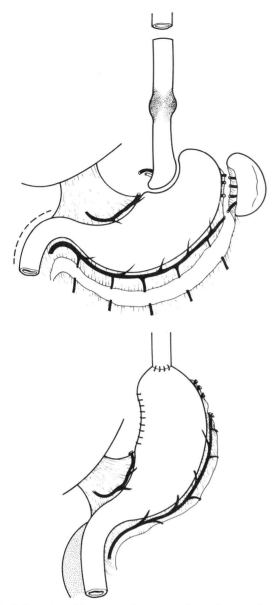

Fig. 18.19 Resection of lower oesophagus, gastric cardia and left gastric vessels for carcinoma of the lower oesophagus. The stomach is mobilized by Kocher's manoeuvre and the right gastric and right gastroepiploic vessels are preserved. Below: after closing the gastric lesser curve, an oesophagogastric anastomosis is fashioned.

carefully preserve the right gastroepiploic vessels intact. Incise the avascular portion of the lesser omentum but carefully preserve intact the right gastric vessels.

3. Carry out Kocher's duodenal mobilization to its full extent (p. 63) in order to allow the pylorus to move upwards and to the left towards the cardia.

4. Ensure that the pyloroduodenal canal is widely patent, testing it by invaginating the bowel with a finger through the pylorus in both directions. If necessary gently stretch the canal by invaginating the anterior antral wall through the pylorus with an index finger. Occasionally, it is necessary to fashion a Heineke-Mikulicz pyloroplasty although this shortens the stomach and therefore anterior

invaded and obstructed by residual microscopic mediastinal deposits of tumour. If possible take it to the neck substernally or subcutaneously provided this does not produce tension.

3. Has the growth proved to be irremovable? Transect the oesophagus above the growth, ligate and oversew the cut lower end. Mobilize the stomach and unite the fundus to the upper cut end. Leave the cardia intact if possible, but if it is fixed by the growth, transect the lower oesophagus below the growth and close the cut lower end in two layers. Unite the upper cut end into stomach, or into a Roux loop of jejunum. Conventionally, the isolated segment of oesophagus is drained into the distal stomach or a second Roux loop of jejunum but if it is closed at both ends it merely forms a mucocele. A satisfactory bypass is achieved by substernal or subcutaneous union of the cervical oesophagus either to colon joined to distal stomach or to a Roux loop of jejunum (see p. 305).

4. If the growth is very extensive, abandon attempts to resect or bypass it. Through a small upper gastrotomy pass a bougie up to the pharynx, have the anaesthetist attach it to the tail of a Mousseau-Barbin or Celestin tube. Draw the bougie and attached tube through the growth, cut off the tube end and close the gastrotomy. Mark the extent of the growth with metal clips if radiotherapy is envisaged.

Check list

1. Make sure the oesophagogastric anastomosis is perfectly fashioned without evidence of tension or ischaemia. An intrathoracic leak is usually fatal.

2. Has all the bleeding stopped? The extensive raw areas ooze considerably so it is worth taking extra care now.

Closure

1. Insert an underwater seal drain into the left pleural cavity through a separate stab incision near the costophrenic angle in the posterior axillary line.

2. Close the diaphragm using non-absorbable sutures. Do not close the hole too tightly around the stomach or bowel passing into the chest.

3. Close the abdominal wound in your usual manner.

4. Close the chest wound, catching the intercostal muscles above and below. Repair the muscles to the shoulder girdle before closing the skin.

IVOR LEWIS RESECTION FOR MIDOESOPHAGEAL CARCINOMA

This two-step operation of Ivor Lewis is the classic method for dealing with midoesophageal carcinoma.

Abdominal operation

1. The anaesthetized, intubated patient lies supine.

2. Explore the abdomen through a midline or left paramedian incision. Ensure that the liver, cardia and coeliac axis are uninvolved.

3. Mobilize the stomach (Fig. 18.20), dividing the short gastric and left gastroepiploic vessels but retaining intact the right gastroepiploic vessels. The greater omentum usually survives, but if it is very bulky and ischaemic do not hesitate to excise it. Divide the left gastric vessels as close to the coeliac axis as possible but preserve the right gastric vessels (see p. 301).

4. Carry out a full Kocher's mobilization of the head of

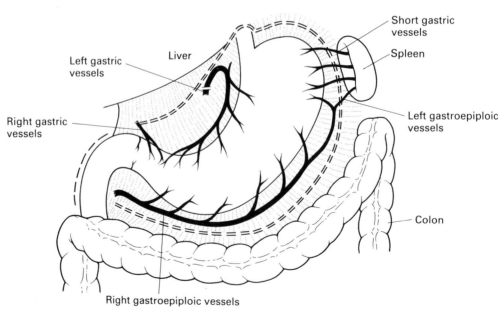

Fig. 18.20 Mobilization of stomach in Ivor Lewis' operation. The double broken line shows the division of the short gastric, left gastroepiploic and left gastric vessels, leaving intact the blood supply to the stomach through the right gastric and right gastroepiploic vessels. The single broken line shows the incision for Kocher's duodenal mobilization.

pancreas and duodenal loop so that the pylorus can be swung on the free edge of the lesser omentum up to or through the diaphragmatic hiatus.

5. Ensure that the pyloroduodenal canal is adequate by invaginating the anterior antral wall through the pylorus with a finger tip and reversing the manoeuvre to prolapse the duodenal wall through into the stomach. Dilate a narrow canal or carry out a pyloroplasty or a gastroenterostomy.

6 Carefully cut through the attachments at the hiatus to free the stomach and lower oesophagus. If necessary enlarge the hiatus by incising the right crus anteriorly between ligatures, after gently freeing the pericardium from the superior surface.

7. Gently free the lower oesophagus and push the upper stomach into the posterior mediastinum. Ensure that the lower stomach lies untwisted in the abdomen.

8. Close the abdomen.

Thoracic operation

1. Turn the patient onto his left side, hands brought up in front of his face, left leg flexed at hip and knee, right leg extended.

2. Carry out a right thoracotomy at the level of the right fifth or sixth rib (Fig. 18.21).

3. Divide the arch of the azygos vein between ligatures to display the oesophagus.

4. Mobilize the oesophagus from its bed throughout the thorax, together with the adventitia and mediastinal glands.

5. Draw the stomach through the hiatus into the chest until the fundus comfortably reaches the level of the proximal oesophagus. Transect the lower oesophagus at the cardia and close the hole in the stomach in two layers. Alternatively, use the TA55 stapling device, and invaginate the staple line with a continuous catgut suture.

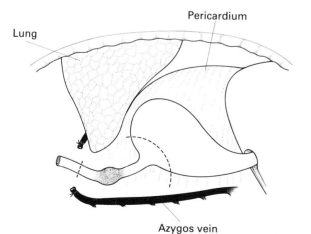

Fig. 18.21 Ivor Lewis' operation. Right thoracotomy with division of the vena azygos. The oesophagus is mobilized and the stomach drawn up into the chest. The gastric cardia and oesophagus are divided along the broken lines. The upper cut oesophagus is joined to the gastric fundus.

6. Transect the oesophagus at least 5 cm above the growth and remove the specimen for histology.

7. Incise the fundus of the stomach so that the hole can be joined to the oesophagus. Insert an all-costs stitch with a second layer to cover the anastomosis. Alternatively, use a stapling device inserted through a temporary anterior gastrotomy. If a nasogastric tube is used, ensure that the tip lies in the stomach.

8. Make sure that the anastomosis lies comfortably and that the stomach is untwisted and is a good colour.

9. Close the chest after inserting an underwater seal drain through a stab wound into the costophrenic region in the posterior axillary line.

MCKEOWN'S TECHNIQUE

In this three-stage modification of the Ivor Lewis operation, the whole thoracic oesophagus is excised and the mobilized stomach is anastomosed to the cervical oesophagus. It is appropriate for all growths above the lower third of the oesophagus.

Action

1. Complete the gastric mobilization through the abdomen, and close the abdomen.

2. Turn the patient on to his left side. Mobilize the oesophagus through a right thoracotomy. Dissect free the whole thoracic gullet. Draw the stomach into the chest, taking the fundus to the thoracic inlet. Ensure that it is not twisted.

3. Close the chest after inserting an underwater seal drain.

4. Place the patient supine. Expose the cervical oesophagus through an incision along the anterior border of the right sternomastoid muscle (p. 283). Divide the omo-hyoid muscle and middle thyroid vein, but if possible preserve the inferior thyroid artery.

5. Gently free the cervical oesophagus from the trachea, taking care to preserve the recurrent laryngeal nerve from damage. By exerting gentle traction on the cervical oesophagus, draw the oesophagus and upper stomach into the wound.

6. Transect the lower oesophagus and close the cardia of the stomach with two layers of sutures or with a TA55 stapler, reinforcing the staple line with a continuous invaginating suture of catgut. Transect the lower cervical oesophagus and remove the specimen.

7. Make a small incision in the gastric fundus.

8. Carry out a two-layer oesophagogastric anastomosis. Alternatively, use a circular stapling device introduced through a temporary anterior gastrotomy. Newer curved circular staplers can be passed downwards through the mouth and pharynx.

9. Close the skin over the anastomosis.

RESECTION OF THE THORACIC OESOPHAGUS WITHOUT FORMAL THORACOTOMY

Radical resection of lower oesophageal tumours and cardiac, gastric adenocarcinomas can be achieved through the abdomen and enlarged oesophageal hiatus.

Abdominal dissection

1. The anaesthetized, intubated patient lies supine with neck extended, head turned to the left. Gain access through an upper midline incision, excising the xiphoid process if necessary.

2. Explore the abdomen and assess the intra-abdominal spread of the growth.

3. If resection if feasible, mobilize the left lobe of the liver and fold it to the right (Fig. 18.22).

4. Incise the peritoneum and transversalis fascia over the front of the oesophageal hiatus. Insert a finger into the posterior mediastinum and separate the pericardium from the upper surface of the diaphragm. Incise the diaphragm forwards for 7–8 cm from the hiatus, ligating and dividing the inferior phrenic vessels.

5. Assess the growth in the lower oesophagus.

6. Mobilize the lower oesophagus keeping well clear of the growth, excising a cuff of diaphragmatic crus, posterior pericardium, mediastinal pleura and posterior connective tissue as necessary. The gullet can be mobilized under vision almost up to the level of the tracheal carina.

7. Now keep close to the oesophagus, carefully separating it from the back of the trachea. Hook branches of the vagus nerves within the flexed index and middle fingers, cutting them with long scissors within the protection of the fingers.

Neck dissection

1. Incise along the anterior border of the sternomastoid muscle, preferring the right side to avoid damaging the thoracic duct. Access is increased if necessary by excising the medial clavicle, a portion of the right first rib and the right half of the manubrium sterni.

2. Expose the cervical oesophagus (see p. 283) between the anterior border of sternomastoid muscle and carotid sheath laterally, and the trachea and oesophagus medially. Divide the middle thyroid vein and omohyoid muscle, preserving if possible the inferior thyroid artery.

3. Separate the oesophagus from the trachea, preserving the recurrent laryngeal nerve from damage.

4. Continue the separation downwards into the superior mediastinum. The final mobilization is best achieved by inserting the fingers of one hand through the neck, passing the other hand up from the abdomen.

Resect

1. Apply a ligature around the cervical oesophagus as low as possible.

2. Transect the oesophagus above the ligature and allow the lower ligated cut end to drop into the mediastinum.

3. Transect below the growth with as wide a margin as possible, ideally 12 cm. This implies total or near total abdominal gastrectomy for growths at the cardia. For higher growths, a cuff of cardiac stomach may suffice, allowing the fundus to be preserved for anastomosis in the neck. Do not risk recurrence by transecting too close to the tumour.

4. Remove the specimen for histology.

Unite

1. If the stomach is to be preserved, mobilize it fully (see p. 302) so the fundus can be brought to the neck through the posterior mediastinum, retrosternally or subcutaneously (see p. 305). Unite the cervical oesophagus to the gastric fundus.

2. If the proximal or whole stomach must be excised, fashion a Roux loop of jejunum (see p. 95) sufficiently long to reach up to the neck, for anastomosis to the cervical oesophagus. It is sometimes difficult to prepare a Roux loop of sufficient length to reach the neck by the subcutaneous route. If so, select the substernal or posterior mediastinal route.

3. Alternatively, use a loop of colon taken out of circuit to unite oesophagus to the distal stomach or duodenum (see p. 305).

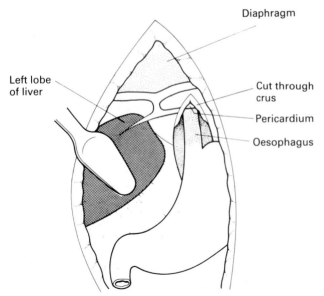

Diaphragm

Left lobe of liver

Cut through crus

Pericardium

Oesophagus

Fig. 18.22 Oesophagectomy without formal thoracotomy. The diaphragm has been incised anteriorly from the hiatus to facilitate dissection within the lower part of the posterior mediastinum.

OESOPHAGEAL BYPASS

1. Resection may not be possible, or is contraindicated because the growth is extensive. Bypass is preferable to intubation in patients with a prognosis of months rather than weeks. Bypass does not preclude radiotherapy, and the conduit lies at a distance from the field or irradiation.

2. The mobilized stomach may be taken above the unresected growth when left thoraco-abdominal or the Ivor Lewis operations were planned. It is taken above the growth as high as possible and anastomosed to the side of the oesophagus. If possible, leave the lower oesophagus in continuity with the stomach. Sometimes it is necessary to divide the lower oesophagus to free the stomach, so that it can be joined well above the growth. Conventionally the lower cut oesophagus should be drained into a Roux loop of jejunum, although some surgeons merely close and drain it.

3. Kirschner's operation is preferable to bypass unresectable middle third growths (Fig. 18.23). Mobilize the stomach through the abdomen. Confirm that the pylorus is widely patent by invaginating the anterior antral wall through it with an index finger. Transect the oesophagus at the cardia and close the lower end. Elevate the skin at the upper end of the wound. Use long-handled scissors to create a track 7–10 cm wide in the subcutaneous tissue plane over the sternum and manubrium. Use a combination of blunt and sharp dissection. The upper cut end of oesophagus is joined to a Roux loop of jejunum. Mobilize the cervical oesophagus through an incision in the right side of the neck (see p. 283). Use this incision to complete the subcutaneous track into the neck. Place a ligature around the mobilized cervical oesophagus as low as possible. Transect the oesophagus above the ligature and allow the lower cut end to drop into the superior mediastinum. Gently manoeuvre the stomach through the subcutaneous track by a combination of pushing and traction. Avoid tension and twisting. If necessary, excise the xiphisternum. Now unite the upper cut end of the oesophagus to the gastric fundus. If the stomach is too short to reach the neck by the subcutaneous route, it may do so if taken substernally. Cut the xiphoid and medial costal slips of diaphragm to allow the fingers to enter the anterior mediastinum. Gently separate the pericardium posteriorly from the sternum. Continue upwards taking care not to tear the pleura laterally. Eventually the hand in the 'main d'acoucheur' position reaches up to the neck, aided by fingers passed down behind the manubrium. The stomach is now drawn and pushed along this tunnel.

4. Carcinoma at or near the cardia can be bypassed using a Roux-en-Y loop of jejunum taken subcutaneously or substernally to the neck or by a segment of isoperistaltic jejunum taken out of circuit but with its blood supply intact, which unites the cervical oesophagus to the distal stomach. Using microvascular anastomotic techniques, a loop of jejunum may be excised, transferred, and given a new local blood supply. A segment of colon (see below) taken out of circuit can also be used as a conduit between the cervical oesophagus and the distal stomach. Most operators with experience of both methods prefer isoperistaltic colon to jejunum for ease of management, because it has a marginal vasculature.

COLONIC REPLACEMENT OR BYPASS OF THE OESOPHAGUS

Appraise

1. The colon usually has a good marginal blood supply (Fig. 18.24). It makes an excellent oesophageal replacement.

2. An antiperistaltic loop can be created by swinging up the mobilized left colon after dividing the left colic vessels, so that it is supplied through the middle colic vessels. It does not always function well (Fig. 18.25).

3. An isoperistaltic loop of right colon can be swung up, based on the middle colic vessels after dividing the right colic and ileocolic vessels (Fig. 18.25).

4. An isoperistaltic loop can be fashioned based on the left upper colic vessels.

5. The colon may be taken to the upper end of the oesophagus through the posterior mediastinum, substernally through the anterior mediastinum or subcutaneously.

Prepare

1. The colon must be prepared beforehand by giving the patient daily small disposable enemas for 4–5 days, reducing the diet to fluids only for 2 days before operation and by giving oral neomycin 1 g every 4 hours and

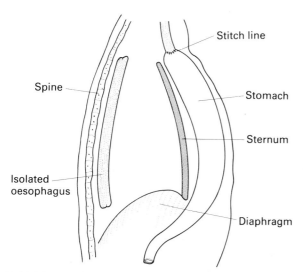

Fig. 18.23 Diagram of side view of Kirschner's operation. The isolated intrathoracic oesophagus is closed at each end. The mobilized stomach is drawn subcutaneously to be joined to the cervical oesophagus.

Labels on figure: Stitch line; Spine; Stomach; Sternum; Isolated oesophagus; Diaphragm

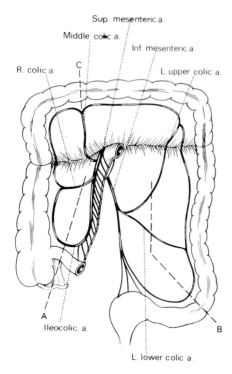

Fig. 18.24 Mobilization of the colon. The right colon survives on the blood supply from the middle colic vessels if the right colic and ileocolic vessels are divided (a). The left colon survives on the blood supply from the middle colic vessels if the left upper and lower colic vessels are divided (b). The bowel is taken out of circuit by transecting it at C and at either A or B.

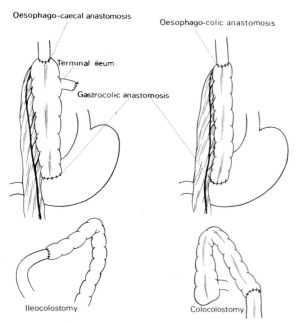

Fig. 18.25 Colonic replacement of oesophagus. On the left is shown the use of the proximal colon, and on the right is shown the distal colon.

metronidazole 1 g 8 hourly for 24 hours before operation. Alternatively, a nasogastric tube can be passed and orthograde lavage can be carried out using physiological saline the day before operation.

2. Some surgeons perform preoperative angiography to delineate the vascular supply to the colon. This is not usually necessary except in patients with features of generalized vascular disease.

Action

1. Carefully study the vasculature of the marginal vessels.

2. To create a subcutaneous track for the colon over the chest wall, gently dissect in the subcutaneous layer, using long-handled scissors and retractors to produce a wide tunnel through which a hand can be passed, from the upper end of the abdominal incision, along the sternum. Dissect downwards in the same plane from the neck.

3. A substernal tunnel can similarly be created by blunt dissection after incising the diaphragmatic slips to the xiphoid process and costal margin. Gently separate the anterior mediastinal contents from the posterior surface of the sternum with a hand inserted through the defect. Dissect downwards behind the manubrium using the fingers of one hand.

4. Mobilize the caecum, ascending and right transverse colon onto the primitive mesentery. They are adequately supplied by the right branch of the middle colic vessels and the marginal vessels. Doubly ligate and divide the ileocaecal vessels near their origin from the superior mesenteric vessels together with the right colic vessels. Divide the terminal ileum and the transverse colon. Unite the proximal cut end of the terminal ileum to the distal cut transverse colon. Close the distal cut end of the terminal ileum. Swing the caecum upwards and gently push and pull it through its track. Long-handled swab-holding forceps make excellent grasping instruments. Unite the caecum to the cervical oesophagus in two layers (see p. 287). Unite the proximal cut end of the transverse colon to the distal stomach. Ensure that the bowel and blood vessels are untwisted and not under tension before closing the incisions. Close the diaphragm or anterior abdominal wall slackly around the colon so that it is not constricted.

5. A loop of left colon supplied by the middle colic vessels may be similarly elevated on its primitive mesentery. Isolate, doubly ligate and divide the left colic vessels. Transect the bowel in the middle of the transverse colon and above the segment supplied by the upper sigmoid artery. Unite the proximal cut end of transverse colon to the distal cut end of the sigmoid colon. Swing the proximal cut end of descending colon upwards to be united to the oesophagus while the proximal cut end is united to the distal stomach. This is an anti-peristaltic loop, and does not usually function well, at least initially.

6. Belsey has described an isoperistaltic loop of transverse colon based on the left colic vessels. If necessary the left branch or even the right branch of the middle colic

artery can be divided. The continuity of the large bowel is re-established between ascending & descending colon. The proximal cut end of colon is taken up to the oesophagus and the distal end of the interposed segment is united to the distal stomach.

Assure

1. Assure yourself that bleeding and oozing from the many raw surfaces has been controlled, before closing the wounds.

2. Although oral feeding will be postponed, the patient must swallow saliva and air. Do you wish to pass a naso-visceral tube through the anastomosis for decompression now, and possible enteral feeding later? If so, consider using a pharyngostomy. Pass a long curved artery forceps orally into a pyriform fossa, push the points outward until they feel almost subcutaneous, and well clear of the carotid pulsations. Nick the skin over the closed tip, project the forceps tip to grasp a thread and draw it upwards and out through the mouth. Attach this end of the thread to the upper end of an oro-visceral tube and use the thread to draw the tube out to project as a pharyngostomy. This is comfortable and safe for the patient, and the fistula will close immediately the tube is withdrawn.

3. Insert a basal and, if necessary, an apical underwater seal drain whenever the pleural cavity has been breached. It is easier to remove them later than insert them in a conscious patient.

4. Has the patient a good central venous catheter in place? If not arrange with the anaesthetist to have one inserted.

5. Maintain the urethral catheter drainage to monitor urinary output.

Aftercare

1. Following major oesophageal surgery nurse the patient in an Intensive Therapy Unit for at least the first 24 hours, so that cardiorespiratory, urinary and cerebral functions can be monitored with early correction of any abnormalities. Some patients benefit from initial respiratory assistance on a mechanical ventilator attached to an endotracheal tube. Arrange regular chest X-rays to ensure full pulmonary expansion. Order chest physiotherapy, and aspiration of bronchial secretions per-orally or through the endotracheal tube.

2. Order adequate regular analgesics, continue antibiotics and venous thrombosis prophylaxis.

3. Aspirate the visceral tube regularly, but as bowel function recovers, the tube may be used for feeding if its position has been checked with X-rays. After 4–5 days, screen the patient following a swallow with water-soluble contrast to exclude leakage. Withdraw the tube and start oral feeding, progressing to solids over a day or two. Stop parenteral feeding. If a jejunostomy was created, give small volumes of dilute fluids as soon as bowel sounds return, increasing to larger volumes of full strength feeds until oral feeding is established. Then remove the jejunostomy catheter.

4. Remove the chest drains after 24–48 hours unless they produce fluid. If they have failed to function, and fluid or air persists, do not hesitate to insert further suitably placed underwater sealed drains.

5. Study the pathologists' report carefully. Is adjunctive radiotherapy or cytotoxic treatment justified?

Further reading

Akiyama H, Tsurumaru M, Kawamura T, Ono Y 1981 Principles of surgical treatment for carcinoma of the oesophagus. Annals of Surgery 194: 438–446

Atkinson M, Ferguson R, Parker G C 1978 Tube introducer and modified Celestin tube for use in palliative intubation of oesophagogastric neoplasms at fibreoptic endoscopy. Gut 19: 669–671

Barrett N R 1964 Achalasia of the cardia: reflections upon a clinical study of over 100 cases. British Medical Journal 1: 1135–1140

Earlam R, Cunha-melo J R 1980 Oesophageal squamous cell carcinoma. I. A critical review of surgery. British Journal of Surgery 67: 381–390

Hopkins R A, Alexander J C, Postlethwaite R W 1984 Stapled esophagogastric anastomosis. American Journal of Surgery 147: 283–287

Huang G, Zhang D, Wang G, Lin H, Wang L, Liu J et al 1981 Surgical treatment of carcinoma of the esophagus: report of 1647 cases. Chinese Medical Journal 94: 305–307

Kirk R M 1983 Oesophagoscopy. In: Rob and Smith's Operative Surgery 4th Edn. Dudley H, Pories W J, Carter D C (eds) Alimentary tract and abdominal wall. Vol 1. Butterworths, London p. 8–16

Kirk R M 1983 Double indemnity in oesophageal carcinoma. British Medical Journal 286: 582–583

Kirk R M, Stoddard C J 1986 complications of surgery of the upper gastrointestinal tract. Baillière Tindall, London

Merendino K A, Dillard D H 1955 The concept of sphincter substitution by an interposed jejunal segment for anatomic and physiologic abnormalities at the esophagogastric junction — with special reference to reflux esophagitis, cardiospasm and esophageal varices. Annals of Surgery 142: 486–509

Nissen R 1961 Gastropexy and 'fundoplication' in surgical treatment of hiatal hernia. American Journal of Digestive Diseases 6: 954–961

Skinner D B, Belsey R H R 1967 Surgical management of esophageal reflux and hiatus hernia. Long term results with 1030 patients. Journal of Thoracic and Cardiovascular Surgery 53: 33–54

Starling J R, Reichelderfer M O, Pellett J R, Belzer F O 1982 Treatment of symptomatic gastroesophageal reflux using the Angelchik prosthesis. Annals of Surgery 195: 686–691

Thal A P 1968 A unified approach to surgical problems of the esophagogastric junction. Annals of Surgery 168: 542–550

Tytgat G N, den Hartog Jager F C 1977 Non-surgical treatment of cardio-esophageal obstruction role of endoscopy. Endoscopy 9: 211–215

Williamson R C N 1975 The management of peptic oesophageal stricture. British Journal of Surgery 62: 448–454

Wu Y K, Huang K C 1979 Chinese experience in the surgical treatment of carcinoma of the esophagus. Annals of Surgery 190:361

Thoracic surgery

Cardiothoracic surgery demands a precise knowledge of the topographical anatomy of the thorax when viewed from the lateral, anterior or posterior aspect; this knowledge is necessary for the accurate dissection which is required. It is essential that no vessel is sacrificed other than those of the diseased area because of the consequent increased loss of lung function and the risk of lung infarction.

The safety margin during intrathoracic dissection is small. The bronchi and vessels are short and their branches close together and therefore vulnerable. In addition, the respiratory reserve of the patient is often compromised.

Although the main pulmonary veins have strong walls, the pulmonary arteries are very thin-walled and there is always the risk of producing a hole with sudden heavy loss of blood. It is vital to learn how to deal with such an acute bleed, using the appropriate vascular clamps and fine atraumatic cardiovascular sutures. Most vessels are dissected inside the adventitial layer because this allows the encircling ligatures to be passed more readily. Secure ligation or suture of the main vessels is essential. A satisfactory intravenous infusion must be available from the beginning of the operation to allow rapid replacement of blood or plasma expanders.

Accurate bronchial closure is perhaps the most vital step in pulmonary resection, to avoid the risk of breakdown of the suture line with the formation of a bronchial fistula and secondary empyema. In pneumonectomy, this is the most important risk to the patient now that reactionary haemorrhage has been largely overcome.

The accurate placing of good calibre drainage tubes is essential to secure rapid and full re-expansion of the lung, by removing fluid and air in the postoperative period. Meticulous and accurate technique, coupled with prophylactic antibiotic therapy, minimizes the incidence of infection which can cause secondary haemorrhage and interfere with bronchial and chest wall healing.

While the range and frequency of pulmonary surgery has shown little change and may have decreased numerically, there has been a great increase in the number of cardiac operations performed. This increase is almost entirely due to the rapid expansion in surgery for coronary artery disease and its complications whereas the incidence of valvular and paediatric disease is static.

In cardiovascular surgery, similar techniques are employed, coupled with the ability to perform accurate leak-free anastomoses and blood tight closure of openings in the cardiac chambers. It is vital to learn how to preserve the functional efficiency of the heart as a pump, during bypass, by avoiding chamber distension, especially of the left ventricle, by avoiding ventricular fibrillation with its deleterious effect on myocardial perfusion and by the use of cardioplegia combined with local cardiac and moderate systemic hypothermia.

Accurate control of cardiopulmonary bypass with pressure monitoring, serial blood gas, pH and serum potassium measurement is essential to preserve cerebral, pulmonary, hepatic and renal function which may be impaired pre-operatively.

The prevention of air embolism, knowledge of the use of inotropic agents and anti-arrhythmic drugs is required, as is the speedy and efficient management of cardiac arrest if it occurs.

DIAGNOSTIC BRONCHOSCOPY

Appraise

1. This procedure is used extremely commonly as the initial diagnostic procedure in thoracic surgery.

2. The assessment of tumours both for operability and the scale of operation required for their attempted cure.

3. There are almost no contraindications, since bronchoscopy can be carried out under local anaesthesia augmented with intravenous diazepam sedation.

RIGID BRONCHOSCOPE

This is the instrument usually used by surgeons although the fibrescope may be used to extend the range of observation. Straight and right angled telescopes are routinely used with the rigid bronchoscope.

Prepare

1. *Adults*: use local or general anaesthesia. If a relaxant is used oxygen is ideally supplied through a venturi jet on the bronchoscope.

2. *Children*: use general anaesthesia.

3. *Infants*: halothane anaesthesia is often preferred to the use of a relaxant.

4. Make sure good suction is available.

Action

1. Pass the bronchoscope with the bevel facing posteriorly over the middle of the tongue until the tip of the epiglottis is seen.

2. Elevate the epiglottis so that the cords come into view, then rotate the scope 90° and pass it through the vocal cords.

3. Keep pressure off the gums and teeth by inserting a moist swab or guard and supporting the bronchoscope with the left thumb, whilst manipulating it with the right hand.

4. Take care not to catch the lips between the teeth and the bronchoscope.

Difficulty

It is very easy to pass the bronchoscope too far posteriorly, entering the postcricoid region and thus the oesophagus instead of the larynx, i.e. only the epiglottis is elevated. (Fig. 19.1)

Assess

Note the presence of:
1. Endobronchial tumour and its site.
2. Stenosis, which may be circular, oval or irregular and is due to extrinsic compression.
3. Vocal cord paralysis.
4. Prominence and rigidity of the lower tracheal wall.
5. Evidence of subcarinal widening.

3, 4 and 5 are evidence of extensive disease and indicate inoperability.

Difficulty?

1. Haemorrhage is the most important and dangerous complication. It is due to bleeding from a vascular tumour

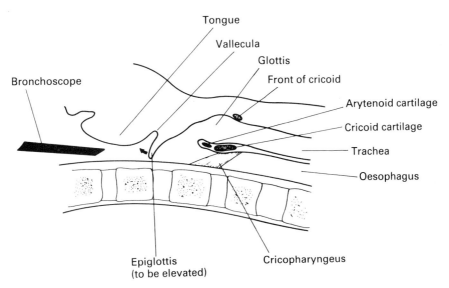

Fig. 19.1 Passage of rigid bronchoscope.

or a vascular area of diseased bronchial wall. Rarely it is due to biopsy of a branch of the pulmonary artery lying adjacent to a segmental bronchus. Keep the bronchoscope in position and suck out the blood. Apply through the bronchoscope a swab soaked in 1 : 1000 adrenaline solution. Place the patient in the head down position. Keep the bronchoscope in place until the patient is coughing again. Then remove the scope and place the patient in the lateral position with the bleeding side underneath. In cases of severe bleeding from the pulmonary artery, pass a Thompson blocker or Fogarty catheter into the bronchus. If the bleeding continues when the blocker is released after 10–15 minutes, perform a thoracotomy.

2. Cardiac arrest may occur due to anoxia in the elderly patient or in the patient with cardiac disease. Atropine in the premedication may act as a preventive. Cardiac monitoring is essential in this type of patient and the arrest can usually be treated successfully in routine fashion. For anaesthetic related techniques, see chapter 12.

3. Laryngeal oedema usually occurs in children. Never force too large a bronchoscope through the small larynx.

FIBREOPTIC BRONCHOSCOPE

Appraise

1. Diagnostic. The fibrescope increases the range of examination out to the branches of the segmental bronchi. It is particularly favoured by physicians. It is especially useful to examine the left and right upper lobe bronchi or their sub-divisions. It can be passed in patients with jaw deformities or rigid cervical spine in whom the rigid scope cannot be used. (Fig. 19.2).

2. Intensive Care Unit. Although the suction capacity is limited when the sputum is viscid, fibreoptic bronchoscopic suction is valuable in artificially ventilated patients, especially when localised clearance is needed, for example, of the left upper lobe.

Transbronchical biopsy of lung parenchyma can be obtained and distal sputum specimens can be aspirated. The fibrescope is valuable in bronchitis research and for photography.

4. Unless you are expert, avoid using the fibreoptic bronchoscope in children where the small calibre airway creates difficulty.

5. The rigid bronchoscope is better for removing a foreign body.

6. Prefer the rigid instrument when investigating active bleeding, because it offers more effective suction.

7. This applies also to tracheal strictures and obstructing neoplasms.

Prepare

Use local anaesthesia and intravenous diazepam sedation.

Action

1. Pass the fibrescope through the nostril or the mouth.

2. Examine the bronchial trees systematically including all the segmental orifices and their branches.

3. During rigid bronchoscopy the fibreoptic instrument can be passed through it to view the more peripheral bronchi.

4. Remove biopsies, cytology brushings or carry out bronchial washing to obtain histological or cytological diagnosis.

Complications

The risk of haemorrhage is very small as the biopsies are tiny.

THERAPEUTIC BRONCHOSCOPY

FOREIGN BODY IN THE BRONCHIAL TREE

Appraise

1. If any doubt exists about the possibility of a foreign body having been inhaled, perform bronchoscopy at once to prevent complications such as bronchiectasis, lung abscess, empyema.

2. In infants, peanuts are commonly inhaled and special forceps are required because the nuts tend to fragment. It is often necessary to withdraw the bronchoscope and the foreign body together, because the calibre of the bronchoscope is so small.

3. Thoracotomy and bronchotomy are indicated when

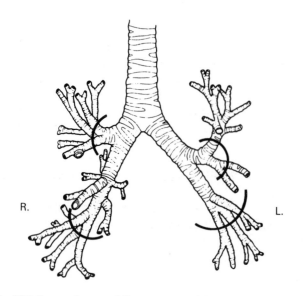

R.   L.

Fig. 19.2 Increased range of fibrescope over rigid scope plus telescopes.

the foreign body is stuck and cannot be extracted with special grasping forceps.

4. Lobectomy or segmental resection are required should the foreign body be out of reach of the bronchoscope, if intensive physiotherapy fails to expel it.

PULMONARY ATALECTASIS

Appraise

1. If physiotherapy and transnasal or peroral suction have failed to clear the retained secretions, bronchoscopy is indicated.

2. Inhalation of vomit warrants immediate bronchoscopy, and often lavage with saline or sodium bicarbonate solution, 1.4%.

Prepare

1. For adults, local anaesthesia is the usual form, after premedication with pethidine or omnopon, but not atropine. Give a benzocaine lozenge or lignocaine 2% viscous solution to anaesthetize the mouth and pharynx; instil 2 ml 4% lignocaine into the larynx through a special curved cannula, while holding the tongue forward.

2. Have available oxygen and resuscitation facilities especially when bronchoscopy is carried out in cardiac patients who may suddenly develop cardiac arrest.

3. Use general anaesthesia for children.

4. Position. Preferably sit the patient up.
In postoperative patients in whom drainage tubes are in situ, connect them to the underwater seal bottles, especially if an air leak is present.

5. If bronchoscopic suction has been repeated but is ineffective, consider tracheostomy or artificial ventilation.

OTHER THERAPEUTIC USES

1. Bronchoscopy may be used for dilatation of tracheal or bronchial strictures.

2. Excess granulation tissue can be removed, or obstructing tumour palliated with lasers or cryotherapy.

MEDIASTINOSCOPY

Appraise

1. This is valuable in the pre-operative assessment and staging of carcinoma of the bronchus. Patients with involved ipsilateral para-tracheal nodes are unlikely to have a long survival and so are usually deemed inoperable.

2. Mediastinoscopy permits the investigation and assessment of a mediastinal mass or a mass due to lymphnode pathology in the mediastinum or the hilum of the lung. A

diagnosis of tuberculosis, lymphoma, sarcoidosis may readily be made.

3. Avoid mediastinoscopy in the presence of superior vena caval obstruction as there is a high risk of severe haemorrhage.

4. Anterior mediastinal pathology is not amenable to mediastinoscopy as this lies anterior to the vessels and the plane of dissection. Subaortic and left anterior hilar nodes are also inaccessible. (Fig. 19.3)

5. A large goitre interferes with access.

Prepare

1. Lay the patient supine with the table tilted head up. Place a pad behind the shoulders.

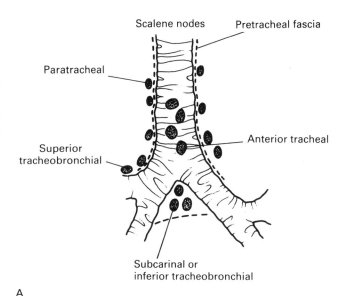

A

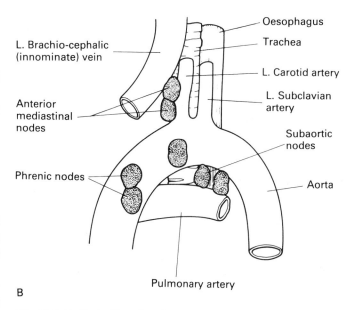

B

Fig. 19.3 Mediastinal lymph nodes.

2. Make a short, slightly curved incision in the suprasternal notch.

Action

1. Dissect and separate the strap muscles to expose the pretracheal fascia which is opened. Avoid the thymus isthmus and inferior thyroid veins.

2. Dissect inside the fascia each paratracheal region digitally down to the level of the upper lobe bronchus on the right and behind the aorta on the left to the same level. (Fig. 19.4)

3. Introduce the mediastinoscope into the created space and use blunt dissection with a swab, pledgelet, large artery forceps or blunt sucker end to visualise the gland masses previously palpated, which are outside the fascia.

4. Aspirate if in doubt, before taking a biopsy.

5. Key manoevure: it is important to stay deep to the vessels, especially the innominate artery.

Difficulty

1. Take care not to damage the pulmonary artery, especially the right upper lobe branch, the superior vena cava or the azygos vein. There is less risk of damage to the innominate artery unless it is densely hidden in a gland mass and not palpable. If bleeding occurs, try inserting gauze packing. If this does not stop the bleeding, perform thoracotomy, not a sternal split, to control it.

2. The pleural cavity may be opened anteriorly to produce a pneumothorax. Detect it with post operative routine chest X-ray. Insert a tube connected to an underwater seal drain.

3. The recurrent laryngeal nerve may be damaged, usually on the left. This usually recovers.

ANTERIOR OR PARASTERNAL MEDIASTINOTOMY

Appraise

1. This allows the diagnosis of an anterior mediastinal mass or lymphnode mass, in the mediastinum.

2. Some surgeons regard this procedure as safer and easier than mediastinoscopy. Larger biopsy specimens can be removed under direct vision and the upper lobe can be palpated and biopsied if indicated. It is especially useful in evaluating left sided bronchial carcinoma with anterior hilar or subaortic spread.

Access

Make a short incision over the second or third costal cartilage

Action

1. Deepen the incision then resect the costal cartilage.

2. Avoid, or ligate, the internal mammary vessels. Dissect the parietal pleura extrapleurally to expose the mediastinum and lung root.

3. Biopsy the mediastinal mass or mediastinal and hilar nodes.

4. If necessary, open the pleura to inspect the lung or obtain a further biopsy.

Closure

1. Insert a drainage tube through a lower intercostal space.

2. Routinely close the wound in layers.

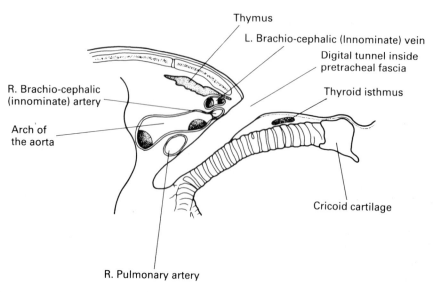

Thymus

L. Brachio-cephalic (Innominate) vein

Digital tunnel inside pretracheal fascia

Thyroid isthmus

R. Brachio-cephalic (innominate) artery

Arch of the aorta

Cricoid cartilage

R. Pulmonary artery

Fig. 19.4 Mediastinoscopy.

PRE-OPERATIVE MANAGEMENT

It is vital to spend a few days in routine preparation, to facilitate the post operative progress of the patient. If necessary, spend up to 2 weeks in preparation, before, for example, resection for bronchiectasis.

Appraise

1. Carefully assess patients with carcinoma by history and examination, looking for evidence of metastatic disease.
2. Order postero-anterior and lateral films of the chest. Screen the diaphragm if phrenic palsy is suspected.
3. Tomography in the postero-anterior or lateral plane may offer a more accurate assessment of a mass or of hilar nodes.
4. Carry out bronchoscopy. Check for recurrent nerve palsy from infiltration by growth, usually on the left.
5. Perform mediastinoscopy but not necessarily as a routine procedure.
6. To exclude metastases, order a CT scan of the brain, and radioactive isotope liver and bone scans in carcinoma patients. Ultrasound of liver is a useful alternative.
7. Check the haemoglobin, blood film, and group. Exclude platelet abnormality and the presence of hepatitis B antigen. Order liver function tests in patients with carcinoma.
8. Exclude diabetes or other general disease.
9. Respiratory assessment is vital and clinical judgement is paramount. The clinical history of exercise tolerance and simple testing is often adequate, when coupled with the clinical state of the patient. Note the presence of obesity, the body build, blood pressure and evidence of coronary artery disease. Radiological evidence of lung or lobar collapse suggests shunting may be present. The simple measurement of forced vital capacity and forced expiratory volume in 1 second (FEV 1) provides evidence of airways obstruction. When more precise evidence is required, order a ventilation perfusion scan coupled with blood gas estimations. A raised P_{CO_2} level is significant and a contraindication to operation.
10. Order ECG

Prepare

1. Stop smokers from continuing.
2. Correct poor oral hygiene and dental disease.
3. Treat sinus disease, especially in the presence of bronchiectasis.
4. Physiotherapy is particularly vital for the postoperative care of the patient. Breathing exercises are taught beforehand to improve lung function and increase diaphragmatic movement. Reduction of sputum is desired and this may be aided by exhibition of an antibiotic after sputum culture. Bronchodilators may also be helpful to relieve bronchospasm, e.g. salbutamol.
5. Start prophylactic digoxin therapy, 0.25 mg daily in older patients to control atrial fibrillation which may develop in the post-operative period and cause cardiac failure.

POSTOPERATIVE CARE

Aims

1. Restore full expansion of the residual lung or ipsilateral residual lobes.
2. Clear bronchial secretions and prevent infection.
3. Prevent pneumothorax or air space.

Action

1. Order routine daily X-rays to assess progress.
2. Pain relief is achieved by repeated small i.m. doses of papaveretum (Omnopon) 5 or 10 mg or pethidine 25 mg titrated to relieve pain. Do not give doses that depress respiration, especially in the elderly, or depress the consciousness level, and so prevent co-operation with the physiotherapist. After 24 hours, less potent drugs such as Distalgesic may be adequate. Cryoanalgesia is valuable in relieving post-thoracotomy pain. A special probe uses the rapid expansion of nitrous oxide to produce a small, 3–4 mm diameter ice ball at minus 60°C. At operation, apply the probe to the intercostal nerve at the level of the incision and those of the two spaces above and two below it. Apply the probe as near to the vertebral body as possible to include the collateral branch. If necessary strip the parietal pleura locally to accurately identify the nerve. Analgesia lasts for up to approximately 3 months and greatly reduces the need for narcotic drugs.
3. Chest drainage: site the drainage tubes in the cryo-treated zone and connect them to underwater seals. Apply gentle suction of 10–15 mmHg or cmH₂O. Milk the tubes frequently to maintain their patency. Measure the drainage daily and take especial care in the immediate post operative period (see p. 314). The basal tube can be removed after 48–72 hours, the apical tube when the air leak has ceased. Occasionally this is a long period of up to 2 weeks. Try instilling streptomycin 1 gm in 10 ml saline through the tube to cause irritation of the pleura if the air leak persists. A small residual air space may have to be accepted, especially if there is no clinical evidence of a significant bronchial fistula from a lobar or segmental bronchial stump leak. Persistent air leaks are usually due to 1–2 mm calibre bronchi on the raw surface of the lung.
4. Pulmonary function can be restored by a number of methods. Physiotherapy aims to help remove sputum and so maintain full lung expansion. Tipping of the patient and inhalation of medicated steam are also helpful. Mucolytic

agents such as bromhexine (Bisolvon) are valuable even if the sputum is very viscid. If these methods fail, try tube suction via the larynx. If this is ineffective bronchoscopic suction is necessary. This is best performed using the rigid scope (see p. 310–311).

5. Early ambulation is possible even when the patient is still connected to a drainage tube. He is usually out of bed the next day and walking as soon as possible. Encourage active breathing exercises and leg exercises. TED stockings are useful in preventing venous thrombosis.

6. Observe for cardiac arrhythmias and continue daily digoxin 0.25 mg in case atrial fibrillation, flutter or supraventricular tachycardia occur. If arrhythmia is not controlled congestive failure may supervene.

7. Antibiotic prophylaxis is indicated for several days. Change the antibiotic if there is clinical evidence of failure to improve, and if X-rays display pulmonary consolidation.

8. Surgical emphysema of lesser degree is common in pneumonectomy patients. More marked emphysema may be caused by a blocked drainage tube, or a delayed air leak after the tube has been removed. Commonly the lung is adherent so that it does not collapse fully and the pressure in the space builds up rapidly. The remedy is to unblock an existing tube, or insert a new one into the space, after radiological assessment.

9. Diuretic therapy may be required using intravenous frusemide 20–40 mg. There is a risk of circulatory overload, especially in the elderly, and after pneumonectomy. Intravenous fluid infusion is not normally required after 12 hours postoperatively, since oral fluids can be taken.

Difficulty?

1. *Bleeding.* If more than 200–300 ml of blood per hour drains during the first 2–3 hours, check the blood coagulation for platelet or clotting factor deficiency. Replace the blood loss and consider exploring the chest if the bleeding continues and there is no apparent haematological cause. The bleeding is usually from a bronchial artery or pulmonary venous branch.

2. *Empyema.* This is due to infection of retained pleural fluid, serous or blood, and the presence of organisms unresponsive to the prophylactic antibiotic. Full re-expansion of the lung obliterates the space and is usually sufficient. After pneumonectomy, this is a major complication which is treated by emptying the space and instilling appropriate antibiotics. If these simple measures fail, institute open drainage by rib resection or the fenestration procedure. The latter involves resection of short lengths of three ribs anterolaterally over the base of the space. Then suture the skin margins to the pleural edge to make a permanent window which will not close in the absence of a tube. After some months it may be possible to close the window. Exclude the presence of a small bronchopleural fistula.

3. *Broncho-pleural fistula* is a rare complication after segmental or lobar resection and is now very uncommon following pneumonectomy. Treat by draining the space, and either resuture the bronchus stump or apply caustic soda 20% followed by acetic acid 30% to the site of the fistula through the bronchoscope. Several applications may be required to produce closure.

4. *Atelectasis* should respond to physiotherapy. If it does not, perform bronchoscopic suction.

5. *Respiratory failure* is more likely in the elderly chronic bronchitic, the emphysematous patient and the heavy smoker. It may be due to spill of blood or infected sputum into the lower lung at operation. Observe closely for clinical evidence of CO_2 retention, such as tiredness, sweating or rising blood pressure and monitor progress with blood gas estimations. If respiratory failure is confirmed, if the patient is hypoxic or becoming exhausted, ventilate him temporarily. Continued assisted respiratory interferes with the healing of the bronchus stump especially in the pneumonectomy patients.

UNDERWATER SEAL DRAINAGE

1. Connect the drainage tube from the patient to the long tube which passes well below the level of a measured amount of water in the bottle so that the fluid provides a seal preventing entry of air into the chest. If necessary, connect the short tube which allows escape of air in a source of suction; this is usually increased up to a negative pressure of 20 cm of water or 20 mmHg (Fig. 19.5)

2. Check free drainage by noting a free swing of fluid in the long tube on inspiration, if no suction is connected.

3. When suction is used the apparatus must not be turned off and left joined to the bottle or the escape of air and fluid ceases.

4. The drainage tube arrangement must not be reversed (i.e. the short tube connected to the patient) as, again, obstruction results.

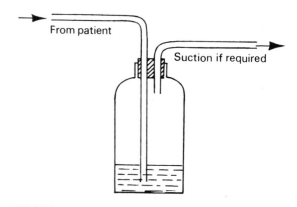

From patient

Suction if required

Fig. 19.5 Underwater seal drainage.

5. Clamp the tubing when movement of the patient is intended which would cause the bottle to be raised above the level of the patient's diaphragm, as fluid could enter the chest through the tubing.

POSTEROLATERAL THORACOTOMY

Appraise

This is the usual route of access for:
1. Pulmonary operations
2. Some oesophageal operations
3. Posterior, middle mediastinal and mainly unilateral anterior mediastinal lesions.
4. Repair of coarctation, division of patent ductus arteriosus, and thoracic aneurysms.

Access

1. Place the patient in either the lateral or the prone position.
(a) The prone position has the advantage of decreased risk of spill of bronchial sections to the opposite lung, but allows poor exposure of anterior hilar structures.
(b) The lateral position gives access from any aspect of the chest and is preferable if the necessary endobronchial anaesthetic tubes are available. In this position, the chest is arched over a soft pad — a Holmes Sellors support is ideal. The arms and legs are positioned as in Figure 19.6.
2. Approach the upper lobe through the fifth interspace or the fourth, if apical difficulty is expected. Approach the lower lobe through the sixth or seventh space. The site of the incision may be modified according to the intended operation, but the ribs are not counted until the muscle layers have been divided.
3. Cut the skin in a smooth curve, running from midway between the midline and medial border of the scapula posteriorly, skirting the angle of the scapula by 2.5 cm. and passing forward to the anterior axillary line.

Action

1. Divide the muscles, using the diathermy point with coagulation of the vessels as required. The muscles are arranged in two layers; the superficial layer consists of the trapezius and latissimus dorsi muscles; the deeper layer is composed of the rhomboid and serratus anterior muscles. Preserve the serratus anterior muscle almost intact by dividing this layer through the aponeurosis below the muscle fibres. (Figs. 19.7 & 19.8)
2. Count the ribs from the apex by passing a hand up under the scapula and the muscle layers posteriorly.
3. Divide with the diathermy point the periosteum of the rib selected.
4. Strip the periosteum from its upper border, using a curved rougine, and work postero-anteriorly.
5. With a costotome or rib shears resect a small portion 1–2 cm of rib posteriorly to increase the exposure. It is not necessary to remove a rib. The portion of rib may be removed from the rib which has been stripped or the one above or below, depending on the direction of access required. Alternatively, the ligaments of the appropriate costo-transverse joint may be divided with a chisel.
6. Open the pleura along the length of the wound after warning the anaesthetist to allow the lung to fall away. The

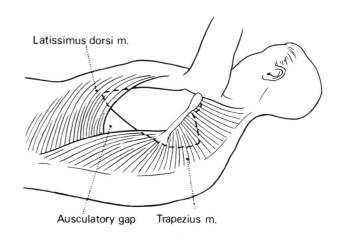

Latissimus dorsi m.

Ausculatory gap   Trapezius m.

Fig. 19.7 Arrangement of superficial muscle layers.

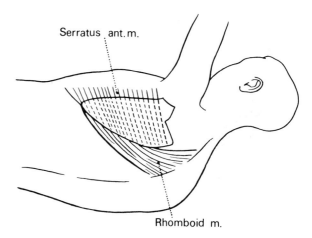

Serratus ant. m.

Rhomboid m.

Fig. 19.8 Arrangement of deep muscle layers.

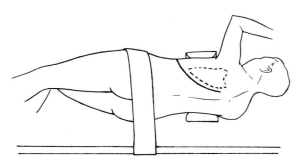

Fig. 19.6 Position for posterolateral thoracotomy.

periosteal separation may be extended anteriorly deep to the wound.

7. Insert the customary rib spreader (Finochietto) after pads have been placed over the wound edges.

8. It is usually obvious that the nerve and the intercostal bundle are placed on stretch as the ribs are spread, and the intercostal nerve may be divided to prevent a traction injury; the intercostal vessels may be ligated and divided. If the cryoanalgesia apparatus is available (see p. 313), do not divide the nerve.

9. If light or filmy adhesions are present, divide them with scissors or diathermy.

10. When widespread and marked adhesion is present, use a mounted gauze swab and blunt dissection to strip the lung in the extrapleural plane. Use a hot pack to control the diffuse oozing and, later, bleeding points may require coagulation with diathermy. Sometimes the extrapleural strip need only be over an area of dense localized adherence, the rest of the lung being free.

Closure

1. Insert apical and basal drains posterolaterally through the second intercostal space below the wound after muscle layers have been put on stretch with Lane's forceps. Pass the apical tube up to the apex of the chest. It may be tethered to the chest wall with a light catgut suture looped around it. This tube is usually sited anterior to the basal drain, the lowest side hole of which is level with the dome of the diaphragm. (Fig. 19.9).

2. Insert two or three pericostal sutures of No. 1. nylon (doubled) when healing is likely to be poor. Pass the pericostal sutures around the upper rib and, to avoid the intercostal nerve, through an awl hole in the lower rib, or around the rib hugging the bony groove. (Fig. 19.10)

3. Using a Holmes Sellors approximator to bring the ribs together, close the intercostal layer with a continuous suture of No. 1 catgut, approximating the edge of the stripped intercostal layer above to the intercostal muscle below the rib which has been stripped.

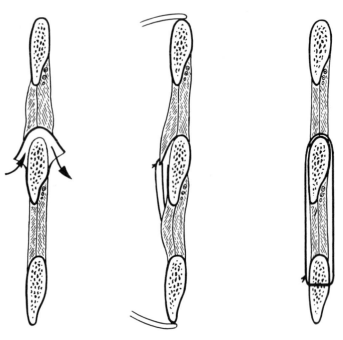

Fig. 19.10 Technique of opening and closing modified intercostal incision and insertion of pericostal suture.

4. Unite each muscle layer with a continuous suture, (No. 1. catgut) which must pass through the whole thickness of the muscle to ensure haemostasis. Suture the superficial fascia with a fine (00) catgut suture.

ANTEROLATERAL THORACOTOMY

Appraise

1. This route gives access to the heart, pericardium and lung. It was the exposure for closed mitral valvotomy but is not often used for cardiac operations as most are performed with cardiopulmonary bypass using median sternotomy.

2. It may be used for open cardiac massage in cardiac arrest and for pericardial drainage.

3. Use a shorter version for open lung biopsy in diffuse pulmonary disease.

Access

1. Lay the patient rotated obliquely with the ipsilateral hip and shoulder supported on pillows or sandbags. Elevate the ipsilateral arm carefully avoiding nerve traction.

2. Use the fifth intercostal space on most occasions. Follow the line of the appropriate rib which can readily be counted anteriorly but, in the female, curve the incision below the breast.

3. Begin your incision close to the midline and extend it to the axilla, to pass 2.5 cm below the angle of the scapula if additional length is required.

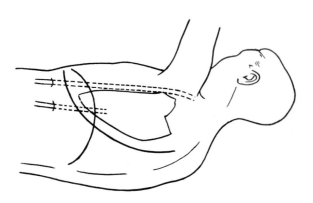

Fig. 19.9 Siting of drainage tubes.

Action

1. Divide the pectoralis major muscle in the line of the incision and split the serratus anterior muscle along the line of the rib selected. If the incision is taken well posteriorly, it may be necessary to divide the lowest portion of the long thoracic nerve. Anteriorly, the upper rectus abdominis muscle is divided.

2. Divide the periosteum using the diathermy point and strip it from the upper border of the rib postero-anteriorly.

3. Open the pleura in the depth of this layer. Take care to avoid the internal mammary vessels close to the sternum.

4. Open the pericardium anteriorly to the phrenic nerve, as this gives better access.

Closure

1. Suture the intercostal layer with 1 catgut. The medial portion is difficult to close because the muscle layers are thin and attenuated at this site.

2. If the costal cartilage should fracture while the chest is opened with the spreader, it is best to resect a small portion to avoid local friction.

3. Close the muscle layers with continuous sutures of 1 catgut. Insert a drainage tube through a separate incision laterally below the level of the main wound.

MEDIAN STERNOTOMY

Appraise

1. This is commonly performed for cardiac operations using cardio-pulmonary bypass, as it provides the best overall access. Postoperative pain is less and least respiratory upset is caused.

2. A shorter version of this incision allows exposure of the trachea for resection of a stricture or tumour.

3. The incision is used for removal of anterior mediastinal tumours such as thymomata, germ cell tumours, and rarely for retrosternal goitre. A shorter incision may be adequate.

4. Excision of bilateral pulmonary metastases may be performed by this route. Access to the left lower lobe is limited by the heart.

5. Bilateral bullous lung disease may be operated on by this access.

Prepare

1. Place the patient supine with the arms by the side on a soft mattress or water blanket.

2. Attach ECG electrodes to shoulders and chest wall.

3. Insert percutaneously a radial artery catheter for arterial pressure monitoring. Insert a central venous pressure line via the internal jugular vein.

4. Insert a urinary catheter, rectal and nasopharyngeal temperature probes.

5. Prepare the skin to allow access to groins and also leg if for coronary artery bypass operations.

Action

1. Make an incision from the lower margin of the suprasternal notch to 2 inches below the xiphoid process.

2. Divide the subcutaneous tissue with the diathermy point down to the periosteum of the sternum to obtain haemostasis. Keep in the gap between the pectoralis major muscles and precisely mark the midline of the sternum with the diathermy point. The sternum is least wide at second space.

3. Divide the linea alba for a short distance below the xiphoid process.

4. Free tissues from the deep surface of the manubrium, the xiphoid process and lower sternum by blunt dissection using a finger, Roberts forceps or scissors.

5. Divide the sternum longitudinally with an electric or pneumatic Stryker saw, hugging the posterior surface to avoid damage to the heart, ascending aorta or the left innominate vein. If this is not available, a Gigli saw may be used, which is withdrawn from above after an extra long Roberts forceps has been passed upwards behind the sternum hugging its posterior surface. With the latter method it is possible to open the pleura, especially on the right, which often lies well across the front of the mediastinum. In emergency, and for the shorter divisions, a Lebsche chisel may be used from above.

6. Secure haemostasis on both aspects of the sternum by diathermizing the periosteal vessels and using bone wax to control the bleeding from the exposed marrow.

7. Insert self retaining retractor and incise the pericardium in the midline. Extend the incision up to the reflection on the aorta, avoiding the left innominate vein, and down to the diaphragm. Sew the pericardial edges to the skin to form a well and improve the exposure of the heart.

Closure

1. If the pericardium has been opened, introduce pericardial and anterior mediastinal drains (24–28FG) catheter through separate skin incisions below the xiphoid process and through separate openings in the rectus sheath.

2. Using an awl or heavy trocar-pointed needle, pass stainless steel wire sutures through each side of the sternum; make a firm closure by twisting the wire to obtain close approximation. Alternatively, pass the needle close to the edge of the sternum, from the second space caudally, avoiding the internal mammary vessels.

3. Approximate the muscle and the subcutaneous layers with catgut sutures, 1 and 00 respectively. Suture the linea alba accurately in the lowest portion of the wound to minimise the risk of an incisional hernia.

THYMECTOMY

Appraise

1. Myasthenia gravis is the important indication for this operation. Its basis is, however, empirical, although the condition is now thought to be due to an auto-immune disease affecting the motor end plates, possibly related to antibody formed in the thymus. The operation is not offered to all patients but is particularly indicated in younger patients with a short history who are not responding well to medical treatment. The gland may be of normal size, hyperplastic, or, in 10% of patients, a thymic tumour may be present.

2. Thymic tumours or cysts are the other indications for surgery. Thymic tumours, of which 10% are cysts, are the commonest form of mediastinal tumour. Approximately 30% of the tumours are malignant and approximately 25% of thymic tumours are associated with myasthenia.

3. Rarely, thymic tumours are associated with red cell aplasia and with immunoglobulin deficiency. The response to surgery is variable.

Assess

1. Perform full clinical assessment, postero-anterior and lateral chest radiographs and CT scans of the mediastinum.

2. The presence of pain, dyspnoea, superior vena caval obstruction and pericardial or pleural effusion suggest advanced disease.

Action

1. Perform a midline sternotomy, beginning the incision at or just below the upper margin of the manubrium, and extending down to approximately the third costal cartilage.

Use diathermy to mark the midline of the sternum and divide the bone either with a lebsche chisel from above or with the Stryker saw. Spread the bone with a self-retaining retractor which will continue the sternal division for a short distance.

2. Gradually mobilise the thymus which overlies the pericardium by a combination of blunt and sharp dissection. The arterial branches come laterally from the internal mammary artery or its pericardiophrenic branch (Fig. 19.11)

3. Dissect each lower pole from the pericardium and the mediastinal pleura. Take care not to damage the phrenic nerve as the gland may extend deeply into the mediastinum around the ascending aorta.

4. Turn the gland superiorly after each lower pole has been mobilised. Find the thymic vein, or sometimes two veins, where they enter the left innominate vein on the posterior aspect of the gland. Divide and ligate the vein.

5. Dissect out the superior poles, which are smaller and may be supplied by small branches of the inferior thyroid artery.

6. Close the sternum with two or three wire sutures. Drain the wound with a small catheter brought out superiorly in the neck. Close the muscle and soft tissue over the bone with catgut sutures. Insert pleural drains if either pleura is opened.

7. The presence of a malignant tumour is suggested by marked adherence or invasion of surrounding tissues. Remove the tumour if at all possible by resecting the pericardium or locally involved lung.

8. Thymectomy for thymic tumours may be performed through a midline sternotomy but in some instances where the tumour is markedly projecting into a hemithorax, a posterolateral thoracotomy may be indicated. With this approach, if the tumour is not accompanied by myasthenia, there is no need to perform a complete thymectomy.

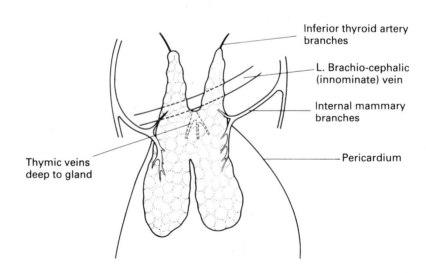

Fig. 19.11 Anatomy of thymus.

PNEUMONECTOMY

Appraise

1. The operation is commonly performed for carcinomata involving the main bronchi or for peripheral carcinomata which have spread more extensively.

2. Occasionally, pneumonectomy is indicated when tuberculosis has destroyed a lung perhaps with an associated chronic empyema.

3. Extensive unilateral bronchiectasis may be an indication provided the other lung is at most, minimally affected.

4. An occasional indication is gross destruction of a lung by infection superimposed on collapse due to a foreign body, a stricture due to trauma or tuberculosis, or a bronchial carcinoid tumour.

Access

1. Perform a posterolateral thoracotomy, usually through the sixth space.

2. For bronchial carcinoma, intrapericardial dissection is commonly used to allow more radical clearance of the pulmonary vessels.

Assess

1. Inspect the site and note the local extent of the tumour, including the attachment to or involvement of the chest wall.

2. Check especially for involvement of the main pulmonary artery, either pulmonary vein or even the left atrium by direct tumour extension or involved lymphnodes.

3. Resectability of the tumour may sometimes only be established after opening the pericardium to ascertain that proximal control of the main vessels is possible.

4. Check for involvement of the oesophagus posteriorly by infiltrated nodes or direct tumour extension.

5. Look for infiltrated subcarinal nodes which may be involving the origin of the opposite bronchus.

6. Check for involved right paratracheal nodes with secondary involvement of the superior vena cava and phrenic nerves.

7. Palpate for enlarged nodes in the aortic hollow involving the recurrent laryngeal nerve or the aortic wall on the left side.

8. Palpate the liver on the right side through the diaphragm.

Action

1. Secure the pulmonary veins first to minimize the risk of tumour dissemination.

2. Open the pericardium in front of the hilum and enlarge the incision to allow access to the superior and inferior pulmonary veins as they enter the left atrium. (Fig. 19.12)

3. Divide the veins between ligatures. If proximal extension of the tumour is marked divide the veins after applying a vascular clamp, such as a Brock atrial, to the left atrium which is then sutured with 2/0 non-absorbable suture.

4. Dissect inside the adventitia and divide the pulmonary artery between ligatures or preferably oversew with 3/0 non-absorbable suture. If necessary divide the left artery close to the main trunk after dividing the ligamentum arteriosum while preserving the recurrent laryngeal nerve.

5. Free the oesophagus from the bronchus posteriorly. Isolate and divide the bronchus close to the carina between clamps.

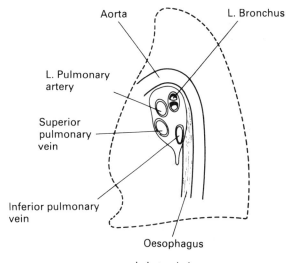

L. Lateral view

A

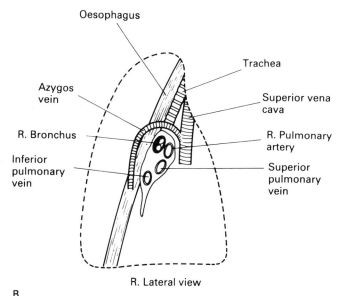

R. Lateral view

B

Fig. 19.12 Anatomical relations of the hila of the lungs.

6. Divide the remaining posterior pericardium, free the lung from the oesophagus posteriorly and divide the inferior pulmonary ligament.

7. Dissect and remove the subcarinal, hilar and right paratracheal nodes. On the left side clear the glands in the aortic hollow with preservation of the recurrent laryngeal nerve. Ligate the bronchial artery to minimize the risk of reactionary haemorrhage.

8. Trim the bronchus back after removing the clamp so that the closure will be flush with the trachea internally. Use non-absorbable suture such as Mersilene, polyester 3/0 or stainless steel, placed as interrupted sutures. Alternatively, use a stapling device. Reinforce the closure by lightly suturing the oesophagus, or on the right side a local mediastinal pleural flap, over the stump.

9. Dissect the lung hilum extra-pericardially for non-malignant disease. Expose the superior vein and the main pulmonary artery anteriorly. Free them on the right side from the superior vena cava which lies antero-medially. Dissect the inferior vein below the main bronchus posteriorly. The distal ties are often on the venous branches.

10. Crush the phrenic nerve to reduce the size of the haemothorax if desired.

11. Pleuro-pneumonectomy. Free the lung extrapleurally in the presence of extensive pleural disease and expose the hilum. Avoid damage to chest wall vessels and the superior vena cava on the right and the aorta and innominate vein on the left.

Closure

Close the intercostal layer with great care, especially posteriorly to prevent leakage of fluid into the muscle layers post operatively, causing wound dehiscence. Routinely no drain is inserted but some surgeons prefer to use a basal drain which is released for half a minute at hourly intervals over the first 12 hours. The mediastinum is maintained centrally with a pneumothorax apparatus, such as a Maxwell box if drainage is not instituted.

LOBECTOMY

Appraise

1. This is the preferred operation for bronchial carcinoma, ideally when the lesion is sited peripherally in the lobe.

2. For the resection of localised bronchiectasis not controlled by conservative measures.

3. For the resection of tuberculous disease which has not responded fully to antituberculous chemotherapy.

4. For chronic lung abscess.

5. For metastatic tumours.

6. Each lobectomy has individual variations dependent upon the relevant anatomical features. The principles of the operation can best be illustrated by a description of a right upper lobectomy.

Access

Perform a right posterolateral thoracotomy through the fifth intercostal space, with the patient in the lateral position.

Assess

Check the paratracheal area for enlarged nodes; palpate the lobar hilum for pathological lymphnodes.

Action

1. The area of the disease may be adherent to the chest wall and may require local extrapleural separation.

2. Dissect the hilum anteriorly and expose the superior pulmonary vein. Find the middle lobe vein inferiorly and isolate the main portion of the upper lobe vein superiorly for ligation. Ligate the segmental branches distally and divide the vein. Take care posteriorly in the dissection as the main right pulmonary artery trunk lies deep to the vein. (Fig. 19.13)

3. Display the upper branch of the right pulmonary artery superiorly to the vein, separating it from the superior vena cava anteriorly. Dissect the artery in the sub-adventitial plane and divide it between ligatures; this branch supplies the apical and anterior segments. Display the main trunk and look for the recurrent branch to the posterior segment. If visible, divide it between ligatures. If it is not visible secure this vessel after division of the right upper lobe bronchus.

4. Rotate the lung anteriorly and expose the right upper lobe bronchus by dissecting the pleura over its posterior aspect. The bronchial artery branch to the upper lobe bronchus will be divided and should be ligated or diathermized. Pass an O'Shaughnessey forceps around the upper lobe bronchus as close to the main bronchus as possible for ease of passage and to avoid the recurrent pulmonary artery branch, which lies in front of the bronchus. Apply bronchus clamps, the non-toothed clamp being applied proximally. Divide the bronchus and find the recurrent artery branch, if it has not been secured previously.

5. Separate the lobe from the lower lobe posteriorly and the middle lobe anteriorly. The ease of separation depends on the degree of development of the fissures. This is most easily done by having the anaesthetist lightly inflate the remaining lobes while you apply light traction on the distal bronchus clamp and at the same time separate the lobes.

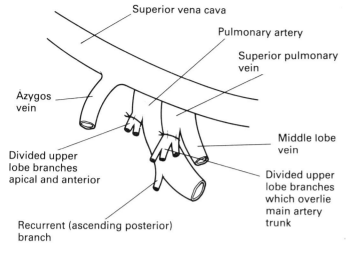

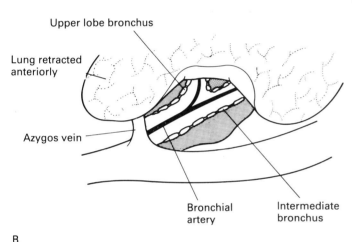

Fig. 19.13 Right upper lobectomy.

Take care to keep in the correct plane and to pick up minor venous or arterial branches which may cross the lobar plane. Apply a warm pack to the raw surface of the lung while the bronchus stump is trimmed so that the internal closure will be flush with the main bronchus. Use simple interrupted sutures of 3/0 polyester material. Test the bronchus stump for airtight closure, using water or saline, and search for small bronchial openings on the raw surface which may require suture or ligation. Reinforce the bronchial closure by suturing the adjacent mediastinal pleura over the stump.

6. Remove the lobar and anterior hilar lymphnodes for biopsy. Remove the paratracheal nodes also if a preliminary mediastinoscopy was not performed. Divide the inferior pulmonary ligament if necessary to allow easy upward rotation of the remaining lobes. Lightly suture the middle lobe, if it is freely mobile, to the lower lobe to prevent rotation and therefore necrosis.

SLEEVE RESECTION OR SLEEVE LOBECTOMY

1. This is a useful procedure to extend the scope of lobectomy and avoid pneumonectomy, especially if lung function is compromised. It is indicated for carcinoma of the right or the left upper lobe which is too close to the main bronchus to permit the bronchial clearance (1.5 cm) necessary for lobectomy (Fig. 19.14). Lobar gland involvement should be absent or minimal unless palliative operation is attempted perhaps combined with local pulmonary artery resection.

2. The technique may also be indicated for the removal of bronchial carcinoids or a tuberculous stricture.

SEGMENTAL RESECTION

Appraise

1. These operations are less commonly performed now that resections for tuberculous disease have become rare.

2. Small (1–2 cm) peripheral bronchial carcinomata may be satisfactorily removed by this operation in the elderly

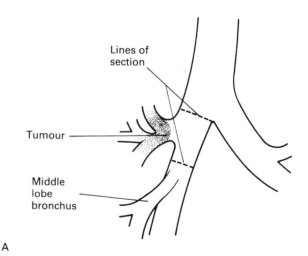

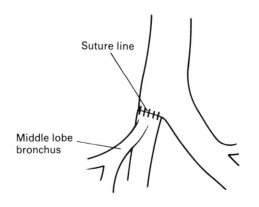

Fig. 19.14 Sleeve lobectomy.

with reduced respiratory reserve. The lesion should be in the centre of the segment.

3. Occasionally metastatic lesions may be removed by segmental rather than lobar resection.

4. Bronchiectatic disease may be localised to segments, e.g. the lingula.

5. Chronic inflammatory disease, e.g. abscess may be resected.

6. A detailed knowledge topographically of the segmental bronchi and arterial branches is required.

Action

1. These resections require only isolation and division of the relevant segmental pulmonary artery branches and the segmental bronchus. The segmental veins course between the segments and are not dissected nor divided, except for the apical segment of the lower lobe and the lingula.

2. The operation is easier in those segments where the segmental bronchus can be isolated first, e.g. in the right upper lobe as the corresponding arteries can then be found and confirmed while the segment is being stripped out.

3. In the left upper lobe segments the arterial branches require ligation before access can be obtained to the corresponding segmental bronchi.

4. Preserve any arterial branch in doubt until it is clear that it is passing to the relevant segment, so that no pulmonary infarction occurs.

5. The apical lower and lingular segments are exceptions and treated as a lobe with division of the corresponding segmental vein. (Fig. 19.15)

6. Strip the segment while exerting traction on the distal bronchus with the lung gently inflated. The intersegmental vein acts as a good guide to the correct plane.

7. Deal with the raw lung surface as described in lobectomy.

COMPLICATIONS OF CHEST INJURY

Patients with chest injuries frequently have multiple injuries which all require assessment. The pulmonary and cardiovascular systems however merit the highest priority in resuscitation and treatment. First secure an adequate airway but promptly perform intubation or bronchoscopy if the lesser measures are unsuccessful.

HAEMOTHORAX

The diagnosis is based on the physical signs of fluid, coupled with a chest X-ray in the **erect** position and confirmed by aspiration of the chest.

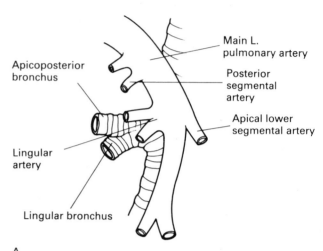

A

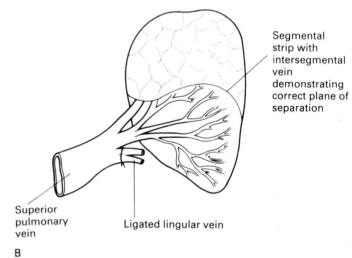

B

Fig. 19.15 Dissection of lingular segmental resection.

Action

1. Aspiration. This treatment is satisfactory if the blood has not clotted and the volume is small, i.e. less than 1 litre, if it is repeated each day, and if the chest is aspirated as dry as possible on each occasion. The use of streptokinase does not usually help to remove older clotted blood.

2. Insert an intercostal tube postero-laterally in a lower space. This is the usual, very satisfactory method and is combined with underwater drainage and preferably low pressure suction. Leave the tube until drainage ceases, usually by 48–72 hours.

3. Thoracotomy. This is required for:
(a) Massive bleeding from a large vessel such as the subclavian or internal mammary artery.
(b) Persistent or recurrent bleeding after aspiration or insertion of an intercostal tube. Deal with the bleeding site by ligation or suture. The source of haemorrhage

is more likely to be an intercostal vessel or vessel on the diaphragm than from the pulmonary vessels.

(c) Clotted haemothorax. Occasionally, large masses of clot form at an early stage, i.e. after 24–48 hours, particularly on the right side and if there is associated abdominal injury, for example, to the liver. Remove the clot from the chest wall and the lung by gentle swabbing, if the operation is performed in the first 7–10 days. Decortication of the lung is required if a longer period has elapsed and is more readily effected after six weeks. By this time the partially organized clot can be removed as a definite layer from the visceral pleura. Remove the parietal pleura with its covering adherent clot by dissection in the extra pleural plane. Removal over the diaphragm is often incomplete.

(d) Infected haemothorax. Some patients develop a low grade infection and are best dealt with by decortication as above.

PNEUMOTHORAX

Appraise

This is the most common cause of inadequate respiration following chest trauma. It is due to injury of the lung by the sharp rib ends at the fracture site. The diagnosis is made by noting reduced or absent air entry, subcutaneous emphysema and by chest X-ray in the erect position. There is often accompanying haemothorax. The air leak continues until the collapse of the lung obstructs the bronchus leading to the leak, when an equilibrium is reached with gas absorption, until the area which is leaking, heals.

Actions

1. Insert an intercostal catheter (20–28 FG) through the second or third intercostal space, preferably through the axilla or anteriorly. Underwater seal drainage with low pressure suction, i.e. 20 cm of water or 20 mmHg is instituted and the tube left in situ until the air leak has ceased for 24 hours.

2. Remove the catheter after clamping it for 24 hours and taking a further X-ray to chck no air space has developed.

TENSION PNEUMOTHORAX

Appraise

This severe degree of pneumothorax is due to a valvular mechanism which may be caused by an adhesion near the site of the tear preventing collapse of the lung, or possibly to pre-existing peripheral bronchial disease, causing a partial inspiratory obstruction which becomes complete on expiration. When the intrapleural pressure becomes greater than atmospheric in expiration, venous return is decreased. The diagnosis is made by noting the marked distress, dyspnoea and often cyanosis of the patient, and supported by evidence of mediastinal displacement to the opposite side on palpation of the trachea and apex beat.

Action

1. Insert a large-bore needle in the axilla or anteriorly in the second space to treat the emergency.

2. Insert an intercostal catheter in hospital. Wait until the lung has partially re-expanded before using suction, as the mediastinum may be sucked over to the injured side.

3. Rarely, a gross air leak continues with marked surgical emphysema; the condition may be due to trapping of the injured lung between the rib fragments. Establish the diagnosis by thoracotomy when marked improvement occurs after freeing the lung.

4. *Note*. A severe air leak coupled with severe surgical emphysema may indicate a ruptured bronchus and indicate the need for bronchoscopy to establish the diagnosis.

FLAIL CHEST

Appraise

1. This is caused by the isolation of a segment of the chest wall of varying size by fracture, at two sites along their length, of several ribs.

2. The lesion is extremely important because of the dangerous and sometimes fatal effect of paradoxical movement of the flail segment, which causes impaired pulmonary function, inability to cough properly and some reduction in venous return. Paradoxical movement becomes more marked as the condition of the lungs deteriorates and greater respiratory effort is required.

Assess

1. Emergency treatment is difficult and not completely satisfactory, so patients should be moved to hospital as rapidly as possible. The most useful emergency measures are to lie the patient on the affected side, combined with support from strapping or sandbags and, occasionally, traction on the flail segment with a large towel clip.

2. Assess the patient clinically on admission. Take erect chest X-rays and suck out bronchoscopically blood and secretions prior to intubation.

UNILATERAL LESIONS

1. Use intermittent positive pressure respiration (IPPR) or operative fixation of the fractured ribs. Decide the need

for ventilator support by measuring pH, Pa_{CO_2}, and Pa_{O_2}, and respiratory rate.

2. Surgical treatment avoids the use of a ventilator and requires less demanding nursing care.

3. Expose the rib fractures through a modified thoracotomy wound and fix them in position using special flat pins or Kirschner wire, which is bent over after inserting it obliquely across the fracture site.

4. Drain the chest.

BILATERAL LESIONS

1. These must be treated by IPPR until the chest wall has become stable enough to allow unaided respiration, which usually takes about 3 weeks. IPPR restores adequate ventilation and provides mechanical support of the rib cage.

2. These severe injuries are commonly associated with haemothoraces or haemopneumothoraces on one or both sides.

3. Insert intercostal catheter drains to prevent tension pneumothoraces.

CHEST WOUNDS
OPEN WOUNDS

These cause an open or sucking type of pneumothorax with embarrassment of ventilation and venous return.

Action

1. Treat the emergency by applying a firm cover with chest drainage by a Heimlich valve. Alternatively, lift the cover from time to time to allow escape of pent up blood and air.

2. Intubate promptly if severe respiratory distress exists.

3. Debride the wound and perform thoracotomy to investigate and assess the extent of the intrathoracic damage and exclude the presence of a foreign body.

4. Segmental resection or lobectomy may be necessary but often suture of the lung or a major blood vessel may suffice.

5. Institute adequate drainage and routine chest closure.

PENETRATING STAB WOUNDS OR PERFORATING WOUNDS

These usually seal quickly and do not result in suction pneumothorax.

Action

1. Such wounds may not necessarily demand a thoracotomy. Treat the patient conservatively and deal with the wounds locally if there is no clinical evidence of serious internal damage, absence of bleeding and a satisfactory chest X-ray. Note the direction of the wound.

2. Remember that stab wounds in the lower half of the chest may be associated with diaphragmatic puncture and intra-abdominal injury to the spleen, liver or hollow viscera.

3. Undertake thoracolaparotomy if in doubt after very careful assessment. Fatal results have followed strangulation of an incisional hernia resulting from an overlooked penetration of the diaphragm, sustained a long time before.

WOUNDS OF THE HEART AND PERICARDIUM
Appraise

1. Many gunshot wounds are rapidly fatal but some patients, especially those who sustain stab or knife wounds, reach the surgeon with a haemopericardium and evidence of cardiac tamponade.

2. Diagnose by the clinical picture of falling cardiac output — peripheral vasoconstriction, tachycardia, low blood pressure associated with rising venous pressure. Intravenous resuscitation increases the venous pressure further.

The site of the wound is likely to be atrial or a minor ventricular injury for the patient to survive.

3. Confirm the clinical diagnosis with X-ray and ultrasonography.

Prepare

Establish a good intravenous infusion and order adequate blood replacement. This is mandatory because on opening the pericardium rapid and profuse bleeding may occur.

Action

1. Aspirate the pericardium to confirm the diagnosis. This may be adequate to relieve the condition.

2. Expose the heart through a left anterolateral thoracotomy via the fifth space if bleeding persists, recurs, or is obviously severe and requires emergency operation. Median sternotomy may be preferable for central or right sided penetrating wounds especially if bypass is available and indicated.

3. Control atrial wounds by finger pressure or an appropriate atraumatic clamp, such as a Brock's mitral clamp, or occasionally, a Duval forceps. Suture with 2/0 or 3/0 vascular sutures. Restore adequate blood volume once bleeding is under control.

4. Control ventricular wounds by finger pressure and then suture with 2/0 sutures. Use a pad of Dacron, Teflon or pericardium to reinforce the closure if the muscle is friable.

5. Injured coronary vessels. Suture an injured artery if possible but trauma to a large branch is likely to be rapidly fatal. Coronary artery bypass may be possible. Ligate a bleeding coronary vein.

6. Some penetrating wounds may be associated with valvular damage which requires investigation and may need treatment later.

7. Drain the pericardium adequately and close the chest in routine fashion.

ASPIRATION OF THE PERICARDIUM

This is performed to treat cardiac tamponade due to the accumulation of blood following trauma or fluid due to inflammation of the pericardium.

Prepare

Sit the patient up at 45° (see Fig. 19.16) Confirm the clinical diagnosis with ultrasonography.

Action

1. Infiltrate the skin below the xiphisternum and to the left of the midline with local anaesthesia.

2. Advance the needle obliquely upwards to just touch the back of the sternum and then guide it more deeply

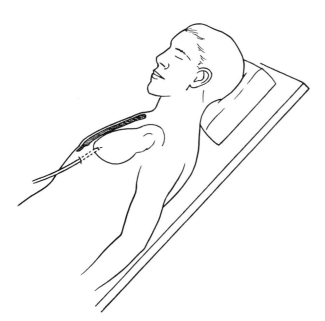

Fig. 19.16 Technique of aspiration of the pericardium.

(approximately at an angle of 45°) until the inferior aspect of the pericardium is felt as a definite resistance.

3. Push the needle through the pericardium and aspirate the fluid.

4. It is possible to introduce a plastic catheter of the intracath variety through a larger bore needle or a small cannula if aspiration needs to be maintained.

EMPYEMA THORACIS

Appraise

A collection of pus in the pleural cavity may follow pneumonia, oesophageal perforation or thoracic operations. Antibiotic therapy has modified the presentation of this condition. Confirm the diagnosis radiologically and by aspiration.

INSERTION OF INTERCOSTAL CATHETER

This may be satisfactory treatment if the pus is thin and is often suitable for post operative patients.

Prepare

1. Use the chest X-ray to count the anterior ends of ribs overlying the pocket. The lateral film determines the location in the coronal plane, e.g. anteriorly, mid-axilla etc.

2. Sit the patient up, leaning comfortably forward over a bedrest or pillows for the usual posterobasal collection.

3. Use 0.5 or 1% lignocaine local anaesthesia. Raise a skin weal then infiltrate the subcutaneous muscle and especially the pleural layer.

Action

1. Make a short transverse incision (1.5 cm) over the lower portion of the cavity and insert two stitches, a central one for the later closure of the wound and the other laterally to hold the catheter in situ.

2. Insert an Argyle catheter, usually size 24 or 28 FG. This combined plastic catheter plus metal trocar is rather blunt and needs considerable pressure so care must be taken not to damage the lung due to precipitate entry. It is helpful to first make a track with a small Spencer Wells forceps.

The classical alternative is a metal trocar and cannula through which an appropriately sized open end catheter is passed after removing the trocar.

3. Connect the catheter to the drainage bottle and underwater seal. Suction may be used if thought beneficial (see p. 314).

OPEN DRAINAGE BY RIB RESECTION

Appraise

1. This is indicated in the presence of thick pus which will block an intercostal catheter.

2. If the pus remains infected despite antibiotic treatment.

Prepare

1. It is essential that the lung should be adherent to the chest wall around the cavity. Determine this partly by the length of time the empyema has been present and by measuring the amount of deposit in specimens of aspirated pus. A level of desposit of one-half or more in the testtube indicates pleural adhesion.

2. Check for the presence of a bronchopleural fistula by noting the expectoration of identical pus and the presence of an airfluid interface in the cavity, not produced by air introduced at aspiration.

3. Determine the site of the pocket as described for catheter insertion. The usual site is posterobasal when the empyema is due to lower lobe pneumonia.

4. Sit the patient up comfortably supported as for catheter insertion.

Use local anaesthesia because of the danger of a bronchopleural fistula which may not always be obvious.

Action

1. Make a short 2 inch vertical incision which prevents pocketing under the wound edges, and allows the choice or more than one rib for resection.

2. Insert a mastoid self-retaining retractor and divide the muscles with diathermy to expose the ribs.

3. Resect the lowest appropriate rib after checking by aspiration. This is usually the 10th rib for the common posterobasal empyema.

4. Infiltrate the intercostal nerve with local anaesthetic.

5. Divide the periosteum with diathermy and strip it from the rib, working forwards along the upper border and posteriorly along the lower edge of the rib.

6. Excise approximately 2–3 cm of rib. The site is just anteriorly to the angle in the posterobasal empyema.

7. Ligate the intercostal vessels at each end of the wound to minimize the risk of secondary haemorrhage. Cleanly divide the intercostal nerve or use cryoanalgesia.

8. Open into the cavity and excise a block of the outer wall, to provide good drainage and tissue for histological examination and pus for bacteriological culture.

9. Suck out the pocket and remove any large fibrin masses using sponge holders and swabs.

10. Inspect the cavity with a malleable light if a bronchopleural fistula is suspected.

11. Insert the drainage tube at the *base* of the cavity with approximately 1–2 cms. projecting internally. No side holes should be made in the tube as granulation tissue may grow in and obstruct the lumen.

12. Fix the tube with a suture and lightly close the wound if the pus is sterile.

Aftercare

1. Apply suction initially but after a few days cut off the tube leaving 2 cm projecting beyond the skin, and institute open drainage into dressings or use an adhesive bag.

2. Institute intensive physiotherapy which is essential to aid rapid re-expansion of the lung and quick obliteration of the cavity.

3. Maintain the tube in situ until serial pleurograms have shown no cavity remains.

4. To maintain adequate drainage, occasionally it is necessary to lengthen the tube because the diaphragm has risen.

EXCISION OF THE EMPYEMA AND PULMONARY DECORTICATION

Appraise

This operation is the alternative to open drainage and is preferred:

1. If the patient is young.

2. If the cavity is large.

3. If lung disease is present which requires concurrent lung resection, e.g. carcinoma, bronchiectasis, tuberculosis.

4. The pus in the cavity should preferably be sterile or have been rendered sterile by antibiotic therapy (systemic and locally).

Action

1. Perform a posterolateral thoracotomy.

2. Free the lung and empyema in the extrapleural plane. This may be a very difficult procedure if the empyema has been present for some weeks or months. Over the diaphragm, the strip is difficult to achieve and often incomplete. Considerable force may be required using finger pressure or blunt dissection with instruments. There is danger of damage to the superior vena cava on the right and the aorta or left innominate vein on the other side. Take care stripping the apex of the thorax.

3. Remove the pellicle of partially or well organised fibrin overlying the visceral pleura linking with the outer wall of the empyema cavity, which has been freed by the extrapleural strip. It is vital to obtain full expansion of the lung by achieving a complete decortication (Fig. 19.17).

4. Institute adequate drainage of the pleural space and intensive physiotherapy as air leak from the lung surface may be considerable.

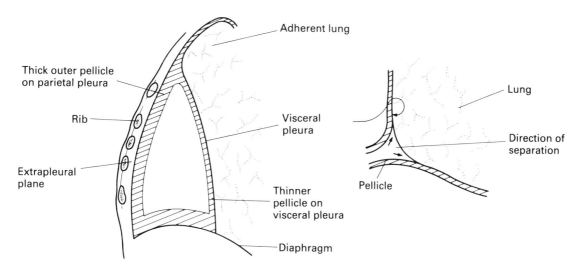

Fig. 19.17 Excision of empyema and decortication.

SPONTANEOUS PNEUMOTHORAX

Appraise

This is relatively common condition due to the rupture of a superficial bleb or bulla in late adolescence and young adults, usually males. The patients are often thin and shallow chested and may have a positive family history. The condition less commonly occurs in older patients with emphysema.

Action

1. Insert an intercostal catheter unless the pneumothorax is a very shallow one, when it may be left to absorb spontaneously.

2. Surgical treatment is indicated (a) after three to four recurrent pneumothoraces on the same side, to prevent further attacks; (b) if the other lung becomes affected, surgery is recommended urgently in case bilateral pneumothoraces occur simultaneously; (c) a severe leak which persists after intercostal drainage.

PLEURECTOMY

1. This is preferred to the older procedure of chemical pleurodesis when insufflation of iodised talc powder is used.

2. Make a short postero-lateral thoracotomy and remove the parietal pleura, after freeing it by gauze dissection, from the apex, upper mediastinum and the posterolateral aspect of the chest.

3. Control the bleeding with hot packs.

4. Inspect the lung and determine the site of the air leak.

5. Preferably ligate the bullae with 1 thread but a large cyst may be unroofed and sutured.

6. Close the chest in routine fashion with underwater seal drainage.

CHRONIC PNEUMOTHORAX

Decortication of the lung is necessary to ensure full re-expansion of the lung.

SPONTANEOUS HAEMOPNEUMOTHORAX

Sometimes a pneumothorax is associated with a marked haemothorax from tearing of an adhesion. The treatment is usually by operation (see Haemothorax, paragraphs 2 and 3 p. 322).

TUBERCULOSIS

Appraise

1. Operations for thoracic disease are seldom performed as the current indications for surgery are limited.

2. Disease due to drug resistant organisms may demand resection of cavitated disease. Occasionally thoracoplasty is chosen as the safer procedure. The most effective second line chemotherapy is used to cover the operation and post operative period.

3. Elective operations are occasionally undertaken for patients with special social or environmental problems to reduce or stop their drug treatment, for example, emigrants to countries requiring a clear X-ray, patients in the Forces or patients who fail to take their drugs regularly. Localised pulmonary resection by segmental resection or lobectomy combined with drug treatment is indicated.

4. Diagnostic operations are chiefly undertaken when the chest X-ray shows a single peripheral lesion of which carcinoma is the most common cause.

5. Rupture of a tuberculous cavity in to the pleural space is a rare but potentially lethal complication.

6. Development of aspergillomata. A mycetoma develops in about 40% of patients with a residual cavity. Resection is indicated if troublesome and severe haemoptyses develop.

7. Tuberculous empyemata are treated on the general lines outlined in the section on excision of empyema and pulmonary decortication. The empyema is excised, together with the diseased portion of lung, e.g. segment, lobe, or lung, and the preserved portion of lung is decorticated.

8. Primary tuberculosis. Extensive glandular spread from the primary Ghon focus may cause bronchostenosis and secondary bronchiectasis which require pulmonary resection. Removal of the gland mass is indicated in some patients to relieve bronchial or tracheal obstruction. Sometimes the disease destroys the bronchial wall and caseous material extrudes into the lumen. Resection and bronchoplasty is required. A calcified broncholith may ulcerate into the lumen and cause obstruction with secondary infection. Appropriate resection is performed.

9. Cold abscesses of the anterior chest wall are usually due to caseous disease of the internal mammary lymphnodes and not tuberculous rib disease. Incision and curettage of the cavity is employed.

HYDATID DISEASE

This is common in New Zealand, Australia and the Middle East where sheep farming is widespread.

Appraise

1. Exclude associated liver disease by CT scanning or ultrasonography.

2. Asymptomatic pulmonary disease presents as a smooth dense spherical opacity radiologically. The indirect haemagglutination test (IHA) is more reliable than the Casoni test for confirmation.

3. Cysts may become infected and others may be expectorated sometimes in large numbers when a large mother cyst has ruptured into a bronchus. Occasionally a fistula may connect with a liver cyst through the diaphragm. The cyst wall consists of a germinal layer inside a gelatinous

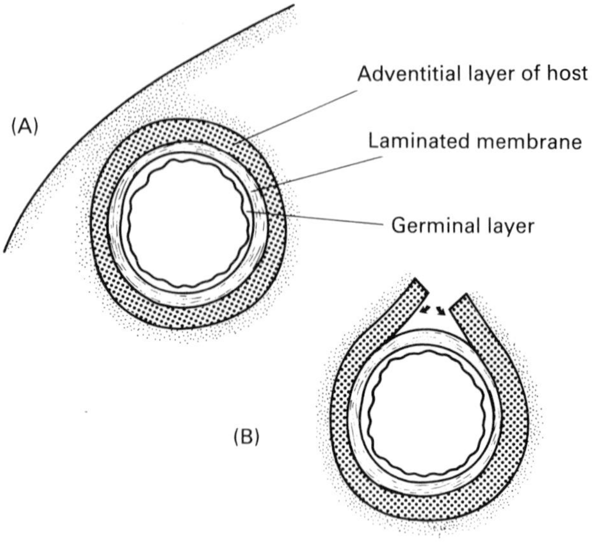

Fig. 19.18 Hydatid cyst of lung.

white laminated membrane and is surrounded by the adventitial layer of the host (Fig. 19.18).

UNCOMPLICATED CYSTS

Action

1. At thoracotomy, incise the overlying visceral pleura to expose the cyst. Incise the adventitia and separate the adventitial and laminated layers using gentle blunt dissection. Gentle lung inflation aids delivery of the cyst.

2. Pack the surrounding area with formalin soaked swabs in case the cyst ruptures.

3. Aspirate some of the fluid using a fine needle and inject formalin or hypertonic saline solution if the cyst is large and likely to rupture.

4. Suture the tiny bronchial holes usually present at the base of the cavity which is then obliterated with pursestring sutures in the lung.

INFECTED OR COMPLICATED CYSTS

These require the minimal pulmonary resection possible, i.e. segmental resection or lobectomy. Occasionally if extensive disease is present, a pleuropneumonectomy is required.

Further reading

Aletras H A 1968 Hydatid disease of the lung. Scandinavian Journal of Thoracic and Cardiovascular Surgery 2: 218–224
Blalock A, Mason M F, Morgan H J, Riven S S 1939 Myasthenia Gravis and Tumours of the Thymic Region. Report of a case in which the tumour was removed. Annals of Surgery 110: 544–560
Carden E 1978 Recent improvements in techniques for general anaesthesia for bronchoscopy. Chest (Suppl 5) 73: 697–700
Carlens E 1959 Mediastinoscopy. Diseases of the Chest 36: 343–352

Clagett O T, Eaton L M, Glover R P 1949 Thymectomy for myasthenia gravis. Surgery 26: 852–860

Clagett O T, Geraci J E 1963 A procedure for the management of postpneumonectomy empyema. Journal of Thoracic and Cardiovascular Surgery 45: 141–145

Cooper J D, Nelems J M, Pearson F G 1978 Extended indications for median sternotomy in patients requiring pulmonary resection. Annals of Thoracic Surgery 26: 413–420

Dorman J P, Campbell D, Grover F L, Trinkle J K 1973 Open thoracostomy drainage of postpneumonectomy empyema with bronchopleural fistula. Journal of Thoracic and Cardiovascular Surgery 66: 979–981

Evans D S, Hall J H, Harrison G K 1973 Anterior mediastinotomy. Thorax 28: 444–447

Keynes G 1955 Investigation into thymic disease and tumour formations. British Journal of Surgery 42: 449–462

McNeill T M, Chamberlain J M 1966 Diagnostic anterior mediastinotomy. Annals of Thoracic Surgery 2: 532–539

Saidi F 1976 Surgery of hydatid disease. W B Saunders Co, Philadelphia

Sanders R D 1967 Two ventilating attachments for bronchoscopes. Delaware Medical Journal 39: 170–175

Seremetis M G 1970 The management of spontaneous pneumothorax. Chest 57: 65–68

Shackford S R, Virgilio R W, Peters R M 1981 Selective use of ventilator therapy in flail chest injury. Journal of Thoracic and Cardiovascular Surgery 81: 194–201

Takita H, Merrin C, Podolkar M S, Douglass H O, Edgerton F 1977 The surgical management of multiple lung metastases. Annals of Thoracic Surgery 24: 359–364

Trinkle J K, Marcos J, Grover F L, Cuello L M 1974 Management of the wounded heart. Annals of Thoracic Surgery 17: 230–236

Surgery of the breast

BREAST ABSCESS

ACUTE LACTATIONAL ABSCESS

Appraise

1. Breast abscess develops most commonly during lactation, though it may occasionally be associated with trauma in a non-lactational patient. Empty the affected breast by manual pressure but permit the child to continue feeding on the opposite breast.

2. Examine the breasts daily. Do not wait for fluctuation, as widespread destruction of the underlying breast tissue may then be found. Ascertain pre-operatively the point of maximum tenderness and mark the point with a skin pencil. As soon as there is such a point, the time is ripe for operative intervention.

3. Antibiotic therapy complicates the clinical picture, in that the abscess is walled-in and may present less acutely.

Access

Operate under general anaesthesia with the patient lying on her back and with the arm on the affected side stretched on an arm board. Do not allow traction on the brachial plexus. The arm should not be above a right angle, and the hand and forearm should be supine.

Action

1. Place the incision over the point of maximum tenderness. If this is near the nipple where the 12–15 major ducts are lying, make a radial incision. If you make a deep periareolar incision in a young woman, you may damage many of the ducts and cause problems in later pregnancies.

2. If pus does not at once pour out, deepen the incision or introduce a syringe with a wide-bore needle attached at varying angles until you obtain pus. Send some pus for culture and antibiotic sensitivities. If necessary, you can later give the appropriate antibiotic.

3. Introduce a gloved finger into the abscess cavity and break down all loculi in the breast tissue by moving the finger in a circular manner. This manoeuvre is necessary since the abscess may be multiloculated.

4. If the cavity allows, introduce a retractor and examine the walls. Stop any bleeding points with diathermy.

5. If there is any possibility of the condition being a carcinoma of pregnancy instead of the expected abscess, then take an adequate biopsy of the cavity wall and send it for histological examination.

6. Ensure that the original incision is long enough to allow the wound to heal from the deepest parts upwards, otherwise there is a risk of the development of a chronic abscess.

7. Drain the cavity from its most dependent part.

8. Apply a dressing such as elastic strapping, provided the patient is not allergic to it. This supports the breast(s) and renders the patient more comfortable. It also diminishes the risk of subsequent development of a haematoma.

RETROMAMMARY ABSCESS

Appraise

Check that this is purely a retromammary abscess clinically and not an abscess which has ruptured through the posterior sheath of the breast. More commonly, although it is rare, it has formed in this deep position as a result of trauma to the chest wall, causing a haematoma which has become infected. Even more rarely nowadays, an empyema of the lung may rupture through the anterior chest wall.

Action

1. Make an incision along the inframammary fold.
2. Insert long sinus forceps until they reach the abscess cavity.
3. Take a specimen of pus for culture and sensitivities to antibiotics.
4. Make sure the abscess is widely opened and fully drained.
5. Drain the cavity to ensure healing from within out.

PLASMA CELL MASTITIS AND MAMILLARY DUCT FISTULA

Appraise

1. In any women developing the signs and symptoms of inflammation of the breast outside lactation or the puerperium, suspect either plasma cell (periductal) mastitis, or less commonly, inflammatory carcinoma of the breast. Plasma cell mastitis is associated with duct ectasia, as a result of which, intraductal lipid material is extravasated through the duct wall into the periductal tissues producing a subacute chemical inflammation. The condition is characteristically of sudden and relatively painless onset. In most cases it resolves spontaneously over 1–2 weeks without active intervention.
2. When there is any doubt as to the diagnosis do not fail to take a biopsy.
3. Occasionally, liquefaction occurs within the area of inflammation, and pus may then discharge spontaneously at the areolar margin. A mammillary duct fistula ensues between the skin surface and one of the terminal lactiferous ducts.
4. If the woman is post-menopausal with recurrent episodes of plasma cell mastitis, and recurrent mamillary duct fistulae, then Hadfield's operation is indicated (see below).
5. Treat a solitary mamillary duct fistula by fistulectomy.

Action

1. Pass a probe through the fistula at the areolar margin and push it out through the duct in the nipple.
2. Incise the skin across the nipple and areola onto the probe.
3. Excise the fistulous track and all granulation tissue.
4. Ensure adequate haemastasis, then pack the wound and leave it to heal by second intention.

NIPPLE DISCHARGE AND BLEEDING

Appraise

1. If the nipple discharge is serous, sero-sanguineous, or frank blood arising from a solitary duct, then manage as below.
2. Test for blood, unilateral or bilateral discharge from multiple ducts. If positive, then the whole duct system needs to be explored for a possible underlying cancer, using Hadfield's procedure. This operation can also be used when a woman is embarrassed by the volume of discharge staining her underclothes in cases of severe duct ectasia.

Action

1. Make a circumareolar incision not extending more than three-fifths around the circumference of the areola, but including the orifice of any sinus or fistula.
2. Cut the subcutaneous tissue down to the duct system.
3. Use blunt dissection to dissect in the plane circumferentially around the terminal lactiferous ducts, just deep to the areola and nipple.
4. Divide the ducts close to the nipple and remove them with a conical wedge of tissue including the distal 1–2 cm of the sub-areolar tissue, which includes the major lactiferous ducts and sinuses.
5. Send equivocal tissue for frozen section examination.
6. Insert a small vacuum drain and close the wound with 3/0 subcuticular Dexon sutures.

NIPPLE BLEEDING

Appraise

1. When first seen, press at different points round the areola between finger and thumb, and mark on a diagram the exact position of the duct from which blood is obtained (Fig. 20.1)
2. If there is no bleeding at the time, ask the patient to return when the nipple is bleeding so you may localize the affected area.
3. If possible take a smear of the blood for cytological examination, as papilloma or carcinoma cells may be demonstrated.
4. Unless the bleeding occurs during pregnancy (when it is frequently bilateral and stops spontaneously after parturition), this symptom requires surgical exploration.

Prepare

1. Mark the site of the affected duct on a diagram.
2. Discuss the operation and the possible implications with the patient.

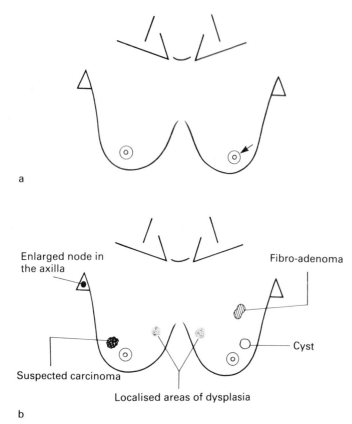

Fig. 20.1 (a) Routine breast stamp used to indicate position of a breast lesion. The arrow shows a suspected duct at 2 o'clock. (b) Methods of marking on the breast stamp where lesions appear clinically.

3. Mark the site and side of the lesion on the patient herself with a skin pencil before the operation.

Access

1. If the discharge can be obtained on the table, attempt to introduce a probe into the affected duct.

2. Pick up the nipple between finger and thumb and you may feel thickening along one duct, or you can feel the probe as it travels along the duct.

Action

1. Make a radial incision to expose the duct and continue until you reach the papilloma or intraduct lesion causing the bleeding; you can usually find this quite easily.

2. Excise the duct and a small amount of surrounding breast tissue. Send for frozen or paraffin section as deemed necessary.

3. Obtain haemostasis.

4. If no other lesion is palpable, close the incision. Drainage is not usually required.

BREAST BIOPSY

Appraise

1. Before describing operative techniques for breast lumps it is important to have a scheme of management in mind for patients presenting with a complaint of a breast lump to the clinic. Figure 20.2 illustrates a scheme that would be widely acceptable in most surgical clinics.

2. At the first stage you must make up your mind whether or not a truly discrete lump is present. If, after careful examination, you cannot detect a lump or a diffuse nodularity, then re-examine a younger woman at a different point in the menstrual cycle and re-assure her.

3. Refer women over the age of 30 if repeat examination is negative, for mammography, if available, to complement clinical examination of the 'difficult' breast.

4. By contrast, if a discrete lump is detected, it is almost always worthwhile to attempt aspiration.

5. Breast cysts can occur at any age but are common in the 35–55 age range. Drainage of the cyst in most cases establishes the diagnosis, 'cures' the condition, and offers immediate re-assurance to the patient. It is therefore both efficient and humane. It must be emphasized, however, if the fluid from the cyst is bloody, or if there is a residual lump, then you should perform excision biopsy. Cytology of the cyst fluid is no longer considered a worthwhile procedure.

6. If the discrete lump is solid, then admit the young lady with the clinically obvious fibroadenoma for excision biopsy (see below.)

7. Carry out excision biopsy of a small lump of uncertain diagnosis on the first convenient operating list.

8. Solid lumps more than 2 cm in size should be subjected to an out-patient Tru-cut needle biopsy under local anaesthesia. As there are no false-positives using this technique, a diagnosis of cancer enables one to speak frankly with the patient and to prepare her for mastectomy on the first convenient list. Again it must be emphasized that a negative biopsy does not exclude cancer and the patient will need to be admitted for excision biopsy to establish a firm diagnosis.

9. Frozen section. Until recent years, the convention for the management of a breast lump was to admit the patient, request permission to proceed to mastectomy, establish a diagnosis by excision and frozen section histology of the suspicious lump, and perform mastectomy if cancer was confirmed. Many surgeons now consider such a process insensitive as well as inefficient, and the number of cases on operating lists labelled, 'Frozen section? proceed' is declining. There is still a place for such a strategem when the lump is clinically suspicious of cancer and mammography is equivocal and where you have failed to achieve an adequate Tru-cut biopsy. These instances should continue to diminish as more and more centres

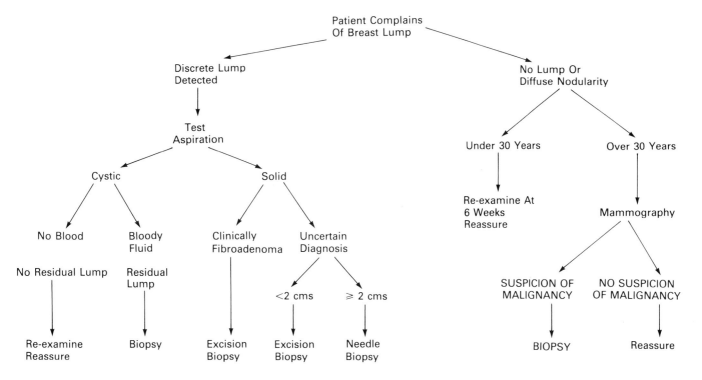

Fig. 20.2 Scheme of management for patients presenting with complaint of breast lump.

become confident with aspiration cystology as a way of establishing a pre-operative diagnosis.

ASPIRATION CYTOLOGY

Aspiration cytology for outpatient diagnosis has the advantage of being applicable for the smallest of breast lumps and requiring the minimum of special equipment. It has the disadvantage of requiring the special skills of an experienced cytologist and these are few and far between. Furthermore, it has been judged that before a diagnosis of cancer can be made with sufficient confidence to recommend mastectomy, experience with over 200 cases of cancer is required. This notwithstanding, many clinicians find the increased suspicion from a 'positive' smear useful in preparing the patient and planning operation lists. As the technique used varies widely with different centres and cannot be described as an 'operation', refer to the section on 'Further reading'.

'TRUCUT' NEEDLE BIOPSY (see Fig. 20.3)

Action

1. Infiltrate the skin over the lump with 1% lignocaine and introduce the needle into the breast, injecting the local anaesthetic deep into the breast tissue until it is judged to have entered the tumour.

2. Make a small nick in the skin with the tip of a sharp pointed scalpel.

3. Fix the tumour yourself or have an assistant fix the tumour within the breast between finger and thumb, to provide a static target.

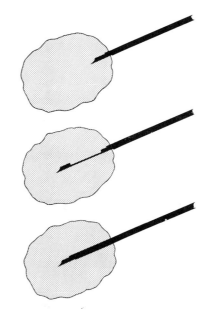

Fig. 20.3 Trucut needle

4. Push the needle in its closed position, through the skin incision until the edge of the tumour is encountered. Advance the inner needle until it is judged to have entered the main tumour mass.

5. Advance the outer sheath of the cutting needle over the inner needle, which is steadied in position, until the closed position of the assembly is re-established.

6. Remove the whole needle and open it to reveal a core of tissue measuring 2×0.1 cm.

7. If no adequate core of tissue is obtained, repeat the manoeuvre once.

EXCISION BIOPSY

Prepare

1. Check the patient's haemoglobin level.

2. Have a sickle test done if the patient is coloured.

3. Did you check that the lesion was still present on admission? Occasionally lesions disappear. Did you check, also, that no new lesion has appeared in either breast?

4. Mark the exact site of the lesion on the breast with the patient lying in the position she will be on the operating table. Otherwise you may be unable to find the mass once the patient has been anaesthetized.

5. Always check you have the right patient in the anaesthetic room and are operating on the correct side. You are responsible for taking every possible safety measure on each patient on whom you operate, to avoid later distress and possible litigation through carelessness.

Access (Fig. 20.4)

1. Incise over the region of the lump. Adequate excision of the lesion is the first priority, but secondly comes the placement of the incision in the most aesthetic position. If possible, place the scar where it will be invisible when the patient is wearing a brassiere.

2. Incisions in the medial half of the breast are more likely to develop keloid scars, but this is of secondary importance to adequate excision.

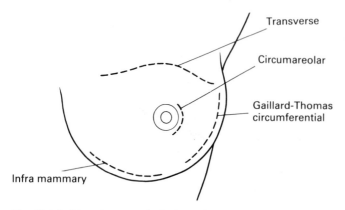

Fig. 20.4 Incisions for removal of a lump from the left breast.

3. Periareolar incisions heal with least visible scars, but may not always be suitable.

4. Avoid radial incision whenever possible.

5. Always make your incision for local excision within the area of skin which will be removed if you proceed to mastectomy at a later date, so that no unnecessary scar is added to the mastectomy scar.

Action

1. Excise the lump completely without cutting into it. Use sharp dissection with scissors or knife.

2. Cut the specimen to see if you can identify a benign or malignant condition. This improves your own diagnostic expertise. A benign lesion is encapsulated, and when cut in half the cut surface is convex. If a knife is drawn across the cut surface of a carcinoma there is a 'gritty' feeling and sound, as though the knife were scratching small pieces of calcium. A benign lesion does not 'extend' into the surrounding tissues. A cancer sometimes exudes a juice when squeezed. You cannot of course, diagnose an in situ carcinoma of the duct with the naked eye.

3. Discard the scalpel blade in case you have incised through malignant tissue.

4. Introduce a finger into the cavity and place your thumb on the overlying skin. Move your thumb radially through 360° so you can feel the breast tissue between finger and thumb to see if there is any more abnormal tissue which should be removed.

5. In mammary duct ectasia, a toothpaste-like substance may issue from numerous ducts. Sometimes it is impossible to remove all the affected tissue unless a simple mastectomy is performed. Under these circumstances, remove the most severely affected tissue.

6. Be obsessional about haemostasis.

Closure

1. Always drain the wound following breast excision. Haematoma formation is lessened and the possibility of development of infection from the haematoma is also reduced. Large cavities are best drained with a 'Redi Vac' vacuum system whilst small cavities are conveniently drained with a test tube 'Mini flap' system.

2. To achieve a good cosmetic result give as much thought to the manner of closure as to the position of the incision. Wherever possible use subcuticular sutures. For short incisions, I favour 3/0 Dexon, and for longer incision 3/0 Prolene on a straight cutting needle. The ends of the sutures can be knotted or held in place with a lead shot. Circumareolar incisions always heal well with an almost invisible scar, so 3/0 interrupted black silk sutures can be used.

CARCINOMA

Assure

If mastectomy is necessary, reassure the patient about the availability of a prosthesis. Tell her that it will be the same weight as her breast, changing shape with her own position and taking on body temperature, and it will thus be almost impossible to tell which breast is the natural one when she is fully dressed. This reassurance of the patient is a very important part of the operation.

Appraise

If invasive cancer is reported, be prepared to follow one of the accepted methods of treatment.

1. Wide excision plus radiotherapy; performed in some centres.
2. Simple mastectomy, plus node biopsy when necessary.
3. Simple mastectomy, plus removal of the pectoralis minor to dissect the axillary nodes (Patey's operation, see p. 336). It is not essential to remove this muscle in order to explore the axilla.
4. Radical mastectomy. This involves removal of the breast plus muscles and nodes.
5. Subcutaneous mastectomy with immediate implant: increasing numbers of surgeons are exploring the role of a silicone implant following a very conservative simple mastectomy or a subcutaneous mastectomy preserving the nipple. Implanting the prosthesis can cause problems, and most clinicians prefer to implant it in the sub-pectoral plane, stitching down the lateral edge of the pectoralis major muscle to retain the prosthesis in a good position. This procedure is also of value in the management of extensive intraduct carcinoma, or the rare sarcoma. Great uncertainty remains concerning the relevance of this procedure (immediate versus delayed) and the best technique to use. It is my view therefore that reconstructive procedures should be left to the specialists and not be undertaken by general surgeons.

PAGET'S DISEASE

When this disease is suspected, take a biopsy of the nipple area under local anaesthesia to prove the diagnosis histologically. When Paget cells are demonstrated histologically, there is always an underlying intraduct carcinoma which is invasive in approximately 50% of cases. Mastectomy may therefore be required.

LUMPECTOMY (TYLECTOMY)

1. Excise the cancer as for wide local excision of a breast lump.

2. Close the cavity with drainage as described under breast lumps.
3. Arrange for the radiotherapist to see and treat the breast and nodal drainage. In ideal circumstances, surgeon and radiotherapist should consult together before surgery is performed.

SIMPLE MASTECTOMY

Prepare

1. Check the side of the lesion is correct.
2. If you think it advisable, have crossmatched blood available in the theatre for transfusion. This is rarely required if the surgery is gentle and the bleeding points are caught as the operation proceeds.

Access

1. Place the patient on the table lying on her back, with the arm on the operative side extended on an arm board, and the forearm supine.
2. Clean the skin with a suitable preparation such as 10% povidone-iodine or chlorhexidine in spirit.
3. Place the incision transversely if possible (Fig. 20.5) and encompass approximately 5 cm of skin round the lesion and also the nipple. If the lesion is in such a position as to make transverse incision impracticable, then make an oblique incision — but there is no need to take it up as far as the clavicle, and certainly not across the axilla or down the arm (this type of scar is still seen on elderly patients who have had a mastectomy many years ago, and is mutilating both physically and psychologically).

Action

1. Elevate the skin flaps so they include the subcutaneous fat. This dissection can be facilitated by subcutaneous infiltration with 1 : 400 000 adrenaline in saline.

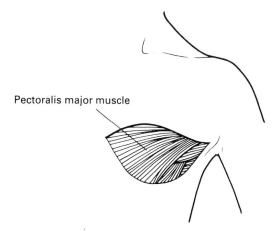

Pectoralis major muscle

Fig. 20.5 Simple mastectomy

2. Have your assistant hold up the skin flaps with an abdominal pack as you make them. This causes the least trauma to the skin. The assistant should also tell you if you are making a flap too thin, which might cause 'button-holding' of the skin. Check this yourself after every few sweeps of the scalpel.

3. Raise the upper flap to the upper limit of the breast. This is usually 2–3 cm below the clavicle but the level varies from patient to patient.

4. Do not allow traumatizing tissue forceps to be placed on the skin flaps but apply Allis forceps to the rolled back edges of the skin if necessary .

5. Catch any bleeding points with fine forceps. Tie these with fine plain catgut or diathermize them. Take care not to burn the skin itself by contact with the diathermy needle. If this does inadvertently happen, cut away the burnt area, bevelling it off so it will not be demonstrable later (Fig. 20.6). Burnt skin takes many weeks to heal and is painful.

6. Raise the lower flap in a similar manner to the lower limits of the breast.

7. Place a large tissue forceps, such as Lane's, on the breast which is to be removed, handing it to an assistant to hold, thus facilitating the subsequent dissection.

8. Return to the uppermost part of the breast and dissect down until you see the fascia of pectoralis major. Introduce a finger covered by a swab and find a plane of cleavage between the fascia and the breast.

9. Proceed in a downward direction. You can see the main blood vessels as they enter or leave the fascia. Catch and tie them before cutting them so they do not actually bleed. This reduces the amount of operative bleeding considerably. It also saves clipping and tying each perforating vessel three times — as it pierces the fascia, the muscle and at the subcutaneous level.

10. Continue downwards, elevating the breast alternatively laterally and medially, until you reach the lower limits.

11. Remove the breast and send it for further histological examination.

12. Obtain haemostasis. Tie or diathermize the bleeding points.

Closure

1. Approximate the skin edges. Introduce sutures half-way along the incision, then half-way between these

lengths. Thus you will not end up with 'dog ears' which might happen if you start suturing at one end of the incision and work to the other end.

2. Leave in two vacuum drains at the medial and the axillary ends of the incision.

3. Rarely you may have to use a split skin graft if the wound edges cannot be opposed without tension. If so, the surgery has probably been too radical or the case selection inappropriate.

4. After suturing is complete and the wound is sealed, activate the vacuum drains and squeeze out all the fluid and air from beneath the skin flaps so that they adhere to the chest wall. Failure to do this leads to the development of a seroma postoperatively.

5. If skin tension is not excessive a better cosmetic result can be achieved with subcuticular 3/0 prolene.

PATEY MASTECTOMY

In this modification of a simple mastectomy, the pectoralis minor muscle is removed. It is dissected from the coracoid process which can be felt just inferior to the clavicle and then it is dissected from its insertion to the ribs (see Fig. 20.7). In any of the above operations where the tumour is attached to the pectoralis major muscle, a portion of this muscle should be removed with the original excision biopsy or at the time of the mastectomy.

Access

1. Position the patient as for a simple mastectomy. Prepare and towel the upper arm on the ipsilateral side so

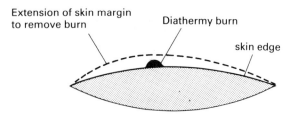

Fig. 20.6 Removal of accidental diathermy burn

Extension of skin margin to remove burn
Diathermy burn
skin edge

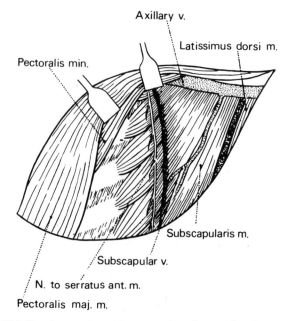

Axillary v.
Latissimus dorsi m.
Pectoralis min.
Subscapularis m.
Subscapular v.
N. to serratus ant. m.
Pectoralis maj. m.

Fig. 20.7 Patey's operation with preservation of pectoralis minor

that it may be flexed and abducted during the operation.

2. Make a transverse elliptical incision and perform total mastectomy, but leave the breast still attached to the axillary contents.

Action

1. Identify the lateral border of the pectoralis major throughout its length by sharp dissection. Have it retracted upwards by an assistant.

2. Facilitate exposure of the subpectoral area by flexing and abducting the shoulder and flexing the elbow so that the forearm lies across the patient's towelled-off face, where it may be supported by the assistant or slung from the cross bar of the anaesthetist's drape support.

3. Separate the acromio-thoracic trunk from the medial border of pectoralis minor muscle by blunt dissection. Clearly define both borders of the muscle using dissecting scissors. Pass a finger under the insertion of the pectoralis minor muscle to protect the underlying structure, and separate the muscle from its insertion into the coracoid process by cutting diathermy.

4. Define the upper limits of the axillary dissection by identifying the axillary vein as it crosses the first rib. This is most safely achieved by blunt dissection using a Lahey 'peanut' swab. Identify the inferior border of the axillary vein along its whole length. Control all vessels passing from its inferior surface into the axillary contents by surgical clips or fine silk ligatures. Make no attempt to clear the structures above the vein.

5. 'Stroke' the axillary contents away from the chest wall and off the subscapularis muscle using a gauze swab wrapped round the finger. Take care to identify and avoid the long thoracic nerve to serratus anterior which is closely applied to the chest wall at the posterior-medial limit of the dissection and the nerve to latissimus dorsi as it runs with the vascular pedicle to subscapularis.

6. Remove the axillary contents, pectoralis minor muscle and breast en bloc, sacrificing the intercosto-brachial nerve as it runs across the mid-axillary region. Ligate and divide any residual vessels arising from the intercostal arteries and veins supplying the insertion of pectoralis minor muscle and the inferolateral portions of the breast disc.

Closure

1. Close as for the simple mastectomy. Insert one vacuum drain for the flaps and a second draining the axilla. Most recently, I have discovered that a subcuticular Prolene suture on a straight cutting needle gives the best cosmetic results.

2. It is your responsibility to supervise the dressing of the wound and in particular, to squeeze out all blood and air from under the flaps into the vacuum containers in order to avoid the subsequent development of a seroma.

RADICAL MASTECTOMY

Appraise

1. This procedure is now rarely used in the United Kingdom, as most surgeons believe that an adequate clearance of cancer within the breast and axillary nodes can be achieved by Patey's modified radical mastectomy.

2. The following procedure is described in some detail, however, both for historical reasons and for the occasional case where the operation is indicated for local control of a relatively advanced cancer that has become resistant to treatment with radiotherapy, or systemic therapy.

Access

1. Make the incision (Fig. 20.8) encompassing the excision line which has been suitably placed, the nipple and 5 cm. of skin overlying the tumour. The incision is thus elliptical. It is sometimes possible to make the incision transversely, which is aesthetically preferable.

2. Make sure you can reach the upper part of the rectus abdominis muscle, the midline of the sternum, the insertion of the pectoralis muscle, the clavicle, and the anterior border of the latissimus dorsi muscle.

Action

1. Raise the skin flaps in turn and protect them with abdominal packs, dissecting half the subcutaneous fat with the flaps as for a simple mastectomy. The medial flap extends 1 cm. beyond the midline and the lateral flap to the anterior border of the latissimus dorsi muscle in the posterior axillary line.

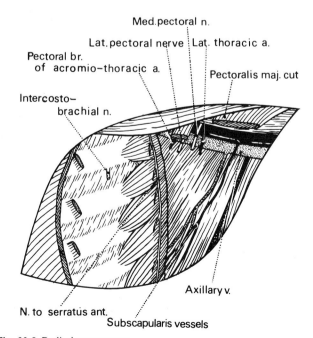

Fig. 20.8 Radical mastectomy

2. Expose the upper part of the pectoralis major muscle and separate the sternal from the clavicular heads with the blunt end of a scalpel handle.

3. Expose and ligate the acromiothoracic vessels as they are thus exposed.

4. Pass your index finger round the tendon of the sternal portion of the pectoral major muscle while your assistant retracts the lateral skin flap, so you can cut the tendinous insertion as near as possible to the bicipital groove of the humerus. This exposes the pectoralis minor muscle lying deep to the major muscle.

5. Cut the pectoralis minor tendon close to the coracoid process. The axilla is now exposed.

6. By careful swab dissection, clean the axillary vessels from the apex laterally and downwards, taking all the fat, lymph nodes and fascia. Divide the lateral thoracic vessels and the intercostobrachial nerve. Avoid damaging the main vessels and brachial plexus branches. Palpate and visualise the long thoracic nerve of Bell on the lateral chest wall, and carefully avoid it. Clean the subscapularis muscle on the posterior axillary wall. The first digitation of serratus anterior muscle marks the extent of the medial clearance.

7. Dissect the whole mass downwards while the assistant clips the branches of the internal mammary vessels as they pierce the intercostal membrane and enter the pectoral muscles.

8. Apply the artery forceps in a plane parallel to the chest wall, not vertically, because it is possible to penetrate the pleural cavity and produce a pneumothorax. Dissect the tissues to just beyond the midline, down to the uppermost fibres of the rectus abdominis muscle, and laterally to the anterior margin of the latissimus dorsi muscle.

9. The complete specimen is now free. Send it for histological examination.

10. Secure haemostatis.

Closure

1. Close the skin flaps as previously described on page 336 for simple mastectomy, to avoid leaving 'dog ears'.

2. If the flaps will not approximate without tension with the arm abducted, take a split skin graft (see. p. 540) from the previously prepared site in the thigh. First estimate the size of the deficit after apposing the wound edges with sutures so far as is easily possible without producing tension. Cut a gauze swab the size of the deficit and have it available when taking the graft as this helps to tell when you have cut an adequate strip. Use fresh gowns, gloves and instruments to take this graft. Apply dressings and bandages to cover the graft area completely before returning to the main operation site.

3. Place the graft on petroleum jelly gauze (skin surface next to the gauze) and gently stretch it to its full size. Turn it upside down over the area to be grafted so the epithelial surface is now in the normal external position, and suture it in position with interrupted skin sutures, leaving one of the ends of each suture long. Each of these will be tied to its opposite number over a wad of paraffin gauze at the completion of the operation.

5. Leave suction drains to the axillary region and to the central portion of the wound and proceed as described for simple mastectomy.

AFTERCARE

1. Supplying and arranging the fitting of a breast prosthesis for the patient is really within the operation manifesto. Artificial breasts are now available which are of a weight and consistency comparable with the removed breast. They change shape with the patient's change of posture and they take on body temperature. It is almost impossible to tell which is the side of the mastectomy when feeling through a patient's clothes, and this is of very great importance to her as a woman. She can buy clothes as anyone else does, and also wear swimsuits and evening dresses without calling attention to her deficiency. Make yourself aware of the range and variety available. In the United Kingdom, under Health Service regulations, any women is entitled to the type and size of prosthesis of her choice. In addition these may be replaced as frequently as necessary. If you are not willing to learn of the variety available, then at least approach the Appliance Officer at an early stage in your career to delegate this responsibility. Some centres now employ mastectomy counsellors who, as well as providing psycho-social support, are also responsible for the physical rehabilitation of the patient. This includes the prescription of a soft temporary prosthesis immediately postoperatively, which can be worn for about 6 weeks until the wound is no longer sore, and then replaced by the permanent prosthesis worn within the brassiere.

2. Finally, no woman should be allowed to leave hospital with a stiff shoulder following mastectomy. Commence active physiotherapy on about the fifth postoperative day and provide the patient with a list of exercises fo abduction of the arm. Encourage her to brush her hair and fasten the back of her dress. Premature or over-enthusiastic physiotherapy may provoke the development of a seroma.

DEVELOPMENTAL ABNORMALITIES

Appraise

1. Mastitis neonatorum occurs in the first few days of life, is associated with maternal hormones, and subsides

spontaneously. Rarely, infection supervenes, requiring surgical drainage.

2. Extra or supernumerary breasts are encountered along the nipple line from midclavicular region to groin. Do not intervene unless they become involved with a disease process such as may affect normal breast tissue. Lactation may occur with pregnancy, and carcinoma occasionally arises in a supernumerary breast. Treatment is as for any breast disease.

3. With the onset of puberty, one breast disc may enlarge in a young girl, from the age of 8 onwards. Do not excise this thinking it is a neoplasm for this is almost unknown before the age of 12. See the child again in 2 months and usually the other breast disc has begun to enlarge. Reassure the mother and child. If the disc is excised, no breast will develop on this side of the body, if biopsied the developed breast may be deformed.

GYNAECOMASTIA

Appraise

1. This is frequently unilateral and may occur in boys and young men, either following minor trauma or spontaneously. It usually settles without treatment.

2. If it does not settle, excise the breast disc on one or both sides, as indicated. The whole breast disc can be excised through a periareolar incision without leaving a noticeable scar.

3. Gynaecomastia also occurs in old age associated with drugs given for hypertension or congestive cardiac failure. Less frequently nowadays it is seen in men treated with high doses of oestrogens for prostatic cancer and rarely amongst men suffering from alcoholic cirrhosis. Occasionally subcutaneous mastectomy is indicated if the condition is an embarrassment or causing pain and tenderness.

Further reading

Adair F E 1974 Cancer 33:1145
Azzopardi J C 1979 Problems in breast pathology. Saunders, London.
Baum M 1980 Carcinoma of the breast. In: Selwyn Taylor (ed) Recent advances in surgery 10. Churchill Livingstone, Edinburgh p. 241
Baum M 1976 The curability of breast cancer. British Medical Journal 1:439
Editorial 1976 Management of early cancer of the breast. British Medical Journal 1:1035
Editorial 1976 Benign proliferative lesions of the breast. British Medical Journal 1:1106

Editorial 1976 Hormone receptors and breast cancer. British Medical Journal 3:67
Editorial 1976 Treating breast cancer — true light or false dawn? British Medical Journal 3:263
George P 1974 Swellings of the breast. Practitioner 212:199
Taylor H B, Norris H J 1967 Cancer 20:2245
Thomas W G, Williamson R C N, Davies J D et al 1982 The clinical syndrome of mammary duct ectasia. British Journal of Surgery
Trott P A 1983 Cytological investigation. In: C. A. Parsons (ed) Diagnosis of breast disease. Chapman and Hall, London. p. 203–213

Surgery of the thyroid and parathyroid glands

General considerations
Biopsy of the thyroid
Exploration of the thyroid
Thyroidectomy
Parathyroid reimplantation
Parathyroidectomy
Thyroglossal cyst

GENERAL CONSIDERATIONS

1. It is common knowledge that many operations are performed on the thyroid gland for other than endocrine disturbances, but it is convenient to consider the total range of thyroid surgery here. The surgical management of thyroglossal cyst and fistula is also included.

2. Many general surgeons wish to undertake the investigation of thyroid problems and perform thyroidectomy; a minority are dealt with by laryngologists and head and neck specialists. Parathyroidectomy is a special case. It can be a difficult and tedious procedure, so is best delegated to general surgeons with a special interest in endocrine disease.

3. For toxic goitre and hyperparathyroidism, close clinical association with an endocrine physician is essential. Expertise can work in both directions. Not only will the physician present patients properly prepared but, with the surgeon's help, he may avoid clinical disasters in problem goitres which are unsuitable for medical treatment.

4. Head and neck surgery is best suited to surgeons who enjoy careful anatomical dissection and are able to handle the tissues, especially fine nerves, with gentleness. For parathyroid exploration, visual acuity is critical and some surgeons employ magnifying spectacles. The surgical approach for thyroidectomy and parathyroid exploration is very similar; it is occasionally necessary to perform partial thyroidectomy in the course of seeking a parathyroid adenoma.

5. Since exploration of the neck follows a similar pattern in most thyroid (and parathyroid) operations, this procedure will be described in detail before the various types of resection are considered. Closure and aftercare are similar after most of these operations.

6. It is a sensible routine to request a laryngologist to check the mobility of the vocal cords by indirect laryngoscopy before and after any operation on the thyroid gland.

BIOPSY OF THE THYROID

PRE-OPERATIVE BIOPSY

1. In the preliminary assessment of goitres, this technique can provide invaluable information especially in the identification of 'cold' lesions on isotope scanning, such as a cyst or tumour, and the differentiation between follicular adenoma and carcinoma. Lymphocytic thyroiditis in nodular or generalised form can also be recognised.

2. Needle biopsy involves three alternatives: drill biopsy and a large cutting needle (e.g. Tru-cut) obtain histological material, whereas fine needle aspiration biopsy obtains cytological material. The large needle techniques require local anaesthesia.

3. Take the biopsy from the most prominent or significant part of the goitre. Sit the patient on a couch with the neck slightly extended, so that puncture may be made directly into the goitre either anteriorly, or laterally through the sternomastoid. It may be necessary to biopsy more than one site.

4. After withdrawing the needle, apply firm pressure over the puncture site for at least 5 minutes to prevent haematoma.

5. The tissue core is fixed and sent for histological examination. With fine needle biopsy, the 'sludge' or fluid material is smeared, air-dried and stained as for bone marrow.

OPEN BIOPSY

1. General anaesthesia is required. If lymphocytic thyroiditis is suspected and other biopsy techniques are not available, then excision of the isthmus is helpful.

2. Through a short collar incision (see below), reflect the platysma and divide the deep cervical, infrahyoid and pretracheal fascias vertically in the midline to separate the strap muscles.

3. Expose the isthmus by gentle pledget dissection. Using blunt clearance with curved artery forceps, free the whole isthmus from the trachea.

4. Mark the limit of resection with artery forceps and remove the isthmus by scalpel or scissors, including the pyramidal lobe. Trim the edges of the lateral lobes so that a cosmetic inversion is possible.

5. Secure haemostasis with fine ligatures (3/0 silk) or diathermy, and suture the edges of each lobe to the tracheal fascia, using interrupted 2/0 chromic catgut stitches. Close the wound in layers (see below): drainage is unnecessary.

EXPLORATION OF THE THYROID

Access

1. Pay careful attention to the position of the patient on the operating table. The patient lies supine with a wide sandbag placed between the scapulae. The head is placed on a sponge-rubber ring, and the neck is supported with a soft cushion. A foot-piece is fixed in place, so that the head-end of the table may be raised by 20° or so.

2. After preparing the skin towel up with either a 'head set' or a four-towel 'square' placed over two large gamgee pads at the side of the neck. Secure the towels with towel clips or skin sutures. Stand initially on the right side.

3. Consider the skin incision, which should be placed transversely in a skin crease (Fig. 21.1). As a rule, site it just below the mid point between thyroid cartilage and suprasternal notch, about 3 cm above the clavicular level. However, if the goitre extends high in the neck, adjust the incision upwards. Mark the incision on the skin by pressing a 2/0 silk suture across the neck and maintaining pressure for several seconds.

4. Make the transverse cervical 'collar' incision, extending at least half way across the width of the sternomastoid muscles. Deepen the incision through fat, which is deepest close to the midline. Divide the platysma, and achieve haemostasis by diathermy coagulation.

5. Elevate the upper flap. Apply two Allis tissue forceps or skin hooks to the platysma layer and develop the plane between the platysma and deep cervical fascia. Using a scalpel with a No. 10 blade and a teasing movement, reflect the upper flap to above the thyroid cartilage in the midline. Finger gauze dissection is useful for the upper part of this

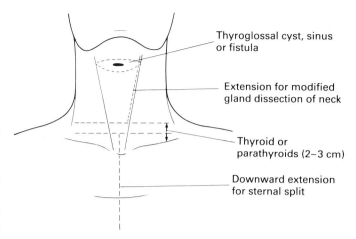

Fig. 21.1 Incisions for operations on the thyroid, parathyroids and thyroglossal lesions. The higher thyroid incision is suitable for large goitres.

freeing. Control minor arterial and venous bleeding by fine ligatures.

6. Change your position to face towards the feet. Elevate the lower flap and dissect it in an identical manner down to the suprasternal notch. Firm elevation will help to reveal the correct plane, dividing the small veins as before. If a venous ostium retracts beneath the fascia, open up this layer and secure the vessel by ligature. Because of the head-up tilt, an incised vein may bleed intermittently.

7. Place skin towels and fix a Joll's self-retaining retractor from the left-hand side, approximating towel and wound edge in the pincers of the instrument. Open the retractor, widely displacing the wound edges.

8. Define the midline and pick up the deep cervical fascia on either side with small artery forceps. Incise the fascia in the midline and separate the two sternohyoid muscles, coagulating small blood vessels in the way. Lift up the left sternohyoid muscle and gently dissect between it and the underlying sternothyroid to reach the lateral border. The nerve supply to sternothyroid from the ansa hypoglossi is now identified.

9. Lift up the medial border of the sternothyroid muscle and fully incise the infrahyoid fascia which connects it with its fellow. The sternothyroid muscle is closely applied to the surface of the thyroid gland. Deepen the dissection to incise the pretracheal fascia, and expose the surface of the thyroid gland enclosed in a thin fibrous capsule (Fig. 21.2). Thus after opening the skin and platysma, three layers of fascia must be divided vertically.

10. Using small artery forceps to lift the muscle edge, gently dissect between the sternothyroid muscle and thyroid. Small veins traverse this interval and require diathermy coagulation. Insert a retractor (Langenbeck or Joll) beneath the sternothyroid to facilitate separation of the muscle from the gland surface. At this stage decide

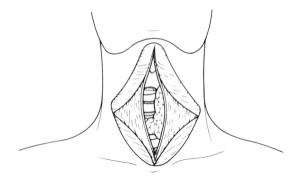

Fig. 21.2 Separation of strap muscles to expose isthmus and larynx-trachea.

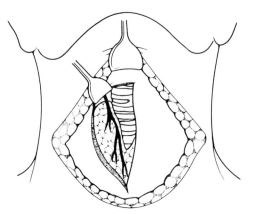

Fig. 21.3 Retraction of strap muscles to expose superior pole and blood supply.

whether you need to divide the strap muscles transversely. In most cases this step will not be necessary (Fig. 21.3).

11. If the goitre is very big, divide the 'strap' muscles on the side of the larger lobe. Identify the anterior border of sternomastoid. Insert two large Kocher's or Sawtell's artery forceps across the sternohyoid and divide the muscle between them. Run an 2/0 chromic catgut suture to each corner and fold the muscles back over the Joll's retractor, having ligated any bleeding veins. Repeat this manoeuvre for the sternothyroid muscle. Divide both muscles towards their upper end to avoid damage to the nerve supply. By retracting the muscles, exposure of the left lobe is partially achieved.

Assess

1. This important phase is greatly facilitated by pre-operative scintiscan and biopsy. If examination of the left lobe alone is inadequate to allow a clear decision regarding the appropriate operation, then change places with the first assistant and expose the right lobe.

2. A solitary nodule provides the greatest challenge in management, although the findings at operation may refute the clinical impression. Many solitary nodules prove to be the most prominent part of a multinodular goitre.

3. If a solitary nodule feels solid and the remainder of the gland appears normal, with pre-operative evidence in favour of adenoma, then perform near-total lobectomy including the isthmus. If in doubt, request frozen section examination of the lobectomy specimen. If follicular carcinoma is reported, carry out near-total removal of the opposite lobe with some form of parathyroid preservation. If the report is of benign disease or is equivocal, do no more.

4. If papillary carcinoma is suspected from preliminary nodal or gland biopsy and the operative findings confirm a solitary lesion with or without enlarged lymph nodes, proceed to near-total thyroidectomy. If pathological nodes are found in the absence of an obvious thyroid tumour, undertake the same operation.

5. The nodule may be cystic or colloid in nature, probably representing a unilateral manifestation of nodular goitre. Perform sub-total removal of the affected lobe and isthmus, taking care to excise the lesion completely. If the opposite lobe is normal leave it alone.

6. If the nodule is part of a multinodular goitre, proceed to bilateral subtotal thyroidectomy.

7. In any of the above presentations, excise any enlarged or otherwise suspicious lymph nodes.

Further reading

Wade J S H 1974 Solitary thyroid nodule. Annals of the Royal College of Surgeons in England 55: 13–20

THYROIDECTOMY

Appraise

1. Simple excision of a thyroid nodule may be appropriate in two instances: firstly if a small, less than 2 cm diameter, neoplasm is suspected in one lobe, and secondly if unilateral lobectomy has been performed for nodular colloid change and there remains a single dominant nodule in the other lobe.

2. The indications for unilateral subtotal lobectomy include adenoma or benign degenerative disease such as a cyst, or nodular goitre confined to one lobe. The isthmus should be included in the resection specimen.

3. Subtotal thyroidectomy, bilateral subtotal lobectomies, may be performed for thyrotoxicosis, multinodular goitre or Hashimoto's disease which has failed to shrink on thyroxine therapy. For thyrotoxicosis the amount of tissue preserved is critical.

4. Total or near-total thyroidectomy is performed only for malignant disease, usually primary carcinoma of the thyroid but occasionally for secondary carcinoma, lymphoma or as part of a total pharyngolaryngo-oesophagectomy. As described in the previous section, papillary or follicular carcinoma require total resection of

the affected lobe plus near-total resection of the opposite lobe to remove multicentric foci and facilitate adjuvant therapy, if needed. For medullary carcinoma of the thyroid, provided a firm diagnosis is forthcoming, it is widely accepted that total thyroidectomy with implantation of all isolated parathyroid glands is correct. For lymphoma and anaplastic carcinoma, if resection is feasible, as much of the tumour as possible should be removed.

SIMPLE EXCISION OF NODULE

1. Mobilise the lobe in the standard manner having ligated the main arterial supply (see below). Place curved artery forceps at the margin of the nodule and totally excise it with knife or scissors.

2. Secure any bleeding points with 3/0 silk ligatures. Coagulation diathermy is also useful and perfectly safe in this instance.

3. Close the defect in the lobe with interrupted 2/0 or 0 chromic catgut sutures.

4. Inspect the excised specimen and submit it to frozen section examination if appropriate.

UNILATERAL LOBECTOMY

1. Decide whether to divide the strap muscles. Stand on the right side of the table to deal with the left thyroid lobe and vice versa. Adjust the assistant's Langenbeck, Czerny or Joll retractor to elevate the strap muscles from the upper pole. Clear the surface of the lobe from the overlying sternothyroid muscle, dividing and ligating the middle thyroid vein(s) at this stage if they prevent mobilisation of the upper lateral border of the gland.

2. Place an Allis tissue forceps on the upper pole, draw it gently downwards and rotate it slightly laterally. Once the fascial layers are totally cleared at the upper pole, the interval between the medial surface of the pole and the lateral wall of the laryngo-pharynx appears (Fig. 21.3). Widen the interval delicately with pledget or forceps. Sometimes vessels pass into the larynx from the superior thyroid vessels; divide and ligate them with 3/0 silk. Clumsy dissection at this stage can damage the external laryngeal nerve and impair the subsequent timbre of the voice.

3. Identify the anterior branch of the superior thyroid artery (and vein) and do not confuse it with the crico-thyroid artery (Fig. 21.4). By means of artery forceps develop a space behind these vessels. Using an aneurysm needle, pass three 0 silk ligatures around the vessels. Tie two above and one below on the gland. Pass an artery forceps through the interval and divide the vessels with a No.15 Blade. Adjust the position of the tissue forceps to ease the pole downwards and display the posterior branch of the superior thyroid artery and vein. Secure and divide these in a similar manner. The upper pole should now be completely mobilised. The right upper pole is higher and more difficult to isolate than the left.

4. Dissect the loose areolar tissue lateral to the thyroid and lift the lobe downwards, ligating and dividing the middle thyroid vein(s) as encountered. Dissect by separating and teasing with a small artery forceps, and find the inferior thyroid artery arching forwards from behind

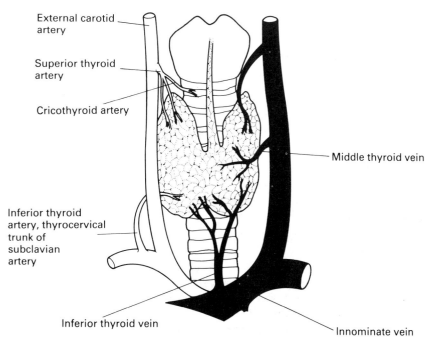

Fig. 21.4 Arterial supply and venous drainage of thyroid.

the carotid sheath; pass a 2/0 silk ligature behind and elevate the artery. Move back to midway between the superior pole and inferior thyroid artery. There is a prominence on the posterior border, and the superior parathyroid usually lies there surrounded by a little fat (Fig. 21.5).

5. Dissect carefully below the artery in the interval between oesophagus and trachea. If the recurrent laryngeal nerve is not immediately found, palpating the region may reveal it. The nerve may lie rather more anteriorly on the lateral surface of the trachea. Trace the nerve for at least 2 cm up to its relationship with the artery and above this point if necessary.

6. On the left side the nerve lies posterior to the artery, whereas on the right side it lies anterior to the artery or passes through its branches (Fig. 21.6). The right recurrent laryngeal nerve is rather more difficult to locate.

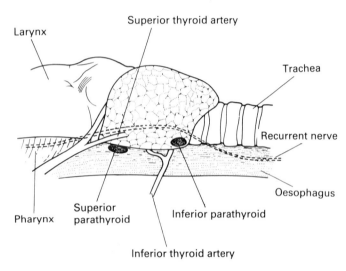

Fig. 21.5 Side view right side to show entry of superior thyroid and inferior thyroid arteries and their relation to the parathyroids.

Remember that it may be aberrant and arise high up from the vagus, passing downwards towards the inferior artery.

7. Make a brief exploration to seek the inferior parathyroid gland in the region where the nerve approaches the inferior thyroid artery, including the surface of the thyroid and around its lower pole.

8. Turning to the pretracheal region, dissect, clamp, divide and ligate (with 2/0 silk) the inferior thyroid veins.

9. Mark the proposed line of section of the gland with small artery forceps, avoiding the recurrent nerve and parathyroid glands. Unless you suspect carcinoma, aim to leave a remnant of about 5 × 1 cm.

10. With scalpel or scissors cut through the thyroid gland from below upwards, extending from the lateral side to the trachea and clamping any vessels encountered. It is sometimes helpful to elevate the thyroid with tissue forceps to facilitate exposure.

11. Separate the isthmus from the trachea and divide it between forceps applied at its junction with the opposite lobe. The specimen can now be removed for examination.

12. The raw surface of the residual thyroid will tend to ooze. Haemostasis is achieved by careful diathermy and multiple ligatures of 3/0 silk. To render haemostasis complete and leave a neat closure of the remnant, suture the lateral edges of the thyroid tissue and capsule to the fascia on the side of the trachea with continuous or interrupted 2/0 chromic catgut sutures.

SUBTOTAL THYROIDECTOMY

1. Commence by mobilising the left lobe of the thyroid from the right-hand side of the table. Ligate the vascular pedicles but do not resect any tissue at this stage.

2. Now move to the opposite side of the table and

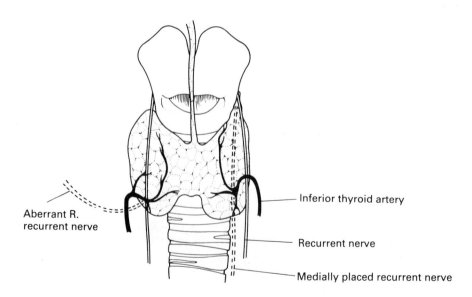

Fig. 21.6 Position of recurrent nerves in relation to inferior thyroid artery and some variations.

mobilise the right lobe in a similar fashion. Remember that the right recurrent laryngeal nerve can be more difficult to locate, but try and identify both nerves before proceeding to resection.

3. Having returned to the right side of the table, remove both lobes together with the isthmus and pyramidal lobe as far as the hyoid bone. The blood supply of the isthmus and pyramidal lobe is from the crico-thyroid branches, which must be secured and ligated with 3/0 silk.

4. For thyrotoxicosis and nodular colloid goitre, preserve a strip of thyroid on each side measuring 5 × 1 cm. For Hashimoto's goitre, nodular thyroiditis and thyroiditis superimposed upon nodular goitre, preserve a larger remnant consistent with parathyroid preservation.

TOTAL THYROIDECTOMY

1. Once the thyroid lobes have been fully mobilised, identify as many parathyroid glands as possible; the superior glands are by far the easier to find. Operate entirely from the right side.

2. Elevate the lower part of the right lobe with tissue forceps. Identify the right recurrent laryngeal nerve and keep it in constant view. Using small curved artery forceps remove the lobe from the nerve. This necessitates clamping and ligating small blood vessels until the nerve is exposed as far as its genu, where it passes posteriorly to enter the larynx deep to inferior constrictor. If it is possible to preserve the right superior parathyroid with a small fringe of thyroid capsule and vascular attachments then do so (Fig. 21.7). However if the parathyroid appears to be totally isolated, it is safer to remove and re-implant it. If the inferior parathyroid has been found it should also be removed for implantation (see below).

3. At the exit of the recurrent nerve, the deep surface of the lobe is adherent to the upper lateral trachea and cricoid by the thyrotracheal and laryngeal 'ligaments' (ligaments of Berry). Clamp these attachments carefully and divide them with scalpel or scissors. Keep the recurrent nerve under constant view. Detach the right lobe with the isthmus and proceed to the left recurrent laryngeal nerve.

4. Develop the tissue space superficial to the nerve with artery forceps and lift the left lobe off the nerve as for the right side, apart from the region of the superior parathyroid. Unless there is macroscopic tumour it is reasonable to preserve the left superior gland with a thin fringe of thyroid tissue, about 10 × 2 mm. Save the inferior gland for implantation. Use 3/0 silk ligatures for vessels and be very precise and sparing with coagulation diathermy.

5. Pursue a careful search for enlarged lymph nodes. They should be excised singly or in groups ('node picking') without necessarily resorting to block dissection of the neck. If a group of nodes lies laterally close to the carotid sheath, it is acceptable to divide sternomastoid trans-

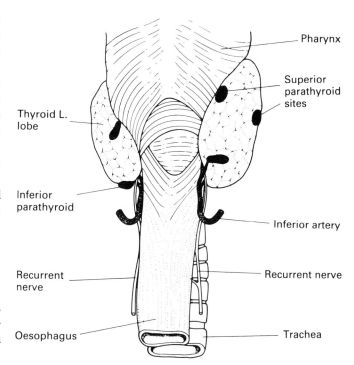

Fig. 21.7 Thyroid and parathyroids seen from behind. Variable positions of parathyroid glands.

versely, remove the nodes and repair the muscle carefully with interrupted 0 chromic catgut sutures.

Difficulty?

1. Adequate exposure is the sine qua non of thyroid surgery. Pay particular attention to the interval between sternothyroid muscle and thyroid gland. Do not hesitate to divide the strap muscles and allow easy exposure. Sometimes separation of the medial upper attachments of sternothyroid to the oblique line of the thyroid cartilage for 3–4 mm allows improved isolation of the upper pole.

2. Remember that the right thyroid lobe is naturally slightly larger and placed higher than the left. Hence mobilisation of the right upper pole may be technically difficult.

3. Venous bleeding from a torn middle thyroid vein can usually be avoided by care with delivery of the lateral border of the lobe; but the vein(s) are unpredictable and bleeding can arise from minimal digitation. Pack the bleeding area with dry gauze for 5 minutes; be sure to have an adequate suction cannula and improve the exposure. After removing the pack the bleeding sites can usually be secured.

4. Retrosternal goitre should be detected in the course of pre-operative investigations and should therefore not come as an operative surprise. Most retrosternal goitres lie anteriorly in the superior mediastinum. The general rule is to mobilise the cervical thyroid and deliver the retrosternal portion from above by traction and gentle

digitation. If the goitre is so large that it is jammed within the mediastinum, a sound manoeuvre is to break the thyroid capsule and remove the gland piecemeal by digital dissection. All the retrosternal goitre is cleared and the capsule may be left in situ to avoid the risk of uncontrolled bleeding.

5. In rare instances, where the transverse diameter of the retrosternal thyroid exceeds that in the neck, some surgeons prefer a sternal split in addition to cervical exposure to remove the gland.

6. Repeat operations on the thyroid are hazardous, as the sternothyroid becomes adherent to the remaining lobe or remnants. Make sure that the vocal cords are checked beforehand. Expose the thyroid in the standard manner, and separate the sternothyroid from the gland with great care. Next pass immediately to the region of the recurrent laryngeal nerves and find them. Trace the nerves up to the thyroid and then proceed to thyroidectomy avoiding injury to the nerve.

Closure

1. Check the operative field for haemostasis, then ask the anaesthetist to remove the interscapular sandbag, thereby reducing the degree of neck extension. Re-examine the total operative field for bleeding.

2. Insert one or two (Redivac) suction drains into the para-tracheal spaces. Pass the drains through the sterno-mastoid muscle and bring them through the skin 2 cm below the incision.

3. Repair the strap muscles with interrupted 2/0 chromic catgut sutures, similarly for the deep cervical fascia. The platysma is conveniently closed with a split continuous 4/0 plain catgut stitch, commencing in the midline and suturing to each corner.

4. The skin is cleaned with saline and dried before metal clips are applied. Some surgeons like to stretch the incision with Allis tissue forceps or skin hooks to assist the accurate application of the skin clips.

Aftercare

1. After recovery from the anaesthetic, the patient is kept well propped up in bed. The drains can usually be removed 24–48 hours postoperatively and the skin clips at 1–3 days.

2. Reactive haemorrhage beneath the deep cervical fascia can cause acute asphyxia. If this emergency is suspected re-open the wound immediately, if necessary in the ward, to allow evacuation of the clot. Be sure that a pair of clip-removing forceps is available in the recovery room or surgical ward in which thyroid cases are nursed.

3. Unsuspected damage to both recurrent laryngeal nerves can also cause respiratory embarrassment in the early postoperative period. Neurapraxia may lead to adduction of the affected cord. Suspect nerve damage if stridor and cyanosis develop without swelling of the neck. Unless endotracheal intubation is rapidly successful, emergency tracheostomy should be performed after reopening the incision.

4. Beware of hypocalcaemia following inadvertent parathyroid injury or excision during total thyroidectomy. Test for latent tetany and monitor serum calcium levels on the first few postoperative days. Give 10 ml calcium gluconate by intravenous injection if required. Oral supplements of calcium and vitamin D may subsequently be needed.

5. Thyroxine treatment is mandatory following total thyroidectomy. It may also be given to suppress growth of glandular remnants after operations for carcinoma or multinodular goitre, or to correct borderline endocrine insufficiency.

Further reading

Beaugie J M 1975 Principles of thyroid surgery. Pitman, London.
Chiu-An Wang. Thyroid cancer treatment. In: Werner S C, Ingbar S H (eds) The thyroid. A Fundamental and Clinical Text, 4th edn. 1978, Harper and Row, Maryland. p. 558–583
Lennox S C 1981 Mediastinal cysts and tumours. In: Wilson J S P (edn) Operative Surgery, Fundamental International Techniques, 3rd edn. Head and Neck Part 11 Butterworths, London, p. 812–829
Rosswick P 1981 Thyroidectomy. In: Wilson J S P (ed) Operative surgery. Fundamental international techniques, 3rd edn. Head and Neck Part II. Butterworths, London. p. 802–811
Sedgwick C E, Cady B 1980 Surgery of the thyroid and parathyroid glands, 2nd edn. Saunders, Philadelphia
Taylor S 1980 Thyroid tumours. In: De Vischer M (ed) The thyroid gland. Raven, New York. p. 257–278
Wade J S H 1972 Clinical research in thyroid surgery. Annals of the Royal College of Surgeons in England 50: 112–127

PARATHYROID REIMPLANTATION

1. This procedure may be indicated during total or near-total thyroidectomy, when radical resection of the gland is required for malignant disease.

2. Identify and remove the glands, placing them on a swab soaked in normal saline. Trim off excessive fat.

3. Choose either the left sternomastoid muscle or the brachioradialis in the non-dominant forearm. Open the overlying fascial layer, and by scissor dissection fashion a space in the muscle about 10 mm deep.

4. Delicately slice the parathyroid glands into cubes or slivers of around 1 mm thick.

4. Place the parathyroid fragments into the muscular nidus and close the fascia with fine silk sutures or arterial clips.

PARATHYROIDECTOMY

Appraise

1. The operation is indicated for autonomous hyper-parathyroidism, whether primary adenoma, carcinoma,

hyperplasia or tertiary adenoma of the parathyroid is suspected.

2. Precise pre-operative investigation is imperative, and this may include selective venous sampling and parathormone assays. Arrange for peroperative frozen section examination and warn the histopathologist that the vigil may be lengthy.

Access

Proceed as for exploration of the thyroid gland. It is not usually necessary to divide the strap muscles unless there is a coexistent nodular goitre.

Action

The search

1. Mobilise the superior pole of each thyroid lobe very carefully, ligating the blood supply. Inspect the medial surface of the upper pole then move down the posterior border of the lobe. Isolate the inferior thyroid artery with a 2/0 silk ligature and find the recurrent laryngeal nerve.

2. Return to the posterior border midway between the superior pole and entry of the inferior thyroid artery. The superior parathyroid gland is most commonly found there either on the surface of the thyroid or close to it (Fig. 21.7). Look for fatty tissue and the parathyroid is usually within it. Normal parathyroids measure approximately 6 × 4 × 2 mm; they are orange-brown in colour and are ovoid or elongated in shape.

3. Elevate the lateral lobe with a tissue forceps and closely inspect the region of the inferior thyroid artery insertion and the recurrent nerve, seeking the inferior parathyroid. Check also the lower pole of the thyroid lobe especially on its superficial and deep aspect.

4. Change your position to face the suprasternal notch. On the left side is a thin tongue of lymphoid tissue passing from the lower pole of thyroid towards the thymus; this is the thyro-thymic axis. Lying just deep to the manubrium sterni and extending upwards for a variable extent are the upper poles of the thymic lobes. Dissect between thymus and thyroid, seeking the inferior glands.

5. Open the fascial capsule of the thymic lobes and seek parathyroids within or on the surface of the thymus. Parathyroids contrast sharply with the paler cream colour of thymus.

6. Inspect other sites (Fig. 21.8). Check the carotid sheath (vascular trunks) from the root of the neck to the upper border of the thyroid cartilage. Look carefully into the tracheo-oesophageal groove over the same extent. Elevate the larynx and trachea from the cervical spine, to allow dissection behind the oesophagus. Inspect the surface of the oesophagus. Check carefully the surfaces of the lower pole of the thyroid; a parathyroid can be plastered

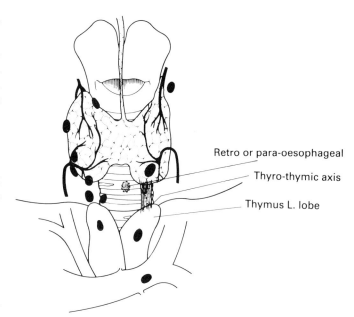

Retro or para-oesophageal
Thyro-thymic axis
Thymus L. lobe

Fig. 21.8 Various positions for parathyroid glands.

over the natural contour, and if bruised it may closely resemble thyroid tissue. Trace any aberrant branches of the inferior thyroid arteries; they may lead to a parathyroid adenoma.

Resection

1. If a probable parathyroid adenoma is found, remove it and send it for frozen section examination. Seek the other parathyroid glands. Select one parathyroid and try to ascertain the site of entry of the blood supply. Using either fine dissecting forceps, skin hook or 25-gauge hypodermic needle lift up the non-vascular pole and excise about a third of the gland for frozen section examination. If the report indicates normal parathyroid tissue, then establish haemostasis and close the wound as for thyroidectomy.

2. If parathyroid hyperplasia is found this will be obvious macroscopically and is easily confirmed by frozen section examination. It is customary to remove $3\frac{1}{2}$ glands and to mark the site of the remaining gland with silk sutures or metal clips.

3. Occasionally nodular goitre coexists with a parathyroid adenoma; there is no contraindication to thyroidectomy in such circumstances. If the adenoma has not been found and thyroidectomy is necessary, the pathologist should be requested to section the thyroid very carefully, as the adenoma may lie within it.

RE-OPERATION

1. If an adenoma or hyperplasia was confidently expected by none found, then after an extended search in the neck

the wound should be closed and the diagnosis checked. If substantiated, then a further operation is probably required. Selective venous catheterisation and estimation of parathormone levels may help to decide whether the adenoma lies in the neck or the mediastinum. If mediastinal exploration is required proceed as follows:

2. Re-open the previous transverse cervical scar and make a vertical downwards extension in the midline about 3 cm below the manubriosternal angle. Deepen the incision to the sternum. At the notch divide the small vein and interclavicular ligament in the space of Burns. Gently open the space behind the manubrium by pledget or digital dissection. Stay close to the bone and in the midline. Split the sternum down to the manubriosternal angle by mechanical saw, large bone shears or Lebsche chisel. Place gauze over the divided bone edges and retract them enough to allow a self-retaining retractor to be inserted and opened to expose the contents of the superior mediastinum. Achieve haemostasis by diathermy and bone wax.

3. Dissect out the thymic lobes and remove them, paying particular attention to the short posterior veins which drain into the brachiocephalic vein. Slice the thymic tissue with great care. If the adenoma is not there seek further, around and between the great vessels (Fig. 21.8). As for cervical exploration, frozen section facilities must be available.

4. Following successful removal of the thymus and adenoma establish haemostasis. Insert a suction drain brought out through the neck and approximate the sternal edges. Use peri-sternal stainless steel sutures, twisting the knots into the interval between the bone edges.

Aftercare

This is as for thyroidectomy. Special care chould be taken in the clinical assessment of hypocalcaemia; serum calcium levels must be measured daily for at least 5 days.

Further reading

Katz A D, Kaplan L 1973 Parathyroidectomy for hyperplasia in renal disease. Archives of Surgery 107: 51–55
Krementz E T, Yeager R, Hawley W, Weichert R 1971 The first 100 cases of parathyroid tumour from the Charity Hospital of Louisiana. Annals of Surgery 173: 872–883
Wells S A Jr, Ketcham A S, Marx S J, Powell D, Bilezikian J P, Shimkin P M et al 1973 Pre-operative localisation of hyperfunctioning parathyroid tissue: radioimmunoassay of parathyroid hormones in plasma from selectively catheterized thyroid veins. Annals of Surgery 177: 93–98

THYROGLOSSAL CYST

Appraise

1. These interesting lesions develop from embryological failure of the thyroglossal tract to obliterate. Thyroglossal cyst is far more common than a fistula, where a track exists between the upper surface of the tongue and the cervical skin.

2. At least 65% of thyroglossal cysts present as an upper cervical swelling before the age of 30 years.

3. Most cysts are subhyoid in position and may present not directly in the midline but to one or other side. Laterally-placed thyroglossal cysts are rare.

4. Infection is common in thyroglossal cysts because of the lymphoid tissue which lies in the cyst wall. Spontaneous or operative drainage of an infected cyst to the exterior is likely to result in a chronic discharging sinus. A near-midline upper cervical abscess should never be incised for fear of extensively disrupting the cyst wall and rendering subsequent elective excision unsuccessful. The infected cyst may be aspirated with a fine needle and treated at length with a broad-spectrum antibiotic.

Access

1. The position of the patient on the operating table is similar to that used for thyroidectomy but with increased extension of the neck. A four-towel arrangement with gamgee neck pads at the sides is convenient, and the towels may be sutured in position.

2. Make a transverse incision across the neck at the level of the cyst. Reflect the upper and lower skin flaps for at least 5 cm each way. Hold the skin edges apart with some form of self-retaining retractor (Joll's is very suitable).

Action

1. The platysma may be divided transversely or preferably split vertically. Retract the platysma and separate the sternohyoid muscles by dividing the deep cervical fascia.

2. Clear the underlying fascial layers to expose the cyst and carefully dissect around it. Take great care to avoid breaching the wall.

3. Inferiorly define the lower limit of the cyst; this will usually involve ligating the fibrous upper limit of the pyramidal lobe.

4. Dissect laterally, detaching the cyst from the thyrohyoid muscles. If a possible lateral track is found, trace it to its limit.

5. Clear both sides of the cyst, and use pledget dissection deep to the cyst to separate it from the thyrohoid membrane.

6. Palpate at the level of the hyoid to identify the greater cornu, which is obscured by muscle attachments. Incise along each greater cornu with a No. 15 scalpel blade and gently scrape the muscle away from the bone, taking great care not to breach the cyst.

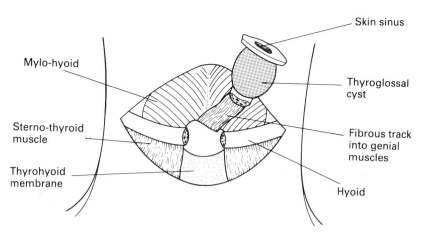

Fig. 21.9 Excision of thyroglossal cyst with sinus showing excision of hyoid bone.

7. Using small bone nibblers, carefully divide the hyoid lateral to the cyst and isolate the portion of the hyoid body attached to the cyst (Fig. 21.9).

8. Dissect into the mylohyoid muscle above the hyoid and remove any fibrous track which may seem to pass from the hyoid into the genial muscles. A significant connection is rarely present. Digital pressure on the tongue by the anaesthetist may assist access to the uppermost portion of the thyroglossal tract.

11. Establish haemostasis especially in the depths of the wound. Close the muscles without distortion, using 2/0 chromic catgut, and insert a small corrugated rubber drain into the depths. Close the platysma with interrupted 4/0 plain catgut sutures. Approximate the skin with clips.

Difficulty

If any aberrant track is found it should be dissected out and ligated with a 3/0 silk suture to help identify the site in case further exposure is required. Operations on thyroglossal cysts or fistulas may be difficult. Careful painstaking dissection is required.

Further reading

Ellis H 1981 Thyroglossal sinus or fistula, thyroglossal cyst. In: Wilson J S P (ed) Operative surgery. Fundamental international techniques, 3rd edn. Head and neck part II. Butterworths, London p. 798–802
Sistrunk W E 1920 The surgical treatment of cysts of the thyroglossal tract. Annals of Surgery 71: 121–122

Surgery of the head and neck

GENERAL PRINCIPLES

INTRODUCTION

Details of anatomy tend to be more important in the head and neck than in operations in other regions, because in the head and neck many structures are crowded into a small volume, and because many of them, such as the facial nerve, are vital to important functions, or even (e.g. the recurrent laryngeal nerve, the internal carotid artery) to life itself.

Maintenance of the airway may be threatened by the accumulation of blood, by laryngospasm, etc. and so endotracheal intubation is mandatory for all but the simplest procedure.

Complications of the type resulting from operations on the gastrointestinal tract — peritonitis, paralytic ileus and disturbances of water and electrolyte balance are conspicuous by their virtual absence, and thromboembolic complications are also uncommon. Postoperative chest complications, although they certainly occur after direct interference with respiratory passages or after long oper-ations, are less common than in abdominal or thoracic surgery. Even massive resections of tissues are therefore well tolerated. Infection is uncommon and healing is usually by first intention. When skin grafting is necessary to repair a defect, the grafts take well. Good healing is evidence of the good blood supply enjoyed by the territory. Unfortunately, the good blood supply also determines that the principal operative hazard (after the risk of damage to important anatomical structures) is primary haemorrhage.

MINIMIZE BLOOD LOSS

1. Before the operation, discuss with the anaesthetist if you think that blood loss is likely to be excessive. The anaesthetist may decide to use hypotensive anaesthesia, lowering the arterial blood pressure by such agents as ganglion-blockers (suxamethonium) or sodium nitropruss-ide. If you do operate under hypotension, remember the increased risk of reactionary haemorrhage shortly after the wound has been closed; delay the closure until you are certain that the blood pressure has been restored to the normal range (see p. 355).

2. Venous bleeding is more difficult to control than arterial. Venous pressure, and therefore venous bleeding, can be minimized by paying careful attention to posture. The patient should be positioned so that the area being operated on is at a higher level than the heart. Carefully avoid direct pressure on local veins from clumsy positioning of the head, neck or shoulders, presence of supports or towels etc. If it is necessary to divide a large vein draining the operative area, postpone this step in the operation to the latest possible moment. The anaesthetist helps to reduce venous pressure by maintaining the clearest possible airway, and by keeping arterial carbon dioxide tension normal or below normal.

3. Control blood vessels before dividing them: in this way excessive blood loss due, for example, to a haemostat slipping off the cut blood vessel is obviated. For sizeable vessels, use an aneurysm needle to pass ligatures around

the vessel, and tie the ligatures before dividing the vessel between them. A detailed knowledge of anatomy, so that one sees the vessels before cutting them, pays particular dividends here.

4. Many surgeons infiltrate the skin and subcutaneous tissues with a dilute solution of adrenaline, thereby producing vasospasm and reducing bleeding. I do not find this method valuable, but you should make up your own mind.

5. Diathermy is a very useful aid to haemostasis, but you must use it carefully. Remember that diathermy stops bleeding by coagulating the tissues in the immediate neighbourhood of the active electrode through the very high temperature (greater than 1000°C) produced. Haemostasis is achived at the expense of destruction of tissue. Because of the great vascularity of tissues in the head and neck, it is easy to produce extensive tissue necrosis. There are two forms of current available, 'cutting' and 'coagulating'. The cutting current produces a high intensity of energy over a sphere of small radius from the active electrode; the coagulating current produces a lower intensity over a sphere of larger radius. It is traditional to use the cutting current to incise tissues and the coagulating for producing haemostasis, on the principle that the larger zone of action of the coagulating current compensates for any small inaccuracy in identifying the bleeding point. It is better, however, to use the cutting current for haemostasis, having first made sure that each bleeding point has been accurately identified, and this discipline reduces unnecessary tissue destruction to a minimum.

6. After the operation, use suction drainage (see p. 365) to obliterate the dead space under the skin flaps, thereby reducing the risk of reactionary haemorrhage and haematomas. Note that in the neck a haematoma is a potentially lethal complication, because of its possible effect upon the patency of the airway.

REPLACE BLOOD LOSS

1. Before operation, ensure that *every* patient has been asked about any history of a bleeding tendency, that a haemoglobin estimation has been performed and that blood has been taken for grouping and serum saved in case crossmatching becomes necessary.

2. With regard to which cases require blood to be crossmatched before the operation, it is difficult to lay down rules. Much depends upon the experience of the operator, and particularly upon that of the anaesthetist. Conservative parotidectomy under good hypotensive anaesthesia should not need a blood transfusion, but an inexperienced operator performing this procedure under normotensive anaesthesia would be well advised to have two units of blood crossmatched before the operation. I ask for four units to be crossmatched before any extensive resection involving

bone and/or block dissection of the cervical lymph nodes.

3. Normally the anaesthetist controls blood replacement, should it become necessary during the operation. The principles are accurate measurement of the blood loss (weighing swabs, measuring the volume of the contents of the sucker bottle), and complete and rapid replacement, preferably monitored by the measurement of central venous pressure or of urine output.

AIRWAY

1. After any extensive procedure, especially any involving resection of the lower jaw, ask yourself whether such factors as an unstable tongue or laryngeal oedema might be a particular threat to the maintenance of the airway in the postoperative period.

2. Be prepared to perform a temporary tracheostomy in such circumstances.

APPLICATION

1. Much of the advice in this introduction is applicable to operations on regions other than the head and neck. Surgical technique is a subject whole and indivisible. Nevertheless, attention to the points stressed here yields particular dividends in the surgery of this region.

2. The importance of a detailed knowledge of anatomy cannot be overemphasized. There is no substitute for such knowledge. Before doing a new or unfamiliar operation, refresh your memory of the anatomy, not only of the immediate operative area but also of neighbouring areas: one never knows beforehand exactly how extensive a dissection will be dictated by the findings in, or difficulties of, a particular operation.

3. Remember that the head and neck in particular is a region of overlap with other specialities. Before embarking on any major procedure, it is a good idea to ask yourself whether it may be useful to seek advice from, or the collaboration of, a plastic, thoracic, dental or neurosurgeon, or an otolaryngologist.

PAROTIDECTOMY

Appraise

1. The facial nerve and its five main branches run through the substance of the parotid salivary gland, and are at risk in any operation designed to remove parotid tissue (parotidectomy).

2. Expose the facial nerve and its branches at an early stage of any parotidectomy, and over a sufficiently wide area to ensure that the required resection of parotid tissue is done without cutting the nerve (conservative parotidec-

tomy). However, if the object of your operation is to remove a lump in the parotid with a wide margin of normal tissue, you will sometimes find that this condition is impossible to fulfil; an adequate margin cannot be achieved unless you sacrifice the whole nerve (radical parotidectomy) or one or more of its branches (semi-conservative parotidectomy).

3. If the decision whether to sacrifice the main nerve is not clear-cut, you should lean towards radicalism in the elderly male, conservatism in the young female. Biopsy of the lump, and an immediate opinion on its histological nature following examination of frozen sections, can help, but only with the following provisos.

(a) Take extreme precautions against spreading the tumour in taking the biopsy; parotid tumours are notorious for their tendency to implant.*

(b) Your pathologist must be an expert in the histopathology of parotid lesions.**

4. Repair any gap you have produced in the facial nerve system by immediate primary suture, if possible, or by bridging the defect with a free cable graft from the great auricular nerve, taken as a routine at the beginning of the operation. Ignore any damage to the fifth (cervical) branch.

Prepare

1. Check that male patients are clean-shaven on the side of the operation, and that all patients are shaved for 5 cm around the external ear in all directions.

2. Tilt the top half of the operating table upwards till the external jugular vein collapses. Turn the patient's head away from you and extend his head on his neck (use a head-ring to achieve a stable position), but ensure that the patient is lying close to your side of the operating table.

3. Ask the anaesthetist to provide hypotension if possible. Ensure that he has protected the patient's eyes from possible damage by lotions used in the skin preparation. Clean the skin over the area shown in Figure 22.1.

4. Sew the towels in place to leave exposed only the area shown in Figure 22.1. Twist a small piece of cotton wool, and push it into the external auditory meatus with a pair of artery forceps; discard the artery forceps as no longer sterile. Ask the theatre nurse to add the piece of cotton wool to the swab count.

Access

1. The standard S-shaped cervico-mastoid-facial incision is shown in Figure 22.1. The lower (cervical) part lies in

  * Stevens K L, Hobsley M 1982 The treatment of pleomorphic adenomas by formal parotidectomy. British Journal of Surgery 69: 1–3
  ** Hobsley M 1981 Sir Gordon Gordon-Taylor: two themes illustrated by the surgery of the parotid gland. Annals of the Royal College of Surgeons of England 63: 264–269

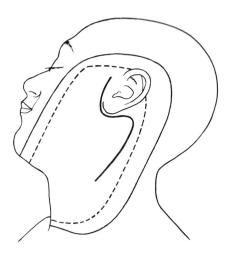

Fig. 22.1 The standard S-shaped cervico-facial incision for parotidectomy. Clean the skin of the area enclosed in the continuous line: towel up so as to leave exposed the area enclosed by the dotted line.

the upper skin crease of the neck, extending forwards to the external jugular vein. The upper (facial) part lies in the skin crease at the anterior margin of the auricle, extending upwards to the zygoma. Between these two parts, the mastoid part of the incision curves gently backwards over the mastoid process; but if the operation is being performed to remove a lump in this posterior part of the gland, exaggerate the posterior curve so that the incision lies clearly posterior to the lump.

2. Start by making the cervical part of the incision. If you make the incision in three parts from below upwards, stopping all bleeding before proceeding to the next part, you will have much less trouble with bleeding from the upper part of the wound obscuring your field lower down. Incise through skin, fat and platysma. Identify the external jugular vein near the anterior end of the wound, and two branches of the great auricular nerve vertically below the anterior margin of the auricle (Fig. 22.2). Preserve the vein; sacrifice the thinner (usually the more anterior) branch of the nerve; dissect free a convenient length of the thicker branch of the nerve (usually 4 cm can easily be obtained) and excise it. The nerve runs upwards towards the ear, and breaks up into two or three branches; it is advantageous to include a centimetre of each branch with the segment of steam excised. Ask the theatre nurse to preserve the excised nerve in a bowl of sterile physiological saline until the end of the operation.

3. To facilitate your dissection, put a row of artery forceps on the subcutaneous fat of the upper margin of the wound and get your first assistant, standing opposite you, to lift the forceps. Identify the anterior border of the sternomastoid muscle. Follow the border upwards and posteriorly towards the mastoid process, as far as the incision permits. Deepen the dissection to expose in turn the

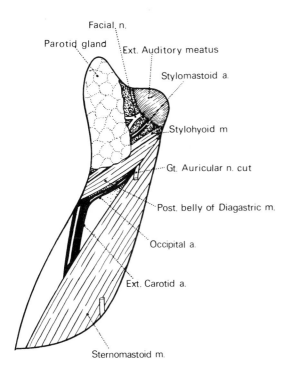

Facial. n.

Parotid gland

Ext. Auditory meatus

Stylomastoid a.

Stylohyoid m

Gt. Auricular n. cut

Post. belly of Diagastric m.

Occipital a.

Ext. Carotid a.

Sternomastoid m.

Fig. 22.2 The S-shaped incision has been deepened in its upper third (in front of the ear) to the bony external auditory meatus, and in its lower third in the neck to the stylohyoid muscle. This leaves a bridge of tissues in front of the mastoid that must be whittled away to expose first the stylomastoid artery, then the facial nerve.

posterior belly of the digastric and the stylohyoid muscles, proceeding at this stage only as far as is convenient.

4. Make the mastoid part of the incision and deepen it on to the sternomastoid muscle. Continue the exposure of the anterior border of the muscle right up to the mastoid process. Put more artery forceps on the upper subcutaneous border of the wound, and get your assistant to pull the superficial part of the lower pole of the parotid forwards and superficial from the anterior border of the sternomastoid. Friable, yellow parotid tissue forms the visible aspect of the anterior margin of the incision. Continue the exposure of the posterior belly of the digastric and the stylohyoid muscles upwards towards the mastoid process for as far as convenient at this stage.

5. Make the *facial* part of the incision, and deepen it along the anterior surface of the cartilaginous external auditory meatus by pushing in an artery forceps and opening the blades in an anteroposterior plane. Deepen this plane until you can feel the junction where the cartilaginous becomes the bony external auditory meatus (Fig. 22.2).

6. You now have a large S-shaped incision in which two deep cavities, one in the neck and one in front of the ear, are separated by a bridge of tissues where the dissection has not been deepened to the same extent, in the region of the front of the mastoid process. Whittle away these tissues piecemeal; push a closed, curved artery forceps from the upper cavity, downwards at 45° towards the lower

cavity so that the tips emerge, separate the tips and cut the tissue between them. Concentrate on defining the region where the anterior border of the sternomastoid, and the two deeper muscles, reach the anterior surface of the mastoid process. As this dissection proceeds and you approach the region of the facial nerve, take increasing care; take smaller bites of tissue and ask for the diathermy apparatus to be turned down to the lowest mark.

7. Your best warning that you are close to the facial nerve is given by the stylomastoid artery. This runs downwards and forwards in the same general direction as the facial nerve: control it with ligatures or with diathermy and divide it. Continue the dissection and about 3 mm deeper you will find the facial nerve trunk. It is 3–6 mm in diameter, white but with fine red vessels visible on its surface, and it bifurcates 1–2.5 cm from the base of the skull.

8. Further steps depend upon the exact operation you wish to perform.

SUPERFICIAL PAROTIDECTOMY

Appraise

1. You cannot set out with a stated intention to do a superficial parotidectomy if you are operating to remove a lump in the parotid; because clinical evidence cannot prove that the lump is confined to the superficial part of the gland.

2. The definite indications for superficial parotidectomy are therefore (a) recurrent parotitis due to a stone in the parotid duct at a site inaccessible from the mouth* (see p. 357) and (b) recurrent parotitis of unknown aetiology, usually in the group of conditions called Sjögren's syndrome or keratoconjunctivitis sicca.

3. For both indications, you *must* remove as much parotid tissue and as long a length of parotid duct as you can achieve with reasonable effort; otherwise there is a risk of recurrent flare-up of the residual infected tissues.

Access

A full description is given on page 352.

1. Make the usual cervico-mastoid-facial S-shaped incision.

2. Expose the main trunk of the facial nerve and its primary bifurcation.

Action

1. Choose either the upper or the lower main division of the nerve to start the dissection, whichever seems the

---

* Suleiman S I, Thomson J P S, Hobsley M 1979 Recurrent unilateral swelling of the parotid gland. Gut 20: 1102–1108

most convenient. Your aim is ultimately to reflect forwards the parotid tissue superficial to the facial nerve and its five branches until the anterier margin of the gland is reached.

2. Take a pair of find-bladed, gently curved artery forceps (e.g. mosquito forceps), and place their closed blades, with the convexity of the curvature facing superficially, along the exposed division of the nerve and in *immediate* contact with the nerve.

3. Push the points along the surface of the nerve for about 5–10 mm into the region where the nerve is still unexposed, and use the curve of the blades to make the points surface through the parotid tissue (Fig. 22.3). Parotid tissue is tough and you may be surprised at the amount of force needed. Separate the points of the artery forceps, elevate the whole instrument to make the overlying bridge of tissues taut, and divide the bridge with a pair of scissors. This act brings another few millimetres of the nerve into view.

4. Repeat the process, following the *more posterior* nerve at any bifurcation, until you are beyond the margins of the parotid (at the zygoma, if you have followed the upper division, beyond the external jugular vein if you have followed the lower division).

5. Next, repeat this process with the other main division of the facial nerve and its most posterior branch. You now have the facial nerve trunk and its temporal and cervical branches exposed.

6. The zygomatic branch arises from the upper division, the mandibular from the lower division, and there are at least two buccal branches, one from each division, and

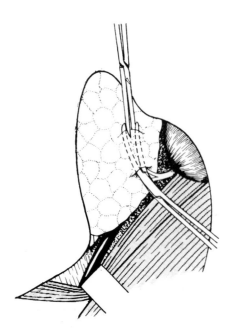

Fig. 22.3 The trunk of the facial nerve and its primary bifurcation have been exposed. When the scissors divide the bridge of tissue covering the blades of the forceps, a further segment of the upper division of the nerve will become visible.

sometimes a third (usually from the lower division). Working from the periphery towards the centre of the gland, follow the other main facial nerve branches forwards to the anterior margin of the parotid, i.e. along a vertical line halfway between the anterior and posterior borders of the masseter muscle.

7. Reflect the skin off the anterior flap until you reach the superior and anterior margins of the gland. A little more dissection along the nerve branches now frees the gland except for the parotid duct. Note that you should not reflect the skin flap at an earlier stage. This point is not important if you are removing an inflamed parotid, but certainly is if you are operating for a lump i.e. presumably a neoplasm. Should the lump be in the deep part of the gland, it may by the pressure of its expansion have caused the superficial part of the gland to atrophy and the facial nerve may be lying very close to the skin. I have seen the nerve cut during early reflection of the skin flap in such circumstances.

8. Dissect the parotid duct forwards to the anterior border of the masseter muscle, where it turns medially to perforate the cheek and reach the mouth. At this stage the dissection is facilitated by freeing the closely applied buccal nerve branches. Tie it at the anterior border of the masseter with an absorbable suture and cut the duct. The excision is complete.

Caution

1. If there is a bleeding point so close to the facial nerve that you are afraid that an attempt at stopping the bleeding with artery forceps or diathermy may injure the nerve, ask your assistant to press on the bleeding point with a swab and turn your attention to dissecting another part of the facial nerve system. When you return to the original spot the bleeding will probably have stopped.

2. The fifth, cervical, branch is not cosmetically important as it only supplies a part of the platysma. However, do not be tempted to sacrifice it at an early stage of the operation; the fourth, mandibular, branch often arises very far forwards from the fifth branch. You must make quite certain that you have identified and preserved the fourth branch before you can consider sacrificing the fifth. The fourth branch takes a very long route, dipping behind the angle of the jaw into the submandibular region of the neck before turning upwards and medially to reach the lower lip. Damage to this branch produces the ugly deformity of loss of the Cupid's bow of the lower lip.

3. You will meet several cross-communications between the five branches of the nerves. Preserve these if you find it easy to do so, but otherwise do not hesitate to cut them.

4. Two of the buccal branches are intimately related to the parotid duct and need particular care if you are to avoid damaging them as you dissect the duct.

Check list

1. Bleeding. Make sure that the anaesthetist has raised the blood pressure to a level reasonably comparable with the patient's normal level, and at least greater than 100 mmHg. If you fail to insist on this precaution, you will find a high incidence of reactionary haemorrhage. Restore the table to the horizontal position, to ensure that any tendency to bleeding becomes immediately manifest.

2. Have you removed the cotton wool from the external auditory meatus?

Closure

1. Close the skin with a continuous blanket suture. There is no need for a subcutaneous stitch.

2. Always use a drain. Use suction drainage via a stab incision 5 cm below the cervical end of the incision.

PAROTIDECTOMY FOR A LUMP IN THE PAROTID REGION

Access

A full description is given on page

1. Make the usual cervico-mastoid-facial S-shaped incision.

2. Expose the main trunk of the facial nerve and if possible, its primary bifurcation.

Assess

Start to dissect forwards along the nerve or along its upper and lower divisions, as described in detail on pages 352–3. Before long you will be able to decide whether the lump is in the part of the gland superficial to the facial nerve or the part deep to the facial nerve, and whether the nerve trunk or its main divisions are running straight into the lesion rather than being pushed aside by the lesion.

Action

Superficial (conservative) parotidectomy is performed if the lump is superficial to the facial nerve (details on page 353).

Total conservative parotidectomy is performed if the lump is deep to the facial nerve.

1. Perform superficial parotidectomy as described in detail on pages 353–4.

2. Dissect under the trunk, divisions and branches of the facial nerve, lifting the nerves very gently — fingers are safest — off the underlying deep part of the parotid gland until there is clear space between the nerves and the whole of the deep part of the gland.

3. Find the external carotid artery (and its companion

vein if there is one) at the upper border of the stylohyoid muscle. Make sure the artery is the external and not the internal carotid artery by (a) identifying the occipital branch that arises from the external carotid artery at this level and runs backwards and upwards along the upper border of the stylohyoid muscle, and (b) noting that the artery enters the lower pole of the deep part of the parotid gland. Divide the external carotid artery (and its companion vein) between ligatures.

4. Mobilize the deep part of the parotid and its contained lump by working from the anterior and posterior parts of the gland towards the centre, and from its lower pole upwards. You may aim at mobilizing the deep part in such a way as to remove it above, or below, the facial nerve system, or even between the two main divisions in the region of the bifurcation, whichever route seems most convenient (Fig. 22.4).

5. You will find that mobilization of a lower pole containing a large tumour is greatly facilitated by dividing the stylomandibular ligament, of which the anterior insertion is into the angle of the jaw. If necessary, fracture the styloid process to gain more room.

6. As you continue the mobilization of the deep parotid off the masseter muscle and mandible anteriorly and the bony external auditory meatus posteriorly and approach the upper part of the gland, look out for the termination of the external carotid artery at the upper pole where it bifurcates into the superficial temporal artery and the maxillary artery. When you have tied and divided these arteries and their accompanying veins, the deep parotid is free and you can remove it.

Radical parotidectomy, i.e. with sacrifice of the facial nerve, is performed if the nerve or its main divisions are surrounded by the tumour.

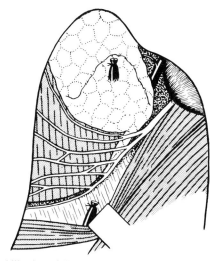

Fig. 22.4 Mobilization of the deep lobe of the parotid gland. The external carotid artery (and companion veins, not shown) have been divided at the lower pole of the gland, and the latter has been turned upwards to be delivered (in this case) **above** the main trunk of the facial nerve.

1. Reflect the skin forwards to the anterior margin of the gland.

2. Find the external carotid artery at the lower pole of the gland, and divide the artery and its companion vein between ligatures.

3. Divide the trunk of the facial nerve and mobilize the posterior aspect of the whole gland off the cartilaginous and bony external auditory meatus.

4. Divide the facial nerve branches at the anterior border of the gland, and mobilize the whole gland backwards off the masseter muscle and the posterior border of the mandible.

5. Mobilize the whole gland from below upwards, divide (between ligatures if possible) the superficial temporal and maxillary arteries at the upper pole of the gland, and remove the freed whole gland with its contained facial nerve system.

Semi-conservative parotidectomy, i.e. with sacrifice of one or more branches of the facial nerve but with preservation of at least one of the upper four branches, is performed if necessary to preserve an adequate margin round the lump. Carry out primary repair of the cut branches by end-to-end apposition if the cut ends will meet, or bridge the gap or gaps with the segment of greater auricular nerve obtained earlier in the operation. Use the finest available suture material for joining the nerves.

Difficulty?

1. The whole point of the operation is to remove the lump with an adequate margin of normal tissue. The preservation of an adequate margin demands your constant concentration; at frequent intervals as the operation progresses, feel the part of the parotid being removed with its contained lump and make sure that you are not getting too close to the lump.

2. To assist in preserving the margin, always modify the incision as necessary to avoid cutting down through skin straight on to the swelling. If in doubt, take a layer of extraparotid tissues such as sternomastoid or other muscles, a slice of cartilage or sliver of bone of the external auditory meatus, and so on.

3. Bleeding from the maxillary veins may be very troublesome if you are unable to control the veins before dividing them. They retract under cover of the zygoma. Use deep sutures to obliterate this plexus of veins.

EXPLORATION OF THE LOWER POLE OF THE PAROTID

Appraise

This operation is indicated:
1. To determine whether a lump in the neck is or is not in the lower pole of the parotid salivary gland. The lower pole of the gland extends well down into the neck behind the angle of the jaws and is separated anteriorly from the submandibular salivary gland only by a thickened sheet of fascia, the stylomandibular ligament.

2. To obtain a large piece of tissue from the gland as a biopsy for histological examination.

Access

1. Make an incision in the upper skin crease of the neck, starting just in front of the external jugular vein and extending backwards to a point vertically below the lowermost tip of the mastoid process.

2. Define the external jugular vein and the two divisions of the greater auricular nerve. Sacrifice the thinner division of the nerve; mobilize the thicker division but preserve it for the moment (you may find it necessary to sacrifice the thicker division later).

3. Define the anterior border of the sternomastoid muscle. Put a row of artery forceps on the subcutaneous fat of the upper margin of the wound and get your assistant to raise this margin off the muscle.

Assess

1. If you are exploring for a lump that is possibly in the lower pole, it should now be obvious whether the lump is moving upwards with the parotid in the upper leaf of the incision, or whether it lies on a deeper place between the sternomastoid and the posterior belly of the digastric (or deeper) muscles.

2. Should you still be unable to decide, extend the incision upwards, with a curve that is convex posteriorly, across the mastoid process to reach the point where the anterior margin of the lobule of the auricle reaches the face (see Fig. 22.2). Continue raising the flap of skin and superficial parotid forwards off the anterior border of the sternomastoid muscle. The greater exposure provided will certainly enable you to decide the position of the lump.

Action

1. If the lump is in the parotid, continue the operation as a parotidectomy for lump (p. 355). Even if the lump seems very superficial, do *not* be tempted to excise it locally; it is far safer, from the viewpoint both of the safety of the facial nerve and of ensuring complete removal of the lump, that you do a formal parotidectomy after exposure of the trunk of the facial nerve.

2. If the lump is not in the parotid, continue the operation by removing the lump, ignoring the parotid.

3. If your aim is to take a generous biopsy of the parotid, undertake (access) step 1. Deepen this cervical part of the dissection to expose the posterior belly of the

digastric muscle and the stylohyoid muscle. Define these muscles up to the region of the mastoid process.

4. You will find that a large portion of the lower pole of the parotid is now elevated with the anterior skin flap, and you can take a large biopsy of this mobilized portion without any risk to the facial nerve.

Closure

1. Check haemostasis.
2. Close the skin only.
3. Always use a drain. Insert a suction drain by a separate stab, 5 cm below the midpoint of the cervical part of the incision.

OPERATIONS ON THE PAROTID DUCT ORIFICE IN THE MOUTH

Appraise

1. Stomatoplasty is used to enlarge the parotid duct orifice*, either to enable a calculus in the parotid duct to be passed more easily or to prevent a stricture forming at the orifice after the duct has been explored, for example to remove a stone from the duct.

2. Two branches of the facial nerve are closely applied to the parotid duct in the cheek, and may even wind around the duct. Therefore, do not pass ligatures round the duct to prevent a stone escaping or to assist retraction (contrast with the procedure for removal of stone from the submandibular duct, p. 359).

Access

1. Ask the anaesthetist to use a per-nasal endotracheal tube, thereby leaving the mouth free for your manipulations. Also ask him to pack the pharynx around his tube, as a precaution against blood from the mouth being aspirated into the lungs.

2. Fix the patient's mouth open with a dental prop or Ferguson's forceps inserted between the teeth (or gums) of the jaws on the side opposite to your operation. Insert a towel clip (with its jaws in the horizontal plane) into the tip of the tongue and ask your assistant to retract the tongue towards the opposite side also.

3. Identify the papilla on which the parotid duct opens on the inside of the cheek, immediately opposite the second upper molar tooth. Take an atraumatic 00 catgut stitch on a half-circle (30 mm) cutting needle and put a stitch into the mucosa and underlying muscle of the cheek, about 5 mm above the papilla. Do not tie this stitch; cut the

* Hobsley M 1981 Sir Gordon Gordon-Taylor: two themes illustrated by the surgery of the parotid gland. Annals of the Royal College of Surgeons of England 63: 264–269

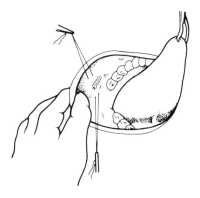

Fig. 22.5 The approach to the right parotid duct orifice. The dental prop in the left side of the mouth is not shown. The tongue is retracted to the opposite side with the towel clip. The operator pulls the angle of the mouth towards himself and at the same time pushes the cheek inwards to make the papillary region prominent inside the mouth; the assistant helps in achieving the latter effect by pulling on the two stay sutures. The dotted line indicates the incision to be made through the mucosa of the cheek and the mucosa of the wall of the duct.

catgut so that each end is 15 cm long, and grip the ends of the stitch with a pair of artery forceps (Fig. 22.5).

4. Insert a similar stitch about 5 mm below the papilla. Get your assistant to pull on the two stitches via the artery forceps, thereby elevating the region of the papilla towards you.

Access

1. Feel the region of the papilla with two fingers of one hand, exerting counterpressure with the fingers of the other hand applied to the external aspect of the cheek. Can you feel a stone?

2. Try to identify the parotid duct orifice. To find the hole, use a lacrimal duct dilator (a fine probe with a slight bend at each end in the shape of an elongated letter S). To facilitate this manoeuvre, use one hand to guide the dilator and, with the other, pull the angle of the mouth forwards towards you with your thumb working against the metacarpophalangeal joint of your index finger, and push the cheek inwards with the fingertips.

3. At this stage, you are ready to remove a stone from the parotid duct, or to proceed immediately to stomatoplasty, as indicated by your findings.

REMOVAL OF STONE FROM PAROTID DUCT — INTRAORAL APPROACH

Action

1. If you can feel the stone at the orifice, keep the papillary region pushed inwards into the mouth by the manoeuvre just described and cut down on the stone with a short-bladed, long-handled scalpel. Start the incision at

the orifice of the duct, and carry it horizontally backwards for 1 cm.

2. When you have deepened the incision sufficiently, the stone will become visible. Grasp it with any convenient instrument, such as fine-toothed dissecting forceps, and lift it out of the duct. You will find that your incision has divided *two* layers of mucosa, the lining of the inside of the cheek, and the inner lining of the wall of the parotid duct.

3. If you cannot feel a stone in the duct, pass the lacrimal duct dilator into the orifice and along the duct for 2 cm. Get your assistant to hold the dilator steady, keep the papillary region of the cheek pushed inwards into the mouth with your other hand, and cut down on the dilator, carrying the incision from the orifice of the duct horizontally backwards for 1 cm.

4. Explore the duct as far back as possible by passing the lacrimal duct dilator; you may be able to feel a stone grating on the tip of the probe. If you can, try milking the stone forward by digital pressure on the parotid gland and duct from outside. This manoeuvre is not often successful, but is worth trying.

5. Whether or not a stone has been found and removed, the operation must be completed by fashioning a larger parotid duct orifice (stomatoplasty — see below). After you have done the stomatoplasty, complete the procedure by going through the check list for that operation.

PAROTID DUCT STOMATOPLASTY

Action

Enlarge the orifice of the parotid duct. To do this, pass a lacrimal duct dilator into the duct for 1–2 cm, get your assistant to hold it steady, keep the papillary region of the cheek pushed inwards into the mouth with your other hand, and cut down on the dilator. Take the incision from the orifice of the duct horizontally backwards for 1 cm. Remove the dilator.

Closure

You will find that your incision has divided two layers of mucosa, the lining of the inside of the cheek, and the inner lining of the wall of the parotid duct. Unite these two layers with a series of interrupted, 000 chromic catgut sutures around the margins of the incision (Fig. 22.6).

Check list

1. Make sure all bleeding has stopped.
2. Remove the stay sutures above and below the duct orifice and the towel clip from the tongue, and check that bleeding does not continue from the puncture wounds.
3. Ask the anaesthetist to remove the pharyngeal pack.

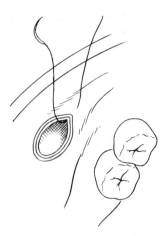

Fig. 22.6 Sewing together the two layers of the mucosa, of the cheek and of the duct. The stitch shown is the first of six or eight that will be inserted at intervals all round the periphery of the now enlarged stoma of the parotid duct.

If the pack has been effective, there will be no blood on the deeper part of the pack.

4. Remove the dental prop or Ferguson's forceps.

REMOVAL OF STONE FROM THE SUBMANDIBULAR DUCT

Appraise

1. Do not attempt this operation unless the stone is easily palpable well forward in the floor of the mouth, and its presence has been confirmed by radiological investigation.

2. If the stone is more posterior, and can only just be felt in the floor of the mouth, or if the submandibular salivary gland is clearly chronically infected, then the whole gland should be removed together with the stone and as much duct as possible (see the description of excision of submandibular salivary gland for calculous disease, p. 359). Clearly if there is any possibility of this situation arising, the patient's consent to this larger procedure must be obtained.

3. A stone easily accessible in the anterior part of the duct may slip back into the gland during manipulations in the region of the duct. To prevent this happening, gain control of the duct behind the stone with a ligature under-running the duct at an early stage of the operation.

Access

1. Ask the anaesthetist to pass a nasal endotracheal tube and to pack off the pharynx.

2. Keep the patient's mouth open with a dental prop or Ferguson's forceps, inserted between the teeth or gums of the molar region of the contralateral side of the mouth.

3. Grasp the tip of the tongue with a towel clip, closed

with the jaws in a horizontal plane, and get your assistant to retract the tongue towards the contralateral side.

Assess

1. Inspect and feel the submandibular duct in the floor of the mouth. Make sure that the stone is present and where you expect it to be, well forward in the duct.

2. If you cannot feel the stone, do not explore the submandibular duct. Either the stone has passed spontaneously or it has fallen back along the duct into the gland. In the latter circumstance, you should be able to feel it by bimanual palpation via the neck and the floor of the mouth simultaneously. If you can feel the stone in the gland, try to milk it forwards into the duct. If you fail to milk the stone forwards, the only method of removing the stone safely is to remove the whole salivary gland with it, by the cervical route. In this larger operation justified by the duration and severity of the patient's symptoms? Have you the patient's signed consent for the larger operation? If the answer to both these questions is 'yes', proceed to submandibular sialoadenectomy for calculous disease (p. 360).

3. If the stone is palpably, and maybe visibly, present well forward in the submandibular duct, proceed as below.

Action (Fig. 22.7)

1. Take an atraumatic 00 catgut stitch on a 30 mm half-circle cutting needle, and run the stitch under the submandibular duct, immediately proximal to the stone. Do not tie this stitch; cut it so that each end is 15 cm long, grasp the two ends in the jaws of a pair of artery forceps, and ask your assistant to pull the stitch upwards and proximally along the duct. This manoeuvre obliterates the lumen of the duct by kinking and prevents the stone from slipping backwards along the duct into the gland.

2. Put a similar stitch, with a deep bite, vertically into the floor of the mouth in the midline between the terminations of the ridges marking the right and left submandibular ducts. Grip this stitch similarly with a pair of artery forceps, and get your assistant to pull towards you and towards the contralateral side.

3. Identify the orifice of the ipsilateral submandibular duct by passing a fine lacrimal duct dilator through the orifice. With the dilator in place, try to ensure that you leave the terminal 0.5 cm of the duct intact.

4. With a small-bladed, long-handled scalpel, cut boldly down on to the stone along the length of the duct.

5. Lift the stone out of the duct with any convenient instrument, e.g. fine-toothed dissecting forceps.

6. Leave the linear incision in the anterior wall of the duct open.

7. If the stone is impacted at the orifice of the duct, try to milk it backwards along the duct so that you can preserve the integrity of the duct at its orifice. However, if you are forced to slit open the orifice, complete the operation by performing a stomatoplasty, sewing the mucosal lining of the duct to the mucosa of the floor of the mouth to leave an enlarged (0.5 cm) orifice (exactly as in the operation of parotid duct stomatoplasty, p. 358).

Check list

1. Make sure all bleeding has stopped.

2. Remove the two stay sutures, and the towel clip from the tongue, and check that bleeding does not continue from the puncture wounds.

3. Ask the anaesthetist to remove the pharyngeal pack. If the pack has been effective, there will be no blood on the deeper part of the pack.

4. Remove the dental prop or Ferguson's forceps.

SUBMANDIBULAR SIALOADENECTOMY FOR CALCULOUS DISEASE

Appraise

1. The mandibular (fourth) branch of the facial nerve dips down into the neck behind the angle of the jaw, and then curves upwards and medially to cross superficial to the posterior part of the submandibular salivary gland on its way to the angle of the mouth. This branch is therefore at risk during submandibular sialoadenectomy.

2. The facial artery and vein lie in a groove on the deep aspect of the posterior pole of the superficial lobe of the gland. The vessels are so intimately bound to the gland that you should not try to dissect them away from it.

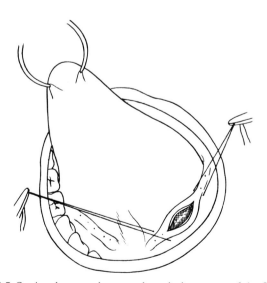

Fig. 22.7 Cutting down on the stone through the mucosa of the floor of the mouth and the muscle and mucosa of the wall of the duct. The duct is steadied, and counter-pressure exerted against the scalpel blade by the two stay sutures, while traction on the proximal one prevents the stone slipping proximally into the gland.

3. The gland has a superficial and a deep lobe; the separation is not complete, the two portions being continuous around the posterior edge of the mylohyoid muscle.

Access

1. Ask the anaesthetist to provide hypotension if possible.

2. Position the patient with a head-up tilt from the waist, sufficiently steep to cause collapse of the external jugular vein. Turn the patient's head away from you and extend his head on his neck, but make sure that he is lying close to your side of the operating table. Use a head-ring to get a stable position.

3. After cleaning the skin and applying towels, make an incision through skin and platysma in the upper skin crease of the neck (about 5 cm below the lower border of the mandible), extending from a point 2 cm lateral to the anterior midline of the neck to a point vertically below the angle of the jaw.

Action

1. Identify by palpation the inferior border of the submandibular salivary gland.

2. Deepen the cervical incision in the direction of the inferior border of the gland till the border is exposed.

3. Keeping as closely as possible to the surface of the gland, dissect all round the superficial lobe until it is free except for the area where it becomes continuous with the deep lobe. During the course of this dissection, you will meet the facial artery and vein both at the lower and upper borders of the posterior pole of the superficial lobe (Fig. 22.8). Divide the vessels, preferably the artery and vein separately, between ligatures, both at the upper and the lower border. A segment of each vessel then remains attached to the gland, to be removed with the gland. If you keep very close to the superficial surface of the gland, you stand little chance of injuring the mandibular branch of the facial nerve, which will be retracted upwards by your assistant within the superficial flap of tissues.

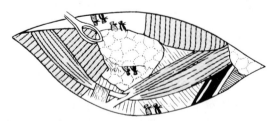

Fig. 22.8 Excision of submandibular gland for calculous disease. The superficial lobe of the submandibular salivary gland has been mobilized by dividing the facial vessels above and below the gland (they are adherent to the deep aspect), and the beginning of the deep lobe can be seen. The deep lobe extends forwards deep to the mylohyoid muscle, and the duct starts at the anterior end of the lobe. Deep to the deep lobe lies the lingual nerve.

4. Apply a pair of tissue forceps to the gland as it dips deep to the posterior border of the mylohyoid muscle. Get your assistant to pull the gland laterally and retract the posterior border of the mylohyoid medially, while you free by blunt dissection the deep part of the gland from the deep surface of the mylohyoid. You will probably at this stage be able to feel the stone stuck in the duct at the point where the duct leaves the anterior pole of the deep lobe. Do **not** proceed further forwards with the dissection at this stage, even if it seems technically easy, since you may damage the lingual nerve where it crosses the lateral (superficial) aspect of the duct.

5. Now get your assistant to retract the deep portion of the gland medially, i.e. round the edge of the mylohyoid muscle. Dissect by blunt dissection along the deep surface of the deep lobe, separating it from the hyoglossus muscle on which it lies. Keep very closely to the gland, because it also lies in contact with the lingual nerve. You can recognize the nerve as a rather broad (7.5 mm) thin band of white tissue, running forwards and medially on the hyoglossus and a little above the level of the submandibular duct.

6. At the anterior pole of the gland you will again probably feel the calculus (this is the commonest site), and see the commencement of the duct. You must now dissect forwards along the duct, taking special care not to damage the lingual nerve as it crosses the superficial aspect of the duct from above downwards, and then winds right round the lower border of the duct to cross its medial aspect from below upwards.

7. Free the duct as far forwards as possible, i.e. practically to its termination in the mouth. Tie the duct distally with a catgut ligature, and cut it across. Duct and gland can then be removed, with the contained stone.

Closure

1. Check haemostasis. Make sure that the anaesthetist has raised the blood pressure sufficiently (see p. 355).

2. Close the skin only. Some surgeons repair the platysma as a separate layer, but judging by results this step is unnecessary.

3. Always use suction drainage via a separate stab incision, 5 cm below the middle of the wound.

SUBMANDIBULAR SIALOADENECTOMY FOR TUMOUR

Appraise

1. If a submandibular salivary gland swelling is not due to calculous disease, it must be assumed to be due to a tumour. If there is clear-cut evidence that the tumour is malignant, see the 'commando' operation (p. 374) for details of treatment.

2. If there is no evidence of malignancy, assume that the tumour is a mixed salivary tumour. You should then aim to remove the submandibular salivary gland with a wide margin of normal tissue, so as to ensure completeness of the excision and guard against any implantation recurrence (see p. 352).

3. Warn the patient before the operation that he may develop weakness of the angle of the mouth and the lower lip, lose general sensation and taste from the ipsilateral half of the anterior two-thirds of the tongue, and develop wasting and paralysis of the ipsilateral half of the tongue.

Access

1. Make a skin crease incision through skin and platysma in the upper skin crease of the neck, extending from 2 cm lateral to the anterior midline of the neck to a point vertically below the angle of the jaw. Do not hesitate to extend this incision in either direction to facilitate removing a large tumour.

2. Deepen the incision towards the lower border of the submandibular salivary gland, but stop a few millimetres short of actually exposing the gland.

Assess

By palpation, bimanually if necessary, determine the exact site and extent of the tumour in the gland. In particular, decide whether the tumour reaches the superficial aspect of the superficial lobe.

Action

1. Dissect free the superficial aspect of the superficial lobe. If the tumour does not reach this aspect, it is acceptable to dissect close to the gland, preserving the mandibular branch of the facial nerve in the overlying platysmal flap as described in the similar operation for calculous disease (p. 360). If the tumour does reach this superficial aspect, perform the mobilization in a plane more remote from the gland. Try to identify the mandibular branch of the facial nerve, and preserve it, provided that this does not jeopardize your margin around the tumour. Divide the facial vessels between ligatures, well above and below the posterior pole of the gland.

2. Continue the mobilization of the superficial and deep lobes as described in the corresponding operation for calculous disease, but wherever the tumour reaches the surface of the salivary gland make certain of your margin by excising the neighbouring normal tissue. This policy usually only entails the sacrifice of fibres from such muscles as the anterior belly of the digastric anteriorly, the intermediate tendon of the digastric and the stylohyoid muscle inferiorly, the stylomandibular ligament posteriorly, and

the mylohyoid, stylohyoid, hyoglossus and posterior belly of the digastric medially.

3. Remember that an intimate deep relation of the deep lobe is the lingual nerve. It is nearly always possible to preserve all or part of this nerve, but occasionally the nerve has to be sacrificed to ensure completeness of excision of the tumour.

4. Very occasionally, the hypoglossal nerve is so intimately related to the inferior border of the gland that it has also to be sacrificed to maintain a margin around the tumour.

5. Dissect the submandibular duct forwards as far as possible, tie and divide it, and lift out the block of tissue.

Closure

1. Check that the anaesthetist has restored the blood pressure to an acceptable level (p. 355).

2. Close the wound with one layer of skin sutures.

3. Always use a drain. Insert a suction drain via a separate stab incision, 5 cm below the middle of the wound.

EXCISION BIOPSY OF A RODENT ULCER OF THE FACE

Appraise

1. A rodent ulcer may be treated by surgery or by radiotherapy. If surgery is chosen, the ulcer must be excised with a wide margin of normal tissue, both around the lesion and deep to it. A 'wide margin' means preferably 1 cm, but in regions where skin is precious, for example near the eye, 0.5 cm is acceptable.

2. Sometimes the ulcer is small and occurs in a region where there is plenty of redundant skin. In these circumstances, primary closure of the elliptical wound may be possible. Often, however, a skin graft is needed. A full-thickness graft is desirable; the cosmetic result of a split skin graft on the face is unacceptable. The description below includes two sites for obtaining a free full-thickness skin graft. Plastic surgeons can rotate flaps to cover large defects, but it is not ideal that the general surgeon should attempt these.

Assess

1. The extent of the lesion, and of the area of excision required, is carefully assessed by inspection and palpation. The **depth** of excision required may be difficult to assess at this stage.

2. In planning the incision, remember to take into account the direction of Lange's lines of skin tension. After the excision, you may find it is possible to close the defect

by primary suture, and the scar will then lie in the skin crease.

Action

1. Mark out the oval of skin that you have decided to excise.

2. Cut vertically through the skin along the oval line, until the superficial fat is clearly visible everywhere in the wound. It is not possible to make a curved incision with a straight knife-blade, but a series of short linear incisions will permit your incision to approximate closely to the oval you have marked.

3. Deepen the incision at one end of the longer diameter of the oval. Raise the skin at the end of the diameter with a pair of toothed dissecting forceps, and using either a clean scalpel or a pair of scissors start raising the oval of skin and some subcutaneous tissue towards the region of the lesion.

4. At this stage you will find it easier to decide by palpation how deeply the lesion extends. Make sure that your plane of cutting is sufficiently deep to give a wide margin of normal tissue below, as well as all round, the tunour.

5. Complete the excision. You may find it more convenient to do this by starting again at the opposite pole of ellipse, the two planes of section meeting deep to the lesion.

6. Inspect the wound for bleeding and stop it with diathermy.

7. Take a single sheet of vaseline gauze, lay it on the wound, and cut out a piece the shape and size of the wound. This piece of gauze will serve as a pattern for cutting a full-thickness (Wolfe) graft of skin.

8. Lay the piece of vaseline gauze on the skin at the site you have chosen for supplying the skin graft. Suitable areas, where even a large oval defect can be closed by primary suture without tension, are the loose skin immediately below the clavicle, or the groove between the side of the head and the medial aspect of the posterior part of the pinna. Cut out an area of skin corresponding in size and shape to the pattern; take the full thickness of the skin, but as little as possible subcutaneous fat. Clean off any subcutaneous fat adhering to the deep surface of the skin, using a sharp scalpel for this purpose. Sew up the defect in the donor area.

9. Lay the full-thickness skin graft on the defect produced by the excision of the rodent ulcer, having first made certain that there is no bleeding. Stitch the edges of the graft to the margins of the defect with a series of interrupted non-absorbable sutures, tying the knots so that they lie on the surrounding intact skin rather than on the skin graft. You must arrange these sutures to achieve sufficient tension in the graft to discourage the formation of a haematoma beneath it, but less tension than will produce a strangulation effect on the graft and cause its death.

10. Spray the grafted area with an artificial skin preparation such as Nobecutane. Use the spray sparingly and allow the liquid film to harden, then repeat the procedure several times to get a firm dressing. Protect the eyes, nostrils, mouth and hair during the spraying.

Check list

1. Do not forget to dress the donor site.

2. Check that the specimen, properly labelled and accompanied by the appropriate request forms, is sent to the histopathologist.

LOCAL EXCISION OR BIOPSY OF AN INTRA-ORAL LESION

Appraise

1. Small lesions in the surface of the oral mucosa, whether on cheek, tongue, palate, floor of mouth or inner surface of the lips, are best dealt with by excision biopsy, i.e. excision with a sufficiently wide margin of normal tissue to ensure that excision is complete.

2. Make sure, however, by careful palpation beforehand, how deeply the lesion penetrates beneath the mucosa. Remember that you must achieve an adequate margin of normal tissue on the *deep* aspect of the lesion as well as around it.

3. The oral tissues are very vascular, and special precautions are advisable to minimize haemorrhage and to prevent aspiration of blood into the lungs.

Access

1. Ask the anaesthetist to pass a per-nasal endotracheal cuffed tube and to distend the cuff. As a further precaution against aspiration of blood, ask him to pack the pharynx with 2.5 cm ribbon gauze.

2. Fix the patient's mouth in the open position by means of a dental prop or Ferguson's forceps inserted between the teeth or gums of the molar region on the side opposite to the lesion.

3. Position the patient with a head-up tilt of about 15°, sufficient to cause the external jugular vein to collapse. Use a head-ring to stabilize the position of the head.

Assess

1. Palpate the lesion carefully again to assess its depth. Tissues often feel different when the patient is anaesthetised, and you may occasionally change your decision about the depth of penetration of the lesion.

2. If you are still sure that you can remove the lesion with a wide margin of normal tissue on all aspects, and

without producing deformity or serious loss of function, proceed to excision biopsy (see below). If you are not sure, however, change your plan of action to biopsy of the lesion (see below).

EXCISION BIOPSY

Action

1. Form a mental picture of the exact position and shape of your incision.

2. Using a 3/0 absorbable suture on a half-circle 30 mm or 50 mm cutting needle (according to the depth of bite required), insert a stitch through the tissues near each end of your proposed incision. The stitches must traverse the tissues far enough from the incision that they will not be cut when you make the incision. Bear in mind particularly the *depth* of stitch you will require if you are to get the depth of excision that you need. Leave the two ends of each untied but held in four artery forceps.

3. Excise the lesion with at least a 5 mm margin in all directions. Make the wound roughly oval, the direction of the long axis of the oval being dictated by the need to minimize damage to neighbouring structures. Do this as speedily as possible, as you cannot control bleeding till the excision is complete.

4. Pull each stitch end across the wound towards the opposite end of the other stitch i.e. the stitch ends form a cross. This should control the worst of the bleeding. Get your assistant to maintain traction on the stitch ends.

5. Inspect the excised specimen to make sure that, at least to the naked eye, the excision is complete. If it does not seem to be complete, you must consider taking more tissue from the appropriate region of the wound.

6. Assuming that the excision did appear complete, tie the stitches in the form of the cross, as your assistant has been holding them.

7. Complete haemostasis with diathermy and/or further sutures. Suction is a valuable aid to maintaining a clear field while you do this.

BIOPSY

Appraise

Decide where you will take your biopsy. Plan to get from the rim of the lesion a piece of tissue that includes a generous portion of the lesion in continuity with a generous portion of the neighbouring normal tissue. In general, the piece of tissue removed will be an oval with its long axis at right angles to the margin of the lesion.

Action

1. Insert one or two deep sutures of 3/0 absorbable material through normal tissues on either side of your proposed excision, and leave the ends untied. Do not put sutures into the lesion itself, since such a procedure may spread neoplasm.

2. Excise the specimen, taking care not to cut your sutures.

3. Tie the suture or sutures. Usually this stops all bleeding, but if it fails to do so, use diathermy or more sutures.

Check list

1. Was there any blood on the deeper parts of the pharyngeal pack? If there was, pay special attention to the possibility of chest complications later.

2. Are you sure that the specimen has been correctly bottled and labelled, that the request form for the pathology department has been accurately filled out, and that you are satisfied with the arrangements for conveying the specimen to the laboratory?

3. Should you send part of the specimen for bacteriological examination (e.g. if the lesion may be tuberculous)? Remember that any such sample must be sent in a sterile container **without formalin**.

PARTIAL GLOSSECTOMY

Appraise

Small lesions of the anterior two-thirds of the tongue are easily dealt with by excision biopsy. Larger lesions can also be excised with a wide margin. Remember, however, that the functions of the tongue in speaking, mastication and deglutition demand that it is a long mobile structure. Large excisions must be so planned as to preserve length, therefore, rather than width or thickness. To illustrate this principle, a wedge excision of the tip of the tongue is described.

Access

Prepare the patient in the same way as for a local excision biopsy of an intraoral lesion (p. 362).

Assess

1. Palpate the lesion and its surroundings carefully.

2. Decide the width and length of wedge that you have to remove to ensure a wide margin of normal tissue around the lesion.

Action

1. If you are right-handed, stand on the patient's right. If you are left-handed, you should reverse all references to side in these instructions.

2. Lay the index finger of your left hand long the

dorsum of the tongue, your thumb along the ventral aspect, to the right of the right-hand margin of your proposed excision. Squeeze the tongue (Fig. 22.9a).

3. Get your assistant, standing on the patient's left, to squeeze the tongue between the index and thumb of his right hand, to the left of the left-hand margin of your proposed excision.

4. Excise the wedge carrying the lesion. The digital pressure of your assistant and yourself minimizes bleeding.

5. Insert a series of interrupted absorbable 3/0 sutures to approximate the muscles in the deeper parts of the defect (Fig. 22.9b). A temporary relaxation of the fingers, first on one side and then the other, allows the efficacy of these sutures in stopping bleeding from the deeper parts of the wound to be assessed. Further sutures are inserted to close the mucosa along the dorsal and ventral surface of the tongue, and to stop bleeding from the superficial layers.

WEDGE EXCISION OF THE LIP

Appraise

Early tumours of the lip can be removed with a wide margin by this operation. Particularly in elderly people, up to one-third of the length of the lip can be removed in this way with an acceptable functional and cosmetic result. If the patient is young, or if a length of lip greater than one-third must be sacrificed, various plastic operations are available (see Ch. 31). These plastic operations are more difficult than they look, and should be done only by the expert. If such an expert is not immediately available, do

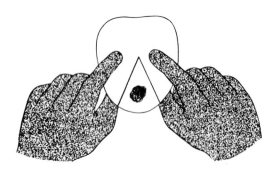

Fig. 22.9a Digital pressure method for controlling bleeding. The index finger and thumb on each side are applied just outside the margins of the proposed excision (indicated by the dotted lines).

Fig. 22.9b The start of the repair: the deepest suture has been inserted (the squeezing fingers have been omitted in the interests of clarity).

a simple wedge operation — carcinoma of the lip must be treated urgently. Subsequently, refer the patient to a plastic surgeon for correction of the disability and deformity.

Assess

1. Inspect and palpate the lesion and its surroundings with care.

2. Decide on the width and length of wedge necessary to excise the lesion with a clear margin, 0.5–1.0 cm, of normal tissue.

Action

1. Cut out the wedge, taking the full thickness of the lip. The method of digital pressure along the margins of the excision, as described in the operation of wedge excision of the tip of the tongue (see above), can be used to control bleeding. Another method is to use non-crushing intestinal clamps.

2. Close the defect with three layers of interrupted sutures: 3/0 absorbable sutures for the muscle, the same for the mucosa, and very fine non-absorbable sutures for the skin and the vermilion border. Pay special attention to the accuracy with which you make the two edges of the vermilion border, and of the mucocutaneous junction, meet.

EXCISION OF SUPRAHYOID (SUBMENTAL) CYST

Appraise

1. A cystic, subcutaneous swelling in the midline of the neck, above the level of the hyoid bone, may be a thyroglossal cyst or some simpler lesion such as a dermoid cyst. If the lump moves on swallowing, and on protrusion of the tongue, it is thyroglossal; if it does not, it is dermoid.

2. The distinction between the two types can be difficult. Therefore, when operating on a lump you have diagnosed as a dermoid cyst, always look for evidence of a track upwards towards the tongue, or downwards towards the hyoid. If you find such evidence, you must alter your diagnosis to thyroglossal cyst and change your operation accordingly (p. 367).

Access

1. The patient lies supine, with the upper half of the table angled sufficiently upwards to cause the external jugular veins to collapse. The head is extended on the neck, but the cervical spine is flexed on the thoracic spine. This position facilitates access to the front of the neck, without putting the strap muscles and the superficial

tissues on stretch. It is easy to obtain this position if the head-piece of the table is separately adjustable. If this facility is not available, you may find that a soft cylindrical object about 12 cm in diameter (e.g. an unopened roll of cotton wool), placed transversely under the neck, gives the right position.

2. Clean the skin from the level of the mouth to the clavicles, and from the anterior midline of the neck to the posterior border of each sternomastoid muscle laterally. Tuck a pad of sterile wool beneath the neck and scapular regions.

3. Towel up to leave exposed the lesion and a surrounding margin of 5 cm in all directions. Fix the towels to the skin of the neck around the exposed area, using No. 2 silk sutures inserted with a curved, cutting 50-mm needle.

4. Make a transverse (skin crease) incision centred over the lump and extending 2 or 3 cm past its borders on either side. Deepen this incision through the skin and superficial fascia, obtaining haemostasis with diathermy.

5. With a clean knife-blade, deepen the incision through the platysma, and then through the fascial layers until you reach the surface of the lesion.

6. Raise flaps of skin and the other superficial tissues upwards and downwards until the whole of the superficial aspect of the lump is exposed.

Action

1. Using fine, curved artey forceps, open up the plane between the surface of the lump and the surrounding fascial tissues. Continue this dissection, which should prove relatively bloodless, in all directions until you come to the deep aspect of the lesion.

2. In the region of the deep aspect, be particularly careful not to miss any fibrous extension of the wall of the cyst, either penetrating the median raphe between the underlying right and left mylohyoid muscles on its way to the tongue, or passing downwards towards the hyoid bone.

3. Assuming that you find no such extensions, complete the dissection of the deep aspect. The lump is now free.

Closure

1. Check haemostasis. Ask the anaesthetist to flatten the table so as to encourage bleeding points to become manifest immediately, while you are watching, rather than later when you have closed the skin.

2. Insert a suction drain 2.5 cm below the incision near either the right or the left extremity of the wound, and arrange the tube to lie along the length of the wound. To ensure an airtight fit of the tissues around the tube, pass it through the lower flap from the inside by screwing the tube on to the end of a special sharp introducer (shaped rather like a bootmaker's awl) and pushing the introducer

through the tissues. Make sure that there are several side-holes in the part of the tube that is left lying within the wound, and that there are no side-holes in the part of the tube lying outside the skin. Stitch the tube to the skin to maintain the optimal position: you must, of course, not transfix the tube with this stitch as this would result in an air leak and prevent efficient suction inside the wound. If the ends of the stitch are tied around the tube as a clove-hitch, the tube will be firmly anchored in position.

3. Close the skin with a continuous blanket stitch (Fig. 22.10). Remember that apposition must be made perfect along the whole length of the wound, not only to promote healing but to ensure that the wound is airtight so that the suction drainage can work efficiently.

4. Connect the drainage tubing to the suction apparatus — suction pump, evacuated bottle or Canny-Ryall syringe (Fig. 22.10). Check that after the air has been evacuated from the wound the system is airtight.

EXCISION OF THYROGLOSSAL CYST, SINUS AND FISTULA

Appraise

1. Much of the thyroid gland (the isthmus and part of the lateral lobes) originates at the foramen caecum at the junction of the posterior third and anterior two-thirds of

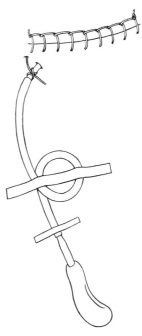

Fig. 22.10 Some details of the closure. Blanket-stitch gives firm, side-to-side apposition along every millimetre of the incision, ensuring that the incision is airtight. The suction-drain tubing is stitched to the skin using a clove-hitch to ensure that the tube cannot slip in or out. Two strips of Elastoplast strapping or paper tape are used to fix the tubing. The first fixes a loop so that pulling on the end of the apparatus does not pull the tube out of the wound. The second fixes the end of the tubing when the Canny-Ryall bulb syringe is inserted.

the tongue, and during foetal life migrates downwards to reach its definitive position anterior to the thyroid cartilage and overlapping the upper end of the trachea. The course of this migration is midline, first through the tongue itself and the muscles of the submental region, then closely applied to the anterior aspect of the hyoid; at this stage it loops upwards and backwards for a short distance before again turning downwards to the isthmus of the thyroid gland (Fig. 22.11).

2. Any part or all of this track, the thyroglossal tract, may persist. Persistence of the whole tract produces a fistula between the mouth and the neck, but this is very rare. The sinus is more common; an opening in the skin near the level of the thyroid isthmus connects with a track which proceeds upwards for a variable distance towards the foramen caecum. The most common lesion is the cyst, which may lie at any point in the track but most often in the region of the hyoid bone, and which may have associated with it a variable stretch of persistent track both upwards and downwards.

3. Whatever the exact lesions, you must ensure that all persistent portions of the track are excised, because otherwise recurrence is inevitable.

4. The intimate relationship between the track and the back of the body of the hyoid necessitates excision of a segment of the bone from the midline to make sure that this portion of the track has been excised.

5. Operations are described separately for (a) a thyroglossal sinus, and (b) a thyroglossal cyst lying just below the body of the hyoid.

EXCISION OF THYROGLOSSAL SINUS
Access

1. Make a symmetrical elliptical collar incision at the

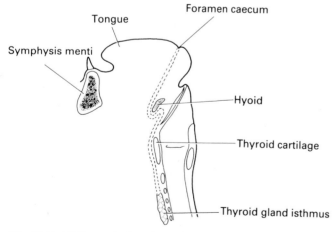

Fig. 22.11 Midline sagittal section through the mouth and neck to show the path taken by the thyroid between the foramen caecum at the base of the tongue and the definitive position of the gland. Note the intimate relationship between the track and the posterior aspect of the body of the hyoid, and the angle at which the suprahyoid portion of the track inclines.

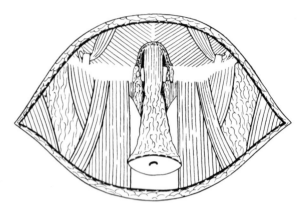

Fig. 22.12 Flaps of skin with platysma have been raised, leaving the opening of the sinus surrounded with an ellipse of skin. The track has been cored out to the body of the hyoid, the central portion of the bone has been detached in continuity with the track, and a cylinder of muscle is cored out in the midline from the submental muscles in a direction backwards and upwards at 45° (See Fig. 22.11)

level of the opening of the sinus, circumcising the sinus with an oval of skin and also excising any skin scarred by infections of the track.

2. Raise flaps of skin and platysma together; the lower flap need only be raised for 2–3 cm, but the upper flap must be raised to a level (in the midline) at least halfway between the hyoid and the symphysis menti (Fig. 22.12).

Action

1. Dissect the oval of skin and superficial fascia and the fibrous tissue around the upward track from the sinus opening, raising a tube of tissues containing the track. At this and every subsequent stage, be careful to keep a margin of tissue between your instruments and the track itself.

2. The opening of the sinus may be situated above the thyroid isthmus, in which case you may be able to feel a fibrous cord, representing the lowest part of the track, running downwards from your dissected tube. Cut across this cord and follow its lower end downwards to the thyroid isthmus to excise this part of the track as a separate item.

3. Continue coring out the upper part of the track upwards till you reach the level of the hyoid bone. Pass a blunt dissector (such as Macdonald's) deep to the body of the hyoid and gently separate the bone from the attached muscles and the underlying thyrohyoid membrane for a distance of about 1 cm centred on the midline. Use bone-cutting forceps to excise this segment of bone, leaving it in continuity with the track.

4. Above the hyoid, the track plunges through the median raphe of the mylohyoid muscles in a direction sloping at 45° backwards and upwards. It traverses the deeper submental muscles to reach the foramen caecum.

Get your assistant to put his index finger in the mouth and push the base of the tongue downwards towards you. Core out a cylinder of muscle in the direction described to complete the dissection of the track. The uppermost part of the track is practically never patent, and indeed may not be palpable even as a fibrous cord, but it is wise to extend this procedure for 2 cm deep to the mylohyoid. If necessary, you must be prepared to continue till you are separated from the mouth (and your assistant's finger) only by the mucous membrane covering the tongue. Cut across the core of muscle and remove the whole dissected track.

Closure

1. Achieve haemostasis.
2. Suture the defect in the submental muscles in one or more layers. Repair any midline defect in the strap muscles produced by coring out the track.
3. Insert a suction drain via a separate stab incision in the lower flap (see p. 365).
4. Close the skin.

EXCISION OF THYROGLOSSAL CYST

Access

1. Make a symmetrical collar incision, centred over the cyst.
2. Raise flaps of skin with platysma downwards to the lower margin of the cyst and upwards to a point (in the midline) halfway between the body of the hyoid and the symphysis menti.

Action

1. Dissect all round the superficial aspects of the cyst. As you approach the deep aspect, separate the sterno-hyoid muscles in the midline so that you can get a good view of the deep aspect.
2. Search for any downward extension of the track as a fibrous cord in the midline. If you find one, follow it as far downwards as you can feel it, or to the isthmus of the thyroid gland, and excise it separately.
3. Mobilize the cyst upwards on its deep surface. You will find that it is intimately adherent to the body of the hyoid bone in the midline.
4. Resect 1 cm of the body of the hyoid as described above, in continuity with the cyst.
5. Complete the excision by the coring-out procedure of the muscles of the submental region as described above.

Closure

This is the same as after the excision of a thyroglossal sinus (see above).

OPERATIONS FOR BRANCHIAL CYST, SINUS AND FISTULA

Appraise

1. Portions of the first or second branchial clefts may remain patent. This happens more commonly with the second cleft; the complete lesion is a fistula, with one opening in the pharynx in the region of the posterior pillar of the fauces, and the other in the skin at the junction of middle and lower thirds of the anterior border of the sterno-mastoid muscle. The complete fistula is not as common as a branchial sinus, where the lower opening and the main track are present but the track does not communicate at its upper end with the pharynx.

2. The branchial cyst occurs when the central portion only of the second cleft remains patent. There is then a cystic spherical swelling deep to the junction of the upper and middle thirds of the sternomastoid muscle, and becoming superficial at the anterior border of the muscle. A large branchial cyst encroaches on what is clinically the parotid region. In such cases, you must be careful to proceed in such a manner as to enable you to carry out a formal parotidectomy if necessary (see exploration of the lower pole of the parotid, p. 356). The description given in this section assumes that the clinical diagnosis of branchial cyst is straightforward and that there is no possibility that the swelling is a parotid tumour.

3. Finally, the first arch remnant may give rise to a cyst in the parotid region, or the cyst may communicate as a sinus posteriorly with the cartilaginous external auditory meatus or anteriorly with an opening in the skin of the submandibular region, or there may be a complete fistula between the submandibular region and the external auditory meatus. The simple cyst will not be distinguishable clinically from other lumps in the parotid region, and you will remove it by formal conservative parotidectomy. If the cyst communicates with the external auditory meatus, you may find during the parotidectomy that a cartilaginous extension from the external auditory meatus runs into the cyst. You can cut across this funnel of cartilage and leave the resulting defect open, then proceed with the parotidectomy, and after the facial nerve is well exposed you can close the cartilaginous defect by sewing soft tissues together over the defect and without danger to the facial nerve.

4. The really difficult technical problem is the sinus in the submandibular region with a track extending into the parotid region, with or without a palpable cyst in the parotid region. The surgeon who operates only occasionally in the parotid region should not attempt to operate on this condition, and the operation will therefore not be described in detail here. The principle of the operation is that a superficial parotidectomy is commenced and taken up to the stage where the cervical and mandibular branches of the facial nerve have been exposed well forwards along their course, at least to the anterior border of the parotid

gland itself, and that the submandibular sinus is then circumcised and the track dissected backwards into the parotid region. If, as is usual, the track is superficial to the facial nerve, the operation is completed by completing the superficial parotidectomy. Occasionally, however, as one dissects the track backwards it is seen to run into the deep part of the parotid and a deep or total conservative parotidectomy must be performed (p. 353).

5. The operations described in detail in this section are those for a typical (second cleft) branchial sinus or fistula and branchial cyst.

EXCISION OF BRANCHIAL SINUS OR FISTULA

Access

1. Position the patient supine, with the upper half of the operating table tilted upwards sufficiently to cause the external jugular vein to collapse. Turn the patient's head to the opposite side.

2. Clean the skin from the level of the mouth to the clavicle, and from the anterior midline of the neck to as far posteriorly as can be reached. Tuck a pad of sterile wool beneath the neck and scapular regions.

3. Towel up to leave exposed an area from the jaw above to 5 cm below the opening of the sinus below, and from the anterior midline of the neck to the anterior border of the trapezius posteriorly.

4. Make an elliptical incision (Fig. 22.13) in the skin

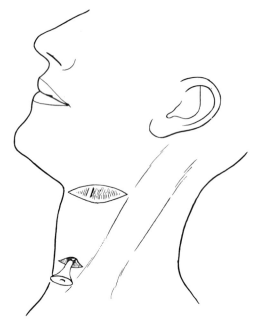

Fig. 22.13 The opening of the sinus or fistula low in the neck is circumcised with an elliptical incision, and the track cored out upwards by incising the deep fascia. At the level of the hyoid, a second incision is made and the mobilized track drawn upwards through the second incision.

around the opening of the sinus; the long axis of the incision should be horizontal (i.e. in the skin crease) and about 5 cm long, while the short axis should give 1 cm clearance above and below the margins of the opening.

5. With a clean knife-blade, deepen the incision through the subcutaneous tissue and the platysma. Put traction on the skin ellipse with tissue forceps or a stitch, and you should be able to feel the track from the lower aspect of the wound as a fibrous cord running upwards along the anterior border of the sternomastoid, deep to the deep (investing cervical) fascia.

6. Dissect upwards on all aspects of the track, coring it out from the fascial planes of the neck. To facilitate this dissection, raise the upper skin flap in the plane deep to the platysma, and incise the deep fascia upwards along the anterior border of the sternomastoid, superficial to the track.

7. If the track can be palpated to ascend higher in the neck than you can comfortably expose through your incision, make a further skin crease (horizontal) incision with the skin knife at the level of the hyoid bone, extending from 2 cm short of the anterior midline of the neck to the anterior border of the sternomastoid. Use the clean knife to deepen this incision through subcutaneous tissue and platysma, and then elevate the lower flap in the plane deep to the platysma until you can pass a pair of long curved artery forceps downwards through the upper incision to grasp the skin ellipse at the lower end of the track. Pull the skin ellipse upwards under the skin-bridge between the two incisions so that it presents at the upper incision. You now have comfortable access for completing the dissection.

Action

1. Continue the dissection of the track upwards. Remember that the most efficient way of finding the direction of the track is to feel the fibrous cord with your fingers.

2. The usual course of the track is to pass between the external and internal carotid arteries and then deep to the posterior belly of the digastric muscle. Divide the digastric at its intermediate tendon anteriorly, and 2 cm behind the track posteriorly. When you have excised the segment of muscle between these points, it is easy to follow the track upwards to its termination.

3. Deep to the posterior belly of the digastric, the track lies superficial to the middle constrictor muscle of the pharynx (Fig. 22.14). Take care not to damage the hypoglossal nerve, which runs forwards between the track and the middle constrictor at the level of the lower border of the digastric. Also look out for the glossopharyngeal nerve, which runs a similar course about 1 cm higher up and must also be preserved.

4. Immediately above the glossopharyngeal nerve, the

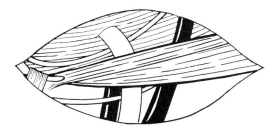

Fig. 22.14 The track is now followed further upwards, passing between external and internal carotid arteries deep to the posterior belly of the digastric, to merge with the fascia covering the middle constrictor. The glossopharyngeal and hypoglossal nerves run between the track and the middle constrictor.

track swings forwards and its fibrous sheath blends with the aponeurosis covering the middle constrictor. At this point there may be a connection between the interior of the track and the lumen of the pharynx, but it is not important to discover whether such a connection exists. Simply apply two pairs of artery forceps to the track where it blends with the muscle, cut between the forceps, and tie off the pharyngeal end.

Closure

1. Insert a drain through skin and platysma via a point just below the lower incision, and lay the part of the tube within the wound up through the bed of the track to the middle constrictor.

2. Repair the vertical incision in the deep fascia with fine silk or chromic catgut ligatures. Check haemostasis carefully, especially in the tunnel between the upper and lower incisions.

3. Close the skin incisions, fix the tube to the skin, and attach the tube to suction as described for the excision of supra-hyoid (submental) cyst (p. 365).

EXCISION OF BRANCHIAL CYST

Access

1. Make a horizontal (skin crease) incision at the level of the lesion, i.e. at the junction of upper and middle thirds of the sternomastoid, extending from 1 cm anterior to the anterior margin of the lesion to halfway between the anterior and posterior borders of the sternomastoid.

2. Deepen the incision through subcutaneous tissue and platysma, and reflect the flaps upwards and downwards in the plane deep to the platysma, to the upper and lower margins of the lump.

3. Incise the deep (investing cervical) fascia over the lump in a direction parallel to the anterior border of the sternomastoid.

4. Use a self-retaining retractor to separate the upper and lower flaps of skin and platysma. Ask your assistant

to retract the anterior border of the sternomastoid posteriorly. You now have excellent access to the swelling.

Action

1. By careful blunt dissection, wipe away the intervening areolar tissue to display the wall of the cyst. Continue the dissection around the superficial aspect of the cyst, and then proceed around the deep aspect of its lower pole.

2. Immediately deep to the cyst lies the beginning of the external and internal carotid arteries. Be careful not to damage these or the vagus nerve lying behind the internal carotid artery.

3. The cyst wall is often very thin; try not to damage the wall, as it is easier to be certain that you have removed the whole cyst if it remains intact throughout the operation. If you leave fragments of the wall behind, the lesion may recur.

4. Continue the dissection upwards behind the cyst, mobilizing it from the middle constrictor muscle. Note and preserve the hypoglossal nerve, running forwards between the cyst and the middle constrictor at the level of the lower border of the posterior belly of the digastrict, and 1 cm higher up the glossopharyngeal nerve, running in the same direction and in the same plane (Fig. 22.14 shows the relevant anatomy of this area).

5. Sometimes the cyst does not extend much above the level of the posterior belly of the digastric, but often it does extend considerably upwards, deep to the posterior belly. In such cases, it is necessary to excise a segment of the posterior belly, from the middle tendon in front to the posterior margin of the cyst behind, so that the dissection can proceed safely upwards on both superficial and deep aspects of the cyst.

6. Occasionally, at the deep aspect of the cyst above the level of the glossopharyngeal nerve, you will find a fibrous track arising from the cyst and blending with the fascia covering the middle constrictor, rather like the top end of a branchial fistula. Divide this track between two pairs of curved artery forceps, and tie the end attached to the muscle. Usually, you will find no evidence of this track and the simple blunt dissection around the cyst is sufficient to free it. Remove the cyst.

Closure

1. Check for bleeding. Use diathermy to stop bleeding points, with special care not to damage the nerves you have demonstrated during the dissection. Insert a drainage tube via a skin puncture 5 cm below the incision (see p. 365).

2. Repair the deep fascia along the anterior border of the sternomastoid with fine silk or catgut stitches.

3. Close the skin and apply suction to the drain.

EXCISION BIOPSY OF CERVICAL LYMPH NODE

Appraise

1. Never attempt this operation under local anaesthesia if general anaesthesia is available. Cervical lymph nodes may feel superficial yet lie deeply in the neck, and the dissection to remove them may be much more difficult than you expect.

2. Depending on the position of the lymph node, neighbouring structures may be at risk during the operation. An example commonly encountered is the accessory nerve, either in the anterior triangle of the neck at the junction of upper and middle thirds of the anterior border of the sternomastoid muscle, or in the posterior triangle at the junction of the middle and lower thirds of the sternomastoid.

3. A lymph gland must be handled very gently during the dissection. Rough handling is likely to distort the internal structure of the node and make histological interpretation difficult.

4. The operation described here is for a lymph node lying under cover of the anterior border of the sternomastoid muscle near the junction of its upper and middle thirds. The principles illustrated can be applied to an operation on a lymph node anywhere else in the neck.

Access

1. Position the patient supine with the upper half of the operating table tilted upwards sufficiently to cause the external jugular vein to collapse. Turn the patient's head to the opposite side.

2. Clean the skin from the level of the mouth to the clavicle, and from the anterior midline of the neck to as far posteriorly as can be reached. Tuck a pad of sterile wool beneath the neck and scapular regions.

3. Towel up to leave exposed a circular area of radius about 5 cm around the palpable lymph node. Fix the towels to the skin of the neck around the exposed area by No. 2 silk sutures, inserted with a curved, cutting 50 mm needle.

4. Make an incision across the palpable lump and extended for 1 cm beyond its margins in both directions, in the direction of the lines of skin tension (in this case roughly horizontally, with a slight convex curve downwards). Deepen this incision through skin and platysma.

5. Achieve haemostasis with diathermy.

Assess

1. Feel the lump carefully again. Is it covered only with fascia or is any other structure between your fingers and the swelling?

2. If the intervening tissues are fascia only, deepen your incision through these tissues with a clean scalpel until you can see the surface of the lymph node itself.

3. If there is some structure other than fascia in the way, you must move it out of the way, excise it or cut through it so as to reach the surface of the lymph node. Exactly what you do will depend upon the nature of the structure. The commonest in this particular site is the anterior border of the sternomastoid muscle. Usually it is easy to spread apart the edges of the wound in the skin and platysma with retractors, to divide the fascia where it joins the anterior border of the muscle over a distance of about 3 cm, and to retract backwards the anterior border of the muscle. The fascia overlying the lymph node can now be incised.

Action

1. Dissect the lymph node free from its surroundings. A good way to do this is to lay a small, curved artery forceps along the surface of the node, with the curve of the forceps corresponding with the curvature of the surface. Insert the tips of the blades of the forceps between the gland and the free edge of investing fascia where you have cut the fascia in order to reach the swelling. Gently push the forceps further along this plane and then separate the blades, thereby stripping the fascia off the lymph node. Cut the fascia with scissors between the separated blades of the forceps, so as to increase the exposure.

2. Repeat this process of combined blunt and sharp dissection all over the superficial aspect of the lymph node. Minimize bleeding by the use of diathermy on vessels before you cut them, if that is possible. A really dry field facilitates the dissection.

3. During this superficial clearance, there is no need to handle the lymph node at all. As you approach the deep aspect, it becomes necessary to push the gland in one direction so that you can free it in that area of its bed from which you are displacing it. This manipulation is likely to damage the gland; be very gentle, and use a finger rather than a metal instrument.

4. Somewhere in this deep aspect you will nearly always find a fairly large feeding artery to the gland. In this region, also, it is easy to damage neighbouring important structures such as the accessory nerve, because the exposure is limited by the overhanging gland. The safe rule is to cut only tissues that you can see perfectly.

5. When you have completed the dissection deep to the lymph node, it will be lying free. Remove the node, cut it into two equal parts, put one into a container which will later be filled with formol-saline and sent for histological examination, and put the other into a sterile empty container so that it can be sent for culture (including for tuberculosis).

Closure

1. Ensure complete haemostasis. Ask the anaesthetist to flatten the operating table; this change of posture raises venous pressure and sometimes starts bleeding, and it is

better that this should happen while you have the wound still open rather than after you have sewn up.

2. Ask the instrument nurse whether swab and instrument counts are correct.

3. Sew up any deep muscle that you have had to divide, using 2/0 absorbable sutures.

4. Some surgeons put a similar layer of sutures in the platysma. I find this unnecessary.

5. Sew up the skin wound.

Check list

1. Is there any sign of a haematoma forming?

2. Are the two portions of the specimen being properly dealt with?

SCALENE NODE BIOPSY

Appraise

1. The pad of fat lying superficial to the lower end of the scalenus anterior muscle contains a number of small lymph nodes which are often involved (even if they are not palpably enlarged) by diseases of the lungs or mediastinum.

2. If the nodes on the left side are palpable, or if the intrathoracic disease being investigated involved only the upper lobe of the left lung, do the biopsy on the left side. In all other cases, do the biopsy on the right side, since the glands on the right side are much more likely to be involved.

Access

1. Position the patient and drape as for cervical lymph node biopsy, page 370.

2. Make a 5 cm horizontal skin-crease incision 2.5 cm above the clavicle, extending from the anterior border of the trapezius muscle to the posterior (lateral) border of the sternal head of the sternomastoid muscle. Deepen the incision through the platysma.

3. Divide between ligatures the external jugular vein and its tributaries. The main vein runs vertically just deep to the platysma, about the middle of the incision.

4. Divide the clavicular head of sternomastoid by passing a blunt dissector (e.g. Watson-Cheyne's) gently deep to the muscle and cutting down upon the dissector. Do the cutting in small portions, so that you can prevent troublesome bleeding from veins within the muscle. Remember also that your dissector is close to the internal jugular vein, and accordingly take care over this manoeuvre.

Action

1. Retract the margins of the wound with a self-retaining retractor. The fat pad lying superficial to the scalene

anterior muscle is now visible, but it may be overlain by the transverse cervical vessels just above the clavicle. Push these vessels downwards, grasp the fat pad with plain dissecting forceps immediately above the vessels, and cut horizontally into the fat pad till the fascia covering the scalenus anterior becomes visible. Lift the fat pad upwards, and with scissors or knife elevate the fat pad off the fascia from below upwards (Fig. 22.15).

2. Important structures form the bed of the fat pad and you must take care not to damage them. Lying on the anterior surface of the scalenus anterior muscle, but deep to the fascia, is the phrenic nerve, running more or less vertically downwards but with a trend from lateral to medial. Medial to the scalenus anterior is the internal jugular vein, lateral to the muscle lies the brachial plexus.

3. As the elevation continues, the omohyoid muscle must be retracted upwards: the muscle crosses the upper part of the field obliquely, running in a superomedial direction.

4. When you have freed the fat pad as far as you can conveniently push the omohyoid, cut through the upper end of the pad to remove it completely.

5. Check haemostasis. Note whether lymph is accumulating in the wound. This complication is of course more likely on the left side. Try to find the damaged lymphatic duct (thoracic duct) and tie it off.

Closure

1. Repair the clavicular head of sternomastoid with fine sutures.

2. Drain the wound by a suction drain via a separate stab incision.

3. Sew up the skin.

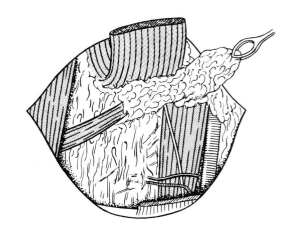

Fig. 22.15 Scalene node biopsy. Flaps of skin with platysma have been raised, the clavicular head of sternomastoid divided. The fat pad covering the scalenus anterior is excised between the transverse cervical vessels below and the omohyoid muscle above. Damage to the brachial plexus, phrenic nerve and internal jugular vein must be avoided.

OPERATIONS ON TUBERCULOUS CERVICAL LYMPH NODES

Appraise

1. You may encounter tuberculous cervical lymph nodes in three main surgical situations: the undiagnosed lump, the mass that is biopsied to establish the diagnosis but does not disappear with chemotherapy, and the **cold** abscess.

2. The operation to remove an enlarged, undiagnosed lymph node in the neck is described on page 370. Remember to send half of the specimen for culture, including culture for acid-fast organisms, as well as the other half for histology. If the histological report comes back as tuberculosis, consult with a physician about chemotherapy. If a physician is not available, start the patient on triple therapy with a combination of three common drugs such as streptomycin, isoniazid and rifampicin, while awaiting the culture of the organisms and sensitivity tests upon them.

3. A larger mass of lymph nodes should be biopsied. When a histological report of tuberculosis has been received, start chemotherapy. Usually under the influence of chemotherapy the mass shrinks and disappears. Occasionally this does not happen, and you should then suspect that the organisms are not sensitive to the combination of drugs that you are using. Should the mass of infected glands become larger, the centre of the mass become fluctuant (cold abscess), or the skin become involved and threaten to break down, surgery is indicated. Aspirate a cold abscess, inserting a hypodermic needle through uninvolved skin at some distance from the lesion so as to produce a long oblique track with a valvular effect that should minimize the risk of sinus formation. Remember to send the material from the abscess for culture and sensitivity tests. However, if all or most of the lesion is solid, an open operation is indicated as described later.

4. Sometimes (not often these days in countries with a high standard of primary health care) you may see a lesion that has already progressed to the stage of a cold abscess, or skin involvement with inflammatory changes and scar formation or even sinuses, by the time you first see the patient. The important point about this particular situation is that no matter how typical the clinical picture, the diagnosis of tuberculosis must be confirmed by biopsy. It is unthinkable to subject a patient to several months of chemotherapy without a definite diagnosis. In these circumstances, and since the material obtained by aspiration of a cold abscess often fails to clinch the diagnosis, an open operation is also indicated.

PRINCIPLES OF OPEN OPERATION

1. Make a horizontal (skin-crease) incision over the swelling, of a generous length to provide adequate exposure.

2. Modify the incision where necessary to excise all affected skin.

3. Reflect flaps of skin and platysma upwards and downwards to the limits of the involved lymph nodes.

4. Divide the investing fascia of the neck in the region of any fluctuant area or areas, enter the abscesses and evacuate their contents.

5. If the main purpose of the operation is to confirm the clinical diagnosis, scrape the walls of the abscess cavity with a curette to obtain generous portions of the granulation tissue for culture and histology.

6. If the main purpose of the operation is to excise infected glands that have proved resistant to chemotherapy, dissect out as much of the involved lymph nodes as is technically possible. This is a difficult operation, because the lymph nodes tend to be adherent to neighbouring structures that are functionally important and must be preserved.

7. This section is called the 'principles of open operation' because it is not possible to specify in detail all the difficulties and dangers that you may meet. These depend on the exact site of the involved lymph nodes. For example, the lymph nodes of the anterior triangle may be adherent to the jugular vein, the common carotid artery and its two branches, and the vagus nerve; the jugulo-digastric group may be adherent to the hypoglossal, accessory and glossopharyngeal nerves; and there may be involved lymph nodes in the posterior triangle around the lower part of the accessory nerve.

8. When you have completed the excision, ensure that you have achieved meticulous haemostasis and then close the skin, if possible without drainage. If much skin has been excised, some rearrangement of the skin flaps may be necessary to achieve primary closure.

BLOCK DISSECTION OF CERVICAL LYMPH NODES

Appraise

Many carcinomas of the head and neck metastasize to the cervical lymph nodes. Whatever the best mode of treatment for the primary, whether surgery or radiotherapy, control of affected cervical lymph nodes is best obtained by excising them. The aim is to remove a block of connective tissue containing the nodes from the anterior and posterior triangles, extending from the clavicle below to the base of skull above. However, remember that the operation is futile unless (a) the primary growth is cured or curable, and (b) there are no metastases at more distant sites.

Access

1. If you are removing the primary growth at the same

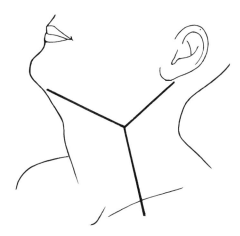

Fig. 22.16 Block dissection of the neck. The incision.

time, the standard approach for parotidectomy, glossectomy, mandibulectomy, laryngectomy, etc. is extended appropriately to make flaps which lay open the neck on the side of the growth. (See, for example, p. 355).

2. If the block dissection is done as a separate procedure, after apparent cure of the primary tumour, make an inverted Y-shaped incision with equal limbs (Fig. 22.16). Reflect the flaps to expose the entire neck from clavicle to mandible and mastoid, and from midline backwards to trapezius.

Action

1. Divide the clavicular and sternal heads of the sternomastoid just above their insertions. Very gently dissect the lower end of the internal jugular vein, separating it from the common carotid artery and, deep to that, the vagus nerve. Be careful on the left side not to damage the thoracic duct. Ligate and divide the vein, placing two stout non-absorbable ligatures on the lower stump: for extra safety, let one of these be a transfixion ligature.

2. Divide the inferior belly of the omohyoid and extend the dissection laterally just above the clavicle to the anterior border of trapezius. Watch out for an unusually high subclavian vein and deepen the dissection to the prevertebal fascia covering the scalenus muscles and brachial plexus.

3. In front of the trachea divide the thyroid isthmus and inferior thyroid veins, so that the hemithyroid gland and strap muscles (first divided above the clavicle and sternum) can be stripped upwards. Ligate and divide the inferior thyroid vessels, (preserving the recurrent laryngeal nerve unless a laryngectomy has already been done). Some surgeons do not perform hemi-thyroidectomy unless the primary tumour was close by, e.g. laryngeal.

4. Now dissect the block upwards, taking the hemithyroid gland, sternomastoid, internal jugular vein and all connective and lymphoid tissues from the anterior and posterior triangles. Clean the tissues off the trapezius border and leave the brachial plexus, prevertebral fascia, scaleni, vagus and phrenic nerves, thoracic duct, carotid vessels, trachea and oesophagus intact. The accessory nerve will be divided entering the trapezius. At the top of the wound divide the sternomastoid again, and carefully divide the deeper fascial planes until, drawing the specimen forwards, you can find and dissect again the upper end of the internal jugular. Ligate and divide it as near as safely can be to the skull base.

5. Cut the deep fascia close to the lower border of the mandible and clear the contents of the submental and submandibular triangles. Divide Wharton's duct so that the submandibular gland can be removed as part of the block excision. If necessary be prepared to take the lower pole of the parotid, but remember that the cervical branch of the facial nerve will then probably be lost. Lingual and hypoglossal nerves are of course left intact.

6. Sundry large veins — common facial, posterior facial — will need individual ligation, and as the block is worked downwards, the remaining vascular attachments (near the external carotid) to be divided after double ligation are the facial and sternomastoid arteries. The upper attachments of the sternohyoid and sternothyroid muscles are divided, and the accessory nerve at its entry into the sternomastoid. A few residual shreds of carotid sheath are divided and the specimen is free. (Fig. 22.17)

Technical

1. If it is not necessary to remove the thyroid gland, the sternothyroid and sternohyoid muscles can be preserved.

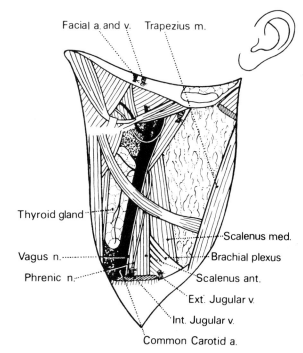

Fig. 22.17 Neck dissection completed.

2. In selected cases of 'floor of mouth' cancer, the procedure is limited by some surgeons to the upper half of the neck.

3. In case of bilateral metastases, the internal jugular vein should be preserved if possible on one side. Separate the two block dissections by a period of not less than 6 weeks.

4. 'Conservative' neck dissection preserves the sterno-mastoid muscle and accessory nerve — a more difficult but commendable procedure.

Closure

Meticulous haemostasis is essential. Ensure the adhesion of the skin flaps by meticulous skin closure, and use continuous vacuum drainage to encourage primary healing.

RADICAL PAROTIDECTOMY WITH BLOCK DISSECTION

1. Patients with proven malignant disease of the parotid gland require a formal block dissection in continuity with the parotidectomy. The posterior end of the upper skin flap is modified by prolonging it as the mastoid-facial part of the standard parotidectomy incision (Fig. 22.18).

2. Frequently in such cases the disease spreads posteriorly to involve the external ear, and anteriorly to involve the mandible in the region of its angle. The pinna and the posterior part of the mandible, including the ramus and the body as far forwards as the second molar tooth, are then removed in continuity with the rest of the excised tissue. The modification of the skin incisions is shown in Figure 22.19. Any area of skin infiltrated by the tumour must be widely sacrificed. The upper flap is reflected well

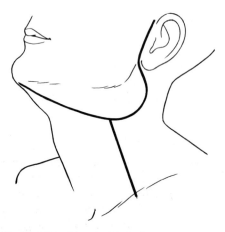

Fig. 22.18 Modified Y-incision for block dissection to include radical parotidectomy. The posterior limb becomes prolonged as the upper two-thirds of a formal parotidectomy incision (see Fig. 22.1) This incision is also suitable for the commando operation, provided that the anterior limb is extended fully to the symphysis menti.

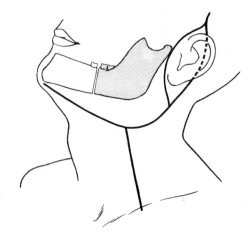

Fig. 22.19 Modified Y-incision for block dissection with excision of the pinna and radical parotidectomy. The portion of mandible to be removed if the tumour extends close to that bone is indicated.

forwards to expose the masseter muscle and the mandible cleared of the buccinator muscle forwards to the second molar socket.

If the patient is edentulous, the medial aspect of the body can now be cleared without opening the oral mucosa; if the molars are present, the mucosa must be cut in their vicinity to free them from the mouth. The body is divided through the socket of the second molar.

The inner aspect of the ramus is then freed from the temporalis muscle (attached to the coronoid process) and the pterygoid muscles (the lateral attached to the mandibular condyle, the medial to the mandibular angle). Division of the masseter from the zygoma at the upper border of the coronoid and condylar processes frees the bone and attached lower portion of the masseter, and then the dissection proceeds posteriorly to remove the whole parotid. If indicated, the zygomatic arch can be resected as well. Closure of the skin flaps can be difficult after this operation, if much skin infiltrated by disease has been sacrificed.

RADICAL SUBMANDIBULAR SIALOADENECTOMY WITH RESECTION OF SEGMENT OF MANDIBLE AND BLOCK DISSECTION

1. An operation involving resection of a segment of the body of the mandible in continuity with a block dissection of the servical lymph nodes is often called a commando operation.

2. Proven malignant disease of the submandibular gland requires resection of the neighbouring segment of mandibular body to achieve a wide clearance. Carcinoma of the floor of the mouth or of the tongue, adjacent to the mandible, is another indication.

3. The incision should be of the type shown in Figure

22.18 without the posterior parotid extension and with the anterior end of the upper incision prolonged to reach the symphysis menti. Wide elevation of the upper flap to the upper border of the body of the mandible gives good exposure.

4. After the excision, the mucosa and muscles of the floor of mouth and submandibular region are repaired. The defect in the body of the mandible can be immediately repaired with a titanium prosthesis, provided that the area has not been X-irradiated; alternatively, the defect is accepted. Provided that the region of the symphysis menti is intact, a gap in the body does not produce a severe deformity, or instability of the lower jaw.

Further reading

Ballantyne J, Groves J 1971 Diseases of the ear, nose and throat, 3rd edn. Butterworths, London

Cook H P, Ranger D 1969 A technique for excision of para-pharyngeal tumours. Journal of Laryngology and Otology 83: 863–871

Hobsley M 1973 Salivary tumours. British Journal of Hospital Medicine 10: 553–562

Hobsley M 1983 A Colour Atlas of Parotidectomy. Wolfe Medical Publications, London

Arterial surgery

INTRODUCTION

Any competent general surgeon should be able to open, repair and join an artery during the course of an operation for something else. There are three reasons for operating directly on an artery:

1. *Injury*. This may result from assault or road or industrial accident or from a mishap following deliberate puncture.
2. *Aneurysm*. Nowadays this means dilatation due to atherosclerosis.
3. *Blockage*. Most arterial occlusions occur from thrombosis of a diseased vessel and are part of a generalised aging process which needs careful assessment before surgery is planned. More rarely, a normal vessel is blocked by an embolus arising from elsewhere. Management of these two events is quite different.

The sections which follow are devoted to techniques of arterial reconstruction and make the assumption that the patient has already been critically evaluated and the need for operation established. The operations described are those which the general surgeon should know about; there are plenty of more detailed works for the intending specialist.

PRINCIPLES OF ARTERIAL SURGERY

EQUIPMENT

Instruments

Most vascular operations can be done with the naked eye, but it is useful to practice with ×2 magnifying spectacles and for very fine work a microscope is essential.

As well as a general surgical set, including small scalpels and self-retaining retractors, the following special instruments are necessary.

1. Obtain a set of lightweight vascular clamps. The DeBakey 'atraugrip' range provides a good selection, and a few minature clamps of the Castañeda or similar type designed for paediatric cardiac surgery are useful. The springs should be light and gentle, because arteries are damaged by tight clamping. Vessels can be usually controlled by light traction with a nylon tape. Coloured plastic loops cost more, and have no particular advantage.
2. Use Potts' scissors, angled in two planes, for extension of arterial incisions.
3. Use a Watson Cheyne and James MacDonald dissector for elevating the core of an endarterectomy.
4. Always have available a complete set of Fogarty embolectomy catheters ranging from 3F to 6F.
5. Long tunnelling instruments such as the Taylor tunneler, together with introducing forceps, are necessary for conveying grafts between the unconnected incisions.

Sutures

1. Arteries are always sewn with nonabsorbable stitches. These are of two types. Fine monofilament material such as polypropylene ('Prolene'), has the advantage of being very smooth and slipping easily through the tissues, so that a loose suture can be drawn up tight. It does have a slight tendency to stretch and so become spiral if it is pulled hard. The other types of suture is braided material coated with an outer layer of polyester, to render it smooth. Examples of such sutures are 'Ethiflex' and 'Ethibond'.

Sutures of this type do not slip so easily through the arterial wall, but are pleasantly floppy to handle and knot easily. Tough atraumatic needles are suaged to each end of the suture.

2. In general, use the finest suture which is strong enough for the job. Most surgeons use 3/0 or 4/0 on the aorta, and 5/0 or 6/0 on the popliteal and tibial vessels. An endarterectomized artery can be closed with a finer suture than is necessary for a vessel of full thickness. For very fine work, a monofilament stitch is always necessary.

Solutions

Use 5000 units of heparin in 500 ml normal saline as an irrigating fluid to keep host and graft tissues moist, to flush out suture lines, and freshen the operation field.

Arterial substitutes

The best arterial substitute is the patient's own vein. Other biological materials such as arterial or venous allografts or xenografts have been tried and abandoned. However, quite often there is no vein available, because it is absent, too small or thrombosed. Under these circumstances a prosthesis has to be chosen and three are available.

1. *Dacron* is the longest established and best known material and is available in the form of tubes from 5 to 25 mm in diameter, straight or bifurcated, knitted or woven. In general, the knitted material with a velours lining is preferred, as its porosity leads to better anchoring of the internal surface. Knitted grafts need to be carefully preclotted (see below), and in an emergency such as a ruptured anaeurysm it is better to use a woven graft, which leaks less.

2. *Expanded PTFE ('Gore-Tex')* is about three times more expensive than Dacron, but appears to behave rather better in the long-term. This difference in performance is not important in large arteries such as the aorta, but may become crucial in operations below the inguinal ligament. As yet, it is difficult to be certain whether the extra expense incurred by the routine use of this material rather than Dacron is justified by better long-term patency rates.

3. *The Dardik Human Umbilical Vein* 'Biograft' is again very much more expensive than synthetic material, but experience to date suggests that it performs almost as well as autogenous vein. Most surgeons would wish to have one or two of these grafts on hand, for use in the exceptional case where a distal anastomosis has to be carried cut in a patient who has lost his saphenous vein.

Preclotting technique

It is important when using all forms of Dacron synthetic to carry out a meticulous preclotting procedure, so as to produce a graft which is both leak-proof and antithrom-

bogenic. For the theory underlying the method, refer to the work of Lester Sauvage. The practical procedure is as follows:

1. Before the patient is heparinised, withdraw 20 ml of blood from a convenient artery or vein, and pass it through the graft. The blood is then left in a receptacle and the graft emptied and placed in a dish to one side. The blood is allowed to coagulate and the time taken noted (usually about 4 minutes).

2. Following this, withdraw a further 20 ml of blood and pass it through the graft, which is again laid in a separate receiver. Because fibrin precursors have accumulated on the inside, this second 20 ml of blood clots much more rapidly than the first, usually in about half the time.

3. Withdraw a further 20 ml of blood and repeat the process. The graft is by this time intensely thrombogenic, and often the blood coagulates so quickly that it is almost impossible to pass it through. Once again the graft is squeezed dry and placed aside.

4. At this stage, the prosthesis is virtually leak-proof, because its pores have been sealed by fibrin and platelets. However, it is thrombogenic, because of the mass of unneutralised thrombin which has accumulated on its inner surface. The final step involves neutralisation of this thrombin with heparin. Withdraw 50 ml of blood, mix it with 20 000 U heparin and flush it repeatedly through the graft, while testing its integrity by the use of a syringe and a clamp. We now have a tube which will neither leak nor clot, and is ready to put into the patient. Wrap it in a sterile swab and place it carefully on one side.

TYPES OF OPERATION

1. Repair of arterial trauma (see below).

2. Removal of an embolus. This is a comparatively simple procedure, because it involves clearance of what is in most cases a normal arterial tree. The basic instrument used is a Fogarty catheter.

3. Correction of an aneurysm. Aneurysms are dangerous because they enlarge in exponential relation to their diameter. A small aneurysm enlarges slowly but a large one enlarges fast, and rapidly approaches the point of rupture. Surgical treatment of an intact aneurysm is simple whereas that of rupture or embolus is dangerous and difficult, so that all aneurysms need prompt surgery. It is not usually necessary to remove the aneurysm, which can more safely be dealt with either by exclusion and bypass, or a prosthetic inlay.

4. Relief of arterial thrombosis. Blocked arteries are part of the aging process and only require treatment if they involve a threat to the life, life-style or limb of the patient. The obstruction is dealt with by endarterectomy (see below) or by bypass, using the patient's own vein or if necessary a prosthetic tube. Endarterectomy is suitable for

short localized strictures in large arteries such as the carotid or the aortic bifurcation, but long blocks are better treated with a bypass.

5. More recently, transluminal angioplasty has been introduced. This technique involves dilating the block with a rigid balloon catheter, under X-ray control. The precise indications for the technique are not yet worked out, but it appears promising, particularly in the case of a short, readily-passable arterial stenosis. Close cooperation between the surgeon and radiologist is essential, so that treatment can be decided at the first angiography, and balloon dilatation carried out immediately if it seems indicated. Failure may require an urgent operation.

GENERAL CONSIDERATIONS

Anaesthesia. Most patients with arterial disease have associated heart problems. In a patient who is desperately ill from cardiac failure, angioplasty or embolectomy, even of the aortic bifurcation, can be carried out under local anaesthesia, but on the whole, general anaesthesia is better and is well tolerated. It is obviously risky to attempt a delicate arterial suture on a restless patient, and the apprehension involved imposes great stress on the myocardium.

Antibiotics. Infection is disastrous in arterial work and antibiotic cover is essential, particularly if a prosthesis is to be used. Since the main organism involved is the staphylococcus, the usual regime is to give a large parenteral dose of a cephalosporin, when anaesthesia is induced, and two further doses at 12 and 24 hours.

Anticoagulation. Once an artery is clamped, a stagnant pool of blood is created below the level of the clamp, which is liable to clot. Clotting is prevented by heparin, which interferes with the conversion of fibrinogen to fibrin. At the same time, the integrity of the arterial suture line is not compromised, because this depends on platelet activity, which heparin does not directly influence. Therefore it is a fundamental principle in arterial surgery to give a large dose of heparin 2 minutes before clamps are applied. Once the reconstruction is complete, the heparin is reversed so as to prevent venous and capillary oozing from the operative field.

Osmotic diuresis. Clamping the aorta below as well above the level of the renal arteries can lead to renal tubular damage. This can be mitigated by infusing an osmotic diuretic such as mannitol (20G in 200 ml) which promotes renal plasma flow.

Drainage. Operations on arteries usually cut across lymph vessels. Lymph in the wound leads to infection which can be catastrophic. Suction drainage is therefore needed in most cases, particularly if the groins are involved.

Smoking. The chances of an arterial reconstruction staying open for a useful length of time are greatly reduced if the patient continues to use tabacco. Some surgeons take the extreme view that they will refuse to operate on a person who has not stopped smoking. This is not usually socially practicable, but every effort should be made to explain the situation clearly and induce the patient to cooperate in his treatment.

ARTERIAL DISSECTION

The planes

1. There are two constant and essential tissue planes to bear in mind. The first is the plane of dissection *outside* the artery, which lies close up to the outer layer of the adventitia. Atheromatous arteries stick firmly to their surrounding veins, and unless care is taken in defining this plane, a thin-walled vein can be torn, which is of nuisance value in small vessels such as the popliteal, but can be disastrous where the vena cava or iliac vessels are involved. Major arteries have an investing layer of vascular lymphatic tissue, which must be cut through, in order to get right up to the arterial wall. This particularly applies to the aorta.

2. The other important plane of dissection lies *within* the artery. This is the plane of disobliteration, which occurs in mature atheroma. Fortunately for both patient and surgeon, the main strength of the arterial wall is contained in the outer half of the media and the adventitia, so that the inner media and pathological intima, cholesterol and thrombus can be removed, leaving a smooth tube which withstands arterial pressure without weakening into an aneurysm. This is the basis of the operation of endarterectomy. The plane is unmistakable, but difficult to describe. Working with an experienced arterial surgeon is the best way to discover it.

Control

Incisions for arterial operations must be generous, so that normal artery above and below can be controlled before the lesion itself is approached. This particularly applies to aneurysms, which can often be bypassed, without actually being exposed. Also, it is important to have a good length of artery on both sides of the suture line so that clamps do not get in the way.

Arterial repair

1. Arteries are best opened longitudinally. This is for two reasons. In the first place a longitudinal incision is easier to close, and secondly, the clot which forms on the suture line will have less effect on the lumen (Fig. 23.1). Any tendency to narrow the artery can always be corrected by a patch of autogenous vein or synthetic material (see below). A transverse arteriotomy is difficult to close because the intima retracts away from the outer layers.

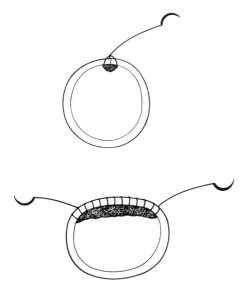

Fig. 23.1 Clot on longitudinal and transverse suture lines.

2. It is important to use as fine a suture material as is compatible with the quality of the arterial wall, and to draw each bite tightly so as to produce a smooth leak-proof anastomosis, without at the same time constricting it by a 'purse string' effect.

3. The aim is to produce an everted suture line, so that intima meets intima. This is quite different from the technique used in sewing bowel, where the mucosa is deliberately inverted into the lumen. There is no need to use mattress everting sutures, which narrow the vessel. A simple over-and-over stitch is adequate (Fig. 23.2), provided that care is taken to see that the intima comes upwards. Every bite must include the entire arterial wall including the intimal lining, and must pass from within outwards. Failure to do this will produce a flap, which can be stripped up by the blood steam and block the artery.

4. The prettiest anastomoses are achieved by the close apposition of fine sutures giving a completely smooth line of contact. However, much arterial surgery deals with irregular, dilated, thickened and calcified vessels, which do not lend themselves to this delicacy. It is much better to have a strong and dependable, albeit rugged, suture line, than one which will leak. The surgeon is often obliged to use a coarse technique which involves driving strong needles around calcified plaques in fragile vessels, taking large bites so as to correct difference in calibre. Much major vascular surgery is of this nature, and in fact, the quality of lumen produced is usually better than of the original artery. The skilled vascular surgeon is capable of changing gear between 'coarse' and 'fine' work, and takes pride in both.

End-to-end anastomosis. This is most easily accomplished by a modification of the original Carrel 'triangulation' technique. Place one double-ended suture at the back, being careful to tie the knot on the outside, and then place two additional sutures so as to divide the circumference of the vessels roughly into three. Any disparity of calibre can be corrected at this stage. The two back suture lines are then completed, leaving the easiest portion at the front to be finished last (Fig. 23.3–6). This method has the advantage of being applicable to almost any situation, especially where the arteries lie deeply and cannot be rotated. There are of course other methods available.

End-to-side anastomosis. This should always be oblique, and in the direction of blood-flow, so that there is a 'heel' and 'toe' to the anastomosis. The simplest way of completing it is to use two running sutures and to finish at the toe (Fig. 23.7). However, the four quadrant technique, has the advantage of keeping the inside of the suture line continuously in view. Start by inserting a double-

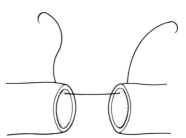

Fig. 23.3 End-to-end anastomosis by the triangulation technique.

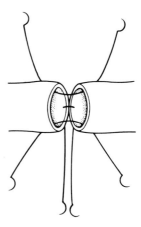

Fig. 23.4 End-to-end anastomosis by the triangulation technique.

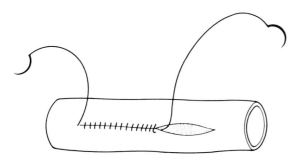

Fig. 23.2 The everting arterial suture line.

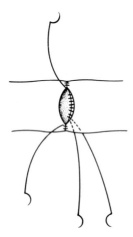

Fig. 23.5 End-to-end anastomosis by the triangulation technique.

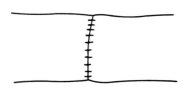

Fig. 23.6 End-to-end anastomosis by the triangulation technique.

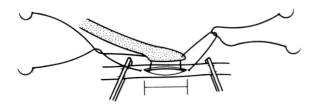

Fig. 23.7 End-to-side anastomosis using two running stitches.

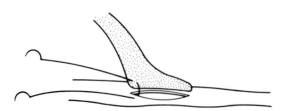

Fig. 23.8 End-to-side anastomosis using a four quadrant technique.

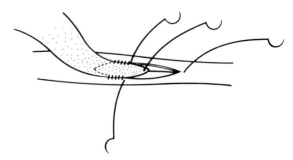

Fig. 23.9 End-to-side anastomosis using a four quadrant technique.

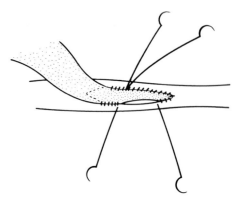

Fig. 23.10 End-to-side anastomosis using a four quadrant technique.

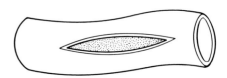

Fig. 23.11 Endarterectomy.

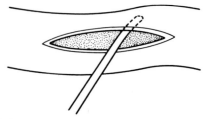

Fig. 23.12 Endarterectomy.

ended suture at the heel of the graft, tying the knot on the outside and bringing the needle through so that it lies on the correct side. The anterior and posterior suture lines are then carried up to the mid-point, finished there and trimmed, leaving the ends long. A further stitch is now inserted through the toe, and each quadrant carried up again to the middle point, where the remaining threads are tied (Figs. 23.8–10). Before the suture line is complete flush the vessels from below and above to make sure there is no retained clot or debris. The type of anastomosis is applicable for artery-to-artery, vein-to-artery or prosthesis-to-artery junctions. It is particularly useful in aorto-femoral and femoro-popliteal bypass (see below).

Endarterectomy. The 'open' technique will be described. After heparinization, lightly clamp the artery above and below the occluded segment, leaving as much room as possible. Incise the artery for 2 cm over the middle of the occluded segment, and deepen the incision until the core is reached, with circular fibres of media running on the outer coat (Figs. 23.11–16). Dissect all round the core

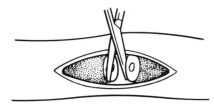

Fig. 23.13 Endarterectomy.

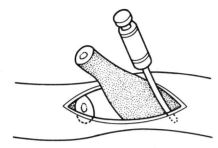

Fig. 23.14 Endarterectomy.

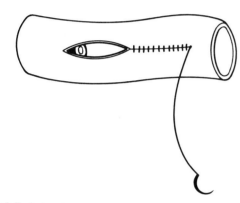

Fig. 23.15 Endarterectomy.

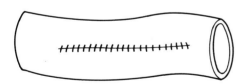

Fig. 23.16 Endarterectomy.

with a Watson-Cheyne or similar instrument, being careful *not to make a hole in the back-wall*. Elevate the core with a blunt curved (James MacDonald) dissector. Develop the plane up and down and extend the arteriotomy with Pott's angled scissors. Bisect the core and remove the two halves. Remember that the vital part of an endarterectomy is the *distal end*, and the whole finesse of the operation consists in knowing how and when to finish the distal dissection. Thus the incision must always extend downwards beyond the zone of endarterectomy, so that the distal intima can

if necessary be pinned down and incorporated in the closure. Having completed the endarterectomy, flush the area thoroughly with heparin saline, remove any loose flaps or tags, and close the incision with one running fine (4/0 or 5/0) suture. If it looks as though simple closure will narrow the lumen, apply a patch (see below).

The closed technique of endarterectomy, whereby ring strippers are inserted through short arteriotomies and run up and down the plane of dissection, removing the core blindly, are much less used nowadays and are dealt with in more specialised texts.

Bypass. This is the preferred method of dealing with a long occlusion in a medium-sized or small artery, such as the femoral or popliteal. The details are explained below in relation to individual operations. Saphenous vein is the ideal bypass material; failing this another vein such as the cephalic can be used or, as second bext, a synthetic tube.

Patching

1. Apart from endarterectomy and bypass, the application of a 'patch' is a very useful technique in arterial surgery. The principle is different from that of endarterectomy, in that the lumen of the vessel is left intact, but its circumference is enlarged. Patches may be of autogenous vein or artery, or of synthetic material. As already explained, it is better to use the patient's own tissues.

2. A venous patch is usually taken from the saphenous vein. Take the vein from the ankle, so as to preserve the upper saphenous vein, (Fig. 23.17) which may be required later.

3. An arterial patch is obtained by carrying out an endarterectomy (see above) on an occluded artery, such as the upper part of the superficial femoral, removing the diseased interior and using the external layers to repair a lesion elsewhere, be it in the carotid or, more commonly, the profunda area (Figs 23.18, 19).

4. A prosthetic patch is almost always of Dacron, as the

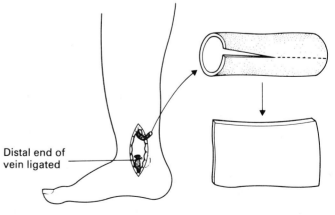

Distal end of
vein ligated

Fig. 23.17 Taking a patch from the saphenous vein at the ankle.

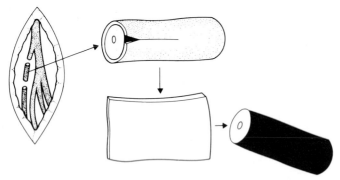

Fig. 23.18 A disobliterated arterial patch.

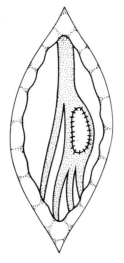

Fig. 23.19 Applying a patch to the profunda origin.

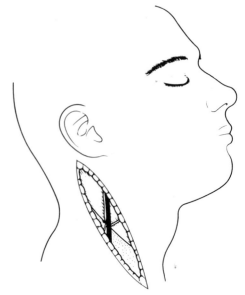

Fig. 23.20 Exposure of the carotid arteries.

more expensive synthetics have not been shown to be better. The patch is shaped, and preclotted according to the principles outlined above. The patch is stitched into the artery as already described. It is important, before finally completing the suture line, to flush out any clot or debris. With correct preclotting, haemostasis should not be a problem, and any ooze usually responds to a few minutes' light pressure with a swab.

EXPOSURE OF THE MAJOR ARTERIES

CAROTID ARTERIES

1. The best exposure of the carotid system is via a long incision from the mastoid process to the sternoclavicular joint, running along the anterior border of the sternomastoid. Deepen the incision through the platysma, divide the tributaries of the internal jugular vein, together with the great auricular nerve, and reflect the sternomastoid backwards to expose the carotid sheath. Open the sheath with great care, paying particular regard to the vagus which lies behind, because traction on this trunk can produce prob-

lems with the recurrent laryngeal nerve (Fig. 23.20). It may be necessary to split the lower pole of the parotid gland at the top of the incision, but this does not seem to matter.

2. Gently elevate the common carotid artery and pass a tape around it, so as to gain proximal control. Following this mobilize and tape the external carotid artery, which can be identified by its branches, and control the proximal one or two branches with snares. Before approaching the internal carotid artery it is customary to inject 0.5–1.00 ml of 1% lignocaine into the region of the sinus nerve, so as to block the nerve and prevent fluctuations in blood pressure which can occur when the sinus area is stimulated (Fig. 23.21). Then clear and mobilize the internal carotid

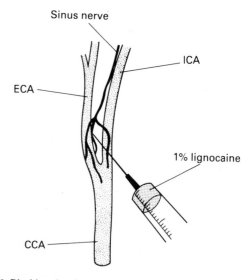

Fig. 23.21 Blocking the sinus nerve.

at the uppermost limit of the dissection, and lift it away. It is important to identify both the hypoglossal nerve, which passes obliquely across both carotid arteries just deep to the parotid gland, and its ansa, which runs down on the lateral surface of the jugular vein.

3. The three main carotids can now be lifted up and the back of the bifurcation mobilized completely, so as to make certain that no uncontrolled branches remain. During this dissection avoid handling the bifurcation, because this may dislodge small platelet emboli into the cerebral vessels.

SUBCLAVIAN ARTERY

1. The distal half of this artery can be exposed quite easily by a standard approach as for a cervical sympathectomy, through a supraclavicular incision, dividing the platysma, sternomastoid and scalenus anterior (Fig. 23.22). The two main structures at risk are the phrenic nerve and (on the left side) the thoracic duct. Injury to the duct is signalled by a flood of clear fluid into the wound and unless it is found and ligated a serious chylous fistula may develop.

2. For more extensive exposure of the artery, it is better to remove the inner two-thirds of the clavicle by subperiosteal dissection and disarticulation of the sterno-clavicular joint. This gives excellent access to both artery and vein, and allows resection of an aneurysm or correction of subclavian steal by a carotido-subclavian bypass. Removal of the clavicle produces no symptoms.

3. Approach the origin of the subclavian by means of a costo-sternal flap (Fig. 23.23), or a postero-lateral thoracotomy through the bed of the second or third rib. This is particularly useful on the left side, where the subclavian springs far backwards from the aortic arch.

AXILLARY AND BRACHIAL ARTERIES

1. The axillary artery can be exposed just below the lateral third of the clavicle by splitting the fibres of the pectoral mucles (Fig. 23.24). This manoeuvre gives perfect access for an axillo-femoral graft.

2. The brachial artery is found in the groove between biceps and brachialis on the medial side of the upper arm (Fig. 23.25). It is here enlaced by the roots of the median nerve, which must of course be carefully separated and preserved. This approach is sometimes needed in the correction of injuries to the vessel, following left heart catheterization.

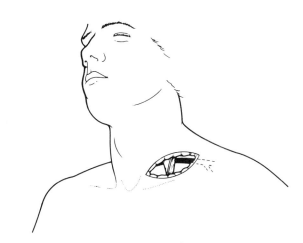

Fig. 23.22 Exposing the distal subclavian artery.

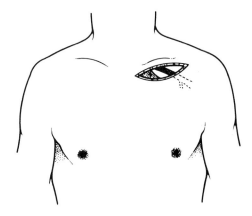

Fig. 23.24 Exposure of the axillary artery below the clavicle.

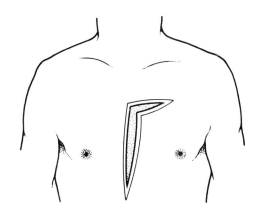

Fig. 23.23 Costo-sternal flap to expose the proximal subclavian artery.

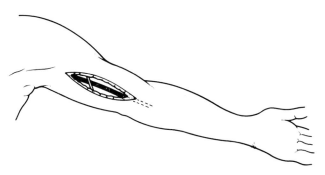

Fig. 23.25 Exposure of the brachial artery.

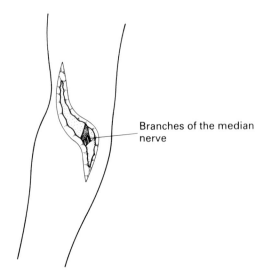

Fig. 23.26 Exposure of the brachial bifurcation.

3. The brachial bifurcation can be exposed by a 'lazy S' incision in the antecubital fossa (Fig. 23.26), followed by division of the lacertus fibrosus of the biceps tendon. The radial and ulnar arteries can be followed down between the muscles of the forearm through an extended incision. This exposure may be useful in supratrochlear fractures or for extraction of an embolus.

FEMORAL ARTERY

1. The femoral bifurcation needs to be exposed more frequently than any other vessel in the body, and it is important to know how to do this swiftly and correctly.

2. The surface marking of the artery is at the mid-inguinal point, i.e. half-way between the anterior superior iliac spine and the pubic symphysis. This marking is important to remember, because the artery cannot always be identified by pulsation, as for instance in a fat patient with a blocked aorta.

3. Provided that the saphenous vein will not be required during the operation, make the incision directly over the artery, deepen it through the subcutaneous fat, medial to sartorius, taking care to avoid cutting across lymph-nodes. The femoral sheath is exposed, and the artery is identified by the plexus of vessels on its wall. The vein lies medially and must be carefully protected, but the femoral nerve is on a much deeper plane and is not usually at risk.

4. Identify, and if necessary cut, the inguinal ligament early on so as to gain maximum upward length of vessel. Encircle the common femoral artery with a tape and lift it up.

5. Mobilize its superficial and deep branches in the same way. When controlling the profunda branch, take care not to injure the profunda vein which runs immediately across its origin (Fig. 23.27).

6. If the saphenous vein is to be exposed, make the incision *medial* to the femoral artery, straight down to the vein, and then elevate the pad of fat and lymphatics laterally. If an incision is made over the artery and the vein is then 'burrowed out' by undermining the medial flap, the skin may slough and lead to infection.

7. Any vascular exposure in the groin divides lymphatics, which may lead to a lymph fistula. Various expedients have been tried to avoid this, including preliminary injection of Patent Blue dye into the foot so as to outline the lymphatic vessels and enable the surgeon to avoid them, or the construction of a sartorius flap, which involves cutting the origin of the sartorius muscle and swinging the entire flap with its lymphatic contents medially away from the femoral sheath. However, neither of these procedures has gained general acceptance, and most surgeons prefer to rely on simple naked eye avoidance of the lymphatics.

8. The entire extent of the femoral artery can be exposed

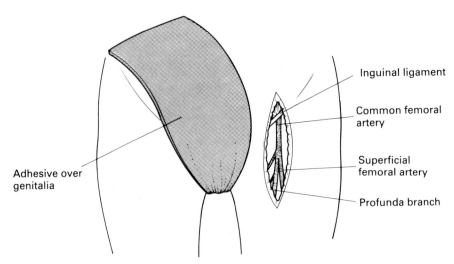

Fig. 23.27 Exposure of the femoral bifurcation.

by prolonging the incision downward, if necessary to below the knee, so as to expose the popliteal trifurcation. This is done in long femoral endarterectomies or for 'in situ' saphenous vein grafts. There are however, many snags to this total thigh incision, apart from purely cosmetic ones, such as oedema, flap necrosis and wound infection. It is much better if possible to expose the femoral and popliteal arteries through separate incisions.

9. The most inaccessible part of the artery is just above the knee-joint, where it runs through the tendon of the adductor magnus to enter the popliteal fossa, deeply placed against the femur. It is often wiser to leave this segment untouched and to expose the popliteal artery lower down.

POPLITEAL ARTERY

1. This can be exposed through either a medial or a posterior approach.

2. For the medial approach make a curved incision, centred on the adductor tubercle, on the inner side of the knee, its length depending on the arteriographic findings. Deepen it between the sartorius-behind and the origin of the gastrocnemius in front (Fig. 23.28), through the popliteal pad of fat, where the neurovascular bundle will be easily found. Remember that the artery lies next to the bone, and the nerve some distance away, with the vein in between. The artery is surrounded by a plexus of veins which are easily injured and can cause haemorrhage. These must be peeled carefully away, and tied or coagulated individually, so as to mobilize 4–5 cm of normal patent vessel.

3. It is easier to expose the artery below the knee-joint. To do this, deepen the incision between the medial head of the gastrocnemius and the tibia. The artery lies next to the bone and passes downwards in front of the soleus arch,

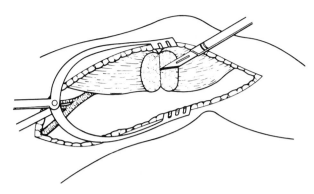

Fig. 23.29 Division of the medial head of the gastrocnemius.

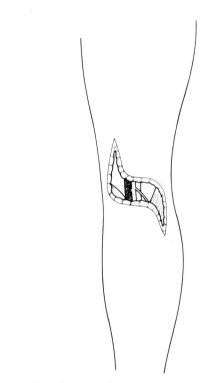

Fig. 23.30 Posterior approach to the popliteal artery.

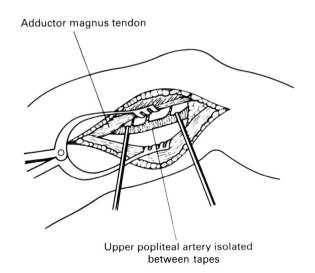

Adductor magnus tendon

Upper popliteal artery isolated between tapes

Fig. 23.28 Exposure of the popliteal artery.

where it divides into anterior and posterior branches. If necessary the entire medial head of the gastrocnemius can be cut through (Fig. 23.29), which gives excellent access, and the tendons of sartorius, semimembranosus and semitendinosus can be divided in the same way, with little effect on the stability of the limb. It is elegant, though perhaps not necessary, to resuture the muscles on the way out.

4. The posterior approach, which is used to gain full access to the upper tibial vessels, is carried out through a 'lazy S' incision in the popliteal fossa, with the patient lying prone (Fig. 23.30). Deepen the incision through the popliteal fat, opening the diamond between the hamstrings above and the two heads of the gastronemius below then follow the short saphenous vein into the neurovascular bundle.

ARTERIAL TRAUMA

Appraise

1 Arterial injury may be an isolated event, but more often it complicates head and chest trauma or fracture of a long bone. The artery and if necessary, the vein should be dealt with before the limb has been stabilized by an orthopaedic surgeon.

2. In uncomplicated stab or blast wounds, observe the general principles of wound toilet, including arterial repair. Delayed primary suture should be used provided that the arterial suture line is covered by vascular tissue (which in practice usually means a muscle flap). Antibiotic cover and antitetanus prophylaxis are required.

3. When operating on an injured artery expose the normal vessel well above the wound, and extend the incision below, so as to gain vascular control. The injury is always worse than suggested by physical examination or X-rays.

4. Beware of the concept of 'arterial spasm'. It is of course true that the smooth muscle of arteries contracts protectively when injured, so that an important vessel which has been cut across may appear quite small. However, to treat an injured artery with local or systemic drugs is a mistake, because there is always a mechanical fault, varying between abrasion of the intima to total loss of continuity. Absent pulses in an injured limb indicates such a fault and demands repair.

Access

1. Provide ample exposure, as advised above, across the site of the injury.
2. Tape the normal vessel above and below, before entering the haematoma.

Assess

Mobilize the damaged vessel and assess the severity and length of the lesion.

Action

1. If the artery is completely severed, apply light clamps above and below, cut back the injured segment until normal artery is exposed and interpose an appropriate length of long saphenous vein removed from the ankle or calf.

2. If the artery is still in continuity but does not conduct blood and appears bruised, open the bruised segment between light clamps and inspect the interior. Almost always there will be a rolled-up flap of intima with associated clot, which needs to be removed. It is usually necessary to resect the damaged segment. If the lesion is short, it may be possible simply to join up the ends. More often an interposed vein graft is needed (Fig. 23.34).

3. With very limited injuries, one can sometimes simply remove the flap of intima and pin it back, closing the arteriotomy with a patch (see above).

EMBOLECTOMY

Action

1. Under full heparin cover, expose and open the artery as already described.

2. Select a balloon catheter of the Fogarty type (there are now many varieties on the market) appropriate to the size of the vessel: either 3F (axillary or popliteal), 4F (femoral) or 5F (aortic bifurcation). Measure the length of catheter required against the patient (Fig. 23.31).

3. Pass the uninflated catheter upwards beyond the clot. Inflate the balloon and pull gently downwards, while the assistant controls the arteriotomy. Resistance will be encountered at natural bifurcation points or at areas of atheroma; adjust the balloon pressure accordingly. Finally, pull the inflated balloon through the arteriotomy, so as to retrieve the embolus.

4. Repeat this procedure until full forceful flow is achieved, then gently reclamp the artery and carry out the same procedure distally.

5. Fill the vessels with heparin/saline and repair the arteriotomy. Close the wound with drainage.

CAROTID ENDARTERECTOMY

Prepare

Assemble the instruments so that everything is in readiness before the artery is occluded:
1 fine scalpel blade (No. 22)

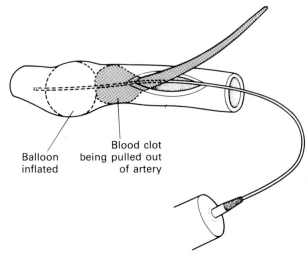

Balloon inflated

Blood clot being pulled out of artery

Fig. 23.31 Embolectomy using the Fogarty catheter.

3 lightweight arterial clamps of the Castañeda type
2 pairs of Potts' scissors, angled in two planes
2 pairs of MacIndoe fine dissecting forceps without teeth
1 Watson-Cheyne and 1 James MacDonald dissector
1 fine vascular needle-holder, Mayo or Holmes-Sellors type
1 20 cm length of 00000 vascular suture with one needle attached
2 20 ml syringes filled with dilute heparin/saline.

Access

Under general anaesthesia, expose the carotid bifurcation as already described.

Assess

Carefully and gently palpate the vessels above and below the lesion to determine its limits. Usually there is a reasonable length of internal carotid lying above the plaque, which allows application of a clamp.

Action

1. When everything is ready, completely heparinize the patient and allow 2 minutes to elapse.

2. Apply clamps to the external, common and internal carotid arteries in that order.

3. Make a 1.5 cm incision over the lesion and develop the plane in the common carotid artery.

4. Cut the 'core' across proximally. Separate it upwards into the bifurcation and cleanly sever it at the origin of the external carotid; take it up beyond the abnormal segment into the internal carotid. Almost invariably, the intima becomes abruptly normal 1 cm or so beyond the internal carotid origin and 'feathers' nicely so that no additional sutures are needed.

5. Take down the proximal half of the core into the common carotid origin and cut it across.

6. Wash the area with dilute heparin/saline and trim away any tags or flaps.

7. Starting at the top, immediately above the arteriotomy, insert a fine running suture and carry it straight down to the lower end, picking up the intima at each extremity. As the suture is completed the external, common and internal carotid clamps are momentarily removed, in order to flush out air and debris. Before the final stitch is inserted and tied, release the external and common carotid artery clamps and allow blood to flow through them for a few seconds, before finally removing the internal carotid clamp, so that any contained air will go into the face rather than the brain.

8. Haemostasis is usually no problem and is complete after a few minutes of gentle pressure. If there is any undue oozing, reverse the heparin; otherwise it is allowed to neutralize naturally.

9. Arrange suction drainage through the skin of the lower neck via the sternomastoid, and then close in layers.

10. Check the superficial temporal pulse.

Technical points

1. The simple technique described here avoids the use of a shunt, which some surgeons insist upon, but has it own complications.

2. The results of endarterectomy are acceptable, if it is carefully and neatly performed. Provided that the patient has been acurately assessed before the operation and the state of the other carotid and vertebral arteries is known, the maximal occlusion time does not appear to be of very great importance, but in practice it is almost always possible to complete the endarterectomy and closure within 10 minutes.

3. It is unusual to narrow the artery by this procedure, but if necessary a patch can be applied (see above).

ABDOMINAL AORTIC ANEURYSM

Appraise

1. The abdominal aorta is the commonest site for aneurysms. As already explained, these are dangerous lesions and should be treated aggressively. Unless the patient is gravely ill from other causes, any aneurysm broader than 5 cm should be operated upon.

2. Estimate the diameter by clinical examination, lateral X-ray of the lumbar spine and ultrasound. Aortography is unnecessary and may be both dangerous and misleading.

Prepare

1. The patient is fully anaesthetized, with total muscular relaxation and lies supine on the operating table. The arms are at the sides, with arterial and venous lines in place.

2. Insert an indwelling bladder catheter.

3. The entire area from nipples to mid-thigh is prepared, a small towel is placed over the genitalia, and an adhesive drape is applied so as to allow access to the whole of the abdomen and both inguinal regions.

Access

Make a midline incision from xiphisternum to pubis, skirting the umbilicus.

Assess

1. Check the abdominal contents to exclude the presence of some other condition which would alter the de-

cision to operate on the aneurysm. These patients are of an age where abdominal problems are common and it is of course a stupid mistake to embark on a complicated vascular procedure in the presence of cancer of the colon or ovary.

2. Note gallstones or a peptic ulcer, but do nothing further.

3. Assess the size of the aneurysm and its relation to the renal and common iliac arteries. Aneurysms which involve the renal arteries are rare and their treatment is beyond the scope of this chapter. If the common iliac arteries are grossly dilated, it is better to take the graft down to femoral level: hence the importance of preparing both groins at the beginning of the operation.

Control

1. Pack away the abdominal contents. This makes all the difference to the subsequent course of the operation and it is essential that it is done correctly. One assistant stands opposite the surgeon on the patient's right, and lifts up the right edge of the wound. Pack the small bowel carefully and gently away into the right upper quadrant, and cover it with a large moist pack, which is held in place by a Deaver retractor. Insert two more packs if necessary.

2. If necessary, free omental adhesions and partially mobilize the caecum in order to visualize the whole of the aneurysmal sac from where it is crossed by the third part of the duodenum down to the bifurcation (Fig. 23.32). On the left side, pack away the sigmoid colon.

3. Next mobilize the neck of the aneurysm. Pick up and incise the peritoneum on the front of the aneurysm and gently mobilize the duodenum off it. Continue the dissection close to the aortic wall, until the left renal vein is exposed. If this gets in the way it can quite safely be transfixed and divided, provided that this is done well over to the right, so as to preserve the outflow from the kidney via the adrenal and gonadal veins.

4. By careful blunt dissection with the finger tips and curved instruments, free the neck of the aneurysm from the inferior vena cava and pass tapes around it. Fortunately, because of the elongation of the aorta, there is almost always a gap between the aorta and cava at this level.

5. Having defined the neck, next isolate the iliac arteries. Some surgeons omit this and simply apply massive clamps to both arteries and veins, without any preliminary dissection. This can be a life-saving manoeuvre when dealing with a rupture, but it is not generally recommended. It is much safer formally to isolate the iliac arteries and to divide them under direct vision. To do this, pick up the peritoneum just below the aortic bifurcation and dissect the right common iliac artery downwards for a few centimetres. At the back, it is firmly adherent to the left common iliac vein and this particular 'dangerous angle' is one of the trickiest parts of the operation (Fig. 23.33). It is very easy to tear a hole in the thin iliac vein, which leads to very troublesome haemorrhage. Meticulously separate the artery and vein with small dissecting pledgets and scissors, until the artery can be lifted clear with a tape. Once this has been achieved, the plane becomes much easier to identify and the operation proceeds without difficulty. Repeat the manoeuvre on the left side, but here artery and vein are usually less adherent and easier to isolate. Remember that the ureter crosses the iliac bifurcation on each side and should be seen and protected during this dissection. It is not necessary to control the median sacral or lumbar arteries.

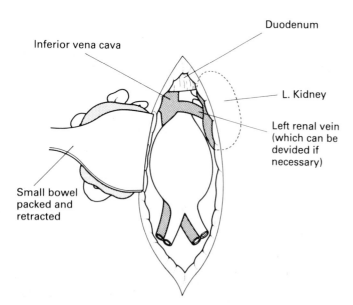

Fig. 23.32 Abdominal aortic aneurysm — exposure.

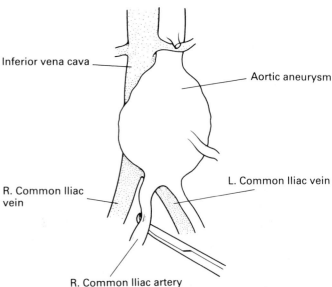

Fig. 23.33 Isolation of the right common iliac artery.

6. With three tapes in position the aorta is now under control, and one of the most crucial stages of the operation is completed. Now decide whether to use a bifurcation graft, and if so of what size and whether it will be attached to the iliac arteries or to the femorals. Having selected the appropriate prosthesis, preclot it by the Sauvage technique (see above).

Action

1. Systemically heparinize the patient and allow 2 minutes to elapse before applying clamps to the neck of the sac and the iliac arteries. Apply the clamps with the least force needed to secure complete occlusion, and incise the sac of the aneurysm.

2. Rapidly evacuate into a receiver the contents, which are degenerate atheromatous material, laminated clot and liquid blood, and clean out the interior of the sac. Sometimes the material in the aortic wall bears an alarming resemblance to pus, and indeed there is a certain incidence of spontaneous infection in aortic aneurysms. Always send a specimen for culture, though in most cases it will prove to be sterile. A certain amount of bleeding occurs from the lumbar and sacral vessels on the back of the sac, and these are controlled with mattress sutures of nonabsorbable material.

3. Having secured complete haemostasis, finally decide whether a straight inlay graft can be used or whether it will be necessary to use the whole bifurcated tube. This depends on the anatomy of the lower end of the sac. If there is a well developed 'ring' above the origins of the iliac arteries, to which a large tube can easily be sewn, then the inlay technique is certainly better. If, however, the aneurysm involves the iliacs or the bifurcation is heavily diseased and will not take sutures, then it is better to use a Y-shaped tube either on to the cut ends of the iliac arteries, or via tunnels to the common femorals. If the iliac arteries are grossly diseased and a downward extension appears necessary, have the assistant expose both common femoral arteries in the groin, while you continue with the upper anastomosis (see above for method of exposing femoral arteries).

4. Trim the prosthesis so that only 3–4 cm of it lies above the bifurcation, and pull a 'sleeve' of material over it. (Fig. 23.34).

5. Then transfix the neck of the aorta well below the clamp, so as to leave as long a stump as possible for anastomosis.

6. Perform the anastomosis using 4/0 suture material as already described (Fig. 23.35) and slip up the prepared sleeve over the suture line. Apply a soft mitral clamp to the prosthesis immediately below the sleeve and, having warned the anaesthetist, cautiously open the upper clamp. There should be very little in the way of haemorrhage, but if loss appears excessive, immediately reclamp the aorta,

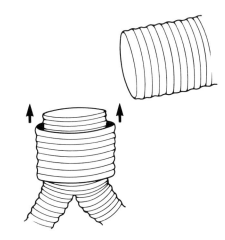

Fig. 23.34 Trimming the prosthesis and applying the sleeve.

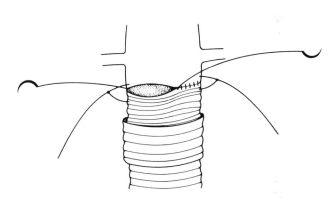

Fig. 23.35 The upper anastomosis.

draw the sleeve downwards and inspect the suture line for any holes, which are promptly repaired.

7. Bring down the left limb of the prosthesis, and anastomose it either to the cut end of the left common iliac artery, or as a side-to-side anastomosis to the common femoral artery, via a previously contructed tunnel (for details of this see section on aorto-iliac occlusion, below). The end-to-end iliac anastomosis is most easily carried out using a modified triangulation technique. If there is any doubt about satisfactory backflow, pass a Fogarty catheter down to the foot before the suture is completed.

8. Next remove the mitral clamp and flush out the aorta, so as to remove any clot which has accumulated above the clamp. Complete the suture line and release the aorta and left iliac artery, allowing flow into the left leg. There may be a sudden drop of blood pressure at this stage, owing to reduction in peripheral resistance, so warn the anaesthetist in advance.

9. Deal with the right limb of the prosthesis in exactly the same way, and remove the clamps so that blood now runs into both legs.

Inlay technique

1. Use this where there is a well-defined 'ring' at the lower end of the aneurysmal sac or where the aneurysm ends well above the bifurcation.

2. Trim the aortic prosthesis so as to leave adequate length to span the length of the sac. Do not transect the upper aorta but carry out the anastomosis from within (Fig. 23.36).

3. Draw the prosthesis down under tension, trim it, and attach it to the lower aortic wall on the right and left sides, using 3/0 or 4/0 vascular suture material and deal with it in the same way. Take strong deep bites of the posterior aortic wall, avoiding as far as possible areas of plaque formation and calcification. The anterior layers usually require some trimming of the front of the sac.

Closure

1. Clean the remains of the sac of debris and trim it back so that it can be comfortably approximated over the graft (Fig. 23.36), without tension, using interrupted sutures of nonabsorbable material. Carry the stitches upwards and downwards as far as possible, so as to keep the duodenum and small bowel separate from the suture lines. The sleeve materially lessens the incidence of aorto-duodenal fistula. Rescue the small bowel from the right upper quadrant and gently position it over the closed sac. Pull the greater omentum down over the sac.

2. These patients invariably develop a degree of ileus, and intestinal decompression is necessary either through a nasogastric tube, or better via a small gastrostomy through

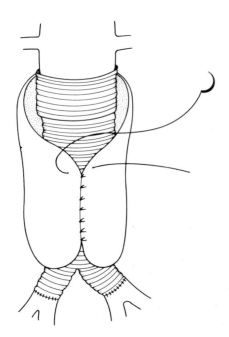

Fig. 23.36 Closing the sac.

the left hypochondrium. This gives much better postoperative comfort and aids respiratory function. Provided it is done as a final step in the operation, when the prosthesis has been excluded from the peritoneal cavity, no contamination arises.

Aftercare

Remember four potential complications in particular:

1. Haemorrhage. If the anastomoses have been properly sutured, breakdown is rare. If it occurs, it demands immediate re-operation and correction of the fault. 'Haematological' bleeding due to inadequate reversal of heparin or the development of intraoperative clotting problems is commoner, but can usually be promptly corrected with 1–2 units of fresh blood or fresh frozen plasma.

2. Occlusion. This results either from embolization of material trapped above the aortic clamp, which was not flushed out, or from a technical fault at one of the suture lines. Try passing a large Fogarty catheter as a first measure, but re-exploration is usually necessary.

3. Renal tubular necrosis. This complication has become much less common by regularly using mannitol and minimizing the period of aortic occlusion. It usually removers spontaneously but rarely may require haemodialysis. Total anuria imediately after the operation suggests the possibility of occlusion of both renal arteries. Request immediate aortography to confirm the problem, and re-explore the patient.

4. Infection. An untreated infected prosthesis results in the death of the patient or the loss of one or both limbs. It may become manifest anything from days to months after the operation. The symptoms are fever, backache and perhaps a purulent discharge from the wound. If nothing is done, a fatal haemorrhage will sooner or later occur. Once the diagnosis has been made, remove the graft. This of course involves re-establishing the circulation through an extra-anatomical route such as an axillo-bifemoral bypass (see below).

AORTO-ILIAC RECONSTRUCTION

Access

Explore the abdomen as for an aneurysm.

Assess

1. Palpate the aorta and the iliac arteries to determine the exact limits of the block. There are two crucial points. Above is the relationship of the upper limit of the block to the renal and the inferior mesenteric arteries. Below is the state of the external artery, which can be felt easily as it runs along the brim of the pelvis to the internal inguinal ring.

2. At this point decide whether to carry out an endarterectomy, a bypass procedure or a combination of both.

3. If the block extends to the origins of the renal and superior mesenteric arteries, a local endarterectomy is necessary at the top, whatever technique is to be used below. On the other hand, when there are 2–3 cm of patent aorta below the renal arteries endarterectomy may not be required.

4. If the disease process stops abruptly at the iliac bifurcation, with a patent and supple external iliac artery below, most surgeons prefer to perform endarterectomy, which involves less surgery than a prosthetic bypass. However, if the external iliac arteries are occluded or extensively diseased, there is no doubt that it is much better to bypass the whole segment and carry blood directly from the aorta to the femoral arteries by means of an implant.

AORTO-ILIAC THROMBOENDARTERECTOMY

Action

1. Mobilize the aortic bifurcation as already described by incising the parietal peritoneum over the aortic bifurcation in the region of the origin of the inferior mesenteric artery. Control the lumbar vessels with thread 'snares'. Dissect the iliac vessels clear and take care not to injure the sympathetic plexus which crosses them; cutting this plexus leads to impotence.

2. Assuming the upper limit of occlusion is well below the renal arteries heparinize the patient and clamp the aorta as high as possible so as to be well clear of the suture line. Clamp the external and internal iliac arteries in the same way, and make a small vertical incision into the aortic wall 1 cm below the upper limit of the block. Deepen it until the plane of disobiliteration is reached. Develop the arteriotomy up and down for a few millimetres (Fig. 23.37), transect the isolated core with Potts' scissors

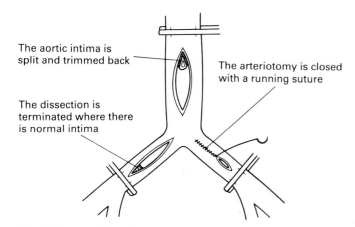

The aortic intima is split and trimmed back

The arteriotomy is closed with a running suture

The dissection is terminated where there is normal intima

Fig. 23.37 Aorto-iliac endarterectomy.

and mobilize it downwards. The upper end can be left for the time being.

3. Achieve mobilization by a combination of blunt dissection, injection of saline through a wide-mouthed cannula, and finger pressure. Continue the process downwards to a point as near as possible to the aortic bifurcation.

4. Make a small, 1–2 cm, incision in the wall of the right common iliac artery near its bifurcation. The obstructing core is similarly developed and transected. Carry the dissection up as far as possible towards the already mobilized aortic segment. At this stage do not attempt to repair the distal intima. Make a similar incision in the left common iliac artery, if necessary, freeing the sigmoid mesocolon. Take the core upwards in the same way.

5. Once the obstructing lesion is mobilized from these three points of attack, it is generally possible to use simple digital pressure to express the lesion in the shape of an inverted Y upwards through the aortotomy. When the segment is freed, it leaves behind a thin but strong aortic wall, which has a smooth and glistening lining representing the outer half of the arterial media. Sometimes a few circular flaps of outer media remain. Trim them away, always bearing in mind that the back of the vessel must never be torn because a defect in this situation is dangerous and difficult to repair.

Closure

1. Before closing the arteriotomy, trim the upper end to ensure continuity of the lumen. Mistakes here do not matter too much, because the aorta is very broad and the direction of blood flow tends to stick the inner layers down rather than to raise a flap. The distal end of the reconstruction is quite different. Here the repositioning of the intima is absolutely crucial because the bloodstream can reflect up a flap so that the lumen of the artery is blocked and the entire operation fails. The difficulty with any endarterectomy is to know when to stop. This is the main reason why the operation described here is unsuitable for a patient with gross disease of the external iliac artery. This vessel must be reasonably normal so that the endarterectomy can be terminated by bevelling off a normal intima.

2. When the intima of the aorta and of one iliac vessel has been trimmed in this way, briefly remove the clamps to ensure that there is adequate flow and to flush out clots. Inject heparin saline into the iliac artery and reapply the clamp.

3. Close the aortic wall with a running 4/0 stitch, taking care to pick up the detached intima at the upper end. Repair the common iliac arteriotomy in the same way, with corresponding attention to the intima at the lower end. Before final closure release the iliac clamp again to free any clot and to ensure that there is adequate back bleeding. If

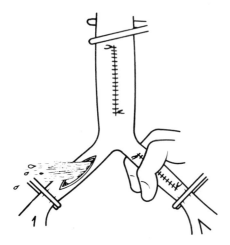

Fig. 23.38 Flushing the suture line.

doubt exists, pass a 4F Fogarty catheter downwards to retrieve thrombus and ensure patency. Occlude the repaired iliac artery with the fingers while the aortic clamp is briefly released to flush out any retained clot through the open side (Fig. 23.38).

4. When it is certain that there is good aortic pulsation down to the upper clamp, a completely empty reconstructed segment and a patent distal tree, clamp the other, open, iliac artery at its origin while the other clamps are removed to allow blood to flow into that leg. Trim the intima on the remaining side in the same way and repair the arteriotomy.

AORTOBIFEMORAL DACRON BYPASS

Appraise

1. This is the method of choice if the disease extends for any distance beyond the iliac bifurcation.

2. The exposure of the aorta need not be as extensive as for endarterectomy. It is only necessary to isolate 5–6 cm of aorta at a conveniently accessible point above the bifurcation.

Action

1. While you expose the aorta, have your assistant expose the contralateral femoral artery in the groin as already described. He tapes the common, superficial and profunda femoris arteries.

2. To connect the abdominal and groin incisions, pass a finger up besides the femoral artery on its lateral side, so as to avoid the vein, under the inguinal ligament and into the extraperitoneal space. Pass the index finger of the other hand in the same plane under the leaf of peritoneum at the aortic bifurcation and gently burrow through the intervening areolar tissue until the two finger-tips meet. After carefully stretching the tunnel introduce a 'tunneler'

through the inguinal incision to emerge within the abdomen. Pass a strong thread through its eye. Withdraw the tunneler so that the thread lies along the prepared track, connecting the abdomen and groin (Fig. 23.39). Repeat this procedure on the other side.

3. Heparinize the patient. Clamp the aorta twice and transect it. Oversew the lower end with a strong vascular suture (Fig. 23.40). Clear the upper end of thrombus. Quite strong pressure may be needed against the vertebral column to get the aorta completely clear and this is verified by momentarily removing the upper clamp, which should result in forcible pulsatile flow.

4. Anastomose the trimmed and pre-clotted prosthesis end-to-end to the aortic stump. Slip the sleeve over the suture line (Fig. 23.41) and re-apply the clamp below.

5. Following this, draw down the two limbs of the prosthesis into the groin incisions, and anastomose them end-to-side to the common femoral arteries (Fig. 23.42).

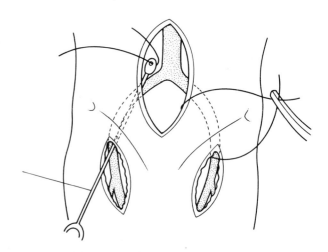

Fig. 23.39 Making the tunnels.

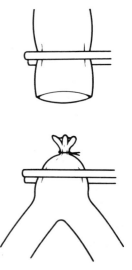

Fig. 23.40 Clamping and dividing the aorta.

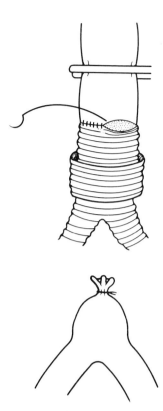

Fig. 23.41 The upper anastomosis.

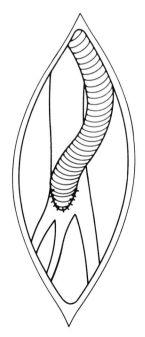

Fig. 23.42 The lower anastomosis.

Flow is now restored to both legs and also to the pelvis, as shown by pulsation of the closed lower aorta.

6. Check the anastomoses in the usual way and close the abdomen after creating a gastrostomy.

Technical

The end-to-end anastomosis described here is the one most often performed, but some surgeons prefer the on-lay or 'piggy-back' pattern, illustrated in Figure 23.43.

FEMORO-POPLITEAL SAPHENOUS VEIN BYPASS

Prepare

1. The leg is shaved together with the pubic area and lower abdomen.

2. Mark the course of the long saphenous vein in the thigh with indelible ink.

3. The patient lies supine on an X-ray tunnel which is covered with a foam mattress. The knee of the affected leg is flexed to 45°, with the hip slightly flexed and externally rotated; the knee must not overlap the edge of the film cassette. Soft foam cushions support the knee and ankle.

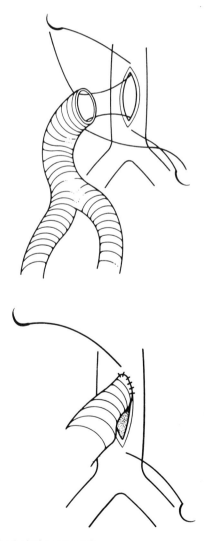

Fig. 23.43 The 'onlay' anastomosis.

Male genitalia are drawn aside from the field of operation with a strip of adhesive.

4. Swab the whole area from the umbilicus to the upper calf with antiseptic, and wrap the foot in a sterile towel. Place towels to expose an area from well above the groin to below the knee and hold them in position with an adhesive drape. Plenty of exposure is needed at the top; the common femoral artery lies much higher than one might suppose and it is a common fault to make the incision too low.

Action

1. The operation takes less time if two surgeons work together.

2. Expose the long saphenous vein through separate upper and lower incisions (Fig. 23.44). As already explained, it is important to make the skin incision over the vein and not along the course of the artery.

3. The extent of the lower incision depends on whether the lower anastomosis will be made above or below the knee. If the popliteal artery above the knee appears on the arteriogram to be smooth and of good calibre, it is better to make the anastomosis there. If, on the other hand, it is rough and irregular it is preferable to go lower down and to accept the slight disadvantage of a graft that runs across the knee.

4. Dissect out the long saphenous vein from the groin to the knee, or below the knee if necessary. Divide each tributary and tie it with fine material a millimetre or so away from its junction with the main trunk to avoid the possibility of narrowing the graft. Tie the peripheral ends of the divided veins and expose the portion of vein in mid-thigh beneath the intact skin bridge by lifting the skin with retractors. Transfix the sapheno-femoral junction with a stitch.

5. One operator now takes the vein-graft aside to prepare it, while the other exposes the popliteal artery as described above. Distend the vein with heparinized blood, (5000 U heparin in 50 ml blood), using a syringe and cannula and as each segment is distended move the clip

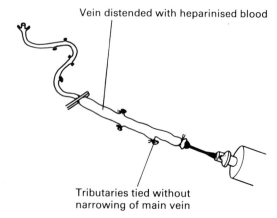

Fig. 23.45 Preparing the vein as an arterial substitute.

further upwards, while tying any tributaries that have been missed with 5/0 ligatures (Fig. 23.45). Finally place the prepared vein in a jug of heparin and lignocaine in saline to await use.

6. If the vein is inadequate with less than 5 mm lower diameter, something else must be done such as an endarterectomy, a bypass using the cephalic vein or a prosthesis, or a combination of these methods.

7. Following heparinization, isolate about 5 cm of popliteal artery between clamps at the chosen site and control the branches by snares. Incise the medial side of the artery longitudinally for about 2 cm, making the initial incision with a scalpel through the whole thickness of the arterial wall, and extending it with Potts' scissors. Do not separate the intima from the outer layers and resist the temptation to carry out a local endarterectomy at this site. Flush the lumen of the artery and its distal branches with heparin in saline.

8. Prepare the upper end of the reversed long saphenous vein for anastomosis. Split the vein longitudinally with scissors for about 2 cm and trim the corners to make it suitable for oblique end-to-side anastomosis, which is then carried out as already described (Fig. 23.8–10). When the anastomosis is complete, attach the cannula at the other end of the vein to a syringe and inject heparinized blood forcibly to test the suture line and irrigate the distal arterial tree. Place a soft bulldog clip across the vein graft immediately above the anastomosis, and remove the arterial clamps.

9. While the lower anastomosis is being performed (Fig. 23.46), the operator who prepares the vein graft completes the exposure of the femoral artery in the groin (Fig. 23.27). A tunnel is then made deep to the sartorius using one of the special instruments available and the vein is drawn through to emerge in the inguinal incision.

10. Before the proximal anastomosis is started, flush the vein again with heparin in saline to confirm that there is free flow down to the lower anastomosis with no obstruction or kinks. Remove the bulldog clip from the

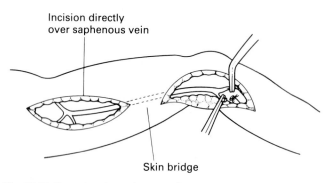

Fig. 23.44 Removing the saphenous vein.

Point A: the vein must not be narrowed
where the suture starts

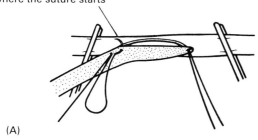

(A)

Point B: needle takes a small bite of artery,
great care being taken to include the intima

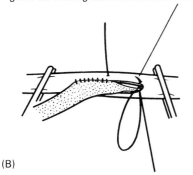

(B)

Fig. 23.46 The lower anastomosis.

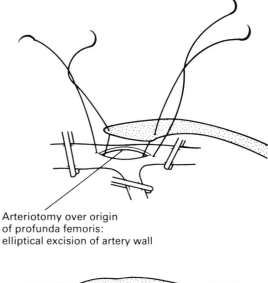

Arteriotomy over origin
of profunda femoris:
elliptical excision of artery wall

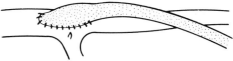

Fig. 23.47 The upper anastomosis.

lower part of the vein graft while this is being done. Place the vein under moderate tension, cut off the end containing the cannula and split the vein lengthwise to prepare it for an oblique anastomosis in the same way as before.

11. Clamp the common, superficial and deep femoral arteries and make a 2.0 cm incision over the origin of the deep branch. Carry out a standard end-to-side anastomosis (Fig. 23.47).

12. Check both anastomoses and confirm pulsation in the popliteal artery below the reconstruction. In case of doubt perform an operative arteriogram.

Closure

If the tendons of the semitendinosus and gracilis have been divided, approximate them by tying the stay sutures and then repair them. Close the subcutaneous parts of both incisions with interrupted sutures. Close the skin incision with drainage to the inguinal area.

Aftercare

1. As soon as the towels have been removed, seek the foot pulses and mark them so that the nurses can note at intervals whther they are still present. Even if the vessels are open, the foot pulses are not always felt immediately after the operation, but reactive hyperaemia usually becomes evident within a few hours.

2. If pulses that have been palpable or detectable with the Doppler probe in the early postoperative period later become impalpable or undetectable, or if the state of the foot deteriorates, consider re-exploration.

3. Keep the knee slightly flexed for 24 hours to avoid tension on the graft. Allow the patient out of bed after 48 hours. Allow him to take a few steps on the third post-operative day. Some swelling of the lower leg is almost invariable after successful reconstruction and this may be controlled by gentle bandaging. The patient is usually ready for discharge from hospital after 10–12 days.

POPLITEAL ANEURYSM

Appraise

1. After the abdominal aorta, the popliteal artery is the second commonest place for aneurysms to occur. 60% of these aneurysms are bilateral. They are dangerous lesions,

because of their strong tendency to rupture or thrombosis. Thrombosis of a popliteal aneurysm usually leads to amputation, because this is an end artery with little collateral circulation. Haemorrhage is rarely so great as to endanger life, but it is often followed by distal blockage.

2. For this reason, popliteal aneurysms should always be operated upon, even if asymptomatic. The only ones that do not require surgery are those which are already thrombosed, and where enough collateral circulation has remained to preserve the limb.

Prepare

Position the leg as for a femoro-popliteal bypass. Identify and remove the saphenous vein, and prepare it for use as an arterial substitute as described above.

Access

1. Deepen the incision to expose the tendon of adductor magnus, and identify the neuro-vascular bundle as it emerges.

2. The popliteal artery will be found to be large and tortuous. Mobilize 3–4 cm of it and tape it, if necessary dividing the adductor tendon to increase exposure.

3. Pass a strong non-absorbable ligature, such as No.1 nylon, twice around the popliteal artery immediately above the neck of the aneurysm, but do not tie it (Fig. 23.48).

4. Next, deepen the lower part of the incision to expose the medial head of the gastrocnemius, which is drawn backward or if necessary cut through to reveal the neuro-vascular bundle.

5. Separate the popliteal artery from it concomitant veins and deal with in the same way, placing a strong nylon ligature around it below the aneurysm, but leaving it untied.

6. Note that the principles outlined above have been observed, in that access has been achieved above and below, but that the aneurysm itself has not been interfered with. It is a mistake to attempt to dissect the aneurysm which can easily result in damage to the nerves or to profuse venous haemorrhage which is difficult to control.

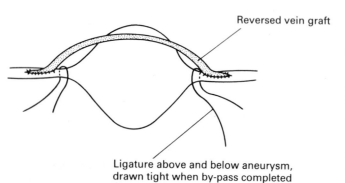

Reversed vein graft

Ligature above and below aneurysm, drawn tight when by-pass completed

Fig. 23.48 Bypassing a popliteal aneurysm.

Action

1. Heparinize the patient.

2. After 2 minutes have elapsed, lightly clamp the upper popliteal artery and incise it for approximately 1 cm.

3. Trim the reversed saphenous vein and anastomose it to the incision with a standard four-quadrant technique (see above).

4. Lightly cross-clamp the vein immediately below the anastomosis. Lead it downwards into the popliteal fossa, deep to the major tendons (Fig. 55) and across the medial side of the gastrocnemius to reach the popliteal artery below the aneurysm, to which it is attached in the same way.

5. Remove the upper and lower clamps and allow flow to proceed through the vein graft around the clamped aneurysm. When the suture lines are dry and satisfactory flow has been established, draw tight the nylon ligatures, thus excluding the aneurysm from the circulation and bypassing it completely.

6. Reverse the heparin and close the wound. If there is any significant oozing insert a suction drain.

AXILLOFEMORAL GRAFT

Appraise

The usual indication for this operation is failure from thrombosis or infection of an aortic or aorto-bifemoral reconstruction.

Access

1. Expose the axillary and femoral arteries as already described.

2. Preferably expose *both* femoral arteries, because an axillobifemoral graft has a higher flow-rate than a one-sided reconstruction and remains open for longer.

Prepare

The long 'Y' shaped prosthesis is not readily available and may have to be made up on the spot.

Action

1. Measure out and pre-clot a length of prosthesis corresponding to the dimensions of the patient's abdominal wall. Cut off a length and join it end-to-side to the main stem.

2. Introduce a tunnelling instrument from axilla to groin, with if necessary one small accessory incision (Fig. 72). Make a subsidiary tunnel from right to left, for the side-arm.

3. The anastomoses are conveniently carried out by two

surgeons working simultaneously, the right limb being opened first, and the left when the first anastomosis is seen to be functioning. It is possible that the recently introduced rigid non-compressible prosthesis confers some advantage.

INTESTINAL ISCHAEMIA

Acute, Massive Ischaemia

This may be due to (rarely) a mesenteric embolus, an acute thrombosis or sudden decompensation of an already narrowed mesenteric artery or, in about one third of cases, the so-called 'non-occlusive infarction' where no vascular blockage is responsible.

Appraise

1. Is the gut infarcted or viable? If the former, then the only possible course is resection, which may have to be massive (see Ch. 6). Make no attempt to construct a primary anastomosis, but exteriorise the ends and close the abdomen. If the patient survives, continuity may be restored at a later date.

2. If the gut appears ischaemic but recoverable, consider vascular reconstruction. If from the history and antecedents, the case appears to be one of *embolism*, then open the ileocolic artery at a convenient point and pass a catheter up into the aorta to remove as much of the embolus as possible. If this is successful and pulsation returns to the bowel, the ileocolic artery can be ligated at this point. If not, then a side-to-side anastomosis between ileocolic and right common iliac artery can be carried out and the gut irrigated 'upstream'. This avoids approaching the inaccessible area of the origin of the superior mesenteric artery. If this is unsuccessful it may be necessary to lift the transverse colon upwards and dissect the vascular trunk beneath the neck of the pancreas. The artery can then be opened directly and attempts made to clear it. Successful revascularisation usually results in abrupt fall in the blood pressure, due to loss of fluid into the ischaemic loops, and perhaps also 'washout' of toxic material from the bowel. Warn the anaesthetist and ask him to transfuse liberally at this stage.

3. Book the theatre for the next day. A 'second look' operation is always worthwhile and very often you will find ischaemic loops of bowel which were not obvious at the first operation.

CHRONIC INTESTINAL ISCHAEMIA

Appraise

1. While genuine cases of 'intestinal angina' due to chronic obstruction of the visceral arteries do certainly exist, they are not easy to define or identify, because there is no exact relationship between arteriographic abnormalities and symptoms.

2. Elective reconstruction of the visceral arterial trunks is a highly specialised procedure, which is probably best carried out in centres with a particular interest.

3. In practice, most patients with arterial disease and abdominal pain prove to have straightforward organic problem in the gastro-intestinal tract, unrelated to the blood supply.

Further reading

Bell P R F, Barrie W W 1982 Operative arterial surgery. Butterworths, London
Gardham J R C, Marston A 1975 Femoro-popliteal saphenous vein by-pass grafting. British Journal of Hospital Medicine 14:679
Marston A 1977 Reconstruction of the blocked aorta. British Journal of Hospital Medicine 18:69
Marston A 1986 Vascular diseases of the gut. Edward Arnold, London In Press
Slaney G, Ashton F 1971 Arterial injuries and their treatment. Postgraduate Medical Journal 47:257
Yates S G, Barros d'Sa A A B, Berger K et al The preclotting of porous arterial prostheses. Annals of Surgery 188: 611–622

Surgery of the veins and lymphatics

Varicose vein surgery
Operations for deep vein thrombosis
Operations for venous ulcer and post-phlebitic syndrome
Lymphatic surgery

VARICOSE VEIN SURGERY

Appraise

1. Most patients seek treatment for their varicose veins because they dislike the appearance of the large, tortuous veins on their exposed legs.

2. Many patients also complain that the veins ache; a symptom which is often worse at the end of the day or after prolonged standing. The greater number of varicose vein operations carried out in women may reflect the greater importance that they attach to attractive legs.

3. The severe pre-ulcerative skin changes of liposclerosis may be reversed and venous ulcers prevented by appropriate surgery to all the sites of superficial valvular incompetence in patients with normal deep veins.

4. Recurrent attacks of superficial thrombophlebitis or extensive bleeding from a ruptured varix are further clear cut indications for surgical treatment.

5. Surgical ligation and stripping remains the treatment of choice if there is major venous incompetence since injection therapy only provides short term benefit. Varicose branch veins may be avulsed through local incisons at the time of saphenous surgery or in the absence of saphenous incompetence treated equally well by injection compression.

6. Persistent or recurrent varicosities after saphenous surgery are also satisfactorily treated by injection compression unless a groin or popliteal recurrence is the underlying cause.

7. Many patients presenting with painful or swollen legs are erroneously diagnosed as having 'varicose veins' although these are often co-incidental and not the cause of the symptoms. You must therefore exclude arterial disease, lymphatic oedema, arthritis of hips and knees and referred pain from the back in many patients with 'varicose veins'.

8. Most patients with uncomplicated and clear cut varicose veins require little in the way of investigation beyond a careful history and an examination of the legs to determine the competence or incompetence of the major sites of communication between the superficial and deep venous system. Inspection and palpation with cough, percussion and tourniquet tests provide this information.

9. Patients who have had past ulceration or those who show marked pre-ulcer skin changes should undergo bipedal ascending phlebography to enable an accurate assessment of both the deep and perforating veins to be made.

10. Patients with bizarre, complicated or recurrent varicose veins may be more accurately assessed by varicography, in which low osmolity contrast material is injected directly into the surface veins to demonstrate their course and deep connections.

11. Doppler examination of venous reflux may give useful additional information but an overall examination of calf pump function provided by ambulatory pressure measurements, plethysmography and foot volumetric studies is more useful in research than in clinical assessment.

Prepare and carefully re-examine all patients admitted for operations on their varicose veins. Mark the major sites of communicating vein incompetence and all the large branch varicosities with an indelible pen. Confirm or exclude long and short saphenous incompetence, and incompetent calf perforating veins. Suspect the latter in patients with lipodermatosclerosis.

HIGH SAPHENOUS LIGATION (TRENDELENBURG'S OPERATION) AND STRIPPING OF THE LONG SAPHENOUS VEIN

Appraise

1. Perform the operation on patients with varicose veins and evidence of long saphenous reflux at the groin on clinical or Doppler examination.

2. Avoid the operation if the long saphenous is acting as a collateral to an obstructed femoral vein.

Position

1. Place the patient supine in Trendelenburg's position with approximately 30° of head down tilt.

2. Abduct both legs by about 15° from midline and place the ankles on a padded board which can be held under the rubber of the operating table. This position facilitates access and reduces bleeding.

Access

1. Make a short oblique incision parallel to and below the inguinal ligament over the sapheno-femoral junction. This lies approximately 2 cm lateral and 2 cm below the pubic tubercule.

2. Deepen the incision through the subcutaneous fat, which is spread by the insertion of a self-retaining retractor such as Traver's, West's or Cockett's.

Assess

1. The long saphenous vein normally appears in the centre of the dissection as the fat is spread by the teeth of the retractor, but if it is difficult to find, trace a small tributary back to the main trunk.

2. Do not divide the long saphenous until the sapheno-femoral junction has been identified.

Action

1. Disect out the long saphenous vein from the surrounding fat and follow it up towards the sapheno-femoral junction.

2. A variable number of tributaries join the vein near its termination. These must be dissected free before they are ligated with 2/0 catgut and divided. The superficial inferior epigastric vein, the superficial circumflex iliac vein, the superficial and deep external pudendal veins all join the saphenous trunk near its termination. In addition the postero-medial and antero-lateral thigh veins also terminate close to the sapheno-femoral junction (Fig. 24.1). One or more of these veins may join up before emptying into the saphenous trunk.

3. After these tributaries have been divided the sapheno-femoral junction is approached as the long saphenous dips down through the cribriform fascia over the foramen ovale. Display the femoral vein for approximately 1 cm above and below the sapheno-femoral junction and clear it of any small branches entering from either side.

4. Ligate the long saphenous vein in continuity, with 0 chromic catgut and divide it. The saphenous stump may be doubly ligated or transfixed for greater safety.

5. Place a ligature around the long saphenous trunk and

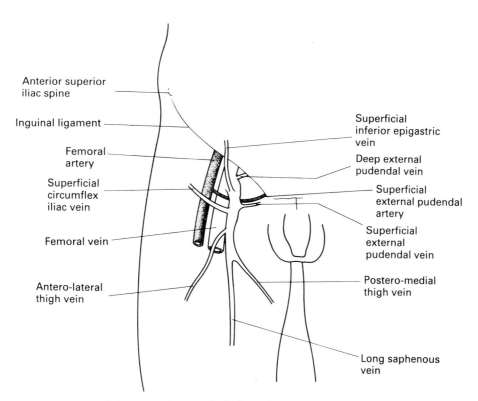

Fig. 24.1 The termination and tributaries of the long saphenous vein in the groin.

hold it up to occlude the flow of blood from below, while a small side hole is made in the vein above the tie to introduce the tip of the stripper. Use either a flexible steel stripper or a plastic disposable stripper with a suitably sized head. Gently manipulate the tip of the stripper into and down the vein while controlling the bleeding by the ligature placed around the vein.

6. The end of the stripper can usually be seen passing down the saphenous vein around the knee. Advance it to approximately a hand's breath beyond the knee where it may remain in the saphenous vein or pass into a similar tributary.

7. At a convenient spot make an oblique 1–2 cm incision in Langer's lines over the end of the stripper. The incision must be large enough to allow the head of the stripper to pass.

Dissect out the vein containing the stripper, which is easily found by palpation and free it from the accompanying nerves before tying it off distally. Place a ligature around the vein and stripper and tie it down to prevent blood loss when the vein is incised to deliver the stripper.

8. Strip the long saphenous vein from the groin to knee by steady downward traction on the wire, after attaching the T-shaped handle to aid traction. Ease the stripper and bunched-up vein through the lower incision.

9. Prevent excessive bleeding from the stripper track either by tightly applying a sterile crepe bandage while the stripper is withdrawn or by expressing the blood by gently rolling a swab along the course of the vein until all the bleeding has stopped before applying bandages.

Closure

1. Insert interrupted 2/0 plain catgut to the subcutaneous tissue and fascia.
2. Close the skin with interrupted 4/0 nylon or subcuticular sutures with steristrips.

Difficulty?

1. The retrograde passage of the stripper may be impeded by competent valves, varicosity of the saphenous vein or false passage into small tortuous tributaries. Attempts at forced passage often result in the stripper passing out through the vein wall and if difficulty is encountered withdraw the stripper and repass it. Successful passage of the stripper may be helped by twisting the free portion so rotating the tip to negotiate irregularities. If hold-up occurs around the knee, passage may be aided by flexing and extending the joint and gentle external compression over the tip of the stripper which prevents passage into superficial tributaries.

2. If all these measures fail, leave the stripper in situ and pass a second stripper into the long saphenous vein below the knee. If this passes up without difficulty to the first stripper, gradually withdraw it is front of the advancing stripper passed from below.

3. If neither will bypass the obstruction cut down over the tips of the strippers. One stripper may be re-directed through the cut down incision and passed on down the vein but if this fails, strip out the two halves of the vein leaving a short residual portion between the two incisions. Alternatively this segment of residual vein may be forcibly avulsed.

Aftercare

1. Keep the legs elevated to 30° above the horizontal in bed.
2. Encourage early mobilisation after applying extra blue-line or elastocrepe bandages over the sterile crepe bandages put on in theatre. This reduces haematoma formation, and provides better support when the patient stands. Patients should walk when up and not stand still or sit with their feet down.
3. Discharge fit patients between 24 and 48 hours postoperatively, to re-attend for removal of sutures a week later.

SHORT SAPHENOUS LIGATION AND STRIPPING

Appraise

1. This operation is indicated if there is gross dilation of the short saphenous trunk or its tributaries.
2. The termination of the short saphenous vein in the popliteal or femoral vein is extremely variable so take care to accurately identify this point.
3. Pre-operative varicography or on table saphenography both provide accurate information on the termination of the short saphenous vein and its proximal tributaries.

Position

1. Place the anaesthetized, intubated patient prone with pillows under the chest, midriff and pelvis, with 30° of head down tilt.
2. Slightly abduct the legs to ease access.

Access

1. Make a short transverse incision behind the lateral malleolus.
2. Make a longer transverse incision in the popliteal fossa over the sapheno-popliteal junction.

Assess

1. The short saphenous vein needs to be identified and carefully separated from the sural nerve behind the ankle.

2. A stripper passed up the vein may 'flick' as it enters the popliteal vein giving an indication of the level of the sapheno-femoral junction, although more accurate information is provided by the radiographic techniques described above.

Action

1. Find the short saphenous vein at the ankle by dissecting it from the fat and accompanying sural nerve.

2. Insert the stripper and pass it up the vein in an identical manner to that described for the long saphenous vein.

3. Make a transverse incision 3–5 cm long in the popliteal fossa at the level of the sapheno-popliteal junction, which has been identified by one of the three methods described.

4. Divide the deep fascia and define the short saphenous vein containing the easily palpable semi-rigid stripper. Pull the stripper back slightly before ligating and dividing the vein.

5. Gently dissect free the proximal end of the vein from the surrounding fat until the T-junction with the popliteal vein is identified. Then doubly ligate the stump of the short saphenous vein with 0 chromic catgut.

6. Strip out the vein, bandage the leg and close the incisions.

Aftercare

Manage the patient in the same manner as described in the section on the long saphenous stripping.

INCOMPETENT PERFORATING OR COMMUNICATING VEIN LIGATION

Appraise

1. Communicating veins between the branches of the saphenous system and deep veins of the leg cross the deep fascia of the lower leg. Blood normally passes from the superficial veins to the deep but reversal of flow occurs if the valves in these veins have become incompetent. Three almost constant communicating veins in the medial calf are particularly important in the development of venous ulceration. These veins are the medial calf perforating veins.

2. Ligation of the perforating veins is indicated in patients with clinical or radiographic evidence of incompetent perforating veins who have severe liposclerosis or healed ulceration without evidence of severe post-phlebitic damage of their deep veins.

3. Re-ulceration or future ulceration may be prevented by this procedure in these patients.

4. Perforating veins may be incompetent without any associated skin changes.

Position

As for long saphenous surgery.

Access

1. Make a long vertical incision from the medial malleolus to the upper calf, placed about a finger's breath behind the posterior subcutaneous border of the tibia.

2. Carry the incision directly down and through the deep fascia of the leg, ligating and dividing superficial venous channels on the way down (Fig. 24.2).

Assess

1. A number of vascular bundles will be found passing from the muscles to the deep surface of the divided fascia (Fig. 24.2).

2. Develop the plane between the posterior calf muscles and deep fascia by finger separation of losse areolar tissue and sharp division of the fascial planes.

3. Dissect free these vascular bundles then ligate and divide them. All perforating veins are accompanied by a small artery which is usually tied with the vein.

4. Incompetent veins are wide and, when divided, bleed from the muscle end showing that the valve is defective.

5. Confirm back-bleeding by forced plantar and dorsal flexion of the ankle which works the calf muscle pump and increases perforator reflux (Turner-Warwick test). It is however often difficult to assess the degree of incompetence

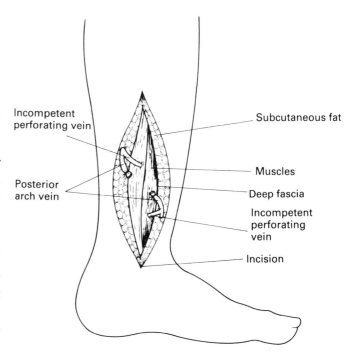

Fig. 24.2 The subfascial operation for ligation of the medial calf perforating veins.

of these veins and it is better to tie all vessels crossing the fascial envelope.

Action

Dissect and ligate any vascular bundle passing from the muscle compartment through the deep fascia.

Closure

Close the deep fascia with continuous 2/0 chromic catgut and the skin with interrupted 4/0 nylon or a subcuticular stitch with steristrips.

Aftercare

Retain sutures for 10 days and mobilise patients more slowly than after simple saphenous surgery. Otherwise the management is identical.

Difficulty?

Thickened vascular subcutaneous tissue makes the sub-fascial approach of Linton (1938) described above much easier than the extra-fascial approach of Cockett (1955). If you choose the extra-fascial approach injudicious under-mining of skin flaps will result in a high incidence of skin necrosis and wound problems. You may miss incompetent perforating veins if all the fascial compartments are not opened. Difficulty may also be experienced in finding veins coming through close to the posterior subcutaneous border of the tibia and around the ankle joint where the incision may need to be extended.

Alternatives

1. Insert the Edward's phlebotome (Fig. 24.3) beneath the deep fascia via a transverse incision in the upper calf. Then push the instrument down towards the ankle, 'shearing' off any perforating veins. Take care to keep the blade of the instrument held up against the deep fascia to ensure that it does not dig into the muscles and soft tissues

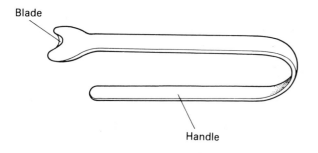

Blade

Handle

Fig. 24.3 The 'Edwards' phlebotome.

of the leg causing vascular and soft tissue damage. Trouble-some bleeding may result from side tears in the deep veins.

2. Place smaller incisions over individual perforating veins suspected to be incompetent on clinical, radiological or doppler ultrasound testing. This results in better healing but there is a risk of missing other unsuspected perforating veins.

3. Place the incision in more normal skin down the back of the calf if the skin over the medial calf is severely damaged.

AVULSIONS OR LOCAL TIES

Appraise

1. Large branch veins which are not in close proximity to the saphenous or perforator systems must be occluded or excised to prevent unsightly local recurrences and provide a satisfactory cosmetic result.

2. A number of alternative techniques have been used to achieve this, including surgical avulsion, transcutaneous suturing and transcutaneous diathermy.

Action

1. Make minute stab incisions in Langer's lines directly over the course of the tributaries. Draw out a loop of vein by gentle, blunt dissection with an artery forceps.

2. Divide the loop between artery forceps and tease out the vein in either direction by steady traction and gentle blunt dissection under the skin flaps, with fine mosquito forceps.

3. Ease out the vein by gentle rotary movements during maintained traction using a similar technique to a bird delivering a worm from a hole in the ground.

4. Stop traction when the vein starts to stretch and at this point tie off both ends with catgut. Alternatively, continue the traction until the vein breaks. Control bleeding by local pressure until traumatic venospasm develops.

5. Place incisions about 5 cm apart along the course of each tributary. The whole vein may be satisfactorily avulsed by using the technique described above.

Difficulty?

1. Thin walled 'blue' veins avulse poorly compared with thick 'white' veins, and if the veins tear easily with exten-sive blood loss, use local ligations in preference to avulsion.

2. Careful pre-operative marking of branch veins ensures that they are easily found through the small stab incisions.

Closure

Use single 4/0 monofilament nylon mattress sutures or subcutaneous catgut and steristrips.

OPERATIONS FOR DEEP VEIN THROMBOSIS

Appraise

1. These are of two types. Thrombectomy is designed to remove loose non-adherent clot. Alternatively, ligation, plication and insertion of filters are designed to 'lock-in' clot and prevent proximal embolisation.

2. Confirm the presence of thrombosis by adequate bilateral ascending phlebography to assess both the type and extent of the thrombus.

3. Operations are not indicated in patients with thrombus that is shown to be old, fixed or totally occlusive. Surgery is also inappropriate in patients with minor calf vein thrombosis and all these patients are best treated by anticoagulation.

4. Surgery is indicated if anticoagulation is dangerous or ineffective, especially if repeated embolisation occurs despite adequate anticoagulation.

5. Treat the rare complication of venous pre-gangrene or gangrene, by venous thrombectomy if possible.

6. Operations are thought to lower the mortality from pulmonary embolism in patients with large quantities of loose propagated clot extending into the femoral or abdominal veins although this has never been tested in a prospective randomised trial.

7. Many surgeons continue to treat all patients with deep vein thrombosis with anticoagulants unless these are contra-indicated.

FEMORAL AND ILIAC VENOUS THROMBECTOMY

Prepare

1. Employ general anaesthesia unless it is contraindicated.
2. Place the patient supine, with the legs again abducted from the midline on a board.

Access

1. Make a vertical incision over one femoral vein extending from the mid-inguinal point down the centre of the thigh for 15–20 cm.

2. Divide the subcutaneous fat lateral to the long saphenous vein which may be traced down to the sapheno-femoral junction.

3. Incise the deep fascia over the femoral vein in a vertical direction and gently dissect the femoral vein from the femoral artery on its lateral border. Use sharp dissec-

tion and take care to avoid handling the vein if it contains loose thrombus.

4. Gently pass silastic tubing around the femoral vein, above and below the profunda branch which is also snared.

5. Carry out a similar dissection on the opposite groin if the thrombus is bilateral or iliac in position.

Assess

Confirm the presence of thrombus within the femoral vein by gentle finger palpation.

Action

If distal thrombus is present:

1. Give 5000 units of heparin intravenously and place bulldog clamps on the proximal femoral and profunda veins. Pass a Fogarthy catheter of appropriate size (4 or 5 F) through a transverse venotomy, as far distally as competent valves allow.

2. Pull up silastic tubing to prevent bleeding around the catheter.

3. Inflate the catheter balloon and slowly withdraw the catheter, pulling out loose thrombus in advance of the balloon.

4. If the catheter will not pass competent distal valves, distal compression or limb-bandaging should be used to force out the thrombus.

5. When no more thrombus can be obtained, close the venotomy with a continuous 6/0 polypropylene suture. Remove the clamps and close the wound in layers with Redivac suction drainage.

If thrombus is present in one iliac vein:

1. Give the patient 5000 units of heparin and make a short transverse venotomy on the unaffected side.

2. Pass a large Fogarthy catheter (size 6 F) up into the inferior vena cava and blow up the balloon to prevent proximal embolisation during the attempted removal of thrombus from the other side. Tighten the silastic tubing around the catheter to prevent troublesome back-bleeding.

3. Make a second venotomy in the femoral vein of the affected side after obtaining control of the femoral and profunda veins with bulldog clamps.

4. Carefully insert a second large Fogarthy catheter (size 6 F) past the iliac thrombus into the vena cava before inflating and withdrawing the balloon and extracting loose clot from the iliac segment (Fig. 24.4).

5. Remove any distal thrombus by the technique described above and close the venotomy with a continuous 60 prolene suture.

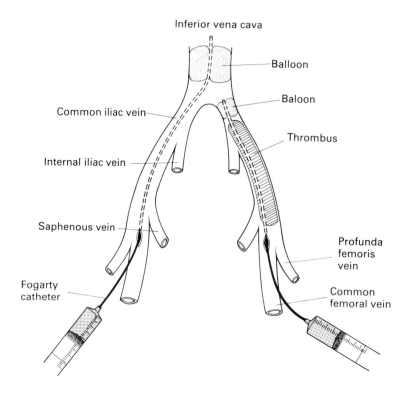

Fig. 24.4 Iliac venous thrombectomy.

6. Now remove the blocking catheter from the other side and close the second venotomy in an identical manner.

7. Close the wounds with Redivac drainage.

Difficulty?

1. Retrograde passage of the catheters may prove difficult past competent valves and thrombectomy may have to be abandoned in favour of simple ligation.

2. Loose thrombus trapped by the blocking catheter may be lost if it slips into the opposite iliac vein when the blocking catheter is withdrawn. Nothing can be done to prevent this complication.

FEMORAL VEIN LIGATION

The access and dissection are identical to those for iliac thrombectomy with which ligation may be combined. Femoral clot may be removed above the profunda vein by the techniques described above and distal clot is then prevented from embolising by ligation of the femoral vein below the profunda insertion. Ligation may be used as the sole manoeuvre if thrombus is present below the profunda origin.

CAVAL CLIPPING OR PLICATION

Position

Place the anaesthetised patient supine with a sandbag under the right buttock.

Access

1. Make a transverse muscle splitting incision just above the umbilicus, lateral to the right rectus abdominis muscle, extending to the costal margin.

2. Split the external and internal oblique muscles in the direction of their fibres and carefully separate the transverse abdominis muscle from the underlying peritoneum, which is pushed medially to expose the retroperitoneal tissues.

3. Insert two Pozzi retractors to hold the peritoneum medially, and expose the inferior vena cava lying on the lumbar vertebrae.

Action

1. Using a combination of sharp and blunt dissection, carefully dissect free and snare a segment of vena cava between the two sets of lumbar veins.

2. Place a plastic clip around the vena cava and hold it closed by a silk ligature as shown (Fig. 24.5a). Alterna-

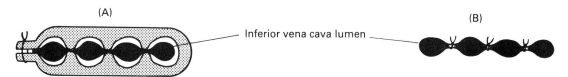

Fig. 24.5a The caval clip.   **Fig. 24.5b** Caval plication.

tively pass three or four mattress sutures across the vessel from front to back and tie them down (Fig. 24.5b). Both techniques produce a number of small channels incapable of allowing a large clot to pass into the lungs.

Difficulty?

Take care to ensure that the clipping or plication is performed above the upper limit of the thrombus. Access may be difficult in a fat patient with a large malignant liver, or with retroperitoneal spread of tumour.

Closure

1. Close the deep part in layers with 1. Dexon.
2. Insert interrupted nylon to skin.
3. Arrange Redivac suction of the retroperitoneal tissue.

INSERTION OF UMBRELLA FILTER

Both Mobin-Uddin and Greenfield-Kimway umbrella filters may be inserted into the inferior vena cava via a venotomy in the interal jugular vein under local anaesthesia. The filter is held closed inside an introducing catheter and passed under X-ray screening using an image intensifier into the inferior vena cava. When the catheter lies in the vena cava below the renal veins the filter is ejected and it fixes into the side wall of the vessel by a series of tiny barbs around its periphery. These are designed to prevent the filter from migrating, which is the major complication of the procedure. Incorrect siting of the filter may also be a problem. Umbrella filters may obviate the need for caval clipping in the future.

Aftercare

1. Maintain intravenous heparin for a minimum of 48 hours postoperatively after all these procedures unless there is a strong contraindication to its use.
2. More prolonged oral anticoagulation may be required after femoral vein ligation to prevent the development of proximal or profunda thrombosis.
3. Encourage all patients who have had a severe deep vein thrombosis to wear graduated compression elastic stockings for support, to prevent the development of severe postphlebitic ulceration in the future. There is a need for a controlled clinical trial to provide clear guidance as to the best treatment of deep vein thrombosis, and the subsequent management of the postphlebitic limb.

OPERATIONS FOR VENOUS ULCER AND POST-PHLEBITIC SYNDROME

Appraise

1. Hopes that saphenous and perforating vein ligation would prevent recurrent ulceration in post-phlebitic limbs have not been fulfilled and a plethora of new operations have been developed in an attempt to improve ulcer-prophylaxis. None of these operations have proved consistently successful as yet.

2. Superficial femoral vein ligation. This is described above. It is theoretically useful when there is isolated femoral vein incompetence with a normal profunda. It is of doubtful value.

3. Saphenous transposition in which the contra-lateral saphenous vein is dissected down until it can be swung across in a supra pubic tunnel and anastomosed to the opposite common femoral or profunda vein to provide a collateral channel for a single blocked iliac segment (Fig. 24.6a). It is only of value if there are no suprapubic collateral channels and patency may be improved if it is combined with an arterio-venous fistula.

4. Valvular repair in which the valve cusps are tightened with reefing sutures in an attempt to render incompetent valves competent (Fig. 24.6b). This operation is only of value in the rare condition of primary valve incompetence which appears to be common in Hawaii.

5. Long saphenous or profunda femoris vein transposition. The femoral vein is divided below the profunda and the distal end is anastomosed end to side to the profunda or end to end to the long saphenous vein below a competent valve (Fig. 24.6c). Results so far are disappointing and the operations chief protagonists have abandoned its use.

6. Autograft insertion. The opposite saphenous vein is used to bypass obstructed segments of vein or a competent valve in a segment of brachial vein may be transplanted into a femoral vein with gross venous reflux (Fig. 24.6d). Early results from a single centre appear encouraging but must be confirmed elsewhere before the operation can be recommended.

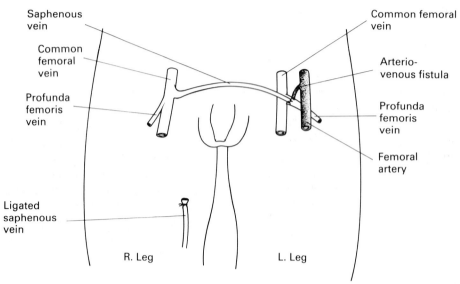

Fig. 24.6a Saphenous transposition bypass.

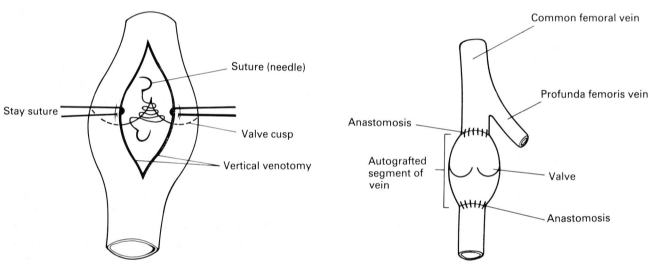

Fig. 24.6b Venous valvuloplasty.

Fig. 24.6d Brachial vein orthograft valve transfer

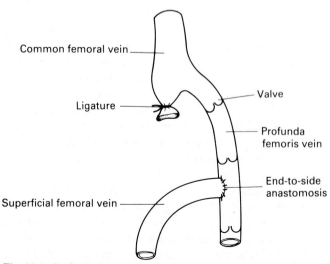

Fig. 24.6c Profunda femoris transposition.

Comment

All these techniques are of doubtful value at present and require careful controlled evaluation against permanent elastic support before they can be accepted into standard clinical practice.

VENOUS ULCERATION

Prepare

1. Following bedrest and intensive antiseptic cleaning, healthy granulations form the base of the ulcer. Direct split skin grafts or pinch grafts are now used to promote ulcer healing.

2. Dirty ulcers with poor granulations require curettage

or excision down to healthy tissue before skin grafting is attempted.

Aftercare

1. If investigation shows the deep veins to be normal, surgery to sites of superficial vein incompetence provides good ulcer prophylaxis.

2. When the deep veins are shown to be severely damaged on phlebography, permanent elastic support or one of the operations described above must be considered.

LYMPHATIC SURGERY

Appraise

1. You must confirm lymphoedema by contrast or isotope lymphography before operations are considered. This ensures that other causes of the swelling are not misdiagnosied and may effect subsequent management.

2. Many patients with mild primary or secondary lymphoedema require little in the way of active treatment and sensible advice on elevation, elastic support and massage is all that is needed to maintain an acceptable level of swelling.

3. A few patients develop severe limb swelling which interferes with limb function and mobility, despite adequate attention to the conservative measures outlined above. Many of these patients show evidence of proximal nodal disease, or the rarer problems of obstruction or megalymphatics. A number of surgical procedures are available to reduce the size of such severely swollen limbs.

REDUCING OPERATIONS

Prepare

1. Order a period of bedrest with limb elevation and intermittent compression using a lymphopress to reduce the size of the limb and make subsequent surgery easier.

2. Eradicate sites of sepsis in the affected leg, paying particular attention to areas of athlete's foot.

3. Access to massive limbs is best provided by inserting a Kirschner wire through the calcaneum and connecting it to its metal stirrup before elevating the leg on a block and tackle suspended from the ceiling of the operating room. The limb is then elevated and abducted, the end of the operating table is lowered and the contra-lateral knee flexed to allow easy access to the medial side of the affected limb. The contra-lateral leg should be fixed to a standard wind-up stool to provide extra support.

4. Ensure a bloodless operating field by applying an Esmarch bandage and tourniquet.

CHARLES OPERATION

Action

1. Fully excise the skin, subcutaneous tissue and deep fascia from the leg between the ankle and knee. Retain existing skin cover over both joints to allow satisfactory post-operative joint mobility (Fig. 24.7).

2. Cover the exposed muscles with split skin grafts taken from the trunk or unaffected contra-lateral limb, using a mechanically operated dermatome, set at an appropriate thickness.

3. Take darts out of the skin around the knee and ankle to prevent a marked 'step' effect. This produces an ugly appearance similar to 'pantaloons'.

4. Suture the skin grafts in place and cover them with non-adherent dressings and thick cottonwool which are held on with crepe bandages.

5. Plan to maintain elevation for one week when the leg is inspected.

Results

1. The reducing effect of the operation is good but the final appearance is often bizarre, with swollen feet and thighs joined by a narrow calf. Severe keloid scars may develop between the sheets of split skin grafts.

2. Delayed healing may be a problem with failure of

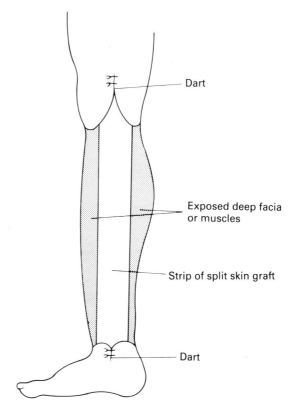

Fig. 24.7 'Charles' leg reduction operation.

'skin graft take'. It is wise to take spare skin at the initial operation to cover unhealed areas in the ward.

HOMANS' OPERATION

This may be performed on both the medial and the lateral sides of the leg.

Action

1. Raise 10–12 cm flaps of skin in an anterior and posterior direction along the whole length of the calf from a hand's breath below the knee-joint to a similar distance above the ankle (Fig. 24.8).

2. Excise the underlying subcutaneous tissues down to the deep fascia and trim excess skin from the flaps to narrow the limb and allow accurate closure.

3. Excise darts at the ankle and knee to avoid dog-ears. The upper dart may be extended up on to the thigh to allow a simple wedge excision of the subcutaneous tissues, as shown in Figure 24.8.

4. Insert several Redivac drains under the skin flaps before carefully closing the wounds with multiple 4/0 nylon sutures.

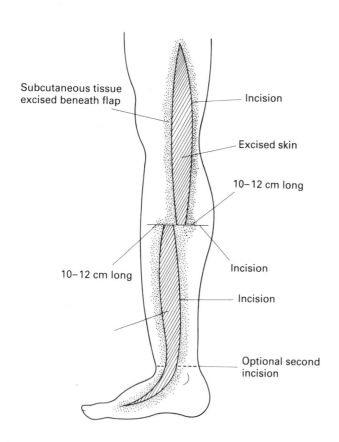

Fig. 24.8 'Homans' medial leg reduction operation.

Subcutaneous tissue excised beneath flap

Incision

Excised skin

10–12 cm long

10–12 cm long

Incision

Incision

Optional second incision

THOMPSON'S OPERATION

1. It was argued that buried skin would contain cutaneous lymphatics capable of anastomosing to the deep lymphatics of the leg, producing better lymphatic drainage of the subcutaneous tissues. The outer layer of skin is excised to prevent pilonidal sinus formation in the buried skin. Later examination of the skin flap has however failed to show consistent development of lymphatic connections and at re-operation little evidence of the buried flap can be found in many patients.

2. Mark out similar flaps to those described above for a Homans' operation. Using a dermatome, denude the anterior part of the posterior flap of its outer epithelium before raising it (Fig. 24.9).

3. Excise the subcutaneous tissue that lies exposed under the skin flaps.

4. Suture down the posterior flap to the divided deep fascia with a number of interrupted 3/0 nylon sutures.

5. Bring the anterior flap over the top of the denuded posterior flap and sew the flap to it with interrupted nylon sutures (Fig. 24.9).

6. Complications include unslightly wounds, delayed healing and pilonidal sinus formation as the result of inadequate excision of hair follicles.

THE MESENTERIC BRIDGE OPERATION

Appraise

1. Patients with obstructive femoral or iliac lymphatics may be helped by means of a mesenteric bridge.

2. This operation is only for use in frankly obstructed lymphatics when the thoracic duct and proximal lymphatic drainage has been shown to be normal. It carries the risks of major abdominal surgery and has only a limited sphere of application.

Action

1. Isolate a short segment of small bowel on its lymphatic and vascular pedicle. Bring it into apposition with the site of the lymphatic block (Fig. 24.10).

2. Split the bowel open along its antimesenteric border and open it out. Dissect the mucosa from the submucosa after injecting 1: 400 000 adrenaline in saline solution to open up the plane. Archieve haemotasis using diathermy.

3. Now sew the submucosa over the divided nodes or lymphatics below the site of obstruction.

4. Subsequent investigation has shown that lympho-lymphatic connections may develop between the obstructed lymphatics and the lymphatics of the submucosa. These drain via the mesenteric lymphatics into the cisterna chyli and thoracic duct.

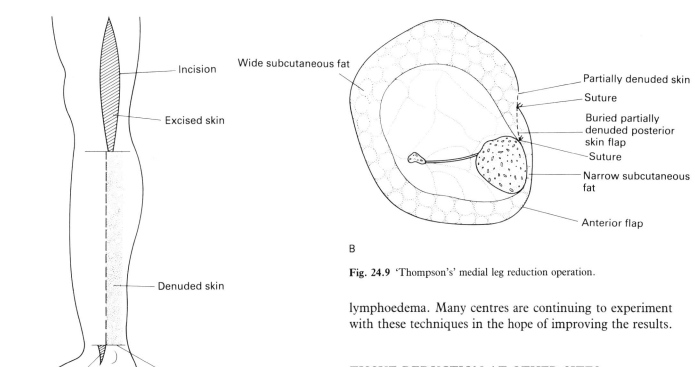

Fig. 24.9 'Thompson's' medial leg reduction operation.

lymphoedema. Many centres are continuing to experiment with these techniques in the hope of improving the results.

TISSUE REDUCTION AT OTHER SITES

The technique already described above can be used to reduce lymphoedema of the upper limb, genitalia and eyelids.

Technical

1. Take care to achieve viable skin flaps and avoid haematoma formation which delays healing in up to 20% of all reduction operations.

LYMPHO-VENOUS ANASTOMOSIS

Microsurgical anastomosis of lymph nodes or individual lymphatics to local veins has failed to produce a significant reduction in limb size in patients with severe long-standing

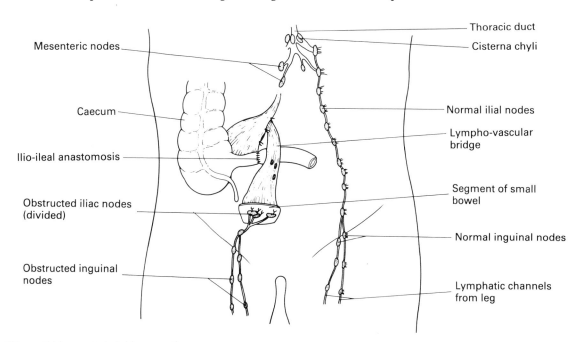

Fig. 24.10 'Kinmonth's' mesenteric bridge operation.

2. When the tourniquets are released achieve haemostasis with catgut ligature, sutures and diathermy to reduce the risk of haematoma.

3. Insert Redivac drains and plan a prolonged period of postoperative bedrest with limb elevation to reduce the risk of haematoma formation.

Results

Although early results appear good, many patients develop recurrent limb swelling which may approach pre-operative dimensions. Repeated reduction surgery combined with good elastic stocking support often produces an acceptable limb although its size rarely matches normal.

Further reading

Browse N L, Lea Thomas M, Solan M J, Young A E 1969 Prevention of recurrent pulmonary embolism. British Medical Journal 3: 382–6

Burnand K G, Lea Thomas M 1983 The value of varicography in the assessment of primary varicose veins of the lower limb. Proceedings of the Union Internationale de Phlebologie, 8th World Congress, Brussels

Burnand K G, O'Donnell T F, Lea Thomas M, Browse N L 1977 The relative importance of incompetent communicating veins in the production of varicose veins and venous ulcers. Surgery 82: 8–14

Charles H 1912 In a system of Treatment, Vol 3, edited by Latham and English, Churchill, London

Cockett F B 1955 The pathology and treatment of venous ulcers of the leg. British Journal of Surgery 43: 260–78

Doran F S A, Barkat S 1981 The management of recurrent varicose veins. Annals of the Royal College of Surgeons of England 63: 432–6

Edwards J M 1976 Shearing operation for incompetent perforating veins. British Journal of Surgery 63: 885–6

Eiriksson E, Dahn I 1968 Plethysmographic studies of venous distensibility in patients with varicose veins. Acta Chirurgica Scandinavica Supplement 398

Fogarty T J, Krippaehne W W 1965 Catheter technique for venous thrombectomy. Surgery Gynecology and Obstetrics 121: 362–4

Greenfield L J 1979 Technical consideration for inspection of vena caval filters. Surgery, Gynecology and Obstetrics 148: 422–6

Hobbs J 1974 Surgery and sclerotherapy in the treatment of varicose veins. A random trial. Archives of Surgery 109: 793–5

Hobbs J T 1980 Preoperative venography to ensure accurate saphenofemoral ligation. British Medical Journal 280: 1578–9

Homans J 1934 Pulmonary embolism caused by thrombosis of deep veins of the lower leg. New England Journal of Medicine 211: 993–7

Homans J 1936 Treatment of elephantiasis of legs. New England Journal of Medicine 215: 1099–1104

Hurst P A, Kinmonth J B, Rutt D L 1978 A gut and mesentery pedicle for bridging lymphatic obstruction. Journal of Cardiovascular Surgery 19: 589–96

Johnson N D, Queral L A, Flinn W R, Yao J S T, Bergan J J 1981 Late objective assessment of venous valve surgery, Archives of Surgery 116: 1461–9

Kinmonth J B 1982 The Lymphatics, 2nd edn. Edward Arnold, London

Kistner R L 1975 Surgical repair of the incompetent femoral vein valve. Archives of Surgery 160: 1336–42

Linton R R 1938 The communication veins of the lower leg and the operative technique for their ligation. Annals of Surgery 107: 582–93

Miles R M, Chappell F, Renner O 1964 A partially occluding vena caval clip for prevention of pulmonary emboli. American Surgeon 30: 40–7

Mobin-Uddin K, Trinkle J K, Bryant L R 1971 Present status of the inferior vena cava umbrella filter. Surgery 70: 914–9

Norgren L 1974 Functional evaluation of chronic venous insufficiency by foot volumetry. Acta Chirurgica Scandinavia Supplement 444

Palma E C, Esperon R 1980 Vein transplant and grafts in the surgical treatment of the post-phlebitic syndrome. Journal of Cardiovascular Surgery 1: 94–7

Scott A, Dormandy J 1976 Outpatient percutaneous ligation of varicose veins. Proceedings of the Royal Society of Medicine 69: 852–3

Stewart G, Gaunt J, Croft D N, Browse N L 1984 The use of radioactive colloid clearance in the diagnosis of lower limb oedema. British Journal of Surgery

Taheri S A, Lazar L, Elias S 1982 Status of vein valve transplant after 12 months. Archives of Surgery 117: 1313–7

Thompson N 1962 Surgical treatment of chronic lymphoedema of the lower limb. British Medical Journal 2: 1567–73

De Weese M S, Hunter D C Jr 1963 A vena cava filter for the prevention of pulmonary embolism. Archives of Surgery 86: 852–68

Werner G, Alexander H A, McPheeters H O 1964 Electrofulguration. New surgical method for varicose veins. Minnesota Medicine 47: 255–7

Wolfe J H N, Kinmonth J B 1981 The prognosis of primary lymphoedema of the lower limbs. Archives of Surgery 116: 1157–60

Sympathectomy

The sympathetic nervous system
Cervicodorsal sympathectomy
Operation for axillary hyperhidrosis
Lumbar sympathectomy

SYMPATHETIC NERVOUS SYSTEM

1. The arteries to the skin and muscle of the limbs have a sympathetic innervation. The sympathetic nerves to the skin of the hands and feet are predominantly vasoconstrictor, but both vasoconstrictor and vasodilator fibres are present to the arteries in muscle. At rest there is a dominant vasoconstrictor tone to skin and muscle. Following sympathetic blockade, skin flow increases markedly and sweating is inhibited, and there is a modest rise in muscle flow. However, the increase in muscle flow during sympathetic blockade is only one-tenth the increase in flow seen during exercise of the muscle. This exercise-induced increase is mediated by the liberation of local metabolites from the contracting muscle fibres.

2. The preganglionic sympathetic fibres, which are myelinated ('white') rami communicantes, pass through the ventral roots of the spinal nerves, travel in the sympathetic chain and synapse in the ganglia. Post ganglionic, unmyelinated ('grey') rami communicantes pass from the ganglia to the corresponding spinal nerves to enter the limb in one or other of the major nerve trunks.

3. The commonest indications for sympathectomy are to relieve vasospasm and control excessive sweating (hyperhidrosis). Operation should be reserved for patients with hyperhidrosis who fail to respond to topical applications of 20% aluminium chloride (Anhydrol Forte).

CERVICODORSAL SYMPATHECTOMY

Appraise

1. The sympathetic fibres to the arm synapse in ganglia T2 to T5 (T2 and T3 for the hand and T4 and T5 for the axilla). The uppermost (T1) ganglion usually fuses with the inferior cervical ganglion to form the stellate ganglion and should be left intact to avoid producing a postoperative Horner's syndrome. The aim of the procedure is to remove the upper thoracic or dorsal sympathetic chain. The title 'cervical sympathectomy' refers to the cervical approach: no part of the cervical sympathetic chain is excised in this operation.

2. Employ cervical sympathectomy for intractable hyperhidrosis of the hands and axillae. If the hyperhidrosis is confined to the axilla, it can be adequately controlled by the more conservative Hurley-Shelley operation.

3. Cervical sympathectomy is effective in severe cases of primary Raynaud's phenomenon (Raynaud's disease) where there is no demonstrable occlusive arterial disease and no necrotic changes in the fingers. It is seldom beneficial in secondary Raynaud's disease, in which there is an identifiable cause such as scleroderma. The results are particularly satisfactory for the first 6 months and for this reason I usually perform the operation in late autumn. Symptoms gradually return, though they are usually less severe than before the sympathectomy.

4. Prolonged exposure of the hand to a temperature below −1°C will cause freezing of the tissues and frostbite. During exposure to the cold there is arterial spasm, and prompt sympathectomy will reduce gangrene and tissue loss of the fingers.

5. Sympathectomy is often of benefit in a variety of ill-understood vasospastic conditions, particularly the severe post-traumatic pain of causalgia, erythromelalgia, acrocyanosis and trophic changes following poliomyelitis.

TRANSAXILLARY APPROACH

Access

1. Place the patient in a lateral position with the operated side uppermost and hold secure with restrainers, as for a nephrectomy. Widely display the axilla by abducting the arm and flexing the forearm, which is then secured to

an arm rest by a crepe bandage. Stand behind the patient.

2. The highest rib that can be felt in the axilla is the second. Make an 8 cm oblique incision from latissimus dorsi, running forwards and down across the third rib roughly in the mid-axilla, as far as the posterior border of pectoralis major.

3. Divide the skin and fatty tissue down to the rib. Divide the periosteum longitudinally with cutting diathermy and reflect it from the superior surface, thereby exposing the costal pleura. It is not necessary to excise a section of rib.

4. Divide the pleura along the upper border of the rib. Insert a rib retractor and open it widely.

5. Displace the apex of the lung downwards with a cloth-covered lung retractor.

6. Always insert a retractor with attached fibreoptic light or a sterile fibre light to illuminate the pleural cavity.

Action

1. Define the ganglia and interconnecting chain as they run beneath the costal pleura over the *necks* of the corresponding ribs (Fig. 25.1). The neck of the first rib is palpable, but the stellate ganglion may be difficult to visualise.

2. Open the pleura over the sympathetic chain from the second to the fifth ribs.

3. Grasp the chain immediately above the second thoracic ganglion with long artery forceps. Divide the chain above the T2 ganglion after clamping the chain above and below with haemostatic clips, such as liga clips. Lift the chain forwards to expose the rami communicantes. Divide the rami between haemostatic clips or with diathermy.

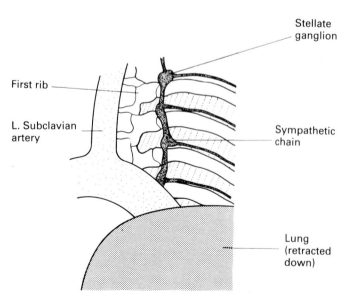

Fig. 25.1 The upper dorsal sympathetic chain on the left has been exposed by division of the costal pleura and retraction of the lung down. It runs over the necks of the ribs.

4. Put a final haemostatic clip across the chain below T5. Divide the chain and lift it out.

5. Do not repair the costal pleura. If you are anxious about the control of bleeding or lung expansion, bring out a chest drain through a separate stab incision in the third intercostal space. Connect the drain to an underwater seal.

6. Perform an intercostal nerve block at the end of the operation to reduce the likelihood of intercostal pain.

7. Tie strong absorbable sutures around the second and third ribs. Ask the anaesthetist to re-expand the lungs. Close the muscles in layers. Close the skin by a standard technique.

8. The opposite sympathetic chain can be excised after repositioning the patient, provided the lung is fully expanded on the operated side.

Aftercare

1. Order a chest X-ray immediately after the operation in order to determine whether the lung has re-expanded satisfactorily.

2. Haemothorax following damage to intercostal veins will stop. If there is no intercostal drain, aspirate the blood and insert a drain if blood re-accumulates.

3. Aspirate air from a pneumothrorax only if it is symptomatic.

4. Post-operative Horner's syndrome caused by damage to the stellate ganglion cannot be treated.

ANTERIOR APPROACH

Access

1. Place the patient supine, with a sandbag under the shoulders, the head turned to the opposite side and the table tilted feet down to about 30°.

2. Make a 5 cm incision placed 1 cm above the clavicle, so that the medial 1 cm overlies the lateral border of the sternomastoid. Divide the platysma with the skin.

3. Divide the lateral fibres of sternomastoid. Locate and divide any large veins in this area, including the external jugular vein, if they are in the way. Insert a small self-retaining retractor.

4. Locate the scalenus anterior muscle which runs down the centre of the field to be inserted into the first rib. It is obscured by fatty areolar tissue, which can be teased aside. Carefully avoid the thoracic duct on the left-hand side.

5. Identify the phrenic nerve passing obliquely over the anterior surface of the scalenus muscle (Fig. 25.2). Tape the nerve and gently retract it medially.

6. Transect the scalenus muscle in line with the skin incision, by grasping the muscle bundles with toothed forceps and dividing them with scissors. Divide the posterior surface of the muscle which is tendinous. Avoid

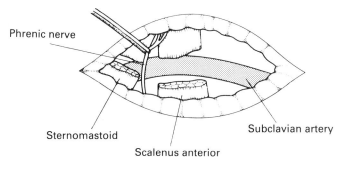

Phrenic nerve

Sternomastoid

Scalenus anterior

Subclavian artery

Fig. 25.2 The lateral fibres of sternomastoid have been divided, the phrenic nerve retracted and scalenus anterior divided to expose the subclavian artery.

damaging the subclavian artery which lies immediately behind these fibres.

7. Expose the arch of the subclavian artery. Place a tape around it and mobilize it as far as possible. Gently tear through the suprapleural (Sibson's) fascia immediately below the subclavian artery.

8. Push the pleura downwards and laterally with swabs, from the necks of the first four ribs. Seal damaged intercostal veins with diathermy or haemostatic clips.

9. Retract the subclavian artery upwards or downwards.

10. The sympathetic chain can now be excised. Identify the stellate ganglion which lays over the neck of the first rib. The chain runs downwards from this.

Action

1. Pick up the chain with a nerve hook or artery forceps between the stellate ganglion and the second thoracic ganglion. Maintain tension on the chain and divide the rami of the second and subseqent ganglia between haemostatic clips.

2. Divide the chain below the T4 ganglion and below the stellate ganglion. Lift it out.

3. Allow the lung to re-expand. Do not repair the scalenus anterior or sternomastoid muscles.

4. Close subcutaneous tissues with absorbable sutures. Close the skin routinely.

5. If necessary, remove the contralateral sympathetic chain immediately.

Difficulty?

1. If a cervical rib is present, retract the subclavian artery forwards to expose the band or rib. Excise the band or remove the rib with bone nibbling forceps, until there is no projection left above or at its articulation with the first rib.

2. Avoid injury to the phrenic nerve by ensuring that it is retracted gently.

3. If injury to the thoracic duct is recognised during the operation, repair it if possible or ligate it.

Aftercare

1. Treat pneumothorax and haemothorax in the same manner as following the transaxillary approach (see p. 412).

2. If a chylous leak develops after operation explore the wound, identify the thoracic duct and tie it off.

3. Horner's syndrome arising from damage to the stellate ganglion cannot be corrected.

OPERATION FOR AXILLARY HYPERHIDROSIS

Appraise

The Hurley-Shelley operation is the most suitable operation for hyperhidrosis confined to the axilla.

Prepare

Map out the sweat-bearing area after drying the axilla and then lightly dusting it with quinizarin compound powder. The powder becomes dark blue on contact with moisture. The moist area roughly corresponds to the hair-bearing area of the axilla.

Action

1. Grasp the skin of the apex of the axilla with Lane's tissue forceps. Excise a 2 cm disc of skin and subcutaneous tissue around the forceps.

2. Closely undercut the skin to excise the underlying sweat glands as far as the edge of the previously mapped out area.

3. Insert a suction drain and close the skin.

Aftercare

Some superficial infection and broadening of the scar are usual but do not often cause complaint as the area is inconspicuous.

LUMBAR SYMPATHECTOMY

Appraise

1. The sympathetic outflow from the spinal cord to the lower limbs extends from T12 to L3 roots, though the number of ganglia is variable. The lumbar sympathetic chain can be blocked by a percutaneous phenol injection. The technique does require expertise, but in centres where this is available, the results of chemical block are comparable to operative sympathectomy without the post-operative morbidity.

2. The indications for sympathectomy in a diabetic patient are the same as in the non diabetic, except that

those with a diabetic peripheral neuropathy will have an autosympathectomy and surgical ablation of the sympathetic chain will not influence peripheral flow.

3. The role of lumbar sympathectomy in atherosclerotic arterial disease has been largely eclipsed by direct vascular operations or bypass procedures. Sympathetic block has little effect on muscle blood flow compared to exercise and has no place in the treatment of intermittent claudication. However, sympathectomy increases blood flow to the digits and it has a role in patients who have early ischaemic ulcers and rest pain and in whom no arterial reconstruction is possible.

4. Sympathectomy performed at the time of an arterial graft will increase the flow through the graft and, if the run off is poor, may theoretically reduce the incidence of early graft occlusion. Though it is not my policy, some vascular surgeons carry out a lumbar sympathectomy as an adjunct to reconstructive arterial operations in the legs.

5. Hyperhidrosis of the feet may be sufficiently severe to warrant a sympathectomy if conservative treatment with astringents is unsatisfactory.

6. Primary Raynaud's phenomenon is improved by sympathectomy though there is a tendency for the symptoms to recur, albeit in a milder form, after 12 months.

7. Sympathectomy may temporarily arrest thrombo-angitis obliterans. This is probably an autoimmune disease and it is seen predominantly in Asia. The disease is unsuitable for arterial reconstruction, as the 'run-off' is usually negligible.

8. Vasomotor disorders of the legs, e.g. acrocyanosis, erythromelalgia and causalgia, will be improved by sympathectomy.

9. Freezing of the foot to temperatures below −1°C is associated with arterial spasm and the resultant tissue loss will be diminished by prompt sympathectomy. Sympathectomy is not beneficial for feet exposed to the cold at temperatures above freezing (trench foot).

Access

1. Place the patient supine with a sandbag beneath the flank on the side of operation.

2. Make an 8–10 cm incision at the level of the umbilicus, extending laterally from the lateral margin of the rectus sheath. Incise the lateral border of the rectus sheath.

3. Separate the fibres of external oblique and divide the internal oblique with cutting diathermy. Separate transversalis fascia carefully to avoid opening the peritoneum. Remember that the peritoneum is much tougher on the lateral side.

4. Using swab and finger dissection, sweep the peritoneum from muscle. Place a retractor over the peritoneum to retract it strongly from the quadratus lumborum and psoas muscle.

5. The ilio-hypogastric and ilio-lumbar nerves run downwards over the surface of quadratus lumborum, while the genito-femoral nerve runs over the psoas. These nerves have no ganglia and should not be confused with the sympathetic chain. The ureter is usually lifted forward with the posterior peritoneum to which it is adherent. It runs anterior to the iliac vessels.

6. Separate the peritoneum medially until the aorta or inferior vena cava can be clearly seen (Fig. 25.3).

Action

1. The sympathetic chain is more readily identified by touch than vision, as it lies in a groove between the side

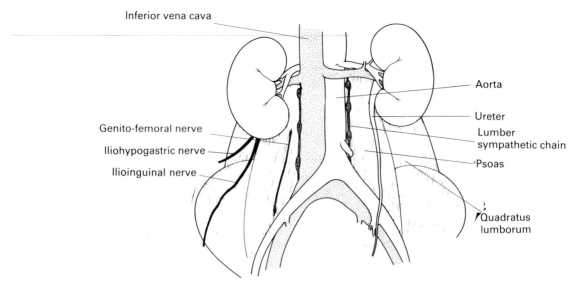

Fig. 25.3 The lumbar sympathetic chain runs down the sides of the bodies of the lumbar vertebra immediately postero-lateral to the inferior vena cava or aorta. The genito-femoral nerve and ureter are important structures that must be avoided.

of the bodies of the lumbar vertebrae and the origins of psoas muscle from the lumbar vertebrae. It passes posterior to the iliac vessels.

2. Lift the chain forwards with a nerve hook and divide the rami after sealing then with diathermy, or between haemostatic clips.

3. Trace the chain inferiorly to the iliac vessels and divide it between haemostatic clips. Then divide the chain superiorly about the level of L2 vertebra and lift out about 7 cm of chain.

4. Repair the muscles separately with absorbable sutures or en masse. Close the skin.

Difficulty?

1. If you accidently open the peritoneum, repair it with absorbable sutures.

2. If you inadvertently get into the wrong plane between psoas and quadratus lumborum, this usually becomes quickly apparent. Retreat and then recommence separating the peritoneum from the anterior surface of psoas.

3. If you accidently injure the ureter, repair it using absorbable sutures across a ureteric catheter. If this cannot be achieved without excessive tension, bring up a tube of bladder (Boari flap) to the proximal end of the ureter (see p. 236). If you are in any doubt, do not fail to ask for the opinion of a urologist if one is available. Alternatively, insert a ureteric catheter to achieve percutaneous drainage of the kidney through the flank and refer the patient to a urologist.

4. Difficulty in identifying the sympathetic chain?

a) The lymphatics lie anterior to the sympathetic chain, they are friable and break easily, unlike the sympathetic chain which is tough.

b) The genito-femoral nerve runs on psoas and lacks ganglia.

c) The anterior longitudinal ligament adheres to the spine and breaks if lifted from the vertebral column.

Aftercare

A curious post-operative pain, post sympathetic neuralgia, extending in to the thigh, occurs in some patients. The explanation is unknown but it passes off in time.

Further reading

Barcroft H 1963 Circulation in skeletal muscle. In: Handbook of physiology, circulation vol 2. American Physiological Society, P P

Campbell W B, Cooper M J 1983 Transaxillary sympathectomy. Hospital Update 9: 533–540

Keane F B V 1977 Phenol lumbar sympathectomy for severe arterial occlusive disease in the elderly. British Journal of Surgery 64: 519–521

Moorhouse J A, Carter S A, Doupe J 1966 Vascular responses in diabetic peripheral neuropathy. British Medical Journal 1: 883–888

de Takats G 1975 Sympathectomy revisited. Surgery 78: 644–659

Terry H, Allan J S, Taylor G W 1970 The affect of adding lumbar sympathectomy to reconstructive arterial surgery in the lower limb. British Journal of Surgery 57: 51–55

Amputations

Amputation, a mainstay of emergency surgery for centuries, was traditionally used as a desperate and often unsuccessful attempt to preserve life. With the advent of modern surgical and anaesthetic techniques, amputation is used less often as an emergency operation and is increasingly carried out as an elective procedure, the object of which is to restore limb function to the maximum possible degree.

Approximately 5000 amputations are performed each year in England. 75% of the patients are over 60 years of age and 70% are men. The indications for amputation are usually vascular and/or diabetic disease (82%). Trauma (10%) and tumours (5%) make up most of the other indications with infection nowadays only responsible for 1.5% of amputations. Major upper limb amputations are rarely required (5%).

GENERAL PRINCIPLES
Appraise

1. The level of amputation (and the type of prosthesis) is influenced by

(a) Cosmetic appearance
(b) Functional requirement
(c) Comfort
(d) Viability of soft tissues

2. Assess the blood supply of the limb clinically by looking at the skin for colour changes, shiny atrophic appearance and lack of hair growth. Feel the skin for temperature changes, check the peripheral pulses and perform Buerger's test. Skin blood flow may be further assessed by transcutaneous Doppler recordings, thermography, radioactive xenon clearance and transcutaneous Po_2 measurement.

3. Assess the bone by taking plain radiographs, tomograms or a radioisotope bone scan. Angiography and CAT scanning are helpful in amputation for bone and soft tissue tumours.

4. Explain the proposed surgery carefully to the patient and obtain consent to amputate if necessary more proximally than you intend.

5. If in any doubt about the necessity for amputation obtain a second opinion from a senior colleague.

6. Clearly mark the limb with indelible marker.

7. Clean the limb and seal off the infected or necrotic areas.

8. Arrange for the disposal of the limb after amputation to the pathology department or straight to the incinerator.

9. Give prophylactic antibiotics, penicillin (or erythromycin) plus one other broad spectrum antibiotic.

10. Proceed under general anaesthesia whenever possible.

Action

1. Use a tourniquet except in peripheral vascular disease. Exsanguinate the limb by elevation for 2 minutes rather than an Esmarch bandage.

2. Prepare the skin and apply the drapes.

3. Mark the proposed skin flaps with methylene blue or similar dye. The flaps should be roughly the same length

with their base at the level of bone section. Leave the flaps too long rather than too short. Wherever possible include underlying muscles in the flap (myoplastic flap) as this greatly improves the blood supply.

4. Cut the muscle with a raked incision angled towards the level of bone section.

5. Double ligate major vessels with strong silk or linen thread. Ligate other vessels with chromic catgut or polyglycolic acid (Dexon).

6. Gently pull down major nerves, ligate any large accompanying vessels, divide the nerve cleanly and allow to retract.

7. Prepare to cut the bone at the appropriate level. Remember that the stump must be long enough to gain secure attachment to the prosthesis and to act as a useful lever but short enough to accommodate the prosthesis and its hinge or joint mechanism. Divide the periosteum and cut the bone with a Gigli or power saw. During bone section, cover the soft tissues with a moist pack and irrigate afterwards to remove bone dust and particles from the soft tissues.

8. Check that the flaps will approximate easily.

9. Release the tourniquet and secure haemostasis.

10. Insert a suction drain.

11. Suture the flaps together without tension starting with the muscle. Handle the skin carefully and close with interrupted nylon sutures.

12. If infection is present, close the flaps loosely over gauze soaked in saline or proflavine. Arrange delayed primary closure at 5–7 days.

Aftercare

1. Apply a well padded compressible but not crushing dressing using either cotton wool or latex foam. Hold this in place with crepe bandage taking care to avoid fixed flexion or other deformity of neighbouring joints.

2. Wherever possible apply a *light* shell of plaster of Paris (maximum four layers) over the dressing. This will make the patient more comfortable and more mobile in bed.

3. Leave the dressing undisturbed if possible for ten days. Increasing pain, seepage of blood or pus through the dressing, rising temperature and pulse are indications for earlier inspection of the wound.

4. Order regular physiotherapy to prevent joint contractures.

5. Encourage mobilisation and use of the stump as soon as the patient is comfortable.

6. When the wound has healed and sutures have been removed, apply regular stump bandaging to maintain the shape of the stump.

7. Refer as soon as possible to the local limb fitting centre.

Complications

1. Haematoma

(a) Avoid this complication by meticulous haemostasis at the time of amputation. Double ligate major vessels and try to prevent infection which may cause secondary haemorrhage. Never close the stump before releasing the tourniquet.

(b) Haematoma in the stump predisposes to infection and greatly delays prosthetic fitting.

(c) Drain collections of blood by aspiration or a small incision. Perform this in the operating theatre under sterile conditions, not on the ward. Local anaesthesia is usually sufficient.

(d) If there is clearly uncontrolled haemorrhage, apply firm compression and elevate the limb whilst you make arrangements to explore the stump under a general anaesthetic.

2. Infection

(a) Amputation stumps are more at risk of infection than most other surgical wounds because of the frequency of poorly vascularised tissues in the stump, infected lesions in the distal extremity and frail, elderly patients with poor resistance to infection.

(b) Give prophylactic antibiotics to all lower limb amputees. The antibiotics should be active against gas gangrene organisms, E. coli and straphylococci.

(c) Handle all soft tissues with care and avoid leaving dead muscle and long sections of denuded cortical bone in the stump.

(d) Treat wound infections promptly with antibiotics. Incise and drain any collection of pus.

(e) If a chronic sinus fails to dry up with a course of antibiotics lasting up to 6 weeks, explore the stump under general anaesthesia. A focus of infection such as a small bony sequestrum or a lump of infected suture material will usually be found.

3. Flap necrosis

(a) Prevent this complication by carefully assessing skin viability prior to amputation and by handling all skin edges and flaps with the utmost care. Use a myoplastic flap whereever possible as this always has a better blood supply.

(b) Treat small areas of wound necrosis conservatively. The wound will granulate beneath the patch of blackened, sloughing skin which will eventually separate spontaneously.

(c) Major flap necrosis will require either a wedge resection down to and including bone or a re-amputation to a higher level.

4. Joint contractures

(a) Particularly important at the hip and knee, contractures are common in the elderly and immobile, in patients with serious head injuries, prolonged coma or chronic pain.
(b) Treat or prevent mild contractures by early active and passive exercises, corrective posturing and prosthetic fitting and mobilisation.
(c) Severe contractures may require serial plasters or surgical release, otherwise the use of a prosthesis is likely to be impossible.

5. Neuroma

(a) All cut ends of nerves form neuromata but they are painful only if trapped in scar tissue or exposed to repeated trauma. It is important that the transected nerves lie deep within the normal tissues of the limb proximal to the end of the stump.
(b) Treat painful neuromata by resecting the neuroma and a length of the affected nerve well away from the area of scar tissue.

6. Phantom limb sensation

(a) Always warn the patient before amputation that after the operation he will have a feeling that the missing part of his limb is still present. Do not introduce the concept of phantom pain however.
(b) After amputation, reassure the patient that this feeling will gradually fade away. Meanwhile warn him of the danger of attempting to use a limb that is not present.

7. Phantom pain

(a) This difficult complication is most common with proximal rather than distal amputations, in patients who had severe pain before amputation and in those who have been in contact with other patients with phantom pain.
(b) The cause is unknown and the pain is untreatable even by nerve section or cordotomy. Be continually optimistic and supportive and remember that this distressing symptom occasionally leads to suicide.

HINDQUARTER AMPUTATION

Appraise

1. This radical operation is usually performed for malignant disease of bone or soft tissue of the pelvis or upper thigh. The aim should be to obtain cure of the disease, rarely palliation.
2. Do not recommend this operation if there are multiple metastases, if the tumour cannot be completely removed, or if the patient is unsuitable due to physical frailty or refusal to accept mutilation.
3. Obtain unequivocal histological proof of the diagnosis by biopsy. Be careful to place the biopsy incision where it will not encroach upon the skin flaps of the amputation.
4. Use X-rays, tomography, arteriography, bone scans, and CAT scans to define as accurately as possible the extent of the tumour.
5. Take bacteriological swabs from the perineum and any open wound. Order prophylactic antibiotic cover accordingly but always include penicillin or other clostridial antibiotic.
6. Clear the rectum with an enema or washout.
7. Ask the anaesthetist to see the patient well in advance. Additional techniques such as spinal or epidural block and hypotensive anaesthesia may be advised.

Action

1. When the patient is anaesthetised, seal off the anus with a small pad plus adhesive surgical drape and insert a catheter into the bladder.
2. Place the patient supine with a long narrow sandbag beneath the shoulder and buttock of the affected side. From this position the patient can easily be rolled into the lateral position at the appropriate stage of the operation.
3. Mark the skin flaps (Fig. 26.1). The incision begins at the symphysis pubis and extends across the iliac fossa to the anterior superior iliac spine. It then continues downwards over the greater trochanter, across the gluteal fold and then upwards into the perineum to meet its point of origin. Make appropriate modifications to allow for previous biopsy scars, proximity of tumour, or skin damaged by radiotherapy.
4. This operation should be performed by an experienced surgeon. The detailed steps in the procedure

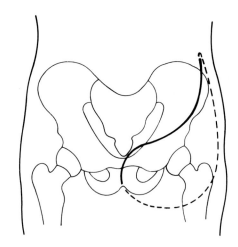

Fig. 26.1 Incision for hindquarter amputation

are best described by Gordon-Taylor and Munro (1962) but the basic principles are as follows:

(a) First, expose the iliac vessels by deepening the anterior incision through the abdominal wall muscles. Ligate the deep epigastric vessels and divide the symphysis pubis taking care not to damage the urethra. Then sweep the peritoneum and ureter medially to expose the common iliac vessels which should be ligated. Cut the femoral, obturator and lateral cutaneous nerves cleanly with a knife. Ligate the iliolumbar tributaries of the common iliac vein.

(b) Secondly, develop the posterior flap by rolling the patient into the lateral position. Preserve as much gluteus maximus muscle as possible. Expose both sides of the greater sciatic notch and using a Gigli saw, divide the posterior ilium at the appropriate site to obtain clearance of the tumour. Divide the remaining soft tissues, sciatic nerve, internal iliac vessel branches, sacrotuberous and sacrospinous ligaments, and remove the hindquarter.

5. Secure meticulous haemostasis.

6. Close the wound with interrupted skin sutures only, over a suction drain. Apply a compression dressing using a crepe bandage spica.

Aftercare

1. Remove the drain at 48 hours and the catheter on the fifth postoperative morning.

2. Give careful fluid and blood replacement initially, and allow oral fluids and food after 24 hours provided there are active bowel sounds (beware of postoperative ileus).

3. Inspect the wound at 10 days and if it is healing well, allow the patient up with crutches. Leave the sutures for about 21 days, particularly if there is any doubt about skin viability.

4. Once the patient is mobile on crutches, consider ordering a prosthesis if the patient is willing and likely to be able to use one adequately.

DISARTICULATION AT THE HIP

Appraise

1. This is a relatively common operation for malignant disease of the thigh and occasionally severe trauma or infection.

2. Obtain unequivocal proof of the diagnosis before proceeding.

3. Consider the possibility of amputating through the lesser trochanter as this will give a better stump.

Action

1. Proceed under general anaesthesia.

2. Place the patient supine with a sandbag beneath the sacrum.

3. Mark the skin flaps. Start the incision just lateral to the anterior superior iliac spine, descend a short distance and then pass medially, parallel to and below the inguinal ligament to the inner thigh about 5 cm below the perineum. Continue posteriorly in a broad curve across the lower buttock 5 cm below the ischial tuberosity and 8–10 cm below the greater trochanter. From there take the incision up to meet the starting point.

4. Expose and ligate the femoral vessels and divide the nerve clearly. Externally rotate and abduct the limb and divide the flexor and adductor muscles in the plane of the incision (cutting diathermy is useful for this stage).

5. Internally rotate the limb and detach gluteus medius and minimus from the greater trochanter. Divide gluteus maximus and the fascia lata in the line of the incision. Divide the sciatic nerve and allow it to retract. Divide the short external rotator muscles and capsule and disarticulate the hip.

6. To preserve the proximal femur leave a longer posterior skin flap, preserve the attachments of gluteus medius and minimus and the short external rotators and section the femur through the lesser trochanter.

7. Secure haemostasis.

8. Close the wound by suturing the muscle and fascia of the posterior flap to the pectineus and adductor muscles using strong interrupted absorbable sutures. Insert a suction drain and suture the skin.

9. Apply a bulky compression dressing.

Aftercare

1. Remove the drain at 48 hrs and the sutures at 14 days.

2. Arrange for a cast to be taken for the socket of the prosthesis as soon as the stump is fully healed and free of all swelling (this often takes about 4 weeks). Remember however, that few elderly patients will have the strength to use the tilting table prosthesis which is required for this amputation.

ABOVE-KNEE AMPUTATION

Appraise

1. Decide on the level of the amputation bearing in mind the following considerations:

(a) The longer the femoral stump the better the control of the prosthesis.

(b) The bone should not be divided lower than 15 cm above the knee joint.

(c) The traditional site of election is 28 cm below the greater trochanter.

(d) If there is fixed flexion deformity at the hip a shorter stump must be fashioned in order to fit into a prosthesis.

(e) A patient who is unlikely to walk after amputation should have a short stump if the hip is stiff.

2. If possible, do not amputate through the femur in children as this would remove the lower, growing end of the femur.

Action

1. Place the patient supine with a sandbag beneath the buttock.

2. Use a tourniquet if there is room to apply it without interfering with the operative area.

3. Operate from the opposite side of the table for better access to, and elevation of, the stump during surgery.

4. Mark out equal anterior and posterior flaps, their bases opposite the proposed level of bone section.

5. Take the incision down to deep fascia and allow the skin to retract slightly. From this level divide the anterior muscles with a raking cut aimed at the level of bone section.

6. Identify the femoral vessels beneath the sartorius and doubly ligate them. Pull down the femoral nerve, cut it cleanly and allow it to retract.

7. Divide the periosteum round the whole femur at the level of proposed section. Cut through the bone with a Gigli or amputation saw, protecting the soft tissues as previously described.

8. Now retract the distal femoral fragment and locate the profunda femoris vessels in the tissues behind the femur. Ligate the vessels then identify the sciatic nerve. Ligate the arteria nervi ischiadii then pull down gently on the nerve, divide it cleanly and allow it it to retract.

9. Complete the division of the posterior muscles using a raking cut to match the anterior flap.

10. Remove the limb.

11. Secure haemostasis.

12. Round off the end of the bone with a rasp.

13. Now turn your attention to the flaps, which should be roughly equal in size and thickness. They are composed of muscle and skin and are called myoplastic flaps. Drill a small hole in the posterior cortex of the femoral stump and using chromic catgut or polyglycolic acid (Dexon), suture the quadriceps over the end of the bone. Then suture the remaining muscles to the quadriceps. Try to achieve roughly equal tension in all the muscle groups.

14. Insert a suction drain.

15. Close the skin with interrupted nylon plus adhesive, e.g. Steristrip tapes.

16. Apply a well padded compression dressing and hold it in place by taking two or three turns of crepe bandage round the waist. Be careful, however, to avoid pulling the stump into flexion with the dressing.

Aftercare

1. Remove the drain at 48 hrs.

2. Encourage maximum mobility as soon as the patient is comfortable. Ensure regular physiotherapy is given which should include prone lying, to prevent a flexion contracture at the hip.

3. Inspect the wound at 10 days and remove the sutures when healed.

4. Apply a firm stump bandage daily thereafter to mould the stump into a roughly conical shape.

5. Arrange for the fitting of a temporary pylon by the third or fourth week and plan for definitive limb fitting between the sixth and twelfth week.

DISARTICULATION OF THE KNEE

Appraise

1. A through-knee amputation provides a better stump for limb wearing than any more proximal amputation. The prosthesis is rather unsightly because of its width and outside hinges but it functions well and is much easier to use than a prosthesis for above knee amputations.

2. Consider this amputation in any frail and elderly patient who is not suitable for a below knee amputation.

3. This is the amputation of choice in children as the growth plate of the distal femur is preserved.

4. Do not perform this amputation in the presence of fixed flexion deformity in the hip.

Action

1. Use a general anaesthetic if possible but epidural or local anaesthesia are also satisfactory at this level.

2. Apply a tourniquet to the thigh with the knee flexed to 90°.

3. Place the patient prone on the operating table.

4. Mark out equal lateral based flaps. Start the incision anteriorly midway between the lower pole of the patella and the tibial tubercle and curve laterally and downwards to mark a flap that runs about 5 cm below the joint line. The incision then curves posteriorly to the middle of the popliteal fossa 2.5 cm above the joint line. Complete the incision by joining the anterior and posterior points with a medial curved flap which should be 2 cm longer than the lateral flap.

5. Incise down to bone medially and laterally and raise the flaps. Handle the flaps with care. Dissect the patellar tendon off the tibial tubercle. Divide the hamstrings close to the bone. Identify and ligate the popliteal vessels. Pull down the popliteal nerves, divide cleanly and allow to retract.

6. Incise the posterior capsule close to the tibia such as

to enter the joint beneath the menisci. Divide the cruciate ligaments and popliteal tendon and remove the limb.

7. Release the tourniquet and secure haemostasis.

8. Suture the patellar tendon to the cruciate ligaments and the remains of the extensor retinaculum to the hamstrings each side using strong chromic catgut or polyglycolic acid (Dexon). Retain the menisci as a cushion over the femoral condyles provided they are healthy and stable.

9. Insert a suction drain.

10. Close the flaps with interrupted nylon sutures.

11. Apply a well padded compression dressing and a light plaster cast which must be well moulded above the femoral condyles. Ensure that the drain tube protrudes through the top of the plaster cast.

Aftercare

1. Remove the drain at 48 hrs by pulling gently on the tube.

2. Mobilise the patient as soon as he is comfortable (48–72 hrs).

3. Remove the sutures at 14 days and thereafter apply a regular stump bandage.

4. Arrange for limb fitting as soon as the wound is fully healed.

GRITTI-STOKES AMPUTATION

Appraise

1. This operation is less satisfactory than a through-knee disarticulation because it rarely provides a useful end bearing stump and as an ischial bearing stump is much worse than an above-knee amputation. It is suitable for patients who are likely to be confined to bed or a wheelchair.

2. Do not perform this operation in the presence of hip flexion contracture, severe osteoporosis (because internal fixation of patella to femur is required) or infection (because of foreign material buried in the stump).

3. Position the patient supine on the operating table.

Action

1. Proceed under general or epidural anaesthesia.

2. Apply a tourniquet to the upper thigh.

3. Mark out the skin flaps. Start on each side at the centre point of the femoral condyle and curve the anterior incision down to cross the tibial tubercle in the mid-point. Join the centre point of each femoral condyle with a straight line posteriorly.

4. Raise the anterior flap by incising down to bone and reflecting the composite flap (skin, fascia, patella ligament, patella and joint capsule) upwards to expose the knee joint. Deepen the posterior incision to fascia but do not raise a flap.

5. Divide the soft tissues at the back of the knee with a knife at the level of the posterior incision. Remove the lower leg. Identify and tie off the main vessels in the posterior flap.

6. Release the tourniquet and secure haemostasis.

7. Transect the lower femur just proximal to the femoral condyles using an oscillating saw. Remove the articular surface of the patella with the saw leaving a flat surface of cancellous bone.

8. Drill a hole transversely across the patella just distal to its midpoint. Drill two further holes obliquely from the cut surface of the femur through the posterior cortex. Pass a length of 20 gauge steel wire through the holes and thus fix the patella onto the cut surface of the femur. Tighten the wires, cut off the twisted ends and bury them in the femur using a punch.

9. Insert a suction drain.

10. Using chromic catgut or polyglycolic acid (Dexon) suture the extensor retinaculum and capsule of the knee joint to the deep fascia of the posterior flap. Close the skin with interrupted nylon sutures.

11. Apply a well padded compression bandage and strap it securely to the thigh.

Aftercare

1. Remove the drain at 48 hrs.

2. Inspect the wound at 10 days and remove the sutures if the skin is fully healed.

3. If the patient is suitable for end bearing, remember that this cannot be considered until the patella has united to the femur. This takes 6–12 weeks.

BELOW-KNEE AMPUTATION

Appraise

1. Assess carefully the viability of the soft tissues of the lower leg when amputation at this level is being considered for peripheral vascular disease, diabetic gangrene or trauma.

2. Use a long posterior flap in peripheral vascular disease, diabetes and trauma. Equal flaps are suitable for amputation for tumours and severe acute infection.

3. Do not consider this amputation in the non-ambulant patient, if the stump will be less than 5 cm long, if there is fixed flexion deformity of the knee greater than 30° or if knee motion is greatly reduced.

4. The traditional site of election is 14 cm from the joint line. Do not make the stump any longer than this.

Action

1. Seal off any infected, gangrenous areas by enclosing in a polythene bag.

2. Use general or epidural anaesthesia.

3. Apply a tourniquet to the thigh unless the amputation is for peripheral vascular disease.

4. Place the patient supine on the operating table with a padded, inverted bowl underneath the proximal tibia.

5. Mark the skin flaps (Fig. 26.2). Start the anterior incision at the base of proposed bone section and pass transversely round each side of the leg to a point two-thirds of the way down each side. Then take the incisions distally on each side passing slightly anteriorly to a point well below the length which is likely to be required. Join the two incisions posteriorly.

6. Dissect the longitudinal incisions down to deep fascia. Anteriorly incise straight down to bone and then onto the interosseous membrane. Ligate the anterior tibial vessels at this point. Elevate the periosteum of the tibia for 1 cm proximal to the level of section. Divide the tibia using a Gigli or amputation saw. Bevel the anterior half of the tibial stump with the saw and a rasp. Divide the fibula 1 cm proximally and bevel the bone laterally.

7. Use a bone hook to distract the distal part of the tibia. Divide the deep posterior muscles of the calf at the same level as the tibia. At this stage identify and ligate the posterior tibial and peroneal vessels and divide the posterior tibial nerve cleanly and allow to retract.

8. Use a raking cut through the soleus and gastrocnemius muscles down to the end of the posterior flap. Remove the limb.

9. Complete the smoothing and bevelling of the tibia and fibula using bone nibblers and a rasp.

10. Pull the posterior flap over the stump and excise excess muscle and skin so as to create a rounded, bulbous stump which can be closed without tension.

11. Release the tourniquet and secure haemostasis.

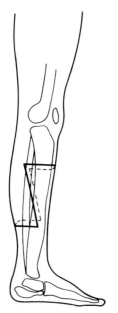

Fig. 26.2 Incision for below-kneea amputation

12. Insert a suction drain.

13. Suture the deep fascia of the posterior flap to the periosteum of the anterior flap using chromic catgut or polyglycolic acid (Dexon).

14. Close the skin with interrupted nylon sutures and adhesive strip such as Steristrip tapes. Do not leave any 'dog ears' laterally.

15. Apply a dressing of gauze and sterile plaster wool and apply gentle compression over the stump with a crepe bandage. Apply a further layer of plaster wool and then a light plaster cast to midthigh level. Mould the plaster over the femoral condyles to prevent it slipping down.

Aftercare

1. Elevate the leg.

2. Remove the drain at 48 hrs by pulling it gently out of the top of the plaster cast.

3. Mobilise early and retain the plaster cast undisturbed for at least 10 days.

4. Remove the sutures at 14 days.

5. Apply a daily stump bandage.

6. Arrange for daily hip and knee physiotherapy.

7. As soon as the wound has fully healed arrange for the fitting of a temporary pylon, either patellar tendon bearing or ischial bearing depending on the quality of the stump. Arrangements for definitive limb fitting may then proceed.

SYME'S AMPUTATION

Appraise

1. Transmetatarsal and tarsometatarsal amputations are occasionally required for severe trauma but should not be elective amputations as the Syme's amputation is functionally superior.

2. Properly performed, Syme's is the best amputation of the lower limb. The stump is end bearing with good proprioception and the modern cosmetic prostheses are very light and comfortable.

3. Ensure that there is adequate circulation in the foot. The posterior tibial pulse must be palpable. The skin of the heel must be of good quality.

Action

1. Place the patient supine with the foot over the end of the table.

2. Apply a tourniquet to the thigh.

3. With the foot and ankle neutral, mark the skin flaps (Fig. 26.3). The plantar flap runs from the tip of the lateral malleolus across the sole (curving slightly forward) to a point just below the medial malleolus. The dorsal flap joins the ends of the plantar incision at an angle of 45° from the line of the tibia.

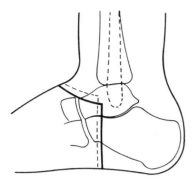

Fig. 26.3 Incision for Symes amputation

4. Incise down to bone in the plantar flap and on the dorsum divide the extensor retinaculum and pull down the extensor tendons, dividing them as high as possible. Open the ankle joint, plantarflex the foot and divide the medial and lateral collateral ligaments from within. Take care to avoid the posterior tibial nerve and artery on the medial side.

5. Dislocate the talus down and open the posterior capsule of the ankle exposing the postero-superior surface of the oscalcis and the anterior surface of the tendo Achilles.

6. Use a periosteal elevator to reflect periosteum and soft tissue from the medial and lateral sides of the os calcis down to the inferior surface of the bone. Continue this dissection so as to free the inferior surface.

7. Detach the long plantar ligament from the tuberosity of the os calcis and continue until the plantar incision is reached and the proximal end of the bone is free except for the insertion of the tendo Achilles. This should then be divided carefully from above downwards keeping close to the bone. Avoid button-holing the skin flap behind the tendon. Now remove the foot.

8. Turn the heel flap backwards and upwards and free the malleoli and distal centimetre of tibia. Remove the malleoli and a thin slice of tibia with a saw. Ensure that your cut is at right angles to the line of the tibia and that you leave the subarticular bone intact. Round off the bone edges.

9. Release the tourniquet and secure haemostasis.

10. Insert a suction drain.

11. Suture the heel flap to the margin of the dorsal incision in two layers with subcutaneous chromic catgut or polyclycolic acid (Dexon) and interrupted nylon to skin. Begin skin closure in the middle and continue to each end.

12. Ensure that the heel flap remains centred over the cut end of the tibia. The flap may be secured with adhesive (e.g. Steristrip) tapes or if very unstable, it should be transfixed percutaneously with a Kirschner wire or Steinmann's pin passed up into the tibia.

13. Apply a well padded pressure dressing and retain this either with adhesive strapping to the upper calf or a lightweight above knee plaster cast.

Aftercare

1. Elevate the leg.

2. Remove the drain at 48 hrs but do not disturb the dressing.

3. If you have not transfixed the heel flap, inspect the wound at 5 days to check the position of the flap. Otherwise, inspect the wound at 14 days when the sutures and the percutaneous pin may be removed.

4. Carefully apply a stump bandage thereafter and arrange the fitting of a prosthesis as soon as the swelling has subsided (2 or 4 weeks).

AMPUTATION OF THE TOES

Appraise

1. Avoid amputating single toes if possible. Neighbouring toes tend to develop secondary deformity and take more weight.

2. Remove all the toes (the 'Pobble' operation) if there are multiple painful, fixed deformities or if several toes are gangrenous.

3. Ray resection of toes may be required for gangrene or diabetes.

Action

1. Use a tourniquet with exsanguination.

2. Mark out a racquet incision for amputation of individual toes. For amputation of all the toes the incision should be transverse, passing across the root of the toes on the plantar aspect (i.e. overlying the proximal phalanx) and across the metatarsophalangeal joints on the dorsum. The eventual scar should lie dorsally.

3. Take the flaps straight down to bone and dissect off the proximal phalanx.

4. Preserve the base of the proximal phalanx where possible, dividing the bone just distal to the insertion of the capsule. A small wound cavity is thereby created which heals quickly and the amputation does not damage the transverse metatarsal ligaments. Otherwise perform a careful disarticulation.

5. Secure haemostasis.

6. Close the skin with interrupted nylon sutures.

7. Apply a bulky compression dressing, passing a few turns of crepe bandage round the ankle to hold the dressing in position.

Aftercare

1. Elevate the leg.

2. Remove the sutures at 10 days and mobilise the patient.

3. Where individual toes have been amputated, ask the chiropodist to supply a toe spacer.

4. Where all the toes have been amputated, order from the surgical appliances department a special insole which incorporates a combined metatarsal and cavus support plus a cork toe-block faced with sponge rubber.

FINGER AND HAND AMPUTATIONS

Appraise

1. Avoid unnecessary delay in starting treatment. The viability of injured tissue can be adversely affected by digital nerve blocks and rubber catheter tourniquets, so use more proximal nerve blocks or general anaesthesia and a pneumatic tourniquet around the upper arm.

2. Assess the full extent of the injury and always take X-rays. Wash the injured area gently and thoroughly with copious sterile saline. Remove all foreign matter and any undoubtedly non-viable tissue.

3. Always consider the possibility of re-implantation of major traumatic amputations. Contact the local micro-vascular unit for advice and transfer the patient with the amputated part preserved in a sterile polythene bag cooled with ice.

FINGERTIP INJURIES

SUBUNGUAL HAEMATOMA

Action

1. Release the haematoma which is under tension by perforating the nail with the red-hot end of a wire paper clip. The attachments of cuticle and skin to the margins of the nail will retain it in place so that it continues to act as a useful splint for the fingertip should the distal phalanx be fractured. Usually such fractures do not require manipulation.

PARTIAL AVULSION OF THE NAIL

Action

1. If the X-ray shows either an intact phalanx or an undisplaced fracture, evacuate all residual blood from beneath the nail.

2. Repair splits in the nail bed with fine catgut sutures. Trim the cuticle and skin from the free margins of the nail and retain it in place with one or two fine nylon sutures.

3. Always try to preserve the nail. Even though it will subsequently be lost, it will act as a biological dressing and splint.

4. Remember that if the distal phalanx is seen on X-ray to have sustained a transverse fracture the injury is really an incomplete amputation with in all probability only the volar pulp and skin still intact.

5. If there is a displaced fracture of the phalanx or a displaced epiphysis, reduce the deformity before stabilising the finger by suturing the nail. Do not forget that this is an open fracture and will require antibiotic prophylaxis.

INCOMPLETE AMPUTATION

Assess

1. Conservation of the tip is justified in slicing injuries particularly if one neurovascular bundle is undamaged and particularly in children.

2. In crushing injuries where the prospect of survival is less good, employ a 'wait and see' approach if there is doubt about viability.

Action

1. Realign the fractured phalanx.

2. Suture the soft tissues with interrupted fine nylon.

3. When there is only a tenuous attachment of the tip, excise much of the contained fibrofatty tissue and the amputated tip of the phalanx before suturing the skin back in place. This skin becomes in effect a full thickness skin graft which even if it fails to take will act as a safe biological dressing. However, if the skin is badly crushed and/or contaminated then discard the tissue and treat as a complete amputation.

COMPLETE AMPUTATION

Assess

1. Decide whether there is skin and soft tissue loss only or whether there is exposure of and damage to bone.

2. Ascertain which of the patient's hands is dominant and what particular hand function is required in his occupation, sports and hobbies.

3. Be conservative when treating children, those to whom cosmesis is important, those who need as much length as can be salvaged and those who have sustained amputation of two or more digits.

4. Decide whether it is in the patient's best interest to conserve length at all cost (e.g. the thumb), to resect just sufficient bone to allow direct closure or grafting or to perform definitive amputation at an appropriate level.

5. Direct closure has the advantages of durability and above all sensibility in comparison with grafted skin.

Action

1. When there is skin and soft tissue loss without exposure of bone, treat small defects by applying a non-adherent dressing. Occasionally, slightly larger defects may be sutured directly with minimal tension to obtain

complete closure or partial closure which will subsequently epithelialize. Larger defects will require a split skin or pinch graft from the medial aspect of the forearm. Suture the graft in place and tie the long ends of the suture over a pad of flavine wool. Alternatively, use a cross finger or thenar flap.

2. Do not use skin grafts for pulp amputations. Either suture the amputated pulp back in place with fine nylon sutures and await healing in children or epithelialization beneath the tip in adults or repair the defect with a V–Y advancement flap as described by Kutler or a cross finger-flap.

3. Amputate fingers that have suffered serious damage to vessels, nerves, tendons and joints proximal to the terminal tissue loss.

DEFINITIVE AMPUTATION OF FINGERS

Action

1. Use an exsanguinating tourniquet.
2. Place the arm on a side table.
3. Mark the incision which should be so arranged that the scar will lie on the dorsal aspect and the stump will be covered by volar skin.
4. Do not suture together the ends of the extensor and flexor tendons over the end of the bone.
5. Identify the digital nerves and isolate them from the vessels before dividing them cleanly 1 cm proximal to the stump.
6. Round off the end of the bone and remove the articular cartilage and prominent condyles when performing a disarticulation.
7. Reduce the bulk of the fibrofatty subcutaneous tissue to allow the skin edges to be brought together without difficulty.
8. Release the tourniquet and secure haemostasis before closure.
9. The skin closure must not be tight otherwise painful and ischaemic torsion may develop during postoperative swelling. Also some soft tissue retraction occurs during the first 2 months. Excessive slackness of the stump should be avoided, however, as this may result in an unsightly unsupported soft tissue mass.
10. Apply a compression dressing of gauze and narrow crepe bandage.

AMPUTATION THROUGH THE DISTAL PHALANX

If less than one-quarter of the length of the nail remains, the patient may be troubled later by an irregular hooked nail remnant. Therefore ablate the nail bed and excise the lateral angles as completely as possible.

DISARTICULATION THROUGH THE DISTAL INTERPHALANGEAL JOINT

1. Incise the skin in the midlateral line on either side of the neck of the middle phalanx. Join these two incisions across the dorsum at the level of the joint and across the volar pulp 1 cm distal to the flexor crease (Fig. 26.4).
2. Dissect back the fibrofatty tissue to reveal the digital vessels and nerves, the extensor expansion and the flexor tendon in its sheath.
3. Divide the extensor and flexor tendons at the level of the neck of the middle phalanx and allow to retract.
4. Ligate the digital vessels and divide the nerves proximally.
5. Divide capsule and collateral ligaments to complete the amputation.
6. Shape the head of the middle phalanx using bone nibblers and close the wound as described above.

AMPUTATION THROUGH THE MIDDLE PHALANX

Proceed as above but retain the attachment of flexor digitorum superficialis to bone.

DISARTICULATION THROUGH THE PROXIMAL INTERPHALANGEAL JOINT

Proceed as above but fashion a volar flap 1.5–2 cm long.

AMPUTATION THROUGH THE PROXIMAL PHALANX

Amputation of a single digit at this level is not advised. Disarticulation at the metacarpophalangeal joint is preferable except in special circumstances, e.g. multiple amputations.

DISARTICULATION THROUGH THE METACARPOPHALANGEAL JOINT

Assess

1. Use this operation normally only for the middle and ring fingers. It is particularly suitable for the hand of a man doing manual labour as a powerful grip is retained.

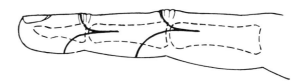

Fig. 26.4 Incision for disarticulation through interphalangeal joints.

2. The two disadvantages are the obvious deformity and a gap between the fingers through which small objects in the hand may fall.

3. Disarticulation of the index or little fingers at this level leaves the metarcarpal head projecting and unprotected. Oblique amputation through the metacarpal shaft is preferable.

Action

1. Mark the skin incisions which should lie over the proximal part of the proximal phalanx on each side leaving sufficient skin to permit full abduction of the other fingers without tension in the cleft.

2. Join the incisions anteriorly just distal to the flexor crease and posteriorly over the metacarpal head with an extension along the line of the metacarpal (Fig. 26.5).

3. Complete the amputation as described above.

AMPUTATION THROUGH THE SHAFT OF THE METACARPAL

Action

1. Use the same skin incision as for a disarticulation in the middle and ring fingers.

2. For the index and little finger use an incision along the midlateral aspect of the radial (or ulnar) border of the hand from the junction of the proximal and middle thirds of the metacarpal to the metacarpophalangeal joint (Fig. 26.5). Fashion a larger palmar flap and a smaller dorsal flap and joint the incisions in the cleft at the level of the web.

3. Amputate the middle and ring fingers by dividing the metacarpal cleanly through the neck taking care not to splinter the bone.

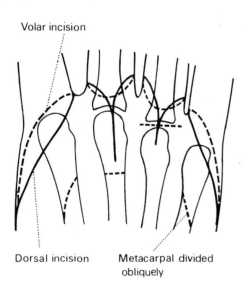

Volar incision

Dorsal incision   Metacarpal divided obliquely

Fig. 26.5 Incision for disarticulation through a metacarpophalangeal joint and for amputation through a metacarpal.

4. Amputate the index and little fingers by exposing the middle third of the metacarpal, stripping the muscular attachments and dividing the bone obliquely with a power saw. Smooth the edges of the bone and allow the muscles to fall back over the stump. Divide the digital nerves to the radial border of the index or the ulnear border of the little finger in the proximal part of the wound.

MAJOR UPPER LIMB AMPUTATIONS

Appraise

1. Fortunately rarely required, these amputations are usually for trauma although occasionally also for malignancy, severe infection and congenital abnormalities or deformities.

2. Upper limb amputation should be considered very carefully and a second opinion sought except in emergency situations.

3. Remember that forearm amputation in children will not grow in proportion to the rest of the body, whereas above elbow amputation will continue to grow and indeed may require revision with time.

Action

1. Use a general anaesthetic with an exsanguinating tourniquet whenever possible.

2. Place the patient supine with the arm on a side table.

3. Rest the arm on an inverted bowl just proximal to the site of the amputation.

Aftercare

1. Remove the drain at 48 hours.

2. Start physiotherapy to the remaining joints in the limb at 48 hours.

3. Remove the sutures at 10 days.

4. Refer to the local limbfitting centre as soon as the wound has healed.

BELOW ELBOW AMPUTATION

1. Mark out equal dorsal and volar skin flaps with their bases at the junction of the middle and lower third of the ulna (approximately 17 cm distal to the olecranon process).

2. Ensure that the arm is supination on the table without any torsional strain below the elbow. Otherwise the flaps, after being cut, are drawn into an oblique position by the elasticity of the skin.

3. Reflect the flaps deep to the deep fascia. Cut the muscles and tendons with a slightly raked incision aimed at the level of bone section.

4. Incise the periosteum circumferentially at the level of

section and divide the bones with a Gigli or a power saw.

5. Identify and ligate the main vessels. Gently pull down the nerves and divide cleanly as high a possible.

6. Release the tourniquet and secure haemostasis.

7. Insert a suction drain.

8. Close the deep fascia over the bone ends using interrupted chromic catgut or dexon. Close the skin with interrupted fine nylon sutures plus steristrip tapes.

DISARTICULATION AT THE ELBOW

1. Mark out equal anterior and posterior skin flaps with their bases level with the humeral epicondyles. Ensure that the forearm is in full supination. Take the anterior flap in a gentle curve to just below the bicipital insertion and the posterior flap to just below the tip of the olecranon.

2. Reflect the skin flaps to the level of the epicondyles.

3. Divide the bicipital aponeurosis and then detach the common flexor muscles from the medial epicondyle and retract distally.

4. Ligate the brachial artery and vein. Draw down the nerve and divide cleanly so that they retract at least 3 cm proximal to the joint line.

5. Detach the biceps tendon from the radial tuberosity and the brachialis from the coronoid process. Divide the common extensor mass 6 cm distal to the joint line and reflect proximally.

6. Detach triceps from the olecranon and complete the disarticulation.

7. Release the tourniquet and secure haemostasis.

8. Leave the articular surface of the humerus intact and cover it by suturing triceps to the distal ends of biceps and brachialis. Further soft tissue cover is produced by swinging the extensor muscle mass (suitably thinned) medially and suturing it to the stump of the common flexors.

9. Insert a suction drain.

10. Close the skin and apply a compression dressing.

ABOVE-ELBOW AMPUTATION

1. Mark out equal anterior and posterior flaps with their bases 20 cm from the tip of the acromion process of the scapula.

2. Reflect the flaps deep to the deep fascia.

3. Divide the muscles with a raking incision down to bone.

4. Divide the bone with a Gigli or power saw.

5. Ligate the main vessels. Pull down the nerves and shorten them by about 2.5 cm so that they retract into the depths of the wound.

6. Release the tourniquet if present and secure haemostasis.

7. Insert a suction drain.

8. Close the deep fascia over bone using chromic catgut or dexon. Close the skin and apply a compression dressing.

FOREQUARTER AMPUTATION

Appraise

1. This mutilating operation should be carried out only after careful consideration, including a second opinion and by an experienced surgeon.

2. Decide whether to use the classic anterior operation described by Berger (1887) or the posterior operation advocated by Littlewood (Fig. 26.6).

3. Contraindications are the presence of secondary deposits or the inability to remove all tumour, the patient's refusal to accept mutilation and medical or mental unfitness for major surgery.

4. Unequivocal histological proof of diagnosis is essential. The biopsy incision must be so placed as not to interfere with the skin flaps of the amputation.

Action

1. Proceed under general anaesthesia with endotracheal intubation. Controlled hypotension helps to reduce blood loss and improve the speed accuracy and safety of the surgery.

2. Employ the anterior operation of Berger which is safer and more straightforward than the posterior approach.

3. Place the patient on his side with the affected arm uppermost. Allow the trunk to incline backwards against a low support or sandbag. This facilitates the approach to the clavicle and vessels. Drape the affected arm free, having sealed off any fungating or infected lesions.

4. Mark out the skin flaps. Start just lateral to the sternoclavicular joint and pass above and parallel to the medial two-thirds of the clavicle. Then divide the incision into anterior and posterior portions. Take the anterior incision

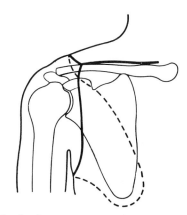

Fig. 26.6 Incision for forequarter amputation.

obliquely downwards over the clavicle and coracoid process then across the middle of the axillary fold, obliquely across the axilla to the inferior angle of the scapula. Complete the posterior incision by passing up across the scapula and over the outer part of the spuraclavicular fossa to meet the bifurcation of the supraclavicular incision.

5. Deepen the supraclavicular incision using cutting diathermy to divide the clavicular portions of pectoralis major and sternomastoid muscles. Reflect the periosteum off the middle third of the clavicle and excise this section of bone using a Gigli saw. This reveals the deep periosteum of the clavicle and the axillary and cervical fascia beneath which lie the axillary and subclavian vessels and the brachial plexus.

6. Divide pectoralis major downwards from its clavicular bed to provide wider exposure of the vessels. Divide the deep periosteum of the clavicle and the fascia with care exposing first the axillary vein. Ligate the supraclavicular and cephalic branches before doubly ligating the axillary vein at the level of the first rib. Then doubly ligate the subclavian artery at the same level having first ligated the superior thoracic and acromiothoracic branches. Divide the trunks of the brachial plexus cleanly with the scalpel.

7. Complete the anterior dissection by dividing pectoralis major and minor close to the chest wall. Dissect axillary fat, lymphatics and clavipectoral fascia downwards and outwards en bloc.

8. An assistant now holds the arm forwards for the posterior dissection. Ligate the suprascapular vessels. Dissect the flap backwards just posterior to the vertebral border of the scapula. Resect as much trapezius, latissimus dorsi and levator scapulae as necessary using cutting diathermy. Divide the rhomboid muscles. Retract the scapula away from the chest wall and divide the lower digitations of serratis anterior close to the scapula. Then allow the patient to roll backwards again, hold the arm out laterally, divide the upper digitations of serratus with attached fascia and remove the limb.

9. Secure meticulous haemostasis.

10. Insert one or two suction drains.

11. Close the skin with interrupted nylon sutures and steristrip tapes.

12. Apply a compression bandage using gauze, wool, crepe and adhesive strapping.

Aftercare

1. Leave the drains for at least 72 hours and up to 5 days if draining actively.

2. Inspect the wound at 10 days and remove sutures about the 24th day.

3. Few patients will wear an upper limb prosthesis but many will be grateful for a light shoulder piece which will disguise the worst of the residual deformity.

Further reading

Angel J C, Weaver P C 1979 Amputation surgery in operative surgery. In: Rob and Smith Orthopaedics, Part 1. Butterworths, London p

Gordon Taylor G, Monro R 1962 Technique and management of hindquarter amputation. British Journal of Surgery 39: 536–

Littlewood H 1922 Amputation at the shoulder and at the hip. British Medical Journal 1: 384–

Thompson R G 1972 Complication of lower extremity amputation. Orthopedic Clinics of North America 3: 323–

Tooms R E 1980 Amputations. In: Edmerson, Crenshaw Compbell's Operative Orthopaedics, Vol. 1. C V Mosby, St. Louis p

Slocum D B 1949 Atlas of amputations. C V Mosby, St. Louis

Westbury G 1967 Hindquarter and hip amputation. Annals of the Royal College of Surgeons of England 40:226–

The surgical management of the severely injured person

INTRODUCTION

The title indicates that there is more to this subject than operations. The majority of severely injured persons, who are most often the victims of road accidents, have only one serious injury for which any necessary operation is easily decided upon, but there may be as many as 10 separate injuries that need to be diagnosed and then treated. These patients need careful and repeated clinical, radiological and perhaps other methods of examination; they also need resuscitation. More than one casualty may require immediate and careful attention.

In addition to surgical operations, important and perhaps life-saving preliminaries are required in order to decide who needs what done when, thus assessing priorities.

The main steps in diagnosis will be considered in outline, after which the necessary surgical operations will be described, not in detail, but as standard procedures that may need to be modified in the circumstances.

ARRANGE

1. Take the seriously injured patient straight from the ambulance to a room that is suitably laid out and equipped for his reception and resuscitation. Radiography on the spot may be less accurate and clear than when conducted in the department but it is much safer for the patient. Sufficient information can usually be found in portable films.

2. Transport the seriously injured casualty from the ambulance on a suitable bed trolley. As a rule, remove all clothing without delay but life-saving measures may be required even before this.

ESSENTIAL STEPS

1. Recognize and deal with any threat to life.
2. Carry out a thorough clinical examination and decide what other investigations are required to identify all the injuries so their treatment can be planned.
3. Carry out definitive primary treatment and such further treatment as is required to enable the patient to make the best possible recovery in the shortest possible time.

THREATS TO LIFE

RESPIRATORY

Choking is caused by obstruction or collapse of normal or injured air passages because of unconsciousness or swelling of soft tissues from injury to the face and jaws. The passages may be blocked by accumulated blood, vomitus, teeth or foreign matter within them, or by swelling caused by inhaling irritant fumes, or by haematoma. Endotracheal intubation may be urgently necessary but requires great skill if the casualty is still more-or-less conscious. Carry out tracheotomy or cricothyrotomy only when a tube cannot be passed through the larynx.

Suffocation results from reduced mechanical efficiency of the bellows from multiple fractures of the ribs with paradoxical movement, from rupture of the diaphragm and from tetraplegia with weakness of the diaphragm and paralysis of the intercostal muscles, which produces see-saw movements of the chest and belly walls. Haemothorax and pneumothorax cause the lung to collapse. The lung may become consolidated following direct injury, the effects of blast and, later, infection. Be prepared immediately to clear the air passages by suitable posture of the patient, by suction, or by endotracheal intubation. If necessary restore stability to the unstable chest wall by internal pneumatic splintage (artificial ventilation). Re-expand the lung by letting out blood and air, using suitably placed drainage tubes with water seals or other valvular arrangements. Ensure adequate ventilation of consilidated lung, by artifical means if necessary. Artifical ventilation in the presence of surgical emphysema, fractured ribs and paradoxical respiration, or blast lung, may lead to a rapidly expanding pneumothorax. Insert air drains as a precautionary measure.

Appraise

1. Carry out a careful bedside examination for marks of injury, which warn of underlying damage, wounds that bubble or hiss, respiratory distress, cyanosis or pallor, and congestion of veins, which suggests obstruction in the mediastinum or pericardium if the breathing is quiet. Surgical emphysema at the root of the neck indicates rupture of the trachea or a large bronchus; elsewhere it comes from a torn lung or peripheral bronchus.

2. Note asymmetry of the shape or movement of the chest, displacement of the trachea or heartbeat, palpable crackling of surgical emphysema, instability of the chest wall, unequal blood pressures in the upper limbs, and marked reduction of breath sounds on one or other side of the chest. It is quite easy to misdiagnose consolidation on the normal side when a pneumothorax weakens the breath sounds on the other. Listen for clicking in time with the heartbeat, which is the sign of mediastinal emphysema. These observations alone often provide the evidence that immediate remedial action is required to save life. Radiography, electrocardiography and other tests are not the first lines of diagnostic approach.

CIRCULATION

1. The most frequent cause of defective circulation is bleeding, which may be external or internal or both. With open injuries, how much blood was lost before the patient reached hospital? How much visible bloodshed is there? A mass of injured tissue corresponding with the bulk of the clenched adult fist or an area of injured tissue corresponding with the area of the outstretched adult hand is associated with the loss of roughly half a litre of blood. With closed injuries the number, site and severity of the injuries give a useful indication of the order of bleeding to plan for (Fig. 27.1).

2. Pericardial tamponade is rare and not always easily recognized. The classical signs of full veins in the neck and reduced pulse pressure may be absent because of oligaemia; the heart sounds may be obscured by surgical emphysema and background noise; the electrocardiogram and X-ray films of the chest may leave doubt about their significance. If tamponade is suspected, aspirate the pericardium.

3. Injury of the heart is also rare, but penetrating wounds occupy an increasingly important place compared with myocardial contusion and rupture of septa and valves. Harsh systolic murmurs, together with signs of acute cardiac failure, suggest damage to the valves or septa of the heart.

Stop bleeding

1. First aider's tourniquets can act as venous congesters and may need to be removed. Do not remove an *effective* haemostatic dressing until you are ready to deal with torrential bleeding.

2. Local pressure and perhaps elevation stop most bleeding. Apply artery forceps only to vessels that can be seen. Small vessels may be clipped but whenever possible do not apply forceps to large ones.

3. Be prepared for urgent exploration to stop bleeding into the chest and abdomen. A patient reaching hospital before signs of life have disappeared after a stab wound of the chest stands a fair chance of surviving, if vigorous resuscitation is combined with thoracotomy within minutes of arrival.

4. If possible, locate bleeding with fractures of the pelvis by angiography and stanch it by therapeutic embolism.

5. Measure pulmonary arterial pressure and cardiac output in severely injured patients.

Restore

1. The exsanguinated patient needs two or even three large intravenous cannulae. Use the upper limbs unless there is profuse bleeding from the root of the neck. Avoid the lower limbs if there has been profuse bleeding into the abdomen or pelvis.

2. In general, if a given quantity of blood is required to resuscitate the patient, the same quantity again should be available for any necessary operation and a further 25% to replace subsequent oozing.

3. Warm and filter blood if more than three or four bags are to be given. Investigate clotting power and give fresh frozen plasma after one blood volume of blood has been given. If necessary, give young women group O Rhesus positive blood; if they are Rhesus negative, protect them

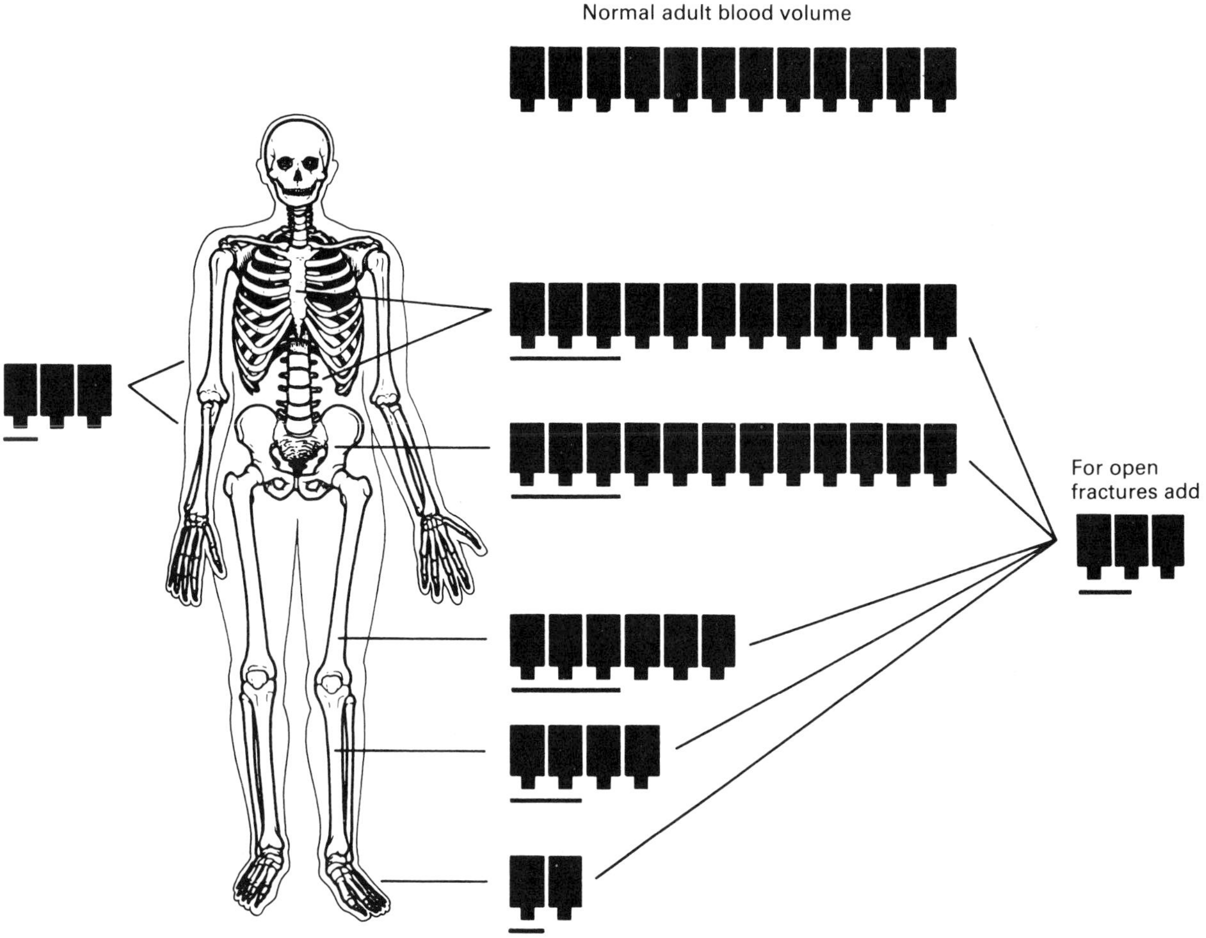

Normal adult blood volume

Fig. 27.1 The quantities shown are based on the assumption that the normal blood volume is the equivalent of 12 donations. The bags underlined represent the loss with mild to moderate injuries of the area concerned and the whole row the loss that may occur. While the proportion remains the same at different ages, the absolute quantities vary a good deal. The order of loss shown occurs within about 24 hours.

against immunization by giving anti-D serum shortly afterwards.

4. Adequate replenishment is indicated by the return of warmth and colour to the skin, improved consciousness in some cases, and a central venous pressure of 5 cm or more of saline, but provide for continuing bleeding.

5. For the exsanguinated patient, the theoretical advantages of colloidal suspensions are of doubtful relevance; 0.9% saline or Hartmann's solution are the most readily available infusates that can be given rapidly, when necessary, in quantities of up to 2 l until blood arrives. Infuse the fluid at first under sufficient pressure to provide a steady stream

6. Record urinary output after passing a catheter.

Check list

1. At some stage, examine limbs used for infusion for injuries that may have been overlooked or ignored at first.

2. Re-examine limbs that were pale and cool because of exsanguination. After resuscitation, failure to become warm and pink and to regain pulses suggests important damage to a main artery. Apply emergency splints with this need in mind.

3. Exsanguinated patients may have full stomachs and need general anaesthesia. Do not pass a stomach tube until after starting the infusion of blood.

CENTRAL NERVOUS SYSTEM

1. Unconsciousness following a blow on the head may have untreatable causes such as concussion or a stroke, which could have caused the accident. Treatable causes include intracranial bleeding and cerebral hypoxaemia resulting from exsanguination, choking, or suffocation.

2. The restless patient may be the victim of concussion, but the aggressive patient may be a victim of cerebral hypoxia, drugs or alcohol (which may have caused the accident), diabetes, fat embolism or meningitis.

Action

1. Always treat the unconscious state, whatever its cause.

2. If the patient does not answer questions or obey simple instructions, ensure that the air passages are clear, that the lungs are adequately ventilated and that the Pa_{O_2} is at least 60 mmHg.

3. Start using the Glasgow coma scale (Fig. 27.2).

TIME	0–24 HOURS
EYE OPENING	Spontaneous To speech To pain None
BEST VERBAL RESPONSE	Orientated Confused Inappropriate Incomprehensible None
BEST MOTOR RESPONSE	Obeying Localising Flexing Extending None

Fig. 27.2 The Glasgow coma scale.

Record the state of the pupils, muscle tone, reflexes, spontaneous movements, respiration, pulse rate and blood pressure.

4. Radiograph the skull.

5. Measuring intracranial pressure is a useful safeguard in the paralysed and ventilated patient.

6. Computerized tomography provides the most reliable evidence of intracranial damage but the patient may not be in a fit state to be subjected to it, especially if he would have to be transferred to another hospital.

7. Later measures include adequate nutrition, care of the skin, lungs, bladder and bowels, and the prevention of contractures.

GENERAL APPRAISAL

1. Once necessary life-saving measure have been taken, remove all clothing and examine the patient thoroughly and repeatedly. Start at the head and work down to the feet. Examine the back, buttocks and perineum, especially in cases of assault, gunshot and explosion.

2. Do not be content to examine the patient to find what injuries have been inflicted. Look for the injuries that may be present in the light of what is known of the degree, nature and direction of injuring forces. If some components of a characteristic pattern of injury are present, look for the others.

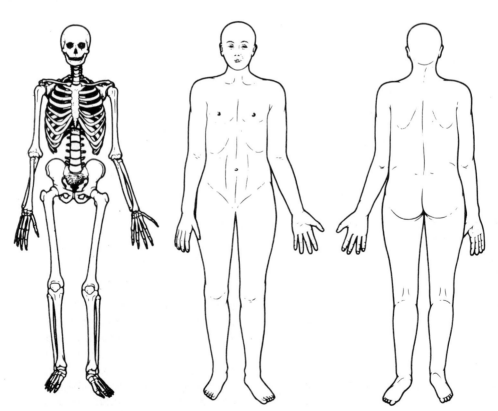

Fig. 27.3 Useful diagrams for showing the sites of multiple injuries.

3. Search for the injuries that are often overlooked. These will be indicated at appropriate stages.

4. Record the findings accurately so that newcomers can know for sure whether or not changes have taken place. Diagrams are helpful for summarizing multiple injuries (Fig. 27.3).

HEAD AND FACE

1. Look for signs of injury of the face and brow. **Warning:** When they are present, radiograph the neck. A good lateral view of the neck is one of the first films to be made in any unconscious person. Make sure that all seven vertebrae are shown. Look particularly at C1 and 2.

2. Look for black eyes, subconjuctival bruising, abnormal posture or movements of the eyes or Horner's syndrome. Use an ophthalmoscope.

3. Look for bruising of the scalp; it may be over an extradural haematoma.

4. Seek bleeding from the ears, nose or mouth, and the puffy dish face of fractures of the middle third. Look also for irregular, missing or broken teeth and torn gums.

5. Feel for boggy swelling of scalp, irregularity of skull and facial bones. Test for mobility of the alveolar margin, the maxilla, and abnormal mobility of the mandible.

6. Test the function of the cranial nerves.

NECK

1. Look for warning injuries of the face and brow, abnormal posture of the head and neck. Detect wounds, especially if penetrating or sucking, and fullness of veins. Punctate bruising of skin that does not have bone close behind it suggests a heavy blow and may be accompanied by surgical emphysema, associated with rupture of the larynx or trachea.

2. Feel for the position of the trachea and for surgical emphysema. In the unconscious patient, it is often possible to put a finger down the throat and feel the irregularity, swelling or abnormal mobility of an extension fracture of the neck. In contrast, palpation of the back of the neck is not usually informative.

3. Listen for bruits near wounds, or swellings over large arteries.

SHOULDERS

1. Look for bruising; in the axilla this suggests a torn artery. Swelling indicates fracture, deformity indicates dislocation while fracture-dislocation causes swelling and deformity. Posterior dislocation is easily overlooked, but the

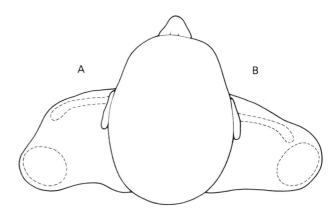

Fig. 27.4 A posterior dislocation of the shoulder showing well the prominence of the outer end of the clavicle (the acromion process has been omitted), the flattening in front and the prominence behind.

characteristic flattening in front and swelling behind can best be seen from above (Fig. 27.4).

2. Look for wounds.

3. Feel for irregularity of the clavicles. Fractures and dislocations can be recognized by picking the bone up between finger and thumb.

4. Listen for bruits near wounds and swelling over large arteries.

CHEST

1. At intervals, repeat the examination carried out immediately after receiving the patient. Respiratory distress, cyanosis, congested veins, surgical emphysema and paradoxical movement may develop hours or even days later.

2. Radiography is sometimes less informative than clinical examination but is always required. Remember that posture affects the distribution of gases and liquids. If the patient cannot sit up, ask for lateral views in the supine posture or antero-posterior views with the patient on his side.

ABDOMEN AND PELVIS

1. Look for wounds and bruising, especially around the pelvis and perineum. Punctate bruising of skin that does not have bone close beneath it nearly always indicates internal injuries. Observe the shape and movement. Measuring the girth is of little value, because important distension can be seen but swelling of an inch or two can be ignored.

2. See-saw (paradoxical) movements of the chest and abdomen suggest tetraplegia or multiple fractures of the backs of ribs on both sides (Fig. 27.5).

3. Look for bleeding from the urethra.

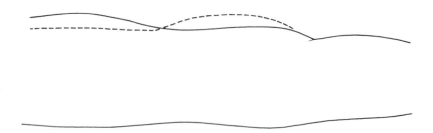

Fig. 27.5a This represents a silhouette of the lateral view of a recumbent person, with the thighs on the right. The solid upper line represents the resting position of the chest and the abdomen and the dotted line the position during inspiration, when the diaphragm draws down the rib cage and pushes down the abdominal viscera, thereby increasing the prominence of the abdominal wall.

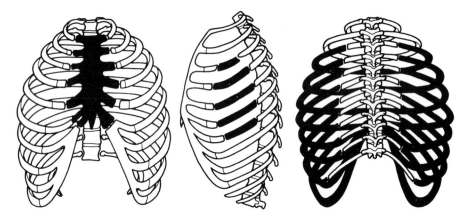

Fig. 27.5b Examples of the main patterns of stove-in chest. The right hand figure shows multiple fractures of the backs of ribs, which is another cause of the paradoxical movement shown in a.

4. Feel for abdominal rigidity and guarding, which is the sudden tensing of a soft abdominal wall as it is gently depressed. Feel also for lumps and swellings and abnormal shape and movement of the pelvis.

5. By rectal examination establish the position and mobility of the prostate gland.

6. Listen for bowel sounds. Occasionally the splashing of liquid in inert bowel is mistaken for sounds of peristalsis but it occurs in time with breathing. Listen for bruits over main arteries. Shifting dullness is usually not worth testing for.

Radiography

1. Plain films may reveal fractures, dislocation of the 12th rib and lumbar scoliosis. A grey, ground-glass appearance is caused by intra- or extraperitoneal blood. The shadows of psoas major and kidney may be lost. Free air may be within the peritoneal cavity or in the tissues as surgical emphysema. Foreign bodies can also be seen.

2. The most frequently used contrast radiography is excretion urography, with, if necessary, continuous infusion. Do not assume that the bladder is normal until it is seen at least moderately filled and with a lateral view. The value of urethrography is disputed; escape of the material is more reliable than an apparently normal appearance. Angi-

ography is most useful to locate the source of continuing bleeding, to settle doubt about the existence or function of a second kidney, and in the investigation of later difficulties. Sinography of stab wounds is not a reliable guide to whether or not the belly should be explored.

Peritoneal irrigation

1. There is no place for tapping the four quadrants of the belly. Instead, run in saline and drain it out for inspection unless the catheter drains frank blood. Irrigation is most useful in the victim of multiple injuries, especially when unconscious, and with injuries of the chest or pelvis.

2. If there is doubt about the significance of the degree of staining, test the effluent for bile and amylase, repeat the test in an hour or so and consider angiography.

BACK

1. No patient is too badly injured to be turned carefully onto one side so that the back can be examined. Always examine the whole circumference of the trunk.

2. Look for marks of injury, bruising and swelling centred on the spine, abnormal contours and irregularity of the spinous processes.

3. Feel for gaps between the spinous processes. These are reliable evidence of a disruptive lesion such as a fracture-dislocation and are accompanied by a palpable gap in the thoracolumbar fascia and an overlying boggy swelling.

LIMBS

1. Remember that limbs in splints and those used for infusion may have sustained injuries of their nerves and circulation and must at a suitable time be examined again.

2. Look for deformity, wounds, abrasions and bruising. Decompress gross blistering on the summit of a bruise by generous incision. Pallor and cyanosis and the state of the veins are other important observations. Observe the characteristic postures of the upper limbs in tetraplegia (Fig. 27.6).

3. Feel for soft-centred bruises. If on firm pressure the skin can be pressed directly against bone, important intervening structures such as ligaments, muscles, nerves and blood vessels must have been crushed through, like the meat in an uncooked sausage. Explore the wound. Note the pulsation of arteries, the temperature of the skin and the presence or absence of sweating.

4. Listen for bruits near wounds and bruising over main vessels.

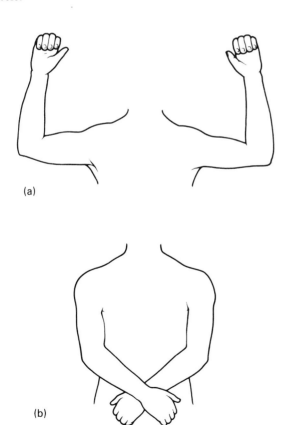

Fig. 27.6 The postures in tetraplegia a) with lesions of C5/6, b) with lesions of C6/7.

PRIORITIES

After fully examining the patient the working set of diagnoses can be made. From this the treatment of the individual patient(s) can be planned. Surgical operations may be grouped into three orders of priority.

FIRST PRIORITY

1. Continuing internal bleeding, which is more often into the abdomen or pelvis than the chest. Intracranial bleeding is small in amount but can be rapidly fatal.

2. Persisting hypoxaemia as from rupture of a bronchus or of the diaphragm with herniated viscera, increasing and impassable laryngeal oedema or because of the carapace-like shell of hard-burnt skin on the trunk.

3. Surgically remediable ischaemia requiring repair of a main artery or decompression of a group or muscles.

SECOND PRIORITY

1. Large wounds of muscle, especially when contaminated.
2. Injuries of bowel, whether open or closed.
3. Flayed limbs with wrinkling and twisting of skin flaps that may be capable of surviving.
4. Increasing bruising and swelling that begins to show blisters on its surface.

THIRD PRIORITY

1. Other wounds and burns.
2. Fractures of limbs with sufficient deformity to blanch skin, impair circulation and compress nerves should be manipulated as soon as possible in order to reduce dangerous pressure; definitive treatment may then be delayed.
3. Deal with large wounds with fractures before mere punctures.
4. Wounds of the face and scalp, even when accompanying fractures, can safely be left for 12 hours or more if carefully dressed and if antibiotics are given.

Timing and order

1. Notwithstanding the foregoing, when it is reasonable to do so, perform operations simultaneously rather than consecutively. When a necessary operation has to be carried out, this may provide an acceptable opportunity to carry out one or more others that would otherwise have been deferred.
2. Careful planning saves time.
3. Those doctors with an overall view must choose the

order of operations on a number of casualties. If you are a member of a surgical team, be content to operate on patients that are selected for you.

Other practical considerations

1. Bear in mind the need to do the best for all that require your services. Do not, therefore, waste time and material on unnecessarily elaborate or over-optimistic procedures.

2. Amputate rather than make a lengthy attempt to repair a limb with little prospect of useful survival.

3. Abandon fruitless efforts to stop torrential bleeding when there are others in need of limited supplies of blood.

4. Leave open wounds that might otherwise have been closed at once; this is in addition to wounds for which delayed primary closure is in any case the right treatment.

5. Confine the first operation to surgical toilet, that is, remove dead and damaged tissue and foreign matter to render the wound fit for repair, then merely dress it. Delayed primary repair (as well as closure) saves a great deal of time and it may allow a suitably skilled surgeon to undertake the most difficult stages without disadvantage or risk to the patient.

EXPLORATION OF THE WOUND

Appraise

1. Practical procedures are described in general terms but with emphasis on the special features appropriate to particular conditions.

2. You should, if necessary, be able to carry out life-saving operations on most parts of the body. One test of judgement is knowing how to modify a standard operation to meet the prevailing requirements. This includes knowing when and how to cut corners safely.

4. Do not hurry, but work expeditiously to avoid delays.

Action

1. This most frequently required surgical procedure for the injured person is a subject on which few surgical apprentices receive formal instruction. The ability to explore a wound successfully is a good test of basic surgical understanding and tissue craft. It is all too often failed by otherwise experienced surgeons with highly developed technical skills. It is the last stage in diagnosis and at the same time it is the first stage in treatment of a wound.

2. Identify the depth and extent of damage inflicted on the tissue. The best exploratory equipment is the eye. The history has provided evidence of the force of injury, the direction and perhaps the patient's posture.

3. Should the wound be enlarged? Not if you can see its full depth and extent by the careful use of retractors and other instruments in, if possible, a bloodless field.

However, it may then be necessary to enlarge the wound in order to carry out the requisite repair.

4. What rules govern the enlargement of an existing wound? Enlarge it if you cannot see or reach all that you need to. A finger or a probe indicates the general direction in which a wound has been inflicted. It is not a reliable indication of its depth. The most direct approach to a track is to cut through the overlying tissues. This may not be advisable because it may jeopardize the survival of some skin, it may cross creases and leave an ugly scar, or it may interfere with any further operations that are required. These considerations govern the choice of incision. Z-plasties and other procedures may avoid undesirable scars, but technical virtuosity is no substitute for the successful use of simple measures.

5. What are the steps of the exploration? Look carefully into the existing wound and identify its extent using retractors, a good light and anatomical knowledge of tissue planes, which are also planes of separation and retraction. Blood marks the site of injury of retracted structures and it also marks the line of their retraction. Avoid dissection until it is unquestionably necesary, because it destroys the natural relationships of tissues that you rely on. Starting with the skin, each layer with a hole in it has another layer beneath it. Explore that deeper layer and if a hole is found it in it, explore the next layer, and so on. When exploring a penetrating wound, in particular, remember that at the moment of penetration the track passed straight through a number of layers but the relationship of the layers may have altered by the time of operation, at which they form a series of baffles.

6. What about foreign bodies? Not all of them need to be removed. Before attempting to remove a foreign body ensure that you have good operating conditions, light, assistance and instruments. Ensure that the field is bloodless if possible. Make sure that anaesthesia can be continued indefinitely. Do not make single-handed attempts under local analgesia unless the object can be seen or felt near the surface. Take films of a radio-opaque foreign body in the operating position. This may be much different from a standard radiographic position and consequently greatly alter the apparent position of the surgical target. Decide in which layer of tissue the object lies. If the object touches bone, first expose the appropriate surface of the bone. Approach long, narrow objects such as needles from the side, not the ends. They do not leave traceable tunnels.

SCALP AND FACE

SCALP

Assess

1. Scalp wounds are frequent and bleed profusely. If a main artery is bleeding hard, clamp it, but otherwise apply

a firm bulky dressing held by two or three 10 cm crepe bandages.

2. Consider the need for blood transfusion after enquiring about blood lost at the time of injury, noting visible loss in the hair, clothing and dressings, and remembering that further blood may be lost during the operations.

Closure

1. The good blood supply enables most wounds of the scalp to heal without surgical toilet, but trim crushed and tattered edges.

2. Close small wounds in one layer unless they are outside the hairy area.

3. Close larger wounds, and those over fractures or outside the hairy area, in two layers.

4. If tissue has been lost, it may be possible to close the defect by extending the wound and rearranging the scalp (Fig. 27.7). Failing this, apply split skin grafts to the epicranial aponeurosis, other fascia, or the pericranium.

5. If there is bare bone, rotation flaps or free flaps are usually required. However, if the outer table must be removed because it has been killed by burning, apply split skin grafts to the diploe. Split grafts also take on dura mater.

FACE

Appraise

1. Use fine materials and take pains over each step and each stitch. A good repair can last a lifetime, a bad one

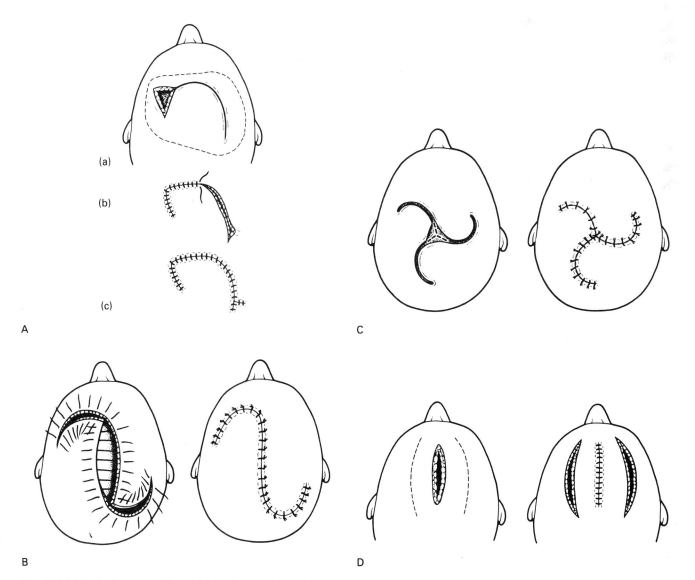

Fig. 27.7 Methods of closing different defects in the scalp following wounding.

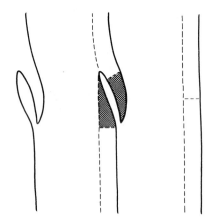

Fig. 27.8 Slicing wounds should be cut square by removing the parts shown in solid black. Undermining may be necessary to allow comfortable closure thereafter.

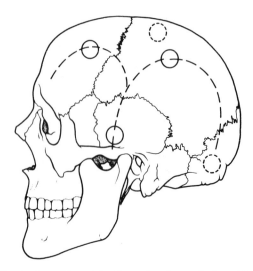

Fig. 27.9 The sites of burr holes for exploration are indicated by the complete circles, together with the flaps that can be raised, having made one or more of these. The dotted circle near the vertex represents a place where a plug for measuring pressure can be screwed in and that in the occiput for the occasional exploratory burr hole.

poses future surgical problems. The face heals well so spare as much tissue as possible.

2. Cut the thin edges of slicing wounds square (Fig. 27.8).

3. Identify key points such as the edges of eyelids, nostrils and the pink margins of the lips, and accurately restore them.

4. Operations on the eye are the province of a specialist.

5. Repair mucous membrane, muscle and skin as separate layers.

6. Preserve cartilage of ears and nose and cover it with living skin.

7. If necessary, bury exposed cartilage of the pinna in the scalp.

8. When destructive wounds of lips or cheeks make simple repair impossible experts may be able to swing flaps; otherwise sew mucous membrane to skin or use a skin graft.

SKULL

BURR HOLES (see Ch. 33)

Appraise

1. These are used to insert a plug for measuring the intracranial pressure, identifying an intracranial haematoma and elevating some depressed fractures.

2. For measuring intracranial pressure, make the incision (Fig. 27.9) near the midline on top, where the projection will not interfere with turning the head. For intracranial haematoma, incise over a bruise or a fracture when either is present. In the absence of localizing signs, make the first hole in the temporal fossa, the second high in the frontotemporal region and, if necessary, make two more on the other side. For depressed fracture, be prepared to make a burr hole to elevate it from its edge.

Action

1. Clip at least half the hair short.

2. Have an assistant press firmly on either side of where the cut will be made.

3. Cut straight down to bone.

4. Scrape the bone clear with a xyster.

5. Insert a self-retaining retractor. This usually stops the bleeding; if it does not, use fine ligatures or unipolar diathermy.

6. Have the head steadied by an assistant.

7. Apply a 1–1.5 cm perforator in the centre of the cut and perpendicular to the skull. When introducing the plug for measuring intracranial pressure, use the matching set of perforator, burr and tap. Wash away bone dust while making the hole.

8. When clot or dura appears, exchange the perforator for a burr and continue as before until it begins to jump or there is only a thin and narrow shelf of inner table left.

9. Apply wax to any bleeding vessels in the bone.

10. Scrape away the thin bony shelf with a sharp-edged tool.

11. If blood is seen outside or inside the dura remove as much of it as possible and then extend the burr hole by nibbling away skull, or make a bone flap to allow the source of bleeding to be found and dealt with.

12. If the dura is bulging but not blue and you are inexperienced, seek advice about what to do next. You may need to tap a ventricle, make more burr holes, raise a flap, or try to reduce pressure by over-ventilation or by injecting mannitol intravenously.

BONE FLAP

Action

1. Site a sufficiently large flap to give comfortable access to the lesion.
2. Cut down to bone for 5–7 cm at a time.
3. Apply clips to the cut edges of the galea aponeurotica and turn them back over a moist pad resting on the scalp.
4. Complete the flap in this way, then separate it from the skull and the temporal fascia when this has to be exposed.
5. Stop any continuing bleeding.
6. Make four, five or six burr holes at the edges of the intended flap.
7. Connect the holes by means of a skull-cutting tool or Gigli's saw. If the flap is in the temporal region, crack the bone at the base of the flap. Do not cut through but leave the temporalis muscle attached to the bone.
8. If the dura has to be opened, first pick it up with a fine hook and cut it with a fine-pointed knife. Complete the flap with scissors or diathermy.
9. Suck out blood, clot and pulped brain; wash away debris and stop bleeding with clips or diathermy.
10. Close the dura, fill any gaps with fascia lata or temporalis fascia.
11. Replace the bone flap.
12. Close the scalp in two layers.

DEPRESSED FRACTURE

Appraise

Closed fractures do not usually need to be elevated. Open fractures must always be explored because of the likelihood of infection arising from hair or other foreign matter that becomes trapped in the fracture, and because the dura may have been torn.

Action

1. A straight incision may be satisfactory, but raise a flap for an extensive depression and to keep scars off hairless areas.
2. Remove and preserve loose fragments of bone.
3. Remove foreign matter. If possible, elevate the fragments in situ; otherwise, make a burr hole at the edge of the depression and pass an elevator through this to elevate the fragments. It is rarely necessary to cut out the depressed area in order to deal with it, but inspect the dura and repair it when necessary.
4. Replace loose pieces to restore the contour and continuity of the skull. Scrub and boil dirty bone and replace it. If a defect remains, close the scalp over a fine suction drain.

PENETRATING WOUNDS OF THE BRAIN

1. Expose the brain adequately.
2. Suck away blood and pulped brain while irrigating the track gently.
3. Remove accessible foreign matter but do not disturb normal-looking brain in pursuit of other matter.
4. If the track keeps closing, suspect haematoma or large foreign body elsewhere.
5. Close the dura and scalp securely and replace bony fragments when possible. If in doubt, keep them until later.
6. Drain the layer beneath the scalp.

Dressings

1. Some suture lines can be left exposed and sprayed with an antiseptic or sealing substance. Do not use antibiotic sprays.
2. When dressings are required pass the bandage low on the brow and well beneath the occiput. Apply it firmly and secure it with sticky tape.

SKULL TRACTION (see Ch. 28)

1. Crutchfield's device is the most generally available but Gardner-Wells's is favoured because it can be applied without cutting the scalp and it is less likely to come out; Cone's is less bulky.
2. Whichever is used, apply it, using local analgesia, on the line drawn vertically through the ear holes. Apply Gardner-Wells's or Cone's device below the widest part of the skull.
3. For Crutchfield's tongs, expose the skull and drill the outer table with the guarded drill, insert the spikes and close them tightly with the clamp. Close the scalp snugly round the spikes and dress lightly.

NECK

SUICIDAL CUT THROAT

1. It is usually sufficient to repair all that has been divided, ligating small vessels and repairing large ones, without extending the incision.
2. If possible, repair the trachea over an internal tube; if necessary convert the wound into a tracheostome.
3. Drain any repair of the pharynx.
4. Close the platysma muscle separately from the skin.

PENETRATING WOUNDS

1. Explore the wound if there has been (or is) more than slight bleeding, a large haematoma, a bruit, surgical emphysema, haemoptysis or signs of peripheral or central neural damage.

2. When in doubt, explore. Arteriography may be helpful in some cases. Choose the incision (Fig. 27.10) that allows most convenient access, both proximal and distal, to any suspected injury of a large blood vessel.

CRICOTHYROTOMY

This offers the quickest way of relieving otherwise untreatable laryngeal obstruction. In case of desperate emergency, push the widest bore needle that is available through the cricothyroid membrane. This is better than nothing.

Action

1. Identify the cricothyroid membrane by feel.
2. Cut the skin horizontally over it. The length of the cut depends on the thickness of the overlying tissues.
3. Insert a self-retaining retractor and open it widely.
4. Expose the membrane by blunt dissection.
5. Make a 1 cm opening with a knife and insert the largest available tube.
6. Suck out the trachea.
7. Connect the tube to a ventilator if necessary.
8. Stop bleeding; it largely ceases when the patient can breathe clearly once more.
9. Close the wound around the tube.
10. Apply a light dressing.

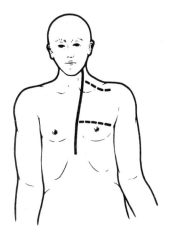

Fig. 27.10 Incisions for exploring injuries of the vessels in the neck. Any part of the solid line may be used with the added extensions as appropriate.

TRACHEOSTOMY

Appraise

1. Regard this as a planned operation; it is rarely necessary to perform it in a hurry.
2. General anaesthesia is much preferable to local.
3. Raise the shoulders in order to extend the neck.
4. **Warning.** A child's trachea can be pulled a long way out of the chest, so choose the level of the cut against the trachea not the suprasternal notch.
5. Make sure that the cuff of endotracheal tube and the syringe are in working order.

Action

1. Make a transverse cut, one (patient's) fingersbreadth below the cricoid cartilage and down to the deep cervical fascia.
2. Stop bleeding.
3. Retract the wound edges upwards and downwards.
4. Cut through the deep fascia vertically between the sternohyoid and sternothyroid muscles and retract them sideways with a self-retaining device.
5. Expose the trachea and free the isthmus of the thyroid gland by blunt dissection.
6. Clamp, cut and ligate the isthmus.
7. Insert a sharp hook below the cricoid cartilage and pull the trachea proximally upwards into the wound.
8. Make a 1.5 cm three-sided rectangular cut between the second and third rings and through the third ring of the trachea, to make a flap based inferiorly. Pass a stitch through the upper part of the flap.
9. Have the anaesthetist withdraw the endotracheal tube.
10. Insert the tracheal tube and connect it to the anaesthetic machine. The hook and stitch usually open the trachea sufficiently, but use a dilator if necessary.
11. Inflate the cuff.
12. Stop any residual bleeding.
13. Close the wound around the tube.
14. Dress the wound lightly and tie the tapes with the knot near the front.

INTUBATING THE TRACHEA

1. Every medical member of an emergency service must have a working knowledge of this procedure and understand that it can be both very difficult and damaging.

2. The greatest need and the greatest difficulty coexist in the conscious or semiconscious patient with a full stomach, a smashed and bleeding face and jaws, with obviously obstructed breathing. Relaxation is necessary but liable to be followed immediately by regurgitation from the stomach.

3. Ensure that the laryngoscope, tube, forceps and sucker are at hand.

4. Ensure that the patient is correctly positioned as the relaxant is injected.

5. Do not pass the tube too far. Most tubes are too long and if inserted fully they enter the right main bronchus and block the left, so causing the left lung to collapse. This is easily recognized once it has been suspected because there is paradoxical movement of the whole of the left side of the chest and breath sounds are absent on this side.

CHEST

Apart from dealing with wounds of the chest wall the most valuable procedure is to drain the pleura. Thoracotomy is rarely required. See Chapter 19.

CHEST WALL

1. Bubbling and hissing mean that the pleura has been breached.

2. Artificial ventilation may expand the lung and is a good first step in treatment.

3. Apply an airtight dressing to a penetrating wound.

4. Insert an intrapleural drain, and if this succeeds, apply a dressing.

EMERGENCY VENTING OF THE PLEURAL SPACE

1. This is usually a planned procedure to remove air or blood. Rarely, it is urgent and life-saving.

2. Massive pneumothorax produces increasing respiratory distress, cyanosis, congestion of veins in the neck, with enlargement, diminished movement and absent breath sounds on one side of the chest. The trachea and heartbeat are displaced.

3. Act at once. Push the largest available needle or cannula through the chest wall in the second intercostal space below the middle of the clavicle.

4. When there is less urgency, insert a trocar and cannula and connect it to a water seal. Heimlich's valve may be used instead to let out air, but if blood is present it will clog the valve.

5. In a man, the second intercostal space is satisfactory. In a woman, use the fourth space behind the anterior axillary fold.

6. Cleanse the skin with an alcoholic disinfectant.

7. Inject 1% lignocaine.

8. Make a 1 cm cut in the skin.

9. Push in the trocar and cannula so that about 5 cm are inside the chest.

10. Withdraw the trocar, clamping the tube when the trocar is clear of the chest wall.

11. Attach the tube to the valve and secure it with a stitch or strapping.

12. If there is no bubbling or movement of the liquid in the tube, examine the system and rectify the fault.

PERICARDIAL DRAINAGE

1. Two routes can be used. Push the needle through the fourth left intercostal space 2.5 cm from the sternum or push the needle upwards and backwards at an angle of about 45° to the skin through the left costoxiphoid notch. It must pierce the diaphragm, which offers recognizable resistance.

2. In order to avoid puncturing the heart, connect the needle to one lead of an electrocardiograph. If the needle touches the heart the trace is deflected.

THORACOTOMY (see Ch. 19)

1. This is rarely needed after injury of the chest.

2. In an exsanguinated patient after a penetrating wound, when the heart is still beating or has only just stopped, start a massive infusion and open the chest from in front. Clamp the aorta above the diaphragm, and identify and deal with the source of bleeding.

3. Thoracotomy may be required to deal with recurrent pericardial tamponade and persistent bleeding from a closed injury. Ruptured aorta, ruptured diaphragm and perforation of the gullet demand thoracotomy, which may also be necessary to fix broken ribs that are causing paradoxical movement. Rib fixation is not widely adopted and the need is not urgent.

4. In general, perform urgent operations from in front. Planned procedures require standard approaches to the heart, aorta, lungs or bronchi.

THORACOLAPAROTOMY

1. This operation is not often necessary.

2. Repair a ruptured diaphragm from above, especially if the guts have entered the chest. Upper abdominal injuries can be repaired from above, but for full exploration of the abdomen this cavity should be opened separately.

3. Explore stab wounds of the chest that have pierced the diaphragm from the abdominal aspect, unless there is obvious serious damage in the chest as well.

4. The reparative procedures within the chest are described in Chapter 19.

ABDOMEN

WOUNDS OF THE ABDOMINAL WALL

Appraise

1. Opinions vary about the necessity for exploring the abdomen when a wound has penetrated the peritoneum. There is clear evidence that up to 50% of wounds that do enter the peritoneal cavity have caused no damaged to its contens, but there is doubt in some surgeons' minds that a decision to explore, or not, can safely be based on signs and symptoms. This applies to low velocity bullet wounds as well as to stab and similar penetrating injuries.

2. Aspiration of the peritoneal cavity by the so-called four-quadrant tap is unreliable.

3. Peritoneal lavage is a useful supplementary test in doubtful cases such as an unconscious patient, or when abdominal injury is suspected following injury of the chest or pelvis, or if the patient has been paralysed by drugs or spinal injury. Inject analgesic solution into the midline of the abdomen about 5 cm below the umbilicus. Expose the peritoneum. Stop all bleeding. Push a dialysis catheter downwards and backwards through the peritoneum. Remove the trocar and insert 20–25 cm of catheter (push the trocar upwards in a woman in the later months of pregnancy.) If blood comes out, explore the abdomen. If nothing comes out, run in 1 litre of saline solution and syphon it back. If there is no blood continue observation, but if there is heavy blood-staining explore the abdomen. Test faint bloodstained fluid for bile and amylase, continue the observation and repeat the test in 1 hour. In case of doubt, consider angiography.

EXPLORATORY LAPAROTOMY (see Ch. 4)

Appraise

1. The diagnosis of damage within the abdomen is made by exploration, not by clinical examination.

2. Relaxation brought about by drugs or by opening the abdomen is sometimes followed by sudden collapse that results from profuse bleeding.

Access

1. Utilize wounds of the abdominal wall extended for exploration only when they are suitably placed.

2. Make a median vertical incision that will admit both your hands. It can be made, and closed, quickly. It can be extended as far as is necessary either upwards or downwards and gives access to all parts of the abdomen, and to the chest if necessary.

Assess

1. Feel for ruptures of the spleen and liver. Deliver the intestines and examine both them and the mesentery. Mop and suck out blood. Look all round the peritoneal cavity.

2. Explore retroperitoneal haematomas adjoining pancreas, duodenum and colon, and large haematomas overlying large blood vessels. Before doing so, prepare for torrential bleeding.

3. Explore retroperitoneal emphysema or bile stains near the duodenum.

Action

1. The management of the individual viscera is dealt with in detail elsewhere and will be merely summarized here.

2. Remove a severely ruptured spleen. There is now a swing of opinion towards repair and retention whenever possible (see Ch. 12).

3. Most injuries of the liver are mild and do not need to be stitched, but drain them all (see Ch. 11). Repair deep rents unless partial hepatectomy has already been almost completed. Formal hepatectomy is rarely justified. Severe bleeding from the large veins taxes the most skilled and experienced surgeons. If you cannot control such bleeding, pack the tear for 2–3 days then remove the pack, or arrange for the patient to be transferred to a specialized unit. Some bleeding can be controlled by ligating one or other of the hepatic arteries.

4. Drain small wounds of the pancreas. Severe injuries may require removal of part of the gland. Removing the body is relatively easy, then oversew and drain the remainder. Removing the head is much more difficult because of the likelihood of coexistent damage to the duodenum and portal vein. If extensive resection is required you must restore continuity of the gut and the biliary tract, and drain the pancreatic remnant into the gut. There is much scope for ingenuity as well as need for surgical skill.

5. Repair and drain an injured duodenum. Place tubes in the stomach and jejunum.

6. Repair stomach and small intestine whenever possible. Resect only if necessary.

7. Repair of injured large intestine is unlikely to succeed unless the wound is fresh, tidy, and on the right side. In case of any doubt, bring it to the surface or remove the damaged part. In either case, make a colostomy. If the rectum is injured, drain it widely after repair. Create a completely diverting proximal colostomy.

8. Do not explore the kidneys without good reason (see Chapter 14). Repair or resect in part whenever possible. Remove only if conservation is impossible.

9. Repair and drain damaged ureters.

10. Repair and drain an injured bladder.

11. Treat all injuries of the urethra by suprapubic cystotomy. A few days later, pass a fine catheter with the aid of a panendoscope. If the abdomen has to be opened it is

reasonable to open the bladder and pass a urethral catheter into it from below. This is not easy. Drain the retropubic space. The place of urethrography and trial of catheter is argued but both can be dispensed with.

12. Repair an injured uterus or vagina. Remove the uterus if necessary. Injury of a pregnant uterus is very rare and Caesarian section or hysterectomy may be necessary. If possible, whether or not the foetus is alive, repair the uterus and await developments. A live foetus may survive and be born naturally, a dead one will be expelled in due course.

PELVIC FRACTURES

Appraise

1. Many fractures can be operated on but few need to be. Internal or external fixation can be used, given the necessary skill and equipment.

2. Bleeding is most simply dealt with by diagnostic arteriography and therapeutic embolism. If this is not available, inflatable trousers may be applied, with or without induced hypotension. If these measures fail obtain plenty of blood, 10 units for a start, and prepare to open the pelvis.

Action

1. Open the pelvis widely.

2. Occlude the aorta. Arteriography on the table may locate the main source of bleeding so that it can be controlled. If it does not, first clear out as much clot and blood as possible. Release the clamp or tape on the aorta and try to identify the bleeding vessel and control it. Repeat this sequence of events if necessary.

3. **Warning.** Ligating one or both internal iliac arteries is not reliable. Fatal bleeding can come from other sites.

LIMBS

WOUNDS

1. Exploration has been dealt with in general terms but the limbs offer some special features that need to be considered.

2. One of the most challenging injuries is a wound that divides many or all of the structures on the flexor surface of the forearm or wrist.

3. Have available a diagram of a cross-section of the part if you are not absolutely familiar with it.

Assess

1. Use a bloodless field.
2. Have the hand and fingers exposed.

3. Enlarge the wound only if necessary and after careful examination with the aid of rectractors.

4. Identify distal ends of tendons by pulling on them and seeing what movements result. Proximal ends may have retracted but may be brought into view by milking the limb proximal to the wound. Look for traces of blood, carefully use retractors to identify the lines of retraction and find the structures.

5. Avoid dissection because it disturbs natural relationships. Blood vessels retract but they leave blood stains in their wake. One end sometimes sticks out. Nerves may also retract and leave blood stains, but one end often sticks out.

Action

1. Repair bones before blood vessels, veins before arteries and nerves before tendons. Repair of nerves, tendons and skin may be better deferred for a few days.

2. If muscles in the limb have been ischaemic for long, carry out extensive fasciotomy. Completely excise dead or doubtful muscle. Living muscle works better without the impediment of scarred and, worse, infected remnants. If proximal division of a muscle divides its neurovascular bundle, remove the muscle.

DELAYED PRIMARY CLOSURE

1. Employ this when there has been extensive damage in a road accident or by high velocity missile wounds, including shotgun injuries at close range.

2. Delay closure if you are in doubt about the viability of tissues or if there has been heavy bacterial contamination. Do not close the wound but fill it lightly with dry gauze, not greasy mesh.

3. If synovial membrane can be closed at once, do so. The skin can be closed later. Nevertheless, an open joint can remain clean and healthy, especially if the profuse synovial flow drains out freely and not by overflowing.

4. Cover the gauze generously with wool and secure it with a conforming bandage.

5. Support the limb comfortably in a suitable plaster or other splint.

6. After 3–5 days examine the wound with the aid of general or regional anaesthesia. If all is healthy, carry out any necessary repairs. Provide suction drainage and close the wound by suture or skin grafting as appropriate.

7. Reapply dressings and support.

FLAYING

1. Skin that has been widely stripped and perhaps badly crushed as well is unlikely to survive. Replacing it is widely condemned, although it has produced some pleasant surprises after careful surgical toilet.

2. After 10–14 days the distinction between living and dead skin is clear. Remove the dead skin and graft the defect.

3. If signs of infection develop, inspect the wound at once. Remove all dead skin, and establish free drainage. If the wound is clean a few days later, apply split skin grafts.

4. Some surgeons recommend cutting off the flaps, removing the fat from them and sewing them back as free, full-thickness grafts.

5. Injection of dyes stains living tissue, including the patient as a whole. It may help to assess viability. Unfortunately a circulation that is present a few hours after injury may cease a few hours later.

INTERNAL FIXATION OF FRACTURES

1. Whether or not fractures should be fixed in this way remains a hotly debated subject. Fixation should be undertaken only by a suitably trained, equipped and experienced surgeon who accepts responsibility for complications and is capable of dealing with them.

2. Make incisions for this purpose well away from crushed, bruised or undermined skin. If it is not possible to keep well away, cut through the injured skin rather than narrowly skirting it.

3. Leave the wound open for a few days if immediate closure is difficult.

EXTERNAL FIXATION

This may be a safer way of restoring skeletal stability while adding little or no damage to the skin. It provides access for later repairs or closure (see Ch. 28).

Further reading

Ackroyd C E, O Connor B T, De Bruyn P F 1983 The severely injured limb. Churchill Livingstone, Edinburgh.
Ayella R J 1978 Radiological management of the massively traumatised patient. Williams & Wilkins, Baltimore.
Demetriades D 1984 Cardiac penetrating injuries: personal experience of 45 cases. British Journal of Surgery 71:95–97
Demetriades D, Rabinowitz B 1984 Selective conservative management of penetrating abdominal wounds: a prospective study. British Journal of Surgery 71:92–94
Du Priest R W Rodriguez A, Khaneja S C, Sodenstrom C A, Maekawa A, Ayella R J 1979 Open diagnostic peritoneal lavage in blunt trauma victims. Surgery Gynecology Obstetrics 148:890–894
Freeland A E, Jabaley M E, Burkhalter W E, Chaves A M V 1984 Delayed primary bone grafting in the hand and wrist after traumatic bone loss. Journal of Hand Surgery 9:22–28

Kirby G K, Blackburn G 1981 Field Surgery Pocket Book. Her Majesty's Stationary Office, London.
London P S 1974 Injury and pregnancy. Injury 6:129–140
London P S ed 1978 Operative Surgery Vol 3, Accident Surgery. Butterworths, London.
Merriam W F, Mifsud R P 1983 Internal fixation in patients with multiple injuries. Injury 15: 78–86
Nance F D, Wennan M H, Johnson L W, Ingram Jc Jr. Cohn 1 Jr. 1974 Discussion of surgical judgement in the management of penetrating wounds of the abdomen. Annals of Surgery 179:639–646
Owen-Smith M S 1981 High velocity missile wounds. Edward Arnold, London.
Reid D A C, Gosset J 1979 Mutilating injuries of the hand. Churchill Livingstone, Edinburgh.
Ronen G M, Michaelson M, Waisbrod H 1974 External fixation in war injuries. Injury 6:94–98

Orthopaedic and trauma surgery: general principles and spine

PRE-OPERATIVE PREPARATION

Appraise

1. Most orthopaedic operations are carried out on otherwise healthy patients but always assess the patient's fitness for operation beforehand.

2. Postpone elective operations until any underlying abnormality such as a chest or urinary infection or hypertension has been corrected, and septic lesions eradicated.

3. Correct blood loss and dehydration before emergency operations.

PROPHYLACTIC ANTIBIOTICS

Infection of bone and non-living implants is a very serious complication. Give prophylactic antibiotics for all but the most minor operations on bone, when an implant is used, and if there is an open wound.

Inject 500 mg of cephradin intramuscularly with the premedication and give two further doses of 500 mg each at 8-hourly intervals.

PROPHYLACTIC ANTICOAGULANTS

There is a wide diversity of opinion on the wisdom of using prophylactic anticoagulants for major orthopaedic operations, particularly on the hip joint. The anticoagulants themselves may lead to serious consequences and are, in my opinion, best avoided.

If there is a previous history of thromboembolic disease, give 400 ml of dextran 80 intravenously during the operation in addition to any blood that may be required, and a further 400 ml before the drip is removed 12–24 hours later.

ANAESTHESIA

Use a general anaesthetic for most orthopaedic procedures, with controlled hypotension when a tourniquet cannot be used, for example, in operations on the spine or proximal part of the limbs. Use regional or local nerve blocks for operations on the limbs when general anaesthesia is contraindicated or unobtainable.

TOURNIQUETS

Appraise

Most orthopaedic operations on the limbs are facilitated if performed in a bloodless field. This can be achieved by using a tourniquet. Never use a tourniquet if the patient suffers from peripheral vascular disease or if the blood supply to damaged tissues is deficient.

Do not exsanguinate the limb with an Esmarch bandage in the presence of infection, suspected calf vein thrombosis, soft tissue damage, foreign bodies, superficial cysts, fractures or dislocations.

Action

1. Apply a pneumatic tourniquet of appropriate size over a few turns of orthopaedic wool around the proximal part of the upper arm or thigh.

2. Exsanguinate the limb either by elevation for 5 minutes or by applying an Esmarch rubber bandage in overlapping fashion from the extremity proximally.

3. Secure the cuff with zinc oxide strapping or a cotton bandage and inflate until the pressure just exceeds the systemic blood pressure for tourniquets on the upper limb, and to twice the systemic blood pressure for tourniquets on the lower limb. Higher pressures are unnecessary and may cause soft tissue damage by direct compression, especially in thin patients. The pressure should never exceed 250 mmHg in the arm or 500 mmHg in the leg.

4. Record the time of inflation of the tourniquet and the duration of its application, which must be kept to a minimum by careful planning of the operation. 1 hour is usually regarded as the maximum tourniquet time, but there is ample evidence that 2 hours is quite safe and indeed preferable to temporarily releasing and then reinflating the tourniquet.

5. If the tourniquet is accidentally deflated or slips during the operation allowing partial or complete return of the circulation, deflate the cuff completely, reposition and re-fasten it and elevate the limb before reinflating the cuff.

6. Release the tourniquet and achieve satisfactory haemostasis before closing the wound unless there is a reason to do otherwise, for example, meniscectomy.

Aftercare

1. On completion of the operation always ensure that the circulation has returned to the limb.

2. Prevent postoperative swelling by using bulky cotton wool and crepe dressings for at least 24 hours after the operation. Encourage and supervise active exercises.

SKIN PREPARATION

Elective surgery

1. There should be no break or superficial infection in the skin of a limb or the area of the trunk which is to be operated on.

2. Instruct the patient to bath or shower within 12 hours of the operation using an antiseptic soap. Then the skin is shaved to remove hair from the area around the operation site.

3. Mark the limb or digit to be operated on with a felt tip pen. Give instructions to re-mark if the mark is accidentally erased before the operation.

4. Iodine is the most effective skin antiseptic but occasionally provokes a reaction in the skin of sensitive patients. Perform a patch test at least 12 hours before operation by painting a small area of skin remote from the site of operation with iodine. If an erythematous reaction develops, prepare the skin with chlorhexidine in spirit and not iodine.

Emergency surgery

1. Prepare the skin in the anaesthetic room after induction of anaesthesia.

2. Cover open wounds with a sterile dressing held in place by an assistant.

3. Clean the surrounding skin with a soft nail brush and warm cetrimide solution, removing ingrained dirt and debris.

4. Remove the dressing and clean the wound itself in similar fashion to remove all dirt and debris, controlling bleeding by local digital pressure.

5. Irrigate the wound with normal saline.

6. Complete the cleansing and irrigation of the wound in the theatre as part of the definitive surgical treatment.

OPEN WOUNDS

Before dealing with the wound, resuscitate the patient if necessary, making sure that the airway is clear. Restore the circulating blood volume and order blood to be cross-matched. Stop bleeding from the wound by local pressure.

Appraise

1. Determine how the wound was sustained and whether it is recent and clean, longstanding and dirty and superficial or deep. The longer the period since the injury, the deeper and dirtier the wound, the greater the need for antibiotics and tetanus prophylaxis.

2. Consider what structures may have been damaged and test for the integrity of arteries, nerves, tendons and bones.

3. Make an initial assessment of skin loss or damage, and look for exit wounds following penetrating injuries.

4. An X-ray will demonstrate bone damage and implanted radio-opaque foreign bodies, but do not delay treatment in severely injured patients to take X-rays.

5. Depending on the extent of the wound, further assessment and treatment may be carried out without anaesthesia or with regional or general anaesthetic. Avoid local infiltration anaesthesia.

Prepare

1. Give a broad spectrum antibiotic (see p. 445), unless the wound is clean, superficial and recent in origin.

2. If the wound is dirty, deep and more than 6 hours old, give 1 g of benzylpenicillin and 0.5 ml of tetanus toxoid intramuscularly if the patient has been actively immunised in the past 10 years.

3. If the patient has not been actively immunised, give 1 vial (250 units) of human tetanus immunoglobulin in addition to the toxoid. Ensure that further toxoid is given 6 weeks and 6 months later.

4. Clean the wound and prepare the skin, as described above.

5. Apply a proximal tourniquet when appropriate.

Assess

1. Gently explore the wound examining the skin, subcutaneous tissues and deeper structures and following the track of a penetrating wound with a finger or a probe to determine its direction and to judge the possibility of damage to vessels, nerves, tendons, bone and muscle. If muscle damage is suspected, slit open the investing fascia and take swabs for an anaerobic bacterial culture. Decide into which category the wound falls since this will determine the subsequent management.

2. *Simple clean wounds* have no tissue loss, although all wounds are contaminated with micro-organisms which may already be dividing; in clean wounds seen within 8 hours of injury, the bacteria have not yet invaded the tissues.

3. *Simple contaminated wounds* have no tissue loss. However, they may be heavily contaminated and if they are seen more than 8 hours after the injury, they can be assumed to be infected. Late wounds show signs of bacterial invasion with pus and slough covering the raw surfaces, and redness and swelling of the surrounding skin. Although there is no loss of tissue from the injury, the infection will result in destruction.

4. *Complicated clean wounds* result when tissue destruction (e.g. loss of skin, muscle or damage to blood vessels, nerves or bone) has occurred, or foreign bodies are present in the wound. Recently acquired low velocity missle wounds fall into this category, since there is insufficient kinetic energy to carry particles of clothing and dirt into the wound.

5. *Complicated dirty wounds* are seen after heavy contamination in the presence of tissue destruction or implantation of foreign material, especially if the wound is not seen until more than 12 hours have elapsed.

6. *High velocity missile* wounds deserve to be placed in a category of their own. For instance, when a bullet from a high powered rifle strikes the body it imparts its high kinetic energy to the tissues as it passes through. Although the entry and exit wound may be small, structures within the wound are often severely damaged. Muscle is particularly susceptible to the passage of high velocity missiles and becomes devitalised. It takes on a 'mushy' appearance and consistency and fails to contract when pinched or to bleed when cut. If the bullet breaks into fragments or hits bone, breaking it into fragments, the spreading particles of bullet and bone also behave as high energy particles. The whole effect is of an internal explosion. In addition, the high velocity missile carries foreign material (bacteria and clothing) deeply into the tissues causing heavy contamination. The risk of tetanus and gas gangrene is increased when the wound is sustained over heavily cultivated ground in which the organisms abound. Devitalised ischaemic muscle makes an excellent culture medium. As haematoma and oedema formation develop within the investing fascia, tissue tension rises, further embarrassing the circulation and causing progressive tissue death. Although hand gun bullets, shot gun pellets, shrapnel from shells and fragments from mine, grenade and bomb explosions have a relatively low velocity, they behave as high velocity missiles when projected into the tissues from nearby. When a shotgun is fired from close to the body, the wad and the pellets are carried in as a single missile.

Action

1. Stop all bleeding. Pick up small vessels with fine artery forceps and ligate them with fine absorbable sutures. Control damage of major arteries and veins with pressure, tapes or non-crushing clamps, so they may be repaired.

2. Irrigate clean simple wounds with sterile saline solution and close them without drainage. Do not attempt to repair cleanly divided muscle with stitches but simply suture the investing fascia. Close the skin accurately.

3. Never close simple infected wounds immediately. Take a swab for culture and make sure there is no foreign material, devitalised tissue or undrained pockets of infection. Systemic antibiotic or local installations may be started but will not make up for poor technique. Pack the wound with gauze soaked in sterile isotonic saline solution, and cover this with an occlusive dressing. Plan to renew the packing daily until the wound is clean and produces no discharge. Provided there is no redness or oedema of the surrounding skin, close the wound by delayed primary suture, usually after 3–7 days. In suitable cases the stitches can be inserted when the wound is first seen and left untied with long ends. After the infection is overcome the sutures are tied and apposition of the skin is aided using strips of adhesive plastic across the wound edges.

4. Complicated clean wounds can be partially repaired after excising the devitalised tissue. Repair damaged segments of major arteries and veins. Arterial injuries often require the insertion of a reversed vein graft taken from the other limb. Loosely appose the ends of divided nerves with one or two stitches in the perineurium, so that they can be readily identified and repaired later when the wound is healed and all signs of inflammation have disappeared. Similarly appose the ends of divided tendons in preparation for definitive repair at a later date. Do not remove small fragments of bone which retain a periosteal attachment, or large fragments whether they are attached or unattached. Excise devitalised muscle, especially the major muscle masses of the thigh and buttock. Remove foreign material

when possible. Some penetrating low velocity missiles are better left if they lie deeply, provided damage to important structures has been excluded. Remove superficial shotgun pellets. Low velocity missile tracks do not normally require to be laid open or excised. Excise damaged skin when the deep flap can be easily closed, if necessary by making a relaxing incision or applying a skin graft. Do not lightly excise specialised skin from the hands; instead leave doubtful skin and excise it later if necessary. If there is a fracture immobilise the limb in plaster of Paris, cutting a window into it so that the wound can be dressed. If the fracture is very unstable, it is preferable to use an external fixator (p. 451).

5. Complicated dirty wounds require similar treatment of damaged tissues such as nerves and tendons, but do not attempt to repair damaged structures other than major blood vessels. Pack the wound and change the dressings daily until there is no sign of infection, then close the skin by suture or by skin grafting.

6. Lay open high velocity missile wounds extensively. Foreign matter including missile fragments, dirt and clothing is carried deeply into the wound, so contamination is inevitable. Explore and excise the track since the tissue along the track is devitalised, lay open the investing fascia over disrupted muscle to evacuate the muscle haematoma and excise the pulped muscle, leaving healthy contractile muscle which bleeds when cut. This leaves a cavity in the track of the missile. Mark divided nerves and tendons for definitive treatment later. Excise the skin edges and pack the wound with saline-soaked gauze. In the presence of a fracture immobilise the limb in plaster of Paris or with an external fixator. Change the packs daily until infection is controlled and all dead tissue has been excised. Only then can skin closure be completed and the repair of damaged structures be planned.

OPERATIVE FIXATION OF BONES

Appraise

1. The fragments of a fractured or osteotomised bone can sometimes only be held together in a satisfactory position by internal fixation using Kirschner wires, staples, screws, plates, intramedullary nails, or by an external fixator.

2. The choice of technique depends on the circumstances, but attempt to hold the bone together without supplementary plaster of Paris fixation if possible.

3. Do not use internal fixation in the presence of infection, heavily contaminated wounds or for open fractures, unless there are extenuating circumstances, such as an associated arterial injury which cannot be repaired unless the bone is completely stabilised.

4. Use an external fixator (p. 451) where rigid fixation is required but when internal fixation is inappropriate, for example in open fractures of the long bones when the skin cannot be closed.

KIRSCHNER WIRES

1. Use Kirschner wires for the definitive fixation of small fragments of bone to the main fragment or to hold small fragments of bone in place temporarily during the reduction of comminuted fractures, until the permanent fixation device is in place.

2. Kirschner wires are available in diameters of 1, 1.5 and 2 mm. Use the largest size which can be inserted without splitting the bone. This is a matter of judgement.

3. Accurately appose the fragments under direct vision or under the image intensifier.

4. Insert the wire either through the wound or percutaneously, with a small hand drill, from the smaller fragment into the larger fragment. When the wire is used for definitive fixation it should penetrate the distal cortex of the main fragment, so that the tip lies in the subcutaneous tissues distal from the point of insertion, to facilitate later removal.

5. Cut the wire 2–3 mm from the surface of the proximal fragment, or flush with the skin if inserted percutaneously. Then tap the wire in deeper with a punch, so that the cut end lies under the skin.

6. Insert a second or third wire if the fragment of bone is large enough, at a different angle from the first wire, to prevent the fragment rotating.

7. Wires used for definitive treatment can usually be removed after 6 weeks. The wire is best withdrawn tip first to minimise possible displacement of the bone fragment. Locate the tip of the wire under the skin and then infiltrate 1 ml of lignocaine around it. Expose it through a small stab wound and withdraw it with pointed nosed pliers or small bone nibblers.

STAPLES

1. Staples are commonly used to hold two cancellous bone surfaces together when performing an upper tibial osteotomy or triple arthrodesis for example.

2. Place the staple in the introducer. Hold it at right angles to both the superficial and cut surfaces of the bone and tap it into place. Remove the introducer and finally drive the staple home with the punch.

3. To remove, insert a Bristow's elevator or a special tool under the staple and lever it out.

SCREWS

Screws may be used for definitive fixation of a fracture of

a long bone in which the length of the fracture surface is more than twice the diameter of the bone, for example in spiral or oblique fractures of the shaft of the tibia. More commonly, screws are used to fix fragments of bone to the two main fragments which are then held together with a plate.

Action

1. Expose the fracture site.

2. Strip the periosteum from only enough of the bone ends to permit manipulation and reduction. Do not detach comminuted fragments from their soft tissue attachments.

3. Reduce the fracture and hold it in place with one or more bone clamps.

4. If there are separate fragments, reduce and secure the pieces to the main fragment first, rather than attempting to reduce all pieces simultaneously.

5. When fixing a comminuted fracture one screw should link the two main fragments if possible. If there is not a reasonable area of contact between the two main fragments, secure the fracture with a plate, combined with screws if necessary, rather than with screws alone.

6. Place at least one screw at right angles to the long axis of the shaft of the bone. Position additional screws such that their direction bisects the angle between the perpendicular to the shaft and the perpendicular to the fracture itself (Fig. 28.1). Do not insert screws at right angles to the fracture itself, as such screws are insecure against longitudinal shearing forces. Arrange screws at different radial directions around the bone (Fig. 28.1). Avoid placing screws too near the pointed ends of the fragments which easily split off.

7. Drill the entire width of the bone piercing both cortices with a twist drill. For the standard 4 mm (5/32″) stainless steel screw use a 3 mm (1/8″) twist drill. For the common 3.5 mm vitallium screw use No. 31 (3 mm) drill. Drill the superficial cortex only with a drill larger than the external diameter of the screw so that there is no grip on this cortex (Fig. 28.1).

8. If it is available use a special C-shaped drill guide and clamp, cannulated to receive twist drills up to 4 mm in diameter, together with a straight drill guide. With this apparatus the twist drill is always directed to the far jaw of the clamp and its alignment is known more accurately than with the free hand technique. Use these guides either as illustrated in Figure 28.2, or insert the straight drill guide down the centre of the C-shaped clamp and drill the far deep cortex with an unguarded drill.

9. Counter-sink the entry hole into the superficial cortex to receive the bevelled portion of the head of the screw.

10. Cut the thread in the hole with a tap. This tool is brittle and easily snaps if an angulating force is applied to it. It should therefore be rotated with care, removing it every two or three turns to clear the bone dust.

11. Select a screw which will engage fully the deep cortex but which will protrude no more than 2 or 3 mm. Screw lengths include the bevelled portion of the head.

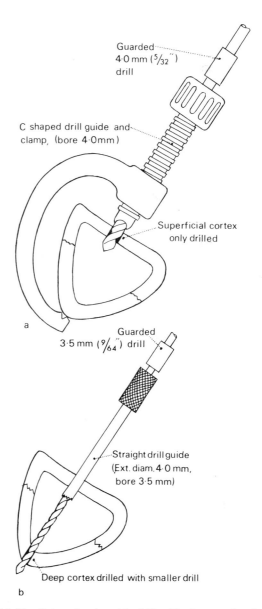

Guarded 4·0 mm (5/32″) drill

C shaped drill guide and clamp, (bore 4·0mm)

Superficial cortex only drilled

a

Guarded 3·5 mm (9/64″) drill

Straight drill guide (Ext. diam. 4·0 mm, bore 3·5 mm)

Deep cortex drilled with smaller drill

b

Fig. 28.2 The C-shaped and straight drill guides for use when inserting compression screws.

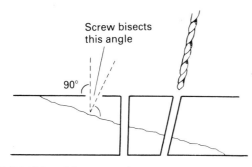

Screw bisects this angle

90°

Fig. 28.1 Principles of the compression screw.

Insert the screws but do not tighten fully until all screws are in place.

12. Since the screws have a grip on one cortex only, they will compress the bone fragments when they are tightened.

PLATES

Action

1. Expose the fracture and an adequate length of bone on either side (see appropriate sections for individual approaches).

2. Strip the periosteum from the fractured ends for 1–2 mm to permit reduction. Do not detach bone fragments from their soft tissue attachments.

3. Reduce the fracture by manipulation under vision using hooks, levers, bone holders and clamps to assist.

4. If there is a large separate bone fragment at the fracture site, first secure it to one main fragment with one or two screws. Place these so that they are in a plane at right angles to the proposed plate and will interdigitate with the screws fixing the plate.

5. Select a plate of suitable size with at least two holes, and preferably more, on either side of the fracture site.

6. Apply the plate to the selected aspect of the bone, preferably its deep surface, so that it does not lie subcutaneously, and hold it in place with one or more clamps.

7. Bend the plate to fit the curvature of the correctly reduced bone using special plate benders.

8. Drill vertical holes for the screws in the centre of each hole of the plate using the drill guide if available.

9. Select a screw of appropriate length using a depth gauge illustrated in Figure 28.3. If the end of the plate lies over cancellous bone use a cancellous screw if possible. Try to fill each hole in the plate with a screw.

COMPRESSION PLATES

Compressing the ends of the bone together improves the apposition and the rigidity of the fixation.

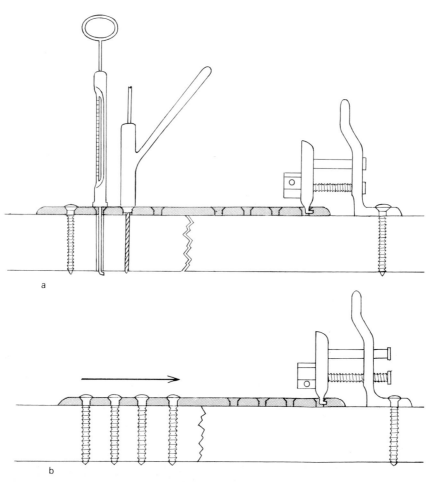

Fig. 28.3 Principles of the compression plate.

Action

1. Secure the plate to one fragment with the full number of screws.

2. With the compression device fully opened engage its hook in the unattached end of the plate and drill a hole in the bone where the hole in the foot plate lies.

3. Secure the compression device to the bone with a single full length screw (Fig. 28.3a).

4. Tighten the device, drawing the fragments together.

5. Secure the remaining half of the plate to the bone with screws.

6. Remove the compression device and discard the single screw which held it to the bone.

7. Insert the final screw into the end hole of the plate.

8. Insert a suction drain.

9. Close the subcutaneous fat and skin but leave the fascia open to avoid a compartment syndrome.

10. Apply a compression dressing.

11. Apply a plaster cast if fixation is inadequate.

INTRAMEDULLARY NAILS

Intramedullary nails are suitable for immobilising fractures of the long bones, such as the femur, tibia and humerus and occasionally the ulna. The nail may be introduced by open or closed techniques and each technique varies with the individual fracture. The description will be found in the appropriate section.

THE EXTERNAL FIXATOR (DENHAM) (Fig. 28.4)

There are many types of external fixator. The essential feature of them all is one or more rigid bars, which are aligned parallel to the limb, to which the threaded pins that are drilled into the fragments of bone are attached. In the more sophisticated apparatus this is done by clamping the pins to universal joints, which allow the position of the fragments to be adjusted before the clamps are finally tightened. In the simplest form, here described, the pins are held to the bar with acrylic cement.

Prepare

1. Treat the wound (p. 446).
2. Reduce the fracture.
3. Maintain the reduction with bone clamps.

Action

1. Make a stab wound through healthy skin proximal to the fracture site.

2. Drill a hole through both cortices of the bone

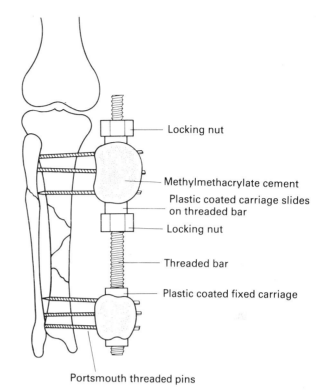

Locking nut

Methylmethacrylate cement

Plastic coated carriage slides on threaded bar

Locking nut

Threaded bar

Plastic coated fixed carriage

Portsmouth threaded pins

Fig. 28.4 The Denham external fixator.

approximately at right angles to the bone with a 3.6 mm drill and measure the depth of distal cortex from the skin surface.

3. Mark the depth on the threaded pin with methylene blue and insert with a hand drill so that both cortices are penetrated.

4. Inset two more pins approximately 3–4 cm apart into the proximal fragment and three pins into the distal fragment in similar fashion.

5. Loosen the locking nuts which hold the carriages on to the rigid bar and hold the bar parallel to the limb and 4–5 cm away from the skin.

6. Place one carriage opposite the protruding ends of each set of three pins and adjust the locking nuts to hold the carriages in position.

7. Fix the pins to the carriages with two mixes of acrylic cement for each carriage, moulding the cement around the pins and the carriage, maintaining the position until it is set.

8. Remove the bone clamps and carry out the final adjustment on the locking nuts to compress the bone ends firmly together.

9. Dress the wound.

Aftercare

1. Remove the device when the fracture is stable and after definitive treatment of the wound is complete, preferably within 6 weeks of applying it.

2. Cut the pins with a hacksaw or bolt cutters and then unscrew them. The acrylic cement can be removed from the carriages which may be used again.

OPEN (COMPOUND) FRACTURES

Appraise

1. The patient (see p. 445).
2. The wound (see p. 446).
3. X-ray to decide whether the fracture can be reduced and stabilised without the use of internal fixation.

Prepare

1. Anaesthetise the patient.
2. Prepare the skin (see p. 446).
3. Clean the wound (see p. 446).

Action

1. Explore and reassess the wound (see p. 447).
2. Examine the fracture. Remove only small and completely unattached fragments of bone.
3. Disentangle the bone ends from the fascia and muscle and wash away any blood clot and other debris.
4. Strip the periosteum for 1–2 mm only from the bone ends to allow accurate reduction without the interposition of soft tissues.
5. Using a combination of traction, bone clamps, levers and hooks, reduce the two main fragments into an anatomical position. If necessary, extend the original wound to improve access.
6. If the fracture is stable, immobilise in plaster of Paris after definitive treatment of the wound (p. 447).
7. If the fracture is unstable, treat by internal fixation only if it is a simple, clean wound (p. 447) which can be closed, or if there are multiple injuries or the limb is severely mutilated and amputation is the only alternative and when the use of an external fixator is impracticable.
8. Apply an external fixator when the wound is contaminated or there is extensive skin loss (see p. 448 for complicated clean and dirty wounds).

SKELETAL TRACTION

Appraise

1. Skeletal traction may be used to immobilise a limb after injury or operation as a temporary measure, as definitive treatment, or as a supplement to treatment.
2. Skeletal traction is most commonly applied through the tibia or calcaneum. Other sites such as the olecranon are occasionally used.
3. There are two types of pin (Fig. 28.5). Each has a

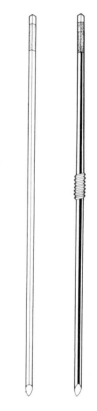

Fig. 28.5 a) Steinmann pin. b) Denham pin.

triangular or square butt which inserts into a chuck, and a trochar point. The Steinmann pin is uniform throughout but the Denham pin has a short length of screw thread wider than the main shaft near its centre, which screws into one cortex of the bone and prevents sideways slip during traction.

Prepare

1. Clean the skin and drape the limb, leaving about 10 cm exposed on either side of the site of entry.
2. Anaesthetise the skin, subcutaneous tissue and periosteum on both sides of the bone at the site of entry and exit of the pin with 1% lignocaine.
3. Make sure that the pin selected fits the sockets in the stirrup (Fig. 28.6).

Action

1. To insert the pin through the upper tibia make a 5 mm incision in the skin on the lateral side of the bone 2.5 cm posterior to the summit of the tibial tuberosity. If the tibial plateau is fractured make the nick and insert the pin 2.5–5.0 cm distally.
2. To insert the pin through the calcaneum make a 5 mm nick in the skin on the lateral side of the heel 2.5 cm distal to the tip of the lateral malleolus.

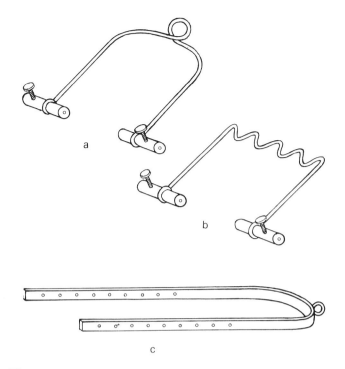

Fig. 28.6 Traction loops.
(a) The Bohler Stirrup.
(b) The Nissen Stirrup.
(c) The Tulloch-Brown 'U' Loop.

3. Introduce the point of the pin through the nick at right angles to the long axis of the limb and parallel to the floor with the limb in the anatomical position. Avoid obliquity in either plane.

4. Drill the pin through both cortices of the bone with a hand drill until the point just bulges under the skin on the opposite side of the limb. Take care that the pin does not suddenly penetrate the skin to impale your hand or the opposite limb. Incise the skin over the point.

5. Adjust the pin until about equal lengths protrude on either side of the limb. When using the Denham pin the threaded section should be screwed into the cortex a further 6–8 mm so that the thread engages the bone.

6. Make sure that the skin is not distorted where the pin passes through. Make tiny relieving incisions if necessary.

7. Dress the punctures with small squares of gauze soaked in tincture benzoin.

8. Attach the traction stirrup to the pin.
Three types are available:
(a) The Bohler Stirrup, for general use (Fig. 28.6a).
(b) The Nissen Stirrup, for more accurate control of rotation (Fig. 28.6b).
(c) The Tulloch-Brown 'U' loop for Hamilton Russell traction (Fig. 28.6c).

9. Put guards on the ends of the pin.

10. Attach a length of cord to the centre of the stirrup through which the traction will be applied.

HAMILTON RUSSELL TRACTION

This is a convenient method for fractures and other conditions around the hip. It controls the natural tendency of the leg to roll into external rotation and avoids the use of a Thomas's splint, the ring of which causes discomfort if the hip is tender.

Action

1. Set up the apparatus as in Figure 28.7, passing the cord through the pulleys as indicated. The sections of string x and y must be parallel to the horizontal and the section z must lead in a cephalic direction. The calf may be supported either on two ordinary pillows or on slings of Domette bandage attached to the 'U' loop with safety pins.

2. Attach between 2–5 kg of weight to the end of the cord and make sure that it is clear of the floor.

3. Keep the point of the heel clear of the bed to avoid pressure sores.

4. Place a foot rest between the bars of the loop to maintain the foot at a right angle to the leg.

SLIDING SKELETAL TRACTION

Sliding skeletal traction with the leg supported on a Thomas's or similar splint is a standard method of conservative treatment for shaft or supracondylar fractures of the femur.

Action

1. Set up the apparatus as in Figure 28.8. Apply 4–8 kg of weight for traction (w).

2. The splint should have a Pearson's or equivalent knee piece attachment so that the knee may be flexed (20° for

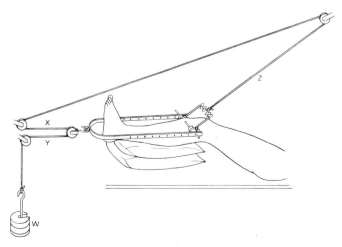

Fig. 28.7 Hamilton Russell skeletal traction.

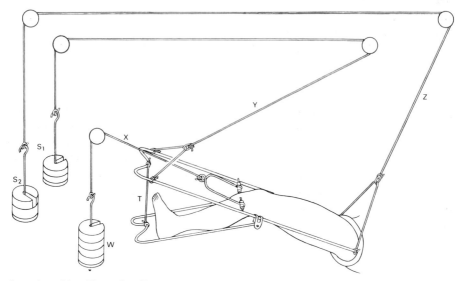

Fig. 28.8 Sliding skeletal traction with a Thomas's splint.

shaft fractures and 40° or more for supracondylar fractures). Tie the distal end of this attachment to that of the main splint with string. Only the string x is concerned with traction. Strings y and z and weights S1 and S2 merely suspend the splint to aid nursing.

3. Support the limb from the sides of the splint with Domette bandage held in place with safety pins. Pad the underside of the limb with sheets of cotton wool.

SIMPLE SKELETAL TRACTION

Simple skeletal traction over a pulley fixed to the end of the bed usually suffices for relatively stable fractures, for example, of the tibial plateau. Unstable fractures need the support of a splint. Support the calf on two or three pillows with the point of the heel clear of the bed. Have the traction string horizontal and apply 2–4 kg of weight.

CALCANEAL TRACTION

Use calcaneal traction with the leg supported on a Bohler-Braun frame in the conservative treatment of unstable fractures of the tibia. If desired it may be combined with a padded plaster of Paris cast to provide more lateral stability. Set up the apparatus as in Fig. 28.9. Apply 2.5–3.5 kg of weight (w). Support the calf and thigh from the side bars of the frame with slings of Domette bandage. Pad under the limb with cotton wool.

SKULL TRACTION

Appraise

1. Skull traction is often employed to immobilise the

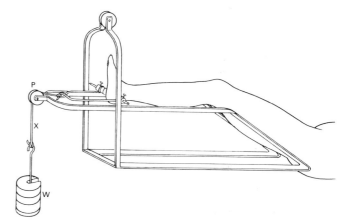

Fig. 28.9 Calcaneal skeletal traction with a Bohler-Braun frame.

cervical spine after injury and sometimes operations on the neck.

2. The traction is applied through skull tongs under local anaesthetic prior to the administration of any general anaesthetic. The anaesthetist then has the benefit of the added security of the traction.

Access

1. Shave a strip of the scalp about 15 cm by 3.5 cm across the vertex in the line of the external auditory meati. Clean the shaved scalp and moisten the surrounding hair to keep it flat.

2. Place a waterproof layer and sterile towel under the head and drape off the bared area. Leave the face of the conscious patient uncovered.

3. Open the Crutchfield tongs to their fullest extent. Place the points symmetrically on either side of the midline

of the scalp on a line joining the external auditory meati and mark the position of the points with methylene blue.

4. Infiltrate the scalp down to the pericranium with 5 ml of 1% lignocaine on each side, anaesthetising an area about 2.5 cm in diameter.

5. Make a straight coronal incision 2.5–3.0 cm long. Carry this down to the pericranium and immediately insert a small self-retaining retractor. Stretch the wound open tightly to control bleeding from the scalp.

Action

1. Make a cruciform incision in the pericranium and with a rougine bare an area of the skull about 1 cm in diameter. With the tongs check the proposed siting of the points.

2. With the guarded perforating instrument mounted on a Hudson's brace, drill a hole in the outer table of the skull at right angles to the surface. There will be slight pain when the diploë is reached, but the outer table itself does not give rise to more than an uncomfortable vibration.

3. Repeat the process on the opposite side.

4. Insert the points of the tongs into the prepared holes and tighten the knob on the outer end of the screw until the apparatus is firm. Lock the tongs in position by tightening the knob on the inner side of the screw.

Aftercare

1. Remove any bone dust from the wound. Remove the self-retaining retractor and immediately suture the scalp with full thickness interrupted stitches which will control bleeding as they are tied.

2. Dress the wound with 2 cm ribbon gauze soaked in tincture benzoin which adheres to both scalp and metal, providing a compact seal. No bandages are required.

3. Apply traction or proceed to manipulation as desired. Tie the traction cord to the ring on the central pivot of the tongs and not to the screw.

BONE GRAFTING

Appraise

1. Bone grafts may be required to promote the union of a fracture or arthrodesis (e.g. spinal fusion) or to fill a cavity in a bone. Cortical bone has no osteogenic potential and so cancellous bone is always used, although on occasions the grafts may include a cortical backing to support the cancellous bone.

2. The usual donor site is the anterior iliac crest, but the posterior iliac crest is more suitable if the patient is prone on the operating table.

3. Small quantities of cancellous bone may also be obtained from the upper or lower end of the tibia, greater trochanter of the femur and the lower end of the radius and olecranon for operations in that area where appropriate. However, for general purposes, the anterior crest is the most suitable source of cancellous bone grafts.

Access

1. Make a 10 cm incision from the anterior superior iliac spine posteriorly as a cord to the curve of the iliac crest. Deepen it to the fascia over the gluteal muscles and secure haemostasis. The oblique muscles of the anterior abdominal wall usually overhang the anterior iliac crest and should be retracted to expose the gluteal attachment.

2. Divide the fascial covering of the muscles attached to the crest along and just inferior to its outer lip for 10–12 cm from the anterior iliac spine posteriorly with the diathermy needle. Leave enough soft tissue attached to the crest for subsequent closure.

3. With a wide periosteal elevator strip the gluteus medius and minimus from the outer surface of the wing of the ilium. Insert a temporary pack to control bleeding.

Action

1. With a straight 20 mm osteotome, make a series of cuts through the outer cortex and into the cancellous bone, but not through the inner cortex, a few millimetres from the outer lip of the crest throughout the extent of the wound. The final cut at each end of the wound should cut through the margin of the crest and then the entire crest may be hinged on its medial intact periosteum like a lid (Fig. 28.10).

2. From the thickest portion of the crest cut a series of vertical slivers of bone, each about 2 mm thick and consisting of a slice of the outer cortex and of cancellous bone leaving the inner cortex intact. The first few slivers removed are usually fragmentary but subsequent ones may be obtained intact. Aim at pieces about 5 cm long.

3. When as much bone as possible has been taken in this way, use a 6 mm gouge or Volkmann's curette to scrape out cancellous bone from the remaining ilium and its lid.

4. Alternatively, a rectangle of cortical bone from the outer table may be elevated and removed after cutting around the margins with an osteotome leaving the iliac crest intact. This may be used as a cortico-cancellous graft either whole or in parts. The underlying cancellous bone may be removed with a Capener gouge.

Closure

1. Turn the iliac crest back into place and suture the fascial covering of the glutei to it with interrupted absorbable sutures.

2. Place a suction drain under the muscles.

3. Close the rest of the wound in layers.

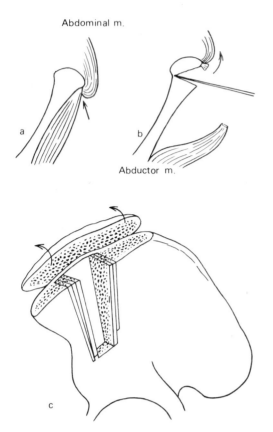

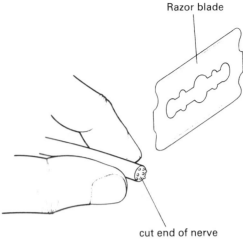

Fig. 28.10 Technique for taking cortico-cancellous bone grafts from the iliac crest.

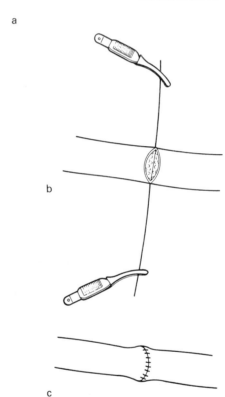

Fig. 28.11 Nerve suture.
(a) Cutting back to pouting fibres with a razor blade.
(b) First and second sutures in place.
(c) Sutures completed.

PERIPHERAL NERVE REPAIR (Fig. 28.11)

Complete disruption of a peripheral nerve may be associated with both open and closed injuries and recovery will not take place unless continuity is re-established surgically.

Appraise

1. A peripheral nerve injury in the presence of an open wound should always be assumed to be a neurotmesis (complete division of the nerve fibres) and the nerve should be identified when the wound is treated (p. 447). If it is divided, appose the ends in their correct orientation for secondary repair later.

2. Primary repair may sometimes be undertaken in specialist centres but secondary repair is safer and easier, when the wound is soundly healed and the danger of infection has passed.

3. An operating microscope may facilitate repair but is not essential and there is no unequivocal evidence to suggest that the results are better.

4. Treat the peripheral nerve injury in the absence of an open wound conservatively at first. A neurapraxia will recover spontaneously in days or weeks, and an axonotmesis in the time it takes for the axons to regenerate. This is calculated by measuring the distance from the site of injury (e.g. a fracture) to the point at which the motor nerve enters the first muscle innervated distal to the lesion. Axons regenerate at a rate of 1 mm per day and so it will take approximately 90 days, for example, for reinnervation of the brachioradialis to occur following an injury to the radial nerve at the distal end of the musculo-spiral groove of the humerus.

5. If recovery fails to occur in the predicted time then explore the nerve and if it is divided repair it.

PRIMARY APPOSITION OF A DIVIDED NERVE

1. Prepare the skin (p. 446).
2. Apply a tourniquet (p. 445).
3. Clean and explore the wound (p. 447).
4. Identify the ends of the nerve and place them in their correct rotational orientation.
5. Appose the ends with two or three fine black silk sutures (for ease of later identification). Pass the needle through the epineurium 2–3 mm from the cut ends.
6. If the ends cannot be apposed without tension, tack them to the underlying soft tissues to prevent retraction until definitive repair is undertaken.
7. Release tourniquet and secure haemostasis.
8. Close the wound when appropriate (p. 448).
9. Carry out secondary suture when the wound is healed and free from induration, ideally 6 weeks later or as soon as possible thereafter.

SECONDARY NERVE REPAIR (Fig. 28.11)

1. Prepare the skin.
2. Apply the tourniquet.
3. Excise the previous scar if necessary, and extend the wound proximally and distally along the course of the nerve.
4. If there was no wound, make an incision 15 cm long along the course of the nerve centred at the site of injury. Use a 'lazy S' incision if the incision crosses the flexor crease of a joint.
5. Expose the nerve through normal tissue on either side of the site of injury.
6. Carefully dissect along the course of the nerve towards the point of injury. In the case of an open wound there may be extensive scar tissue and adhesions. The previously placed marker sutures will help to identify the nerve ends.
7. Free the ends of the nerve from the surrounding soft tissues and place a marker suture through the perineurium 2–3 cm proximally and distally from the site of injury to facilitate later alignment of the ends.
8. Cut transversely across fibrous scar tissue which may be joining the ends together.
9. Holding one end of the nerve firmly between the finger and thumb, carefully cut thin slices of tissue from the exposed end with a sharp razor blade at right angles to the long axis of the nerve until all the scar tissue has been excised and the nerve bundles can be seen pouting from the cut surface (Fig. 28.11a).
10. Repeat the procedure on the other end of the nerve. A centimetre or more may need to be resected from each end of the nerve due to the intraneural fibrosis ('neuroma') caused by the initial injury.
11. Mobilize the nerve from the surrounding soft tissues

proximally and distally as far as is necessary to bring the ends together without tension, carefully preserving and dissecting out the main branches. A neighbouring joint may be flexed if necessary.
12. Release the tourniquet and secure haemostasis.
13. Ensure that the ends of the nerve are correctly orientated by aligning the marker sutures.
14. Place an 8/0 stitch through the perineurium on one side of the nerve. Cut the suture 3 cm from the knot and hold the ends in a small bulldog clip (Fig. 28.11b).
15. Place a second suture directly opposite the first and place another bulldog clip on the ends.
16. Place further sutures through the perineurium, 1.5 mm or so apart, around the circumference of the nerve.
17. After completing the repair of the superficial surface, turn the nerve over by passing one bulldog clip suture under and the other over the nerve.
18. Complete the repair. Cut the first pair of sutures and turn the nerve back to the correct position (Fig. 28.11c).
19. Close the soft tissues and skin without altering the position of the limb if there is any danger of putting tension on the suture line.
20. Apply a padded plaster without increasing the tension on the repair.
21. Remove plaster and skin sutures after 3 weeks and gently mobilize the limb. If joints were flexed to avoid tension they must only be extended gradually over the next three weeks, if necessary by applying serial plasters at weekly intervals, or by incorporating a hinge with a locking device to allow flexion but no more than the set amount of joint extension.

TENDON SUTURE (FIG. 28.12)

Appraise

1. Tendons are relatively avascular structures and heal by the ingrowth of connective tissue from the epitenon. When the tendon is divided within a fibrous sheath on the flexor surface of the hand, for example, the sheath will also be damaged and the connective tissue from the healing sheath grows into the healing tendon causing adhesions. For this reason injuries to the digital flexor tendons within the sheath (see p. 494) should be preferably treated by experienced hand surgeons.
2. Tendons may also require suturing as part of another procedure such as tendon transfer.

Assess

1. Examine the wound. If it is in the vicinity of a tendon, assume the tendon is divided until it is shown to be intact on clinical examination.
2. If no action is demonstrated and there is doubt, explore the wound.

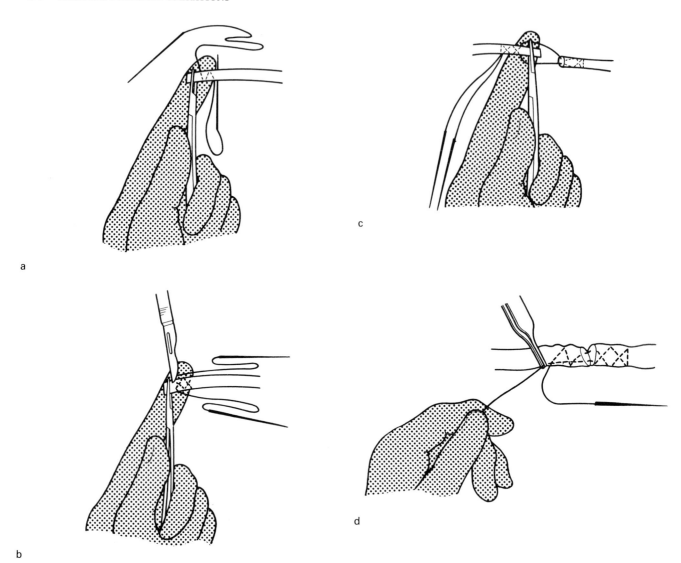

Fig. 28.12 End-to-end suture of a tendon using Bunnell criss-cross stitch.

Action

1. Prepare the skin.
2. Apply the tourniquet.
3. Explore the wound and extend it if necessary in order to identify any divided tendons.
4. If the wound is suitable for primary closure (p. 446) then proceed to repair the tendons. If not, delay the repair until the wound is healed and is no longer indurated, maintaining full mobility of the joints in the meantime by physiotherapy.
5. When several tendons are divided (for example at the wrist) make sure that the cut ends are correctly paired. It is easy to suture the proximal end of one tendon to the distal end of another or even to the cut end of a nerve!
6. Draw the cut ends together after picking up the paratenon round each end of the tendon with fine mosquito forceps, flexing neighbouring joints if necessary.

7. Use a synthetic 4/0 absorbable suture with a straight needle at both ends using a Bunnel criss-cross stitch (Fig. 28.12).
8. Pass one needle obliquely into the tendon and withdraw it through the opposite side 2–3 mm from the cut surface, leaving 10–15 cm of the suture loose (Fig. 28.12a).
9. Pass the needle back obliquely through the tendon to the opposite side and withdraw it before passing it obliquely back to the first side.
10. Pass the needle transversely across the tendon and then back and forth obliquely as before until the needle emerges opposite the point at which it originally entered.
11. Trim the end of the tendon and nick the surface where the sutures emerge with a small knife so that the suture emerges from the cut end (Fig. 28.12b).
12. Draw both ends of this suture tight and then pass first one needle and then the other through the opposite end of the tendon is similar fashion, taking each needle

to opposite sides of the tendon and then back again in turn.

13. Finally, pass one needle transversely across the tendon to emerge alongside the other needle (Fig. 28.12c).

14. Trim the end of the tendon and nick the surface as before.

15. Draw the sutures tight. Cut off the needles and tie the ends of the suture together (Fig. 28.12d).

16. Release the tourniquet and secure haemostasis.

17. Close the wound with suction drainage if necessary.

18. Apply a padded plaster so that the suture line is not under tension and remove after 3 weeks in the upper limb and 6 weeks in the lower limb.

BIOPSY

Biopsy of bone or soft tissue may be taken at an open operation or by aspirating material through a needle (closed biopsy). In both cases take the material from the margin of the lesion, for the tissue in the centre is often necrotic and difficult to identify. Take at least 2 specimens, one for culture and the other for histological examination.

OPEN BIOPSY

Action

1. Apply a pneumatic tourniquet if possible but do not exsanguinate the limb.

2. Incise the skin over the most superficial aspect of the lesion, taking care to place the incision in such a way that it will be excised if amputation is subsequently required, and will not interfere with skin flaps.

3. Incise the deep fascia and split the muscle in the line of its fibres until the margin of the lesion or the bone is reached.

4. Take a wedge-shaped piece of tissue from the margin of the lesion approximately 1 cm long by 0.5 cm thick and 0.5 cm deep. Place it in formal saline unless specific staining techniques are required. Consult the pathologist beforehand if in doubt.

5. Take a further similar specimen for immediate culture.

6. If pus is present, aspirate as much as possible and take a swab for culture.

7. Take a further specimen for microscopic examination and a further specimen for culture from a different part of the lesion if it is large enough.

8. If the lesion is in bone, remove the specimen with a sharp osteotome, and include the periosteum.

9. If the lesion is not obvious, drill a Kirschner wire or a thin twist drill into the suspected site and examine the area under the image intensifier, or take plain X-rays in two planes at right angles. Note the relationship of the lesion to the marker before taking the specimens.

10. Examine radiologically once more to ensure that the specimen has indeed been removed from the lesion.

11. Label each specimen immediately and accurately.

12. Release the tourniquet and stop any bleeding.

13. Close the wound and apply a pressure dressing.

14. Personally ensure that the specimens are sent to the pathological laboratory.

CLOSED (ASPIRATION) BIOPSY (Fig. 28.13)

Several patterns of biopsy needle are available, and the technique using the Harlow Wood needle is described.

Action

1. Premedicate the patient with 10 mg of intravenous diazepam.

2. Prepare and drape the skin as for open biopsy.

3. Infiltrate skin and soft tissues down to the site of the lesion with 1% lignocaine using a fine spinal (e.g. lumbar puncture) needle.

4. Make a stab wound over the most superficial and accessible part of the lesion.

5. Introduce the guide wire (Fig. 28.13a). Advance it slowly towards and into the lesion under biplane radiographic control, preferably using an image intensifier.

6. Remove the guide wire knob and advance the tapered dilator (Fig. 28.13b) over the guide wire to the bone under radiographic control.

7. Remove the dilator knob and slide the trephine guide (Fig. 28.13c) over the dilator to the bone, thus pushing the soft tissues aside.

8. Remove the guide wire and dilator.

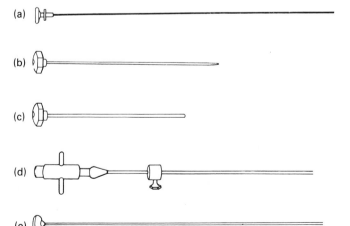

Fig. 28.13 The Harlow Wood Biopsy Needle.
(a) The guide wire.
(b) The tapered dilator.
(c) The trephine guide.
(d) The biopsy trephine.
(e) The obturator.

9. Adjust the collar on the trephine (Fig. 28.13d) so that the end of the trephine will not penetrate more than 0.5–1.0 cm beyond the end of the trephine guide.

10. Pass the trephine through the guide to the bone and then rotate, whilst applying gentle pressure until the collar makes contact with the guide.

11. Check radiographically to be sure that the end of the trephine has penetrated the lesion to a depth of 0.5–1.0 cm. If not, adjust the collar and advance the trephine further.

12. Apply negative pressure to the trephine with a small disposable syringe and then rotate the trephine gently and withdraw it.

13. Pass the obturator (Fig. 28.13e) through the trephine to expel the specimen into formal saline for histological examination.

14. Adjust the collar on the trephine to obtain a second deeper specimen for culture.

15. Close the stab wound if necessary and apply a pressure dressing.

DRAINAGE OF ACUTE OSTEOMYELITIS

Appraise

1. Any unwell infant or child with an area of local bone tenderness has osteomyelitis until proved otherwise and should be treated as such.

2. If an abscess is present on initial clinical examination or if pain, temperature, local swelling and tenderness fail to improve within 12 hours of starting antibiotic therapy, undertake operative treatment immediately.

3. Do not wait until there is radiological evidence of infection. It is then too late.

Prepare

1. Take blood for culture, ESR, WBC and differential white cell count.

2. Arrange a Technetium-99 methylene diphosphonate bone scan, but do not await results before beginning treatment.

3. Give cloxacillin 100–200 mg/kg of body weight daily in divided doses intravenously until there is clinical improvement, usually apparent within 24 hours. If the patient is intolerant of penicillins give cephradine 100 mg/kg of body weight daily.

4. Change antibiotic as necessary when sensitivities are known, as a result of blood culture or operation. Otherwise continue with oral flucloxacillin 50–100 mg/kg, when there is clinical improvement.

5. If operation proves to be necessary, it should be under a general anaesthetic and the most tender point on the limb should be carefully marked before premedication.

Action

1. Apply a tourniquet if possible but do not exsanguinate the limb.

2. Prepare the skin and apply the drapes.

3. Centre the skin incision over the most tender point on the bone and extend proximally and distally for 2.5–3.0 cm.

4. Incise the deep fascia and retract the soft tissues until the periosteum is exposed.

5. Pus may already have escaped into the soft tissues but if not, incise the periosteum and take specimens for culture. Excise obvious dead tissue.

6. If frank pus is not visible, swab the bone surface.

7. Drill a single hole with a 2 mm twist drill, 5 mm proximal to the epiphyseal line which is easily identified under the periosteum. If pus emerges, drill a second and, if necessary, a third hole 5 mm proximal to the preceding hole. Usually a single drill hole is sufficient to ensure that there is no pus in the medullary cavity.

8. Irrigate the wound and insert a suction drain through normal skin. This should be removed after 24 hours or when drainage ceases.

9. Close the skin and apply a padded back splint so that the limb is immobilised and the wound can be inspected. Remove the slab when the wound is healed.

Aftercare

Continue antibiotics for 10 days or longer if necessary, until the clinical signs of infection subside and the ESR falls.

CHRONIC OSTEOMYELITIS

Appraise

1. Chronic pyogenic infection of bone may give rise to a recurrently discharging or permanent sinus and be associated with an underlying sequestrum. Identify a sequestrum radiologically by tomography, and obtain a sinogram to determine the extent of the sinus.

2. Operative treatment is not indicated in the absence of a sequestrum or sinus.

Action

1. Under general anaesthetic apply a tourniquet to the elevated limb but do not otherwise exsanguinate it.

2. Prepare the skin and apply the drapes.

3. Inject methylene blue solution into the sinus through the nozzle of a 5 mm disposable syringe until it oozes from the sinus. Express excess dye with a swab.

4. Centre the skin incision on the mouth of the sinus

and excise it. Extend the incision in the direction of any sequestrum, excising any previous scars.

5. Carefully dissect around the track of the sinus, the blue staining of which is usually visible through the surrounding cuff of normal tissue, down to the bone. Excise the sinus track.

6. The entrance of the sinus into the bone will be stained blue. Strip the periosteum proximally and distally to expose any dead underlying bone, which has a white appearance.

7. Remove dead bone with an osteotome and open the medullary cavity.

8. Remove the sequestrum if present, and unroof the part of the cavity stained blue. Curette to remove all granulation tissue which has been stained by the dye.

9. Irrigate the cavity thoroughly, with half strength hydrogen peroxide and then normal saline.

10. Place one or more chains of gentamicin-inpregnated methyl methacrylate beads into the cavity so that it is completely filled. The chains must not be kinked or intertwined. Leave the last bead of each chain protruding above skin level.

11. Place a perforated drain under the skin before closure, and connect it to a non-evacuated suction bottle.

12. Close the skin leaving the terminal bead of each chain protruding from the wound, and dress the wound.

Aftercare

1. Remove the drain after 24–48 hours, or when the discharge ceases.

2. Remove beads by gentle traction on the protruding bead after 10–14 days. An anaesthetic is not usually required.

3. If the chain breaks, leave the beads in situ and remove them subsequently when the wound is well healed, under a general anaesthetic.

ACUTE SEPTIC (PYOGENIC) ARTHRITIS

Appraise

1. In all cases of acute arthralgia, especially in children, suspect septic arthritis.

2. Do not fail to aspirate the joint when the signs and symptoms of infection are present in association with a leucocytosis or a raised ESR, even if X-rays are normal.

Prepare

1. Take blood for culture, WBC count and differential and ESR.

2. X-ray the joint.

3. Give cloxacillin and methacillin intravenously (see p. 460).

4. Administer a general anaesthetic.

5. Clean and drape the skin.

Action

1. Insert a wide bore needle attached to a syringe into the joint through the site of easiest access, maximum tenderness or fluctuation. Needles should *not* pass through an area of cellulitis because of the risk of infecting a sterile effusion.

2. Aspirate any fluid present for culture, cell counts, and an immediate smear. If the aspirate is free from pus and no organisms are seen on the smear, treat by antibiotics and immobilisation alone, until the results of cultures and all cell counts are available.

3. Open the joint if the aspirate is obvious pus, or organisms are visible on the smear or are subsequently grown and if the cell counts exceed 100 000/mm³.

4. Make an incision 2.5–3.5 cm long at the site of aspiration and approach the joint, if possible through a standard approach (see sections on individual joints).

5. Make a cruciate incision in the capsule and irrigate the joint thoroughly with normal saline, removing all pus, fibrin or other debris.

6. Insert a suction drain and close the skin only.

Aftercare

1. Immobilise the joint in a stable position in a padded plaster with access to the wound.

2. Change the antibiotic if necessary when the cultures of the blood or aspirate are available. Change from intravenous to oral administration after 24–48 hours in the light of clinical improvement.

3. Remove the suction drain after 24–48 hours or when drainage ceases.

4. Continue antibiotics and immobilisation for 6 weeks.

THE SPINE

Most operations on the vertebral column and its contents are highly specialised and intricate. Operations within the dura are usually carried out by neurosurgeons and operations on the spinal column itself by orthopaedic surgeons.

The anterior approach is suitable for operations on the vertebral bodies, particularly the cervical vertebrae. The bodies of the thoracic vertebrae may be approached through the chest and the lumbar vertebrae through the abdomen, particularly for the treatment of spinal tuberculosis; this should only be carried out by experienced surgeons. The lateral or anterolateral approach (costotransversectomy) is the classical approach to a tuberculous spine, allowing decompression of the cord without causing spinal instability.

POSTERIOR APPROACH (Fig. 28.14)

Appraise

1. This is most commonly employed for affording access to the neural arch, the spinal canal and the intervertebral discs. Only this approach will be described in detail.

Prepare

1. Administer a general anaesthetic with controlled hypotension.
2. Position the patient face down on the operating table, on an orthopaedic mattress or suitably placed sandbags, to free the abdomen from pressure.
3. Prepare the skin from the natal cleft to the thorax.
4. Cover the buttocks and lower limbs from the top of the natal cleft distally with a waterproof sheet and a large drape. Cover the head and thorax with a second large drape. Place further drapes on either side leaving the spinous processes exposed, and cover the exposed skin with adhesive plastic film (e.g. Steridrape) to hold the drapes in position.

Action

1. Make a longitudinal midline incision 10–15 cm long, centred on the spine of the vertebra to be exposed, through the skin and subcutaneous tissue over the tips of the vertebral spines. In the lower lumbar region the spine of L4 can be used to locate the incision. It usually lies at the level of the iliac crest but check an anteroposterior X-ray of the patient to be sure.
2. Coagulate bleeding subcutaneous vessels.

3. Strip subcutaneous fat from the deep fascia on either side of the midline for 1.0–1.5 cm with a periosteal elevator, to facilitate closure.
4. Incise the deep fascia along the tips of the spines and then with the cutting diathermy current, separate the attachments of the paraspinal muscles from the sides of the vertebral spines.
5. With a broad periosteal elevator strip the muscles from the posterior neural arches and from the tip of the spines downwards and laterally to the facet joints (Fig. 28.14).
6. Repeat for at least one and possibly two vertebrae above and below the affected one, depending on the exposure required.
7. Insert two large self-retaining retractors down to the neural arches and open as widely as possible.
8. Complete the exposure by removing residual soft tissue with a small periosteal elevator, knife or scissors.
9. Control bleeding by diathermy or packing.
10. After completing the definitive procedure, remove retractors and suture the lumbodorsal (deep) fascia with interrupted synthetic absorbable sutures over a suction drain.
11. Close the subcutaneous tissue and skin.

VERTEBRAL BIOPSY (Fig. 28.15)

Appraise

1. Biopsy of the vertebral bodies for diagnostic purposes is most appropriately performed by closed aspiration. The exact technique varies for cervical, thoracic and lumbar vertebrae, but radiological control with the image intensifier is essential. The close proximity of important anatomical structures in the cervical and thoracic spines makes the technique hazardous for the inexperienced, but needle biopsy below the tenth thoracic vertebra is relatively safe and will be described.

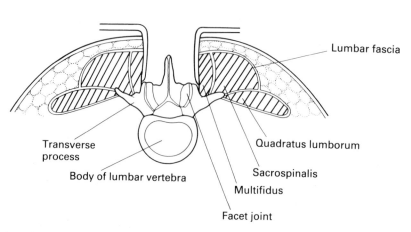

Transverse process

Body of lumbar vertebra

Lumbar fascia

Quadratus lumborum

Sacrospinalis

Multifidus

Facet joint

Fig. 28.14 Posterior approach to the lumbar spine.

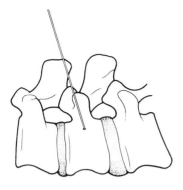

a

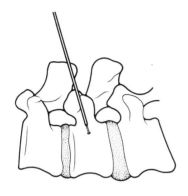

b

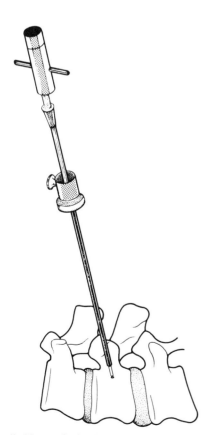

c

Fig. 28.15 Needle biopsy of a lumbar vertebral body.
(a) The introduction of the guide wire to the vertebral body.
(b) The tapered dilator advanced over the guide wire.
(c) Biopsy through the trephine guide with the large trephine.

Prepare

1. Place the patient prone on the operating table.
2. Clean and drape the skin, leaving approximately 6 cm by 6 cm of skin exposed.
3. Under radiological control, infiltrate a track with 1% lignocaine from a point 6–7 cm lateral to the appropriate spinous process, medially at an angle of 35° to the vertical, until the side of the vertebral body is reached (Fig. 28.15a). If a transverse process is encountered, move the needle to pass above or below it.
4. Introduce the guide and proceed as described on p. 459.

REMOVAL OF A PROLAPSED LOWER LUMBAR INTERVERTEBRAL DISC (FIG. 28.16)

Appraise

1. This operation is not technically demanding but the decision to operate frequently requires mature experience and judgement.
2. It should only be undertaken by the junior when there is conclusive clinical and myelographic evidence of a definite disc prolapse.

Prepare

1. Administer a general anaesthetic with controlled hypotension.

Action

1. Expose the neural arch of the appropriate vertebra, and the vertebra above and below, through a posterior approach (see p. 462).

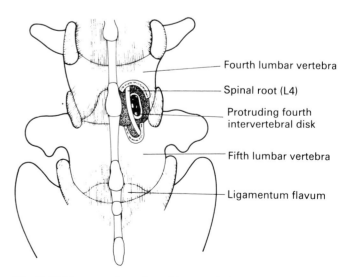

— Fourth lumbar vertebra
— Spinal root (L4)
— Protruding fourth intervertebral disk
— Fifth lumbar vertebra
— Ligamentum flavum

Fig. 28.16 Exposure of a prolapsed intervertebral disc and a spinal nerve root.

2. Check the vertebral level by counting up from the sacrum which can be palpated or visualised. The spine of L5 is mobile, S1 is not, and the lower edge of the lamina of L5 is sharp when compared with the vertebra above.

3. 'Break' the operating table and flex the spine as much as possible.

4. Incise the ligamentum flavum along the margin of the lamina on either side of the space to be explored with a No. 15 blade. Take care not to incise too deeply for the dura may then by punctured.

5. If the ligamentum flavum is barely visible between adjacent laminae, remove 1–2 mm of bone from the margin of the upper lamina carefully with a small osteotome and then remove the ligamentum flavum as above.

6. Note the extradural fat. If present, gently push it towards the midline with a swab or Watson Cheyne dissector, to expose the underlying dura.

7. Retract the dura medially with a dural retractor or a MacDonald dissector, to expose the nerve root as it passes laterally.

8. If the nerve root is not readily visualised, remove more from the laminae above and below with Hajek's angled bone punch forceps (Fig. 28.16).

9. A prolapsed disc is usually visible in the angle between the nerve root and the dura, but on occasions may be seen directly beneath the nerve root or lateral to it. A central disc prolapse lies medially under the dura.

10. Retract the nerve root appropriately with a nerve root retractor.

11. A sequestrated disc can now be removed intact, or piecemeal with pituitary rongeurs.

12. If the annulus is still intact, make a cruciate incision with a No. 15 blade through the apex of the bulge, and insert first straight and then angled pituitary rongeurs through the hole. Open the jaws of the instrument and close them, withdrawing the nucleus pulposus either intact or in fragments. Repeat the process until no more disc material remains.

13. Carefully control any bleeding by diathermy if an obvious bleeding point is seen, or by Gelfoam packing and gentle pressure.

14. If the dura is inadvertently punctured, close it with one or more 8/0 silk sutures.

Closure

1. Close the lumbodorsal fascia and skin. A suction drain is not usually necessary.

Aftercare

1. Nurse the patient flat for 48 hours, turning every 4 hours until pain permits the patient to turn himself.

2. Retention of urine is a common complication. Catheterise.

3. Allow up after 48 hours or as soon thereafter as pain permits.

4. Start gentle spinal flexion and extension exercises.

Further reading

Brown K L B, Cruess R L 1982 Bone and cartilage transplantation in orthopaedic surgery. Journal of Bone and Joint Surgery 64A: 270–279

Dixon R A 1978 Nerve repair. British Journal of Hospital Medicine 20: 295–305

Fyfe I S, Henry A P J, Mulholland R C 1983 Closed vertebral biopsy. Journal of Bone and Joint Surgery 65B: 140–143

Gelberman R H, Berg J S V, Lundborg G N, Akeson W H 1983 Flexor tendon healing and restoration of the gliding surface. Journal of Bone and Joint Surgery 65A: 70–79

Klenerman L, Miswas M, Hughland G H, Rhodes A M 1980 Systemic and local effects of the application of a tourniquet. Journal of Bone and joint Surgery 1980; 62B: 385–388

Lowbury E J L, Lillie H A, Bull J P 1960 Disinfection of the skin of operative sites. British Medical Journal 1960; 2: 1039–1044

Macnab I 1977 Backache. Williams & Wilkins Co., Baltimore. 1–231

Müller M E, Allgöwer M, Schneider R, Willenegger H 1979 Manual of internal fixation. Techniques recommended by the AO group, 2nd edn. Springer-Verlag, Berlin

Nade S 1979 Clinical implications of cell function in osteogenesis. Annals of the Royal College of Surgeons of England 61: 189–194

Nade S 1983 Acute haematogenous osteomyelitis in infancy and childhood. Journal of Bone and Joint Surgery 65B: 109–120

Nade S 1983 Acute septic arthritis in infancy and childhood. Journal of Bone and Joint Surgery 65B: 234–242

Patzakis M K, Gustilo R V, Chapman M W 1982 Management of open fractures and complications. In: Frankel V H (ed) Instructional course lectures. The American Academy of Orthopaedic Surgeons Vol 31 St. Louis Missouri C V Mosby Co, St. Louis. p. 62–88

Seddon H 1975 Surgical disorders of the peripheral nerves, 2nd edn. Churchill Livingstone, Edinburgh

Shipley J A, van Meerdervoort H F, van den Endej 1981 Gentamicin polymethyl methacrylate beads in the treatment of chronic bone sepsis. South African Medical Journal 59: 905–7

Stewart J D M, Hallet J P 1983 Traction and orthopaedic applicances. Churchill Livingstone, Edinburgh

Orthopaedic and trauma surgery: the upper limb

APPROACH TO THE SHOULDER

Most surgical procedures on the glenohumeral and acromio-clavicular joints are required for the treatment of injuries, for these joints are rarely affected by the common orthopaedic conditions.

THE ANTERIOR APPROACH (Fig. 29.1)

Appraise

The glenohumeral joint may be exposed through anterior, posterior or transacromial approaches, but most procedures can be carried out satisfactorily through the anterior approach.

Prepare

1. Operate under a general anaesthetic, preferably with controlled hypotension.
2. Place the patient supine on the operating table in a semi-reclining position with a long narrow sandbag between the shoulder blades.
3. Have your unscrubbed assistant elevate the arm.
4. Clean the skin from the scapula posteriorly, round the axilla and over the chest wall to the midline anteriorly, and from the angle of the jaw to the costal margin and down the arm to the elbow.
5. Towel the head separately (see thyroid p. 341).
6. Tuck a large drape, backed by a waterproof sheet, carefully between the table and the trunk. Cover the trunk with another large sheet, the upper edge of which reaches the lower margin of the head towels. Wrap the arm in a medium-sized towel, from the fingertips to the midpoint of the upper arm, and secure this towel firmly with an open weave bandage.
7. Cover the exposed skin with a transparent adhesive skin drape, taking care to seal the axilla.

Access

1. Incise the skin and subcutaneous fat in an arc from the clavicle above, downwards over the tip of the coracoid process to the anterior axillary fold. Raise the flaps of skin and fat medially and laterally to expose the delto-pectoral groove running obliquely across the wound (Fig. 29.1a).
2. Identify the cephalic vein in the groove and incise the investing fascia throughout the length of the vein.

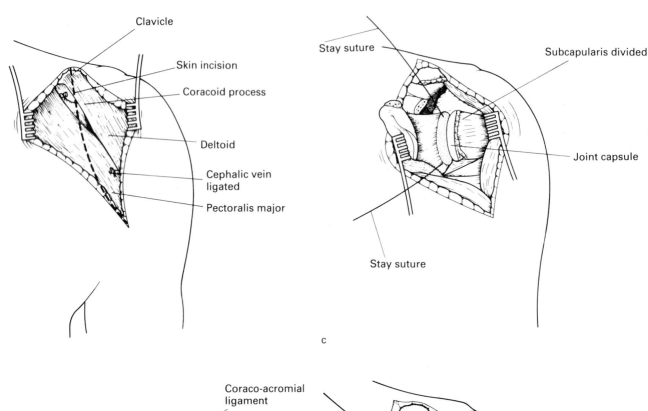

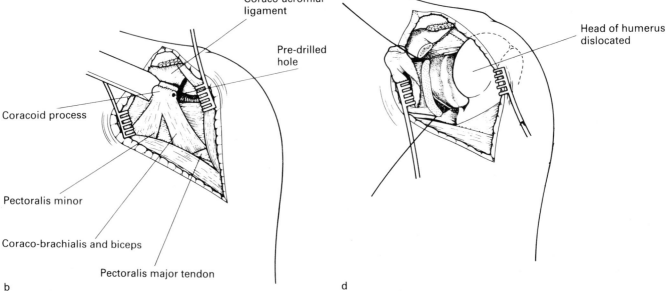

Fig. 29.1 The anterior exposure to the shoulder joint.
(a) The skin incision. Location of the delto-pectoral groove and coracoid process.
(b) Division of the coracoid process with its attached muscle.
(c) Division and retraction of the subscapularis and the capsule.
(d) Dislocation of the head of the humerus.

3. Ligate the cephalic vein, which is often duplicated, at the lower end of the incision, and proximally before it penetrates the clavipectoral fascia immediately below the clavicle.

4. Remove the ligated segment of vein, coagulating the tributaries as they are encountered.

5. Separate the deltoid from the pectoralis major by blunt dissection and retract the muscles with a large self-retaining retractor, exposing the underlying short head of biceps and coraco-brachialis (Fig. 29.1b).

6. Palpate the superolateral surface of the coracoid process and make a hole with a small Paton's burr from the tip along its axis.

7. Divide the coracoid process 1.5 cm from its tip with

a sharp osteotome from the medial side, taking care not to split it. The combined insertion of the coraco-brachialis, short head of biceps and pectoralis minor can now be retracted medially with the tip of the coracoid, so exposing the underlying subscapularis (Fig. 29.1c).

8. Externally rotate the arm and identify the lower border of subscapularis by seeing the branches of the anterior circumflex humeral vessels lying on its surface. Divide these between ligatures.

9. Identify the upper margin of subscapularis and place stay sutures at the upper and lower margins at the musculo-tendinous junction. Divide the muscle just lateral to the stay sutures (Fig. 29.1c).

10. The underlying capsule is usually adherent to the deep surface and is frequently divided at the same time, opening the joint as the subscapularis is retracted medially.

12. The head of the humerus can now be dislocated if required by external rotation and extension of the arm.

Closure

1. Internally rotate the arm. Apply gentle traction on the stay sutures to draw together the divided subscapularis muscle. Suture the muscle with 2/0 synthetic absorbable sutures.

2. Reattach the coracoid process with a 4 mm screw of appropriate length (usually 2.0–2.5 cm).

3. Insert a suction drain.

4. Draw the margins of the deltoid and pectoralis major muscles together with 2 or 3 absorbable sutures.

5. Close the skin and dress the wound.

Aftercare

1. Bandage the arm to the trunk by first placing a length of smooth wood or metal approximately 10–15 cm wide and 1 m long between the patient and the operating table, so that it lies between the shoulder blades and extends from the iliac crest to the top of the head.

2. With the anaesthetist controlling the head, lift the upper trunk from the table by raising the top end of the board.

3. Flex the elbow so that the fingertips touch the opposite shoulder and bandage the upper arm to the chest wall over a layer of wool. Secure the bandages with 10 cm adhesive strapping.

4. Gently withdraw the board from within the bandages and lower the patient to the table.

RECURRENT DISLOCATION OF THE SHOULDER (PUTTI-PLATT REPAIR)

Appraise

1. Operation is required if the shoulder dislocates more than once or twice after the initial acute dislocation.

2. The type of repair will depend on the preference of the surgeon. The Putti-Platt repair is described.

Access

1. Expose the subscapularis through the anterolateral approach and divide it with a knife between stay sutures at its musculo-tendinous junction, as far medially as possible (Fig. 29.1).

2. Open the underlying capsule if it has not been opened already.

3. Insert the tip of a Bankart retractor under the posterior margin of the glenoid, and retract the head of the humerus posterolaterally.

Assess

Carefully retract the subscapularis and capsule medially. Inspect the anterior margin of the glenoid to see if the labrum is detached (Bankart lesion).

Action

1. If the labrum is detached, roughen the anterior surface of the glenoid and adjacent neck of scapular with a small osteotome.

2. Internally rotate the humerus and suture the lateral stump of the subscapularis tendon to the deep surface of the capsule along the anterior margin of the glenoid, with absorbable 2/0 synthetic mattress sutures. Do not tie the sutures until all are in place (Fig. 29.2).

3. Separate the capsule from the under surface of the subscapularis and suture the free lateral edge to the stump of the subscapularis tendon as far laterally as possible (Fig. 29.2).

4. Suture the free edge of the medial part of the subscapularis to the rotator cuff at its attachment to the greater tuberosity, so overlapping the stump.

5. Close the wound (see p. 467).

Aftercare

1. Bandage the arm to the chest for 3 weeks.

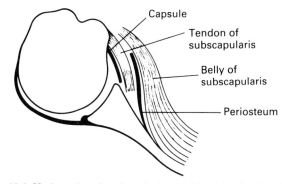

Fig. 29.2 Horizontal section through the shoulder joint showing the double breasting of the capsule and the tendon of subscapularis. The Putti-Platt repair.

2. Mobilise during the next 3 weeks with pendulum exercises progressing gradually. Finally, permit external rotation.

OTHER OPERATIONS ON THE SHOULDER

OPEN REDUCTION AND INTERNAL FIXATION OF FRACTURES OF THE HUMERAL NECK

Fractures of the surgical neck and tuberosities of the humerus rarely require operative treatment. The position of the fragments is almost always acceptable in the elderly patients in whom these fractures usually occur. An exception is a fracture dislocation of the glenohumeral joint, if the head of the humerus cannot be reduced by manipulation. Operative treatment is technically difficult, and the anterior approach is usually appropriate. Three- and four-part fractures require prosthetic replacement.

ARTHRODESIS OF THE SHOULDER

Arthrodesis of a painful stiff glenohumeral joint is best carried out through the posterior approach. It is an operation for the experienced surgeon.

ARTHROPLASTY OF THE SHOULDER

Excision arthroplasty leaves an unstable, weak, albeit pain-free, shoulder and has been superceded by replacement arthroplasty. Leave this to the expert on the rare occasions when there is a need for it.

ROTATOR CUFF REPAIR

The indications for exploration and repair of the rotator cuff are controversial, but when the need arises, a transacromial approach is most appropriate.

DISLOCATION OF THE ACROMIOCLAVICULAR JOINT (Fig. 29.3)

Appraise

Sprains and subluxations of the acromioclavicular joint are treated conservatively, but complete dislocation requires operation.

Prepare

1. Operate under general anaesthesia.
2. Lie the patient supine in a semi-reclining position.
3. Clean the skin from the midline of the neck around the point of the shoulder to include the upper third of the arm, and over the top of the shoulder onto the front of the chest, 10 cm below the clavicle.
4. Towel the head separately (see p. 341) and cover the trunk and arms with a large sheet, leaving the affected shoulder exposed.

Access

1. Incise the skin and platysma along the outer third of the superior surface of the clavicle across the acromioclavicular joint to the tip of the acromion.
2. Strip the trapezius muscle subperiostally from the superior surface of the clavicle and expose the acromioclavicular joint.
3. Palpate the tip of the coracoid process.

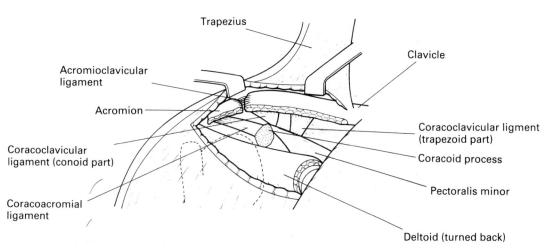

Fig. 29.3 The approach to the acromioclavicular joint.

Action

1. Using a hand drill, carefully drill a hole 3.2 mm in diameter, through the clavicle, directly in line with the coracoid process.

2. Carefully locate the exact position of the coracoid process with the tip of the drill. It is easy to pass the drill to one side or the other. Continue drilling through the coracoid process.

3. Over-drill the clavicle only with a 3.5 mm twist drill.

4. Depress the clavicle to reduce the dislocation and measure the depth of the hole with the depth gauge (see p. 450).

5. Insert a cancellous bone screw and carefully tighten it until the dislocation of the acromioclavicular joint is completely reduced.

6. Close the wound.

Aftercare

1. Immobilise the arm in a sling for 10 days and then gently mobilise.

2. Remove the stitches after 7 days.

3. Remove the screw 6 weeks after the operation and allow full mobility.

APPROACHES TO THE UPPER ARM

Orthopaedic operations on the upper arm are infrequent but access to the humerus is occasionally required for internal fixation of fractures.

ANTEROLATERAL APPROACH

Appraise

1. This approach to the humeral shaft avoids the major neuromuscular structures.

2. The radial nerve is still susceptible to damage as it passes around the lateral aspect of the humerus, so take great care to protect it.

Prepare

1. Have 2 units of cross-matched blood available.

2. Operate under general anaesthetia.

3. Place the patient supine on the operating table with a large arm table in place.

4. An unscrubbed assistant elevates the arm so that it can be cleaned from the neck to the wrist.

5. Place a small triangular towel in the axilla and take it over the tip of the shoulder or around the edge of the tourniquet. Fasten with a towel clip.

6. Place a waterproof sheet and covering towel over the arm board and tuck under the trunk.

7. Place a large sheet over the trunk and head.

8. Wrap the forearm and hand in a small towel and bandage firmly to the forearm with an open weave bandage.

9. Cover the exposed upper arm with a large transparent adhesive drape.

Access

1. Palpate the moveable mass of the biceps muscle overlying the fixed mass of the brachialis.

2. Make a longitudinal skin incision along the lateral border of the biceps from the deltoid above to the elbow below.

3. Retract the biceps and cephalic vein medially, dividing the lateral tributaries to expose the brachialis.

4. Split the brachialis longitudinally down to the bone 1.5 cm lateral to the biceps' edge with the knife directed obliquely towards the midline of the humerus anteriorly (Fig. 29.4).

5. Strip the muscle off the bone with a periosteal elevator. The outer strip of the brachialis protects the radial nerve from direct damage, but avoid forceful retraction.

6. If necessary, extend the wound proximally (after removing the tourniquet if present) by incising the skin in the line of the delto-pectoral groove to the clavicle.

7. Detach the deltoid from its origin to the clavicle as far laterally as the acromioclavicular joint with the cutting diathermy. Leave sufficient tissue attached to the clavicle to take the sutures when closing.

8. Turn back the detached deltoid laterally to expose the tendon of pectoralis major. This may then be cut to allow

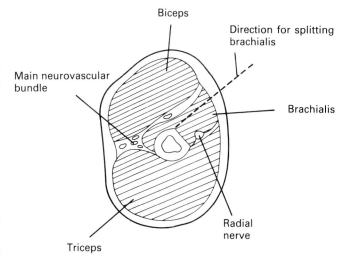

Fig. 29.4 Cross section through the middle third of the arm showing the lateral part of the brachialis which is not covered by the biceps. This is split in the direction of the dotted line to expose the front of the distal half of the humerus. The cut slopes in to reach the midline of the shaft.

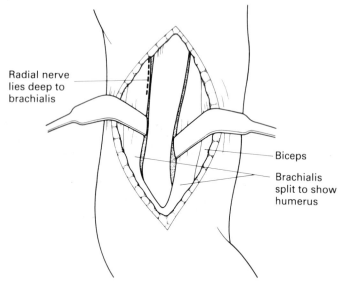

Radial nerve lies deep to brachialis

Biceps

Brachialis split to show humerus

Fig. 29.5 The distal exposure of the humerus.

retraction of the muscle medially, exposing the long and short heads of biceps and the neurovascular bundle.

9. The anterior surface of the lower third of the humerus can be exposed by extending the skin incision distally along the lateral border of the biceps, curling medially and then distally again, to cross the elbow crease in the midline of the forearm (Fig. 29.5).

10. Split the brachialis as far as the elbow joint and flex the elbow to open the wound.

Closure

1. Release the tourniquet if present.
2. Secure haemostasis.
3. Re-attach the deltoid and approximate the margins of the brachialis with 2/0 absorbable sutures.
4. Place a suction drain in a subcutaneous layer.
5. Suture the skin.

Aftercare

1. Apply a firm dressing and elevate the arm for 24 hours.
2. Use a sling until the wound has healed.
3. Encourage the patient to exercise the fingers, elbow and shoulder as soon as postoperative pain permits.

INTRAMEDULLARY FIXATION OF HUMERAL SHAFT FRACTURES

Appraise

1. Fractures of the humeral shaft are usually treated conservatively.
2. If open reduction and internal fixation is necessary

(see p. 448), intramedullary nailing is preferable to plating.

3. Closed nailing is best left to the experienced surgeon with access to an image intensifier.

Access

1. Use the anterolateral approach to expose the fracture, extending the exposure proximally for fractures of the upper third of the shaft of the humerus.
2. Pack the wound.
3. Flex the elbow and make a posterior longitudinal incision in the midline of the upper arm, extending 6 cm proximally from the tip of the olecranon.
4. Split the distal end of the triceps aponeurosis and the underlying muscle to expose the olecranon fossa and the posterior surface of the humerus.

Action

1. Make a hole through the apex of the fossa into the medullary cavity of the humerus with a Paton's burr.
2. Enlarge this hole and elongate it proximally for 1–2 cm with small bone nibblers.
3. Measure the length of a sharp pointed guide wire and pass it through the hole into the medullary cavity of the humerus as far as the fracture site.
4. Reduce the fracture accurately and maintain the reduction with a small Lowman's clamp if necessary.
5. Advance the guide wire through the fracture site until it comes to a halt against the cortex of upper end of the humerus.
6. Take a check X-ray and advance or withdraw the guide wire if necessary.
7. Measure the length of the guide wire protruding from the olecranon fossa and subtract from the total length of the nail required. Add 1 cm to allow for the 'eye'.
8. Replace the guide wire with an olive-tipped guide and ream the medullary canal with a 6 or 7 mm diameter cannulated flexible powered reamer passed over the guide wire. Repeat with reamers increasing in diameter by 0.5 mm until the cavity is 9 or 10 mm in diameter according to the size of the bone.
9. Replace the olive tipped guide wire with a standard guide wire.
10. Introduce a Küntscher nail for calculated length and 1 mm less in diameter than the ultimate reamer. Tap it gently home with the eye of the nail towards the superficial rather than the deep surface of the olecranon. Leave sufficient of the eye protruding to facilitate later removal of the nail.
11. Check the position with X-rays.
12. Insert a screw transversely through the eye into the anterior cortex of the humerus to prevent the nail from backing out.

13. Remove the bone clamp and close both wounds with suction drainage.

Aftercare

1. Support the arm in a sling.
2. Encourage the patient to begin active finger and elbow exercises immediately.
3. Start assisted shoulder exercises after removal of the drains in 48 hours.

APPROACHES TO THE ELBOW

The elbow joint may be exposed from the anterior, posterior, medial or lateral aspects. Avoid the anterior approach except for very special circumstances. The posterior approach gives access to the whole of the lower end of the humerus, whilst the medial and lateral approaches give a more limited access to the corresponding side of the joint, which is sufficient for more limited procedures.

POSTERIOR APPROACH

Appraise

1. This approach gives the widest access to the lower end of the humerus and the elbow joint.
2. Use it for open reduction and internal fixation of the more extensive fractures.
3. It is also suitable for arthroplasty and arthrodesis of the elbow.

Prepare

1. With the patient under general anaesthetic, apply a pneumatic tourniquet high on the upper arm.
2. Position and prepare the arm as if the humerus were to be exposed (see p. 468), leaving 12 cm of skin exposed above and below the tip of the olecranon.
3. An assistant flexes the elbow and holds the arm across the chest.

Access

1. Start the skin incision in the midline 10 cm proximal to the tip of the olecranon and extend it distally in a gentle curve to pass just lateral to the tip of the olecranon, ending 5 cm distal to it over the subcutaneous border of the ulna.
2. Dissect the skin and subcutaneous tissues medially and laterally as far as the epicondyles and hold the edges apart with a self-retaining retractor.
3. Identify the ulnar nerve as it lies in its groove on the posterior surface of the medial epicondyle. Carefully incise the investing fascia and mobilise the nerve proximally and distally until it disappears into muscle.

4. Pass a tape moistened in saline around the nerve, clipping the ends together with artery forceps in order to retract the nerve medially.

5. Identify the attachment of the central portion of the triceps tendon to the olecranon. Turn down a tongue-shaped flap 7 cm long based on the olecranon attachment by incising the tendon and the underlying muscle down to the bone (Fig. 29.6).

6. Sweep the residual attachments of the triceps muscle medially and laterally off the posterior surface of the condyles in continuity with the common flexor and extensor attachments.

7. Clear the olecranon fossa of fat and expose the joint capsule.

8. Incise the collateral ligaments at their attachment to the epicondyles. Dislocate the joint if necessary.

9. To expose the head of the radius in the distal part of the wound, strip the anconeus from its attachment to the ulna and retract it laterally.

10. The ulnar nerve may be transposed anteriorly if desirable (see p. 478) by detaching the common flexor origin from the anterior aspect of the medial epicondyle.

Closure

1. Suture the long head of triceps back into place with interrupted absorbable sutures through the aponeurosis.
2. Release the tourniquet and stop the bleeding.
3. Place a suction drain under the skin before closing it.

Aftercare

1. Apply a padded plaster back slab on the upper arm to the wrist with the elbow flexed to 90° and the forearm in mid-rotation.
2. Remove the drain after 48 hours.
3. Remove sutures in 10–12 days and mobilise the arm according to the basic procedure carried out.

POSTEROLATERAL APPROACH (Fig. 29.7)

Appraise

This approach is particularly suitable for exposing the head of the radius and can be extended distally to expose the upper proximal third of the radius and adjoining ulna.

Prepare

Position the patient and drape the arm as for the posterior approach.

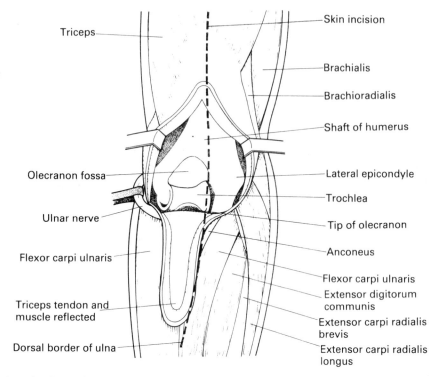

Triceps

Skin incision

Brachialis

Brachioradialis

Shaft of humerus

Olecranon fossa

Lateral epicondyle

Trochlea

Ulnar nerve

Tip of olecranon

Anconeus

Flexor carpi ulnaris

Flexor carpi ulnaris

Extensor digitorum communis

Triceps tendon and muscle reflected

Extensor carpi radialis brevis

Dorsal border of ulna

Extensor carpi radialis longus

Fig. 29.6 Posterior approach to the elbow joint.

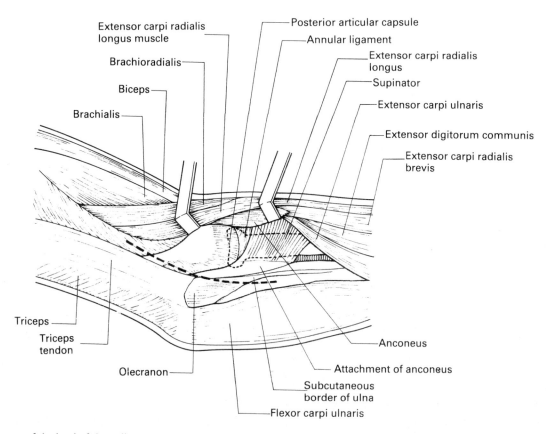

Extensor carpi radialis longus muscle

Posterior articular capsule

Annular ligament

Brachioradialis

Extensor carpi radialis longus

Biceps

Supinator

Brachialis

Extensor carpi ulnaris

Extensor digitorum communis

Extensor carpi radialis brevis

Triceps

Triceps tendon

Anconeus

Attachment of anconeus

Olecranon

Subcutaneous border of ulna

Flexor carpi ulnaris

Fig. 29.7 Exposure of the head of the radius.

Access

1. Begin the skin incision 3 cm proximal to the tip of the olecranon and continue distally between the olecranon and the lateral epicondyle down to the subcutaneous border of the ulna (Fig. 29.7).

2. Divide the subcutaneous tissue and cut the deep fascia between the ulna and the anconeus and the extensor carpi ulnaris muscles.

3. Strip the anconeus from the ulna subperiosteally. Retract it laterally to expose the capsule covering the radial head and in the distal part of the wound the supinator muscle.

Closure

1. Release the tourniquet.
2. Secure haemastasis.
3. Re-attach the anconeus.
4. Close the skin.

Aftercare

Immobilise the elbow with padded back slab as above.

LATERAL APPROACH (Fig. 29.8)

Appraise

This approach is suitable for treating fractures of the lateral epicondyle and for opening the lateral aspect of the joint.

Prepare

Position the patient and drape the arm as above.

Access

1. Flex the elbow and begin the skin incision 3–4 cm proximal to the lateral epicondyle. Continue it distally just anterior to the epicondyle and along the lateral surface of the forearm.

2. Retract the skin edges to expose the lateral epicondyle.

3. Develop the interval between the triceps posteriorly and the origin of extensor carpi radialis and brachioradialis anteriorly to expose the lateral border of the humerus.

4. The radial nerve lies deep to these muscles and must be protected at the proximal end of the wound, especially as it enters the interval between the brachioradialis and brachialis muscles (Fig. 29.8).

5. Detach the common extensor origin from the epicondyle and extend the wound distally between extensor carpi ulnaris anteriorly and flexor carpi ulnaris posteriorly.

Closure

1. Release the tourniquet and stop bleeding.
2. Flex the elbow and re-attach the common extensor origin to the bone with two or three mattress sutures.
3. Close the skin.

Aftercare

Apply a plaster padded back slab as before.

MEDIAL APPROACH (Fig. 29.9)

Appraise

This approach is suitable for operations on the medial condyle, epicondyle and on the ulnar nerve and the common flexor origin.

Access

1. Flex the elbow to a right angle. Begin the skin incision 3 cm proximal to the medial epicondyle and carry it just anterior to the epicondyle for a further 3 cm.

2. Identify the ulnar nerve in the groove on the posterior aspect of the epicondyle and isolate if more than minimal exposure is required (see Posterior Approach).

3. Divide the common origin of the flexor muscles close to their attachment to the medial epicondyle leaving sufficient stump for later re-attachment.

4. Dissect the muscle mass anteriorly towards the front of the elbow joint, taking care not to damage the branches of the median nerve which enter the muscles from the lateral (deep) side.

5. Expose the antero-medial aspect of the capsule which may be incised to open the joint.

Closure

1. Release the tourniquet.
2. Repair the capsule.
3. Re-attach to common extensor muscles to their origin with 2/0 absorbable mattress sutures.
4. Close the skin.
5. Apply a padded plaster back slab as before.

FRACTURES OF THE LOWER END OF THE HUMERUS

SUPRACONDYLAR FRACTURES

Appraise

1. This fracture can usually be treated conservatively by manipulation or olecranon traction.

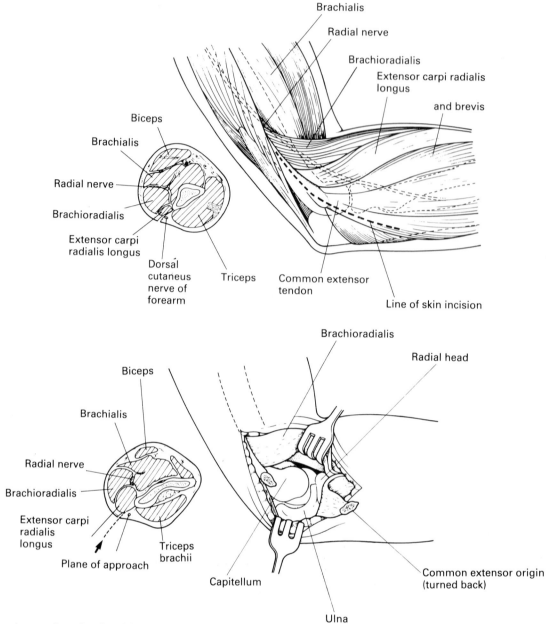

Fig. 29.8 Lateral approach to the elbow joint.

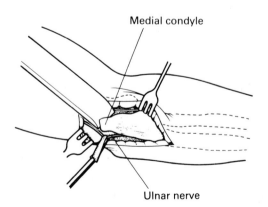

Fig. 29.9 Medial approach to the elbow joint.

2. Take anteroposterior radiographs of both elbows in a comparable position (usually acutely flexed) after closed reduction.

3. Draw a line along the epiphyseal surface of the lower humeral metaphysis, and measure the angle between this and a line perpendicular to the long axis of the humerus. Compare this angle (Baumann's angle) on the two sides (Fig. 29.10).

4. Residual varus or vagus tilt of more than 10° requires operative correction.

5. Circulatory impairment either before or after closed reduction demands immediate exploration of the brachial artery if the circulation cannot be restored by allowing the

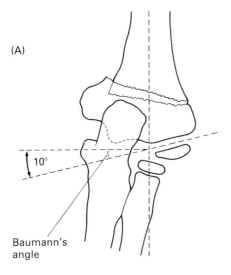

(A)

10°

Baumann's
angle

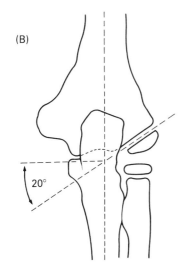

(B)

20°

Fig. 29.10 Measurement of Baumann's angle.

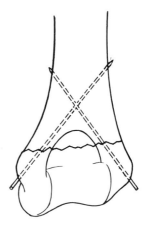

Fig. 29.11 Supracondylar fracture of the humerus held by crossed Kirschner wires.

elbow to extend, but this should not be undertaken by the inexperienced (see vascular injuries, Ch. 23).

Access

1. Expose the fracture through the posterior approach but do not strip the muscles from the epicondyles.
2. Identify but do not disturb the ulnar nerve.

Action

1. Drill a 1 mm Kirschner wire (K-wire) through the fracture surface of the distal fragment at approximately 45° to the long axis of the humerus with a hand drill, so that it emerges through the medial epicondyle and the overlying skin. Take care to avoid the ulnar nerve.
2. Withdraw the wire until only 1–2 mm protrudes from the fracture.

3. Reduce the fracture under direct vision, freeing any interposed soft-tisse.
4. Flex the elbow to 90°, and drill the K-wire back across the fracture to engage the lateral cortex of the shaft of the humerus (Fig. 29.11).
5. Through a small stab wound over the lateral condyle, drill a second wire across the fracture site to engage the medial cortex of the shaft.
6. Drill another wire across the fracture site from either the medial or the lateral side at a slightly different angle, if fixation is not adequate.
7. Take X-rays to check the accuracy of the reduction and the position of the wires.
8. If satisfactory, cut the wires leaving the ends just beneath the skin.

Aftercare

1. Apply a padded plaster back slab.
2. Check the circulation and leave instructions that the radial pulse is to be taken every hour for the next 12 hours.
3. Remove the plaster at 4 weeks.
4. Remove the Kirschner wires at 3 months (see p. 448).

SEPARATION OF MEDIAL EPICONDYLE

Appraise

If the displacement of the medial epicondyle is greater than one half the diameter of its base, open reduction is required.

Action

1. Use the medial approach (see p. 473) but do not detach the common flexor muscles from their bony attachments.

2. Identify the epicondyle which may be rotated through 180° or even lie within the elbow joint.

3. Flex the elbow to relax the flexor muscles which are attached to the fragment.

4. Impale the epicondyle on a Kirschner wire (K-wire). Then reduce it accurately and drill the wire into the lateral cortex of the humerus.

5. Check the position of the fragment and the wire on X-ray.

6. Cut the wire just beneath the skin.

Aftercare

1. Immobilise the elbow at right angles in the padded plaster back slab for 2 weeks.

2. Remove the K-wire at 6 weeks.

FRACTURES OF THE LATERAL CONDYLE

Appraise

1. This injury is essentially a fracture separation of the capitular epiphysis of the humerus and occurs in children.

2. The fragment, being partly cartilaginous, is much larger than it appears on X-ray and includes a portion of the metaphysis.

3. When the fragment is displaced, perform open reduction and internal fixation.

Action

1. Use the lateral approach.

2. Expose the fracture between the triceps posteriorly and the brachioradialis and extensor carpi radialis longus anteriorly, taking care not to detach the extensor muscles from the fragment.

3. Hold the fragment gently with toothed tissue forceps and impale it on a Kirschner wire (K-wire) through the metaphyseal part with a power drill.

4. Replace the fragment accurately in its bed and drill the wire across the fracture site and into the opposite cortex.

5. Insert a second K-wire at a different angle to the first.

6. Check the position of the fragment and the wires on X-ray.

7. Cut the wires off just below the skin.

Aftercare

1. Mobilise the elbow at a right angle and in mid-rotation in a padded back slab for 4 weeks.

2. Remove the wires at 6 weeks.

FRACTURES OF THE CAPITELLUM

Appraise

1. Fractures of the capitellum are often overlooked.

2. Open reduction and internal fixation is invariably necessary.

Action

1. Use the lateral approach.

2. Open the joint and reduce the fracture.

3. Fix the fragments into place with two diverging K-wires. These can only be introduced through the articular cartilage and should penetrate the posterolateral cortex of the lower end of the humerus by at least 0.5 cm.

4. Check the position of the fracture and wires on X-ray.

5. Cut the wires flush with the surface of the articular cartilage and tap the ends so that they lie deep to it with a small punch.

Aftercare

1. Immobilise the elbow at a right angle in a padded plaster back splint for 4 weeks.

2. Remove the wires at 6 weeks from the humeral side (see p. 448).

OTHER INTRA-ARTICULAR FRACTURES

The operative treatment of these fractures is controversial and the result is usually no better than non-operative treatment. Do not attempt operation if you are inexperienced.

FRACTURES OF THE PROXIMAL RADIUS AND ULNA

FRACTURES OF THE OLECRANON

Appraise

1. Displaced fractures invariably require open reduction and internal fixation.

2. Non-comminuted fractures can be fixed with a single screw.

3. Comminuted fractures require more complicated techniques or excision of the fragments and re-attachment of the triceps to the ulna.

Action

1. Use the distal part of the posterior approach and expose the fracture.

2. Remove any small fragments of bone and haematoma from the elbow joint and the periosteum for 1–2 mm from the bone ends.

3. Grasp the olecranon firmly with a towel clip and extend the elbow until the fracture can be reduced.

4. Incise the triceps aponeurosis over the tip of the olecranon. Drill a hole from the point of the olecranon with a 3.6 mm drill towards and into the anterior cortex of the ulna 1 cm distal to the coronoid process (Fig. 29.12).

5. When the tip of the drill is judged to have crossed the fracture site but before it strikes the anterior cortex of the ulna, open the fracture site to make sure that the articular surface of the olecranon has not been breached.

6. Reduce the fracture once more and change the angle of the drill if necessary before drilling through the anterior cortex of the ulna.

7. Remove the drill carefully and enlarge the hole in the cortex of the olecranon with a Paton's burr while maintaining the reduction.

8. Fix the fragment into place with a 3.6 mm screw, taking care not to over-tighten.

9. Check the reduction and the position of the screw with X-rays.

10. Release the tourniquet.

11. Close the skin.

Aftercare

1. Immobilise the elbow in a padded back slab for 3 weeks.

2. Encourage gentle exercises.

FRACTURES OF THE HEAD OF THE RADIUS

Appraise

1. Undisplaced fractures of the radial head can be treated conservatively.

2. Displaced and tilted marginal fractures involving more than a third of the head of the radius should be treated by reducing and fixing the fragment into place.

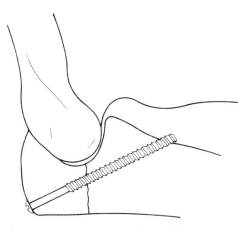

Fig. 29.12 Fracture of the olecranon held by oblique screw.

3. Treat comminuted fractures by excision of the radial head.

Action

1. Use the posterolateral approach (see p. 471).

2. Incise the capsule and the annular ligament in the long axis of the radius as far as the proximal edge of the supinator muscles.

3. If the head is comminuted, remove the loose fragments of bone and assemble them to make up the head of the radius to ensure that none are left behind.

4. Trim the stump of the neck of the radius with bone nibblers to form a flat surface.

5. Reduce large marginal fragments and secure them by drilling two thin K-wires through the circumference of the fragments and into the residual part of the head, taking care not to penetrate the opposite surface.

6. Cut the wires flush with the surface and tap them gently below with a punch.

7. Repair the annular ligament and capsule with 2/0 absorbable sutures.

Aftercare

Immobilise the elbow in a padded back slab at 90° for 2 weeks.

MONTEGGIA FRACTURES

Appraise

Dislocation of the radial head associated with a displaced fracture of the shaft of the ulna usually requires open reduction and internal fixation, except in the child and the very old.

Action

1. Use the posterolateral approach and extend the incision distally along the subcutaneous border of the ulna until the fracture site is exposed.

2. Retract the anconeus and extensor carpi radialis longus anteriolaterally to expose the front of the joint, when the head of the radius will frequently be found button-holing the capsule.

3. Open the capsule. Reduce the head of the radius and the fracture of the ulna by pulling on the arm.

4. Stabilise the fracture with a plate and screws (see p. 450) applied to the posterolateral surface of the ulna.

5. Repair the annular ligament and capsule.

OPERATIONS ON THE ELBOW JOINT

ARTHROTOMY TO REMOVE LOOSE BODIES

Appraise

1. Locate the position of the loose bodies immediately before operation on X-ray.
2. Choose the most appropriate approach according to their position.

Action

1. Use the approach which gives the best access to the loose bodies.
2. Open the joint and remove the loose bodies.
3. Flex and extend the elbow and rotate the forearm to get the inaccessible loose bodies into view.
4. Irrigate the joint with saline to ensure that all the loose bodies have been removed.

Aftercare

1. Immobilise the elbow in 90° of flexion in a padded back slab for 10 days.
2. Remove sutures and mobilise.

SYNOVECTOMY

Appraise

1. Removal of the inflamed synovium from the elbow joint is usually carried out in the early stages of rheumatoid arthritis and is frequently combined with excision of the head of the radius through the lateral approach.
2. If access is insufficient, also open the joint from the medial side.

Action

1. Use the lateral approach.
2. Incise the capsule of the joint longitudinally along the anterior border of the lateral ligament which runs from the lateral epicondyle to the annular ligament.
3. Divide the annular ligament and place a ring-handled spike bone lever around the neck of the radius just proximal to the superior margin of the supinator. Take great care to avoid injury to the posterior interosseous nerve.
4. Divide the neck of the radius immediately distal to the head with an oscillating bone saw (narrow blade). Alternatively, use a 1.5 cm osteotome but take care not to split the bone.
5. Remove as much of the inflamed synovium as possible from the anterior compartment of the joint piecemeal with small long-nosed bone nibblers.

6. Incise the capsule along the posterior edge of the lateral ligament and extend the elbow to give access to the posterior compartment and the olecranon fossa.

Closure

1. Release the tourniquet and stop the bleeding.
2. Close the capsule with 2/0 absorbable sutures and re-attach the common extensor muscles.
3. Insert a suction drain and close the skin.

Aftercare

1. Immobilise the elbow at a right angle in a padded back slab for 10 days.
2. Remove the suction drain after 48 hours.
3. Mobilise the elbow after removal of the stitches at 10 days.

RELEASE OF THE COMMON EXTENSOR ORIGIN

Appraise

Release of common extensor origin is carried out for chronic tennis elbow.

Action

1. Use the lateral approach (Fig. 29.8).
2. Divide the attachment of the common extensor muscles of the forearm to the lateral epicondyle close to the bone, and dissect it off the underlying lateral and annular ligaments.
3. The muscle mass retracts distally leaving a gap of 0.5 cm between the stump and the lateral epicondyle.
4. Re-attach the muscles to the underlying lateral ligament and annulus with 2/0 absorbable sutures.

Closure

Close the wound after release of the tourniquet and haemostasis.

Aftercare

1. Immobilise the elbow in a padded back slab for 2 weeks.
2. Remove the stitches and mobilise.

ANTERIOR TRANSPOSITION OF THE ULNAR NERVE

Appraise

Transposition of the ulnar nerve may be carried out for the treatment of ulnar neuritis, to gain length to repair the nerve following injury, or as part of another procedure.

Action

1. Use the medial approach (Fig. 29.9).
2. Identify the ulnar nerve in the ulnar groove and incise the investing fascia in the line of the nerve, preserving its blood supply.
3. Place a saline-soaked tape around the nerve and gently lift it from its bed.
4. Free the nerve proximally until it passes anteriorly through the intermuscular septum.
5. Excise the intermuscular septum from this point to the medial condyle.
6. Free the nerve distally as it passes between the two heads of flexor carpi ulnaris. Several short small articular branches may be divided, but preserve the nerve to flexor carpi ulnaris.
7. Divide the common flexor origin anterior to the ulnar nerve, leaving a cuff of tissue attached to the bone for later re-attachment.
8. Place the nerve deep to the common flexor muscle mass and ensure there are no kinks in its course.

Closure

1. Re-attach the common flexor muscles with three or four absorbable mattress sutures.
2. Release the tourniquet and close the wound.

Aftercare

1. Immobilise the elbow at 90° of flexion and with the forearm in mid-rotation in a padded plaster back slab for 2 weeks.
2. Then remove the stitches and mobilise the elbow.

EXCISION OF AN OLECRANON BURSA

Appraise

Do not excise the olecranon bursa if it is acutely inflamed. Aspirate it and immobilise the elbow until the inflammation has resolved. Then remove it if necessary.

Action

1. Incise the skin longitudinally over the bursa to include any sinuses within the incision, taking care not to cross the point of the elbow.
2. Find the plane between the wall of the bursa and the surrounding soft tissue on either side of the midline.
3. Identify the ulnar nerve and dissect out the bursa with curved scissors.

Closure

Release the tourniquet, obtain haemostasis and close the wound with a suction drain in situ.

Aftercare

1. Apply a compression dressing with the elbow flexed to 90°.
2. Remove the dressings and sutures after 10 days.

APPROACHES TO THE FOREARM

The shafts of the radius and ulna are best approached through separate incisions, the ulna from behind and the radius from in front.

POSTERIOR APPROACH TO THE ULNA
(Fig. 29.13)

Prepare

1. The patient is under general anaesthesia, lying supine. Have a large arm table attached to the operating table.
2. Apply a pneumatic tourniquet around the upper arm.
3. Prepare the skin from above the elbow to the finger tips.
4. Cover the arm board with a waterproof sheet and towel.
5. Drape off the arm just proximal to the elbow with a triangular towel.
6. Cover the head and trunk with a large sheet.
7. Cover the fingers and hand as far as the wrist with a size 8 surgical glove.
8. Pass the arm through a large sheet with a hole in the centre.

Action

1. Incise the skin along the subcutaneous border of the ulna over that part of the forearm to be exposed.
2. Divide the common aponeurosis which attaches to the bone the flexor carpi ulnaris and flexor digitorum profundus medially and the extensor carpi ulnaris laterally.
3. Separate the muscles from the bone with a periosteal elevator to expose the shaft of the ulna.

THE ANTERIOR APPROACH TO THE RADIUS
(Fig. 29.14).

Prepare

1. Prepare the arm as above.
2. Supinate the forearm.

Access

1. Incise the skin proximally from the radial styloid in

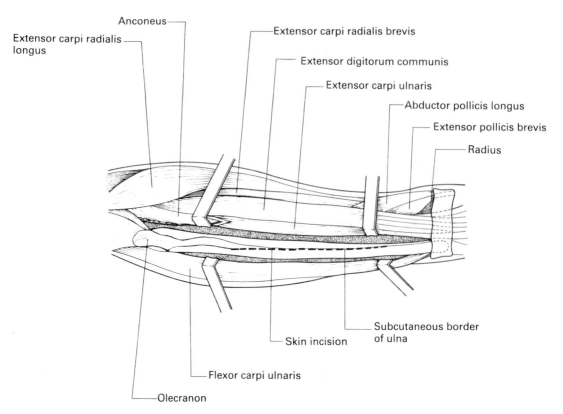

Anconeus

Extensor carpi radialis longus

Extensor carpi radialis brevis

Extensor digitorum communis

Extensor carpi ulnaris

Abductor pollicis longus

Extensor pollicis brevis

Radius

Subcutaneous border of ulna

Skin incision

Flexor carpi ulnaris

Olecranon

Fig. 29.13 Exposure of the shaft of the ulna.

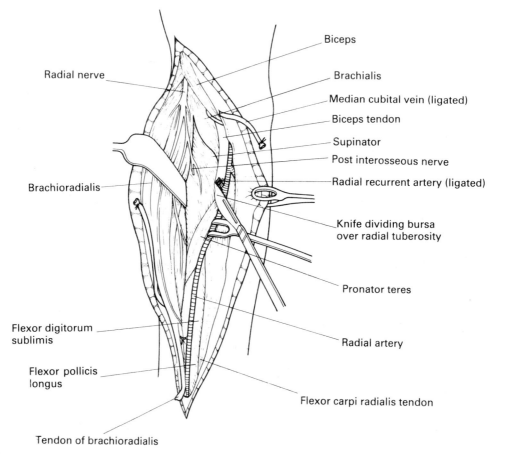

Radial nerve

Biceps

Brachialis

Median cubital vein (ligated)

Biceps tendon

Supinator

Post interosseous nerve

Radial recurrent artery (ligated)

Brachioradialis

Knife dividing bursa over radial tuberosity

Pronator teres

Flexor digitorum sublimis

Flexor pollicis longus

Radial artery

Flexor carpi radialis tendon

Tendon of brachioradialis

Fig. 29.14 Anterior approach to elbow and proximal radial shaft.

the interval between the brachioradialis and the flexor carpi radialis muscles in a straight line as far as the lateral side of the biceps tendon, to expose the whole radial shaft. More limited exposure to any part of the radius is gained by using an appropriate part of this incision.

2. Starting at the distal end of the incision, identify and protect the sensory branch of the radial nerve as it lies beneath the brachioradialis.

3. Mobilise flexor carpi radialis and the radial artery and vein, and retract them medially to expose the flexor digitorum sublimis, flexor pollicis longus and the pronator quadratus in the floor of the wound.

4 Pronate the forearm and elevate flexor pollicis longus and pronator quadratus subperiosteally from the outer edge of the radius. Strip them medially to expose the distal two-thirds of the anterior aspect of the radius.

5. To expose the proximal third of the radius, supinate the forearm and extend the incision proximally. Divide and tie the large superficial vein crossing the middle part of the wound.

6. Expose the biceps tendon and divide the deep fascia on its lateral side with blunt nosed scissors.

7. Retract the belly of the brachioradialis and the long and short radial extensors of the wrist laterally, and the flexors medially, to expose the radial artery. Divide and carefully ligate the fan-shaped leash of vessels passing laterally from the artery (Fig. 29.15).

8. Flex the elbow to 90° to expose the supinator.

9. Cut down to the tuberosity of the radius immediately lateral to the attachment of the biceps tendon.

10. From this point sweep the supinator laterally off the bone with a periosteal elevator. The vulnerable posterior interosseous nerve lies within its substance.

11. Pronate the forearm to expose the lateral aspect of the radius.

Closure

1. Replace the muscles which have been stripped from the bone and tack them into place with absorbable sutures as appropriate.

2. Release the tourniquet and stop the bleeding.

3. Insert a suction drain.

4. Close the skin.

FRACTURES OF THE SHAFTS OF THE RADIUS AND ULNA: OPEN REDUCTION AND INTERNAL FIXATION

Appraise

1. Fractures of both bones of the forearm usually require open reduction and internal fixation because of the difficulty of correcting rotational malalignment of the bones by manipulation.

2. Open reduction and internal fixation is required unless reduction is near perfect.

Access

1. Use the posterolateral approach for fractures of the proximal third of the radius (see p. 471). Extend this distally along the subcutaneous border of the ulna to expose the ulnar fracture.

2. Use the anterior approach to the radius for fractures of the distal two-thirds of the bone and the posterior approach to the ulna for fractures throughout its length.

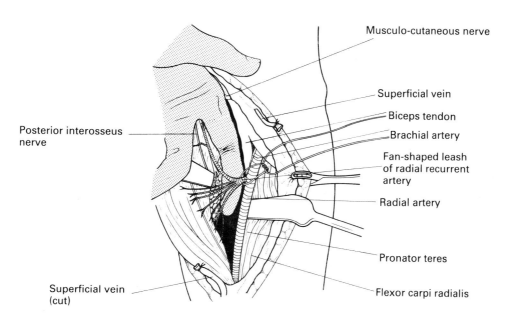

Fig. 29.15 Division of the branches of the radial artery.

Action

1. Expose both fracture sites.
2. Evacuate the haematoma and remove any small detached fragments of bone.
3. Strip the soft tissues from the bone for 3–4 cm on either side of the fracture site.
4. Strip the periosteum for 3–4 mm from the bone ends with a rougine.
5. Place a small Hey Groves bone clamp on the radius on either side of the fracture site and reduce the fracture.
6. Remove the clamps and reduce the ulnar fracture. It is essential to reduce both fractures before either of them is plated, because if one is plated before reduction of the other, then reduction of the second fracture is frequently impossible.
7. Remove the clamps and carefully place a four or six holed plate (depending on the proximity of the fracture to the bone ends) on to the deep surface of the ulna. Bend it to fit the contours of the bone if necessary.
8. Replace the plate and hold it in position with small bone clamps. Before fixing it to the bone make sure that the radial fracture is still reduced.
9. Fix the plate to the bone (see p. 450) and remove the clamps.
10. Bridge the radial fracture with a similar plate on its flexor surface, bending it if necessary before fixing it.

Closure

1. Release the tourniquet. Stop the bleeding.
2. Insert a suction drain into each of the wounds.
3. Allow the soft tissues to fall into place.
4. Close the skin only, to avoid compartment syndrome.

Aftercare

1. Apply a pressure dressing.
2. Remove the drains after 48 hours and start gentle movements of the elbow and forearm.
3. Remove the stitches at 10 days and immobilise the arm in a full arm plaster for 6 weeks.

APPROACHES TO THE WRIST

ANTERIOR APPROACH (Fig. 29.16)

Prepare

1. Position the anaesthetised patient with the affected limb on a large arm table.
2. Use a pneumatic tourniquet on the upper arm.
3. Clean the forearm and fingers and drape the limb as described for the upper arm, but leave the fingers and hand exposed.

Access

1. Incise the skin in a broad curve, skirting the thenar eminence as far as the mid-point of the transverse palmar crease. Continue almost transversally in the skin crease for 1 cm before curving proximally and extending the incision along the radial side of the flexor carpi radialis tendon for 3–4 cm.

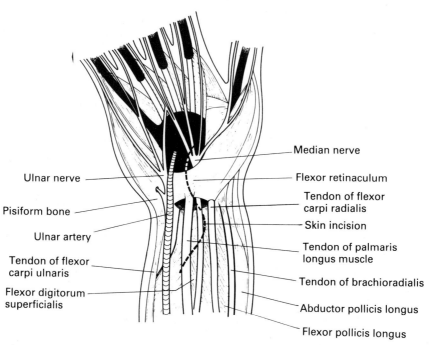

Fig. 29.16 Anterior approach to the wrist.

2. Retract the skin edges with skin hooks. The anterior carpal ligament will be exposed in the distal part of the wound and is continuous proximally with the deep fascia of the forearm.

3. Carefully incise the deep fascia between the palmaris longus (if present) and flexor carpi radialis, exposing the median nerve.

4. Retract the median nerve and palmaris longus towards the ulnar side to expose the tendon of flexor pollicis longus which should also be retracted medially.

5. The pronator quadratus lies in the floor of the wound. Divide this longitudinally to expose the lower end of the radius and the radiocarpal joint.

Closure

1. Remove the tourniquet and stop bleeding.
2. Close the skin only.

POSTERIOR APPROACH

Access

1. Prontate the forearm.
2. Make a straight incision 10 cm long on the dorsum of the wrist centred on Lister's tubercle.
3. Retract the skin edges with skin hooks and expose the extensor retinaculum. Divide this close to its ulnar attachment and turn it towards the radial side of the wound to expose the extensor tendons.
4. Separate the tendons of extensor digitorum on the radial side from extensor digit minimi on the ulnar side to expose the capsule of the wrist joint and the inferior radio-ulnar joint.

Closure

1. Allow the tendons to fall into place.
2. Release the tourniquet and stop the bleeding.
3. Suture the extensor retinaculum.
4. Close the skin.

MEDIAL APPROACH

Access

1. Make a curvilinear incision centred on the ulna styloid, the proximal limb in the line of the ulna and the distal limb curving anteriorly at first and then distally in the line of the fifth metacarpal.
2. Avoid the dorsal branch of the ulnar nerve which passes on to the dorsum of the wrist immediately distal to the head of the ulna.
3. Open the capsule of the wrist joint longitudinally.

LATERAL APPROACH (Fig. 29.17)

Access

1. Make a curvilinear incision 5 cm long centred on the tip of the radial styloid.
2. Curve in a palmar direction towards the tendons of extensor pollicis brevis and abductor pollicis longus and then proximally, parallel to the radius. Curve the distal limb towards the extensor pollicis longus and then parallel to it.
3. Do not fail to identify the dorsal branch of the radial nerve immediately deep to the skin; protect it to avoid a painful neuroma.
4. Retract extensor pollicis brevis and abductor pollicis longus, the radial artery and the dorsal branch of the radial nerve towards the palm. The tubercle of the scaphoid and the lateral capsule of the wrist joint are exposed distally and the lower end of the lateral aspect of the radius proximally.

SMITH'S AND BARTON'S FRACTURES: OPEN REDUCTION AND INTERNAL FIXATION

Appraise

These injuries are often difficult to reduce and immobilise by closed methods. When this is the case, use open reduction and internal fixation.

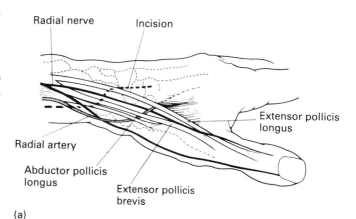

(a)

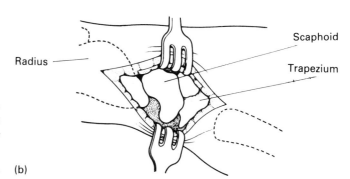

(b)

Fig. 29.17 Lateral approach to the wrist.
(a) Skin incision.
(b) Approach completed.

Access

1. Use the proximal limb of the anterior approach as far as the tranverse crease of the wrist.
2. Divide the pronator quadratus longitudinally and expose the fracture.

Action

1. Reduce the fracture by traction and bone hooks.
2. Bend an Ellis T-shaped plate to fit the contour of the lower end of the radius.
3. Secure the plate to the radius proximal to the fracture site with two screws.

Closure

1. Remove the tourniquet and stop the bleeding.
2. Close the skin only.

Aftercare

1. Apply a padded plaster with the elbow at 90° and the forearm supinated and the wrist in the neutral position.
2. Remove the plaster at 6 weeks and mobilise the wrist.

OPERATIONS FOR SCAPHOID FRACTURE

INTERNAL FIXATION OF A FRACTURE OF THE WAIST (Fig. 29.18)

Appraise

1. Carry out internal fixation of a scaphoid fracture if it is displaced or fails to unite after 8 weeks plaster immobilisation.
2. Treat old ununited fractures by grafting.

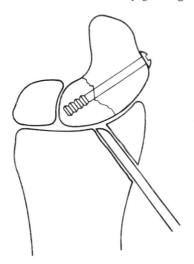

Fig. 29.18 Fracture of the scaphoid treated with a compression screw. The radial styloid is resected.

Access

1. Use the lateral (radial) approach.
2. Expose the tubercle of the scaphoid and the styloid process. Place the hand in ulnar deviation.
3. Open the wrist joint through a mid-lateral longitudinal incision in the capsule and continue the incision 1.5 cm proximally from the tip of the radial styloid through the periosteum.
4. Strip the periosteum and the radial collateral ligament in continuity from the radius.
5. Resect the radial styloid with an osteotome, starting 1 cm proximal from the tip and at an angle of 45° to the long axis of the shaft.
6. Remove the resected bone to expose the articular surface of the scaphoid and the fracture.
7. Reduce and stabilise the fracture with a small bone hook or a McDonald's dissector.
8. Insert a Kirschner wire down the long axis of the bone with a small hand drill.
9. Check the position of the wire with X-rays and adjust if necessary before calculating the length of the screw required.
10. Drill a hole with a special cannulated twist drill (if available) passed over the wire. Otherwise drill a hole alongside and parallel to the wire with an ordinary 3 mm drill.
11. Drill the distal fragment only with a 3.5 mm drill.
12. Insert a cannulated scaphoid screw of appropriate length over the wire using a special cannulated screwdriver; alternatively, use an ordinary screw parallel to the wire.
13. Remove the Kirschner wire.
14. Release the tourniquet and stop the bleeding.

Closure

1. Carefully close the capsule and periosteum and repair the radial collateral ligament.
2. Close the skin.

Aftercare

Immobilise the wrist in a lightly padded scaphoid plaster for 2 weeks only, if the fixation is very secure; otherwise, leave the plaster for 6 weeks before mobilising the wrist.

GRAFTING OF AN UNUNITED FRACTURE

Appraise

Treat ununited fractures of the waist of the scaphoid by bone grafting rather than internal fixation unless there is avascular necrosis of the proximal pole. The approach can be anterior or lateral, but I recommend the latter.

Action

1. Use the lateral approach.
2. Proceed as if the fracture were to be screwed, but pass the K-wire just to one side of the long axis of the bone.
3. Drill a hole with a 3.5 mm twist drill alongside the wire and parallel to it.
4. Fashion a peg 4 mm in diameter from the lateral cortex of the resected styloid process with bone nibblers, retaining as much cancellous bone on the deep surface as possible.
5. Push the peg into the prepared hole and pack fragments of cancellous bone down either side if there is room.
6. Trim the peg flush with the surface of the scaphoid.
6. Remove the K-wire.

Aftercare

Immobilise the wrist and forearm in a padded scaphoid plaster for 3 months.

RESECTION OF THE DISTAL RADIUS OR ULNA

THE STYLOID PROCESS OF THE RADIUS

1. Resection of the styloid process alone often relieves the pain of osteoarthritis secondary to old ununited fractures or avascular necrosis of the scaphoid.
2. The operation is performed as in the description of the internal fixation of a fracture of the scaphoid.
3. Immobilise the wrist and scaphoid in plaster until the stitches are removed at 2 weeks.

THE DISTAL END OF THE ULNA

Appraise

1. If the lower end of the ulna is prominent and wrist movements are limited and painful following malunited fractures of the lower end of the radius, it should be excised.
2. Excise it in patients suffering from painful rheumatoid arthritis of the wrist, and as part of the operation of dorsal synovectomy of the wrist or repair of the extensor tendons of the wrist.

Action

1. Use the proximal part of the medial approach.
2. Incise the periosteum longitudinally in a proximal direction for 2.5 cm from the tip of the ulna styloid; expose the bone subperiosteally.
3. Detach the ulnar collateral ligament from the tip of the styloid process leaving it in continuity with the periosteum.

4. Cut the ulna obliquely in a radial direction at an angle of 45° to the shaft, starting at a point on the medial cortex 1.5 cm proximal to the ulnar styloid.
5. Divide the remaining soft tissue attachments and remove the resected bone.

Closure

1. Release the tourniquet and stop the bleeding.
2. Close the periosteum with a continuous 2/0 absorbable suture.
3. Close the skin.
4. Immobilise the wrist in a padded back slab in a neutral position until the stitches are removed after 10 days.

EXCISION OF THE TRAPEZIUM

Appraise

The indication for this operation is painful degenerative arthritis of the carpometacarpal joint of the thumb.

Access

1. Use the distal half of the lateral approach.
2. Identify positively the articulation between the trapezium and the base of the first metacarpal and the trapezium and scaphoid. It is easy to mistake the scaphoid for the trapezium.

Action

1. Adduct the wrist.
2. Drill a hole with a 3.5 mm twist drill into the trapezium and insert a 2.5 cm long screw for half its length.
3. Apply traction through the screw and at the same time divide the soft tissue attachments of the trapezium to the adjoining bones with a small tenotomy knife which can be inserted into the intercarpal joints.
4. Rarely the bone can be removed in one piece; more frequently it must be removed piecemeal with small bone nibblers after removing the screw.
5. Pull on the thumb and inspect the cavity for residual fragments of bone before packing it with a plug of haemostatic gauze (Oxycel) to preserve the length of the thumb.
6. Release the tourniquet and stop the bleeding before closing the wound.

Aftercare

Immobilise the thumb in a padded scaphoid plaster until the stitches are removed at 10 days.

ARTHRODESIS AND ARTHROPLASTY OF THE WRIST

ARTHRODESIS

Appraise

1. There are many techniques for arthrodesing the wrist. The choice depends to some extent on the reasons for wishing to stiffen the joint.

2. Painful limitation of movement associated with osteoarthritis or rheumatoid arthritis is the usual reason for performing this operation, and the following technique is appropriate.

Access

1. Use the posterior approach. Make a straight longitudinal incision 12 cm long from the third metacarpophalangeal joint along the shaft of the third metacarpal, passing across the wrist joint to the distal end of the radius.

2. Retract the skin edges with skin hooks.

3. Detach the extensor retinaculum from its attachment to the lower end of the ulna and the pisiform and reflect it radially.

Action

1. Drill a hole through the ulnar cortex of the third metacarpal bone at its mid-point and elongate it with bone nibblers.

2. Resect the lower end of the ulna (see p. 485) but from the dorsum.

3. Palmar flex the wrist and carefully de-corticate the articular surfaces of the radiocarpal and inter-carpal joints with small bone nibblers to leave raw cancellous surfaces.

4. Push a Rush reamer through the centre of the proximal surface of the lunate, on through the capitate and into the shaft of the third metacarpal.

5. Insert a Rush pin 20 cm long and 3 mm in diameter through the hole in the third metacarpal and advance it to the radiocarpal joint as the reamer is withdrawn.

6. Push the point of the pin into the lower end of the radius. Then place the wrist in as near neutral position as possible before advancing the pin along the intramedullary canal of the radius until the crook engages the cortex of the metacarpal.

7. X-ray the forearm to be sure that the pin is within the medullary cavity of the radius and reaches the bicipital tuberosity but no further.

8. Firmly impact the carpus against the lower end of the radius, grip the hand and lower forearm firmly, and with both thumbs pressed on the dorsum of the wrist bend the Rush pin so that the wrist is dorsiflexed 10° and is in 10° of ulnar deviation.

9. Tap the pin home and insert a staple into the radius

and the carpus on either side of the pin whilst an assistant holds the wrist firmly in this position.

Closure

1. Release the tourniquet and stop the bleeding.

2. Place the extensor retinaculum deep to the extensor tendons and tack it into place with 2/0 absorbable sutures.

3. Insert a suction drain.

4. Close the skin.

Aftercare

1. Apply a compression dressing and a padded plaster front slab.

2. Elevate the arm in a roller tower suspended from a drip stand and encourage movements of the fingers.

3. Remove the suction drain after 24–48 hours.

4. Remove the plaster and stitches at 2 weeks.

ARTHROPLASTY

1. Excision of the proximal row of the carpus is rarely performed and the place of prosthetic arthroplasty has yet to be confirmed and should be left to the specialist in this field.

2. Excision of the distal end of the ulna, the styloid process of the radius and of the trapezium may be regarded as limited examples of excision arthroplasty.

OPERATIONS ON THE EXTENSOR TENDONS AT THE WRIST

EXTENSOR TENDON SYNOVECTOMY AND SYNOVECTOMY OF THE CARPUS AND WRIST JOINT (Fig. 29.19)

Appraise

Proliferation of the synovium around the extensor tendons and in the wrist and intercarpal joints occurs in rheumatoid arthritis. The 'boggy' swelling is frequently associated with painful limitation of movement and progressive destruction of the articular cartilage and bone and rupture of the tendons which may be prevented by synovectomy. The operation is usually combined with resection of the distal end of the ulna and repair of the extensor tendons if they are ruptured.

Access

1. Use the posterior approach.

2. Retract the skin carefully with skin hooks and avoid dividing the superficial veins if possible.

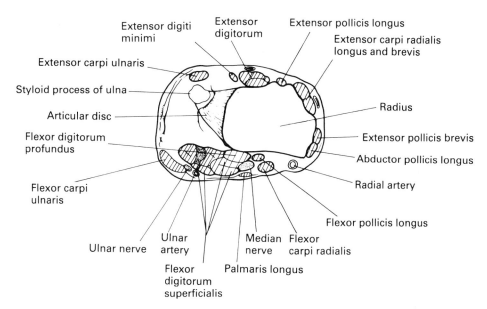

Fig. 29.19 Cross-section through the distal end of the right radius and the styloid process of the right ulna.

3. Detach the extensor retinaculum from the ulna, triquetrum and pisiform bones, and carefully reflect it radially on its attachment to the dorsal tubercle of the radius, exposing the long extensor tendons of the thumb and the extensor tendons of the wrist.

4. Incise the retinaculum overlying the tendons of extensor carpi radialis longus and brevis on the radial side of the wrist.

Action

1. Resect the distal end of the ulna (see p. 486).

2. Pick up each of the extensor tendons in turn with a blunt hook and strip the synovium from it, using a gauze swab and the convex side of the blades of a small pair of curved scissors.

3. Separate the extensor tendons in the midline and retract them to either side to expose the wrist and carpal joints.

4. Palmar flex the wrist and hand and excise the remnants of the dorsal capsule from the radiocarpal and intercarpal joints. Remove the synovium piecemeal with small bone nibblers.

5. With the wrist in neutral position replace the extensor retinaculum deep to the extensor tendons and tack it into place with 2/0 absorbable sutures.

Closure

1. Release the tourniquet and control the bleeding.
2. Insert a suction drain.
3. Close the skin.

Aftercare

1. Apply a firm padded dressing and a plaster of Paris slab to the front of the wrist.
2. Remove the drain and change the dressings after 48 hours.
3. Remove the plaster and stitches on the fourteenth day and mobilise the wrist.

REPAIR OF RUPTURED EXTENSOR TENDONS

Appraise

The extensor tendons of the fingers and thumb frequently rupture in patients suffering from rheumatoid arthritis and cannot be directly repaired.

Access

1. Use the posterior approach.
2. Reflext the extensor retinaculum (see above).

Action

1. Remove the diseased synovium and the distal end of the ulna.

2. Identify the ruptured tendon, the ends of which may be joined by attenuated granulation tissue which should be resected.

3. Suture the distal stump side to side to an adjacent intact tendon, taking care to adjust the tension so that there is no lag.

Closure

1. Release the tourniquet and control the bleeding.
2. Close the skin.

Aftercare

1. Apply a compression dressing.
2. Immobilise the wrist and fingers in full extension with a plaster of Paris front slab.
3. Remove the sutures at 2 weeks and the plaster at 3 weeks and start mobilising the fingers.

TENDON TRANSFER FOR RUPTURE OF THE EXTENSOR POLLICIS LONGUS TENDON

Appraise

Direct suture of the extensor pollicis longus tendon is usually possible if it is divided as a result of a penetrating injury, but when rupture occurs as a result of rheumatoid disease or a malunited Colles' fracture, tendon transfer is usually required.

Access

1. Use the distal part of the posterior approach to expose the distal end of the ruptured tendon which can usually be palpated under the skin.
2. Make a transverse incision 2 cm long over the neck of the second metacarpal.
3. Identify the tendons of the extensor indicis and on its radial side the tendon of extensor digitorum communis which should be divided.
4. Expose the tendons of extensor digitorum communis at the level of the wrist through a transverse incision. By pulling on the cut end of the tendon to the index finger, identify it at the level of the wrist.
5. Grasp the tendon firmly with a swab and pull it out through the proximal wound.
6. Pass the nose of straight artery forceps subcutaneously from the incision over extensor pollicis tendon to emerge at the wrist. Grasp the end of the extensor digitorum communis tendon and pull it gently under the skin to emerge on the dorsum of the thumb.
7. Cut the tendon to the correct length and suture it end to end (see p. 457) to the distal stump of the extensor pollicis longus tendon so that the thumb is extended and the tendon is under slight tension.

Closure

1. Release the tourniquet.
2. Close the skin.

Aftercare

1. Apply a padded plaster with the wrist and thumb in full extension.
2. Remove the plaster and the stitches at 3 weeks and mobilise the thumb.

DE QUERVAIN'S SYNDROME: DECOMPRESSION OF THE EXTENSOR POLLICIS BREVIS AND ABDUCTOR POLLICIS LONGUS TENDONS

Appraise

Tenosynovitis of extensor pollicis brevis and abductor pollicis longus tendons usually resolves following local steroid injections or immobilisation of the wrist and thumb. When conservative treatment fails, operation is required.

Action

1. Use the lateral (radial) approach.
2. Divide the extensor retinaculum covering the tendons on the lateral aspect of the radius.
3. Open the tendon sheaths in the line of the tendon and lift each tendon in turn from its bed with a small blunt hook.
4. Remove as much of the inflamed synovium as possible from the surface of the tendon using the convex side of the blades of a small pair of curved scissors.

Closure

1. Release the tourniquet and stop bleeding.
2. Close the subcutaneous fat and skin.
3. Immobilise the thumb and wrist in a padded plaster until the sutures are removed at 10 days.

GANGLION OF THE DORSUM OF THE WRIST

Appraise

A simple ganglion commonly arises from a synovial joint and rarely from a tendon sheath. The extensor surface of the wrist is a common but by no means exclusive site. Recurrence is common unless care is taken in removing the ganglion.

Action

1. Make an incision in a skin crease over the apex of the swelling.
2. Deepen it carefully until the bluish grey surface of the ganglion is seen.

3. Carefully dissect around the ganglion with small curved scissors.

4. Do not grasp it with toothed forceps to avoid puncturing it.

5. The swelling is often multi-locular and passes between the tendons. With care its attachment to the capsule of the joint can be identified.

6. Remove the small portion of the capsule (or tendon sheath) to which the ganglion is attached, as well as the ganglion itself.

7. Remove the tourniquet and close the skin.

Aftercare

1. Apply a compression dressing for 24 hours and then replace this with a small adhesive dressing.
2. Remove the stitches at 10 days.

MEDIAN NERVE DECOMPRESSION IN THE CARPAL TUNNEL

Appraise

1. The median nerve should be surgically decompressed if conservative treatment fails to relieve the symptoms of carpal tunnel syndrome, or if abnormal neurological signs are present.

2. Combine decompression with flexor tendon synovectomy in rheumatoid arthritis when the proliferating synovium is the cause of compression of the nerve.

Access

Use that part of the anterior approach (see p. 482) distal to the transverse crease of the wrist. This avoids the palmar cutaneous branch of the median nerve.

Action

1. The flexor retinaculum (anterior carpal ligament) is immediately exposed with the insertion of the short muscles of the thumb on the radial side.

2. Incise the retinaculum longitudinally to expose the median nerve.

3. Make sure that the proximal part of the retinaculum has been incised where it disappears under the skin at the proximal end of the wound, by passing a dissector along the surface of the median nerve.

4. Take care not to damage the transverse palmar arch at the distal end of the incision.

5. When the hypertrophied synovial coverings of the tendon are the cause of the compression, strip the synovium from each of the flexor tendons in turn (see p. 482) by pulling first the proximal and then the distal end into the wound.

Closure

1. Release the tourniquet: the nerve will 'blush' at the site of compression.
2. Stop any bleeding.
3. Close the skin.

Aftercare

1. Apply a firm compression dressing and then replace it with an adhesive dressing after 24 hours.

2. Instruct the patient to exercise the fingers immediately after the operation.

3. Remove the stitches at 10 days.

APPROACHES TO THE HAND AND FINGERS

The unique sensibility and mobility of the hand and fingers call for special care whenever surgical treatment is contemplated.

PALMAR APPROACH (Fig. 29.20)

Appraise

Incisions may be made anywhere in the palm of the hand provided that they do not cross the skin creases. As far as possible make incisions parallel to but not within the creases. They will therefore usually be gently curving (Fig. 29.20).

Prepare

1. Use a general anaesthetic or nerve block.
2. Attach the arm table to the operating table.
3. Apply a pneumatic tourniquet to the upper arm.
4. An unscrubbed assistant grasps the forearm immediately below the elbow whilst the skin is cleaned from his fingers to the patient's fingertips.
5. Place the towels as if the operation were to be on the wrist (see p. 482).
6. Supinate the forearm and spread the fingers and thumb apart and hold them extended with a 'lead hand'.

Action

1. Incise the skin and subcutaneous tissue in the line and parallel to the nearest skin crease over the structure to be exposed.

2. Carefully dissect the skin and subcutaneous tissue from the underlying fascia and retract the edges with skin hooks.

3. Expose the deeper structures with incisions made

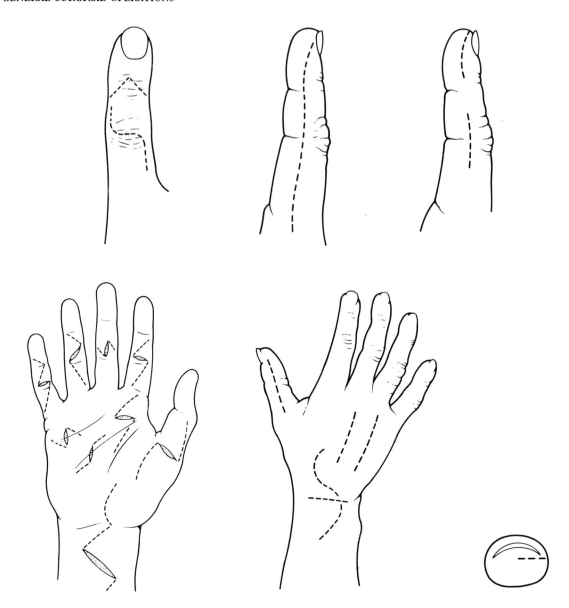

Fig. 29.20 Skin incisions in the hand and fingers.

according to anatomical considerations and not necessarily following the skin incisions.

Closure

1. Release the tourniquet and control bleeding.
2. Close the skin.

Aftercare

1. Apply a fluffed-up gauze pad to the palm.
2. Extend the wrist, flex the metacarpophalangeal joints, extend the interphalangeal joints and bandage the hand firmly over the gauze pad with the fingers in this position.

DORSAL APPROACH TO THE HAND (Fig. 29.20)

Appraise

Placing of incisions on the dorsum of the hand is not so critical and they may be longitudinal or transverse, whichever is most appropriate.

Prepare

As for the palmar approach.

Access

1. Incise the skin over the structure to be exposed.

2. Retract the skin edges.

3. Avoid damaging the superficial nerves and veins.

Closure

1. Release the tourniquet.
2. Close the skin.

Aftercare

1. Apply a padded dressing and elevate the arm in the roller towel if the patient is in hospital, or in a sling for 24 hours.

2. Instruct the patient to move the fingers as soon as possible after the operation, even though this may be painful.

MIDLATERAL INCISIONS ON THE DIGITS
(Figs 29.20 & 29.21)

Appraise

The midlateral incision may be made on either the radial or ulnar side of the digit and gives access not only to the corresponding side but also to the palmar and dorsal aspects of the fingers or thumb. In general, incisions on the radial side are more convenient.

Prepare

1. As for approaches on the hand and wrist.
2. Place the hand on the arm table with the forearm in midrotation and the thumb uppermost.

Access

1. Flex the interphalangeal joints to 45°.
2. Incise the skin longitudinally on the radial side of the digit from the apex of the proximal interphalangeal joint skin crease to the apex of the distal interphalangeal skin crease.
3. Extend the incisions proximally or distally in the same lateral line as required.
4. Carefully deepen the incision towards the shaft of the phalanx between the dorsal and palmar neurovascular bundles which are in the respective flaps.
5. Deepen the wound towards the anterior or posterior aspect of the phalanges as required.

Closure

1. Release the tourniquet.
2. Suture the skin.

Aftercare

1. Apply a pressure dressing (see p. 490).
2. Mobilise the fingers as soon as the underlying condition will allow.

FRACTURES OF THE METACARPALS AND PHALANGES: OPEN REDUCTION AND INTERNAL FIXATION

METACARPAL FRACTURES (Fig. 29.22)

Appraise

Operate upon displaced fractures of the metacarpal shafts which cannot be accurately reduced and stabilised by conservative means.

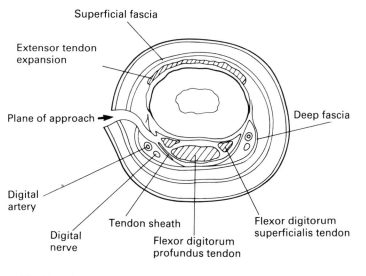

Fig. 29.21 Lateral approach to expose the flexor tendons and phalanges.

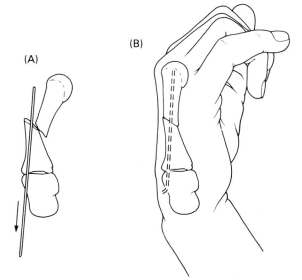

Fig. 29.22 Intramedullary fixation of metacarpal shaft fracture.

Access

1. Use a dorsal approach over the metacarpal shaft.
2. Retract the extensor tendon to one side.
3. Strip the periosteum from the bone ends for 1–2 mm on either side of the fracture site.
4. Flex the metacarpophalangeal joints fully.
5. Lift the proximal end of the distal fragment of the metacarpal out through the wound.
6. Drill a 1.5 mm Krischner wire along the medullary cavity of the metacarpal to emerge through the skin over the metacarpal head.
7. Detach the drill and withdraw the wire distally until the proximal end is level with the fracture.
8. Reduce the fracture accurately and with the wrist and fingers flexed, drill the wire back through medullary canal of the proximal fragment until it emerges through the skin on the dorsum of the wrist.
9. Detach the drill and withdraw the wire until it no longer penetrates the metacarpal head.
10. Cut the proximal end of the wire flush with the skin and allow the skin to retract over the cut end.

Closure

1. Release the tourniquet and stop any bleeding.
2. Suture the skin.

Aftercare

1. Apply a padded dressing.
2. Apply a plaster back slab with the wrist in 20° of dorsiflexion extending from the metacarpo-phalangeal joints to the elbow.
3. Elevate the arm for 24 hours.
4. Mobilise the fingers as soon as possible.

5. Remove the back slab and sutures after 10 days.
6. Remove the wires when the fracture has united.

FRACTURES OF THE SHAFTS OF THE PHALANGES (Fig. 29.23)

Appraise

1. Open reduction and internal fixation is indicated if manipulation fails to reduce the displacement or if redisplacement occurs, particularly with fractures of the proximal or middle phalanges.
2. The repair of soft tissue injuries associated with open fractures is facilitated by internal fixation of the fracture.

Action

1. Use the midlateral approach making an incision 3 cm long centred over the fracture, or utilise an open wound, carefully extending it if necessary, but do not cross the flexor creases.
2. Expose the fracture site and strip the periosteum for 1.5 mm on each side.
3. Drill a 1 mm diameter Kirschner wire into the proximal fragment of the phalanx at an angle of 45° to the long axis, starting in the centre of the open end of the medullary cavity, until it penetrates the skin on the opposite side of the digit.
4. Withdraw the wire through the skin until the tip just protrudes from the medullary cavity of the phalanx.
5. Accurately reduce the fracture and hold the fragments firmly together whilst an assistant drills the Kirschner wire back across the fracture site and into the distal fragment until the tip penetrates the cortex.
6. If the fracture is transverse or short oblique, drill a second Kirschner wire across the fracture site at an angle

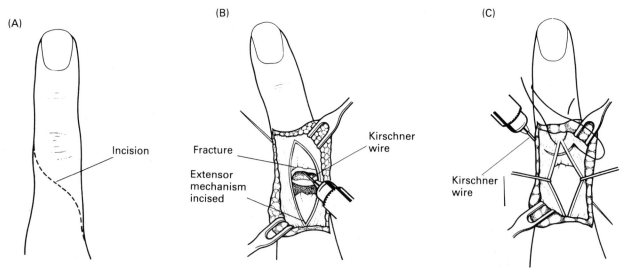

Fig. 29.23 Open reduction and internal fixation of a fracture of a phalangeal shaft.

of 70–80° to the first until it penetrates the skin on the opposite side of the finger, whilst the bone ends are held firmly together.

7. If the fracture is oblique or spiral, place the second wire 2–3 mm from, and parallel to, the first wire.

8. Cut the wires as near to the surface of the bone as possible and flush with the skin on the opposite side.

9. Tap the cut ends deep to the skin with a punch.

10. Release the tourniquet and close the wound.

Aftercare

1. Apply a boxing glove dressing (see p. 490).
2. Elevate the hand for 36 hours.
3. Encourage movements of the fingers within the dressings.
4. Remove the dressings and sutures after 10 days and actively mobilise the fingers.
5. Remove the Kirschner wires after 4–6 weeks, depending on the radiographic evidence of union.

CONDYLAR FRACTURES OF THE PHALANGES

Appraise

Collateral ligaments of the interphalangeal or metacarpophalangeal joints may be avulsed with a fragment of bone from the condyle or the whole condyle may be detached. Open reduction and internal fixation is usually required if the fragment is displaced.

Action

1. Use a midlateral approach 2 cm long, centred over the joint.

2. Take hold of the avulsed fragment of bone in fine toothed forceps and retract it sufficiently to clear any debris from the joint.

3. Take care not to detach it from its soft tissue attachments.

4. Impale the fragment on a thin Kirschner wire and then replace it accurately into its bed.

5. Drill the wire into the phalanx until it penetrates the opposite cortex and the tip is felt beneath the skin.

6. Cut the wire flush with the bone.

7. Release the tourniquet and suture the wound.

Aftercare

1. Apply a boxing glove dressing and elevate the hand for 24 hours.

2. Replace the pressure dressing with a small adhesive dressing. Strap the finger to an adjacent finger with one strip of adhesive strapping proximal and another distal to the joint.

3. Remove the strapping and the stitches after 10 days.

4. Remove the Kirschner wire after 3–4 weeks.

BENNETT'S FRACTURE OF THE THUMB
(Fig. 29.24)

Appraise

Although Bennett's fracture-dislocation of the carpometacarpal joint of the thumb can usually be reduced by traction on the abducted thumb, immobilisation in plaster is usually unsuccessful and operative treatment is preferable.

Action

1. Use a dorsal incision 3 cm long between the tendons of extensor pollicis brevis and extensor pollicis longus, centred on the carpometacarpal joint.

2. Avoid dividing the terminal branches of the radial artery and nerve.

3. Open the capsule of the joint and expose the fracture site by placing the thumb in full opposition.

4. Clear any debris from the joint and assess the size of the triangular fragment which remains in contact with the trapezium.

5. Reduce the fracture by traction on the opposed thumb.

6. Drill a hole of 1.3 mm diameter into the metacarpal shaft 5 mm from and parallel to the articular surface.

7. Insert a 'finger plate' screw.

8. Check the reduction and fixation with X-ray or image intensifier.

Closure

1. Release the tourniquet.
2. Close the capsule with 2/0 absorbable sutures.
3. Suture the skin.

Aftercare

1. Apply a padded plaster from the elbow to the interphalangeal joint of the thumb (scaphoid plaster).

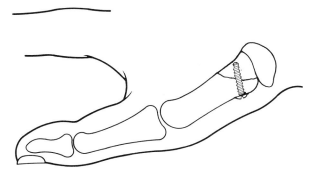

Fig. 29.24 Reduction of fixation of Bennett's fracture with a screw.

2. Remove the plaster at 4 weeks and mobilise the thumb.

REPAIR OF DIGITAL EXTENSOR TENDONS

Appraise

1. If the extensor tendon is divided at the level of the distal interphalangeal joint, direct suture of the ends is impossible; suture the proximal end to the terminal phalanx.

2. If the tendon is divided proximal to the distal interphalangeal joint, repair it as if it were divided on the dorsum of the hand (see p. 457).

Action

1. Use a transverse incision over the dorsum of the distal interphalangeal joint.

2. Find the proximal cut end which may have retracted under the skin and withdraw it into the wound.

3. Trim the end and insert a 2/0 absorbable (Dexon or Vicryl) suture by the Bunnell technique (see p. 457), leaving both ends long.

4. Trim the distal stump; drill a straight needle obliquely through the phalanx from the stump of the tendon until it emerges through the tip of the digit.

5. Drill a second needle parallel and 2–3 mm to the side of the first needle.

6. Thread one end of the suture onto the first needle and the other end onto the second needle.

7. Withdraw both needles through the pulp of the digit and tie the sutures over a padded button.

Closure

1. Release the tourniquet.
2. Suture the skin.

Aftercare

1. Cut a length of padded malleable metal splint long enough to extend from the proximal interphalangeal joint to the tip of the digit.

2. Hyperextend the distal interphalangeal joint and bend the splint to fit the contour of the digit.

3. Attach the splint to the dorsum of the digit (padded surface to the skin) with adhesive strapping.

4. Remove splint and button and as much of the suture as possible after 3 weeks and mobilise the finger.

REPAIR OF FLEXOR TENDONS IN THE HAND

Appraise

1. When the flexor tendons are divided between the distal palmar crease and the proximal interphalangeal joint

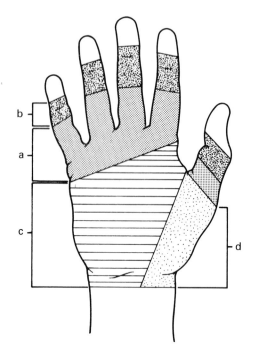

Fig. 29.25 Zones of the flexor surface of the hand and fingers.

of the fingers (Fig. 29.25a), primary repair should only be undertaken by an expert because of the dangers of adhesions between the two flexor tendons and the fibrous flexor sheath. Treat the wound and refer the patient to a specialist hand surgeon for tendon grafting at a later date.

2. When a profundus tendon or the tendon of flexor pollicis longus is divided distal to the proximal interphalangeal joint, primary suture is safe (Fig. 29.25b).

3. Primary suture of the tendons of the flexor digitorum profundus should be performed when they are divided in the palm proximal to the distal palmar crease (Fig. 29.25c).

4. Division of the flexor pollicis longus between the wrist and the interphalangeal joint of the thumb should be treated by an expert or by later tendon grafting (Fig. 29.25d).

Action

1. Excise a minimum of damaged skin from the edges of the wound.

2. Extend the wound when necessary, following the skin creases in the palm or the midlateral line in the digits. Alternatively, the wound should be extended in a zig-zag fashion on the palmar surface (Fig. 29.26).

3. Deliver both ends of the cut tendon into the wound. If the proximal end has retracted, the end can usually be palpated beneath the skin and a small accessory incision can be made over it.

4. Withdraw the end into the wound with fine artery forceps.

5. Trim the ends and suture with a Bunnell's suture (see p. 457).

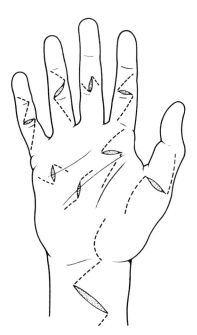

Fig. 29.26 Exposures for the suture of divided flexor tendons. Lacerations (solid lines) may be extended along the dotted lines to provide additional exposure.

6. If the tendon is avulsed from the terminal phalanx, reattach it as described for the extensor tendon (see p. 494), tying the suture over the nail.

Closure

1. Release the tourniquet.
2. Suture the skin.

Aftercare

1. Apply a gauze dressing to the wound and bandage the hand and fingers over a pad of fluffed-up gauze in the palm with the wrist and fingers flexed.
2. Add a plaster back slab from the elbow to the distal interphalangeal joint and bandage over the dressings.
3. Elevate the hand for 48 hours.
4. Allow gentle movements of the digits within the dressings.
5. Remove the plaster and dressings after 3 weeks and mobilise the fingers and hand under supervision.

RELEASE OF TRIGGER FINGER OR THUMB

Appraise

The thickening in the tendon and the flexor sheath usually lies deep to the distal palmar crease or over the metacarpophalangeal joint of the thumb and is easily palpable.

Action

1. Make an incision in the skin over the thickened tendon sheath 1.5 cm long and parallel to the skin crease.
2. Incise the palmar fascia longitudinally to avoid damaging the digital nerves and vessels.
3. The flexor tendon sheath is encountered immediately and the thickened and constricted portion identified.
4. Excise the anterior wall of the thickened part of the sheath.
5. Flex and extend the digit to ensure that the tendon moves freely.

Closure

1. Release the tourniquet.
2. Suture the skin.

Aftercare

1. Apply a boxing glove compression dressing and elevate the hand for 24 hours.
2. Replace the compression dressing with a small adhesive dressing after 24 hours and actively mobilise the fingers.
3. Remove the sutures after 10 days.

DUPUYTREN'S CONTRACTURE: LOCAL EXCISION OF THE PALMAR APONEUROSIS (FIG. 29.27)

Appraise

1. Dupuytren's contracture presents in varying degrees of severity from nodular thickening in the palm to a gross flexion contracture of one or more fingers.
2. Severe longstanding contractures cannot be corrected by excising the affected palmar aponeurosis, and amputation, especially of the little finger, is more appropriate.
3. When the contracture of the metacarpophalangeal or proximal interphalangeal joints exceeds 30°–40°, Z-plasty of the skin is required (see Ch. 31).

Action

1. Prepare for a palmar approach.
2. Incise the skin in the line of the thickened palmar fascia.
3. From one end of the incision make a second incision of equal length in the line of the palmar skin crease at an angle of 50°–60° to the first incision.
4. From the other end of the first incision make a third incision similar to the second but in the opposite direction.
5. Pick up the corner of each skin flap with a small hook and carefully dissect it off the underlying palmar fascia to

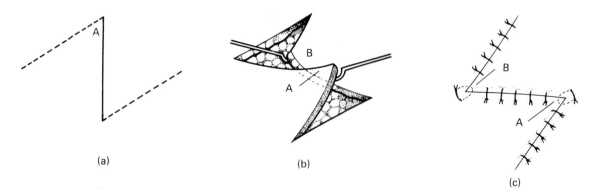

Fig. 29.27 Simple Z-plasty to release a long narrow contracture.
(a) Central limb of the 'Z' is made along the line of the contracture and the other two limbs (broken lines) are made as shown.
(b) Flaps are shifted.
(c) Flaps sutured in their new positions.

which it is attached, with a small knife. Take care not to button-hole the skin.

6. Incise the thickened deep fascia carefully over the flexor tendon and then dissect each portion laterally, looking for the digital nerves running longitudinally and in close relationship to the thickened fascia.

7. Remove the thickened fascia and any deep extensions. If necessary extend the wound proximally or distally in to the adjacent finger by further Z-plasties.

Closure

1. Release the tourniquet and stop the bleeding.
2. Transpose the apex of each flap (Fig. 29.27) and suture the skin edges.

Aftercare

1. Apply a pressure dressing over fluffed-up gauze in the palm with the fingers flexed.
2. Elevate the hand for 24 hours.
3. Inspect the wound after 24 hours and evacuate any haematoma which would prejudice the viability of the skin flaps.
4. Reduce the dressings and begin gentle movements of the fingers, avoiding full extension initially.
5. Remove the sutures at 10 days and encourage full extension of the fingers if the healing of the wound permits.

PYOGENIC INFECTIONS OF THE HAND
(Fig. 29.28)

Appraise

1. Pyogenic infections of the hand are common and most resolve with antibiotics, elevation and rest.
2. Incision and drainage is mandatory as soon as pus is

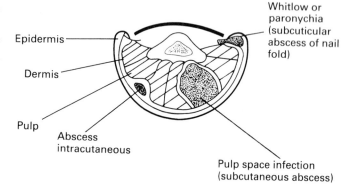

Fig. 29.28 Superficial and deep infections of the digits.

detected either visually or because of increasing pain and tenderness.

3. Open subcuticular, intracutaneous and subcutaneous infections where they are most superficial.

4. Web and palmar space infections are rare. Very little swelling is obvious in the palm, but the back of the hand is oedematous and pain is severe.

5. Tendon sheath infections cause swelling and tenderness along the line of the sheath, and the finger cannot be extended passively because of excruciating pain.

Action

1. Accurately localise the most tender point with the tip of an orange stick before induction of anaesthesia.

2. Prepare the hand for a palmar approach but do not exsanguinate the limb.

3. When the infection is superficial, make a cruciate incision over the most tender point and cut away the corners of the skin to saucerise the lesion.

4. If pus extends under the nail, remove only that portion of the nail that has been raised from the nail bed.

5. Incise in the line of the skin crease over the most

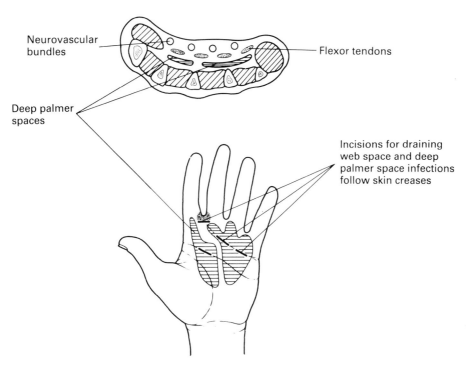

Fig. 29.29 Incisions for the drainage of web and deep palmar space infections.

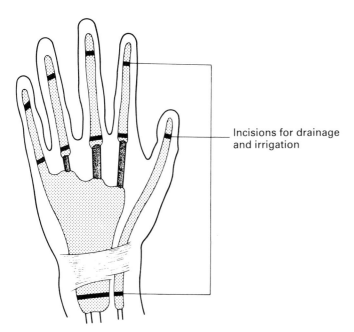

Fig. 29.30 Drainage of tendon sheath infections.

tender part when a web or palmar space is infected. Do not incise the web itself.

6. Carefully explore between the deeper structures (Fig. 29.29) by blunt dissection and follow the track to the abscess cavity.

7. Insert a small latex drain.

8. Drain tendon sheath infections through transverse incisions at either end of the sheath (Fig. 29.30).

9. Irrigate the sheath through a fine ureteric catheter with antibiotic solution until the effluent is clear.

10. Cut back the skin edges to ensure adequate drainage but do not insert a drain.

11. Leave the incision open to ensure drainage.

Aftercare

1. Place the corner of a gauze dressing in the wound to keep it open.

2. Apply Tubigrip to the fingers or a fluffed-up pressure dressing to the palm as appropriate and immobilise the hand with a plaster of Paris back slab with the fingers in semi-flexion.

3. Elevate the hand and redress daily so long as the wound is draining and then leave the dressings until epitheliazation is complete.

OPERATIONS ON THE NAILS

PARTIAL AVULSION OF A NAIL

Appraise

The nail should be preserved as far as possible, to splint any associated soft tissue or bony injury.

Action

1. Remove only that part of the nail that is separated from the nail bed, using fine scissors.
2. Apply a non-adherent dressing and tubigrip.

EVACUATION OF A SUBUNGUAL HAEMATOMA

Make a hole in the nail with a red-hot needle. The blood under pressure will spurt out. Cover the hole with a sterile dressing.

Further reading

Barton N J 1984 Review article. Fractures of the hand. Journal of Bone and Joint Surgery 66B: 159–167

Bailey D A 1963 The infected hand. H K Lewis Co. Ltd., London.

Cofield R H, Briggs B T 1979 Glenohumeral arthrodesis. Operative and long term functional results. Journal of Bone and Joint Surgery 61A: 668–677

Copeland S A, Taylor J G 1979 Synovectomy of the elbow in rheumatoid arthritis. Journal of Bone and Joint Surgery 61B: 69–73

Fisk G R 1984 Review article. The Wrist. Journal of Bone and Joint Surgery 66B: 396–407

Grace T G, Eversmann W W 1980 Forearm fractures. Treatment by rigid fixation with early motion. Journal of Bone and Joint Surgery 62A: 396–407

Henry A K 1957 Extensile exposure applied to limb surgery, 2nd edn. E & S. Livingstone Ltd. Edinburgh & London

Hovelius L, Thorling J, Fredin H 1979 Recurrent anterior dislocation of the shoulder. Results after the Bankart and Putti-Platt operations. Journal of Bone and Joint Surgery 61A: 566–570

Keon-Cohen B T 1966 Fractures at the elbow. Journal of Bone and Joint Surgery 48A: 1623–1639

Lettin A W F 1980 Total Joint Replacement. British Journal of Hospital Medicine 24: 328–345

Lettin A W F, Copeland S A, Scales J T 1982 The Stanmore total shoulder replacement. Journal of Bone and Joint Surgery 64B: 47–52

Macnicol M F 1979 The results of operation for ulnar neuritis. Journal of Bone and Joint Surgery 61B: 159–164

Neer C S 1970 Displaced proximal humeral fractures. Part I Classification and Evaluation. Journal of Bone and Joint Surgery 62A: 1077–1089

Neer C S 1970 Displaced proximal humerus fractures. Part II Treatment of Three-Part and Four-Part Displacement. Journal of Bone and Joint Surgery 52A: 1090–1103

Packer N P, Calvert P T, Bayley J I L, Kessel L 1983 Operative treatment of chronic ruptures of the rotator cuff of the shoulder. Journal of Bone and Joint Surgery 65B: 171–175

Roper B A, Levack B 1982 The surgical treatment of acromioclavicular dislocations. Journal of Bone and Joint Surgery 64B: 597–599

Stern P J, Mattingly D A, Pomeroy D L, Zenni E J, Kreig J K 1984 Intramedullary fixation of humeral shaft fractures. Journal of Bone and Joint Surgery 66A: 639–646

Orthopaedic and trauma surgery: the lower limb

APPROACHES TO THE HIP AND PROXIMAL FEMUR

The hip joint is deeply placed and relatively inaccessible. It may be exposed by several routes which are variations of the anterior, posterior and lateral approaches, which themselves afford good access for most purposes.

ANTERIOR APPROACH

Prepare

1. Order 4 units of cross-matched blood.

2. Operate with a general anaesthetic, preferably with controlled hypotension unless the patient's general condition precludes it; otherwise use an epidural or spinal anaesthetic.

3. Place the patient supine on the operating table with a sandbag under the buttock of the side to be operated on.

4. Have an unscrubbed assistant elevate the leg.

5. Clean the skin distally from the umbilicus to the knee, including the anterior abdominal wall, perineum and as much of the buttock as possible.

6. Place a waterproof sheet under the affected leg and over the opposite leg, tucking it under the buttock.

7. Place a large drape over the waterproof sheet so that the whole of the unaffected leg and foot and the lower part of the operating table are covered. Pull the top edge firmly into the groin to exclude the genitalia from the field.

8. Fold a medium sized towel ('the shut-off towel') corner to corner and place the centre of the long side firmly in the groin. Take one corner under the leg and the other over the iliac crest, and clip the corners together onto the skin at the posterior end of the iliac crest.

9. With the scrubbed assistant, hold a medium towel outstretched by the corners under the leg from the lower third of the thigh to beyond the foot. Direct that the leg be lowered carefully into it and turn the bottom end over the foot before carefully wrapping the lower thigh, leg and foot in the towel. Bandage the towel firmly onto the leg with an open weave bandage.

10. Cover the head and trunk with a large drape.

11. Place the leg through the hole in a large split sheet and pull it firmly into the groin and around the buttock but leaving the anterolateral aspect of the thigh exposed from the iliac crest distally.

12. Cover the exposed skin with a large adhesive drape wrapped around the thigh.

Access (Fig. 30.1)

1. Make an incision through the skin and subcutaneous fat from the midpoint of the iliac crest along the anterior lip of the crest to the anterior superior iliac spine and then distally along the thigh for 10 cm.

2. Divide the attachment of the gluteus medius and tensor fasciae latae muscles along the lateral lip of the iliac crest with the cutting diathermy.

3. With a periosteal elevator, strip the muscles subperiosteally from the wing of the ilium down to the margin of the acetabulum. Pack the interval between the bone and the muscle to control bleeding.

4. Develop the interval between the tensor fascia lata laterally and the sartorius and rectus femoris medially in the upper part of the thigh, taking care to retract the lateral cutaneous nerve of the thigh with the sartorius.

5. Ligate the ascending branch of the lateral circumflex femoral artery in the lower part of the wound.

6. Turn the tensor fasciae latae and the gluteus medius laterally to expose the anterior and superior aspect of the joint capsule. Divide it along its attachment to the margin of the acetabulum and then laterally towards the greater trochanter along the superior and inferior aspects of the femoral neck to open the joint.

7. More limited access to the joint may be obtained by using the distal part of the approach alone.

8. Dislocate the hip by externally rotating the leg. If the hip will not dislocate with moderate force, insert the blades of a large pair of curved scissors between the articular surfaces and divide the ligamentum teres. Then insert the curved blade of a Lane's lever and lever the head out of the acetabulum.

Closure

1. Suture the gluteus medius and tensor fasciae latae to the iliac crest with 0 absorbable sutures.
2. Insert a suction drain.
3. Suture the subcutaneous fat and skin.

POSTERIOR APPROACH

Prepare

1. Order 4 units of crossmatched blood.
2. Operate with a general anaesthetic and controlled hypotension.
3. Turn the patient onto the side on the operating table with the affected hip uppermost. Place a kidney rest firmly against the lumbar spine and a padded post against the anterior superior iliac spines.
4. Have an unscrubbed assistant elevate (abduct) the leg.

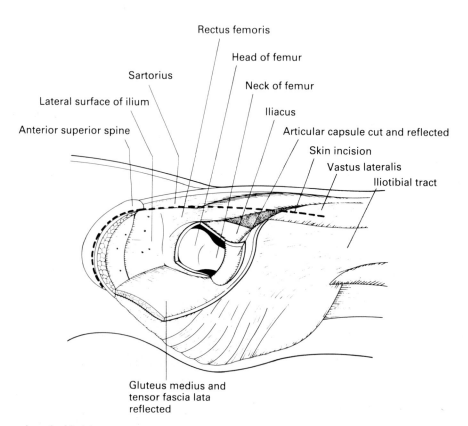

Rectus femoris

Head of femur

Sartorius

Neck of femur

Lateral surface of ilium

Iliacus

Anterior superior spine

Articular capsule cut and reflected

Skin incision

Vastus lateralis

Iliotibial tract

Gluteus medius and tensor fascia lata reflected

Fig. 30.1 Anterior approach to the hip joint.

5. Clean the skin from the costal margin to the knee, from the midline anteriorly to the surface of the table posteriorly.

6. Drape the patient as if the anterior exposure were to be used but leave the buttock and thigh exposed.

7. Cover the exposed skin with a large transparent adhesive drape.

Access (Fig. 30.2)

1. Palpate the postero-superior corner of the greater trochanter and make an incision through the skin and subcutaneous fat in a gentle curve centred on this point. This should extend 10 cm towards the posterior superior

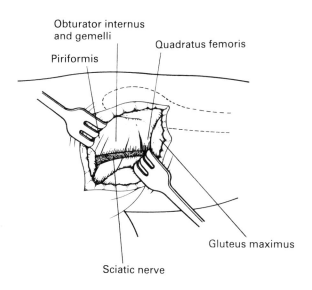

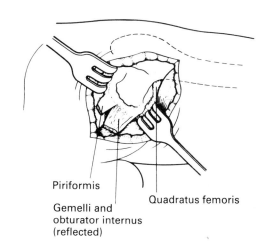

Fig. 30.2 Posterior approach to the hip joint.
(a) Gluteus maximus has been split in the line of its fibres and the edges retracted.
(b) The pyriformis, gemelli and obturator internus have been divided at their insertion on to the femur and retracted medially to expose the exterior aspect of the joint capsule.

iliac spine and 10 cm distally down the posterolateral aspect of the thigh.

2. Split the gluteus maximus in the line of its fibres proximally from the tip of the greater trochanter for the length of the proximal limb of the wound.

3. Cut the thick aponeurotic attachment of the gluteus maximus to the ilio tibial tract distally along the posterior edge of the greater trochanter for 5 cm.

4. Separate the two parts of the gluteus maximus with a large self-retaining retractor, so exposing a mass of fat in the depths of the wound.

5. The sciatic nerve lies embedded in the fat and should be carefully exposed by blunt dissection. The main bulk of the fat may then be safely excised.

6. The sciatic nerve lies on the quadratus femoris and the obturator internus, flanked by the gemelli, before disappearing under the pyriformis in the proximal part of the wound (Fig. 30.2).

7. Have an assistant flex, adduct and internally rotate the leg to put the short external rotator muscles on the stretch. Transfix the combined tendons of the obturator internus and the gemelli with a 2/0 synthetic absorbable suture 0.5 cm from attachment to the trochanteric fossa.

8. Divide the transfixed tendons as close to the bone as possible and turn the muscles posteriorly, using them to retract the sciatic nerve.

9. Divide the proximal 2 cm of the quadratus femoris 1 cm from its femoral attachment with the cutting diathermy to complete the exposure of the posterior capsule. The ascending branch of the posterior circumflex femoral artery is usually divided with the quadratus femoris and must be ligated to avoid troublesome bleeding.

10. Divide the capsule along the margin of the acetabulum and then in the line of the femoral neck to its attachment to the base of the femoral neck. The flaps may be excised or left for later repair, depending upon the nature of the operation.

11. To dislocate the hip, flex, adduct and internally rotate the leg dividing the ligamentum teres if necessary with large curved scissors (see p. 500).

Closure

1. Palpate the trochanteric fossa with the tip of the left index finger and direct the tip of an awl through the trochanter to this point.

2. Thread one end of the stay suture transfixing the tendon of the short external rotator muscles through the eye of the awl and withdraw it through the trochanter.

3. Repeat the process for the other end of the stay suture making the hole 5 mm from the first hole.

4. Draw the sutures tight and tie the ends over the greater trochanter.

5. Suture the divided part of the quadratus femoris.

6. Insert a large suction drain.

7. Repair the aponeurotic part of the gluteal insertion with 2/0 synthetic sutures.

8. Close the skin and subcutaneous tissues.

LATERAL APPROACH TO THE PROXIMAL FEMUR

This exposure may be carried proximally to expose the hip joint if required. The distal part of the approach should be used alone for access to the proximal part of the femur and the femoral neck when treating fractures in this region.

Prepare

1. Crossmatch 3 units of blood.

2. Operate with a general anaesthetic if possible, but epidural or spinal anaesthesia may also be used.

3. Place the patient supine on the orthopaedic operating table with a radiolucent perineal post.

4. Wrap the feet in plaster wool before binding them to the foot pieces of the table (see Fig. 30.3). Abduct the legs fully and tighten the clamps on the table to maintain the position.

5. Place the image intensifier between the patient's legs with the plane of the curved 'C' arm parallel to the sound leg and the X-ray source underneath the affected hip for the AP projection (Fig. 30.3). Rotate the arm to bring the source lateral to the hip for the lateral projection. Screen the hip in both planes and adjust the position of the apparatus as necessary.

When no image intensifier is available, use two portable X-ray machines. Place one between the legs with the beam directed parallel to the sound leg towards the groin of the affected hip. Place a loaded cassette in a carrier and press one edge firmly into the flank immediately above the iliac crest on the affected side, with the plane of the film at right angles to the beam. Make a trial exposure and adjust the position of the beam accordingly.

Place the second X-ray machine with the source vertically above the mid-inguinal point of the affected side. Place a loaded cassette in the carrier below the table and make a further trial exposure.

6. Clean the skin from the level of the umbilicus to the knee, including the perineum and buttock and the circumference of the thigh.

7. Hang a large drape over the sound side from the groin to beyond the toes and include the lateral X-ray machine if it is used.

8. Hang another large drape over the affected leg from the mid-thigh to beyond the toes.

9. Cover the trunk above the iliac crest with a third large sheet.

10. Cover the remaining part of the thigh with two small towels, leaving only a rectangle of skin 30 cm long by 20 cm wide exposed on the lateral side of the thigh. The anterior superior iliac spine is situated at the top corner of this rectangle.

11. Hold the towels in place with a transparent adhesive drape.

12. Cover the heads of the image intensifier (and the second portable X-ray machine if used) separately with purpose-made disposable plastic drapes or towels.

Access (Fig. 30.4)

1. Palpate the postero-superior corner of the greater trochanter and make a straight longitudinal incision from the point distally, through the skin and subcutaneous fat for 15 cm.

2. Split the fascia lata longitudinally posterior to the insertion of the tensor fasciae latae muscle in the line of the incision. Insert a self-retaining retractor to expose the vastus lateralis.

3. Identify the aponeurotic attachment of the vastus lateralis to the anterolateral surfaces of the femur, just below the greater trochanter.

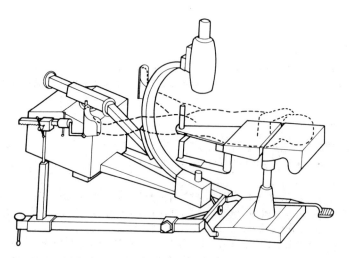

Fig. 30.3 Position and apparatus for internal fixation of a fracture of the left hip, using the image intensifier.

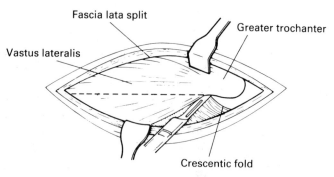

Fascia lata split

Greater trochanter

Vastus lateralis

Crescentic fold

Fig. 30.4 Cutting down on to the femoral shaft.

4. Boldly cut the vastus lateralis in the line of its fibres down to the underlying femoral shaft, starting from the postero-inferior corner of the greater trochanter and continuing distally for 10 cm.

5. Incise the aponeurotic attachment of the anterior part of the muscle to the anterolateral aspect of the femur and strip the muscle off the anterior and lateral aspects of the femur with a periosteal elevator. Insert the tip of the index finger between the vastus lateralis and the anterior surface of the femur and palpate the lesser trochanter on the postero-medial aspect of the bone.

6. Pass a Lane's lever carefully around the femoral shaft with the tip absolutely in contact with the bone so that it lies between the lesser trochanter and the femoral neck. This exposes the anterior and lateral surface of the upper femoral shaft and the base of the femoral neck.

7. Strip the posterior portion of the muscle from the bone in similar fashion and insert a second Lane's lever around the underside of the femoral shaft.

8. Coagulate the several large bleeding vessels in the substance of the muscle.

Closure

1. Insert a suction drain.

2. Suture the vastus lateralis with 0 absorbable sutures, taking large bites of the muscle with a large half-circle needle.

3. Repair the fascia lata with a continuous absorbable suture.

4. Close the subcutaneous fat and skin.

INTERNAL FIXATION OF INTRACAPSULAR FRACTURES OF THE FEMORAL NECK

Appraise

1. There are many devices and techniques which are used for internal fixation of these fractures; the choice is often a matter of individual preference.

2. Use a sliding compression screw for undisplaced fractures (Garden grades 1 and 2).

3. Use a sliding compression screw for displaced fractures (Garden grades 3 and 4), providing the operation can be carried out within 8 hours of the injury and the fracture can be accurately reduced.

4. Displaced fractures which are treated late and which cannot be reduced, especially in patients over the age of 60, require prosthetic replacement (see p. 505).

Prepare

1. Cross-match 3 units of blood.

2. Operate with a general anaesthetic.

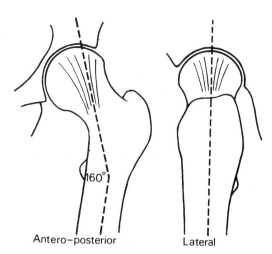

Fig. 30.5 Transcervical fractures of the femur; criteria for reduction.

3. Use an orthopaedic table with X-ray control (see p. 502).

4. Flex the hip and knee on the affected side to 90° and apply gentle traction in the line of the femoral shaft. Bring the leg down into the neutral position, maintaining the traction and at the same time internally rotating and abducting the leg.

5. Bandage the foot to the foot piece with the leg in this position and check the adequacy of the reduction with the image intensifier or X-rays in both planes.

6. On the antero-posterior view, the bony trabeculae of the neck should be disposed symmetrically about an axis making an angle of 160° with the shaft (Fig. 30.5). On the lateral view, the trabeculae of the femoral head and neck should be symmetrical about a line running down the centre of the neck. The head should not be tilted more than 5° either way.

7. If the position is unacceptable, repeat the reduction once more. If the position is still unacceptable, proceed to prosthetic replacement (see p. 505).

Access

Use the lateral approach to the upper end of the femur (see p. 502).

Action

1. Palpate the anterior surface of the femoral neck which should be approximately horizontal with the leg internally rotated.

2. Drill a 3 mm hole in the midline of the lateral cortex of the femur at the level of the lesser trochanter.

3. Load a guide wire of known length into the power drill and slip a 135° fixed angle guide over the wire (Fig. 30.6a).

4. Pass the tip of the wire through the hole in the lateral

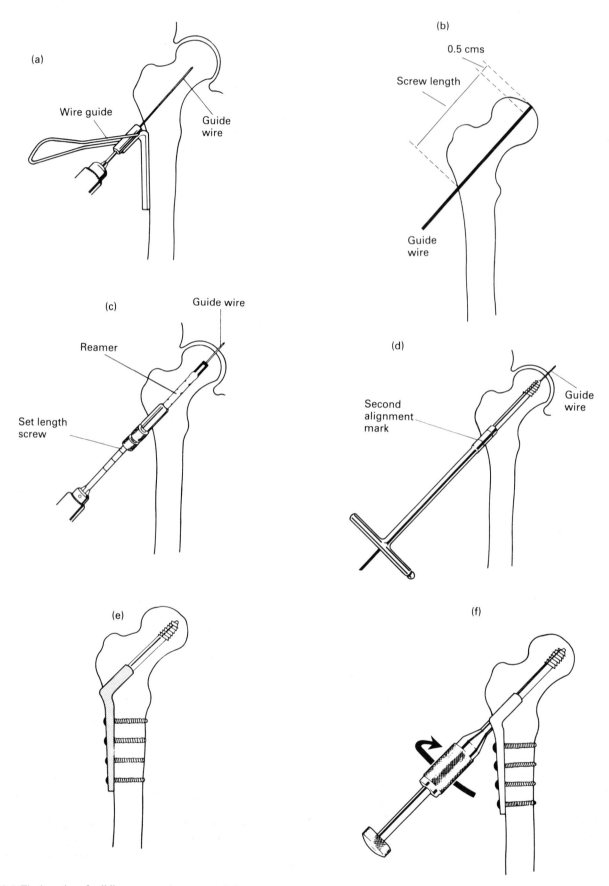

(a)

Wire guide

Guide
wire

(b)

0.5 cms

Screw length

Guide
wire

(c)

Guide wire

Reamer

Set length
screw

(d)

Second
alignment
mark

Guide
wire

(e)

(f)

Fig. 30.6 The insertion of a sliding compression screw and plate.

femoral cortex and hold the wire guide firmly against the femoral shaft. Drill 8–10 cm of the guide wire into the bone parallel to the anterior surface of the femoral neck. (N.B. If the image intensifier is used, check the position and direction of the guide wire immediately it enters the femur.)

5. Remove the drill and check the position of the guide wire in both planes with image intensifier or X-rays. The guide wire should lie within 0.5 cm of the centre of the femoral neck in both AP and lateral planes. Its tip should just penetrate the surface of the femoral head within 0.5 cm of its centre.

6. If the position of the guide wire is unacceptable, insert a second guide wire in appropriate relationship to the first and check the position once more with X-ray.

7. When the position of the guide wire is satisfactory, measure the length that lies outside the bone, and by subtraction calculate the length of wire within the bone (Fig. 30.6b). Reattach the drill and advance the guide wire across the joint into the acetabulum to stabilise the head. Pass a second wire across the joint parallel to the first and 1 cm or so from it to prevent the femoral head from rotating.

8. Set the collar on the reamer 0.5 cm less than the calculated distance between the lateral femoral cortex and the surface of the femoral head and attach it to a power drill. Pass the reamer over the guide wire and ream the channel for the compression screw (Fig. 30.6c).

9. Replace the reamer with the tap and cut the thread for the screw.

10. Select a compression screw the same length as the reamed channel. Screw it into the femoral head over the guide wire with the T-handled impactor as far as the second alignment mark. The 'key way' of the compression screw must finish on the distal side of the channel (Fig. 30.6d).

11. Remove the guide wire and insert a two-holed 135° side plate, the 'key' of which should mate with the 'key way' of the compression screw, and screw it to the femoral shaft (Fig. 30.6e).

12. Compress the fracture surfaces together firmly with the compression instrument and then replace the compression instrument with the small compression screw (Fig. 30.6f).

Closure

(See page 503.)

Aftercare

1. Remove the suction drain when drainage ceases (24–36 hours).

2. Start exercising the hip and knee 24 hours after the operation.

3. Allow the patient to sit out of bed and to walk with

a frame after 48 hours or as soon as the patient's general condition permits.

4. Over the next 14 days, ideally the patient should progress from the frame to crutches and finally to one stick, but this is not always possible.

5. Remove the stitches 10–12 days after the operation and take a check X-ray to be sure that the fracture has not displaced.

PROSTHETIC REPLACEMENT OF THE FEMORAL HEAD

Appraise

Treat displaced intracapsular fractures of the femoral neck by prosthetic replacement of the femoral head if reduction is inadequate or if there is a delay of more than 8 hours between injury and operation. Do not cement the prosthesis into the femur in frail, elderly patients.

Prepare

1. Cross-match 3 units of blood.
2. Operate with a general anaesthetic.
3. Position and drape the patient for the posterior approach to the hip (see p. 500).

Action

1. Open the posterior capsule of the hip joint through the posterior approach.

2. Suck out the blood and bloodstained serous fluid and the fracture will immediately be apparent.

3. Flex, adduct, and internally rotate the leg to open the fracture site.

4. Slip a blunt bone lever into the acetabulum behind the head and lever it out of the acetabulum, dividing the ligamentum teres (see p. 500) and any other residual soft tissue attachments with large curved scissors.

5. Measure the diameter of the femoral head with the calipers or Sillar's template, and select a Thompson prosthesis of the same diameter.

6. Line up the stem of the prosthesis with the femoral shaft. With the centre of the head of the prosthesis opposite the tip of the trochanter, mark the position of the collar of the prosthesis on the stump of the femoral neck with an osteotome.

7. Trim the femoral neck as far as possible to this line with a power saw and bone nibblers. Sometimes more of the neck will have to be removed to provide a suitable flat bed for the collar of the prosthesis.

8. Ream the medullary cavity of the femur with a broach (Fig. 30.7) until it will accept all but the last 0.5 cm of the stem of the prosthesis.

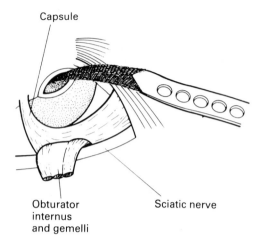

Capsule

Obturator
internus
and gemelli

Sciatic nerve

Fig. 30.7 Posterolateral approach to the hip joint; reaming the medullary cavity of the femur.

9. Tap the prosthesis home with a punch but do not force it into the femur and risk splitting the bone.

10. Place the end of Bristow's elevator between the collar of the prosthesis and the calcar and lever it out of the femur; ream the canal again if necessary.

11. Remove debris and blood clot from the acetabulum and make sure that the prosthesis fits snugly. It should move freely but should not be easily pulled out. Insert the prosthesis into the femur once again and reduce it into the acetabulum by externally rotating, abducting and extending the leg, at the same time applying direct pressure to the trochanter, pushing the prosthesis directly into the acetabulum.

13. Suture the capsule with 0 absorbable sutures if possible.

14. Insert a suction drain.

(N.B. If the patient is a good operative risk, the more experienced surgeon may elect to cement the prosthesis in the femur as described for total prosthetic replacement of the hip [see p. 509]).

Closure

See page 501.

Aftercare

1. Remove the drain after 48 hours and change the dressing.

2. Take an X-ray of the hip to check the position of the prosthesis.

3. Sit the patient out of bed after 48 hours or as soon thereafter as the general condition permits.

4. Allow the patient to walk with a frame, taking weight on the affected leg when pain permits.

5. Ideally the patient should progress to crutches and eventually to one walking stick in the opposite hand, but

this is not always possible and elderly and infirm patients may always need a frame.

EXTRACAPSULAR FRACTURES OF THE FEMORAL NECK

Appraise

1. Treat all extracapsular fractures of the femoral neck operatively unless the patient is unfit.

2. There are many devices available for fixing these fractures. The sliding (Richards) compression screw (see p. 503) is recommended.

Prepare

1. Operate with a general anaesthetic.

2. Cross-match 3 units of blood.

3. Use an orthopaedic table with X-ray control (see p. 502).

4. Do not waste time reducing the fracture. Reduce it later under direct vision.

5. Bandage the foot to the foot piece. Abduct and internally rotate the leg and apply traction through the foot.

6. Clean and drape the patient for the lateral approach (see p. 502).

Access

1. Use the lateral approach (see p. 502) to the upper end of the femur.

2. Pass one Lane's lever anteriorly and another posteriorly around the femur at the level of the lesser trochanter.

Action

1. Place a Hey-Groves bone clamp around the shaft of the femur distal to the fracture site, and use it to control the position of the femoral shaft.

2. If the fracture is comminuted, reduce any large fragments and fix them to the femoral shaft with a further bone clamp, Kirschner wires or screws.

3. Now reduce the two main components of the fracture by manipulating the leg, loosening the traction if necessary.

4. Insert the compression screw under radiographic control as described for intracapsular fractures (see p. 503).

5. Choose a plate long enough to extend beyond any secondary fracture lines and clamp it to the femoral shaft.

6. Screw the plate to the bone and remove any temporary fixation wires that may have been used to attach fragments of bone to the femoral shaft.

Closure

See page 503.

Aftercare

As for intracapsular fractures, see page 503.

OTHER OPERATIONS ON THE HIP

SLIPPED UPPER FEMORAL EPIPHYSIS: PINNING IN SITU

Appraise

1. Pin acute or acute-on-chronic slips of the capital epiphysis of the femur when the slip is less than one-third of the diameter of the head.

2. If the slip is greater, leave it to the expert.

3. Pin the opposite capital epiphysis to prevent this from slipping.

Access

Use the lateral approach to the upper femur.

Action

1. Insert one Newman's pin under X-ray control along the centre of the femoral neck into the capital epiphysis, as if a guide wire were being inserted for treating a fracture of the neck of the femur (see p. 504).

2. Insert two further Newman's pins, one on either side of the first pin but diverging from it by 10–15° in the lateral plane, until the tips are just short of the articular surface.

3. Cut off the protruding portion of the pins with Berkbecker cutters, leaving approximately 1 cm of each pin proud of the cortex.

Closure

See page 503.

Aftercare

1. Repeat the procedure on the opposite hip.

2. Start active and passive hip and knee exercises after 24 hours.

3. Start crutch walking, talking full weight on the 'normal' leg and partial weight on the opposite leg after 24–48 hours.

4. Remove stitches after 10 days.

5. Check position of epiphysis and pins after 6 weeks and allow full weightbearing.

6. Remove pins after epiphyseal plates have fused (6–12 months).

CONGENITAL DISLOCATION OF THE HIP: OPEN REDUCTION

This is carried out through the anterior approach but should be left to the expert.

INTERTROCHANTERIC OSTEOTOMY OF THE FEMUR

Appraise

1. When this operation is used to correct congenital deformities of the upper end of the femur and for the treatment of Perthes' disease in childhood, it should be left to the expert.

2. Intertrochanteric osteotomy for osteoarthritis of the hip is indicated if the hip is mobile and the patient is too young for total hip replacement.

Prepare

1. Operate with a general anaesthetic.

2. Use radiographic control.

3. If an orthopaedic table is available, use it; otherwise use a standard operating table, and replace the centre portion of the mattress that lies under the buttocks with a radiolucent cassette holder.

4. With the patient supine, abduct both hips and flex the knee so that the lower leg and foot on each side hangs over the side of the operating table, with the foot resting on a stool. Pad the leg where it lies against the edge of the table.

5. Position the lateral X-ray machine so that the tube is parallel to the inner side of the sound leg and direct it towards the opposite groin (Fig. 30.8).

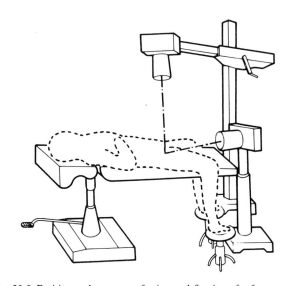

Fig. 30.8 Position and apparatus for internal fixation of a fracture or osteotomy of the right hip using standard X-ray tubes.

6. Position the AP X-ray machine so that the tube is vertically above the femoral point (Fig. 30.8).

7. Clean and drape the affected leg separately in preparation for a lateral approach to the upper femur (see p. 502).

Access

Use the lateral approach to the upper femoral shaft (see p. 502).

Action

1. Place one Lane's bone lever anteriorly between the inferior surface of the neck of the femur and the lesser trochanter (see p. 503) and a second lever posteriorly around the femoral shaft at the same point.

2. Mark the lateral cortex of the femoral shaft at this point opposite the bone levers with an osteotome.

3. Drill a 3 mm hole through the midpoint of the lateral cortex of the femur 1.5 cm above this mark.

4. Drill a guide wire of known length through this pilot hole parallel to the anterior and inferior surfaces of the femoral neck, which can be palpated with the index finger of the opposite hand in the direction of the opposite anterior superior iliac spine.

5. Remove the drill and check the position of the guide wire radiographically in both planes. Advance or withdraw it if necessary until the point is approximately 1 cm from the articular surface of the femoral head.

6. The guide wire should lie within 1 cm of the centre of the femoral neck in both planes. If the position is unsatisfactory, insert another wire using the first as a guide before withdrawing it.

7. When the wire is in a satisfactory position, calculate the length lying within the bone by subtracting the length outside the bone from the total length.

8. Slip the cannulated starting tool over the guide wire and cut the slots in the cortex of the bone for the four fins of a McLoughlin nail.

9. Select a nail equal in length to the interosseous portion of the guide wire and screw the threaded portion onto the introducer.

10. Slip the nail and the introducer over the guide wire and hammer it home taking care not to carry the guide wire in with the nail by frequently checking its length.

11. Remove the introducer and the guide wire.

12. Divide the femur transversly in both planes with the reciprocating saw at the level previously marked between the greater and lesser trochanters.

13. Control the femur with a bone clamp placed around the femoral shaft distal to the lesser trochanter, and rotate the leg to correct any rotational deformity.

14. Remove a wedge of bone from the cut end of the femoral shaft by means of a second saw cut to correct any varus or valgus deformity.

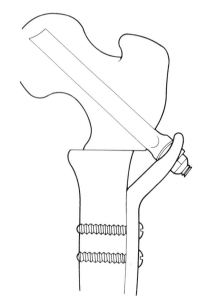

Fig. 30.9 Internal fixation of an upper femoral displacement osteotomy with a nail plate.

15. Place the slot of a 5-holed McLoughlin plate (Fig. 30.9) over the thread of the nail and hold it lightly in place with the introducer. The latter can be used to control the position of the head and neck of the femur.

16. Bring the two cut surfaces of the bone accurately together. Adjust the position of the plate after slackening the introducer until it lies against the lateral side of the femoral shaft.

17. Clamp the plate to the femoral shaft and replace the introducer with the special washer and nut (Fig. 30.9); gently tighten, taking care not to displace the bone ends.

18. Check the position radiographically and, if necessary, carry out any minor adjustments of the plate before tightening the nut with the spanner.

19. Screw the plate to the femoral shaft and remove the bone clamp.

N.B. This technique may also be used for internal fixation of intra-and extra-capsular fractures of the femoral neck, but it is less secure than a compression screw.

Closure

(See p. 503.)

Aftercare

1. Begin active and passive mobilising exercises for both the hip and the knee within the first 24 hours or as soon the patient's general condition permits.

2. Remove the suction drain after 24–36 hours. Allow the patient to walk with crutches, partially weightbearing, as soon as pain permits.

3. Remove sutures and take a check X-ray to be sure the

position is unchanged at 10–12 days, before the patient is discharged from hospital.

4. Allow full weightbearing between 8 and 12 weeks after the operation, depending on radiological evidence of bone union.

TOTAL PROSTHETIC REPLACEMENT OF THE HIP

Appraise

1. Reserve total prosthetic replacement of the hip joint for elderly patients with pain and limitation of movement due to primary and secondary osteoarthritis or rheumatoid arthritis.

2. Avoid prosthetic replacement in patients of less than 55 years of age unless their disability is so severe that failure of the implant would leave them no more incapacitated.

3. There are many different implants which differ only in detail, and the approach to the hip is a matter of personal choice.

Access

I use the posterior approach.

Action

1. Dislocate the femoral head by internally rotating the flexed adducted hip without undue force. N.B. If this proves impossible, remove a sliver of bone 0.5 cm wide from the posterior rim of the acetabulum with an osteotome and repeat the manoeuvre. If the head will still not dislocate, divide the femoral neck with an oscillating saw and remove the head piecemeal.

2. The assistant flexes the knee to a right angle and rotates the leg so that the lower leg is vertical.

3. Place the stem of the trial femoral component of the prosthesis alongside the posterior surface of the femur, and push the tip between the fat and muscle of the lower end of the wound until the centre of the femoral head lies opposite the tip of the greater trochanter, which is easily palpated (Fig. 30.10).

4. Mark the position and the plane of the collar of the prosthesis on the femoral neck with an osteotome.

5. Place Lane's levers around either side of the femoral neck and divide the neck at the level of the mark with an oscillating power saw, the blade of which should be vertical. Remove the femoral head.

6. Place a large bone hook into the medullary cavity of the neck and have the assistant retract the femur anteriorly and upwards to stretch the anterior capsule.

7. Divide the anterior capsule and its attachment to the base of the femoral neck with a knife.

8. Remove the bone hook and slip the end of a Lane's lever under the femoral neck and over the anterior lip of the acetabulum; retract the upper end of the femur anteriorly. Straighten the knee.

9. Excise as much of the capsule as possible after dividing its attachment to the circumference of the acetabulum with a knife.

10. Remove any remnants of the ligamentum teres or other soft tissue from the acetabulum and use a large curved Capener gouge to remove any residual articular cartilage.

11. Deepen the acetabulum if necessary by removing bone from the inner side of the roof, until it will accept a trial cup of appropriate size (usually 45 mm outside diameter). The roof of the acetabulum should cover the cup when its face is anteverted 30° and inclined 30° to the vertical.

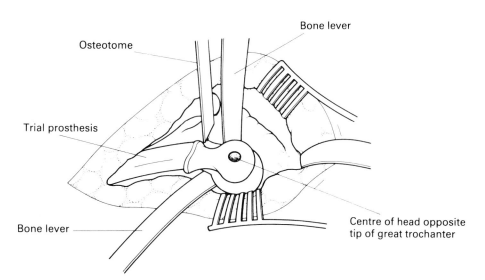

Fig. 30.10 Resection of the femoral head, using the prosthesis as a guide.

12. Ream the acetabulum with graduated powered reamers to leave a roughened surface.

13. Excavate the acetabular pit if present with a sharp curette and remove as much cancellous bone as possible without perforating the inner cortex.

14. If there is no pit, make a hole with a 6 mm drill through the posterior wall of the acetabulum into the ischium and excavate this with a curette.

15. Make two more keyholes through the roof of the acetabulum into the thick part of the ilium at approximately 10 o'clock and 2 o'clock (Fig. 30.11).

16. Enlarge and undercut these holes with a curette.

17. Irrigate the acetabulum with half strength hydrogen peroxide to remove debris and to stop bleeding. Pack the acetabulum with a swab.

18. Remove the bone lever and flex, adduct and internally rotate the leg so that the femoral canal presents in the wound.

19. Remove all loose cancellous bone from the medullary canal with a curette and insert the stem of the trial femoral component. Enlarge the medullary cavity with graduated Charnley reamers if necessary until the femoral component is an easy fit.

20. Irrigate the canal and remove all debris with a 'bottle brush' and sucker.

21. Measure the length of the stem of the prosthesis and plug the femoral canal with a cement restricter placed just beyond the anticipated level of the tip of the stem.

22. Plug the mouth of the medullary canal with a swab and retract the femur with a bone hook to expose the acetabulum.

23. Mix one packet of radio-opaque bone cement; when it no longer sticks to the glove, pack it firmly into the dry acetabulum.

24. Push the acetabular cup firmly into the cement and adjust the final position with the introducer, the short limb of which should be vertical and the long limb 30° anterior to the long axis of the trunk (Fig. 30.12).

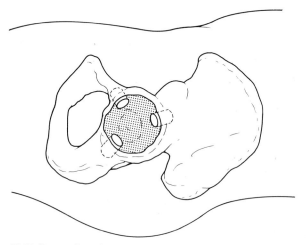

Fig. 30.11 Preparation of the acetabulum, for the acrylic cement. Note the 'key-holes'.

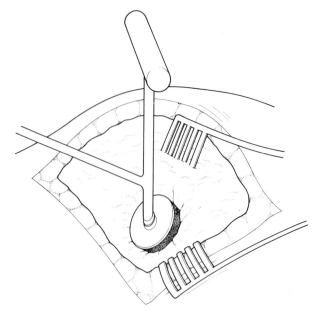

Fig. 30.12 Cementing the acetabular cup, using the cup introducer to hold it in the correct position.

25. Carefully remove excess cement and maintain firm pressure on the introducer until the cement has set.

26. Insert the femoral component into the femur and carry out a trial reduction by extending and externally rotating the leg, at the same time pressing the femoral head firmly into the acetabulum. The reduction should be firm rather than tight.

27. Palpate the knees through the towels and make sure the legs are the same length.

28. Dislocate the hip and remove the femoral prosthesis. Trim the neck if the leg is too long, or use a prosthesis with an extended neck if the leg is too short.

29. Mix one pack of bone cement and whilst it is still runny, pour it into the barrel of the cement gun.

30. Insert the nozzle or the gun as far as possible into the medullary canal and inject the cement. The nozzle is slowly withdrawn. Finally, pack the cement by digital pressure.

31. Insert the femoral component so that it is neither ante-or retroverted, tapping it finally home with a plastic punch. Remove excess cement.

32. Reduce the femoral head as before. Do not move the leg until the cement has set.

33. Wash out any debris and insert a large suction drain.

Closure

(See p. 501.)

Aftercare

1. Place an abduction pillow between the legs and keep it in position for 7 days.

2. Remove the drain after 24–36 hours.

3. Start active and passive knee flexion exercises as soon as possible, but avoid adducting and internally rotating the flexed hip for 3 months, to minimise possible dislocation.

4. Allow the patient to fully weightbear after 2 or 3 days, first using a walking frame and gradually progressing to elbow crutches and finally a stick in the opposite hand.

5. Remove the stitches after 10 days.

6. Dispense with the stick when the patient feels secure.

APPROACHES TO THE UPPER LEG

The femoral shaft may be approached from the anterior, medial or lateral aspects. The posterolateral approach is the most convenient and most commonly used.

POSTEROLATERAL APPROACH (Fig. 30.13)

Appraise

1. Use the posterolateral to approach the femoral shaft unless access to the medial side of the femur is specifically required.

2. The approach may be extended proximally and distally if necessary and is most commonly employed to reduce and internally fix fractures of the femoral shaft.

Prepare

1. Have 3 units of cross-matched blood available.

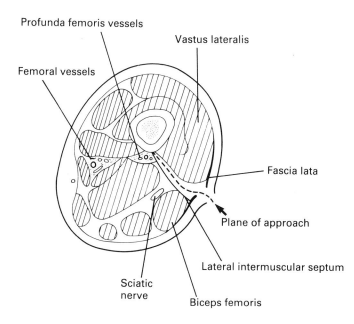

Fig. 30.13 Transverse section of the mid-thigh showing the posterolateral approach to the femoral shaft along the dotted line.

2. Use a general anaesthetic.

3. For operations on the distal two-thirds of the thigh, exsanguinate the leg and apply a pneumatic tourniquet immediately below the groin.

4. Place the patient supine on the operating table with a sandbag under the buttock of the affected side.

5. Elevate the leg and clean the skin from the iliac crest and buttock (or the tourniquet when used) to the upper tibia.

6. Place a large sheet across the operating table and over the sound leg, and pull the upper edge firmly into the groin to cover the genitalia.

7. Place the long edge of the 'shut-off' towel in the groin, or immediately below the tourniquet, and pull it firmly round the thigh; fasten it with a towel clip on the lateral side.

8. Place a medium-sized drape on the table with its upper edge at the level of the knee joint and carefully lower the leg onto the towel.

9. Fold the distal edge of the towel proximally over the foot and then wrap the towel around the leg.

10. Bandage the towel firmly to the leg with an open weave bandage.

11. Cover the trunk with a large sheet and clip it to the underlying sheet on either side of the thigh.

12. Pass the leg through the hole in a split sheet. Clip the margins of the split to the skin at the upper limit of the operating field.

13. Wrap a large transparent adhesive drape round the thigh to cover the exposed skin.

Access

1. Palpate the tendon of the biceps femoris at the level of the lateral femoral condyle and also the posterior margin of the greater trochanter.

2. Incise the skin along the whole or part of the line joining these two points to gain access to the appropriate part of the thigh.

3. Incise the fascia lata in the line of the incision and locate the lateral intermuscular septum immediately anterior to the biceps femoris.

4. Insert a finger between the septum and the bulk of the vastus lateralis lying anteriorly and continue the dissection down to the bone in this plane with a knife.

5. Ligate the perforating branches of the profunda femoris vessels as they are encountered.

Closure

1. Insert a suction drain.
2. Close the fascia lata with 0 absorbable sutures.
3. Close the skin, dress and bandage the wound.

INTRAMEDULLARY FIXATION OF FEMORAL SHAFT FRACTURES

Appraise

1. Transverse or short oblique fractures of the middle third of the femoral shaft are most suitable for intramedullary nailing.

2. The technique may be employed for other fractures at the discretion of the experienced surgeon, but fixation is less secure and may need to be supplemented by support in a Thomas splint.

Access

1. Place the patient on the operating table in the lateral position with the affected leg uppermost.

2. Do not use a tourniquet.

3. Use the posterolateral approach with the incision 15 cm long centred over the fracture.

Action

1. Follow the haematoma down to the fracture site and evacuate it, together with any small detached fragments of bone.

2. Separate the bone ends from the surrounding muscle with a rugine for approximately 5 cm on either side of the fracture site.

3. Grasp the distal end of the bone with large Hey-Groves bone holding forceps and deliver it into the wound.

4. Pass a ball-tipped guide wire down the medullary cavity and ream the bone with flexible side-cutting cannulated reamers passed over the guide.

5. Stop the reamer when it ceases to cut as it enters the expanded distal part of the canal.

6. Repeat, using reamers increasing in diameter by 0.5 mm until the canal is of uniform diameter for 2–3 cm distal to the fracture. Note the size of the final reamer (usually between 12 and 14 mm diameter).

7. With the guide wire in place, measure the length of wire protruding from the bone and calculate the length of the distal fragment.

8. Place the bone clamp around the proximal fragment, delivery this into the wound and ream the medullary canal as before to the same final diameter.

9. Calculate the length of the proximal fragment after pushing the guide firmly into the femur until resistance is felt.

10. Remove the ball-tipped guide and flex and adduct the leg. Push a pointed Kuntscher guide through the medullary canal until the tip can be felt under the skin of the buttock.

11. Make an incision 5 cm long over the point of the guide and retract the skin edges with a self-retaining retractor.

12. Take a Kuntscher nail of the calculated length and 0.5 mm less in diameter than the diameter of the reamed canal; slide it over the point of the guide wire with the eye on the medial side.

13. Hammer the nail into the femoral shaft using the special Kuntscher nail driver until the tip just emerges from the fractured end of the bone.

14. If undue resistance is met, withdraw the nail with the special extractor by means of the eye, and replace it with a nail 0.5 mm smaller in diameter.

15. With Hey-Groves bone clamps on both fragments, and an assistant applying traction to the leg, reduce the fracture accurately, taking care especially to ensure that the rotational alignment is correct.

16. Hammer the nail home until no more than 1 cm protrudes from the tip of the greater trochanter.

17. Remove the bone clamps and make sure the knee bends without grating. If there is any doubt, X-ray the knee to be sure that the tip of the nail has not penetrated the articular surface.

Closure

1. Close the wound (see p. 511).
2. Close the wound in the buttock.

Aftercare

1. Apply a pressure dressing over the wound.

2. Leave the leg free in bed and start qudriceps and knee flexion exercises after removal of the drain 36–48 hours after the operation.

3. Allow up non-weightbearing on crutches as soon as pain permits.

4. Remove stitches and allow partial weightbearing on the affected leg after 10–14 days.

5. Allow full weightbearing when there is X-ray evidence of bone union (6–8 weeks).

APPROACHES TO THE KNEE

Most operations on the knee joint are carried out from the front but many do not require a full and formal exposure of the whole joint, and a more limited exposure is adequate. The posterior approach is used to gain access to the popliteal fossa and occasionally to the posterior part of the knee joint.

ANTERIOR APPROACH (Fig. 30.14)

Appraise

1. Use this approach for operations on the extensor mechanism of the knee joint and to gain wide access to the inside of the joint itself.

2. Use the anterolateral and anteromedial approaches when limited access is required, e.g. meniscectomy, removal of loose bodies.

Prepare

1. Use a general anaesthetic.
2. Apply a tourniquet to the mid-thigh.
3. Place the patient supine on the operating table.
4. Drape the leg as if the distal femoral shaft were being exposed (see p. 511), leaving the skin exposed from the tibial tubercle to the tourniquet.
5. Cover the exposed skin with a transparent adhesive drape.

Access

1. Make a straight incision 15 cm long in the midline, extending proximally from the upper margin of the tibial tubercle.
2. Deepen the incision to expose the patellar ligament, the anterior surface of the patella and the quadriceps tendon and the distal fibres of the rectus femoris (Fig. 30.14).
3. Reflect the skin and subcutaneous fat as a single layer medially to expose the junction of the quadriceps tendon and the vastus medialis, the medial border of the patella and the patella ligament.

4. Make an incision along the medial edge of the quadriceps tendon and through the capsule along the medial margin of the patella and medial edge of the patella ligament into the joint.
5. Turn the patella inside out and retract it laterally, and flex the knee at the same time (Fig. 30.15). Extend the incision proximally into the rectus femoris if this proves to be difficult.

Closure

1. Extend the knee and return the patella to its normal position.
2. Close the incision in the capsule and the quadriceps tendon with 0 interrupted absorbable synthetic sutures.
3. Close the subcutaneous fat and skin.

LIMITED ANTERIOR APPROACHES

These are described with the operations that require only limited access to the knee joint.

POSTERIOR APPROACH (Fig. 30.16)

Appraise

1. Use this approach to gain access to the popliteal fossa.

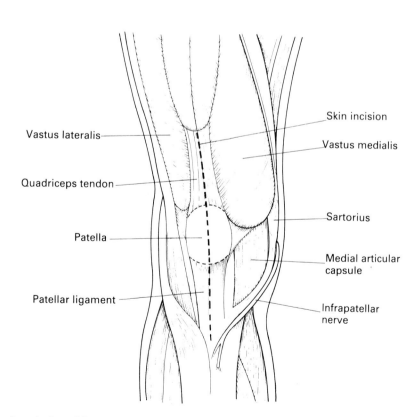

Fig. 30.14 Anterior approach to the knee joint.

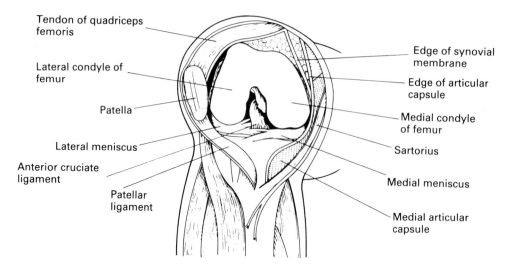

Fig. 30.15 The knee exposed through the anterior approach and flexed.

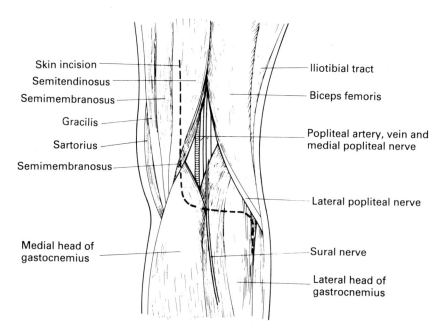

Fig. 30.16 The posterior approach to the knee joint.

2. Use it to gain access to the posterior compartment of the knee joint, for example, to repair the torn posterior cruciate ligament.

3. Use the medial or lateral part of the full approach for more limited exposure.

Prepare

1. Use a general anaesthetic.
2. Apply a mid-thigh tourniquet.
3. Place the patient prone on the operating table.
4. Have an assistant flex the knee to 90° and raise the thigh off the table.
5. Place the drapes as described for the anterior approach.

Access

1. Start the skin incision 7 cm proximal to the medial femoral condyle and take it distally to the transverse skin crease; then curve it laterally and distally again along the medial side of the head of the fibula.

2. Reflect the skin and subcutaneous tissue to expose the popliteal fascia.

3. Identify the posterior cutaneous nerve of the calf (sural nerve) lying beneath the fascia between the two heads of the gastrocnemius.

4. Incise the fascia and trace the nerve proximally to its origin from the posterior tibial nerve.

5. Trace the posterior tibial nerve distally and identify

its branches to the calf muscles; then trace it proximally to the apex of the popliteal fossa where it joins the common peroneal nerve.

6. Follow the common peroneal nerve distally along the medial border of the biceps tendon.

7. Expose the popliteal artery and vein lying anteriorly and medially to the posterior tibial nerve. Gently retract them to expose the superior lateral and superior medial genicular vessels passing beneath the muscles just proximal to the origin of the two heads of gastrocnemius.

8. Retract the semi-tendinosus medially and expose the attachment of the medial head of gastrocnemius to the joint capsule which should be incised longitudinally at this point.

9. Retract the gastrocnemius laterally, using it to protect the nerves and vessels and enter the posteromedial compartment of the joint.

10. Approach the posterolateral compartment between the tendon of biceps femoris and the lateral head of gastrocnemius.

Closure

1. Release the tourniquet.
2. Suture the capsule with interrupted 0 synthetic absorbable sutures.
3. Close the deep fascia and the skin.

OPEN REDUCTION AND INTERNAL FIXATION OF FRACTURES AROUND THE KNEE JOINT

FRACTURES OF THE PATELLA (Fig. 30.17)

Appraise

1. Treat conservatively undisplaced fractures in which the extensor mechanism is intact.

2. Treat displaced transverse fractures by open reduction and internal fixation.

3. Treat comminuted displaced fractures by open reduction and internal fixation or by patellectomy. The choice of treatment requires judgement and experience.

Prepare

1. Apply a high pneumatic tourniquet to the thigh but do not exsanguinate the limb.

2. Use the anterior approach to expose the fracture.

3. Reflect the skin and subcutaneous tissues medially and laterally to expose the medial and lateral patellar retinaculae, which may be torn.

Action

1. Flex the knee and separate the patella into two main fragments. Irrigate the joint with saline and remove blood clot and loose fragments of articular cartilage and bone.

2. If the fracture is comminuted, place the subsidiary fragments in their correct position in relation to the two main fragments.

3. If the fragments are two numerous or too small to reconstitute a smooth articular surface, proceed to patellectomy.

4. Remove each fragment of bone, carefully dissecting those fragments retaining an attachment to the quadriceps tendon and patella ligament.

5. Extend the knee and approximate the central part of the quadriceps tendon and the patella ligament with 0 synthetic absorbable mattress sutures.

6. Excise the ragged margins of the patellar retinaculae and repair the medial and lateral defects in the extensor mechanism in a similar way.

7. If fragments can be reduced, then transfix large fragments of bone with a 1.5 mm Kirschner wire inserted from

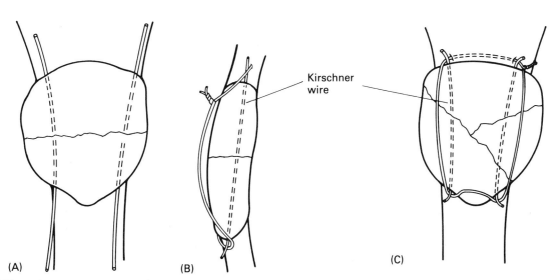

Fig. 30.17 The technique of tension band wiring for the repair of fractures of the patella.

the peripheral margin parallel to the articular surface with a hand drill.

8. Reduce the fragments to the main upper or lower part of the patella as appropriate and drill a Kirschner wire across the fracture line into the main fragment. Cut the wire flush with the margin of the bone.

9. The patella will now consist of two main parts, proximal and distal, and the fracture should be treated as if it were a non-comminuted transverse fracture.

10. When the fracture is transverse or almost so, flex the knee to 45°. Drill a 1.5 mm diameter Kirschner wire through the surface of the fracture into the proximal fragment, parallel to the articular surface and midway between the front and back of the patella and a third of the width of the patella from its medial edge, until it emerges from the superior margin of the bone (Fig. 30.17).

11. Drill a second Kirschner wire through the proximal fragment of the patella parallel to the first wire and a third of the width of the bone from its lateral edge.

12. Reattach the drill to the proximal end of each wire in turn and withdraw until the tip just protrudes from the surface of the fracture.

13. Reduce the fracture accurately by pulling the proximal fragment down with a bone hook and hold the reduction with a towel clip on either side.

14. Make sure the articular surface is absolutely smooth by inserting the tip of the finger through the disrupted patellar retinaculum into the joint.

15. Drill each Kirschner wire across the fracture line from the proximal into the distal fragment until the wires emerge for a centimetre or so on either side of the patellar ligament.

16. Bend the protruding proximal and distal ends of the wires with pliers to a right angle at the margin of the bone.

17. Pass a 25 cm length of 18 SWG (1.2 mm diameter) stainless steel wire through the substance of the quadriceps tendon from lateral to medial and deep to the proximal ends of the Kirschner wires.

18. Bring the wire out over the front of the patella on the medial side and then pass it through the patella ligament deep to the distal ends of the Kirschner wires.

19. Take the end of the wire over the front of the lateral side of the patella, and twist the ends together with a wire tightener to hold the fragments securely together.

20. Cut off the excess wire and turn the stump into the quadriceps tendon.

21. Cut off the protruding ends of the Kirschner wires, leaving 1–2 mm hooking round the circumferential wire.

22. Repair the patellar retinaculae with 0 synthetic absorbable sutures.

Closure

1. Release the tourniquet.
2. Close the subcutaneous fat and skin.

Aftercare

1. Apply a padded plaster of Paris cylinder.
2. Check the reduction and fixation on A.P. and lateral radiographs after 24 hours.
3. Start static quadriceps exercises.
4. Allow full weightbearing with a walking stick if necessary as soon as pain permits.
5. X-ray again after 2 weeks to be sure the fracture has not displaced.
6. Remove the plaster at 6 weeks. X-ray and begin flexion exercises.

FRACTURES OF THE FEMORAL CONDYLES

The management of these fractures is controversial, and operative treatment requires wide exposure and experience.

FRACTURES OF THE TIBIAL CONDYLES AND PLATEAU

Operations on these fractures are rarely straightforward and should not be undertaken by the inexperienced.

PATELLECTOMY

Appraise

1. Comminuted fractures of the patella which require patellectomy are usually associated with complete disruption of the extensor mechanism which must be repaired (see p. 515).

2. Patellectomy for non-traumatic conditions (usually patello-femoral osteoarthritis) can be performed without disrupting the extensor mechanism.

Prepare

1. Use a pneumatic tourniquet.
2. Operate with a general anaesthetic.
3. Position and drape the patient for the anterior approach to the knee.

Action

1. Make an incision in the skin and subcutaneous fat 10 cm long in the midline immediately over the patella.

2. Deepen the incision down to the patella and dissect skin and subcutaneous fat medially and laterally to the patellar margins.

3. Incise the periosteum covering the anterior surface of the patella vertically in the midline from the upper to the lower pole.

4. Dissect this periosteal layer off the bone with a sharp knife keeping it as thick as possible. This layer is thinnest in the midline and is easily perforated.

5. Remove the patella and inspect the inside of the joint, noting the state of the synovium, the menisci, the articular cartilage and the cruciate ligaments.

6. Close the periosteum with interrupted 2/0 absorbable synthetic sutures on a round-bodied needle without tension.

7. Flex the knee to 90° to be sure the sutures do not pull out.

Closure

1. Release the tourniquet.
2. Close the fat and skin.

Aftercare

1. Apply a Robert Jones compression bandage.
2. Start quadriceps exercises immediately and progress to straight leg raising.
3. Allow up on crutches or a stick after 24–48 hours.
4. Start flexion exercises when quadriceps control has been regained (4–5 days).
5. Remove stitches at 10 days, continue quadriceps exercises and progressively increase activities.

MENISCECTOMY

Appraise

1. Although it is possible to remove fragments or even the whole of a torn meniscus through an arthroscope, this is a very specialised and demanding procedure and there is still a place for open meniscectomy.
2. Pre-operative arthrography or preliminary arthroscopy at the time of operation is desirable if there is the slightest doubt about the diagnosis.
3. A limited vertical incision on the appropriate side of the joint provides sufficient exposure.

Prepare

1. Use a general anaesthetic.
2. Apply a tourniquet to the exsanguinated limb.
3. Remove the lower section of the operating table.
4. Position the patient so that the legs hang over the end of the table with the lower edge of the table pressed firmly into the back of the knee.
5. Place a sandbag under the thigh just above the knee.
6. Drape the leg for the anterior approach.
7. Sit at the end of the table with the patient's foot between your knees.

Access

1. Incise the skin on the medial or lateral side of the knee (depending on which meniscus is torn) from the medial or lateral margin of the patella, downwards and slightly backwards to a point 1 cm below the articular margin of the tibia.
2. Incise the capsule in the line of the incision.
3. Pick up the synovium with forceps (in the presence of an effusion it will bulge forward into the wound) and nick it with a knife.
4. Open the synovium in the line of the incision with curved scissors.

Action

1. Retract the patella with a flat bladed Jackson Burrows retractor and then slip the curved blade of the second retractor around the femoral condyle (Fig. 30.18).
2. Adjust the second retractor so that the edge of the blade lies along the synovial attachment of the meniscus.
3. Inspect the inside of the joint, looking especially at the meniscus, the anterior cruciate ligament and the articular surfaces of the patella and femoral condyle.
4. Pass a blunt hook around the free edge of the anterior horn of the meniscus and pull the meniscus forward. This may bring an otherwise unseen tear into view.

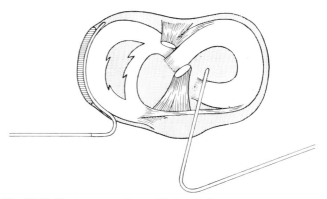

Fig. 30.18 Meniscectomy: the positioning of the retractors.

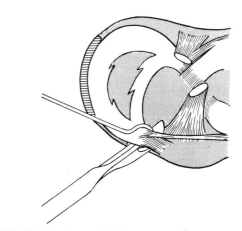

Fig. 30.19 Freeing the anterior horn.

5. Lift the anterior horn off the tibial plateau with the hook and place the blade of a knife horizontally between the meniscus and the bone; cut towards the centre of the joint to detach the anterior horn (Fig. 30.19).

6. Grip the anterior horn with toothed meniscus forceps or small Kocher's forceps and pull the meniscus forward towards the centre of the joint.

7. Divide the peripheral attachment of the meniscus at the synovial reflection using a sharp solid scalpel or a Smillie's meniscus knife keeping the blade vertical (Fig. 30.20). Do **not** use a flimsy, disposable blade. If it breaks, recovery of the fragments may be very difficult.

8. Rotate the lower leg and force it backwards with the knees and with the lower edge of the table as a fulcrum, the tibial plateau will move forward improving access to the posterior part of the meniscus.

9. Divide as much of the peripheral attachment of the meniscus as possible with a Smillie's curved meniscus knife (Fig. 30.21) and then displace the almost completely separated meniscus into the intercondylar notch.

10. Pull the meniscus forward over the cutting edge of a flat bladed Smillie's knife to sever the remaining peripheral attachments and finally the attachment of the posterior horn to the bone (Fig. 30.22).

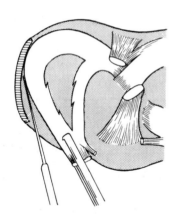

Fig. 30.20 Detaching the periphery of the meniscus.

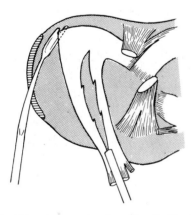

Fig. 30.21 Detaching the posterior rim with a Smillie knife.

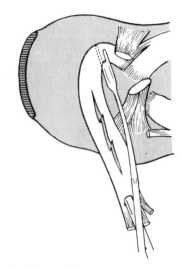

Fig. 30.22 Freeing the posterior horn.

11. If the meniscus ruptures during removal, or inspection of the removed meniscus shows that a sizeable portion has been left behind, this must be removed through a separate posterior incision (Fig. 30.23).

12. On the medial side, it is safe to pass an instrument from the anterior incision along the medial aspect of the joint to the posteromedial corner and then to cut down onto the metal from the skin. Make a 2.5–3.5 cm vertical incision in the skin and a similar one in the capsule behind the medial collateral ligament (Fig. 30.23). The only structure which is at risk is the long saphenous vein.

13. On the lateral side of the knee, the lateral popliteal nerve, the tendon of popliteus and the lateral collateral ligament are all at risk in blind incisions and a formal approach by dissection must be made. Make a posterolateral 3.5 cm incision in line with the anterior margin of the fibular head (Fig. 30.23), and incise the capsule anterior to the lateral collateral ligament; retract the tendon of popliteus posteriorly and superiorly. Remember the lateral inferior geniculate artery which, unlike its fellow on the medial side, runs closely around the edge of the tibial plateau. If damaged, this vessel may be difficult to ligate but its ends can be easily under-run with a pair of sutures.

14. Once the posterior compartment has been entered, insert two small Langenbeck retractors and look transversely across the joint.

15. The posterior rim of the meniscus may be seen and removed using a sharp scalpel and one of the Smillie's knives.

Closure

1. Retract the edges of the capsule and pick up each end of the synovium with fine curved artery forceps.

2. Close the synovium with a continuous 2/0 absorbable synthetic suture on a round bodied needle.

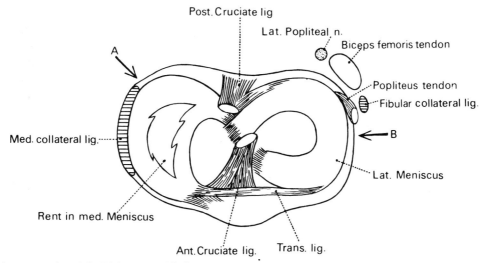

Fig. 30.23 The superior aspect of the left tibial plateau with the approaches to the posterior horns of the medial and lateral menisci arrowed.

3. Extend the knee and close the capsule with 0 interrupted absorbable synthetic sutures.

4. Close the subcutaneous tissue and skin.

5. Apply a Robert Jones compression bandage from the ankle to the lower thigh. Extend the bandage to the upper thigh after removing the tourniquet.

Aftercare

1. Begin static quadriceps exercises immediately the patient recovers from the anaesthetic and progress to straight leg raising exercises as soon as possible. Allow the patient to walk with crutches.

2. Once quadriceps control is achieved, replace the Robert Jones bandage with a crepe bandage and begin knee flexion.

3. Allow full weightbearing at first with a stick when flexion reaches 45°.

4. Remove the stitches in 7 days and allow unprotected weightbearing.

5. Bandage the knee so long as there is any tendency to swell (3–4 weeks), and continue quadriceps exercises until the bulk of the muscle returns.

OTHER OPERATIONS ON THE KNEE JOINT

REMOVAL OF LOOSE BODIES

Appraise

1. Single large loose bodies in the suprapatellar pouch may be palpable and can be removed through a small overlying incision.

2. Single large loose bodies in the main part of the joint should be removed through a 'meniscectomy approach'(see p. 517).

3. A formal exposure is required for multiple and small loose bodies.

Access

1. Apply a pneumatic tourniquet. Do not exsanguinate the leg to avoid disturbing the loose bodies if they are in a favourable position.

2. Prepare the patient for the anterior approach.

3. Open the joint immediately over the loose bodies if possible, or by the anterior approach if not.

Action

1. Retract the wound edges with Langenbeck retractors.

2. Grasp obvious loose bodies with toothed forceps and extract them.

3. Irrigate the joint with saline using a catheter and syringe to dislodge any hidden loose bodies.

4. If the loose bodies cannot be seen or there is a possibility that they have not all been removed, X-ray the knee in both planes, disturbing the joint as little as possible whilst doing so.

5. Flush them out with saline if possible, or remove them through the incisions used to remove the retained posterior horns of the menisci (see p. 518).

Closure

See anterior approach or meniscectomy.

Aftercare

See section on meniscectomy.

REPAIR AND RECONSTRUCTION OF THE CRUCIATE AND COLLATERAL LIGAMENTS

Surgical repair of acute ruptures of the knee ligaments is desirable, but like late reconstruction should be left to the experienced surgeon.

UPPER TIBIAL OSTEOTOMY (Fig. 30.24)

Appraise

1. Varus and valgus deformities occurring at the level of the knee joint may be corrected by removing a wedge of bone from the medial or lateral side of the upper tibia.

2. Treat early osteoarthritis of the knee with or without deformity by upper tibial osteotomy, provided there is no ligamentous laxity and there is a functional range of movement (90° or more of flexion).

Prepare

1. Use a pneumatic tourniquet.
2. Operate with a general anaesthetic.
3. Position and drape the leg for the anterior approach to the knee.

Action

1. Make an oblique incision in the skin from the upper margin of the tibial tubercle laterally to the posterior end of the lateral joint line.

2. Identify the ligamentum patellae and incise the fascia along its lateral edge.

3. Dissect the tibialis anterior off the tibia with a knife, working laterally along the 'flare' of the tibia from the tibial tubercle to the superior tibiofibular joint to expose the upper centimetre of the bone immediately below the lateral condyle.

4. Insert the blade of the knife into the superior tibiofibular joint parallel to the surface of the tibia and divide the joint capsule. Remember the peroneal nerve lies just distal to the head of the fibula.

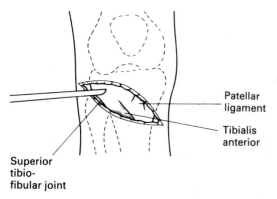

Fig. 30.24 Exposure and division of tibia for osteotomy

5. Place a bone lever under the patellar ligament and retract it medially as far as possible.

6. Divide the tibia transversely from the lateral side with a broad osteotome (2.5–3.0 cm) parallel to the articular surface at the junction of the condyle and shaft (Fig. 30.24).

7. Remove the blade of the osteotome after it has penetrated the bone for a centimetre or two and begin a second cut 0.5 cm distal to the first. Direct it towards the point at which the initial cut will penetrate the medial cortex.

8. Tap the osteotome first into one and then into the other cut as far as the medial cortex. Remove the wedge of bone piecemeal if necessary as the osteotome advances.

9. Apply a valgus force to the knee to close the wedge by cracking of the medial cortex of the tibia. If it fails to close, remove more bone from the medial side. The posterior tibial cortex may also need to be removed separately.

10. Close the wedge and if the alignment of the bone is correct, hammer home two stepped vitallium staples to maintain the position (see p. 448).

11. The upper part of the staple should be inserted midway between the articular margin and the osteotomy.

12. Release the tourniquet.

Closure

1. Suture the tibialis anterior to the periosteum.
2. Insert a suction drain.
3. Close the skin.

Aftercare

1. Apply a Robert Jones bandage.
2. After 24 hrs take a check X-ray and begin quadriceps exercises, progressing to straight leg raising.
3. After 48 hrs remove the drain and allow up partially weightbearing on crutches.
4. Start knee flexion exercises when quadriceps control has been regained (4–5 days).
5. Remove sutures at 10 days, allow partial weightbearing with crutches and continue mobilising exercises.
6. Allow full weightbearing at 6 weeks if check X-ray shows the osteotomy is uniting.

N.B. To correct a valgus deformity, a medial wedge may be removed from the upper end of the tibia in the same way, but in this case there is no need to divide the capsule of the superior tibiofibular joint.

TOTAL REPLACEMENT ARTHROPLASTY OF THE KNEE (Fig. 30.25)

Appraise

1. Total knee replacement is now commonplace but

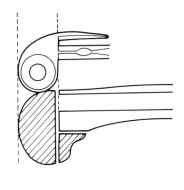

a

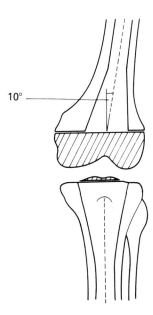

10°

b

Fig. 30.25 Resection of the articular surfaces of the femur and tibia and preparation of the medullary cavities for knee replacement in (a) the lateral and (b) the frontal plane.

should only be used in elderly patients with severe disability resulting from rheumatoid or osteoarthritis.

2. There are many different prostheses which fall into three main groups

(a) Unconstrained or surface replacements

(b) Constrained or hinged replacements

(c) Semi-constrained replacements.

3. It is a matter of personal preference which type is used but the constrained replacements require a less exacting technique and are more suitable for the less experienced surgeon. The technique for the Stanmore prosthesis will be described.

Prepare

1. Have three units of crossmatched blood available.
2. Use a general anaesthetic.
3. Apply a pneumatic tourniquet to the exsanguinated limb.
4. Position and drape the leg for the anterior approach.

Action

1. Use the anterior approach (see p. 512).

2. Flex the knee and at the same time retract the patella laterally turning it inside-out.

3. Place one Lane's lever around the medial and another around the lateral side of the femoral shaft just proximal to the femoral condyles, making sure the tips of the levers are in direct contact with the bone.

4. Divide the femoral attachments of the medial, lateral and cruciate ligaments and remove the remnants of the menisci.

5. Resect the femoral condyles with a hand saw 2 cm from the most distal part of the articular surface. The cut should be at right angles to the long axis of the femur in the anteroposterior plane and at approximately 10° to the long axis in the lateral plane (Fig. 30.25).

6. Trim the posterior part of each condyle (which remains flush with the posterior cortex of the femoral shaft) with the osteotome. (Fig. 30.25).

7. Make a channel through the cut cancellous surface with a curette opposite the groove on the anterior femoral cortex and large enough to take the stem of the prosthesis.

8. Use a power saw to resect the tibial spine and sufficient of the adjacent subchondral bone to provide a flat surface for the plateau of the tibial component of the prosthesis. This surface should be at right angles to the long axis of the tibia in both planes.

9. With a gouge make a hole through the subchondral bone opposite the tibial tubercle just large enough to take the stem of the prosthesis.

10. Remove the cancellous bone from within the medullary canal of the tibia and femur with a curette.

11. Insert the femoral and tibial components and articulate them with the trial axial. Extend the knee. If full extension is impossible, remove more bone from the lower end of the femur with the hand saw.

12. Remove any osteophytes from the margins of the patella with bone nibblers.

13. Remove debris from the medullary canals with water jet and brush (see p. 510). Plug each canal with a cement restrictor so that the tip of the medullary stem will ultimately lie within its centre.

14. Mix the cement (see p. 510), and insert into the femoral canal with a cement gun, packing firmly with the finger before inserting the prosthesis. The articulation for the patella should be opposite the groove on the anterior

femoral condyle. Leave undisturbed until the cement sets.

15. Cement the tibial component into place, making sure the notch on the plateau of the implant lies opposite the tibial tubercle.

16. Articulate the components with the trial axial. Reduce the patella and hold the leg in full extension until the cement sets (7–8 minutes).

17. Flex and extend the knee and make sure that the patella articulates with the parellar articular surface throughout the range of movement, which should be at least 100°.

18. If the patella shows a tendency to dislocate laterally, incise the lateral capsule longitudinally from the patella ligament to the vastus lateralis.

19. Replace the trial axial with the definitive axial and hold this in place with the circlip (Fig. 30.26).

20. Release the tourniquet and stop the bleeding.

21. Wash out the joint with saline and insert a suction drain.

Closure

1. Repair the medial capsule incision with 0 interrupted synthetic absorbable sutures.

2. Reef the medial capsule if the patella shows a tendency to sublux as the knee is flexed and extended.

3. Insert a second suction drain superficial to the patella.

4. Close the subcutaneous fat and skin.

Aftercare

1. Apply a Robert Jones pressure dressing and then a back splint with the knee in full extension.

2. After 24 hrs, take check X-rays and start quadriceps exercises.

3. Change the dressings and remove the drains after 48 hrs.

4. Allow up fully weightbearing with frame or crutches when the pain and quadriceps control permit.

5. Reduce the dressings and begin knee flexion exercises when quadriceps control is regained, providing the wound is healing satisfactorily.

6. Remove the stitches at 10–12 days and allow full weightbearing, progressing from crutches to one stick.

7. Continue with exercises for 3 months.

ARTHRODESIS OF THE KNEE (Fig. 30.27)

Arthrodesis should be reserved for the treatment of stiff painful knees when tibial osteotomy or replacement arthroplasty are inappropriate.

Prepare

1. Use a general anaesthetic.
2. Apply a pneumatic tourniquet to the thigh.
3. Prepare and drape the leg for the anterior approach.

Action

1. With the knee extended and the foot in normal anatomical alignment, drill a Steinmann's pin through the tibia 10 cm below the joint line, at right angles to the long axis of the tibia and parallel to the floor (see p. 453).

2. Drill a second Steinmann's pin through the femur, 10 cm above the joint line at an angle of 10° to the long axis of the femoral shaft, parallel to the floor and in the same plane as the first pin.

3. Make a midline incision through the skin 20 cm long extending proximally from the tibial tubercle.

4. Remove the patella (see p. 516), and extend the incision into the quadriceps tendon proximally.

5. Flex the knee to 90° and retract the extensor apparatus to either side. Pass Lane's bone levers around each side of the femur (see p. 521).

6. Resect the femoral condyles with a hand saw at the level of the intercondylar notch. Keep the saw parallel to

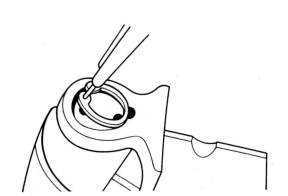

Fig. 30.26 Introduction of the circlip.

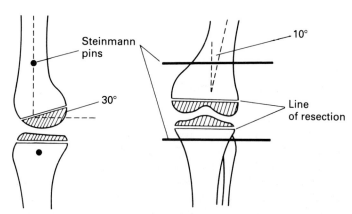

Fig. 30.27 Resection of articular surfaces and placing of the Steinmann pins for arthrodesis of the knee.

the proximal Steinmann's pin in the A.P. plane and angle it at 20° to the axis of the femoral shaft in the lateral plane (Fig. 30.27).

7. Divide the soft tissue attachments to the condyles and remove them.

8. Detach the capsule from the margins of the tibial condyles and expose the proximal 2 cm of the bone, dividing the patellar ligament if necessary.

9. Resect the tibial condyles with a hand saw, removing as little bone as possible to obtain a flat cancellous surface. Keep the saw parallel to the Steinmann pin in the A.P. plane and at right angles to the long axis of the tibia in the lateral plane.

10. Approximate the two cancellous surfaces. If the pins have been correctly placed the alignment of the bones will be correct with the tibia in 10° of valgus (the normal standing angle) and in 20° of flexion.

11. Remove more bone if necessary to obtain this position.

12. Remove the tourniquet and stop bleeding from the soft tissue.

13. Apply Charnley compression clamps to the pins, leaving a space 2.5 cm wide between the clamps and the skin.

14. Tighten each clamp a little at a time, making sure that the bone surfaces sublux neither laterally or antero-posteriorly whilst doing so.

15. Tighten the locking screws holding the clamps to the pins and cut off the ends of the pins with bolt cutters flush with the clamps.

Closure

1. Insert a suction drain.
2. Close the incision in the capsule and quadriceps tendon with 0 synthetic absorbable sutures.
3. Close the subcutaneous fat and skin.

Aftercare

1. Apply a layer of wool around the leg, carefully tucking it between the clamps and the skin.

2. Apply a firm bandage and then a plaster of Paris back slab.

3. Take A.P. and lateral X-rays to check the position of the bones after 24 hours.

4. Remove the suction drain after 48 hours.

5. Check the clamps every day, tightening them if necessary.

6. Remove the stitches at 12–14 days and apply a plaster of Paris cylinder extending from the groin to the ankle and enclosing the clamps which should be smeared with 'Vaseline' beforehand.

7. Mobilise on crutches and allow home.

8. Remove the plaster and loosen the clamps at 6 weeks.

If the arthrodesis feels firm, remove the clamps and pins and apply a plaster cylinder.

9. Allow full weightbearing with a raise on the shoe to compensate for the discrepancy in leg lengths.

10. Remove the plaster of Paris after a further 6 weeks if clinical and radiological union is sound.

APPROACHES TO THE LOWER LEG

The shafts of the tibia and fibula are subcutaneous and may therefore be exposed by incisions through the overlying skin.

ANTERIOR APPROACH (Fig. 30.28)

Appraise

1. Use the anterior approach for access to the shaft of the tibia and the anterior compartment of the lower leg.

2. Expose the fibula through a separate lateral incision if required.

Prepare

1. Cross-match two units of blood.
2. Use a general anaesthetic.
3. Exsanguinate the leg and apply a pneumatic tourniquet to the thigh.

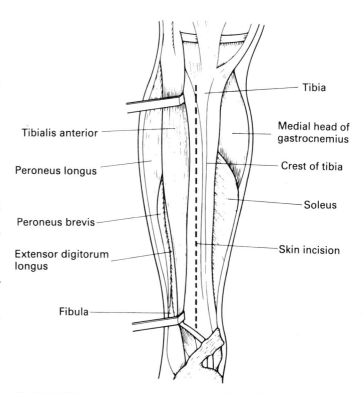

Fig. 30.28 The anterior approach to the shaft of the tibia.

4. Place the patient supine on the operating table.

5. The unscrubbed assistant grasps the ankle and elevates the leg, applying traction at the same time if the tibia is broken.

6. Clean the skin from the tourniquet to the ankle.

7. Place a large sheet across the operating table and over the sound leg.

8. Place the 'shut-off' towel immediately distal to the tourniquet (see p. 511).

9. Fold a small towel corner to corner and place it on the operating table with the long edge transversely just above the level of the malleoli.

10. A scrubbed assistant grasps the leg in a large sterile pack or small towel and lowers it into the triangular 'shut-off' towel.

11. Carefully wrap the ankle and foot in the towel and bandage it securely in place.

12. Continue to drape the leg as described on page 511.

Access

1. Incise the skin longitudinally 1 cm lateral to the crest of the tibia, from the tibial tubercle to the ankle.

2. Reflect skin flaps medially and laterally to expose the subcutaneous surface of the tibia and the tibialis anterior.

Closure

1. Release the tourniquet.
2. Insert a suction drain.
3. Close the skin with 2/0 interrupted sutures.

TIBIAL SHAFT FRACTURES

Appraise

1. Ease of access does not justify indiscriminate operative treatment of fractures of the shaft of the tibia.

2. Operate only when closed methods have failed or are inappropriate (see section on operative fixation of bone, p. 448).

Prepare

Use the anterior approach (see p. 523).

Action

1. Make a skin incision 20 cm long centred over the fracture.

2. Incise the deep fascia along the crest of the tibia.

3. Retract the tibialis anterior laterally to expose the lateral surface of the tibia.

4. Retract the medial skin flap to expose the medial surface of the tibia.

5. Evacuate blood clot and debris.

6. Prepare the bone ends and reduce the fracture (see p. 450).

7. Bend a six-hole plate to the shape of the lateral surface of the tibia and hold it in place with Hey Grove's bone clamps (see p. 450).

8. Fix the plate to the bone with screws with or without compression according to individual preference (see p. 450).

Closure

1. Release the tourniquet.
2. Insert a suction drain deep to tibialis anterior.
3. Do not suture the deep fascia.
4. Close the skin.

Aftercare

1. Apply a padded compression dressing.

2. Apply a plaster back-slab from the toes to the mid-thigh if the fixation is not secure.

3. Start quadriceps exercises immediately.

4. After 36–48 hrs change the dressing and remove the suction drain.

5. Start exercising the knee and ankle as soon as possible in the absence of supplementary external fixation.

6. After 10–12 days, remove the sutures and allow the patient to walk with crutches without taking weight on the affected leg.

7. Allow partial weightbearing after 6 weeks and full weightbearing after 12 weeks, if clinical and radiological progress is satisfactory.

TIBIAL COMPARTMENT FASCIOTOMY

Appraise

Decompress the fascial compartment of the leg:

1. After extensive closed soft tissue injuries of the lower leg.

2. After proximal vascular reconstruction following arterial injury.

3. For chronic exertional compartment syndrome.

Prepare

Prepare for the anterior approach (see p. 523).

Access

1. Make the longitudinal skin incision 4 cm long, lateral to the crest of the mid-tibia.

2. Incise the fascia covering the tibialis anterior muscle and extend the incision in the fascia subcutaneously both proximally and distally with a Smillie meniscectomy knife.

3. Make a second longitudinal incision just medial to the postero-medial border of the tibia.

4. Incise the deep fascia and extend the incision proximally to the level of the tibial tuberosity and distally to a point 5 cm proximal to the medial malleolus, using the same technique.

Closure

1. Close the skin if this is possible without tension.
2. If not, suture the skin 3–5 days later when the swelling has subsided (see p. 448).

Aftercare

1. Apply a compression dressing.
2. Elevate the leg.
3. Mobilisation will depend on the underlying reason for the fasciotomy.

APPROACHES TO THE ANKLE

Operations on the ankle joint itself can usually be accomplished through an anterior approach. Separate incisions are required to gain access to the malleoli and to the posterior aspect of the joint.

ANTERIOR APPROACH (Fig. 30.29)

Appraise

Use this approach to gain access to the ankle joint itself and for arthrodesis or arthroplasty.

Prepare

1. Use a general anaesthetic.
2. Exsanguinate the leg and apply a pneumatic tourniquet to the thigh.
3. The unscrubbed assistant holds the leg just below the knee joint and elevates it.
4. Clean the skin from the assistant's hands to the tip of the toes, paying particular attention to the skin between them.
5. Drape the limb as described on page 523, placing the proximal 'shut-off' towel at mid-calf level and omitting the distal 'shut-off' towel.

Access

1. Make an incision in the skin 10 cm long in the midline, centred over the middle of the ankle joint.
2. Incise the superficial fascia avoiding the superficial peroneal nerve which crosses the wound diagonally. Retract it laterally.
3. Incise the deep fascia and the extensor retinaculum and identify the anterior tibial artery and the deep peroneal

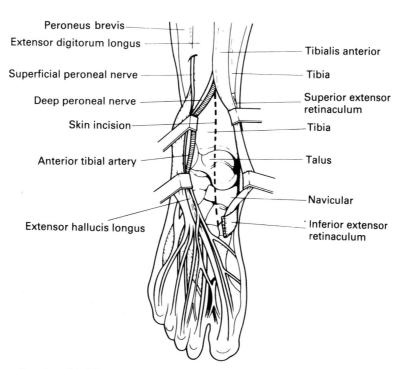

Fig. 30.29 The anterior approach to the ankle joint.

nerve between the tendons of tibialis anterior and extensor hallucis longus.

4. Retract the neurovascular bundle, extensor hallucis longus, and extensor digitorum laterally and the tibialis anterior medially.

5. A pad of fat frequently obscures the anterior capsule of the ankle joint and should be excised.

6. Incise the joint capsule longitudinally and open the ankle joint. Do not confuse it with the talonavicular joint which is unexpectedly close to it.

Closure

1. Release the tourniquet and stop the bleeding.
2. Insert a suction drain.
3. Close the deep fascia.
4. Close the skin.

POSTERIOR APPROACH (Figs. 30.30 & 30.33)

Appraise

Use the posterior approach to gain access to the Achilles tendon and the posterior aspect of the ankle joint and distal end of the tibia.

Prepare

1. Use a general anaesthetic.
2. Exsanguinate the leg and apply a pneumatic tourniquet to the thigh.
3. Place the patient prone on the operating table with the foot hanging over the end.

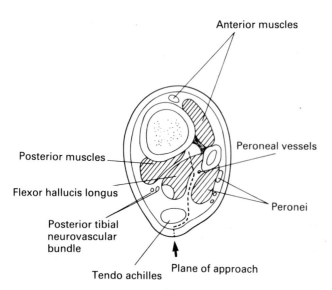

Fig. 30.30 Transverse section of the lower leg just above the ankle joint showing the posterolateral approach to the lower tibia along the dotted line.

4. The unscrubbed assistant holds the leg just distal to the flexed knee.

5. Clean the leg from the toes to the assistant's hands.

6. Place a large drape under the thigh of the affected leg and over the table and the opposite leg.

7. Place a 'shut-off' towel immediately distal to the assistant's hands.

8. Extend the knee and cover the trunk and thighs with a large sheet.

Access

1. Make an incision 15–20 cm long in the midline of the calf ending at the calcaneum.

2. Expose the lateral side of the Achilles tendon, retracting the sural nerve and short saphenous vein laterally with the skin flap.

3. Deepen the incision through the fascia into a fat-filled space, crossed by a branch of the peroneal artery which must be ligated and divided.

4. Locate the peroneus brevis laterally and the flexor hallucis longus medially. Separate these muscles proximally, dividing part of the fibular attachment of the flexor hallucis longus if necessary, taking care to preserve the peroneal vessels running down the back of the fibula.

5. Retract the peroneus brevis laterally and the flexor hallucis longus medially to expose the posterior aspect of the ankle joint and the distal tibia.

MALLEOLAR FRACTURES AND RUPTURED LIGAMENTS

OPEN REDUCTION AND INTERNAL FIXATION OF MALLEOLAR FRACTURES

Appraise

1. Displaced fractures of the medial and lateral malleoli and the posterior lip of the tibia require accurate reduction to restore the articular surface of the ankle joint.

2. When this cannot be achieved by closed methods, operative treatment is essential.

3. The malleoli may be fractured individually or in combination. There are often associated ligamentous injuries, which may be deduced from the radiographs and which should also be repaired.

4. The fibula should always be reduced and fixed before the other fractures.

5. The method of fixation is often a matter of personal preference.

Prepare

1. Operate with a general anaesthetic.
2. Exsanguinate the leg by elevation only and apply a pneumatic tourniquet to the thigh.

3. Clean the skin and drape the leg as described for the anterior approach (see p. 525).

LATERAL MALLEOLUS

1. Make the skin incision along the posterior margin of the distal fibula, starting 7 cm proximal to the tip of the lateral malleolus and curving it anteriorly around the tip of the malleolus for a further 3 cm.

2. Extend the incision proximally if necessary to expose fractures of the distal shaft of the fibula.

3. Dissect the anterior skin flap off the bone and retract it gently with skin hooks.

4. Open up the fracture site and remove any flakes of bone and articular cartilage and blood clot from the ankle joint.

5. Strip the periosteum for 1–2 mm from the bone ends.

6. If the fracture is distal to the inferior tibiofibular joint, reduce it and fix it by tension band wiring (Fig. 30.31).

7. Hold the malleolus in place by gripping it with a towel clip.

8. Drill a 1.5 mm diameter Kirschner wire from a point 4–5 mm anterior to the tip of the malleolus into the medullary cavity of the fibula, crossing the fracture line and extending 4–5 cm beyond it.

9. Insert a second Kirschner wire from a point 4–5 mm posterior to the tip of the malleolus.

10. Bend the protruding ends of each wire to a right angle and cut off the wires 2 mm from the surface of the bone.

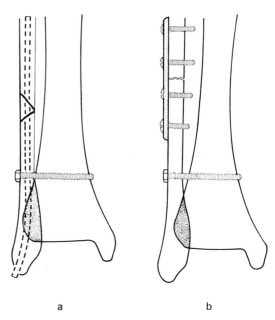

Fig. 30.32 Fixation of fractures of the lower end of the fibula with
(a) an intramedullary nail and
(b) a plate and screws, with transverse screw to close the diastasis.

11. Drill an anteroposterior hole 2 mm in diameter at right angles to the shaft of the fibula, 2–3 cm proximal to the fracture line.

12. Pass a length of 0.7 mm (22 SWG wire) through the hole, cross the ends over the surface of the bone and pass them around the protruding ends of the Kirschner wires before twisting them together with wire tighteners to compress the fracture (Fig. 30.31).

13. Cut off the excess wire and remove the towel clip from the malleolus.

14. If the fracture line is above the inferior tibiofibular joint, fix oblique or spiral fractures with screws (see p. 448), and transverse fractures with small four-hole plates (Fig. 30.32).

15. If there is a diastasis insert a screw transversely through the fibula and into the tibia (Fig. 30.32) proximal to the joint with the ankle in full dorsiflexion. Do not over-tighten.

MEDIAL MALLEOLUS

1. Make a skin incision along the posterior margins of the tibia starting 7 cm proximal to the tip of the medial malleolus, curving anteriorly around the malleolus for a further 3 cm.

2. Retract the anterior skin flap and expose the fracture line.

3. Open the fracture and clear blood clot and debris from the joint.

4. Strip the periosteum from the margins of the fracture.

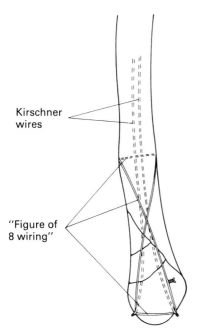

Kirschner wires

"Figure of 8 wiring"

Fig. 30.31 Kirschner wires and figure-of-eight traction absorbing wiring for comminuted fractures of the lateral malleolus.

5. Drill a hole 4.5 mm in diameter retrogradely through the malleolus from the centre of the fracture surface and at right angles to it to emerge through the tip of the lateral cortex.

6. Make a short incision through the deltoid ligament over the tip of the drill before removing it.

7. Accurately reduce the fracture and hold it in place with a towel clip.

8. Pass a 3.5 mm twist drill through the previous hole and extend the hole into the tibia.

9. Carefully remove the drill and insert a self-tapping lag screw and gently tighten.

10. If there is a tendency for the malleolus to rotate, insert a second screw if the fragment if large enough or alternatively a Kirschner wire parallel to the first screw. (N.B. Tension band wiring is also suitable for fractures of the medial malleolus).

11. Take anteroposterior and lateral radiographs of the ankle to check the reduction and the position of the wire or screws, and also the position of any fracture of the posterior malleolus which may now be in a satisfactory position.

12. If the position of the posterior malleolus is unsatisfactory wrap the leg in a sterile towel and elevate it while the drapes are removed.

POSTERIOR MALLEOLUS

1. Turn the patient into the prone position and re-towel for the posterior approach before removing the towel from the lower leg.

2. Expose the posterior capsule of the ankle joint through the posterior approach (see p. 526).

3. Incise the capsule transversely and dorsiflex the ankle to open the joint to inspect the articular surface of the tibia.

4. Reduce the posterior malleolus, inspecting the articular surface to be sure the reduction is complete.

5. Fix the fragment with one or more screws or Kirschner wires according to its size.

Closure

1. Release the tourniquet and stop the bleeding.
2. Insert a suction drain if there is any tendency to oozing.
3. Close the skin.

Aftercare

1. Apply a pressure dressing and elevate the leg.
2. After 36–48 hours inspect the wound and remove the drains. If the fixation was judged to be sound at operation, reduce the dressings and begin mobilising the ankle joint; otherwise immobilise it in a back slab.
3. After 12–14 days remove the sutures and apply a below-knee walking plaster, allowing partial or full weight-bearing according to the security of the fixation.

4. Between 6–8 weeks remove the plaster and allow full weightbearing if clinical and radiographic progress is satisfactory.

REPAIR OF RUPTURED MEDIAL AND LATERAL LIGAMENTS

Appraise

1. Ruptures of the medial and lateral ligaments of the ankle, with or without associated fractures, should be repaired through the incisions used to expose malleolar fractures.

2. Treat isolated ruptures of the lateral ligament in plaster.

3. Ruptures of the medial ligament are usually associated with fractures of the lateral malleolus and should be repaired if the fracture itself requires operative treatment.

4. Repair ruptures of the lateral ligament associated with fractures of the medial malleolus if the fracture requires operation.

Action

1. Expose the ligament as if it were a malleolar fracture.
2. Remove blood clot.
3. Suture the ends together with 0 synthetic absorbable mattress sutures.

Closure

1. Release the tourniquet.
2. Close the skin.

Aftercare

Immobilise the ankle in a padded walking plaster for 6 weeks.

REPAIR OF RUPTURED ACHILLES TENDON

Appraise

1. Ruptures of the Achilles tendon are frequently missed.
2. Immediate repair is desirable but if diagnosis is delayed, wait until swelling and bruising have subsided.

Prepare

1. Use a general anaesthetic.
2. Exsanguinate the leg by elevation only and apply a pneumatic tourniquet to the thigh.
3. Clean and drape the ankle for the posterior approach.

Action

1. Incise the skin in the midline from the mid-calf to the proximal transverse skin crease. Never use curved or flapped incisions (Fig. 30.33).

2. Carefully elevate the skin for 2 cm on either side of the midline and retract the skin gently with skin hooks.

3. Identify and retract the sural nerve and the short saphenous vein laterally.

4. Open the paratenon and expose the ends of the ruptured tendon which are usually very ragged.

5. Turn down two strips of the gastrocnemius fascia 15 cm long and 0.5 cm wide as illustrated in Figure 30.33.

6. Thread each strip on to a Gallie's Fascia Needle and pass each needle through the proximal stump of the tendon to emerge on the rupture surface.

7. Pass each needle through the substance of the distal stump to emerge on the posterior surface of the tendon, 1.5–2.0 cm distal to the rupture.

8. Plantarflex the foot and pull the fascial strips tight to close the gap in the tendon and then cross them over the back of the tendon to the medial and lateral sides.

9. Pass one needle from the lateral and the other from the medial side transversely through the proximal stump 1.5–2.0 cm proximal to the rupture and then down either side of the tendon.

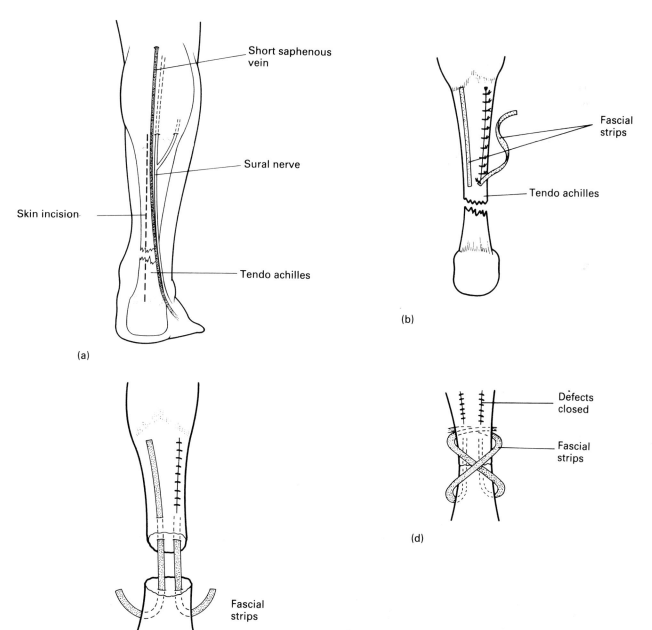

Fig. 30.33(a) Exposure of the ruptured tendo Achillis.
(b) Turning down of fascial strips.
(c,d) Fascial darn.

10. Remove the needles. Pull the fascial strips tight and suture them to the proximal and distal stumps of the tendon with 0 absorbable synthetic sutures.

11. Pass further sutures across the ends of the tendon.

12. Suture the paratenon.

Closure

1. Release the tourniquet and stop the bleeding.
2. Insert a suction drain.

Aftercare

1. Apply a padded compression dressing with the ankle in full plantar flexion.

2. Apply a plaster of Paris slab to the front of the ankle from the upper tibia to the toes and bandage it in place. Elevate the leg.

3. Remove the drain and inspect the wound after 24–36 hours.

4. The skin overlying the tendo Achillis heals badly and has a tendency to slough. Pressure must be avoided by nursing the patient on the side.

5. Remove the sutures when the skin has healed and apply a below-knee plaster with the foot in full plantar flexion. Allow up non-weightbearing.

6. Remove the plaster after 6 weeks and allow full weightbearing with a triple thickness felt pad under the heel. Reduce the raise by one thickness of felt per week over the next 3 weeks.

7. Do not allow full sporting activities for at least 3 months after the repair.

ARTHRODESIS AND ARTHROPLASTY OF THE ANKLE

ARTHRODESIS

Appraise

1. Arthrodesis remains the treatment of choice for unremitting pain arising from the ankle joint, especially if movement is also limited.

2. Arthrodesis allows fixed deformities to be corrected.

3. Arthrodesis will restore stability to the ankle joint.

Prepare

1. Use a general anaesthetic.

2. Exsanguinate the leg and apply a pneumatic tourniquet to the thigh.

3. Position and drape the patient for the anterior approach (see p. 525).

Action (Fig. 30.34)

1. Insert a Steinmann's pin traversely through the tibia from the lateral side 10 cm proximal to the tip of the lateral malleolus, at right angles to the long axis of the tibia and parallel to the floor, with the leg in correct rotational alignment.

2. Insert a second Steinmann's pin through the talus from a point 0.5 cm anterior and 0.5 cm distal to the tip of the lateral malleolus. This pin should be placed in such a way that after subsequent correction of any angular or rotational deformity it will lie parallel to the first pin.

3. After exposing the ankle joint through the anterior approach, incise the capsule transversely and forcibly plantarflex the foot to open up the joint.

4. Place the blade of a forged scalpel between the lateral malleolus and the talus and divide the lateral ligament.

5. Divide the medial ligament in similar fashion.

6. Slip a small bone lever around the medial malleolus and another around the lateral malleolus in contact with the bone and deep to the tendons and neurovascular bundle.

7. With the foot plantarflexed, resect the articular surface of the talus with an oscillating power saw. Make the cut 0.5 cm proximal to the distal Steinmann's pin and parallel to it in the lateral plane, and parallel to the plantar surface of the heel in the anteroposterior plane.

8. Divide the tibia and fibula with the oscillating saw 0.5 cm proximal to the apex of the articular surface of the tibia. The cut should be parallel to the Steinmann's pin in the lateral plane and at an angle of 10° to the axis of the tibia in the anteroposterior plane, so that more bone is removed from the back of the tibia than the front.

9. Take care to protect the structures behind the malleoli with the bone levers, and complete the cut through the posterior cortex of the tibia with a broad osteotome.

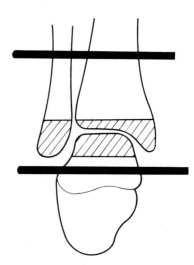

Fig. 30.34 Coronal section through the left ankle joint showing resection of articular surfaces and placing of Steinmann pins for arthrodesis of the ankle.

10. Grasp the resected bone with bone forceps and pull it forward, dividing any remaining soft tissue attachments.

11. Oppose the cut surfaces of the tibia and talus and apply the Charnley bone clamps to the pins (see p. 523); tighten them just sufficiently to hold the bone together.

12. If the pins have been correctly placed and the cuts accurately made, the foot should lie in 10° of plantar flexion with the heel in 5° of valgus. If not, release the clamps and remove more bone.

13. Make sure that rotational alignment is correct, and that the heel is neither too far forward or back when viewed from the side before finally tightening the clamps.

14. Cut off the ends of the Steinmann's pins (see p. 523).

Closure

1. Release the tourniquet.
2. Insert a suction drain.
3. Close the wound (see p. 526).

Aftercare

1. Apply a compression dressing over wool tucked between the skin and the clamps (see p. 523).

2. Apply a plaster of Paris back slab.

3. After 24 hours take a check X-ray and tighten the clamps if necessary.

4. After 48 hours remove the drain.

5. After 14 days remove the stitches and apply a below-knee plaster incorporating the clamps. Allow the patient up non-weightbearing on crutches.

6. After 6 weeks remove the plaster and X-ray. Loosen the clamps and if the arthrodesis is clinically firm, remove the pins and apply a below-knee walking plaster.

7. At 12 weeks, remove the plaster and allow unrestricted weightbearing if the arthrodesis is clinically and radiologically united.

ARTHROPLASTY

Replacement arthroplasty of the ankle is still under trial, but is particularly suitable for patients with rheumatoid arthritis affecting the joints of the hindfoot as well as the ankle.

THE FOOT

Fractures and soft tissue injuries rarely require operative treatment and reconstructive operations require judgement and experience. The common operations on the foot are limited to the toes and each requires an individual approach.

ARTHROPLASTY OF THE FIRST METATARSOPHALANGEAL JOINT (KELLER'S OPERATION)

Appraise

1. Use this operation to treat hallux valgus and hallux rigidus in the middle-aged and elderly patient.

2. The most suitable operation for these conditions in children and adolescents requires judgement and experience.

Prepare

Clean and drape the lower leg and foot as described on page 523, but place the 'shut-off' towel around the instep.

Access

Make a dorsal longitudinal incision 5 cm long in the midline of the big toe, extending proximally from the interphalangeal joint across the metatarsophalangeal joint and in the axis of the first metatarsal.

Action (Fig. 30.35)

1. Incise the deeper layers down to the bone in the line of the skin incision just medial to the tendon of extensor hallucis longus and open the joint.

2. Expose the 'exostosis' on the medial side of the metatarsal head by sharp dissection, cutting the soft tissues off the bone in a single layer and retracting them with a small bone lever.

3. Dissect the soft tissues off the dorsum and the sides of the proximal half of the proximal phalanx.

4. Forcibly plantarflex the toe. Grip the base of the proximal phalanx with a towel clip or Lane's tissue forceps and pull it forward; carefully dissect the flexor hallucis longus tendon from the plantar surface, keeping the knife close to the bone.

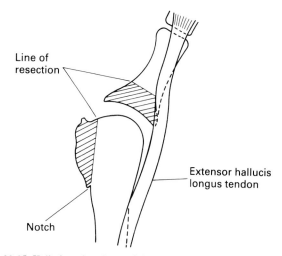

Fig. 30.35 Keller's arthroplasty of the big toe.

5. Divide the proximal phalanx with large double action bone cutters at the junction of its proximal and middle thirds.

6. Trim the cut surfaces of the phalanx with bone nibblers if necessary.

7. Make a small nick in the medial cortex of the first metatarsal just proximal to the exostosis with the 2 cm osteotome.

8. Excise the exostosis with the osteotome in the line of the medial cortex of the metatarsal (Fig. 30.35). Trim the edges of the raw surface with bone nibblers.

Closure

1. Release the tourniquet and stop the bleeding.

2. Pull on the toe and place a pad of haemostatic gauze in the space between the metatarsal head and the proximal phalanx to maintain the length of the toe.

3. Hold the toe in varus and suture the capsule with a continuous 2/0 absorbable synthetic suture.

4. Close the skin.

Aftercare

1. Dress the wound and place a pad of plaster wool between the first and second toes to maintain the over-corrected position of the big toe. Wrap the foot in plaster wool and a crepe bandage from above the ankle to the toes.

2. After 48 hrs allow up non-weightbearing on crutches.

3. Remove the sutures at 10–12 days and allow full weightbearing.

4. Encourage active movements of the toe which will remain swollen for several months.

METATARSAL (HELAL'S) OSTEOTOMY
(Fig. 30.36)

Appraise

1. Pain under the second, third and fourth metatarsal heads is usually associated with clawing of the toes.

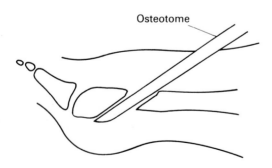
Osteotome

Fig. 30.36 Metatarsal osteotomy. Free the metatarsal head from its plantar aspect with an osteotome after dividing the metatarsal obliquely with a saw.

2. The metatarsal heads are prominent and tender to palpation under the skin of the sole.

Prepare

1. Clean and drape the foot as described for Keller's operation.

2. Manipulate the toes forcibly if necessary to correct any fixed deformities of the proximal and distal interphalangeal joints.

Access

1. Make a dorsal longitudinal incision just lateral to the extensor tendon of the second toe, and extend it proximally for 3 cm from the base of the toe.

2. Make a second incision just medial to the extensor tendon of the third toe.

Action

1. Deepen the first incision down to the distal third of the second metatarsal.

2. Incise the periosteum and strip it to either side with a periosteal elevator and place small bone levers on either side of the exposed metatarsal shaft.

3. Divide the metatarsal with a small oscillating saw at an angle of 45° to the long axis of the shaft, starting 2 cm proximal to the neck (Fig. 30.36).

4. Slide a 1 cm-wide osteotome distally between the bone and the plantar soft tissues to free the metatarsal head, allowing it to displace dorsally and proximally (Fig. 30.36)

5. Trim the dorsal cortex of the distal side of the cut with bone nibblers if necessary.

6. Repeat the procedure on the second metatarsal, making use of the same skin incision.

7. Divide the third metatarsal through the second skin incision.

Closure

1. Release the tourniquet.
2. Suture the skin.

Aftercare

1. Apply a wool and crepe dressing.

2. Elevate the foot for 48 hrs.

3. Start full weightbearing as soon as the pain will allow, usually in 2–3 days.

4. Remove the dressings and sutures after 14 days when loose fitting shoes or sandals can be worn.

5. Allow unlimited walking when the osteotomies have united after 4–6 weeks.

ARTHRODESIS OF THE INTERPHALANGEAL JOINTS OF THE SMALL TOES

SPIKE ARTHRODESIS (Fig. 30.37).

Appraise

1. This operation is suitable for hammer deformities of the proximal interphalangeal joints of the small toes.

2. Passive flexion of the metatarsophalangeal joints is essential, if necessary by extensor tenotomy, otherwise the fixed toe will stick up causing pain.

3. If it is impossible to correct the hyperextension of the metatarsophalangeal joint, metatarsal osteotomy or proximal hemi-phalangectomy should be performed.

Prepare

Clean the skin and drape the leg as described for Keller's operation.

Access

1. Excise an ellipse of skin surrounding the callosity over the dorsal surface of the proximal interphalangeal joint.

2. Divide the exposed extensor tendon transversely at the level of the joint.

3. Flex the joint acutely.

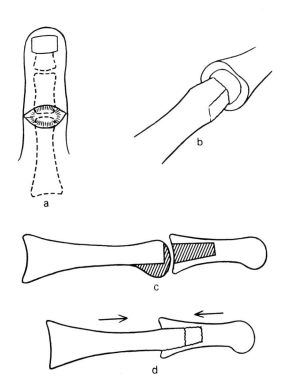

Fig. 30.37 Technique for spike arthrodesis of a small toe joint.

Action

1. With a small scalpel or tenotome dissect on all sides of the head of the proximal phalanx until 1cm of its length is freed.

2. With fine McIndoe bone cutters, resect the sides and under surface and end of the head of the proximal phalanx, converting it into a rectangular peg about 5 mm long and 3 mm in cross-section. Do not resect the cortex on the dorsum of the bone as this is the only part retaining mechanical strength.

3. With Paton's burrs of increasing diameter, bore a hole in the base of the middle phalanx. Begin the hole at the centre of the articular surface and continue in a slightly dorsal direction so that the joint will be fused in the position of slight flexion rather than exactly straight.

4. Impact the peg into the hole.

5. Check that the arthrodesis is sound but do not pull the peg out of the hole once it has been inserted as it will not fit tightly a second time.

6. If the peg breaks or proves too small for the socket in the base of the middle phalanx, retrieve the situation by inserting a Kirschner wire as described below.

Closure

Suture the skin and the transverse cut in the extensor tendon over the joint in a single layer.

Aftercare

1. Fold a gauze dressing into a strip 1.5–2.0 cm wide and place a centre of the strip over the dorsum of the toe. Take each end through the cleft on either side of the toe on to the sole of the foot. Hold the ends in place on the sole with adhesive tape.
(N.B. Do not enclose the toe in a circumferential dressing at this stage to avoid constriction of the toe as it swells.)

2. Wrap the foot in a wool and crepe dressing.

3. After 48 hrs remove the dressings and encircle the toe with ribbon gauze soaked in collodion.

4. Allow full weightbearing and remove this dressing in 6 weeks.

KIRSCHNER WIRE ARTHRODESIS

Appraise

1. Use this technique for the distal interphalangeal joints.

2. Use this technique if difficulties arise whilst performing spike arthrodesis.

Prepare

Clean and drape the foot as for Keller's operation.

Action

1. Excise an ellipse of skin from the dorsum of the joint.
2. Divide the extensor tendon transversely.
3. Plantarflex the joint and divide the collateral ligaments with a tenotomy knife from within the joint.
4. Nibble the articular surfaces of the joint back to cancellous bone, leaving two flat surfaces.
5. Drill a 1.5 mm diameter Kirschner wire of measured length through the cut surface of the distal phalanx and out through the pulp of the toe just beneath the nail.
6. Reattach the drill to the distal end of the wire and withdraw it until the tip protrudes 2–3 mm from the cut surface of the bone.
7. Position the protruding proximal end of the wire opposite the centre of the cut surface of the phalanx proximal to the joint, and push the cut surfaces firmly together.
8. Drill the wire back through the toe, stopping short of the metatarsophalangeal joint.
9. Remove the chuck and measure the length of wire protruding to make sure that the tip has not gone too far, withdrawing the wire if necessary.
10. Cut the wire flush with the skin and then tap the end with a small punch so that it lies subcutaneously.

Closure

Close the wound as described for the spike arthrodesis.

Aftercare

1. Dress the wound as described for spike arthrodesis.
2. Replace the dressings with a small adhesive dressing after 48 hours.
3. At 6 weeks infiltrate the skin over the tip of the wire with 1% lignocaine, and through a small stab incision withdraw the wire with pointed nose pliers or bone nibblers.

PROXIMAL PHALANGECTOMY OF THE SMALL TOE

Appraise

This operation is suitable for those toes which dorsal contracture of the metatarsophalangeal joints makes unsuitable for spike arthrodesis. The cosmetic result is not as good as that after arthrodesis. The toe is left short and flaccid but pressure symptoms are relieved.

Prepare

Clean the skin and drape the foot as described for Keller's operation.

Access

1. Make a 'Z'-shaped incision 2 cm dorso-laterally along the proximal segment of the toe, 1 cm transversely at the metatarsophalangeal joint and 1.5 cm proximally longitudinally along the dorsum of the foot.
2. Divide the extensor tendon in the line of the transverse line of the incision.

Action

1. Deepen the incision to bone and dissect subperiosteally around the midshaft of the proximal phalanx with a scalpel or small rougine.
2. Divide the proximal phalanx transversely at its midpoint with bone cutters.
3. Lift the proximal portion out of the wound with Kocher's forceps and dissect the soft tissues off the plantar surface of the bone to the metatarsophalangeal joint proximally.
4. Remove the proximal half of the proximal phalanx from the wound.

Closure

1. Release the tourniquet.
2. Close the subcutaneous tissues and skin with interrupted sutures.

Aftercare

1. Bandage the toe in the correct position over encircling layers of wool.
2. Reduce the dressings after 24 hrs and cover the wound with a small adhesive dressing.
3. Allow weightbearing as soon as pain will allow.
4. Remove the stitches after 10–12 days.

EXCISION OF PLANTAR DIGITAL NERVE FOR MORTON'S METATARSALGIA

Appraise

Morton's metatarsalgia may be due either to a neuroma on the plantar digital nerve or to an enlarged intermetatarsal bursa pressing on the nerve.

Prepare

1. Warn the patient there will be numbness on the contiguous sides of the two toes after the operation.
2. Clean and drape the patient as for Keller's operation.
3. Raise the foot off the table and sit opposite the sole of the foot which should be at eye level.

Access

1. Make a plantar incision 3 cm long over the affected intermetatarsal space but do not continue the incision proximally into the pad under the metatarsal heads.
2. Insert a small self-retaining retractor.

Action

1. By blunt dissection display the neurovascular bundle. Dissect the nerve and neuroma from their surroundings and excise them from the bifurcation of the nerve as far back into the sole as possible. Do not leave the proximal stump lying distally in the region of the metatarsal heads or the terminal neuroma will cause persistent pain and tenderness.
2. If a bursa is present it is usually about 1.5–2.0 cm in diameter and thick walled. The digital nerve usually runs in one wall of the bursa. Excise both the nerve and the bursa.

Closure

Close the skin only with simple sutures after the release of the tourniquet.

Aftercare

1. Wrap the foot in a wool and crepe dressing.
2. Reduce the dressings after 24 hours and cover the wound with an adhesive strip.
3. Allow up non-weightbearing on crutches.
4. Allow full weightbearing after 2 weeks when the stitches have been removed.

RADICAL RESECTION OF THE NAIL BED (ZADIK'S OPERATION) (Fig. 30.38)

Appraise

1. This operation is suitable for chronic ingrowing toenails.
2. Do not undertake the operation in the presence of sepsis but merely remove the nail and wait for about 2 months until the sepsis has subsided.
3. Do not perform the operation in the presence of peripheral vascular disease.

Prepare

1. The operation may be performed under local ring-block anaesthesia with a rubber band as a digital tourniquet.
2. Clean and drape the leg as for Keller's operation.

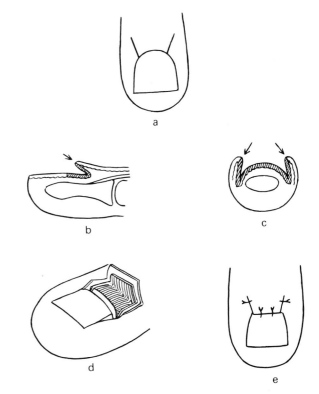

Fig. 30.38 Radical resection of the nail bed.

Action

1. Remove the nail if present by separating if from the underlying nail bed with a MacDonald's elevator.
2. Make two incisions 1 cm long extending proximally from each corner of the nail to the transverse skin crease over the interphalangeal joint.
3. Lift the skin and subcutaneous tissue as a flap and dissect this proximally to the interphalangeal joint.
4. Carry the dissection under the edges of the skin incisions on either side of the terminal phalanx to the mid-lateral line to complete the clearance of the germinal matrix of the nail.
5. Cut across the nail bed transversely at the site of the lunula and join this transverse incision to the dissections under the nail folds.
6. Remove the block of nail bed from the surface of the proximal phalanx as far back as the insertion of the extensor tendon.
7. Check that no fragments of germinal matrix are left behind.

Closure

1. Draw the skin flap distally and suture the end to the nail bed with one or two stitches which must be inserted carefully as they easily cut out.
2. Close the incisions on either side.

Aftercare

1. Dress the wound with a non-adherent dressing.
2. Apply pressure with tubigrip bandage.
3. Release the tourniquet.
4. Elevate the foot for 24 hours.
5. Allow weightbearing with or without crutches as pain permits.
6. Remove the dressings and the stitches after 12–14 days.

Further reading

Antrum R N 1984 Radical excision of the nail fold for ingrowing toenails. Journal of Bone and Joint Surgery 66B: 63–65

Arnold W D 1984 The effect of early weight-bearing on the stability of femoral neck fractures treated with Knowles pins. Journal of Bone and Joint Surgery 66A: 847–852

Barnes R, Brown J T, Garden R S, Nicoll E A 1976 Subcapital fractures of the femur: A prospective review. Journal of Bone and Joint Surgery 58B: 2–24

Blockey N J 1982 Congenital dislocation of the hip. Editorial. Journal of Bone and Joint Surgery 64B: 152–155

Brodie I A O D, Denham R A 1974 The treatment of unstable ankle fractures. Journal of Bone and Joint Surgery 56B: 256–262

Charnley J 1951 Compression arthrodesis of the ankle and shoulder. Journal of Bone Joint Surgery 33B: 180–191

Charnley J 1961 Arthroplasty of the Hip. A New Operation. Lancet 1:1129

Coventry M B 1973 Osteotomy about the knee for degenerative and rheumatoid arthritis. Indication, operative technique and results. Journal of Bone and Joint Surgery 55A: 23–48

Demottaz J D, Mazure J M, Thomas W H, Sledge C B, Simon S R 1979 Clinical study of total ankle replacement with gait analysis. Journal of Bone and Joint Surgery 61A: 976–988

Evans G A, Hardcastle P, Frenyo A D 1984 Acute rupture of the lateral ligament of the ankle: to suture or not to suture? Journal of Bone and Joint Surgery 66B: 209–213

Guiloff R J, Scadding J W, Klenerman L 1984 Morton's metatarsalgia. Journal of Bone and Joint Surgery 66B: 586–591

Helal B, Greiss M 1984 Telescoping osteotomy for pressure metatarsalgia. Journal of Bone Joint Surgery 66B: 213–217

Henry A K 1957 Extensile exposure applied to limb surgery, 2nd edn. E & S Livingstone Ltd, Edinburgh & London

Heyse-Moore G H, MacEachern A G, Jameson Evans D C 1983 Treatment of intertrochanteric fractures of the femur. Journal of Bone and Joint Surgery 65B: 262–267

Hughston J C, Andrews J R, Cross M J, Moschi A 1976 Classification of knee ligament instabilities. Part I. The Medical Compartment and Cruciate Ligaments. Part II. The Lateral Compartment. Journal of Bone and Joint Surgery 58A: 159–179

Joy G, Patzakis M, Harvey J P 1974 Precise evaluation of the reduction of severe ankle fractures. Journal of Bone and Joint Surgery 56A: 979–993

Lettin A W F, Kavanagh T G, Scales J T 1984 The long term results of Stanmore total knee replacements. Journal of Bone and Joint Surgery 66B: 349–355

McKee G K, Watson Farrar J 1966 Replacement of arthritic hips by the McKee-Farrar prosthesis. Journal of Bone and Joint Surgery 48B: 245–259

Miegel R E, Harris W H 1984 Medial-displacement intertrochanteric osteotomy in the treatment of osteoarthritis of the hip. A long-term follow-up study. Journal of Bone and Joint Surgery 66A: 878–887

Mize R D, Bucholz R W, Grogan D P 1982 Surgical treatment of displaced comminuted fractures of the distal end of the femur. Journal of Bone and Joint Surgery 64A: 871–879

Müller M E, Allgöwer M, Schneider R, Willenegger H 1979 Manual of internal fixation. Techniques recommended by the AO group, 2nd edn. Springer-Verlag, Berlin Heidelberg New York

Nister L 1981 Surgical and non-surgical treatment of Achilles tendon rupture. Journal of Bone and Joint Surgery 63A: 394–399

Noble J, Erat K 1980 In defence of the meniscus. A prospective study of 200 meniscectomy patients. Journal of Bone and Joint Surgery 62B: 7–11

O'Brien E T, Fahir J J 1977 Remodelling of the femoral neck after in situ pinning for slipped capital femoral epiphysis. Journal of Bone and Joint Surgery 59A: 62–68

Rasmussen P S 1973 Tibial condylar fractures. Journal of Bone and Joint Surgery 55A: 1331–1350

Rorabeck C H, Bourne R B, Fowler P J 1983 The surgical treatment of exertional compartment syndrome in athletes. Journal of Bone and Joint Surgery 65A: 1245–1251

Salter R B 1984 The present status of surgical treatment for Legg-Perthes disease. Journal of Bone and Joint Surgery 66A: 961–966

Scott J C 1949 Fractures of the patella. Journal of Bone and Joint Surgery 31B: 76–81

Sikorski J M, Barrington R 1981 Internal fixation versus hemiarthroplasty for the displaced subcapital fracture of the femur. Journal of Bone and Joint Surgery 63B: 357–361

Van der Linden W, Larsson K. Plate fixation versus conservative treatment of tibial shaft fractures. Journal of Bone and Joint Surgery 61A: 873–878

West F E 1962 End results of patellectomy. Journal of Bone and Joint Surgery 44A: 1089–1108

Wilson D W 1980 Treatment of hallux valgus and bunions. British Journal of Hospital Medicine 24: 348–361

Winquist R A, Hanson S T, Clawson D K 1984 Closed intramedullary nailing of femoral fractures. Journal of Bone and Joint Surgery 66A: 529–539

Zadik F R 1950 Obliteration of the nail bed of the great toe without shortening the terminal phalanx. Journal of Bone and Joint Surgery 32B: 66–7

Plastic and reconstructive surgery

GENERAL PRINCIPLES

Plastic (*Plassein* — Greek: to mould) and reconstructive surgery is concerned with the restoration of form and function of the human body. This may follow damage or loss of tissue from injury or disease or from treatment of these. Aesthetic or cosmetic surgery is commonly associated with rejuvenating the ageing body including the correction of deformities but this forms only a small part of the practice of most plastic surgeons.

In the past decade there have been many new advancements in plastic surgery which have given rise to a multitude of new methods of reconstruction. The principal development is the application of axial pattern flaps following the recognition of their existance. Many new cutaneous, myocutaneous and other flaps have been described recently but only those used more commonly will be described in this chapter.

PREPARE

1. Plan for repair and reconstruction of tissue defects well in advance of operation where possible. Carry out the simplest procedure to get the wound healed. Reconstruction of a defect may be primary or secondary after repair, often in several stages. Make plans for each stage before embarking on the whole, so that one stage does not jeopardise a subsequent one.

2. Identify the lines of tension within the skin (Langer's lines) in the region of the proposed operation. Try to make all incisions parallel to these lines. When this is not possible, consider using a Z-plasty or local flap in closing the wound to help prevent the formation of scar contracture postoperatively.

3. Mark out a plan of the flap on the patient with a skin marker the day before operation, when using a large flap or a sophisticated reconstruction. For smaller flaps and simple incisions, mark out the area of incision on the patient after preparing the area before incising the skin. Use a fine pen and ink to mark out the lines of incision on the face. Use a broad proprietary marking pen in other areas. Try and follow these lines, as they are a useful guide once the skin has been incised and tension in the surrounding skin has changed. Be prepared, however, on occasions to make adjustments according to the circumstances.

4. Anaesthetic advances in the last two decades have made general anaesthesia a very safe procedure. Do not forget, however, that many operations can be carried out under regional anaesthesia or local anaesthesia (see p. 24). Many operations on the hand can be carried out under regional anaesthesia including cases of replantation. Large areas of split skin graft can be taken from the lateral aspect of the thigh by infiltrating the lateral cutaneous nerve of the thigh in the region of the inguinal ligament with local anaesthetic. Many other procedures can be carried out under regional anaesthesia, with the assistance of a sedative, if necessary. Many simple skin lesions can be excised under local anaesthesia. Use 1% lignocaine for this purpose. For lesions in the head and neck region where the skin is highly vascular, use $\frac{1}{2}$% lignocaine with 1 : 200 000 adrenaline. Wait 5 minutes after injecting the mixture, and this provides a relatively avascular field as well as anaesthesia. Use this mixture for extensive excisions

of the face or scalp even when the patient is under general anaesthesia, but inform the anaesthetist if he intends to use fluothane.

TECHNIQUE

1. Sutures.
(a) On the face approximate the deep dermis of the skin edges with interrupted 4/0 catgut sutures. Accurately appose the skin edges with 6/0 interrupted nylon sutures. Remove them on the third or fourth post-operative day. If they remain longer, suture marks form and these may prove impossible to remove without producing a more ugly scar.
(b) Elsewhere on the body, approximate the deep dermis of the wound edges with chromic catgut sutures and use subcuticular prolene sutures whenever possible, tying a knot at either end to prevent slipping. Leave these sutures in for 10 days or longer if there is a tendency for the scar to stretch because of its site.

2. Instruments.
(a) Respect tissues and their viability by handling them with care and using the appropriate instruments. For surgery of the skin, learn to support the skin with skin hooks or fine toothed forceps. Do not crush it by holding it with non-toothed forceps.
(b) For accurate fine suturing, use a fine needle holder with a clasp which you find comfortable. Needle-holders with their own cutting edges require much practice before they can be used effectively. They are useful when many interrupted sutures are required and the accuracy of these is not crucial to the overall result.
(c) Microvascular surgery requires specialised instruments

3. Drains.
(a) For general principles see page 9.
(b) When moving large flaps use large suction drains at the donor site, which has a large potential cavity.

4. Diathermy.
(a) Beware of the unipolar diathermy when coagulating vessels near the skin. The burnt tissue may be visible and painful.
(b) Always use a bipolar coagulator for fine work and flaps. The current from a unipolar machine could destroy the vessels in the base of a flap as it is being raised.

SKIN COVER

1. Close skin wounds primarily to provide ideal skin cover following incisions of the skin, excisions of skin lesions and simple lacerations.
2. Use split skin grafts to repair wounds with significant skin loss, to avoid skin closure with tension, or following trauma with an appreciable degree of crush injury to the local tissues. Skin graft survival depends on adequate vascularity of the base of the wound.
3. Use skin flaps, which carry their own blood supply with them and are temporarily self-sufficient, in primary or secondary repair or reconstruction. Use them as primary cover for vital structures such as exposed neurovascular bundles or structures which have an inadequate blood supply to support a graft, such as bare bone, bare cartilage, bare tendons and exposed joints.

SKIN CLOSURE

Appraise

1. Employ primary skin closure following simple skin incisions, surgical excision of small skin lesions and to repair simple lacerations. It should not be carried out if the tension in closing the wound causes blanching of the skin.
2. If the skin edges have been crushed, do not further insult them with sutures but carefully trim away dead skin and apply a simple dressing. Close the skin after a delay of 24–48 hours.
3. Beware of skin that has been degloved or torn from its fascial base. Resect it primarily, or if possibly viable, replace and re-examine at 48 hours, resecting it then if there is absence of bleeding when it is cut.

Action

1. Whenever possible make incisions in the direction of the tension lines, particularly on the face.
2. For excisions, mark the skin in ink, planning to excise the minimal necessary amount of tissue. Draw an ellipse with pointed ends around this mark, parallel to the tension lines. (Fig. 31.1 (a)).
3. On the face, inject the surrounding tissue with $\frac{1}{2}$% lignocaine and 1 : 200 000 adrenaline and wait 5 minutes for both components to take effect.
4. Make a vertical cut through the skin along the lines of the ellipse and take adequate clearance of the lesion in depth.
5. Undermine the skin edges beneath the layer of subcutaneous fat to facilitate approximation of the edges without tension. (Fig. 31.1 (b)).
6. Place a skin hook in each end of the wound and ask your assistant to draw them apart. This manoeuvre approximates the edges. (Fig. 31.1 (c)).
7. Close the wound in layers.
8. Apply a small dressing, or use no dressing at all if practical.

SKIN GRAFTS

Appraise

1. A skin graft is a piece of skin detached from its donor

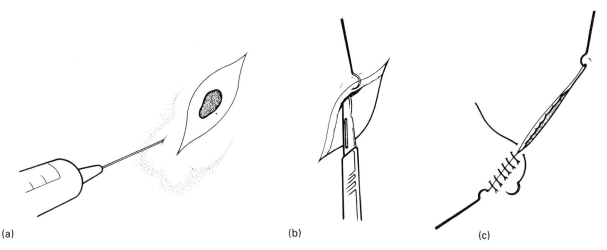

(a)   (b)   (c)

Fig. 31.1 Simple excision of skin lesion. The skin is marked and surrounding skin infiltrated with local anaesthetic (a). Undermining the lateral skin margin (b). The wound ends are distracted with skin hooks to help approximate the edges of the wound (c).

site and transferred to a recipient site. It may contain part of the thickness of the skin (a split skin graft or Thiersch graft) or the full thickness of the skin (a Wolfe graft).

2. A skin graft depends for its survival on receiving adequate nutrition from the recipient bed. Thus, thin split skin grafts survive more readily than thick split skin grafts or full thickness grafts.

3. If there is a poor vascular bed or infection, no graft will survive. In these cases prepare the graft bed appropriately with dressings (see p. 540), or consider using a flap.

4. Choose an appropriate donor site for each individual patient.

SMALL SPLIT SKIN GRAFT

Appraise

1. A split skin graft is a sheet of tissue containing epidermis and some dermis taken from a donor site. It is obtained by shaving the skin with an appropriate knife or blade. A layer of deep dermis is preserved at the donor site, and when dressed appropriately, this is re-epithelialised from residual skin adnexae.

2. Use a small split skin graft to repair traumatic loss of small areas of skin from the hand or fingers, and occasionally in other parts of the body. Avoid using them on the tips of the thumb and index fingers since they tend to become hyper-aesthetic.

3. Choose the donor site carefully. On the upper limb take skin from the medial aspect of the arm where the donor site will be inconspicuous and not from the forearm where an ugly resultant scar may be visible.

Action (see also p. 540)

1. Mark out on the medial aspect of the arm an area of

skin which is more than sufficient to cover the recipient site.

2. Inject $\frac{1}{2}$% lignocaine and 1 : 200 000 adrenaline intradermally into and beyond the marked area and wait for 5 minutes.

3. Lubricate the marked area with liquid paraffin.

4. Grip the arm on the lateral aspect with your left hand so that the skin which is marked out becomes tense, with a convex surface.

5. Cut the graft from the marked area using the Da Silva knife. (Fig. 31.2).

6. Dress the donor site with paraffin gauze, several layers of dressing gauze and a crepe bandage.

7. Apply the split skin graft direct onto the recipient site, spread it, and anchor it using a minimal number of sutures.

8. Apply paraffin gauze, dressing gauze and a crepe bandage.

9. Re-dress the graft at 5 days.

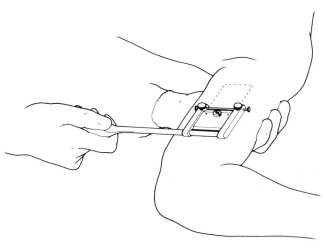

Fig. 31.2 Taking a small split skin graft with a Da Silva knife.

SKIN GRAFTS

LARGE SPLIT SKIN GRAFT

Appraise

1. Use these grafts following extensive skin loss from burns, trauma or radical excisional surgery.

2. The recipient site must be adequately prepared to ensure a good take of the graft. Grafts take best on exposed muscle or well-prepared granulation tissue. They do not take reliably on exposed fat where there is a poor vascular supply.

3. The take of a graft can be improved in certain circumstances by meshing it (see p. 541), quilting it (see p. 541), or by delaying its application and then exposing it (see p. 541).

Prepare

1. Following 'cold' surgical excisions, obtain haemostasis with pressure. Try to avoid using diathermy, as skin grafts do not take over diathermy burns.

2. Where sub-cutaneous fat is exposed, suture the surrounding skin down to the muscle or deep fascia to minimise the area of exposed fat.

3. For infected wounds, take swabs for bacterial culture and prepare the recipient site with dressings of Eusol and paraffin. Change them 3–4 times a day. The recipient site is ready to receive a graft when healthy, compact, red granulation tissue is evident with minimal exudate.

4. Do not apply grafts in the presence of beta-haemolytic streptococci group A. If this organism is present, eradicate it by surgical debridement and appropriate systemic antibiotics before grafting.

5. Choose the donor site most readily available to provide a large area of skin graft; this is usually the thigh. Use the inner aspect of the thigh in young people, where the donor site will be hidden. Use the outer aspect of the thigh in elderly people where the skin is slightly thicker, so that if healing is delayed the wound can be easily managed.

Action

1. Prepare both recipient and donor sites by applying skin antiseptic.

2. Get your assistant to spread a large swab on the side of the thigh opposite to the proposed donor site. With his hand on the swab he supports the thigh and tenses the skin at the donor site by gripping the skin firmly with the swab.

3. Set the blade on the Watson knife to take the appropriate thickness skin graft. Use a medium setting at first and then adjust accordingly.

4. Apply liquid paraffin on a swab to the donor site and along the knife blade.

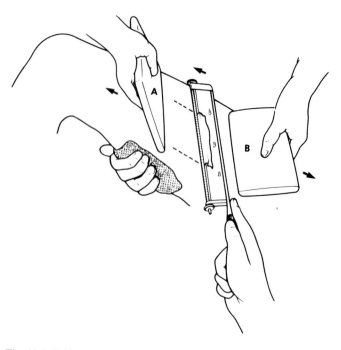

Fig. 31.3 Taking a large split skin graft from the thigh, the surgeon advances board A in front of the knife as it progresses along the thigh. The assistant tenses the skin of the thigh in his right hand, using a large swab to prevent his hand from slipping, and tenses the skin behind the knife using board B.

5. Ask your assistant to hold the edge of a graft board at the starting point with his other hand (Fig. 31.3).

6. Cut a skin graft with the Watson knife, holding a board in the non-cutting hand and advancing this a few centimetres in front of the knife. Start with the knife at 45° to the skin and once the blade has entered the dermis, rotate it axially so that it runs just parallel with the skin surface. Use a 'sawing' action with the knife, advancing the blade only a few millimetres at a time. When an adequate length of skin has been harvested, turn the blade upwards and cut the graft off with one firm movement. If the graft is not detached with this movement, cut along its base with a pair of scissors.

7. Place the skin graft, outer surface downward, on a damp saline swab and make sure that sufficient skin has been harvested. If in doubt take another strip of split skin.

8. Dress the donor site with one or two layers of paraffin gauze, dressing gauze, cotton wool and a crepe bandage.

9. Apply the skin graft to the donor defect. Make sure the graft is placed with its cut surface applied to the wound. The outer surface is opaque, the inner surface is shiny. Spread it, using two pairs of non-toothed forceps.

10. Cut off the surplus skin at the wound edge, leaving a margin of 3 mm around the periphery.

11. If the skin has been applied where a satisfactory compression dressing can be employed, do not use sutures.

12. Dress with several layers of paraffin gauze, dressing gauze, wool and crepe bandage, immobilising the joints above and below the graft with a bulky dressing.

13. In areas where it is difficult to apply a compression dressing, immobilise the graft with interrupted sutures at the edge or insert a circumferential continuous suture around the graft.

14. Dress with paraffin gauze, dressing gauze, wool and strips of elastoplast.

15. Keep the graft site elevated post-operatively.

16. For grafts on the lower limb, do not allow the grafted area to be dependent for 10 days. Then arrange progressive mobilisation with bandage support to the graft.

DELAYED EXPOSED GRAFTS

Appraise

1. Use a delayed graft when the graft in its recipient site can be exposed indefinitely by the patient without being disturbed.

2. Apply them to surgical wounds when haemostasis is difficult to establish per-operatively. Since the graft is exposed, it can be monitored regularly to ensure a good take.

Action

1. Prepare the recipient site during surgery with debridement and haemostasis,

2. Dress with several layers of paraffin gauze, dressing gauze, wool and a crepe bandage.

3. Harvest large split skin grafts adequate to cover the defect and dress the donor site (see p. 540).

4. Spread the split skin graft on paraffin gauze with the external opaque surface on the gauze. Fold and wrap this in a saline-soaked swab and place it in a sterile jar to be stored in a refrigerator at 4°C.

5. On the following day, remove the dressing from the recipient site.

6. Apply the skin graft to the defect and spread it to cover all areas. Trim and store any excess skin at the margin.

7. Remove the paraffin gauze and leave the skin graft exposed.

8. Observe the graft at regular intervals. If serum collects beneath it, roll this out with cotton wool budded sticks soaked in saline, either to the edge or through a small incision made in the graft.

9. Be sure that the exposed area is well protected from any trauma, particularly while the patient is asleep.

MESHED GRAFTS

Appraise

1. Meshed grafts are useful for providing skin cover to large areas, particularly when there is a limited area of donor skin, as often occurs in extensive burns.

2. They are also usefully applied to recipient sites adjacent to an area of chronic infection. An infected discharge would readily lift off a continuous sheet graft, but escapes through the interstices of a meshed graft, leaving the graft elements intact.

Action

1. Prepare the donor site in the usual way.
2. Harvest long, thin strips of split skin grafts, as described above.
3. Dress the donor site.
4. Pass the skin graft through the skin mesher. It may need to be placed on a carrier for this, depending on the type of instrument (Fig. 31.4)
5. Apply the mesh graft directly onto the donor site using two pairs of non-toothed forceps.
6. Spread the skin out appropriately to cover all suitable recipient areas.
7. Suture the graft with continuous sutures at the periphery only if the area is difficult to dress.
8. Dress the area with paraffin gauze, dressing gauze, cotton wool and crepe banadage.
9. Re-dress at 4 or 5 days.
10. Continue to re-dress at approximately 3 day intervals until the interstices have epithelialised.

QUILTED GRAFTS

Appraise

These are most usefully applied to large areas of the tongue or any other highly vascular area. Any method of graft fixation is liable to cause bleeding beneath the graft.

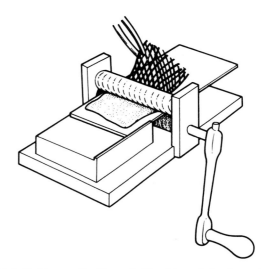

Fig. 31.4 Meshing a split skin graft. The skin graft has been placed on a plastic carrier and is being passed through the skin mesher. The cut skin, elevated at one corner by a pair of forceps, can be stretched to three times its original size or more, depending on the carrier used.

However, at each suture site a small area of graft take is ensured, and epithelialisation subsequently spreads out from each of these.

Action

1. Prepare the donor site.
2. Harvest the skin graft.
3. Put two large sutures in the anterior aspect of the tongue and pull it forward.
4. Apply the skin graft to the tongue and trim the excess at the edges.
5. Place multiple 2/0 silk sutures at the edge of the graft and dotted throughout its surface. (Fig. 31.5).
6. No dressing is required.
7. The sutures can be removed at 10 days if necessary.

FULL THICKNESS GRAFTS

Appraise

1. Full thickness grafts give better cosmetic results than split thickness grafts as they contract less. The quality of the skin is better but they need a very good vascular bed to survive.
2. Their most common application is on the face following excision of small lesions, and the best results are achieved in the eyelid region and around the medial canthus.
3. They can occasionally be used on the hand, but are not generally used elsewhere, as large grafts leave a large primary defect.
4. The best donor sites are those with surplus skin so that the skin can be closed primarily with an insignificant

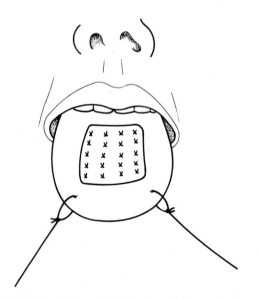

Fig. 31.5 Quilted graft. The graft is fixed to a defect on the dorsum of the tongue with multiple sutures.

scar. The most common donor areas are post-auricular, pre-auricular, upper eyelid, naso-labial and supra-clavicular skin.

Action

1. Mark the area of skin to be removed and measure it.
2. Mark out a similar area in the donor site, allowing an extra 2 mm. at each margin for the contour difference that will be present at the recipient site.
3. Plan an ellipse at the donor site to allow primary closure.
4. Inject local anaesthetic at the excision and donor sites.
5. Create the defect at the recipient site.
6. With a size 15 blade, cut around the margins of the planned donor skin.
7. Raise the full ellipse of skin and subcutaneous tissue.
8. Undermine the skin edges at the donor defect and close this primarily.
9. Place the skin graft onto a wet saline swab, skin surface down.
10. Using small, curved scissors, cut the subcutaneous fat off the skin graft and excise the redundant skin.
11. Place the skin graft into the defect and suture the edges at the periphery. Leave the suture ends long.
12. Use tie-over sutures to fix the dressing of tulle gras and proflavine wool.
13. Apply a pressure dressing for 24 hours, if possible.
14. Dress the donor site.
15. Plan to re-dress the recipient site at one week.

COMPOSITE GRAFTS

Appraise

1. Composite grafts consist of skin and other tissue, usually subcutaneous tissue and some underlying cartilage.
2. They are most commonly used where there is significant loss of a nostril rim.
3. Occasionally, they are used for defects at the periphery of the pinna.

Action

1. Mark out the defect that will be left after excision or debridement of the wound edges.
2. Identify a site on either pinna which corresponds in both size and shape to the planned defect.
3. Mark out this area with ink.
4. Prepare both ears.
5. Plan the reconstruction of the donor defect.
6. Inject 0.5% lignocaine and 1 : 200 000 adrenaline into both sites and wait for 5 minutes.
7. Create the donor defect by excising a lesion or the margins of a wound, and achieve haemostasis.

8. Excise the composite graft and reconstruct the defect.

9. Place the graft into the recipient defect, and suture it with multiple 6/0 nylon sutures inserted at the skin margin only.

10. Leave the graft exposed and clean.

11. Allow the superficial crust which develops after one week to separate spontaneously.

12. If a small part of the graft does not survive, treat it expectantly and re-appraise after separation of necrotic tissue.

SKIN FLAPS

INTRODUCTION

1. Skin flaps are used to repair or reconstruct defects where there is an inadequate blood supply to support a skin graft. They survive on their own blood supply which they bring with them and this may be beneficial to the recipient site. It may help by introducing a new blood supply to an avascular area following irradiation, or to a fracture site where there is delayed union.

2. The quality of the skin in a skin flap is almost normal, and it is cosmetically more acceptable than a graft, although of course a flap may have lost its nerve and lymphatic supply in transit.

3. Until relatively recently, all skin flaps were based on a random vascular pattern. It was recognised that flaps with a length greater than their base would survive in certain areas. It is now realised that the reason for this survival is that these flaps had, unknowingly, been based on an axial pattern basis. If a flap is designed around a recognised artery and vein, with these vessels passing down its central axis, it may be safely transferred with a very large length to breadth ratio. Indeed, the breadth need only be the artery and vein alone, providing they remain patent.

4. Many of the superficial muscles of the body have one principal vascular hilum, and these muscles can be rotated about the hilum on a single pedicle. It has further been realised that the skin overlying these superficial muscles receives its vascular supply from them. Consequently the muscle with its overlying skin can be transposed as a single unit, forming a myocutaneous flap. A large number of these flaps have been described, but only the more commonly used ones will be described below.

5. Special terms are traditionally used in relation to flaps. Delay indicates partial division of a flap at its base and resuturing. This procedure encourages an improved blood supply to the flap from the opposite attachment. Complete division at the base carried out a few days later is then safer. After a flap has been transferred safely, the bridging portion may be divided. The two ends are trimmed and one is sutured into the new recipient area while the other is replaced in the donor site. This is referred to as in-setting.

6. When planning a flap, it is useful to employ a sheet of sterile paper or other similar material to act as a template. This can be cut to shape and used as a trial flap.

Z-PLASTY

Appraise

1. Z-plasties are used for releasing linear contractions. These usually develop along linear scars which traverse Langer's lines.

2. These linear contractions are often most evident when crossing the concavity of the flexor aspect of a joint, but they can occur on extensor surfaces and on other areas unrelated to joints.

Action

1. Draw a line along the full extent of the contracture (Fig. 31.6).

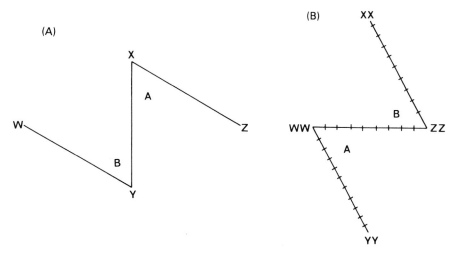

Fig. 31.6 Z-plasty. Contracture along X Y is released to XX YY by raising and interchanging flaps A and B. The distance WZ is shortened to WW Z.

2. From one end, draw a line at 60° to the first line and of the same length.

3. From the opposite end, draw a line at 60° on the opposite side of the line for the same length.

4. Incise along the central line and excise any scar tissue.

5. Incise along the two lateral lines through the full thickness of skin and subcutaneous tissue.

6. Raise the flaps so formed, lifting the skin and subcutaneous tissue as one holding the tip of each flap with a skin hook.

7. Interchange the two skin flaps.

8. If the flaps do not meet comfortably, undermine the skin and subcutaneous tissue around the periphery of the wound to allow them to lie perfectly.

9. Suture the tips of the two flaps into place first.

10. Suture the remaining edges of the flaps.

11. Dress the wound.

Technical points

1. The angle of the Z-plasty can be varied according to circumstances.

2. If the scar contracture is particularly long, use two or more Z-plasties either in series or at intervals along the length of the contracture.

3. For scar contractures across a web space, use a W-plasty (Fig. 31.7). This consists of two Z-plasties, planned in reverse direction to each other, meeting at the base of the web space.

TRANSPOSITION FLAP

Appraise

1. Small transposition flaps on the face have long been used. It is well recognised that in this region, because of the vascularity of the skin, flaps with a large length to breadth ratio can be used safely.

2. Transposition flaps allow skin from an area of abundance to be moved to a defect where primary closure is inappropriate.

3. On the face, there is an abundance of skin appropriate for transposition flaps in the nasolabial area, the glabella area, and the upper eyelid.

4. In other parts of the body, many axial pattern flaps are used as transposition flaps.

Action

1. Mark out the defect in ink.

2. Plan the transposition flap in an adjacent area with superfluous skin and mark this out (Fig. 31.8).

3. Check that the margin of the flap most distal from the defect is long enough from the fulcrum at its base to reach the most distal part of the defect. This is the limiting factor of the flap.

4. Excise the lesion to create the defect.

5. Raise the flap, including skin and subcutaneous tissue, and support the tip of the flap on a skin hook.

6. Transpose the flap into the defect and check that it fits.

7. Undermine the edges of the donor site defect and also the edges of the excision area to allow the flap to sit more comfortably in the defect.

8. Close the donor defect in layers.

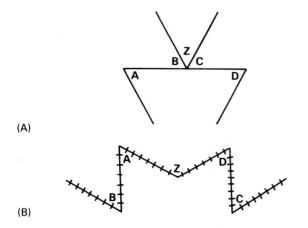

(A)

(B)

Fig. 31.7 W-plasty. This consists of two Z-plasties along the same contracture placed in reverse direction and meeting at the central point. Flaps A and B are interposed and Flaps C and D are interposed. Flap Z stays in the same place but is raised during surgery to allow undermining at its base to allow it to stretch.

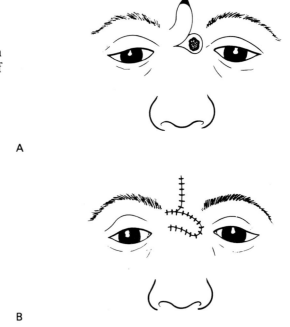

A

B

Fig. 31.8 Transposition flap. A lesion in the region of the medial canthus is excised and a transposition flap from the glabella region is used to reconstruct the defect. A small triangle of skin at the apex of the flap is discarded and the donor site is closed primarily.

9. Suture the flap in place.

10. Leave the flap exposed if possible, to monitor it.

RHOMBOID FLAP

Appraise

1. A rhomboid flap is, as its name suggests, a flap with the shape of an equilateral parallelogram.

2. The rhomboid flap is most useful when the appropriate ellipse for excision of a defect is at right angles to Langer's lines. It has a similar effect to a transposition flap carried through 90°.

Action

1. Mark out the area of the defect.

2. Around this, draw the smallest possible rhomboid with equal sides.

3. Draw two further lines of equal length as shown in Figure 31.9.

4. Excise the lesion.

5. Transpose the flap, as shown in the diagram.

6. Undermine the edges.

7. Close the donor defect.

8. Suture the flap in place.

ROTATION FLAP

Appraise

1. These are large flaps used to close relatively small defects.

2. They use excess skin at a distance from the defect, and borrow small amounts of skin from a large area.

3. Their principal use is for borrowing skin from the neck to take up to the face. They can be used on the scalp, and in treating pressure sores around the buttocks.

Action

1. Mark out the skin defect.

2. Draw an isosceles triangle around the defect, with the apex of the triangle at the centre of the arc of rotation of the flap (Fig. 31.10).

3. Draw the circumference of a semi-circle centred on the apex of the triangle.

4. Raise the skin and subcutaneous tissue of the flap.

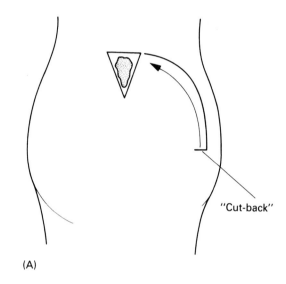

(A)

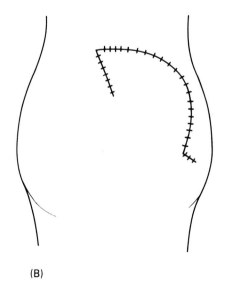

(B)

Fig. 31.10 Rotation flap. A sacral ulcer is created into a triangular defect and a flap from the buttock is rotated into this. A small cut-back allows greater mobility in rotation.

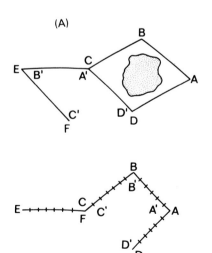

Fig. 31.9 Rhomboid flap. A rhomboid defect is created — A,B,C,D. CE and EF are drawn with equal length making a smaller rhomboid A'B'C'D'. After transposition of the flap to the defect, the donor defect is closed primarily by approximating F to C.

5. Undermine the skin at the edge of the defect and along the skin margin opposite the flap.
6. Rotate the flap into the defect.
7. Suture the flap.
8. If necessary, excise a wedge of tissue along the skin edge opposite the flap to assist rotation. A 'cut-back' into the flap at the opposite end of the arc of the flap from the defect may also help.

ADVANCEMENT FLAP

Appraise

Advancement flaps are most commonly used on the face to preserve feature lines or structures of the face. They can be used on the forehead or for defects of the eyebrow. Frequently, in these situations, bilateral advancement flaps are used simultaneously to reconstruct one defect.

Action

1. Mark out the defect.
2. Mark out the smallest possible square or rectangle enclosing this defect, with lines parallel and at right angles to Langers lines.
3. Extend the marks of the sides running parallel to Langer's lines in each direction from the defect, thus delineating two flaps (Fig. 31.11).
4. Create the defect.
5. Elevate the flaps and advance them towards each other.
6. Suture them together.
7. Suture their sides.

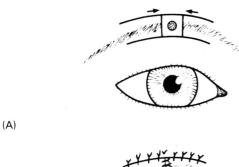

(A)

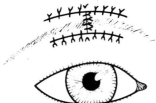

(B)

Fig. 31.11 Advancement flap. A defect in the eyebrow is excised and two advancement flaps one from each side are raised and advanced to meet each other over the defect. The natural lines of the eyebrow are preserved.

EXPANSION FLAP

Appraise

1. These flaps are used specifically for repairing and reconstructing defects of the scalp.
2. Flaps on the scalp are notorious for their inability to stretch because of the inelasticity of the galea.
3. Division of the galea allows some stretching of the skin to take place, especially in younger patients.

Prepare

1. Pay particular attention to the pre-operative planning of the flap. Remember that the scalp flap will move in 3 dimensions.
2. Shave the patient's hair over the whole scalp to a length of 1 cm. Leave long locks of hair only if you can confidently cope with these per-operatively.
3. Make a careful plan of the flap to be used and mark the outline of this.
4. Completely shave the hair for 1 cm on either side of this line and for 1 cm around the outline of the defect.
5. Wash the hair thoroughly to remove all cut and shaved hairs.

Action

1. Place the patient, face downwards, on the operating table. Use a neurosurgical head-rest to support the head, if this is available.
2. Mark out the defect on the scalp.
3. Mark out the flap as previously planned. The flap may be of transposition, rotational or advancement design.
4. Plan a wide base to the flap around the periphery of the scalp to ensure that at least one principal vascular system enters its base.
5. Inject the planned outline of the flap with 0.5% lignocaine and 1 : 200 000 adrenaline and wait at least for 5 minutes.
6. Excise the lesion and create the defect.
7. Incise along the margins of the flap to elevate it with the underlying galea so that this is included with the flap.
8. Reflect the flap backwards exposing the galea.
9. Support the flap on the palm of the hand and make multiple incisions just through the galea with a No. 15 blade (Fig. 31.12).
10. Note the principal vessels beneath the surface of the galea and avoid dividing them.
11. Make multiple transverse incisions at right angles to the first set.
12. Relfect the flap back into the defect.
13. Suture the flap into place with one layer of 3/0 silk.
14. Always insert suction drains under the flap.
15. Dress with paraffin gauze, a large cotton wool dressing and two crepe bandages.

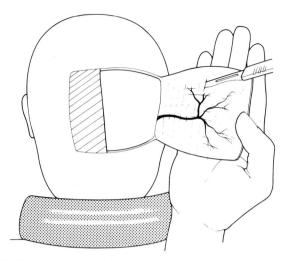

Fig. 31.12 Expansion flap. A knife is used to make multiple incisions in the galea of a scalp flap based on the posterior branch of the superficial temporal vessels which has been reflected back to its base. Following these multiple incisions, the flap can be advanced to cover the defect on the vertex of the scalp.

16. Redress after 48 hours and, if possible, leave exposed.

CROSS LEG FLAP

Appraise

1. Until recently this was the most commonly used flap to cover fractures of the tibia and fibula with extensive overlying skin loss.
2. There are now many flaps described which are more suitable but, on occasions, cross-leg flaps are still appropriate.
3. Cross arm flaps and cross thigh flaps can be created using the same principle.

Preparation

1. Plan the whole operation meticuously 24 hours before hand.
2. Mark out the minimal defect on the leg.
3. Plan a flap from the calf of the donor leg, based medially, preserving the long saphenous vein superiorly. Do not exceed a 1 : 1 length to breadth ratio.
4. Enlarge the defect to a size which will receive a safe flap; i.e. make the defect fit the flap.
5. Using tapes, ensure that with the legs kept closely together, the flap when hinged on its medial axis will stretch to the distal part of the defect, allowing enough tissue to create a bridge between the two legs.
6. Place the patient's legs on top of a bead bag and apply vacuum so the patient's legs are fixed in what will be their post-operative position.
7. Maintain the patient's legs in this bead bag for as

much of the next 24 hours as is practical so that he becomes used to the position pre-operatively.

Action

1. With the patient under general anaesthesia, apply a tourniquet to reduce bleeding.
2. Create the planned defect, obtain haemostasis, then remove the tourniquet from the leg.
3. Elevate the planned flap from the opposite leg, raising the deep fascia with the flap.
4. Check that with the legs in the appropriate position, the flap fits the defect.
5. Take a split skin graft from the thigh of the recipient leg and dress the donor area.
6. Apply and suture the split skin graft to the flap donor site and to the back of that part of the flap which will form a skin bridge between the two legs (Fig. 31.13).
7. Suture the four corners of the flap into place and subsequently suture the edges.
8. Dress the skin graft at the flap donor site and use minimal other dressings.
9. Splint the two legs in the bead bag and apply vacuum.
10. Ensure that there is no tension or torsion on the flap and that it is viable.
11. Monitor the flap postoperatively for any changes.

Complete

1. Take the patient back to theatre after 3 weeks and divide the flap, allowing a generous portion to be inset at the recipient site.
2. Suture the flap lightly into place.
3. Suture the proximal portion to its donor site.

CROSS FINGER FLAP

Appraise

Cross finger flaps are a convenient means of obtaining good quality skin cover for defects on the flexor aspects of the fingers, where split skin grafts would contract. They are taken from the dorsum of an adjacent finger.

Action

1. Mark out the defect on the flexor aspect of the finger.
2. Apply a tourniquet and create the defect.
3. Mark out a flap on the dorsum of the adjacent finger opposite the defect, or as near as possible, avoiding the skin over the joints.
4. Elevate the rectangular flap with its base adjacent to the injured finger.
5. Place the flap over the defect (Fig. 31.14).

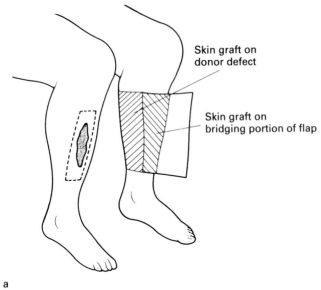

a

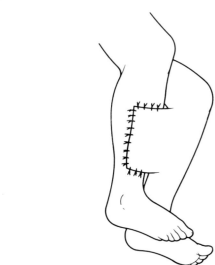

b

Fig. 31.13 Cross leg flap. (a) A skin defect on the front of the right leg is enlarged to accommodate the flap from the calf of the left leg. After the flap has been raised from the left leg, the donor defect and a portion of the bridging part of the flap are grafted before suturing the flap in place. (b) The cross leg flap is sutured in place.

6. Increase the size of the defect to fit the flap.
7. Remove the tourniquet and achieve haemostasis.
8. Take a small split skin graft with a Da Silva knife.
9. Apply the skin graft to the donor defect and the skin bridge.
10. Suture the flap into the defect.
11. Dress the wounds and splint the two fingers together after inserting some dressing gauze between the fingers.
12. Plan to divide the flap at 2 weeks, insetting the skin bridge at both recipient and donor sites, and re-dress the wounds.
13. Remove all sutures one week later.

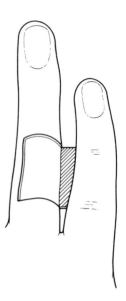

Fig. 31.14 Cross finger flap. A flap from the dorsum of the ring finger is used to cover a defect on the palmar aspect of the little finger.

REVERSE DERMIS FLAP

Appraise

This flap is similar to the cross finger flap but is used for defects on the dorsum of the finger.

Action

1. Mark out the defect.
2. Use a tourniquet to control bleeding and create the defect.
3. Mark out an appropriate flap on the dorsum of an adjacent finger, as with a cross finger flap.
4. Shave the planned flap with a Da Silva knife, removing a thin sheet of epidermis and superficial dermis.
5. Elevate the rectangular flap with subcutaneous tissue leaving it attached at its base adjacent to the finger with the defect.
6. Increase the size of the defect to fit the flap.
7. Remove the tourniquet and achieve haemostasis.
8. Take a small, split skin graft and apply this to the donor site and a portion of the bridge.
9. Suture the flap in place.
10. Splint the two fingers together with some gauze dressing between the fingers.
11. Plan to divide the flap at 2 weeks, and inset the bridge portion of the flap at both donor and recipient sites.
12. Remove all sutures 7 days later.

ABDOMINAL TUBE PEDICLE FLAP

Appraise

1. In this technique a rectangular flap of abdominal skin and subcutaneous tissue is raised, still attached at each end,

the middle part being formed into a tube. After a delay, one end is detached and transferred to a wrist. When it has established a local blood supply, the other end is detached and transferred to the site of a defect. In further stages the whole flap is transferred to the defect and spread over it.

2. Until a few years ago, these flaps were the standard technique for obtaining a large amount of skin and subcutaneous tissue from the abdomen, to be used at a distant site such as the foot, the face, or elsewhere if there had been extensive loss of tissue. They have almost totally been superseded by the introduction of axial pattern flaps, applied either as pedicle flaps or transferred as free flaps using microvascular anastomoses to vessels at the new site.

3. The patient requires approximately 5 months of hospitalisation with many operations, and failure is not uncommon at some stage. However, they remain useful in a few isolated situations.

4. Tube pedicle flaps can be raised from other sites, including the back.

Action

Raising the tube pedicle

1. Mark out a rectangular area 20 cm × 8 cm obliquely on the lower abdomen.

2. Incise along the long edges down to the deep fascia.

3. Dissect along the deep fascia between the two edges to elevate a bridge of skin and subcutaneous tissue.

4. Approximate the two skin edges of the bridge beneath the subcutaneous tissue to form a tube, and suture as far as possible in each direction.

5. At either end suture the skin down to the base to create a closed tube (Fig. 31.15a).

6. Apply a large split skin graft to the residual raw area beneath the skin tube.

Delay of the flap

1. At 2 weeks, using local anaesthesia, partially divide the base of the flap at either end, dividing through three-quarters of the skin and subcutaneous tissue, ligating and dividing the underlying vessels.

2. Re-suture the wound and apply a small dressing.

Division of the tube

1. Three weeks after raising the tube, divide the base of the tube completely, passing through the delay incision.

2. Close the residual defect on the abdomen using a split skin graft if necessary.

3. Place the patient's contralateral arm onto the abdominal wall and find a suitable recipient site at the level of the wrist to insert the tube pedicle.

4. Mark out an appropriate sized circle on the wrist.

5. Elevate the skin and subcutaneous tissue from half of this circle and reflect it backwards as a flap. This produces a circular defect.

6. Suture the free end of the abdominal tube pedicle to the circular defect (Fig. 31.15b).

7. Splint the arm to the chest wall after applying plenty of padding beneath the axilla.

Delay of abdominal tube pedicle

1. This is carried out under local anaesthesia 2 weeks after insertion to the wrist.

2. Make an incision at the base of the flap still attached to the abdominal wall.

3. The technique is the same as that used in the first delay procedure.

Transfer of flap to defect

1. Free the abdominal tube flap from the abdominal wall by dividing the tube at its residual attachment to the abdomen, passing through the delaying incision.

2. Close the donor defect with a split skin graft if necessary, and dress the wound.

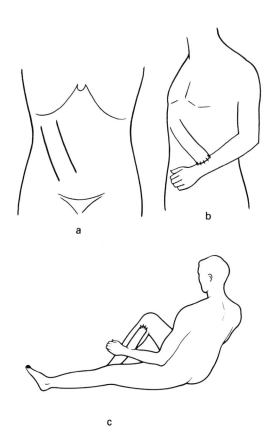

Fig. 31.15 Abdominal tube pedicle flap. (a) The flap is raised on the abdomen (b) The lower end is transferred to the wrist (c). After 3 weeks the abdominal end is detached and sutured around the defect on the contralateral leg.

3. Transfer the arm with its attached pedicle to the site of the defect.

4. Mark out a recipient site for the tube pedicle, preferably on the distal side of the defect, so that the seam of the flap overlies the defect.

5. Elevate a semi-circle of skin and reflect it backwards as a flap, creating a circular defect.

6. Excise any scar tissue from the end of the tube pedicle, and insert the tube pedicle into the skin defect (Fig. 31.15c).

7. Fix the limb appropriately.

Delay of tube pedicle

Carry out a delay of the tube pedicle at the wrist end using the same technique as before.

Transfer of whole flap to defect

1. Divide the flap from the wrist, taking the incision through the delay incision.

2. Return the original skin flap from the wrist to its former site, thus leaving a residual semi-circular wound and suture this.

3. Mark out a circular area on the opposite side of the defect from the initial attachment of the tube pedicle.

4. Elevate a semi-circle of skin and subcutaneous tissue from the adjacent area to the defect and reflect it backwards as a flap, creating a circular defect.

5. Insert the free end of the tube pedicle into this defect.

Insert the flap

1. Allow the flap to 'soften' before insetting. This may involve waiting for 4 or 5 weeks.

2. Debride the underlying defect to leave a healthy base.

3. Excise the seam of the tube pedicle and spread the skin of the tube pedicle over the defect.

4. Suture the edges into the edge of the defect.

5. Do not carry out any further revisions of the flap until it has been allowed to settle for at least several weeks and preferably for several months.

SCALP FLAP

Appraise

1. Scalp flaps are most commonly used for reconstructing defects of the hair-bearing skin on the face. They are usually used for reconstructing the upper lip, lower lip and chin areas in males, but there are many other occasional applications.

2. The flap is based on the posterior branch of the superficial temporal artery.

Prepare

1. Plan the flap on the day before operation

2. Cut all the hair in the area of surgery to less than 1 cm in length.

3. Shave the hair completely in the area of the planned incisions.

4. Check that the posterior branch of the superficial temporal artery is palpable and that there are no significant scars on the scalp, suggesting previous damage to this vessel.

5. Wash the hair thoroughly to remove all cut and shaved hair.

Action

1. Mark out the defect.

2. If appropriate, increase the defect to the shape of a whole cosmetic unit.

3. If appropriate, increase the defect to make it symmetrical on either side of the mid-line.

4. Make a template of the defect with sterile paper.

5. With one end of a tape attached to the template, and a second fixed on the zygomatic arch below the point where the artery was palpated, swing the template up onto the vertex of the scalp using the point on the zygomatic arch as the pivot.

6. Mark out an appropriate area on the scalp behind the anterior hairline around the template.

7. Infiltrate the scalp along the marked line with $\frac{1}{2}$% lignocaine and 1 : 200 000 adrenaline and wait for 5 minutes.

8. Elevate the flap together with the underlying galea, starting at its distal extremity.

9. Identify the posterior branch of the superficial temporal vessels in the pedicle of the flap as it is raised, and adjust the shape of the pedicle if necessary to include these vessels (Fig. 31.16).

10. Taper the pedicle to 2 cm at its base, allowing it to rotate.

11. Transpose the flap into the defect, and inset.

12. Cover the posterior aspect of the flap with paraffin gauze.

13. Close the donor defect primarily. If it is too large for this, cover it with a split skin graft.

14. Plan to divide the flap at 2 weeks, providing there is a large inset. If you are in doubt, divide the flap at 3 weeks and return the pedicle.

FOREHEAD FLAP

Appraise

1. The forehead flap has been used extensively until recently to provide lining of the oral cavity after major

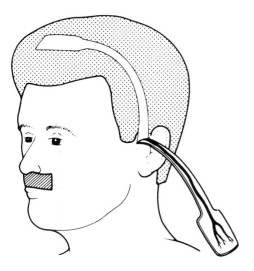

a

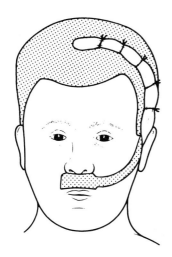

b

Fig. 31.16 Scalp flap. Defect of the upper lip is created and a matching area from the vertex is swung down on a pedicle based on the posterior branch of the superficial temporal artery.

The flap is pivoted above the zygomatic arch and turned to fill the defect (a). A split graft is applied to the donor defect with a tie-over dressing (b).

resections for tumour. It has been used occasionally for resurfacing defects of the scalp and of the cheek. It is the best flap available for total nasal reconstruction.

2. It has been largely superseded by other myocutaneous flaps in its use for oral lining, but it remains an easy, safe and reliable flap to use especially in the elderly and debilitated patient.

3. The main disadvantage of its use is the relatively poor cosmetic defect of its donor site.

4. It is not a true axial pattern flap, but it simulates one surviving on the anterior branch of one superficial temporal artery and its accompanying vein. The distal part of the flap normally acquires its vascular supply from the opposite anterior branch of the superficial temporal artery and the supraorbital and supra-trochlear vessels. When these

vessels to the flap are divided, the vascular network between the branches of the various vessels is adequate to allow the flap to survive on the supply from the single vascular pedicle.

Action

1. Create the defect and measure its dimensions.

2. Mark out the flap on the forehead, making this symmetrical and preferably including the whole of the forehead skin as a cosmetic unit.

3. Increase the defect to accommodate the flap.

4. If the flap is to be used for intra-oral lining, excise the coronoid process of the mandible to allow the flap to pass inside the zygomatic arch.

5. Elevate the flap commencing at the margin distal to the flap pedicle.

6. Identify and ligate the anterior branch of the contra-lateral superficial temporal artery and the supra-orbital and supra-trochlear vessels on both sides.

7. Lift the flap in the plane beneath the frontalis muscle.

8. Identify the anterior branch of the superficial temporal artery and its accompanying veins on the under-surface of the flap, and taper the pedicle to a 2 cm margin, including these vessels (Fig. 31.17).

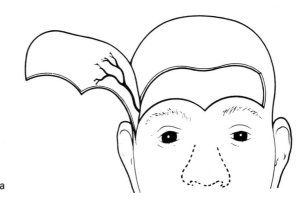

a

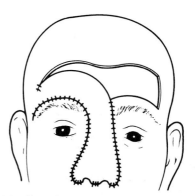

b

Fig. 31.17 Forehead flap. The forehead skin elevated on the anterior branch of the superficial temporal vessels of one side (a). Forehead flap being used for total nasal reconstruction (b). Flap divided and inset at 3 weeks.

9. If the flap is to be used intra-orally, pass this through to the mouth beneath the zygoma.

10. If there is inadequate space to carry this out, excise a segment of the zygomatic arch.

11. To avoid a further operation some 2 weeks later, shave the epithelium from that part of the pedicle that will remain buried between the skin surface and the intra-oral surface.

12. Suture the flap in place.

13. Use chromic catgut sutures to elevate the skin of the eyebrows on either side symmetrically.

14. Lay several layers of paraffin gauze on the donor site.

15. Harvest a large split skin graft to cover the defect in one sheet. In a young person, use the inner aspect of the arm in preference to the thigh as this will give a better colour match.

16. Store the skin.

17. Apply this skin as a delayed graft 24 hours later.

18. After 2 weeks, divide the pedicle and return it, to provide symmetry to the face.

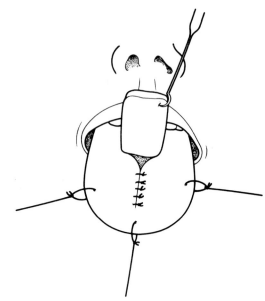

Fig. 31.18 Tongue flap. A posteriorly based tongue flap from the dorsum has been raised for closing a palatal fistula. The donor defect has been closed primarily.

TONGUE FLAP

Appraise

1. Tongue flaps are used for repairing large palatal fistulas, providing mucosa in lip reconstruction, and reconstructing defects of the pharynx and oral cavity.

2. They readily dehisce unless carefully sutured because of the difficulty in splinting them.

3. They are not easily tolerated by young children who cannot provide the necessary co-operation. Tongue flaps are, therefore, rarely useful below the age of 6.

4. Most tongue flaps are not true axial pattern flaps but rely on the rich vascular network within the muscle of the tongue.

5. Flaps for palatal fistulas are taken from the dorsum, those for lining the oral cavity or the pharynx are taken from the lateral aspect, and those providing a vermillion border are taken from the anterior part. In all cases the defect is closed primarily.

Action

1. Create the defect and measure the dimensions.
2. Put a large stay suture in the tip of the tongue and pull it forward.
3. Place two large stay sutures as far to the back of the tongue as possible and use these as the principal stay sutures.
4. Plan and mark out the flap on the tongue. Flaps for palatal fistulas can be based anteriorly or posteriorly, but this depends on the position of the defect.
5. Elevate the flap of mucosa together with a sheet of muscle approximately 4–5 mm thick.

6. Check that the flap fits the defect.
7. Close the donor defect primarily (Fig. 31.18).
8. Suture the most inaccessible part of the flap into the defect first with interrupted sutures.
9. Work proximally leaving the easiest, most anterior suture until last.
10. Observe the flap carefully; it may require resuturing at any time.
11. Divide the flap at 2 weeks, and inset.

DELTOPECTORAL FLAP

Appraise

1. This flap, often known as a Bakamjian flap after its innovator, has its greatest use in providing lining to the oral cavity after resection of intraoral tumours. It is also used for providing skin flap cover to the chin, the cheek, the region of the pinna, and the neck.

2. When raised conventionally there is necrosis of the tip in approximately 15% of cases. Because of this it has been superseded by the pectoralis flap (see below) but may still be used in conjunction with this flap or where a pectoralis flap is inapplicable.

Action

1. Create the defect.
2. Mark out the flap based on the second, third and fourth perforating branches of the internal thoracic artery (Fig. 31.19).
3. Mark the upper margin of the flap along a line

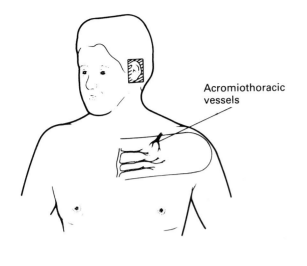

a

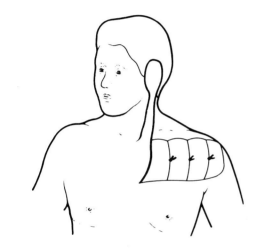

b

Fig. 31.19 Deltopectoral flap. The flap is based on the 2nd, 3rd and 4th branches of the internal thoracic artery (a). The flap being used to reconstruct the skin in the region of the pinna after a pinnectomy (b). The donor defect in this case is covered with a split skin graft and a tie-over dressing. The pedicle is divided and returned at 3 weeks.

parallel with the clavicle, along its inferior margin. Use a line along the superior margin if a block dissection of the neck has been carried out with a McPhee incision.

4. Mark the inferior border of the flap parallel to and 10 cm below the upper border.

5. Mark the distal end of the flap as a semicircle extending to the mid-lateral line over the deltoid muscle.

6. Elevate the flap from its lateral margin including the fascia overlying the deltoid and pectoralis muscle.

7. Divide the vessel from the acromio-thoracic artery, as this perforates the clavi-pectoral fascia.

8. Divide the cephalic vein at the margin of the flap.

9. Reflect the flap medially to within 4 cm of the mid-line.

10. Dissect further medially, very carefully, to avoid dividing the perforating branches on which the flap survives.

11. Pass the flap up to the defect.

12. If the flap passes direct to the defect on the external surface, tube the intervening bridge over the neck.

13. If a block dissection has been carried out and the flap is for intra-oral use, shave the epithelium from the central portion of the flap and pass the flap subcutaneously up to the defect. This manoeuvre converts the reconstruction into a one-stage operation.

14. Suture the flap into the defect.

15. Establish haemostasis on the donor site and cover it with paraffin gauze.

16. Take a split skin graft, store it and apply it to the donor site at 24 hours as a delayed graft.

17. At 3 weeks, divide the pedicle if exposed and inset the flap.

18. Return the remainder of the pedicle to the donor site after excising the split skin graft in the appropriate area.

PECTORALIS FLAP

Appraise

1. This is a most reliable and versatile flap for reconstruction following excision of tumours in the head and neck region. It will reach the oral cavity, the cheek, the pinna and areas on the neck and shoulder.

2. It is myocutaneous flap based on the pectoral vessels supplying the pectoralis major muscle. These in turn supply skin overlying the muscle.

3. Its most useful application is for intra-oral reconstruction, where an island or paddle of skin the size of the defect is transferred from the lower chest wall on the distal part of the flap. The muscle is transposed subcutaneously with this island of skin and protects the carotid vessels when a block dissection has been carried out. The donor site can be closed primarily.

4. It is not so useful in hirsute males where tranposing hairy skin to the oral cavity may prove disadvantageous. The skin island is cumbersome and less reliable in obese individuals and in women with large breasts.

Action

1. Create the defect.
2. Measure the size of the defect.
3. Measure and mark an appropriate area of skin overlying the distal inferior portion of the pectoralis muscle just above the costal margin (Fig. 31.20). Do not include skin across the mid-line nor skin more than 2 cm below the lower margin of the pectoralis muscle.
4. Draw a line from this area direct to the mid-point of the clavicle.
5. Incise along these markings through skin and fat and down to pectoralis muscle. The flap can be dissected without the use of the vertical incision.
6. Identify the lateral margin of the pectoralis muscle and elevate its border.

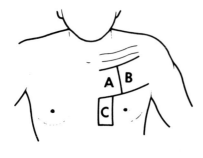

a

b

Fig. 31.20 Pectoralis flap. The pectoralis muscle is used to transfer a cutaneous island of skin (C) from the chest wall into the neck (a). To help exposure, skin flaps A and B with their underlying subcutaneous fat are reflected medially and laterally respectively (b). The muscle flap with its attached paddle of skin (C) is dissected free to the clavicle where it can be passed directly or subcutaneously to a defect above this level.

7. Dissect this distally to the sternal attachment freeing the muscle from its attachments to the chest wall.

8. Dissect the distal element free from the mid-line.

9. Elevate the muscle with its attached skin island up to the clavicle. In doing this, look for and protect the two vascular pedicles on the undersurface.

10. Divide the attachment of the muscle to the humerus at the margin of the deltoid muscle.

11. Pass the flap subcutaneously beneath the neck skin if a block dissection has been carried out and pass the island of skin into the defect. Some rotation of the muscle pedicle may be necessary. Make sure the flap sits comfortably in place, and suture the skin paddle into the defect.

12. Suture the edges of the muscle to adjacent tissue to support it when the patient sits up.

13. If the muscle traverses the neck, take a split skin graft and apply this to the exposed muscle pedicle.

14. Close the donor defect primarily. This may require wide undermining to allow approximation.

15. If the pedicle has bridged the neck, divide it at 3 weeks and inset the pedicle at each end.

LATISSIMUS DORSI FLAP

Appraise

1. The most useful application of this flap is as a myocutaneous flap in breast reconstruction and reconstruction of chest wall defects. It can be used in pharyngeal reconstruction and for defects of the back up to and just above the nape of the neck.

2. It can be used as a muscle flap alone to cover a large defect, or the muscle can be used to transfer a small island of skin (as in breast reconstruction) or a large island of skin. If a large island is transferred, primary closure of the donor site is not possible.

3. The flap has wide application in micro-vascular surgery.

4. The flap is based on the dorsal scapular vessels and these enter the muscle just below its insertion into the humerus.

Action

1. For an anterior chest wall defect, lay the patient on the table in the lateral position.

2. Create and measure the defect on the anterior chest wall.

3. Mark out the island of skin on the back overlying the latissimus dorsi muscle appropriate to the defect (Fig. 31.21).

4. Check that the island will reach the defect, using a tape based in the region of the vascular hilum at the lower margin of the posterior axillary fold. Remember the most posterior point of the flap has to reach the most anterior point of the defect.

5. Incise the skin along the marked lines around the island down to the muscle.

6. Dissect the skin and fascia off the upper surface of the whole muscle proximal and distal to the skin paddle.

7. Identify the anterior border of the muscle.

8. Separate the muscle from the underlying serratus muscles and ribs.

9. Divide the muscle from its attachment, distally and posteriorly.

10. Separate the muscle up to its pedicle, identifying and preserving the principal vessels on the underlying surface.

11. Dissect gently at the hilum to avoid damaging the principal vessels.

12. Identify the vessesls to the serratus anterior arising from the dorsal scapular vessels and divide them.

13. Develop a subcutaneous tunnel between the defect of the flap and the anterior chest wall defect.

14. Pass the flap subcutaneously through this tunnel into the anterior wall defect.

15. Close the donor site defect primarily, if possible, even if this means extensive undermining; insert a large suction drain.

16. Change the position of the patient to prone, re-towelling if necessary.

17. Undermine the skin edges of the defect where appropriate.

18. Suture the latissimus dorsi muscle to the chest wall. A prosthesis is inserted beneath this in breast reconstruction.

19. Suture the skin paddle of the flap to the skin defect.

GROIN FLAP

Appraise

1. This can be used for defects of the lower abdominal wall, but its greatest application is providing skin cover for severe injuries to the hand or wrist. It is therefore, most useful when the skin over the iliac crest is relatively thin.

2. It is an unusual axial pattern flap as the vascular pattern is variable. The flap is based on either the superficial circumflex iliac vessels or the superficial epigastric vessels or a combination of the two. Details of these variations need to be known only if the flap is to be used as a free flap.

Action

1. Create the defect on the hand.
2. Identify the femoral artery by palpation
3. Mark a point 2 cm beneath this.
4. Draw a line from this point to the anterior superior iliac crest which acts as the axis of the flap.
5. Mark an area over the iliac crest close to the mid-axillary line, which is to be used for the definitive skin cover.
6. Mark the flap to include this with parallel lines on either side of the central axis at an equal distance from it (Fig. 31.22).
7. First incise the skin laterally down to the deep fascia and include the fascia with the flap.
8. Reflect the flap medially.
9. At the edge of the sartorius muscle include the fascia overlying it with the flap and so ensure that the superficial circumflex vessels are retained within the flap.
10. Dissect the flap free to within 3 cm of the femoral vessels.
11. Check that the defect on the hand will accommodate the flap.
12. Close the donor defect primarily up to the pedicle of the flap, if necessary flexing the knee and hip.
13. Tube the portion of the flap which will bridge the gap between groin and hand by suturing the two skin edges together.
14. Suture the distal part of the flap into the defect.
15. Immobilise the limb against the trunk after placing padding between the limb and the trunk.
16. Perform a delay procedure at 2 weeks by incising half of the skin at the base of the pedicle opposite the suture line.
17. Identify the axial vessels; ligate and divide them.
18. Resuture the wound.

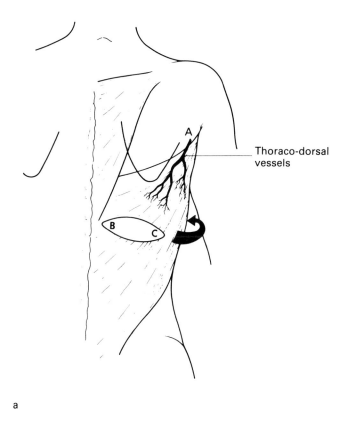

Thoraco-dorsal vessels

a

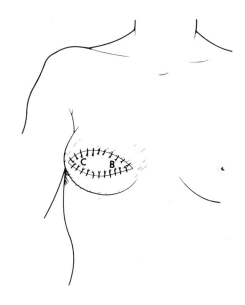

b

Fig. 31.21 Latissimus dorsi flap. The skin overlying the right latissimus dorsi flap is elevated from the muscle leaving a central elliptiform island of skin attached to the muscle. The muscle is freed from its peripheral and underlying attachments and passed subcutaneously to the defect on the anterior chest wall. Pivoted on its insertion A where the thoraco dorsal vessels enter the muscle (a). In breast reconstruction, the muscle is sutured into the region of the reconstructed breast and the island of skin inserted into the mastectomy scar. A prosthesis is inserted beneath the flap (b).

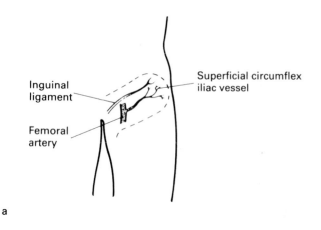

a

b

Fig. 31.22 Superficial groin flap. The inguinal ligament is marked in the groin and the position of the projected line of the superficial circumflex iliac vessels is also drawn. This line acts as the axis of the groin flap to be raised (a). After raising the flap the distal portion is sutured into the defect on the hand and the proximal portion is tubed (b). The donor defect is close primarily.

19. 3 weeks after the initial surgery, divide the pedicle completely at its base and inset into the groin wound.
20. Inset the flap into the hand defect with a few sutures. If tension is apparent in the skin, do not suture it at all but cover the exposed part of the flap with a paraffin gauze dressing.
21. Inset the flap 2 days later.
22. Thin the flap 3 months later, if necessary, by excising the subcutaneous tissue in stages.

TENSOR FASCIA LATA FLAP

Appraise

1. This flap is useful in treating trochanteric and ischial pressure sores. It can also be used for other defects of the upper thigh or lower abdominal wall.
2. It is a myo-fascio-cutaneous flap and is based on the vessels to the tensor fascia lata muscle.
3. Inclusion of the lateral cutaneous nerve of the thigh within the flap converts it into a sensory flap.

Action

1. Place the patient in the lateral position on the table.
2. Create and measure the defect. A pressure sore needs the whole lining and sometimes some of the underlying bone to be excised.
3. Mark the flap.
4. Identify the site of the vascular pedicle 10 cm distal and slightly lateral to the anterior superior iliac spine.
5. Take a line from this point to the lateral margin of the patella and use this as the axis of the flap.
6. Mark the lateral margins of the flap parallel to this line using a width of 6–10 cm (Fig. 31.23).
7. Mark the distal extremity of the flap so that it is not more than two-thirds of the length of the thigh. Check that the flap will reach the defect.
8. Incise the skin distally down to the deep fascia.
9. Incise the skin on the anterior and posterior margins and elevate the flap together with the fascia lata.
10. As the flap is reflected proximally, the tensor fascia lata muscle comes into view. If necessary, divide any small distal vascular pedicle into the muscle after first identifying the large vascular pedicle proximally.
11. Check that the flap will rotate into the defect.
12. Incise the skin between the flap and the defect, and undermine it on either side, allowing the flap to lie in this defect.
13. Excise any excess thigh skin to allow the flap to sit comfortably.
14. Suture the flap into place.
15. Close the donor defect primarily as far as possible.
16. Take a skin graft from the opposite thigh and apply it to the residual flap donor defect.
17. Dress the graft and its donor site with paraffin gauze, dressing gauze cotton wool and crepe bandage.
18. Leave the flap exposed and nurse the patient on his contralateral side.

GASTROCNEMIUS FLAP

Appraise

1. Both heads of the gastrocnemius muscle can be used separately for covering defects on the anterior aspect of the leg.
2. They can be used as simple muscle flaps or as myocutaneous flaps.
3. The flaps are used for covering exposed bone in the upper third of the tibia and for covering the exposed knee joint, sometimes even in the presence of a metal prosthesis.
4. The muscle flap alone is more malleable and versatile than a myocutaneous flap.
5. Although the lateral head is slightly longer use the nearest muscle head to the defect. Do not use both heads simultaneously.

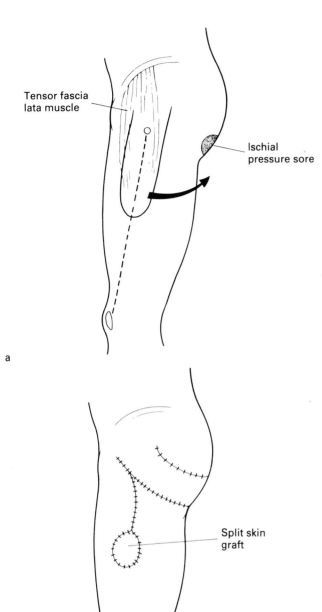

a

b

Fig. 31.23 Tensor fascia lata flap. The axis of this flap based on a line between the greater trochanter and the lateral margin of the patella. It is used to reconstruct ischial pressure sores (a). After transfer, the donor site is closed primarily although the distal portion may require a split skin graft (b).

Action

1. Place the patient in the lateral position with the affected leg uppermost.

2. Mark out and create the defect.

3. Make a vertical incision through skin and subcutaneous tissue down the mid-line of the calf, posteriorly.

4. Identify the muscle bellies of gastrocnemius and their relevant attachments to the tendo calcaneous (Fig. 31.24).

5. Separate the fascia overlying the respective belly of the muscle to be used.

6. Incise the tendon just distal to the muscle attachment.

7. Elevate the muscle belly proximally, laterally and medially dividing its attachment to the opposite belly.

8. Free the muscle belly to the level of the popliteal fossa, preserving the vascular pedicle passing into it.

9. Create a subcutaneous tunnel from the base of the muscle belly to the defect and large enough to accommodate the muscle flap.

10. Pass the muscle belly through this tunnel into the defect.

11. Suture the muscle to the edges of the defect.

12. Close the donor defect in layers and insert a suction drain.

13. Take a thick split skin graft from the thigh and apply it to the exposed muscle in the defect.

14. Splint the leg for 10 days.

15. Allow weightbearing at 10 days and mobilise progressively. Fit an elastic support stocking to cover the graft overlying the muscle. This should be worn for 3 months.

FASCIOCUTANEOUS FLAP

Appraise

1. These flaps have their greatest use in providing skin cover to exposed bone in the middle third of the leg.
They are occasionally used in other sites on upper and lower limbs.

2. They are not true axial pattern flaps but are based on the principle of retaining a rich vascular network lying superficial to the deep fascia, which is retained within the

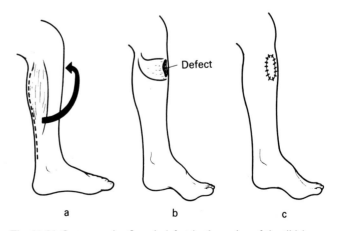

a   b   c

Fig. 31.24 Gastrocnemius flap. A defect in the region of the tibial tuberosity can be covered with the medial head of gastrocnemius (a). The flap is raised through a posterior mid-line incision and passed subcutaneously into the defect (b). A split skin graft is placed over the muscle within the defect.

flap. Flaps of a 2 : 1 and sometimes a 3 : 1 length to breadth ratio can be used.

Action

1. Mark out and create the defect.
2. Mark out the flap based proximally with a 2 : 1 ratio.
3. Check that the flap will reach the defect when transposed (Fig. 31.25).
4. Incise the flap distally, passing through skin, subcutaneous tissue and deep fascia.
5. Elevate the flap proximally, incising along the lateral margins and preserving the deep fascia with the flap.
6. Transpose the flap into the defect.
7. Suture the flap into the defect in layers.
8. Take a split skin graft from the opposite thigh.
9. Apply the split skin graft to the flap donor defect and

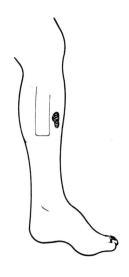

a

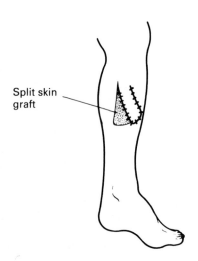

Split skin graft

b

Fig. 31.25 Fasciocutaneous flap. A small defect on the anterior aspect of the leg can be covered with a medially based fasciocutaneous flap (a). The flap is transposed into the defect and a split skin graft is placed on the donor defect. (b).

dress with paraffin gauze, dressing gauze, cotton wool and crepe bandage.

GRAFTS OF OTHER TISSUES
CARTILAGE GRAFTS

Cartilage grafts are used in reconstructing cartilaginous defects of the nose, large defects of the lower eyelids and serious defects of the ear.

NOSE

1. Composite defects of skin and cartilage at the nostril margin can be reconstructed using composite grafts from the ear, as described under composite skin grafts (see p. 542).
2. Most other small cartilaginous defects of the nose can be reconstructed using cartilage from other parts of the nose during a corrective rhinoplasty.
3. If there is extensive cartilaginous loss and the nasal tip requires support, take an 'L' shaped bone graft from the iliac crest and insert it through a mid-columella incision.

EYELIDS

1. Cartilage support for the upper eyelid is rarely required.
2. Large defects of the lower eyelid often require the introduction of cartilage for support and the best donor site for this is the septum of the nose. This provides a composite graft of cartilage and mucous membrane. The latter is used to reconstruct the conjunctival surface.

Action

1. Create the defect and measure it.
2. Mark an appropriate area of the septum using a nasal speculum, commencing at least 3 mm behind the anterior limit of the septum.
3. Infiltrate the marked area with $\frac{1}{2}$% lignocaine and 1 : 200 000 adrenaline.
4. Infiltrate the septum on the opposite side with the same preparation.
5. After allowing at least 7 min for the adrenaline to take effect, incise the mucosa passing through this and the underlying cartilage but avoid penetrating the nasal mucosa on the contralateral side.
6. Separate the contralateral nasal mucosa from the cartilage using a mucosal elevator.
7. Cut around the full margin of the graft and remove it.

8. Stop the bleeding with pressure and avoid using diathermy which can cause necrosis and perforation in the residual mucosal surface.

9. Insert the graft into the defect and stabilise it with a chromic catgut suture through the cartilage at each margin.

10. Suture the conjunctival surface with 6/0 chromic catgut.

11. Suture the skin with 6/0 nylon.

EAR

1. Costal cartilage is used for total ear reconstruction.

2. Reconstruction of a major portion of the ear may be difficult. It is sometimes justifiable to discard those cartilaginous segments already present and perform a total ear reconstruction.

Action

1. Measure the normal ear and make a template for the new ear.

2. Make a straight, oblique incision over the medial end of the seventh and eighth costal cartilages.

3. Retract the skin and subcutaneous tissue and expose an area of cartilage equivalent to the shape of the ear,

4. Mark out an outline of cartilage from the template using the seventh and eighth costal cartilages and excise this.

5. Close the donor defect in layers.

6. Place the graft on a wooden board on a table and carefully shape the cartilage, creating a well-defined helical rim and an anti-helical fold.

7. Make an incision along the hairline of the posterior margin of the auricular skin where it meets hair-bearing scalp skin.

8. Create a subcutaneous pocket beneath the auricular skin to accommodate the cartilage graft.

9. Insert the graft and close the skin.

10. Insert sutures through the skin in the region of the scaphoid fossa. and concha, to highlight the contour of the grafts.

11. After 6 months, reflect forward the cartilage graft together with the underlying subcutaneous tissue and insert a split skin graft onto the posterior surface of the reconstructed ear and the post-auricular region.

VASCULAR GRAFTS

Appraise

1. Large vascular grafts are described on page 377. Small vessel grafts are used in cases of replantation and free-flap transfer. They are occasionally used when limb vessels have been injured.

2. Vein grafts are used to replace both damaged arteries and veins.

3. The size of the vein graft must match the vessel which has been destroyed.

4. Use magnification for the repair. Use a microscope when repairing grafts under 2 mm in diameter.

Action

1. Identify the length of vessel which has been damaged.

2. Place appropriately sized clamps on normal vessel on either side of the damaged section and resect this damaged section.

3. Inspect the cut ends under magnification and check that the endothelium is normal. If it is not, resect further.

4. Check that there is good flow of blood from the cut proximal arterial stump, or the cut distal venous stump, by holding the adventitia of the vessel with jeweller's forceps, and temporarily releasing the clamp.

5. Select a superficial vein of appropriate size and length for insertion as a graft into the defect. For vessels greater than 2 mm diameter, use the long saphenous vein, which is the best available vein graft for both arteries and veins. For vessels smaller than this, use veins from the dorsum of the foot or from the flexor aspect of the forearm.

6. Make an incision through the skin directly over the full length of the chosen vein.

7. By blunt dissection, isolate the full length of the vein to be used.

8. Ligate all branches of the vein graft or use the bipolar coagulator to seal minute branches. Do not use unipolar diathermy which will damage the graft.

9. Isolate a segment of vein graft which is longer than that required. Ligate and divide the vessel proximally and distally.

10. Remove the graft and irrigate it gently with warm heparinised saline to exclude leaks.

11. Place the graft in the site of the defect, ensuring that the blood flow in the graft will be in the usual direction.

12. Choose an appropriate double clamp. Place one portion of this clamp on the proximal end of the divided normal vessel and the other on the vein graft.

13. Under magnification, clean the adventia from the vessel walls of both stumps using small scissors.

14. Flush the stumps with heparinised saline being careful not to grasp the endothelium with forceps.

15. Dilate the vessel with vessel dilators and approximate the ends.

16. Suture the anterior wall with interupted 8/0 or 10/0 nylon sutures. Turn the clamp over and suture the opposite wall.

17. Before the final two sutures are inserted, check that the anastomosis is patent.

18. Carry out a similar anastomosis at the distal end, checking that the graft has been stretched to its original length.

19. Remove the distal clamps first and then remove the proximal clamps.

20. If there is a small leak at either anastomosis, cover it with a warm swab but do not occlude the vessel.

21. If there is a gross leak, re-apply a single clamp to obstruct the flow and insert extra sutures. Remove the clamp and observe.

22. If flow is not established, resect the anastomosis and repeat.

Other grafts

Nerve grafts, tendon grafts and bone grafts are described in the section on orthopaedics (see Ch. 28).

MICROVASCULAR SURGERY

1. Microvascular surgery is a new surgical specialty concerned with the anastomosis and repair of small vessels.

2. It has clinical application in cases of replantation and free tissue transfer.

3. The surgery is highly specialised. Operations may take many hours and require special instruments in addition to an appropriate microscope.

4. This type of surgery should be carried out only in specialised units.

REPLANTATION

Appraise

Replantation may be considered following accidental amputation or devascularisation of any of the following parts.

1. Limbs proximal to the ankle or wrist joints. This is called macro-replantation.
2. Parts of limbs distal to the ankle or wrist joint. This is called micro-replantation.
3. The ear
4. The scalp
5. The penis
6. Composite pieces of facial tissue.

Action

1. Control bleeding from the amputation stump by simple pressure and elevation.

2. Avoid clamping vessels to stop haemorrhage unless essential, as this causes unnecessary damage.

3. Place the amputated part in a polythene bag and lay the bag on ice. The amputated part must be cooled but not frozen as freezing prevents successful replantation.

4. If a part is devascularised and not fully amputated, cool this part by placing polythene bags containing ice around it.

5. Contact the nearest microvascular surgery unit and take advice.

6. Prepare the patient and amputated part for urgent transfer.

MACRO REPLANTATION

Appraise

1. The force required to sever a major portion of a limb is considerable and patients who have suffered such an injury may have other injuries to their body. These may take priority in treatment.

2. Criteria for attempting replanatation are:
a. The patient should be relatively fit.
b. The amputated portion should not be too severely damaged.
c. The 'warm ischaemic time' of the amputated part should not exceed 6 hours. Muscle is unlikely to recover adequately after this period.
d. There should be a reasonable prospect of some functional recovery.

Action

1. Debride and clean both the proximal stump and the wound of the amputated part.

2. Shorten the skeletal structures and fix these. This will allow primary anastomosis of vessels and nerves.

3. Revascularise the amputated part by anastomosing the appropriate artery, or arteries, using vein grafts if necessary.

4. If the warm ischaemic time has been relatively long, revascularise the part prior to skeletal fixation. Allow perfusion of the amputated part for several minutes, discarding the venous blood. Transfuse the patient appropriately. Revise the anastomoses after skeletal fixation if necessary

5. Anastomose twice the number of veins as the number of arteries repaired, again using vein grafts if necessary.

6. Repair the tendons and muscles.

7. Repair the nerves.

8. Carry out extensive fasciotomies incising through skin, subcutaneous tissue and deep fascia on the proximal stump and on the amputated part.

9. Harvest a split skin graft and apply this to the fasciotomy sites and any other residual raw areas where there has been skin loss.

10. Monitor the limb carefully post-operatively, and be prepared to return the patient to theatre at any time if there

is doubt about viability of the replanted or revascularised part.

FREE TISSUE TRANSFER

Appraise

1. Free tissue transfer is used in many forms of reconstruction. It consists of transferring tissue from one part of the body to another.

2. The tissue is isolated on a recognised vascular pedicle and after transfer to its distant site, the vessels of the vascular pedicle are anastomosed to appropriate nearby vessels, either directly or with vein grafts.

3. The arterial supply to the tissue is usually constructed with an end-to-side anastomosis to an adjacent artery, so that the distal supply of this artery is not jeopardised.

4. The venous drainage of the tissue is usually connected to superficial veins or to venae comitantes of a nearby artery.

5. Most free flaps currently used in reconstruction consist of cutaneous or myocutaneous flaps. Apart from those listed above there are many other cutaneous and myocutaneous flaps which are occasionally used.

6. Other free tissue transfers include the following:
a. Vascularised bone grafts from rib, iliac crest, fibula, radius and metastarsal.
b. Osseocutaneous flaps from the iliac crest with adjacent overlying skin, from the radius with overlying skin and metatarsal with overlying skin.
c. Sensory cutaneous flaps.
d. Muscle flaps with motor innervation.
e. Small bowel, for oesophageal reconstruction.
f. Omentum, for soft tissue defects.
g. Testis, resiting a high undecended testicle in the scrotum.

BURNS

Appraise

The treatment of patients with extensive burns is complex and these patients should be treated in a specialised burns unit. There are many aspects of treatment but only the surgical aspects will be considered here.

Assess

1. Assess the depth and extent of the burn. Although pin-prick sensation is usually preserved in superficial burns, detection of sensation is not an absolutely reliable test.

2. The best guide to the depth of burn is found by taking an accurate history of the mechanism of the burn.
a. Thermal burns with gases usually cause superficial burns.
b. Thermal burns with fluids, usually cause deep dermal burns. Boiling water and fat cause full thickness burns. Boiling water which has cooled for 5 minutes causes superficial burns.
c. Contact with hot solids and flames usually cause full-thickness burns.
d. Electrical burns usually cause full thickness skin loss.
e. Radiation burns are usually superficial.
f. Chemical burns are usually superficial.

SUPERFICIAL BURNS

Action

1. Clean the burn wound and remove the roof of all blisters.

2. Expose superficial burns of the face and perineum as these are difficult to dress.

3. Cover superficial burns of other areas with two layers of paraffin gauze and a bulky absorptive dressing. Leave this dressing for 1 week unless it becomes soaked, whereupon you should change it. Change the dressing at 1 week and subsequently twice per week until the wound is healed.

DEEP DERMAL BURNS

1. Tangentially shave with a graft knife or remove the surface of the burn with a dermabrader between the second and fifth day.

2. Continue to shave until punctate bleeding is evident from the surface.

3. Achieve haemostasis with pressure and apply a split skin graft.

4. Redress at 4 days.

5. When fully healed, measure and apply a pressure garment. This is an elasticated garment specifically measured for the individual to cover the area of the burn wound. Advise the patient to wear this for 6 months or longer if necessary to minimise hypertrophy and contracture of the resulting scars.

6. If you do not have facilities or expertise for the above surgery, treat the burn conservatively and redress twice each week.

7. Treat areas which are not healed at 3 weeks as full-thickness burns.

EXTENSIVE FULL-THICKNESS BURNS

Escharotomy

1. Note the areas of full-thickness burns which are circumferential around digit, limb or trunk. If the viability of the distal part is jeopardised, or if respiration is hindered as with partial circumferential burns of the chest wall, carry out an escharotomy.

2. Give an appropriate intravenous dose of diazepam.

3. Take a scalpel and incise along the full length of the full-thickness burn allowing subcutaneous fat to bulge out of the escharotomy wound.

4. Repeat the longitudinal escharotomy at different sites of the circumference until satisfactory perfusion of the distal part is restored.

5. Dress the wounds with paraffin gauze or silver suphadiazine (Flamazine).

Action

1. Identify a suitable area, not exceeding 20% of the body area, to treat primarily.

2. Identify a suitable donor site for the skin graft.

3. Excise the chosen area of full thickness burn with a scalpel and be sure that the resultant bed consists of viable tissue. It is often safer to excise all subcutaneous fat to leave a graft bed of deep fascia. Achieve haemostasis.

4. Harvest a split skin graft and mesh this (see p. 541).

5. Apply the mesh graft to the burn wound site and dress with several layers of paraffin gauze and an absorbent dressing.

6. Re-dress after 4 days.

7. Do not excise burn tissue between the 5th and the 12th day post-burn, as the patient will be in an unsuitable catabolic state.

8. Do not excise further burn until the donor site has healed and is ready for reharvesting, or another donor site is available.

Small areas

1. Operate between the second and fifth day.

2. Excise all burn tissue and apply a split skin graft.

3. If the viability of subcutaneous fat is in doubt, excise this down to the deep fascia.

4. If the viability of the tissues is still in doubt, dress the wound and bring the patient back to the theatre 48 hours later. Re-assess viability at this second operation. Excise further if necessary and graft.

5. Re-dress after 4 days.

FACIAL CLEFTS

CLEFT LIP

Appraise

1. The treatment of clefts of the lip and palate may be very complex and should be carried out where the facilities of many other specialists are available, including a paediatrician, a paediatric anaesthetist, an orthodontist, an ENT surgeon, an oral surgeon, a dentist, an audiologist, a speech therapist as well as the plastic surgeon.

2. The extent of the cleft of the lip is variable and ranges from a slight notch in the vermillion border to a complete cleft of the whole lip.

3. The cleft may be bilateral and there may be an associated cleft of the palate.

4. Mid-line clefts of the lip, with absence of philtrum and columella and associated hypoteleorism, are rare but should be referred to a specialised unit.

5. Rare oblique clefts of the face involving the lip should be referred to a specialised unit for surgical correction.

6. Repair clefts of the lip at 3 months of age.

7. If the cleft is bilateral, repair the two sides separately with a month interval between operations. Repair the more severe cleft first.

8. A prominent philtrum, particularly obvious in bilateral cleft lips, can be corrected pre-operatively with orthodontic appliances. If these are not available, apply simple elastoplast strapping from cheek to cheek across the prominent philtrum, to help reduce it before operation.

9. There are many techniques for repairing a cleft of the lip, but the Millard repair as described below is popular. The steps are outlined.

Prepare

1. Identify the mid point of the philtrum on its vermillion border, and mark (Fig. 31.26, point 1).

2. Identify the vermillion border at the base of the normal philtral column and mark (point 2).

3. Mark the corresponding point on the vermillion border at the base of the projected contra-lateral philtral column (point 3).

4. Mark the mid-point of the junction of the columella with the philtrum (point 4)

5. On the lateral segment of the lip, mark the vermillion border at a point where the white roll disappears (point 5)

6. On the lateral segment, mark the most medial point of normal skin horizontally level with the base of the nostril (point 6).

7. Draw a straight line between points 5 and 6 and a curved line between points 3 and 4 of equal length.

8. Infiltrate the area with local anaesthesia using 0.5% lignocaine and 1 : 200 000 adrenaline.

Action

1. With a size 11 blade cut through the full thickness of the lip along the curved line of the medial segment.

2. Excise the mucosal surface medial to this preserving a small triangular flap of normal skin (the C flap).

3. Excise the mucosa medial to the straight line on the lateral segment.

4. Incise the lateral segment from point 6, laterally around the base of the ala.

5. Reflect back the skin and identify the muscles inserted into the alar base.

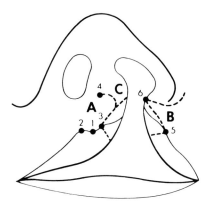

a

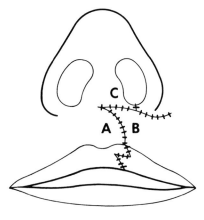

b

Fig. 31.26 Cleft lip — the Millard repair. (1) is the centre of the Cupid's bow. (2) is the peak of the Cupid's bow on the normal side, (3) is the projected point of the peak of the Cupid's bow on the cleft side, (4) is the junction of the mid-point of philtrum and columella, (5) is the start of the mucosal thickening of the cleft side, (6) is the medial extremity of the alar base on the cleft side. The dotted lines indicate the incisions (a). Flaps A and B have been sutured into place and flap C is used to create the nostril sill. A Z-plasty has been introduced into the vermillion mucosa (b).

6. Divide these muscles and dissect them free from their attachment to the alar base.

7. Identify and dissect free the muscle in the medial segment.

8. Suture together the orbicularis oris muscle from each segment with 4/0 chromic catgut.

9. Approximate the skin using 6/0 chromic catgut as a subcutaneous suture.

10. Approximate point 6 to point 4.

11. Approximate point 5 to point 3.

12. Use the 'C' flap to create a nostril sill.

13. Suture the skin with 6/0 nylon.

14. Suture the skin and mucosa within the nostril with 6/0 chromic catgut.

15. Adjust the mucosa of the lip and suture. If necessary incorporate a small Z-plasty.

16. Remove sutures at 3–4 days.

CLEFT PALATE

Appraise

1. A cleft palate often occurs in conjunction with a cleft lip, but may occur separately.

2. The extent of the cleft palate varies from a complete cleft to a submucous cleft where the palate is apparently intact but there has been failure of fusion of the levator palati muscles across the mid-line.

3. Repair the muscle in submucous clefts of the palate to ensure satisfactory function of the palate during speech.

4. Repair clefts of the palate at about 6 months of age to restore the speech mechanism to normal as early as practical.

Prepare

1. Insert a suitable mouth gag such as the Dott or Kilner.

2. Pack the pharynx with ribbon gauze.

3. Mark out bilateral flaps on the palate passing from the uvula along the side of the cleft to its apex and anteriorly along the midline to within 3 mm of the alveolus (Fig. 31.27).

4. Continue marking laterally, keeping just within the margin of the alveolus and passing backwards behind the hamulus to the anterior pillar of the fauces.

5. Ilfiltrate the flaps with 0.5% lignocaine and 1 : 200 000 adrenaline.

Action

1. Incise along the marked edges of one flap, commencing at the tip of the split uvula.

2. Elevate the flap from its anterior margin as a muco-periosteal flap.

3. Scrape the periosteum off the palate using a Mitchell trimmer.

4. On approaching the greater palatine artery, identify this as it emerges through its foramen and dissect the flap away from the bone around its perimeter.

5. Using the Mitchell trimmer, separate the nasal mucosa from the palatal bones.

6. Identify the levator palati muscle inserted into the posterior margin of the hard palate and place a spatula between this attachment and the nasal mucosa.

7. Cut down through this attachment onto the spatula, freeing the levator palati muscle completely from the hard palate.

8. Dissect the levator palati free from both underlying nasal mucosa and its covering palatal mucosa.

9. Repeat the dissection on the opposite side.

10. Repair the nasal mucosa with 4/0 chromic catgut, commencing anteriorly and work posteriorly to reconstruct the uvula.

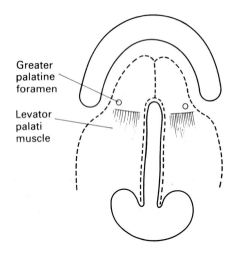

a

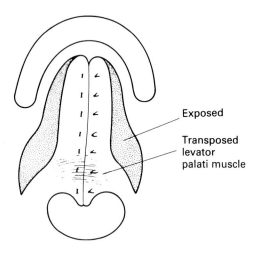

b

Fig. 31.27 Cleft palate repair. The flaps of the two flap repair are shown in fig (a). Note the attachment of the levator palati into the hard palate. This muscle should be dissected off the hard palate and sutured together in the mid-line. The subsequent repair of the mucosa of the soft palate leaves a residual exposed area laterally which epithelialises spontaneously during the first post-operative week (b).

11. Suture the two ends of the levator palati together in the midline with 4/0 polypropylene (Dexon) sutures.

12. Repair the oral mucosa in the midline using 4/0 chromic catgut sutures. Use deep mattress sutures in the central portion.

13. The anterior tip of the two flaps when sutured together may protrude into the mouth. They need not be sutured down as they adhere to the palate very early in the post-operative phase it left free.

ANTERIOR CLEFT PALATE

Appraise

1. A cleft of the anterior palate coexists with a cleft of the lip.

2. It can be partially closed at the time of the lip repair but is usually closed at the time of the palate repair when this is also present.

3. The most effective repair utilises a vomerine flap.

Action

1. Insert a mouth gag.

2. Mark out a flap on the vomer with its base at the vomerine margin (Fig. 31.28).

3. Mark out a lateral flap as for repair of a cleft palate. Infiltrate both flaps with 0.5% lignocaine and 1 : 200 000 adrenaline.

4. Elevate both flaps.

5. Oppose and suture the raw surface of the two flaps together.

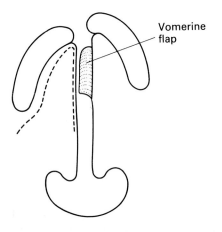

a

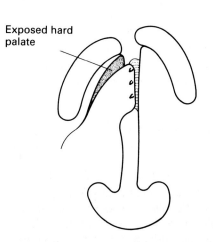

b

Fig. 31.28 Anterior palate repair. Superiorly based vomerine flap is raised off the septum (a). A palatal flap is raised laterally and mobilised. The two flaps are sutured raw surface to raw surface using 3 mattress sutures (b).

PHARYNGOPLASTY

Appraise

1. A pharyngoplasty is necessary to reduce the velopharyngeal space when this is responsible for nasal escape during speech. This is usually due to the soft palate being too short to reach the posterior pharyngeal wall.

2. Carry out pre-operative assessment with a nasendoscope wherever possible.

3. There are many different kinds of pharyngoplasty. Most provide a reduction in the anatomical size of the velopharyngeal space.

4. A few, including the Ortichochea repair described below, attempt not only to reduce the anatomical size of this space but also to provide a dynamic sphincter which helps closure during speech.

Action

1. Insert a Kilner gag.

2. Mark a rectangular pharyngeal flap based inferiorly and reaching as high as can be visualised on the posterior pharyngeal wall.

3. Infiltrate the flap with 0.5% lignocaine and 1 : 200 000 adrenaline.

4. Identify the palatopharyngeus muscle within the posterior pillar of the fauces, and insert a McIndoe scissors behind this after penetrating the mucosa.

5. Separate the blades of the scissors and dissect free the muscle along its length. Dissect it free to its lower limit and divide it at this point.

6. Dissect the opposite muscle free in the same manner, preserving some overlying mucosa.

7. Raise the posterior pharyngeal flap down to its base and achieve haemostasis of its bed.

8. Suture the muscle belly of each of the two flaps to the raw surface of the pharyngeal flap with 4/0 polypropylene sutures.

9. Improve the attachment by suturing the mucosa of the muscle flap to the mucosa of the pharyngeal flap along the various attachments with 6/0 chromic catgut.

CRANIOFACIAL SURGERY

Appraise

1. During the last decade, great advances have been made in the field of craniofacial surgery.

2. Much of this work, pioneered by Tessier, is directed towards treating patients with a bizarre facial appearance due to extensive deformities of the facial bones and the cranial vault.

3. These cases are rare, but much can be done to help them in the specialised centres where this surgery is carried out.

LYMPHOEDEMA

Appraise

1. There are many operations described to treat lymphoedema but the cosmetic result of these is uniformly disappointing.

2. The application of microvascular surgery to the suture of lymphatic vessels in cases of obstructive lymphoedema has not produced the dramatic results initially anticipated.

3. Use pressure garments and other conservative measures before considering surgery.

4. In moderate cases of lymphoedema, where cosmesis is important, use the buried dermis flap operation described by Thompson (Fig. 31.29).

5. In very severe cases of lymphoedema, use the Charles operation.

MODERATE LYMPHOEDEMA

1. When operating on the lower limb, insert a Steinmann pin through the calcaneum and support the limb from above.

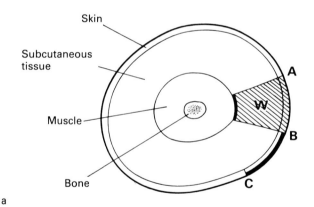

a

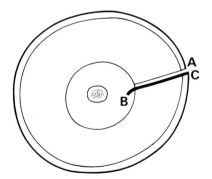

b

Fig. 31.29 Buried dermis flap. Diagramatic cross-section of the lymphoedematous limb shown in fig (a). A wedge of skin and subcutaneous tissue W is excised. The skin B, C is de-epithelialised and turned inwards so B is inserted into the muscle compartment. C is approximated to A (b).

2. Exsanguinate the limb and apply a tourniquet proximally on the limb.

3. Mark a strip of skin a few centimetres across, down the lateral border of the limb. This will be excised.

4. Mark a further strip a few centimetres across, posterior to the first.

5. Shave the second strip with a skin graft knife to remove all epithelial elements.

6. Excise the first strip with underlying fat down to the deep fascia.

7. Elevate the posterior flap and roll it into the wound so the leading edge of de-epithelialised skin meets the deep fascia.

8. Incise the deep fascia and suture the flap into the muscular compartment.

9. Suture the anterior skin flap to the posterior edge of the de-epithelialised skin, using mattress sutures tied over cotton wool bolsters.

10. Insert long suction drains beneath the flaps.

11. Postoperatively, keep the limb elevated for 10 days.

12. Mobilise the limb with a bandage support applied.

13. Remove the sutures at 14 days.

14. Repeat the operation on the medial side of the limb after 4 months if necessary.

15. Repeat the operation on the posterior aspect of the limb a further 6 months later, again if necessary.

SEVERE LYMPHOEDEMA

1. Insert a Steinmann pin through the calcaneum and support the limb from above.

2. Exsanguinate the limb and apply a tourniquet proximally.

3. Take split skin grafts from the surface of the limb to be treated if this is suitable. If it is not, take split skin grafts from another donor area and dress the donor site. Store the skin grafts.

4. Excise all skin and subcutaneous tissue down to the deep fascia, from the limb,

5. Preserve the skin of the sole of the foot and the toes and leave skin to cover the malleoli.

6. Preserve enough skin to flute into the defect at the upper margin of excision.

7. Dress the limb with several layers of paraffin gauze, dressing gauze, absorbant dressings and bandage.

8. Remove the dressings after 24 hours and apply the stored skin with the limb elevated by traction on the Steinmann pin. This manoeuvre allows exposure of the circumferential skin grafts on the limb.

10. Mobilise the limb when the skin grafts are stable, between 10–14 days.

11. Pressure garments should be worn for at least 3 months postoperatively and in most cases indefinitely.

GENITALIA

HYPOSPADIAS

Appraise

1. The male urethral meatus may appear on the surface at any point in the midline between its normal position at the tip of the glans penis and the perineum.

2. In many cases of hypospadias, a tight fibrous band, the chordee, is evident distal to the ectopic meatus which causes curvature of the penis when in the erect position.

3. Reconstructive surgery to place the meatus in its normal position at the tip of the glans aims to produce an apparently normal penis without urethral fistula.

4. Many operations have been designed to treat the condition but none consistently fulfil the above criteria.

5. Experienced surgeons advocate a one-stage procedure, but the less experienced surgeon should proceed with a staged reconstruction.

6. Ideally, carry out surgery in infancy. Some surgeons prefer to wait until the child is continent of urine to release the chordee and then reconstruct the urethra just before the child starts school.

Release of chordee

1. Under general anaesthesia carry out a Horton test. Place some rubber tubing around the base of the penis and pull it tight. Inject the corpora with normal saline to produce an erect penis and note the extent of chordee. Release the rubber tubing.

2. Mark the extent of the chordee in ink. Mark out a Z-plasty for reconstruction following excision of the chordee.

3. Incise down the central line overlying the chordee.

4. Excise all underlying fibrous tissue.

5. Use a bipolar coagulator to achieve haemostasis.

6. Raise the flaps of the Z-plasty, transpose them and suture them with 6/0 chromic catgut. Do not dress the wound.

Distal shaft correction

1. Under general anaesthesia carry out a Horton test as above.

2. If any chordee is still evident, excise this and defer reconstruction for a further 6 months.

3. If no chordee is apparent, mark out a rectangular flap, proximal to the meatus with its base at the meatus. The flap should be 1 cm broad and long enough to reach the glans when turned distally (Fig. 31.30).

4. Mark out a strip of skin distal to the meatus from the meatus to the glans.

5. Catheterise the urethra with a small Foley catheter.

6. Elevate the flap and reflect it distally.

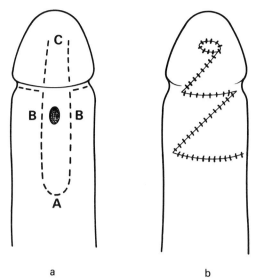

Fig. 31.30 Distal hypospadias repair. A plan of the incisions should be marked pre-operatively. The proximal flap must have adequate length for A to reach C when hinged at the point B adjacent to the external meatus (a). After suturing the lateral margins of this flap, lateral flaps are mobilised using the redundant preputial skin and closed in a Z-plasty fashion (b).

7. Cut along the margins of the strip of skin and elevate the edges.

8. Suture the flap to the cut edges of the strip of skin using 6/0 catgut.

9. Elevate lateral flaps of skin by incising around the attachment of preputial skin to the glans. Mobilise the flaps round to the dorsal surface.

10. Suture the flaps across the reconstructed urethra, so that the suture line between the two flaps traverses the reconstructed urethra. Use 6/0 polypropylene.

11. Suture a foam dressing around the reconstructed penis. This prevents interference from the patient. Suture or strap the catheter to the upper thigh.

12. Remove the dressing and catheter at 10 days.

Proximal shaft, scrotal and perineal hypospadias

1. As with distal shaft hypospadias, there are many operations to correct these deformities. Reconstruct the urethra with flaps of preputial skin from the redundant foreskin or use a free graft of preputial skin.

2. Use local skin flaps to cover the reconstructed urethra.

3. In perineal hypospadias, use the hairless strip of skin in the middle of the scrotum for the urethral reconstruction in this region.

EPISPADIAS AND ECTOPIA OF THE BLADDER

Appraise

1. Epispadias and ectopia of the bladder represent

different expressions of the same basic embryological defect.

2. These rare conditions require highly specialised treatment where one-stage correction is advocated.

Action

1. If specialised treatment is not available do not carry out a pelvic oesteotomy.
2. Close the bladder wall with abdominal flaps.
3. Tighten the bladder neck at a second stage.
4. In a third stage, close the residual epispadias by passing a funnel of mucosa through the base of the penis to the ventral surface and reconstruct the resultant hypospadias.

VAGINAL ATRESIA

Appraise

1. In some patients it is possible to stretch the small dimple at the site of the vaginal orifice with graded dilators up to the average size without surgery. This treatment should be advocated whenever possible

2. Failure of conservative treatment is an indication for surgery.

Action

1. Make a cruciate incision at the vault of the vaginal dimple.
2. Use sharp dissection to open a space up to the perineal membrane.
3. Use blunt dissection above this to create the full vaginal space.
4. Take a large split skin graft from the thigh.
5. Apply the graft to a stent the size of the vagina and suture the edges over the stent.
6. Insert the graft on the stent and then remove the stent.
7. Pack tightly the reconstructed vagina with multiple pieces of sponge foam dressings.
8. Suture the labia together with three sutures of 0/0 silk to retain the foam dressings in place.
9. Redress under general anaesthesia two weeks later.
10. Prevent contraction of the graft by retaining a vaginal dilator in place for 6 months after surgery. Encourage regular dilatation after this time.

SCARS

HYPERTROPHIC SCARS

Appraise

1. These present as red, raised, broad, hard, itchy scars which are unsightly and uncomfortable. They develop a few months after the wound has healed.

2. Beware of excising or revising them unless there was failure of primary healing. Excision of the scar will probably cause a larger one to develop.

3. Inject the scar tissue only with triamcinolone.

4. Repeat the injections at monthly intervals for 3–6 months until the scar is soft.

5. Avoid excessive injections, which may cause skin atrophy.

6. If the scars are extensive, fit and apply a pressure garment as early as possible. Advise the patient to wear this garment for 6–12 months.

Pressure garments

1. A pressure garment is a synthetic elastic garment which is specifically measured to fit part of an individual.

2. In applying pressure to a scar, it modifies the maturation and limits hypertrophic scar formation, provided it is applied early.

3. Pressure garments are most useful in reducing hypertrophic scar formation and preventing the development of contractures particularly from burn wounds.

4. They are also used in controlling progressive lymphoedema.

KELOIDS

Appraise

1. Keloids have a different histological appearance from hypertrophic scars.

2. They are most commonly found in patients of African origin but can be found in all races.

3. Excision of keloids, like excision of hypertrophic scars, only temporarily cures the problem. A larger lesion will develop in its place and this treatment is to be condemned.

4. Some surgeons advocate excision of the keloid followed by treatment of the resultant scar with radiotherapy. Although this usually results in an improved appearance, the long-term effect of the radiotherapy is uncertain.

Action

1. Identify the boundaries of the keloid.

2. Excise its central bulk keeping the margin of excision at the lateral borders and in depth within the keloid tissue. Close the wound primarily preserving a rim of keloid tissue at all margins. Keep all sutures within this rim.

3. Apply pressure to the area for at least 3 months afterwards with a pressure garment specifically fitted for the patient.

4. If the keloid is extensive take a split skin graft from the surface of major bulk of the keloid. Again keep all

sutures within the keloid tissue and apply pressure postoperatively.

AESTHETIC SURGERY

1. Aesthetic operations, like other operations, are best carried out by the specialist.

2. These operations can nearly always be deferred until specialist treatment is available, but a brief outline of the commoner operations is given below.

3. Pre-operative assessment and careful explanation of the expectation of the results of surgery are vital parts of management in this field of surgery.

FACELIFT

Appraise

This operation is carried out to remove redundant skin and subcutaneous tissue in the cheeks, around the mouth and in the neck.

Action

1. Make an incision in the temple hairline. Extend this around the lower two-thirds of the pinna and behind the lateral occipital hairline (Fig. 31.31).

2. Raise the skin anterior to this incision and undermine it to the naso-labial fold, to the chin, and the neck avoiding division of branches of the facial nerves.

3. Retract the skin flap towards the incision line and excise the excess tissue.

4. Suture the flap into place along the original incision margin.

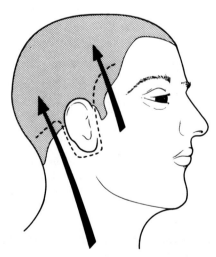

Fig. 31.31 Facelift. The skin incision is marked by the dotted line. After undermining the skin is pulled in the direction of the arrows and after excision of excess skin, the wound is closed.

5. Insert a suction drain.

6. Repeat the process on the opposite side to produce symmetry.

RHINOPLASTY

Appraise

1. Compare and contrast the patient's assessment of his or her nose with your own assessment of the nose.

Action

1. Shave or cut the vibrissae in the nostrils.
2. Make an intercartilagenous incision on each side through mucosa between the alar and lateral cartilages.
3. Extend this incision over the vault of the nostril down to the front of the septum.
4. Through this incision separate the skin on the top of the nose from the underlying septum.
5. Incise the mucosa along the roof of each nostril and divide the upper lateral cartilages from the septum.
6. Reduce the upper lateral cartilages as necessary.
7. Reduce the septal hump with cartilage scissors.
8. Remove the hump of the nasal bones with a chisel and hammer.
9. Make a small incision in each pyriform fossa.
10. Insert a periosteal elevator through this incision on the lateral margin of the nose and elevate the periosteum from the lateral margin of each nasal bone.
11. Insert a nasal saw along each incision in turn and cut half-way through the nasal bone.
12. Insert a chisel along each incision in turn and complete the nasal osteotomy.
13. Manipulate the nasal bones into the new position.
14. Rasp the nasal septum as necessary.
15. Through the intercartilagenous incision, evert the alar cartilages and reduce as necesary.
16. Expose the anterior margin of the nasal septum and adjust as necessary.
17. Suture the nasal mucosa with 3/0 plain catgut.
18. Pack each nostril with paraffin gauze.
19. Dress with tape and a plaster of Paris splint.
20. Remove the nasal packs at 24 hours.
21. Remove the plaster of Paris splint at 10 days.

BLEPHAROPLASTY

Appraise

1. This operation is carried out to reduce the skin and fat tissue in the upper and lower eyelids.

2. Pre-operative assessment should identify the site and volume of the underlying pads of fat.

Action

1. Under local or general anaesthesia, mark the excision margins of the skin of the upper eyelid as an ellipse with an accessory tail laterally.
2. Mark the excision margin on the lower eyelid with a minimal reduction in height.
3. Infiltrate with local anaesthetic, if indicated.
4. Excise the skin from the upper eyelid and excise the underlying fat pads from beneath the orbicularis muscle. Achieve haemostasis and suture with 6/0 nylon.
5. Raise the lower eyelid skin and, with a skin hook, pull the skin upwards and laterally.
6. Excise a triangle of skin at the lateral margin and a minimal amount of skin along the eyelid margin.
7. Reflect the skin flap and excise the fat pads from beneath the orbicularis muscle.
8. Suture the skin with 6/0 nylon.
9. Remove the sutures at 3–4 days.

CORRECTION OF PROMINENT EARS

Appraise

1. This operation is carried out to reduce the prominence of the ears, which may be due to a deep concha but is more commonly due to an absence of the anti-helical fold.
2. The principle of the operation is to remould the shape of the cartilage.
3. Operations which depend on skin and cartilage excisions are unsatisfactory.
4. Defer surgery in children until the age of 6 years, as they do not appreciate a problem before this age.

Action

1. Use general or local anaesthesia.
2. Infiltrate the pinna with local anaesthesia.
3. Mark the site of the proposed anti-helical rim and tattoo the underlying cartilage by passing a needle covered with ink through the full thickness of the pinna at several points along this line.
4. Excise a narrow vertical ellipse of skin from the posterior margin of the pinna.
5. Incise the cartilage posteriorly along the tattoo marks.
6. Dissect the cartilage away from the anterior skin of the pinna.
7. Score the anterior aspect of the cartilage with circumferential and radial incisions, to allow the cartilage to fold backwards.
8. When adequate reduction has been obtained, suture the skin wound with subcuticular prolene.
9. Repeat the process for the opposite ear to provide symmetry.

10. Dress both ears with proflavine wool to ensure apposition of skin to cartilage.

11. Cover both ears with cotton wool and a supportive bandage.

12. Remove the dressing at 10 days and remove the sutures.

13. Maintain a protective dressing over the ears at night for 4 weeks.

BREAST AUGMENTATION

Appraise

1. Breasts can be augmented in size by inserting prostheses in the submammary plane or in the subpectoral plane.

2. Complications are few, except for the development of a fibrous capsule around the prosthesis. When this contracts appreciably, the prosthesis feels hard and uncomfortable and the breast becomes distorted.

3. The size of prosthesis to be used is dependent on the size of the patient and the breast size. A history of previous surgery, previous pregnancy and lactation and weight changes all influence the choice of the size of prosthesis to be used.

Action

1. Incise the skin in the lower outer quadrant along the submammary fold.

2. Dissect a pocket in the sub-mammary plane, sufficient to accommodate the prosthesis.

3. Insert the prosthesis.

4. Close the wound in layers.

5. Keep the breasts well supported in the post-operative phase and for the subsequent 3 months.

6. If a capsular contracture develops, carry out a closed capsulotomy by compression of the capsule in the first instance.

7. If this fails, carry out an open capsulotomy.

BREAST REDUCTION

Appraise

1. Breast reduction is carried out not only for cosmetic reasons but also for physical symptoms.

2. Large breasts may be of sufficient weight to affect the posture of the patient and to cause backache.

3. Pressure marks over the shoulders may be evident where the straps of the brassiere rest.

4. The aim of surgery is to produce an aesthetic breast shape with a viable, sensitive nipple and areola. The latter must be preserved on a vascular pedicle.

5. Breast feeding is rarely possible after breast reduction and should generally be discouraged.

6. There are many operations designed to reduce the mass of the breasts. The inferior pedicle technique devised by Robins is described below.

Action

1. Mark the breasts pre-operatively with the patient sitting.

2. Choose a suitable site for the new position of the nipple near the midclavicular line.

3. Use a keyhole-type breast reduction pattern based on this site and mark the lateral and medial skin flaps (Fig. 31.32).

4. Mark the medial and lateral ends of the submammary crease and the submammary crease itself.

5. Per-operatively, make an intradermal incision through the skin along the patterns marked out pre-operatively so that the skin marks are not lost.

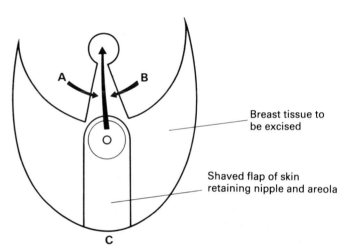

a

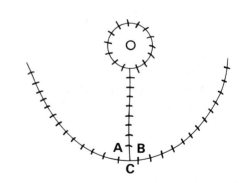

b

Fig. 31.32 Breast reduction. The inferior pedicle technique. The nipple and areolar are preserved on a flap of skin in which the epithelium has been removed. This flap of skin helps to protect the underlying breast tissue which contains the vessels and nerves supplying the nipple. Breast tissue and overlying skin on either side and above this flap are excised (a). The nipple is transferred upwards and flaps (A) and (B) after reflection outwards are brought together in the mid-line below the nipple (b).

6. Shave off the epidermis from the skin between the normal areola and the inframammary fold, and from a rim of skin around the areola.

7. Excise the lateral and medial segments of skin between the lower margin of the skin flaps and the inframammary fold, together with the underlying breast tissue.

8. Excise breast tissue beneath the new site of the nipple and areola.

9. Dissect the inferior pedicle to its base.

10. Elevate the medial and lateral skin flaps with their underlying breast tissue.

11. Suture the nipple and areola into its new site.

12. Approximate the skin flaps in the midline below the new nipple site.

13. Insert a suction drain.

14. Close the wounds in layers, using subcuticular sutures to the skin. Remove these at 3 weeks.

15. Repeat the operation on the opposite side to provide symmetry.

16. Support the breast postoperatively with light dressings.

17. Keep the breasts well supported for 3 months postoperatively.

DERMAL MASTOPEXY

Appraise

1. The breasts of all women have a tendency to become ptotic with increasing age.

2. Ptosis tends to be greater when there has been considerable weight reduction or excessive involution following lactation. It is also marked when the breasts have not been supported with a brassiere over a long period.

3. Dermopexy or correction of the ptosis is appropriate when the nipple can be re-sited at a higher level and the skin envelope of the breast tissue can be reduced without any change in the volume of breast tissue.

Action

1. Mark the patient as for a breast reduction.

2. Carry out the stages as enumerated in a breast reduction, but do not excise breast tissue.

3. In advancing the inferior pedicle to its new site, incise breast tissue at the new site and undermine the skin edges around the new nipple site appropriately.

4. Manage the patient postoperatively as for a breast reduction.

ABDOMINAL REDUCTION

Appraise

1. An abdominal reduction or lipectomy is most appropriate when a patient has lax abdominal skin following multiple pregnancies or substantial weight loss.

2. It is not normally an operation to produce weight reduction.

Action

1. Mark out a symmetrical line traversing the lower abdomen. Start beneath the anterior superior iliac spine on one side and pass through the upper part of the site of the pubic hair to the other.

2. Incise along this mark and cut down to the fascia overlying the muscles.

3. Dissect upwards in this plane.

4. Incise the skin around the umbilicus and separate this from the skin flap.

5. Undermine the skin up to the costal margin on either side.

6. Stretch the skin downwards.

7. Excise the redundant skin and subcutaneous fat.

8. Identify the new site on the skin flap for the umbilicus and excise an oval piece of skin to accommodate it.

9. Break the operating table at the level of the pelvis to flex the hips.

10. Close the lower abdominal wound in layers and suture the umbilicus.

11. Insert a suction drain on each side.

12. Close the skin of the umbilical scar, if still present, in the vertical plane.

13. Post-operatively, keep the hips flexed to reduce tension on the lower abdominal wound for a few days.

14. Remove the sutures at 3 weeks.

Further reading

Barron J N, Saad M N 1980 Operative plastic and reconstructive surgery vols 1–3 Churchill Livingstone, Edinburgh
Converse J M 1977 Reconstructive plastic surgery vols 1–7 2nd edn. W B Saunders Co., Philadelphia, London, Toronto

Grabb W C, Smith J W 1979 Plastic surgery, 3rd edn. Little Brown and Co, Boston
McGregor I A 1980 Fundamental techniques of plastic surgery and their surgical applications, 7th edn. Churchill Livingstone, Edinburgh

Neonatal surgery

General considerations in neonatal surgery
Oesophageal atresia including gastrostomy
Congenital diaphragmatic hernia
Pyloric stenosis
Intestinal obstruction
Malrotation with or without midgut volvulus
Anorectal anomalies
Exomphalos and gastroschisis
Spina bifida aperta (myelomeningocoele)
Intussusception
Inguinal hernia

GENERAL CONSIDERATIONS IN NEONATAL SURGERY

INTRODUCTION

To obtain optimal surgical results, neonatal surgery is best practiced by adequately trained paediatric surgeons working in large regional centres. In such centres the concentration of clinical material offers experience in the management of a wide variety of congenital abnormalities and training programmes can be conducted. Expert support is available in anaesthesia, radiology, pathology, paediatrics and nursing, so essential for a satisfactory outcome.

The two supportive services most vital to the success of neonatal surgery are nursing and anaesthesia. A high level of skilled nursing care, occasionally on a one-to-one basis, is essential for the surgical neonate. High technology monitors, although extremely useful, cannot replace close observation by an experienced nurse. Advances in paediatric anaesthesia have paralleled those in neonatal surgery. Anaesthesia in the neonate, conducted by experts backed by suitable equipment, is now as safe as at any other age.

The neonatal period is defined as the first 28 days of extra-uterine life. The notion that the neonate is merely a scaled down version of the adult is completely out-dated. Both from a physiological as well as anatomical view the

neonate differs widely from the adult. The ratio of surface area to weight in the neonate is twice that of the adult and this exposes the infant to genuine risks of hypothermia from heat loss and dehydration from excessive insensible fluid loss. The neonatal kidney is immature and can only function within a limited homeostatic range. The diuretic response is particularly weak and circulatory overload can easily occur following injudicious intravenous fluid administration. Liver function is likewise restricted, particularly the detoxifying enzyme systems. Finally, the combination of low immunoglobulin levels with reduced leucocyte activity reduces the infant's resistance to infection. From an anatomical point of view, the most important consideration is the fact that congenital anomalies are frequently multiple. The pattern of associated anomalies is generally fairly constant such as renal anomalies in association with anorectal malformations; congenital cardiac anomalies with exomphalos and duodenal atresia; vertebral, anorectal, renal and radial anomalies with oesophageal atresia (VATER association).

RECOGNITION OF A CONGENITAL ANOMALY

External abnormalities are easily recognised at birth and do not merit further discussion. There are, however, a number of clinical features indicative of concealed anomalies which require further amplification.

1. Bilious vomiting. Green bile in the vomitus indicates a mechanical intestinal obstruction unless an alternative cause can be found, such as septicaemia.

2. Respiratory distress merits an X-ray of the chest to exclude a diaphragmatic hernia, oesophageal atresia, pneumothorax or lobar emphysema.

3. Delayed passage of meconium, more than 24 hours after birth, suggests the possibility of Hirschsprung's disease.

4. Failure to pass urine within 24 hours of birth may be due either to inadequate hydration or to urinary obstruction, such as posterior urethral valves.

5. Passage of blood in the stools may be from necrotising enterocolitis or strangulating intestinal obstruction, such as midgut volvulus.

6. An abdominal mass in a neonate is most likely to be a benign anomaly, such as hydronephrosis, or multicystic kidney. Consider hydrocolpos in girls, and an enlarged bladder due to urethral valves in boys. Tumours are rare at this age.

TRANSPORT

1. Newborn infants can be transported safely over long distances provided adequate precautions are taken to maintain body temperature, monitoring facilities are available, and the accompanying staff are fully experienced and adequately equipped to deal with any cardiorespiratory emergency.

2. When resuscitation is required for shock, hypothermia, respiratory insufficiency, and disturbances of fluid, electrolyte or acid-base homeostasis, commence treatment at the base hospital. Delay transfer until the infant's condition has stabilized. If surgery is urgently required for diaphragmatic hernia, intestinal volvulus, gastro-intestinal perforation or profuse haemorrhage, continue resuscitation during transfer.

3. For the safe transfer of a surgical neonate, ensure that
(a) Transport incubator is equipped with facilities for monitoring of heart rate, body temperature, inspired oxygen concentration and has an inbuilt mechanical ventilator.
(b) Cardiorespiratory resuscitation equipment, including laryngoscopes, endotracheal tubes, suction apparatus, chest drainage tubes and a variety of inotropic and respiratory stimulant drugs are available.
(c) Pass a nasogastric tube in all surgical neonates, even if there is no evidence of intestinal obstruction. Leave it freely draining and have it regularly aspirated to keep the stomach empty to avoid pulmonary complications of inhaled vomitus.
(d) Send 10 ml of maternal blood to restrict the amount required from the infant for compatibility studies. All surgical neonates require blood to be available for transfusion at surgery.
(e) Send a valid consent form for surgery.
(f) Send copies of all records regarding the pregnancy, delivery and perinatal period including biochemical results and X-rays.
4. *Special precautions:*
(a) *Oesophageal atresia*: keep the blind upper pouch empty during transfer to prevent aspiration of saliva. Apply continuous or frequent intermittent suction to an indwelling tube, preferably the double lumen Replogle tube, size 10. Place the infant either upright, or prone

with the head slightly depressed to prevent gastric reflux.
(b) *Diaphragmatic hernia*: infants presenting after 12–24 hours of life can usually be managed in a high oxygen atmosphere. Failure to respond, and especially for infants presenting with acute respiratory distress within 6 hours of birth, demands the passage of an endotracheal tube and gentle mechanical ventilation. Do not ventilate the infant with a face mask, as this forces air into the intestines, further compromising respiration. Always pass a large *patent* nasogastric tube. Leave it draining freely to limit the amount of gas entering the stomach. If there is any sudden deterioration during resuscitation or transfer, suspect the presence of a tension pneumothorax. Immediately insert a hypodermic needle into the pleural space through the second intercostal space anteriorly on one or both sides, and aspirate the free air.
(c) *Exomphalos and gastroschisis*: the chief risk to these infants is the loss of heat and large quantities of fluid through the exposed intestine or thin covering membrane. Restrict these losses by wrapping the intestine or intact exomphalos sac in plastic film. Avoid using saline swabs since the water rapidly evaporates and causes hypothermia.

PRE-OPERATIVE PREPARATION

1. Cross-match one unit of fresh whole blood.
2. Administer vitamin K, phytomenadione 1 mg intramuscularly, if this was omitted in the immediate postnatal period.
3. Check the blood glucose using Dextrostix. Correct hypoglycaemia giving 50% glucose intravenously.
4. Keep the infant normothermic.
5. Correct any acid-base and fluid imbalance.

Fluids and electrolytes

1. Use peripherally sited cannulae whenever possible. The umbilical vein appears a tempting alternative but complications such as necrotising enterocolitis and portal vein thrombosis should limit its use except in an emergency.

2. Basic fluids for intravenous infusion should be 10% dextrose in 0.18% saline for neonates, 4% dextrose in 0.18% saline for infants and children.

3. Replace abnormal losses as from nasogastric aspirate and enteric fistula with 0.9% saline (normal saline) adding 20 mmol potassium chloride per litre.

4. Calculate intravenous fluid requirements according to the following scheme:

Intravenous fluid requirements

	Weight	Daily requirement
Neonates	1500 g*	180 ml/kg/24 h
	1500–2500 g*	150 ml/kg/24 h
	2500 g*	120 ml/kg/24 h
	<10 kg	100 ml/kg/24 h
Infants and Children	10–20 kg	1000 ml/24 h **plus** 50 ml/kg/24 h for each kg above 10 kg
	> 20 kg	1500 ml/24 h **plus** 25 ml/kg/24 h for each kg above 20 kg

*at birth

Examples:

An 8.0 kg infant requires 8.0 × 100 = 800 ml/day

A 14.0 kg child requires 1000 mls **plus** 4 × 50 ml = 1200 ml/day.

A 25.0 kg child requires 1500 mls **plus** 5 × 25 ml = 1625 ml/day.

Postoperative

1. Neonates

First 48 hours after operation

⅓ of maintenance requirements

3rd and 4th day after operation

⅔ of maintenance requirements

5th and subsequent days

— full volume maintenance requirements

2. Infants and children

First 24 hours after operation

½ of maintenance requirements

2nd and 3rd day after operation

⅔ of maintenance requirements

4th and subsequent days

— full volume maintenance requirements

OESOPHAGEAL ATRESIA

Appraise (Fig. 32.1)

1. Surgery for the repair of an oesophageal atresia is seldom an emergency so that there is usually adequate time for referrral to a specialist centre where the chances of survival are greater. In the absence of other severe congenital anomalies and pneumonia, nearly all infants weighing over 1500 g survive.

2. Establish the diagnosis with a plain X-ray to reveal arrest of a radio-opaque nasogastric tube in the upper oesophagus. Include the abdomen on the initial radiograph. Air in the stomach indicates a distal tracheo-oesophageal fistula, in which primary repair is usually possible. Absence of gas in the abdomen usually indicates a pure oesophageal atresia in which the distance between the proximal and distal segments is too long to permit a primary oesophageal anastomosis. Plan to perform a

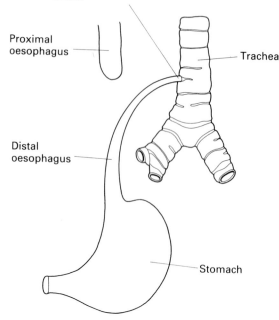

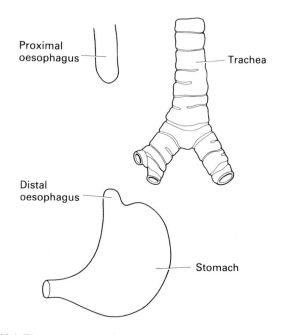

Fig. 32.1 The two main varieties of oesophageal atresia. Above is the most frequent (90%) condition with distal tracheo-oesophageal fistula. Below is the infrequent (5%) state of isolate oesophageal atresia.

feeding gastrostomy and an end cervical oesophagostomy, and transfer the neonate to a specialist centre.

STAMM GASTROSTOMY (Fig. 32.2)

Access

1. Make a transverse incision 3–4 cm long in the left

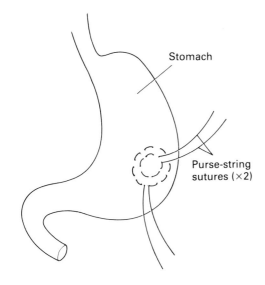

A

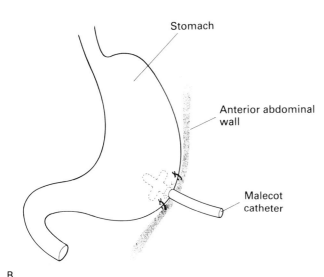

B

Fig. 32.2 The recommended technique of performing a Stamm gastrostomy

hypochrondium, midway between the umbilicus and the costal margin.

2. Incise the subcutaneous tissues, muscles and peritoneum along the length of the incision using cutting diathermy.

Action

1. Identify the stomach and choose the site for the gastrostomy — on the anterior surface of the body of the stomach 0.5–1.0 cm above the greater curvature.

2. Insert two purse-string sutures around the proposed site of the gastrostomy using a 000 atraumatic silk or Nurolon suture. Avoid the gastro-epiploic vessels.

3. Make a small incision in the stomach in the centre of the two purse-string sutures with a pointed scalpel blade

and insert a no. 10–12 F Malecot catheter into the stomach.

4. Tie first the inner and then the outer purse-string suture.

5. Bring the Malecot catheter out through a separate stab incision in the left upper quadrant.

6. Anchor the anterior wall of the stomach to the peritoneum at the site of exit of the tube. This will prevent retraction of the stomach away from the peritoneum and leakage of gastric content.

Closure

1. Close the wound en masse with 000 polyglycolic acid sutures. Suture the skin with interrupted nylon or an absorbable subcuticular suture.

2. Firmly anchor the tube to the skin of the abdomen with one or two silk sutures.

OESOPHAGEAL ATRESIA (Fig. 32.3)

Only the principle steps are outlined. Repair requires special training and facilities.

Access

1. The incision is a right postero-lateral thoracotomy.
2. Gain access via the 4th or 5th intercostal space.
3. Follow a retropleural approach to the mediastinum. This has distinct advantages over the transpleural approach in controlling an oesophageal leak.

Action

1. Isolate the distal oesophagus. The vagus nerve courses on the surface.

2. Trace the distal oesophagus to its proximal connection with the trachea.

3. Divide the oesophagus at this site and suture the defect in the trachea with interrupted 0000 or 00000 Prolene or nylon sutures.

4. Identify the blind-ending upper oesophagus by asking the anaesthetist to apply pressure on the oro- or naso-oesophageal catheter.

5. Excise the tip of the blind-ending upper oesophagus.

6. Construct an anastomosis between the proximal and distal oesophagus using a single layer of interrupted 0000 or 00000 polyglycolic acid, silk or Prolene sutures. It is vital that each suture of the oesophageal wall includes the mucosa which tends to retract away from the cut end.

Closure

1. Insert an underwater seal drain in the retropleural space.

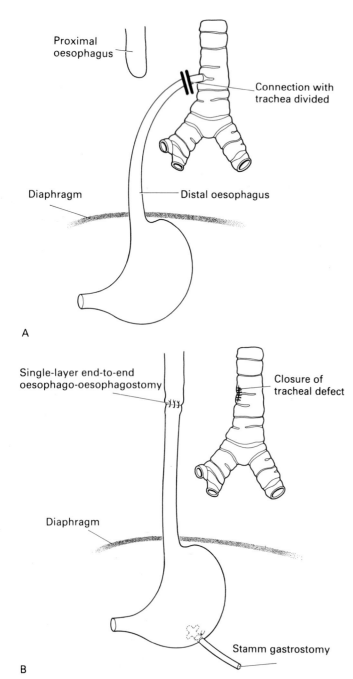

Fig. 32.3 The recommended primary operation for oesophageal atresia with a tracheo-oeosophageal fistula.

2. Close the thoracotomy wound in layers with 00 pericostal and 000 tissue sutures of polyglycolic acid.

CONGENITAL DIAPHRAGMATIC HERNIA (Fig. 32.4)

Appraise

Establish the diagnosis by chest radiograph in an infant displaying signs of respiratory distress with tachypnoea

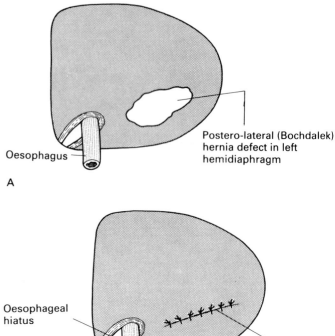

Fig. 32.4 Congenital diaphragmatic hernial defect before and after repair.

more than 60/min, tachycardia more than 160/min, cyanosis, or using accessory muscles of respiration. The X-ray shows bowel gas shadows in the involved hemithorax, with displacement of the mediastinal structures to the opposite side.

Prepare

1. Pass a large No. 10 nasogastric tube. This may be difficult as herniation of the stomach into the chest may produce acute angulation of the gastro-oesophageal junction. Leave the tube patent and aspirate it frequently to prevent accumulation of gas in the stomach, so avoiding further compression of the pulmonary tissue.

2. Nurse the infant in 100% oxygen in the incubator. If an acceptable level of blood oxygenation still cannot be maintained, pass an endotracheal tube for assisted ventilation. Ventilatory pressures should not exceed 12 cm of water, to avoid alveolar rupture with consequent tension pneumothorax.

3. Keep the infant warm in an incubator, or swaddled in warm gamgee with the additional protection of polythene or silver foil where possible.

4. Whenever possible arrange immediate transfer to a regional paediatric surgical centre. The infant should be accompanied by an experienced doctor and nurse with full facilities for cardiorespiratory resuscitation. A police escort

will facilitate the transfer. If transfer from a remote area would exceed two hours, perform the operation locally.

Anaesthesia

1. Employ endotracheal anaesthesia using minimal inflatory pressures.

2. If possible have full monitoring facilities available, including electrocardiography, measurement of blood gases, central venous and arterial pressures, particularly important in the infant less than 12 hours old.

3. The infant's body temperature must be maintained throughout the operation. This is best achieved by wrapping the limbs and head in silver foil, and swaddling its body in warm gamgee while maintaining an ambient theatre temperature of 30°C (85°F).

Access

1. Place the infant supine on the table.

2. The left side is affected in the majority of cases (L : R = 1 : 10). The procedure for right-sided hernias does not differ significantly from that on the left.

3. Perform the operation through the abdomen and not through the chest. There is always an associated intestinal malrotation which can only be corrected via the abdominal approach. Failure to correct the malrotation exposes the infant to the risk of midgut volvulus, which may be difficult to recognise in the early post-operative period.

4. Stand on the right side of the patient.

5. Make a long transverse incision from the most lateral part of the anterior abdominal wall, across the left rectus abdominis muscle to the midline. If you are inexperienced, be prepared to divide the medial half of the right rectus abdominis.

6. Once the dermis has been incised with the scalpel, use cutting diathermy to reduce blood loss. Coagulate the superior epigastric vessels as soon as they appear on the deeper surface of the rectus abdominis muscle.

7. If the incision crosses the midline, remember that the umbilical vein is very large in the neonate, so ligate and divide it as soon as it is exposed.

Assess

1. Frequently, only the right lobe of the liver and left colon are within the abdomen.

2. Often the entire small bowel, the right colon, and the spleen are within the chest.

3. The stomach may or may not be in the chest.

4. In right-sided defects, the only intrathoracic content may be the right lobe of the liver.

Action

1. Identify the edges of the diaphragmatic defect.

2. Slowly and gently withdraw the intestine from the chest.

3. Rarely, the bowel is firmly held within the thoracic cavity. If so, introduce a red rubber or polythene catheter through the defect to allow the ingress of air which frees the trapped viscera.

4. Withdraw the stomach.

5. Leave the spleen within the chest until all other viscera are removed, since this is the most difficult organ to remove through the small diaphragmatic defect.

6. Withdraw the intestines from the abdomen and wrap them in a warm pack.

7. Turn attention now to the edges of the diaphragmatic defect.

8. Incise the peritoneum over the posterior rim of the defect, above the adrenal. Free the edge of the diaphragm. There is nearly always more diaphragm present than at first appears.

9. Insert an underwater seal chest drain to the left thorax. **Do not** attempt to inflate the left lung by increased positive pressure as the lung is hypoplastic and may rupture, producing a potentially lethal bronchopleural fistula. Even worse, the contralateral lung may rupture, producing a potentially lethal tension pneumothorax.

10. Insert several interrupted 00 or 000 silk or Nurolon sutures to unite the edges of the defect. When all the sutures have been inserted, tie them in series, working towards the centre from both lateral and medial corners so as to avoid excessive tension on the central part of the defect.

11. If the defect is excessively large, insert a prosthetic patch consisting of Silastic, Prolene or Teflon, to close the hernial orifice. The mortality rate in these cases is very high.

12. Having closed the diaphragm, direct attention to the intestinal malrotation. Perform a Ladd's procedure as for intestinal volvulus (see p. 581). An inversion appendicectomy may be carried out.

Closure

1. The capacity of the peritoneal cavity is usually severely restricted. In order to be able to accommodate the abdominal viscera, increase the capacity of the abdominal cavity by stretching the muscles of the anterior abdominal wall as for ruptured exomphalos or gastroschisis (see p. 585).

2. Close the abdominal wall en masse using interrupted or continuous sutures of 000 polyglycolic acid, Prolene or nylon.

3. Close the skin with interrupted 00000 nylon or preferably with a subcuticular polyglycolic acid suture.

Aftercare

1. Experienced nursing care, skilled in neonatal intensive care, is essential.

2. Infants presenting within the first 24 hours of life generally require assisted ventilation at least for the first few postoperative days.

3. It is advantageous to insert a radial artery catheter for constant recording of the blood pressure and to facilitate blood gas sampling. Central venous pressure monitoring is also of assistance in estimating fluid requirements.

4. Correct pH of less than 7.2 with small doses of sodium bicarbonate. Remember it is easy to give several days' requirements of sodium with each dose of bicarbonate. Acidosis means poor peripheral circulation with respiratory failure, so improve these rather than giving over-doses of sodium bicarbonate.

5. Peripheral or pulmonary vasodilator drugs may be required, such as dopamine and Tolazoline. When these drugs are used, maintain an adequate cardiac output by expanding the blood volume with infusion of colloid, as estimated by the central venous pressure measurement.

Prognosis

Infants presenting after the first 12–24 hours of life have an excellent prognosis. The mortality rate for infants presenting within 6 hours of birth is very high (40–50%). Death is almost entirely due to associated pulmonary hypoplasia.

PYLORIC STENOSIS (Fig. 32.5)

Appraise

1. This occurs predominantly in first-born male infants (M : F = 4 : 1) around the second to fourth week of life.

2. The cardinal features are projectile non-bilious vomiting, failure to thrive and constipation.

3. The diagnosis is established by palpating the pyloric 'tumour' in the right hypochrondrium.

4. Barium studies to establish the diagnosis are necessary in only 10–15% of cases.

Prepare

1. Measure serum urea and electrolytes and acid-base status.

2. Correct hypochloraemia and hypokalaemia with intravenous infusion of normal saline adding potassium (10–15 mmol KC1/500 ml 0.9% saline).

3. It is unnecessary to correct the alkalosis which resolves spontaneously with the saline infusion.

4. Restrict all milk feeds and perform gastric lavage with warm normal saline until washouts are clear.

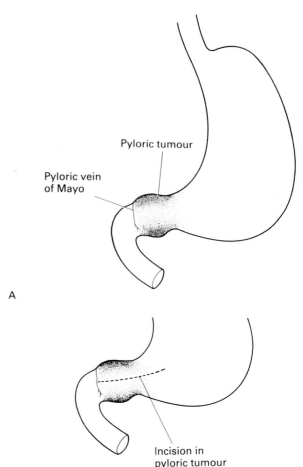

A

B

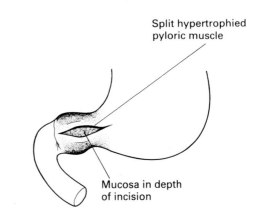

C

Fig. 32.5 Rammstedt's pyloromyotomy

5. The operation for pyloric stenosis is **NEVER** an emergency. Do not hesitate to delay surgery for 24–48 hours while correcting dehydration and electrolyte disturbances.

6. Check that serum potassium levels are above 3.5 mol/l before arranging surgery.

7. Pass a nasogastric tube and aspirate the stomach before anaesthetizing the infant.

Anaesthesia

Although local anaesthesia has been used for pyloromyotomy with great success, if there is an acceptable standard of paediatric anaesthesia available, general endotracheal anaesthesia is smoother and safer.

Access

1. The infant lies prone on the operating table protected from cold.

2. Site the incision, 3–4 cm long, transversely, high in the right hypochondrium midway between the costal margin and the palpable inferior margin of the liver. The medial end of the incision ends 1–2 cm from the midline.

Having incised the skin with the scalpel, divide the subcutaneous tissue and muscles in the length of the incision using cutting diathermy to limit blood loss.

4. Open the peritoneum in the length of the wound.

5. Retract the inferior margin of the liver upwards by means of a broad malleable retractor protected by a moist gauze swab.

6. Identify the greater curvature of the stomach directly or after applying gentle traction on the tranverse mesocolon.

7. **Do not attempt to withdraw the pyloric tumour by applying direct traction on the mass**; this results in serosal tears.

8. Deliver the greater curvature of the body of the stomach into the wound. Apply gentle traction on the greater curvature until the firm, white, glistening pyloric tumour is brought into view. Ease it out of the peritoneal cavity into the wound.

9. Identify the pyloric vein of Mayo. This marks the distal end of the pyloric canal.

Action

1. Make an incision 1–2 mm deep with a scalpel on the anterior surface of the pyloric tumour in the relatively avascular plane midway between the superior and inferior borders. Extend the incision from the pyloric vein of Mayo, through the pyloric canal and onto the hypertrophied body of the stomach.

2. Using firm but gentle pressure on the incised pylorus with a MacDonald dissector, the blunt handle of a scalpel or a blunt artery forceps, split the hypertrophied muscle neatly down to the mucosa.

3. Identify the mucosa as a glistening membrane.

4. Split the pyloric mass from end to end using a pyloric spreader (Denis Browne) or blunt artery forceps. Ensure that all the fibres of the pyloric tumour are split.

5. Introduce air into the stomach through the nasogastric tube and squeeze the air through the pylorus into the duodenum. Escape of air or bile at the duodenal end of the incision signifies a perforation of the mucosa, most common in the duodenal fornix.

6. Close a perforation with a few interrupted 0000 or 00000 chromic catgut or polyglycolic acid sutures.

7. Haemorrhage from the incised pylorus is largely due to venous congestion. Bleeding usually ceases promptly once the pylorus is returned to the abdominal cavity.

Closure

1. Close the wound en masse using interrupted 000 polyglycolic acid sutures to the muscles and peritoneum.
2. Approximate the skin with a continuous subcuticular 00000 polyglycolic acid or chromic catgut suture.

Aftercare

1. Many surgeons commence feeds within 4–6 hours of surgery. There is no evidence that gastric peristalsis is effective so early after operation, and such early feeding increases the incidence of vomiting.

2. Continue intravenous fluids for 12–24 hours.

3. Introduce feeds cautiously 12 hours after surgery starting with 15–20 ml of dextrose saline and gradually increasing the amount of feed until normal oral nutrition is reestablished within 36–48 hours.

4. The infant is ready for discharge from hospital on the third or fourth postoperative day.

5. If a perforation of the mucosa occurred, withhold feeds for 24 hours while continuing nasogastric decompression and intravenous fluids.

INTESTINAL OBSTRUCTIONS

The infant with intestinal obstruction is best managed in a specialist centre for paediatric surgery. This applies not only for the surgical treatment but particularly for the postoperative care which may be complicated and often entails prolonged parenteral nutrition, particularly where massive resections result in a short bowel syndrome.

Appraise

1. The main causes of intestinal obstruction are
(a) Intraluminal causes — meconium ileus
(b) Intramural causes — atresias, stenoses and Hirschsprung's disease.
(c) Extraintestinal causes—malrotation, duplication cysts, and tumours.

2. The precautions required during transfer have been discussed, but the need for efficient nasogastric decompression cannot be emphasised too strongly.

3. Neonates with intestinal obstruction can be safely transported over long distances (transcontinentally and intercontinentally) but local circumstances may dictate that

surgery has to be conducted by a general surgeon. The principles of the operative procedure for laparotomy under these conditions are described below.

Prepare

1. Set up a peripheral intravenous infusion, preferably in an upper limb.
2. Have blood cross-matched and available in the operating theatre.
3. Correct any fluid and electrolyte imbalance and acid-base disturbance.
4. Ensure that the infant is normothermic.
5. Pass a large nasogastric tube.
6. Consider using broad spectrum antibiotics — penicillin, gentamicin, metronidazole.

Anaesthesia

General endotracheal anaesthesia is used, with the infant in the supine position.

Access

1. The best exposure is obtained through an upper abdominal transverse muscle-cutting incision.
2. Incise the skin approximately 1 cm above the umbilical cord. Extend the incision equally across both rectus abdominis muscles.
3. Having incised the dermis, proceed through the fat, anterior rectus sheath and rectus muscles with cutting diathermy in order to limit blood loss.
4. Isolate the umbilical vein in the pre-peritoneal areolar tissue. Clamp the vein, ligate it with 000 silk and divide it.
5. Open the peritoneum in the length of the incision.
6. Take a specimen of peritoneal fluid for culture and antibiotic sensitivity.

Closure

1. Insert en-masse interrupted 000 sutures of polyglycolic acid, nylon or Prolene.
2. Close the skin with subcuticular sutures of 00000 polyglycolic acid, or interrupted fine nylon or silk sutures.
3. It is unnecessary to drain the peritoneal cavity.

MECONIUM ILEUS

The diagnosis of mucoviscidosis is confirmed by sweat tests at the age of 4–6 weeks. Analysis of the sweat reveals sodium levels in excess of 60 umol/l. Since mucoviscidosis is a recessively inherited condition, the implications for the family are considerable.

Assess

1. The small intestine is grossly dilated and packed with thick, tenacious, black meconium. The terminal ileum and colon contain pellets of inspissated, grey mucus.
2. There may be an associated small bowel atresia or the condition may be complicated by perforation of the obstructed intestine.

Action

1. Identify the site of obstruction at the transition between dilated proximal and collapsed distal intestine.
2. Divide the intestine between clamps at the site of obstruction. It may be necessary to sacrifice grossly dilated proximal bowel if its vascular supply is compromised.
3. Endeavour to decompress the proximal and/or distal intestine by irrigating with warm saline, Gastrografin or Tween 80. The latter two substances are strongly hygroscopic and must be used with considerable caution to avoid dehydration and shock.
4. The Bishop-Koop chimney anastomosis is used by many paediatric surgeons, but the simplest and most effective treatment is to perform a standard double-barrelled Mikulicz ileostomy.

INTESTINAL ATRESIA

Assess

1. There is an abrupt transition between proximal, dilated intestine and the narrow, collapsed, 'un-used' distal bowel.
2. The bowel ends may be adjacent to one another, connected by a fibrous strand, or completely separate.
3.In cases of multiple atresias, the more distal atresias may not be obvious.

Action

1. Identify the atretic segment(s).
2. Resect the atretic segment with 1–2 cm distally, the proximal extent of the resection being dependent on the site of the atresia. In high jejunal atresia, resection cannot be carried out proximal to the duodeno-jejunal flexure. In mid-small bowel atresia, resection can be performed into proximal intestine of fairly normal calibre. Avoid extensive resections if possible.
3. Test that the distal bowel is patent by injecting saline through a catheter introduced into the lumen.
4. Join the bowel ends using a single layer of interrupted 0000 or 00000 full-thickness mattress sutures or with interrupted seromuscular sutures. Perform an end-to-end or end-to-back anastomosis and avoid side-to-side anastomoses.

Difficulty?

1. Grossly dilated proximal intestine may have to be 'tapered' in order to achieve an end-to-end anastomosis.

2. 'Tapering' is performed by excising an antimesenteric wedge of proximal bowel.

HIRSCHSPRUNG'S DISEASE

Ideally, frozen section histopathology should be available to identify the transition between proximal ganglionic and distal aganglionic colon.

Action

1. Identify the transition between dilated proximal and collapsed distal colon.

2. Perform a loop colostomy in the proximally dilated ganglionic colon as described in the section on anorectal malformations (p. 583).

3. Excise a narrow ellipse of full-thickness intestine at the site of the colostomy to confirm the presence of ganglion cells on paraffin sections.

Definitive treatment

The definitive treatment of Hirschsprung's disease is highly specialised and should only be performed by experienced paediatric surgeons with full histopathological expertise available.

DUPLICATION CYSTS

These cysts are situated on the mesenteric border of the intestine and cause obstruction by stretching and compressing the adjacent lumen.

Action

1. Identify the duplication cyst.
2. Resect the cyst en-bloc with the adjacent intestine.
3. Perform an end-to-end anastomosis in one layer with interrupted 0000 or 00000 polyglycolic acid sutures, using either full-thickness or seromuscular technique.

MALROTATION WITH OR WITHOUT MIDGUT VOLVULUS

Development

1. The midgut develops within the physiological umbilical hernia in early intrauterine life. Between the 10th and 12th week of development, the midgut loop returns into the peritoneal cavity, rotating in an orderly manner commencing with the small intestine, while the caeco-colic region enters the abdomen last. The duodenum and caeco-colic loops undergo a counter-clockwise rotation of 270°, resulting in fixation of the duodenum and right colon in the retroperitoneum so that the mesentery of the small intestine extends diagonally over a relatively long distance across the posterior abdominal wall.

2. Malrotation results from failure of this normal process and has two effects:
(a) Formation of abnormal bands which cross and may compress the second part of the duodenum.
(b) A narrow base to the midgut which is prone to volvulus. Volvulus may occur at any age but it is particularly likely to occur during the first month of life.

Appraise

1. Consider the diagnosis of malrotation in any infant manifesting bilious vomiting.

2. Plain abdominal radiograph reveals a dilated stomach and duodenum with the rest of the abdomen relatively 'gasless' when volvulus has occurred.

3. The diagnosis can be confirmed by means of either upper or lower gastro-intestinal contrast radiography.

4. Treatment is urgent when volvulus is known to have occurred, producing shock and gastro-intestinal haemorrhage, evidenced by a tender oedematous abdomen. The blood supply to the entire midgut may be obstructed and delay in treatment serves only to increase the amount and extent of intestinal necrosis. Nevertheless, a short, intensive period (1–2 hours) of active resuscitation to correct fluid and electrolyte loss and acid-base inbalance is well worthwhile.

Prepare

1. Correct dehydration with intravenous plasma (20 ml/kg) as rapidly as possible.

2. Administer preoperative antibiotics — penicillin, gentamicin and metronidazole.

3. Consider giving steroids for the severely shocked infant.

4. Effect urgent transfer to a specialized paediatric surgical unit ensuring that full resuscitative measures continue en route.

5. Where specialized facilities are unavailable within a reasonable distance, prepare to undertake surgery locally.

Anaesthesia

Use general endotracheal anaesthesia with the infant in the supine position.

Access

1. Use a long transverse incision placed midway between the umbilicus and costal margin, extending from the medial half of the left rectus abdominis, across the midline and the right rectus abdominis to the transversus abdominis and oblique muscles of the right side.

2. After incising the dermis, use cutting diathermy to reduce blood loss.

3. Ligate and divide the umbilical vein.

4. Send some peritoneal fluid for bacteriological studies. Sometimes there is marked chylous ascites resulting from compression of the lymphatics in the mesenteric base.

Assess

1. Inspect the bowel for obvious areas of gangrene. These should be handled very gently as the intestinal wall is extremely friable and prone to perforation.

2. Assess the direction of rotation and untwist the volvulus. Usually a counter-clockwise manoeuvre will release the volvulus.

3. Whilst awaiting return of circulation to compromised bowel, inspect the root of the mesentery for evidence of a malrotation.

4. In a typical case, the root of the mesentery between the duodeno-jejunal flexure and the ileo-caecal junction is very narrow and fibrotic. The caecum lies below the liver and may be attached to the gall bladder by peritoneal bands.

Action

Ladd's procedure is recommended.

1. Divide the avascular peritoneal bands between the caecum and liver.

2. Once all the bands are divided, the caecum may be placed in the left upper quadrant of the abdomen.

3. See that the duodeno-jejunal flexure is to the right of the midline. Adhesions anchoring the flexure may have to be divided.

4. Mobilize the duodenum by Kocher's manoeuvre and divide all peritoneal folds so that all kinks in the duodenum are straightened.

5. Incise what is now the anterior layer of peritoneum at the root of the mesentery and divide all fibrous bands so that the caecum may be moved as far to the left as possible, away from the duodeno-jejunal flexure so that the base of the mesentery is broadened.

6. Inspect the duodenum carefully, searching for areas of duodenal stenosis. This is uncommon except in those cases presenting in early infancy. Correct a duodenal stenosis by performing a duodeno-duodenostomy. Do not incise the annular pancreas, as this increases the morbidity and mortality and achieves little.

7. Return attention to the small bowel. Measure the length of the ischaemic bowel and assess the blood supply.

8. Resect all truly gangrenous areas unless this would leave the child with less than 30–50 cm of small bowel. Consider whether it would be better to perform a primary anastomosis, or to bring out both ends as temporary stomata. In underdeveloped countries it may be wiser to perform a primary anastomosis. In advanced countries, elect to perform enterostomies and maintain the child by parenteral nutrition until the general condition is improved. In this way it may be possible to preserve more intestine than would be possible with a primary anastomosis.

9. When most of the intestine is ischaemic, return it to the abdomen, having untwisted the volvulus and divided constricting bands and adhesions. Close the abdomen in one layer. Continue intensive medical treatment, and re-explore the abdomen after 24 hours. At the 'second look' laparotomy in young infants one is often surprised at how the blood supply has improved. At the second operation, resect all bowel which is obviously gangrenous, but retain all bowel of doubtful viability. Bring the two ends out as temporary stomata. An anastomosis in compromised bowel is not advised as it is prone to disruption.

10. If all the bowel is viable, consider performing an appendicectomy. The appendix would otherwise lie below the left costal margin and could cause diagnostic confusion at a later date. Appendicectomy is best performed by the inversion method so as not to spill intestinal bacteria in an otherwise 'clean' operation.

Closure

1. Close the deep layers en masse with continuous or interrupted 000 polyglycolic acid, Prolene or nylon.

2. Suture the skin with subcuticular 0000 chromic catgut or use interrupted sutures of 00000 nylon or Prolene placed 1.5–2 mm from the skin edge, so as to avoid cross-hatching.

3. A wound drain is rarely required.

Aftercare

1. Postoperative mechanical ventilation may be necessary especially in the infant with massive intestinal necrosis.

2. In such cases, close monitoring of arterial oxygenation and central venous pressure is essential. Maintain central venous pressure by infusing plasma or fresh whole blood as required. Peripheral vasodilator drugs may be necessary. Administer diuretics to maintain an adequate urinary output (minimum of 1–2 ml/kg/hour).

3. In uncomplicated malrotation with or without volvulus, there is commonly a period of prolonged ileus, up to 10–14 days, during which parenteral nutrition is necessary.

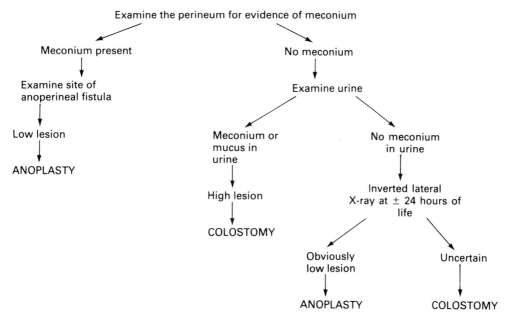

Flow chart showing management of male infants with anorectal anomalies.

4. Following massive intestinal resections, the period of parenteral nutrition will have to be considerably prolonged. Oral nutrition is introduced with considerable caution as there is frequently intolerance to lactose, lipids and proteins.

ANORECTAL ANOMALIES

Appraise

1. It is vital for future continence to differentiate the high (supralevator) anomaly from the low (translevator) lesion. The high lesion requires an initial colostomy while the low lesion can be managed very successfully by an anoplasty.

2. In case of uncertainty perform a colostomy. Do not explore the perineum in search of the rectum. This may result in permanent incontinence.

3. Male infants: see flow chart above.

4. Female infants: in female infants, determine the number of orifices present on the perineum. If 3 orifices are present this is a low lesion, so perform an anoplasty or cutback procedure. If there are 2 orifices, or only 1 from which meconium is being passed, this is a high lesion, so perform a colostomy.

ANOPLASTY

Action (Fig. 32.6)

1. Make an inverted 'V' incision in the skin, the apex being centred on the pin hole opening on the perineum at the anal site.

2. Undermine the skin by sharp dissection.

3. After placing stay sutures, incise the rectal mucosa vertically for 1–2 cm.

4. Suture the inverted 'V' shaped flap into the rectal incision using 0000 polyglycolic acid or 0000 silk sutures.

5. The success of the operation depends upon the construction of a relatively large anus which must be dilated daily for several months. Failure to carry out regular dilatation results in anal stenosis and consequent acquired megacolon which is extremely refractory.

COLOSTOMY

The technique to be described is based on the original description of a skin-bridge colostomy as recommended by Nixon. This avoids the use of a glass rod to prevent retraction of the intestine back into the peritoneal cavity.

Action (Fig. 32.7)

1. Make a 'V'-shaped incision either in the left iliac fossa, for a sigmoid colostomy, or in the right hypochondrium for a transverse colostomy. The latter colostomy has the advantage of leaving sufficient colon distally for secondary surgery to be performed without disturbing the colostomy.

2. Carry the V-incision through skin and subcutaneous tissue.

3. Raise the flap of the V exposing the underlying muscle.

4. Excise two shallow ellipses of skin and subcutaneous tissue immediately adjacent to the V-flap in order to avoid

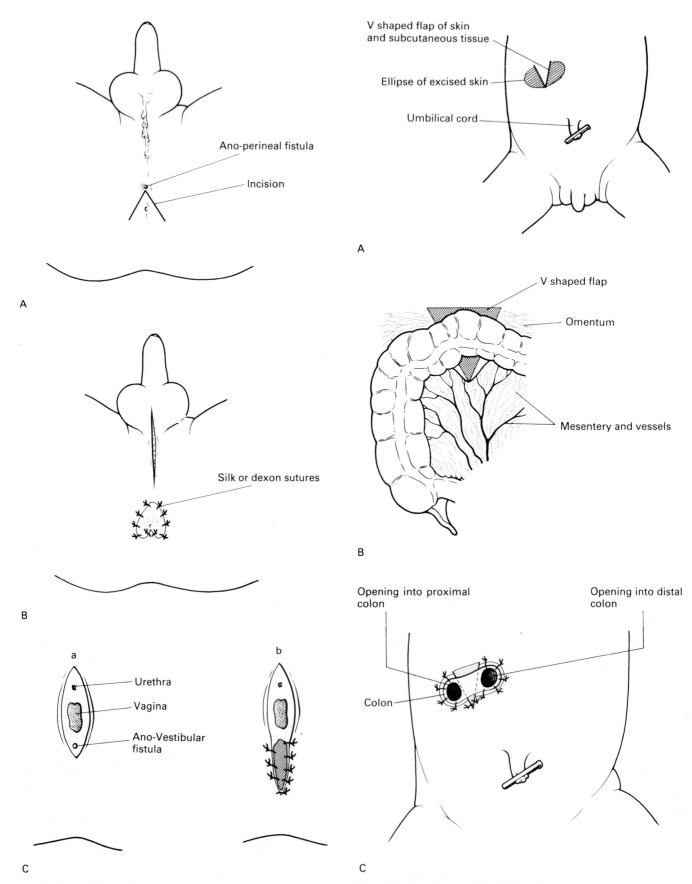

Fig. 32.6 Anoplasty procedures: male and female infants

Fig. 32.7 Transverse loop skin bridge colostomy.

compression of the colon immediately proximal and distal to the stoma.

5. Incise the muscle transversely, perpendicular to the V-incision, using cutting diathermy.

6. Open the peritoneum in the same direction as the muscle incision.

7. Locate the part of the intestine which will form the colostomy. Remember that the sigmoid loop may be greatly dilated, appearing in the right upper quadrant where it is easily confused with the transverse colon. The lack of an omental attachment serves to differentiate it from the transverse colon.

8. Ensure that the bowel is not twisted as it is withdrawn onto the surface. Twisting may produce intestinal obstruction.

9. Make a small opening in the colonic mesentery.

10. Pass the apex of the V skin flap through the mesenteric defect and suture it to its original position with 2–3 loosely tied 000 or 0000 silk or nylon sutures.

11. Suture the peritoneum and muscular fascia to the colonic serosa with a few interrupted 0000 polyglycolic acid or silk sutures. This prevents prolapse of small intestine alongside the colostomy.

12. Incise the colon longitudinally with cutting diathermy.

13. Suture the full-thickness of the opened colon to the surrounding skin with interrupted 0000 polyglycolic acid sutures.

Aftercare

1. The infant should be referred to a specialised paediatric surgical unit for further investigation to determine the precise anatomy of the anorectal malformation and to exclude additional congenital anomalies particularly of the urinary system.

2. The definitive pull-through procedure requires experience and skill if there is to be any chance of the child developing an acceptable degree of faecal continence.

EXOMPHALOS AND GASTROSCHISIS

Appraise

1. Exomphalos is a herniation of abdominal viscera into the persistent 'physiological umbilical hernia'. The contents, which may include liver in addition to intestine, are covered by a thin transparent membrane consisting of peritoneum on the inside, amniotic membrane on the outside, with Wharton's jelly between the two layers.

2. Gastroschisis is an evisceration of peritoneal contents, usually only intestine, through a defect in the anterior abdominal wall. The defect is generally immediately to the right of an apparently normal umbilical cord. The

intestines are thickened, oedematous and frequently matted together.

3. The mortality rate of major exomphalos, where the defect in the anterior abdominal wall measures more than 5 cm in diameter, is high due to the presence of additional congenital anomalies such as major cardiac defects and renal abnormalities. In gastroschisis the eviscerated intestine is matted together with a thick serosal coat and is foreshortened, but other major anomalies are uncommon.

4. Recently improved techniques and postoperative management have significantly improved the survival rates in gastroschisis and ruptured exomphalos. These include the use of elective postoperative mechanical ventilation and of prolonged parenteral nutrition.

Transfer

1. Transfer to a specialised centre as soon as possible.

2. Before transfer, wrap the lesion, or ideally the lower half of the body of the infant, in plastic wrap. This applies particularly to the ruptured exomphalos and gastroschisis where the plastic prevents excessive loss of fluid and heat from the exposed intestine. Do not use sterile, warm, moist gauze as these swabs rapidly become cold and dry and accelerate heat and fluid loss.

3. Swaddle the rest of the infant, including the abdomen, in warm gamgee wool to avoid hypothermia.

4. Always pass a nasogastric tube and keep the stomach empty.

Principles

1. *Exomphalos minor.* The defect is repaired primarily with attention to the associated intestinal malrotation.

2. *Unruptured exomphalos major.* Conservative treatment is by applying an antiseptic, such as povidone iodine, to the exomphalos sac two or three times daily. This serves to prevent infection and rupture of the membrane and aids in shrinkage and contraction of the defect. After several weeks the membrane separates leaving a well-epithelialized surface. The infant may be left with a large ventral hernia which should be closed at 12–18 months of age. Surgical closure of the defect with or without the use of prosthetic material should only be attempted by experienced surgeons with full availability of ancillary services as in a regional centre.

3. *Gastroschisis.* Primary closure of the abdominal wall follows enlargement of the peritoneal cavity by stretching the muscles of the abdominal wall. Using this method of management, postoperative mechanical ventilation is invariably required and for this reason this method should only be attempted in specialist centres. The alternative method of management consists of inserting a prosthetic material into the abdominal wall to cover the eviscerated bowel, such as Silastic, Teflon or Prolene mesh as

described by Schuster. Silastic separates from the abdominal wall after 7–10 days so full repair of the abdominal wall should be possible at that stage.

4. *Ruptured exomphalos major.* Primary repair is frequently impossible. The use of prosthetic material to create an artificial umbilical hernia is the most practical means of dealing with this difficult problem.

SPINA BIFIDA APERTA (MYELOMENINGOCOELE)

All infants with spina bifida should be transferred to a specialised unit for assessment and management since they require the expertise of a team consisting of paediatric surgeons experienced in urology, neurosurgery and orthopaedics, as well as skilled nurses and specialised physiotherapists.

Remember that the initial neonatal operation has little influence on the long-term prognosis which depends upon the site and size of the myelomeningocele. The operation on the back simply rids the infant of the myelomeningocele, so facilitating nursing and ensures a more rapid healing of the lesion than would occur naturally. Whether or not the infant survives depends more on whether or not the concomitant hydrocephalus is treated.

Appraise

1. Relative indications for operation are a small defect that is easily closed, absence of neurological deficit, or a robust infant with some neurological deficit. The parents may demand surgery despite knowing that the infant will have moderately severe handicaps.

2. Relative contraindications for surgery are a large lesion which will be difficult to repair and may break down, an infant in poor general condition, or the presence of other severe congenital anomalies. Surgery is unlikely to be profitable for a neonate in an underdeveloped country with inadequate facilities for treating hydrocephalus, urinary tract complications, or complex orthopaedic abnormalities. An extensive neurological deficit, severe kyphoscoliosis, and gross hydrocephalus also militate against surgery.

Closure

1. Puncture the membrane between the neural plaque and the skin, allowing some of the cerebrospinal fluid to drain. It is difficult to assess the full extent of the lesion until the fluid has ceased to flow.

2. Using a scalpel, make an incision round the circumference of the neural plaque at its junction with the membrane, ensuring continually that there is no damage to the underlying nerve roots.

3. Having freed the neural plaque, excise the whole of the membrane back to healthy skin.

4. Make an incision round the outer limits of the dural layer of fascia, starting on either side and taking particular care both superiorly and inferiorly to avoid damage to the underlying spinal cord.

5. Close the dural layer with a continuous suture of 00000 polyglycolic acid.

6. If the defect is relatively small, make an incision in the thoracolumbar fascia, on either side, at the medial borders of the bifid spinal processes. Elevate the muscles by blunt dissection and suture the fascia together in the midline using 00 polyglycolic acid. If the lesion is very wide it is probably wiser to omit this step.

7. Having brought the musculo-fascial layers together in the midline it is usually possible to do likewise with the skin edges. There is often a distinct fibrous ring round the edges of the defect and this can be sutured with a continuous stitch of 000 polyglycolic acid, so taking tension off the skin edges. Suture the skin with interrupted sutures of 0000 nylon. It should be seldom necessary to perform relaxing incisions in the flanks in order to achieve apposition of skin over the defect.

Aftercare

1. Nurse the infant in the prone position until the wound has healed. Leave the skin sutures in situ for 10–14 days.

2. Measure the head circumference regularly to anticipate the early onset of hydrocephalus.

3. Fully investigate the urinary system.

4. Long-term problems include shunt dysfunction, urinary incontinence and/or renal damage and orthopaedic problems.

INTUSSUSCEPTION

Appraise

1. Between the ages of 6 months and 2 years, most intussusceptions are 'idiopathic', possibly caused by viral infections. The vast majority originate in the ileo-caecal region. The condition is rare in the neonatal period and is less common after the age of 2 years. In the 'idiopathic age group', and in the absence of radiological evidence of intestinal obstruction or perforation, initial treatment is attempted using hydrostatic reduction by means of a barium enema. If this is unsuccessful, operation is required.

2. Outside the usual age range there is more likely to be a leading point such as a Meckel's diverticulum, polyp,

duplication cyst or tumour causing the intussusception, and operation should be advised at an early stage.

Prepare preoperative

1. The sick infant should be resuscitated and then transferred to a specialised unit, resuscitation continuing on the way. These infants often deteriorate rapidly after operation and may not survive unless there are adequate facilities for intensive care.

2. If the child is in reasonable condition and there are adequate local facilities, prepare the child for operation.

3. Ensure that a well-placed, adequately running, intravenous infusion is set up.

4. Most infants will have reduced intravascular volume and will need pre-operative rehydration. Many require replacement of 10% or more blood volume with plasma or whole blood.

5. Unless you are experienced, do not operate before blood is cross-matched and available.

6. Do not operate unless an experienced anaesthetist is available.

7. Do not operate unless a sufficient number of experienced nurses are available. Transfer the child to a specialised centre.

8. Remember that the child may deteriorate suddenly when it is anaesthetized because of hypotension from reduced peripheral vascular resistance.

9. Consider the use of preoperative antibiotics and steroids to prevent intra-operative gram negative shock.

10. Pass a large nasogastric tube.

Access

1. An expert may be able to reduce an intussusception through a short Lanz incision as for appendicectomy. Otherwise, it is wise to use a transverse incision placed just above the level of the umbilicus, extending from the midline laterally across the right rectus abdominis muscle and into the oblique muscles.

2. Having incised the dermis, cut the subcutaneous fat, fascia and muscle with needle diathermy, so as to reduce blood loss.

3. Send a sample of peritoneal fluid for bacteriological studies.

Assess

1. There should be an obvious sausage-shaped mass, usually in the midline, but possibly along the course of the left colon.

2. The anatomy of the right colon will be distorted; being drawn towards the transverse colon.

3. The appendix may not be visible.

Action

1. Withdraw the colon distal to the mass and gently attempt to push out the intussusceptum by squeezing the intussuscipiens in an antiperistaltic direction towards the caecum. **Never** try to pull out the intussusceptum by traction upon it for if the bowel is ischaemic it will perforate or tear away in your hand.

2. Patience and gentleness will succeed in the vast majority of cases.

3. Reduction becomes increasingly difficult as it proceeds towards the starting point (apex), the last few centimetres being the most difficult. Proceed very slowly if the serosa of the intussuscipiens begins to split.

4. Continue the assessment during reduction. If the reduced intussusceptum is obviously gangrenous or perforates, abandon the reduction and proceed to a modified right hemicolectomy.

5. If the reduction is successful, examine the distal ileum to ensure there is no ileo-ileal intussusception. The antimesenteric border of the ileum 5–10 cm from the ileocaecal valve is the usual starting point of the intussusception and it is to be expected that there will be a thickened patch in the bowel wall 2–3 cm long at that site. This is not an indication for intestinal resection. This patch of oedematous bowel is not to be confused with a polyp or tumour.

6. If the bowel is viable, perform an appendicectomy, either by the inversion method or by the routine method of appendicectomy. If there is doubt about the viability of the caecum, leave the appendix in situ and cover the intestine with hot packs for 5–10 minutes. If there is still doubt, it is probably safe to return the intestine to the abdominal cavity and suture the wound. The intestine has remarkable powers of healing in this age group.

7. If the bowel is non-viable, resect the affected areas. A standard right hemicolectomy is rarely necessary. Excise only the gangrenous areas and perform an end-to-end ileocolic anastomosis with a non-absorbable suture of silk or Prolene or use polyglycolic acid.

8. Check for a Meckel's diverticulum. If present, excise it and re-establish intestinal continuity with a one-layer anastomosis.

9. Ensure that there is no polyp, duplication cyst or tumour acting as a 'lead point'.

Closure

1. Close the peritoneum and muscles 'en masse' with polyglycolic acid, nylon or Prolene.

2. Approximate the skin with a subcuticular stitch, or 0000 nylon or Prolene, placed no more than 2 mm from the wound edge so as to avoid 'cross-hatching' marks.

3. A wound drain is rarely required, even after 'hemicolectomy'.

Aftercare

1. Treat the patient routinely as following any intra-abdominal procedure.

2. Observe closely for hypovolaemic or septicaemic shock, especially following gangrenous intussusceptions.

3. Hyperpyrexia is not uncommon in the first 24–48 hours. Measures to reduce body temperature may be required.

INGUINAL HERNIA

Appraise

1. As it is virtually impossible to control an inguinal hernia in a child with a truss, operation is indicated in all cases.

2. Inguinal hernias become irreducible in up to 30% of infants, the peak incidence being between the ages of 6 weeks and 3 months. Strangulation is rare in the neonatal period, but when it occurs, there is an appreciable morbidity, and a not insignificant mortality, rate.

3. If the hernia becomes irreducible, pressure upon the spermatic cord causes testicular ischaemia, and infarction may occur after as little as four hours. At least 25% of infants with an irreducible hernia develop severe testicular ischaemia.

4. Premature babies are particularly prone to develop complications. We recommend that herniotomy in premature infants should be carried out at a stage when the infant has gained sufficient weight to warrant discharge from hospital or as soon as complications occur.

5. In infants under the age of 6 months, surgery is difficult as the tissues are thin and friable and is best left to paediatric surgeons.

6. Before embarking upon surgery for an inguinal hernia, ensure that the ipsilateral testis is in the scrotum, otherwise an orchidopexy is indicated at the same time as the herniotomy.

7. Performing an orchidopexy on an infant under the age of 6 months with an irreducible hernia is a particularly difficult operation which must not be attempted by a surgeon without special training unless there are exceptional circumstances.

8. Except in children with neuromuscular disorders, herniotomy rather than herniorrhaphy is the surgical treatment of choice.

HERNIOTOMY AT THE EXTERNAL RING

This was described by Mitchell Banks of Liverpool in 1882.

1. Make an incision, 2 cm long, in a skin crease over the external inguinal ring.

2. Dissect through the subcutaneous fat, Camper's and Scarpa's fascia to reveal the spermatic cord as it passes from the external inguinal ring.

3. Split the external spermatic fascia in the long axis of the cord and also the cremasteric fascia or muscle.

4. Deliver the cord, surrounded by the internal spermatic fascia, from the wound.

5. Rotate the cord to bring its posterior surface into view.

6. Split the internal spermatic fascia longitudinally, allowing the vessels and vas to be separated from the sac.

7. Exert traction upon the sac to withdraw as much of it as possible from within the inguinal canal, through the external inguinal ring.

8. Doubly transfix and ligate the sac with 000 silk or polyglycolic acid suture. The neck of the sac is divided distal to the last suture.

9. Bring together the superficial fascia with one or two sutures of 000 chromic catgut or polyglycolic acid.

10. Close the skin with a subcuticular suture of 0000 chromic catgut or polyglycolic acid. Alternatively, skin closure tapes may be applied. Non-absorbable sutures or skin clips are not necessary and their removal causes unnecessary discomfort and anxiety.

Difficulty

1. Many surgeons in training find this a difficult operation. It is easy to lose the landmarks in the suprapubic fat pad of the young child.

2. It often appears that there are innumerable layers of fascia around the cord and in the confusion the sac may be missed altogether.

3. Having become 'lost' it is easy to find one's-self dissecting the femoral canal or causing damage to the femoral vein.

4. It is possible to miss the spermatic cord altogether, dissect through the conjoined tendon and subsequently excise the lateral corner of the bladder, mistaking it for the peritoneal sac.

5. During the operation, the testis may emerge out of the scrotum and into the wound. Then it may be difficult to get the testis back into the scrotum in the correct layer. In these circumstances, convert the operation into an orchidopexy and secure the testis into a dartos pouch in the scrotum. Otherwise, the testis may be gradually expelled from the scrotum and become adherent to the scar tissue of the superficial inguinal pouch, necessitating a subsequent orchidopexy.

6. The concept of this operation depends on the fact that, in the infant, the external ring is placed almost immediately anterior to the deep ring, the inguinal canal being very short. This is not correct, and it is almost impossible to ligate the sac 'flush' at the deep ring when pulling the sac medially to the external ring. Hence, there

is a small, but definite recurrence rate from this operation, even in the best hands. For these reasons herniotomy is best performed through the inguinal canal, according to the method described first by Turner of Guy's Hospital in 1912 and subsequently by Potts in 1948.

HERNIOTOMY THROUGH THE INGUINAL CANAL

1. Make an incision 2 cm long in a skin crease midway between the anterior superior iliac spine and pubic tubercle.
2. Divide the subcutaneous fat and Camper's fascia using scissors.
3. Incise Scarpa's superficial fascia with scissors, and retract.
4. Clear a small patch of external oblique aponeurosis over an area of 2 cm², at least 1 cm above the inguinal ligament.
5. Incise the external oblique aponeurosis with scissors or a scalpel and retract the edges. Do not open the external inguinal ring.
6. Dissect into the inguinal canal, keeping close to the posterior surface of the external oblique aponeurosis.
7. Shortly, the ilio-inguinal nerve will come into view, and this provides a useful landmark.
8. Using a mosquito artery forceps, split the fibres of the cremaster muscle overlying the spermatic cord just inferior to the ilio-inguinal nerve.
9. Gently grasp the internal spermatic fascia with a mosquito forceps and use this to deliver the spermatic cord from its bed. At the same time, push away the adherent fibres of the cremaster muscle with delicate non-toothed dissecting forceps.
10. Pass the index finger of the left hand behind the cord and use it and the thumb to rotate the cord so that its posterior aspect comes into view.
11. Using a non-toothed dissecting forceps, split the internal spermatic fascia overlying the vas and vessels in a longitudinal direction.
12. Gently sweep the vas and vessels away from the sac. Do not squeeze the vas or vessels with the forceps.
13. Place an artery forceps across the sac, and divide the sac distal to the forceps. Allow the distal part of the sac to fall back into the wound.
14. Dissect the vas and vessels from the proximal part of the sac, until the inferior epigastric vessels are seen.

15. Rotate the artery forceps so as to twist the neck of the sac, so ensuring that there is no bowel or omentum within it.
16. Ligate the sac flush with the deep ring using a 000 polyglycolic acid suture, and then transfix the sac just distal to this tie. Ligation prior to transfixation and ligation prevents the needle from causing a split in the sac which may spread across the deep ring and onto the peritoneum of the anterior abdominal wall, and so prevents the embarrassing escape of intestines or omentum at a difficult site to repair.
17. Allow the vas and vessels to drop back into the inguinal canal.
18. Close the inguinal canal with two or three sutures.
19. Approximate the Scarpa's fascia with one central suture.
20. Close the skin with a subcuticular stitch. If 000 polyglycolic acid is used, the whole operation may be accomplished using but one suture. Alternatively, close the skin with adhesive skin tapes.
21. Gently pull the testis to the bottom of the scrotum to ensure that it does not become caught in the superficial inguinal pouch, necessitating a subsequent orchidopexy.

Difficulty?

1. Do not panic: think rationally.
2. The ilio-inguinal nerve is a good landmark.
3. If lost, keep close to the deep surface of the external oblique, and track down to the inguinal ligament; the cord lies between the ligament and the ilio-inguinal nerve.
4. Remember that the inguinal canal has definite boundaries and the cord must lie between the external ring, which is palpable, and the deep ring which is delineated medially by the inferior epigastric vessels, which should be visible.
5. If still in doubt, check that you are in the inguinal canal, and check that the incision is placed between the landmarks of the deep and superficial inguinal rings.
6. As a last resort, extend the incision, identify the external inguinal ring and proceed from there, possibly by incising the ring and laying open the anterior inguinal wall.

Aftercare

The procedure is carried out on a day-case basis and there are no special postoperative precautions. A slight fever on the first postoperative night is a normal response to surgery.

Further reading

Hatch D J, Sumner E 1981 Neonatal anaesthesia, London, Edward Arnold
Holder, T M, Aschraft K W (eds) 1980 Pediatric surgery, W.B. Saunders, Philadelphia
Ravitch M M, Welch K J, Benson C D, Aberdeen E, Randolph J G (eds) 1979 Pediatric surgery vols I and II, 3rd edn. Year Book Medical Publishers, Chicago
Rickham P P, Lister J, Irving I M (eds) 1978 Neonatal surgery, 2nd edn, Butterworths, London

Neurosurgery

GENERAL PRINCIPLES

Before operating on the brain or spinal cord, remember that central nervous tissue is easily damaged and, once damaged, cannot regenerate. Although patients may make remarkable recoveries from injuries to the central nervous system, these recoveries are mediated by the compensatory action of intact neural tissue, rather than by local repair of the damaged areas.

These characteristics make neurosurgery different in several important respects from general surgery. The surgeon must not inflict any unnecessary damage on nervous tissue. Every stage of the operation must be carried out with meticulous care. The surgeon cannot afford any complications at all. Even in the simplest neurosurgical procedure, a complication such as wound haemorrhage or infection may have appalling consequences. Complete haemostasis must be achieved before a neurosurgical wound is closed. Packs cannot be used and in general drains cannot be inserted into wounds except for brief periods and to superficial tissue layers.

If you are a general surgeon, avoid neurosurgical operations if at all possible. In most western countries, expert neurosurgical advice can be obtained over the telephone in a matter of minutes. Very few neurosurgical emergencies deteriorate while they are being transferred to a neuro-

surgical centre, which is unlikely to be more than 2–4 hours' travel away. About the only emergency that will not travel and that should be dealt with as soon as possible is the rapidly-developing extradural haematoma of arterial origin. This rule does not of course apply to under-developed countries, where the primary surgeon may be required to carry out a wider range of neurosurgical operations.

Appraise

1. If the situation clearly demands neurosurgery on the spot, discuss the situation on the telephone with the neurosurgeon at the nearest available centre before you start operating. If you do this, elementary mistakes will be avoided, and if you run into any problems there will be someone standing by to give you further advice and help and perhaps accept the patient for transfer.

2. Do not rush at the problem but spend a few minutes carefully assessing the clinical situation and think about what you are going to try and achieve by the emergency operation. Are further investigations or information required before you start operating? Is there any reasonable prospect of the operation benefiting the patient? Inappropriate over-treatment may result in an outcome for which on-one will thank you, particularly in the case of trauma to the brain. If the patient has clearly received a very severe primary brain injury from which a useful recovery is unlikely, there is no point in performing multiple exploratory burr holes. Patients with very severe head injuries commonly have extradural and subdural haematomas which are incidental to the main injury to the brain. The removal of an intracranial haematoma in such a patient may result in the survival of a hopelessly-disabled person.

Prepare

1. Blood

Have blood cross-matched in adequate quantities before you start. In inexperienced hands, intracranial operations are often accompanied by substantial blood loss. Patients with head injuries may have lost a considerable amount of blood before the operation starts, either from scalp lacerations or from injuries elsewhere in the body.

2. Anaesthesia

(a) Use general anaesthesia if at all possible. You may be tempted to use local anaesthesia in a deeply unconscious patient, but such a patient may quite suddenly become restless and uncontrollable when the intracranial tension is lowered by release of a haematoma.

(b) The anaesthetist should have the patient paralysed and ventilated to lower the intracranial pressure and he should be in a position to lower the blood pressure if this is necessary to control bleeding. However, he should not lower the systolic blood pressure below 70–80 mmHg because control of the cerebral circulation is defective in the injured brain and blood pressures below this level may result in ischaemic cerebral damage.

3 Dehydrating agents

(a) When the patient has been prepared for anaesthesia, he should receive intravenous 20% mannitol. 250 ml will suffice for a teenager or an adult, whereas a child aged between 3–10 should receive 100 ml. Mannitol should be given over a period of 5–10 minutes. If it has crystallised out of solution, warm the bottle to dissolve it before administration. Mannitol will lower the intracranial pressure, the effect lasting for up to 3–4 hours. It will also cause brisk diuresis, so insert a catheter into the bladder.

(b) Intravenous mannitol is an invaluable method of 'buying time' on the way to the theatre if the patient's neurological condition is deteriorating rapidly from rising intracranial pressure. However, if you have already decided to operate, do not be tempted to delay merely because the mannitol has produced a dramatic improvement of conscious level, for when the effects of the mannitol wear off, the rebound rise in intracranial tension may cause a very sudden deterioration.

4. Positioning the patient

(a) For operations above the tentorium, lie the patient on his back with his head supported in a horseshoe-shaped head-ring. Access to either side of the head can then be provided by turning the head from side to side. More rotation of the head to the opposite side can be given by placing a sandbag under the appropriate shoulder.

(b) To reduce the venous pressure in the head and thereby minimise cerebral swelling, tilt the patient foot down by 20° but not by more than this or there will be a risk of producing air embolism if a major venous sinus is opened inadvertently during the operation. Make sure the neck is not so twisted by the position of the head that the neck veins are compressed, for this will increase cerebral congestion.

(c) For access to the posterior fossa, position the patient prone, with his face lying in the head ring. In order to open up the atlanto-occipital angle and thus give enough room to work in the posterior fossa, the neck should be flexed as much as possible. Make sure that the eyes are well padded and that the position in the head ring is such that no pressure can be exerted on them. Place foam rubber padding between the ring and face and forehead to prevent disfiguring areas of pressure oedema and necrosis.

5. Preparation of the head

(a) The whole head should be shaved. Although you may feel confident that surgery is required in one area of the head only, unexpected negative findings are common and further exploratory burr holes may then be required elsewhere. Remove the hair with clippers and then carry out a close shave with a sharp blade in a holder of the type used for skin incision.

(b) Clean the whole scalp with an appropriate antiseptic solution: hibitane in spirit is satisfactory. Make sure that any debris on the scalp surface is cleared away and also make sure that the eyes have been covered with tulle gras and sealed off with waterproof adhesive tape before you start.

(c) Mark out intended incisions with a light scratch on the scalp, and then infiltrate the scalp beneath them with adrenaline 1 : 200 000 in physiological saline. The scalp has a profuse blood supply and this is an important means of reducing blood loss during surgery. Insert the infiltrating needle up the skull vault so the injection is made into the loose areolar tissue between the galea and the pericranium. If injection through the needle appears to require a lot of force, then the tip of the needle is outside the galea and further insertion is needed.

(d) After marking the incisions clean the head once more with antiseptic, then dry it and cover it with a Steridrape before towelling up around the area that needs to be exposed. Secure the drapes to the scalp with towel clips. Place clips into the skin just above the eyebrows and then allow the clip handles to bridge the eyes and rest upon the prominences of the cheeks, thus shielding the eyes from inadvertent pressure during the operation.

ACCESS TO THE BRAIN

1. Burr holes

These can be carried out rapidly but are mainly of diagnostic value. Use them to establish whether there is any haematoma on the brain surface in that part of the head or whether the brain is under tension. Realise that a burr hole exposes only a tiny part of the surface of the intracranial contents and that nearby or deep pathology may be present without anything abnormal being found. Burr holes seldom give sufficient access to allow definitive treatment of important lesions. For this reason, always place your scalp incisions and burr holes so that they can be coverted either into an osteoplastic flap or into a craniectomy, if more room is needed.

Apart from the use of multiple exploratory burr holes after a head injury, a single burr hole may be used to biopsy a cerebral tumour, drain a cerebral abscess or tap the lateral ventricles in acute hydrocephalus.

2. Craniotomy

An osteoplastic flap is turned and is replaced at the end of the operation (see p. 597). A craniotomy is the best way of exposing a wide area of the intracranial contents above the tentorium.

3. Craniectomy

A burr hole is extended by removing bone around it, leaving a defect which remains at the end of the operation. Avoid a craniectomy on the skull vault as the bone defect will require a plastic repair later. There are two situations where a craniectomy can be fashioned without the need for later surgery:

(a) A craniectomy is the usual mode of exposing the posterior fossa contents. The bone defect is covered over by the thick sub-occipital muscles.
(b) The outer wall of the middle fossa may be removed by a 'sub-temporal craniectomy', to provide access to an arterial extradural haematoma or a swollen temporal lobe. At the end of the operation the defect is concealed by suturing the temporalis muscle over it.

MULTIPLE EXPLORATORY BURR HOLES

Appraise

Multiple burr-holes may be required after a head injury, when a deteriorating level of consciousness and/or the appearance of focal neurological signs leads one to suspect an expanding intracranial haematoma.

Even if the type and site of the haematoma seem certain, always mark out for multiple burr holes on each side of the head (Fig. 33.1). If a haematoma is present, it will not

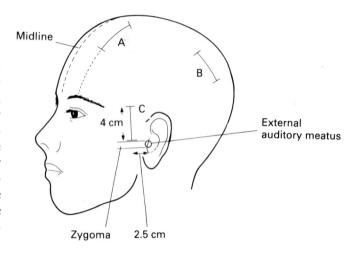

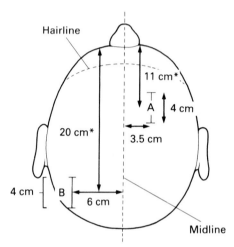

Fig. 33.1 Surface markings for exploratory burr-holes. A: Frontal, B: Parietal, C: Temporal

necessarily be on the side of the fracture or dilated pupil or contralateral to a hemisparesis. Furthermore, there may be bilateral haematomas.

Access (Fig. 33.2)

1. Mark with an indelible pencil the midline of the skull vault from the nasion to the external occipital protuberrance.
2. Mark out three burr holes on each side.

(a) Frontal

Incise the scalp antero-posteriorly just within the hairline and in line with the pupils when the eyes face forwards. The centre of the skin incision should lie 3.5 cm lateral to the midline and 10–11 cm back from the nasion.

(b) Parietal

These should lie over the parietal eminences, the skin incisions running antero-posteriorly. Thus the centre of the

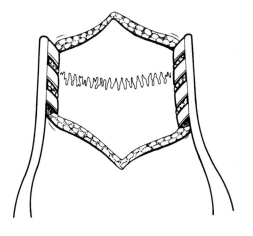

a

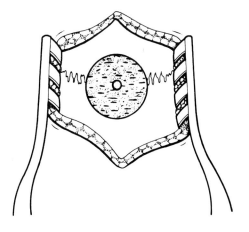

b

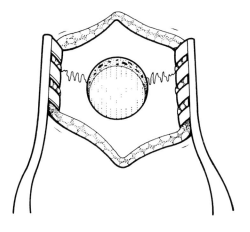

c

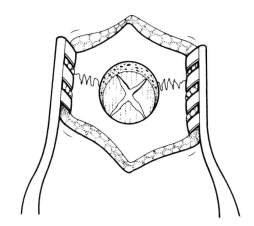

d

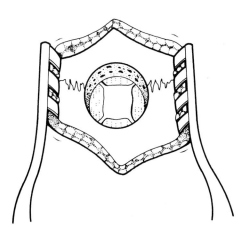

e

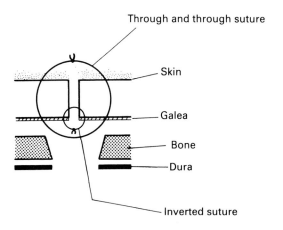

f

Fig. 33.2 Stages of making a burr-hole
(a) Scalp cut down to bone
(b) After use of perforator to expose a small area of dura
(c) After use of conical burr to expose dura more widely
(d) Dura opened in cruciate fashion
(e) Dura burnt back with the diathermy
(f) Closure of scalp

incisions should lie 6 cm lateral from a midline point, which lies 20–21 cm back from the nasion.

(c) Temporal

The incisions should run vertically to end just above the upper edge of the zygoma, 2.5 cm anterior to the external auditory meatus. Do not place the incision further forwards than this or run it below the zygoma, or there will be a danger of cutting the branches of the facial nerve which run to the orbicularis oculi. Each temporal burr hole gives access to the region of the squamous temporal bone where an arterial extradural haemorrhage often originates.

3. Incise the scalp for 3–4 cm for each burr hole. Cut straight to the bone with one incision, then scrape the scalp away from the bone with a periosteal elevator. Hold the scalp edges tightly apart with a self-retaining retractor, so that the bone surface is exposed. In the temporal region, make the incision longer, as it needs to pass through the temporalis muscle to reach the bone.

4. For drilling, use the widest diameter set of perforator and burr available. Make sure that the perforator and burr are of matching size. A burr which is smaller than the perforator may break through into the intracranial contents. Instruct the assistant to hold the head firmly in the ring during drilling.

5. Exercise great caution if drilling near a fracture line, as the skull vault may suddenly give way allowing the drill to penetrate deeply into the brain!

6. First drill with the perforator in the Hudson Brace (the perforator is the drill piece with the flat blade). Drill at 90° to the skull vault drilling cautiously but firmly, until you feel the tip of the perforator begin to wobble slightly. When this happens the tip of the perforator will have penetrated just inside the inner table, exposing a small patch of dura, perhaps covered with a thin flake of bone. Remove the perforator and check that this is so.

7. When you have confirmed that the perforator has penetrated the inner table, drill next using either the rose-shaped or conical burr until you feel the sensation that the burr is being gripped by the bone edge. Remove the burr and a wide area of dura should be exposed, slightly narrower in diameter than the outer part of the burr hole.

8. Clear bone dust from the incision. Arrest bleeding from the diploe by the firm application of bone wax. Bleeding from the surface of the dura may be stopped by diathermy. Do not use a strong current for coagulation or this will cut the dura and cause more bleeding.

Assess

1. An extradural haematoma will be apparent immediately inside the bone when the burr hole has been fashioned. A thin film extradural clot of only a millimetre or two in depth is of no clinical significance. An appreciable extradural haemorrhage will be at least 1 cm deep and will be extruded from the burr hole under pressure. Although a burr hole may be sufficient to reduce the head of pressure from a tense extradural haemorrhage and thus 'buy time', if an extradural haemorrhage is to be evacuated adequately and the source of bleeding secured, you will need to convert the burr hole either to a craniectomy (if the extradural haemorrhage is in the middle fossa) or a craniotomy (if the extradural haematoma is situated elsewhere beneath the vault). For details of carrying out a craniectomy or craniotomy see the separate sections below.

2. If there is no appreciable extradural haematoma, you must open the dura. If a subdural haematoma is present, the dura will be bulging and probably bluish in colour. If an extradural haematoma has been removed and the dura is slack then it need not be opened, but if the dura is tense it should be opened as there may be a co-existing subdural haematoma.

3. To open the dura, lift the centre of the exposed disc of dura with a sharp hook and incise it with a sharp pointed blade. Once a small nick has been made in the dura, insert a dural guide between the dura and the brain surface and cut down on it so that the dura is opened back to the bone in a cruciate fashion. Diathermy the tips of the four small dural flaps so that they are well burned back to the bone surface.

4. If subdural blood is found, your course of action will depend upon its consistency and how long it has been present.

An acute subdural haematoma resulting from a torn artery in a cortical laceration received only a few hours before may still be fluid at the time of operation, and adequate removal may be possible through multiple burr holes alone. However, if the haematoma is partly or wholly clotted or if brisk fresh bleeding occurs when the clot is disturbed, convert the burr holes into a craniotomy to permit the haematoma to be thoroughly cleared out and the bleeding point secured.

A sub-acute subdural haematoma present for several days and most probably originating from a torn cortical bridging vein will be at least partly clotted, and it too will require conversion of burr holes to a flap for thorough removal.

A chronic watery subdural collection can usually be removed through burr holes alone.

Action

1.   If burr holes alone appear adequate for evacuating a subdural haematoma then remove the haematoma by a combination of suction and irrigation. Raised intracranial pressure will usually force out any fluid blood, and any residual small clots should be washed out of the subdural space by a firm jet of normal saline at or just below body temperature.

Direct the saline through each burr hole in turn, thus achieving a fairly thorough wash-out of the subdural space. Do not suck on the brain directly. Keep the sucker tip just on the bone edge or, if you wish to suck within the burr hole, interpose a small square of lintine (a lintine patty) held in the tips of a pair of forceps, between the sucker tip and the brain surface. Make sure that the subdural space is in communication between the burr holes on each side. If the burr holes communicate, saline squirted into one will escape through the others.

2. After a subdural haematoma has been evacuated, the brain will usually expand and largely obliterate the subdural space, but in the case of a chronic watery subdural collection expansion may not occur. The brain surface may then remain well below the inside of the dura, and left alone, the space will just fill up again with fluid and the patient's symptoms will recur. To obliterate a persisting subdural space, you may either tip the patient's head down on the operating table, or if this does not work, insert a lumbar puncture needle into the lumbar sac and slowly inject normal saline at body temperature until the brain has re-expanded almost to the dura. This procedure must only be done under direct vision, i.e. before you close the wounds. Usually between 60–120 ml of saline are needed to reinflate the brain.

3. If brisk bleeding continues from inside the dura after a subdural haematoma has been removed, convert the multiple burr holes into a craniotomy to find the bleeding point.

4. If multiple burr holes have revealed no surface haematoma and the brain surface is not tense, then it is most unlikely that there is any intracranial pathology requiring surgical treatment and the wounds may be closed. If the brain surface is tense and bulging out through the burr holes then clearly there is some mass effect within the brain. In the case of trauma, this will probably be due to cerebral oedema, either diffuse or focal, or it may be due to a haematoma within the brain. There is no way in which you can differentiate between these possibilities without the special investigations such as C.T. scan or cerebral angiography, which will be available only in special centres. Under these circumstances therefore, the only satisfactory course is to transfer the patient, if this can be done, and if the patient's clinical condition justifies it.

Closure

1. Before closing make sure that you have perfect haemostasis. Oozing from the brain surface can be arrested with a patch of Surgicel laid inside the dura and pressed down onto the brain surface by a wet piece of lintine. Bleeding from the dura can be stopped with light diathermy current. Bleeding from the scalp vessels is stopped by the through-and-through skin stitches.

2. Do not insert any drains.

3. Close the scalp in two layers of interrupted 3/0 silk sutures.
(a) The wound edges are held together by galeal sutures, 1 cm apart, inverted so that the knots face inwards. Cut the loose ends very short so that they cannot work their way out through the skin.
(b) Insert skin sutures 1.0–1.5 cm apart, passed through all the layers of the scalp and tied fairly tightly to arrest bleeding from the scalp layers. These sutures may be removed on the fifth postoperative day. Do not insert small sutures closer together than 1 cm or you may produce necrosis of the wound edges.

BURR HOLE FOR VENTRICULAR DRAINAGE

Appraise

This procedure is indicated for acute hydrocephalus.

Access

Make a burr hole in the right frontal region as described above (see p. 592).

Action

1. Open the dura. In acute hydrocephalus, the brain will then bulge out under tension.

2. Find a small area of cortical surface which is free of vessels and diathermise its surface for 2–3 mm.

3. Make a small cut in the coagulated cortex.

4. Run a brain cannula into the brain, holding it gently between thumb and index finger. The needle should be aimed slightly medially towards an imaginary line joining the external auditory meati.

5. At a depth of 4–5 cm inside the brain you will feel a slight 'give' as the needle enters the ventricle. Check that the needle is within the ventricle by removing the stylette from the cannula, when cerebrospinal fluid should squirt out under pressure. Advance the cannula for another 1 cm into the ventricle and then remove it from the brain.

6. Insert a fine soft rubber catheter (maximum diameter 3 mm) along the needle track, introducing its tip for 2–3 cm into the ventricle. Check that the C.S.F. still flows out and then spigot the end of the catheter.

Closure

1. Close the wound around the catheter, while your assistant holds it firmly to prevent it retracting out of the ventricle.

2. Suture the catheter to the wound so that it cannot pull out. Remove the spigot to make sure that C.S.F still flows from the catheter.

BURR HOLE FOR TAPPING CEREBRAL ABSCESS

Appraise

The diagnosis is supported by symptoms of raised intra-cranial pressure developing in a patient with neglected otitis media or frontal sinusitis.

Access

Make a burrhole according to the clinical situation, *either*:

1. Through a vertical incision in the temporal region just above the top of the pinna in line with the external auditory meatus.

or:

2. Via a horizontal incision in the forehead just above the line of the affected frontal sinus. Frontal sinuses vary considerably in size and configuration, and it is important to take a pre-operative anteroposterior skull X-ray and place your burr hole so as to avoid entering the sinus.

Action

1. Diathermise the tense brain surface, avoiding any vessels, and incise the coagulated cortex.

2. Holding it between thumb and index finger, gently, run the widest brain cannula that you possess towards the expected position of the abscess. This will be either just behind the frontal sinus or just above the tegmen tympani.

3. The wall of the abscess will be rubbery in nature and will be felt as a definite resistance to the cannula tip. Push the cannula through into the centre of the abscess.

4. Remove the stylette and gently suck out the pus through the cannula, using moderate suction until the pus no longer freely comes out. Then inject into the empty abscess cavity 5 ml of normal saline in which has been disolved 20 000 units of penicillin and 50 mg of strepto-mycin. Also inject 1 ml of sterile barium sulphate to outline the abscess cavity.

Closure

Withdraw the cannula and close the scalp in two layers of interrupted silk as already described, without drainage.

SUBTEMPORAL CRANIECTOMY FOR EXTRADURAL HAEMATOMA

Indications

If an exploratory temporal burr hole has revealed an appreciable extradural clot, removal of the haematoma will require extension of the burr hole into a craniectomy.

Access (Fig. 33.3)

1. Extend the vertical temporal burr hole skin incision upwards to make a skin incision of total length 8–9 cm,

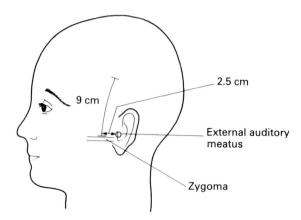

Fig. 33.3 Incision for extradural haematoma

which curves very gently backwards above the tip of the pinna.

2. Hold the skin edges apart with two self-retaining retractors. Arrest with diathermy any bleeding from branches of the superficial temporal artery.

3. Using the cutting diathermy, incise the temporalis muscle to the bone in the line of the skin incision. Scrape the muscle off the bone and reinsert the self-retaining retractors in the muscle incision so that a wide area of the squamous temporal bone is exposed.

4. Nibble away the bone around the burr hole to pro-duce a circular or oval bone defect 4–5 cm across. Fashion-ing this bone defect will usually involve removing the fracture line, which has crossed the path of the middle meningeal artery.

Action

1. Remove the extradural clot with the sucker, breaking up the clot by irrigation with normal saline at body temperature.

2. When this has been done, the bleeding middle meningeal artery can generally be seen on the surface of the dura. Sometimes arterial bleeding will already have been stopped by the pressure of the clot and arterial spasm. Stop any bleeding from the meningeal vessels or the dura with diathermy coagulation, but do not use too fierce a current or the diathermy will cut through the vessel and produce more bleeding.

3. If the bleeding cannot be stopped by coagulation, under-run the responsible dural vessel with a silk suture. Sometimes the bleeding arises from the artery close to the point where the vessel enters the skull through the foramen spinosum. In this situation the match-stick tip of popular legend is of little use and the bleeding is more easily arrested by coagulating within the foramen, perhaps aided by a plug of bone wax firmly pushed into it.

4. If the dura is tense and blue after the extradural haematoma has been removed, there may be an associated

subdural haematoma. Lift the dura with toothed forceps and incise it to exclude subdural clot. If the dura is not tense or discoloured, there is no need to open it.

5. Residual oozing from the surface of the dura can be arrested by a sheet of cellulose mesh (Surgicel), which may be left in situ. Prevent further bleeding into the extradural space opened up by the haematoma by suturing the dura to the temporalis muscle around the edge of the bone defect with interrupted 3/0 silk sutures at 2 cm intervals.

Closure

1. If the dura has been opened, close it with interrupted 3/0 silk sutures. Do not worry if the dural edges have retracted from diathermy coagulation so that a tight dural closure is impossible. Merely cover the defect in the dura with a piece of surgicel.

2. Approximate the separated fibres of the temporalis muscle with interrupted 3/0 silk sutures.

3. Close the scalp in two layers as described in the section on burr holes.

4. If haemostasis has been difficult and the dura has not been opened, the extradural space may be drained for 24 hours by a suction drain on low suction brought out through a separate stab incision.

CRANIOTOMY

Appraise

This approach gives wide access to the intracranial contents above the tentorium. Most traumatic intracranial haematomas require a craniotomy for their effective removal.

Access (Figs. 33.4 & 33.5)

1. Mark out the scalp flap. The base of the flap should be towards the base of the skull as the blood vessels of the scalp come from below. The flap should be in the shape of an inverted 'U'. To ensure an adequate blood supply to the scalp flap, its widest part should be the open mouth of the 'U' and the length of the flap should not exceed its width. The scalp flap should be placed so that the lines of the bone flap do not enter the frontal sinus or overlie the great sinuses (the superior sagittal and transverse sinuses). In order not to become involved in the draining veins and the venous lakes which project from the sides of the superior sagittal sinus, mark out the scalp incision so that it does not come closer than 3 cm to the midline.

2. Incise each of the three sides of the scalp flap in turn. Incise almost to the bone, while your assistant firmly compresses the scalp on each side with the tips of his fingers to minimise bleeding.

3. As each section of the scalp flap is incised, place the tips of artery forceps onto the galea on each side at 2 cm

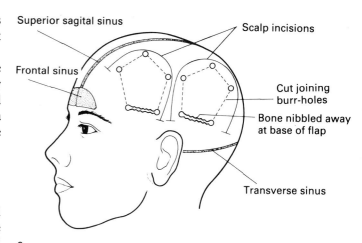

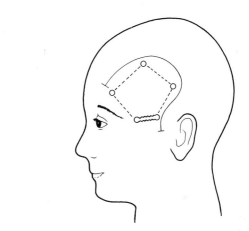

b

Fig. 33.4 Incisions for craniotomy
(a) Frontal and parietal osteoplastic flaps
(b) Flap to expose temporal lobe

intervals, securing any obvious bleeding points as you do so. The galea is a well-defined layer which you should have no difficulty in finding.

4. On each limb of the scalp flap, on either side of the incision, tie the artery forceps' handles together with rubber bands and allow each bundle to fall back. This procedure inverts the galeal edges and reduces bleeding.

5. Reflect the scalp flap by opening up, with sharp dissection, the plane of loose areolar tissue which lies between the galea superficially and the contiguous pericranium and temporalis fascia deeply. Place a rolled-up swab behind the reflected scalp flap, so that the bundles of artery forceps can turn back the edges of the galea to which they are attached. Secure the bundles of artery forceps in position with towel clips to the surrounding drapes.

6. The next stage is to fashion an osteoplastic (bone) flap, which is hinged on the temporalis muscle. With cutting diathermy, cut to the bone a horseshoe-shaped flap of the conjoined pericranium and temporalis muscle,

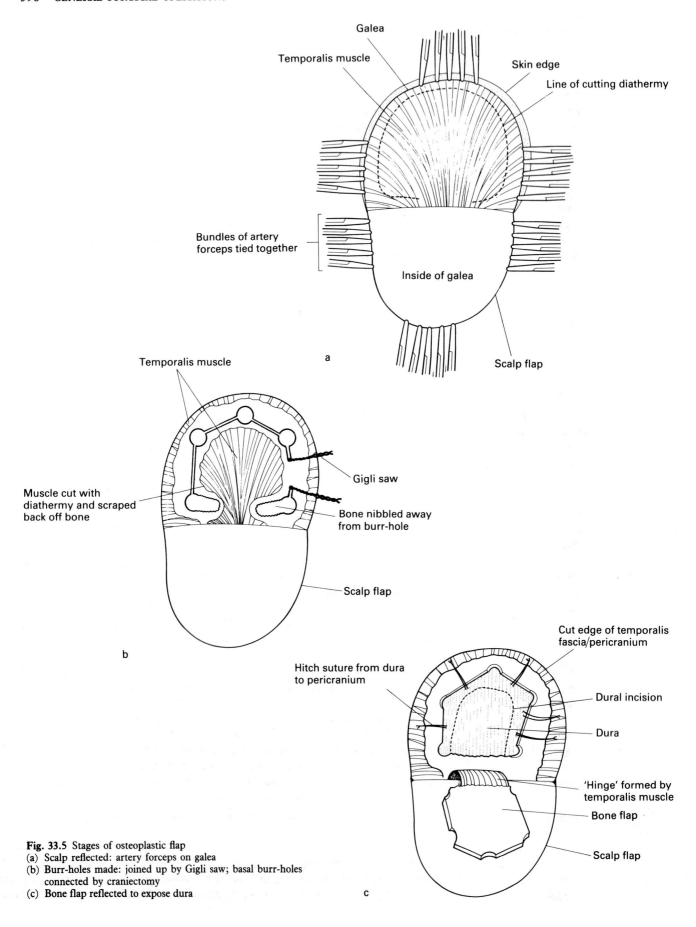

Fig. 33.5 Stages of osteoplastic flap
(a) Scalp reflected: artery forceps on galea
(b) Burr-holes made: joined up by Gigli saw; basal burr-holes
connected by craniectomy
(c) Bone flap reflected to expose dura

keeping intact a band of temporalis muscle 3–5 cm wide to form the hinge.

7. Scrape the pericranium and muscle back widely to expose the bone surface.

8. Drill the burr holes which are to be linked up to form the bone flap. Four or five holes will be needed, spaced out according to the size of the defined flap with about 6–7 cm between each hole. The two burr holes which are to be linked to form the base of the flap should be placed somewhat closer together (5 cm apart).

9. Separate the dura from the bone between the burr holes by running an Adson's periosteal elevator against the inside of the bone surface from one hole to the next. Do this carefully or you may lacerate the dura.

10. Saw the bone between the burr holes with a Gigli saw. When running the blade of the saw between the burr holes on its special protective guide, be sure to keep the blade fairly taut or it may project sideways from the guide and tear the dura. Bevel outwards the cut made by the saw, so that the bone flap will slot into place at the end of the operation.

Do not cut the bone between the two burr holes at the base of the flap with the Gigli saw, but nibble it away with bone cutters to complete the flap.

11. Hinge the bone flap backwards on the stalk of temporalis muscle to expose the dura. Suture the dura to the pericranium round the edges of the bone defect with interrupted 3/0 silk sutures at 3 cm intervals. This will prevent bleeding into the extradural space around the flap.

12. Coagulate any large vessels on the dural surface.

13. Open the dura as a flap with its base toward the base of the skull. To incise the dura, lift it with a sharp hook or toothed forceps and make a small cut in the raised area, so that you enter the subarachnoid space without damaging the cortex. Gently lift the dura and cut the dura with fine scissors in sections. Before cutting each section, gently push a piece of wet lintine between the dura and the brain surface to separate them. When incising the dura near the great venous sinuses or at the frontal or temporal poles, make sure that you do not cut through a bridging vein.

14. Bleeding from vessels on the brain surface may be stopped with diathermy coagulation or metal clips. Oozing from areas of haemorrhagic contusion can be stopped by patches of cellulose mesh (Surgicel) or pieces of fine muslin, pressed into place under patches of wet lintine. They may be left in place when the lintine is taken off.

Closure

1. Do not close any layer until you have perfect haemostasis.

2. Close the dura with interrupted 3/0 silk sutures. Areas where the dural edges will not come together can be covered with Surgicel.

3. Replace the bone flap, holding it in place with inter-rupted 3/0 silk sutures to the pericranium/temporalis muscle layer.

4. Close the scalp in two layers.

5. If you have achieved good dural closure, but still have troublesome bleeding below the scalp flap, drain the subgaleal space with a low tension suction drain brought out through a separate stab wound and removed after 24 hours.

SCALP LACERATIONS

Appraise

1. An unsutured small scalp laceration can pump out a great deal of blood over a short period of time, so arrest any bleeding from the scalp as soon as is practicable after injury with a temporary single layer of through-and-through sutures.

2. If the patient has been struck on the head with a heavy object, X-ray the skull to ensure that the laceration does not cover a depressed skull fracture.

Action

1. Shave adequately and closely round the laceration before exploring it.

2. The scalp is very vascular and heals well, seldom getting infected, so do not excise the contused edges of the laceration in such an enthusiastic manner that you produce a scalp defect or cannot get the edges together without tension.

3. If the galea has been breached, always close the scalp laceration in two layers, one for the galea and one a through-and-through skin layer, as previously described (see p. 595).

4. Transfer a patient with severe scalp loss to a special unit where plastic and neurosurgical facilities are available.

DEPRESSED SKULL FRACTURE

Appraise

1. The purpose of elevating a depressed skull fracture is to reduce the risk of infection, so only *compound* depressed skull fractures require elevation.

2. Depressed fractures with the overlying scalp intact should be left alone. In occasional cases, the dislocation of the skull contour may be so great that elevation is required for cosmetic reasons, but these more severe injuries will invariably be compounded, so that the customary indication for operation is present as well.

Access

1. Excise the overlying scalp laceration if it is badly contused. Extend the incision to give access to the whole

depressed area. Scrape the scalp off the underlying bone and hold the incision wide open with self-retaining retractors.

2. Clear the pericranium away with a periosteal elevator to reveal the whole depressed area.

3. The inner table will be driven in over a much wider area than the visible area of depressed outer table. Make a single burr hole just outside the edge of the visibly depressed region in order to expose dura not involved in the depression.

Action

1. Insert a periosteal elevator into the burr hole, slide it gently between the bone and the dura and ease out the depressed fragments, so that the dura beneath them is fully exposed. Remove dirt, debris and any small flakes of bone from the wound and send them for bacteriological culture.

2. If the dura is intact, do not open it. If it is lacerated, carefully extend the laceration to inspect the brain beneath. If the brain surface is torn, probe gently in the tear for any indriven debris and bone and remove them. Pulped and clearly necrotic brain tissue should be cleared away by a combination of gentle suction and irrigation with normal saline at body temperature. Bleeding points in the brain can be arrested with gentle diathermy coagulation, diffuse oozing by applying patches of Surgicel compressed into place beneath lintine strips.

3. If the depressed bone fragments have been driven through the dura, their removal may tear large cerebral vessels as the fragments are disimpacted from the brain. A large cerebral vessel, not visible on the brain surface, may be picked up and held in the tip of a fine sucker under fairly strong suction while it is coagulated with diathermy or occluded with a metal clip.

4. Be very cautious about elevating a depressed fracture which overlies the superior sagittal or lateral sinus. If the dura over the sinus is torn, there will be torrential venous bleeding as the bone is removed. If a sinus is torn, do not try and effect a closure with sutures. Reduce the pressure in the sinus by tilting the patient foot down, then cover the sinus with several layers of Surgicel and hold them firmly in place under lintine strips for 5–10 minutes. When the pressure is released and the lintine removed, bleeding will have stopped. Do not now disturb the Surgicel. If the bleeding is absolutely uncontrollable, it is permissible to suture a small piece of gauze in place beneath the scalp, which is closed over it, as a temporary measure to reduce bleeding while the patient is tranferred to a special centre.

Closure

1. Before closing, irrigate the whole wound with hydrogen peroxide solution and 20 ml of normal saline containing 20 000 units of penicillin and 50 mg of streptomycin.

2. Close the dura with interrupted 3/0 silk sutures. Cover any gaps in the dura with two layers of Surgicel.

3. Unless the wound is neglected and obviously infected, replace the removed bone fragments on the dura to fill in the skull defect. Before replacing the fragments, scrub them thoroughly in aqueous Savlon.

4. Close the scalp in 2 layers without drainage.

MISSILE WOUNDS OF THE BRAIN

Appraise

1. The energy of a missile is transmitted to the object it strikes. As the energy carried by the missile is related to the square of its speed, even a small high-velocity missile may release an enormous quantity of energy as it passes through the body, causing tissue destruction which extends far beyond its track. The small size of an entry hole may conceal massive disruption of the intracranial structures.

2. Decide whether active treatment is likely to lead to a worthwhile outcome. Through-and-through missile wounds of the brain are almost always fatal. The prognosis is very poor if the patient has been deeply unconscious with fixed dilated pupils from the time of the injury or if he has persistent hypotension which cannot be explained by blood loss, because these features suggest damage to the central structures of the brain.

3. Do not operate until the patient has been resuscitated and his condition is stable. Early bleeding into the intracranial contents is not a common complication of missile wounds of the brain, and a delay of 3–4 hours will allow replacement of any blood loss, adequate assessment of the extent of neurological damage and an interim assessment and treatment of other injuries. As soon as the neurological assessment has been carried out, anaesthetise, intubate and hyperventilate the patient to reduce any cerebral oedema. Before surgery obtain good quality skull X-rays to show the position of fragments of missile, bone and debris. Cross-match adequate quantities of blood: the blood loss during surgery may be considerable. Start a parenteral broad-spectrum antibiotic at high dosage and anticonvulsant medication.

Access

1. The underlying principle of treatment is to minimise the risks of infection and of cerebral swelling by removing all indriven debris and all devitalised brain tissue. The primary debridement must be adequate.

2. Do not try to operate through an approach which limits access. Turn a generous scalp flap which encompasses the entry wound well inside its boundaries. This will allow exposure of any damaged tissue and will provide a scalp flap which can be turned at a later date for cranioplasty.

3. Turn a separate periosteal/temporalis muscle flap which, like the scalp flap, should be based downwards. Clear this flap away from the skull vault to expose the entry hole and the surrounding intact bone.

4. Drill a burr hole 3 cm away from the edge of the entry hole in the bone to expose undamaged dura. From the burr hole nibble away damaged bone so as to produce a craniectomy extending 3–4 cm in each direction outwards from the entry point. This large craniectomy should give adequate access to damaged tissue.

Action

1. Open the dura widely. Excise damaged dura. Pick out indriven bone and debris. Using saline irrigation and gentle suction clear debris, bone fragments and pieces of missile from along the track. Clear surrounding pulped brain. Coagulate bleeding vessels. Very deeply indriven missile fragments may be left if they cannot be removed readily.

2. Irrigate the debrided track with hydrogen peroxide solution and with 20 000 units of penicillin dissolved in physiological saline.

3. Control cerebral swelling by hyperventilation and intravenous mannitol.

Closure

1. Close the dura with interruped 3/0 silk sutures, replacing deficient dura with a patch of fascia lata sutured in place.

2. Excise any contaminated wound edges from the scalp and pericranial tissue.

3. Close the scalp wound edges and the scalp flap in two layers of 3/0 silk sutures.

Aftercare

1. Control cerebral swelling by continuing intubation, sedation and hyperventilation for at least 48 hours. This procedure will obscure the signs of postoperative intra-cranial bleeding, but oedema is the greater risk.

2. Continue a broad spectrum antibiotic fot at least 7 days.

3. Continue anticonvulsant medication: for an adult phenytoin 150 mg b.d. or phenobarbitone 60 mg b.d.

BRIEF NOTES ON OTHER MAJOR NEUROSURGICAL PROCEDURES

SUBOCCIPITAL CRANIECTOMY TO EXPOSE THE CONTENTS OF THE POSTERIOR FOSSA

This may be carried out either in the sitting position or with the patient face down. The sitting position provides easier access for the surgeon, reduces the tension of the posterior fossa contents and allows blood and cerebrospinal fluid to drain away from the wound. Its disadvantage is the risk of air embolism, the negative venous pressure in the head sucking in air if a large vein is opened. To counteract this risk the legs should be compressed by bandages or rubber cuffs to elevate the intracranial venous pressure.

To expose the central part of the posterior fossa, a midline skin incision is made. To expose one side, an 'inverted hockey stick incision' is used, the short limb of the incision extending from the midline to the relevant side. The muscle and nuchal ligament are incised directly to the bone with the cutting diathermy. Again using the cutting diathermy the soft tissues are cleared from the posterior fossa wall and the arch of the atlas, and the wound is held widely open with self-retaining retractors.

One or more burr holes are made in the posterior fossa wall, and these are extended to form a craniectomy. The mastoid air cells should not be opened or there is a risk of postoperative cerebrospinal fluid rhinorrhoea, the fluid leaking via the middle ear cavity and the eustachian tube to the nose. Taking care not to damage the vertebral artery which runs over it on each side, the arch of the atlas should be removed to prevent compression of the medulla if there is any postoperative swelling of the cerebellum.

The dura is widely incised to expose the contents of the posterior fossa. At the end of the operation the dural edges should be approximated with interrupted silk sutures, any gap in the dura being covered over with a sheet of Surgicel or Gelfoam. The wound is closed in layers of interrupted silk sutures without drainage.

REMOVAL OF BRAIN TUMOURS

Exposure is by craniotomy (for supratentorial tumours) or suboccipital craniectomy (for posterior fossa tumours). Tumours within the substance of the brain (e.g. gliomas and metastases) are exposed either by incising the overlying cortex or by excising a disc of cortex after the cortical vessels have been diathermised and divided. The tumour is broken up and removed piecemeal with the sucker and pituitary rongeurs. Haemostasis is achieved by diathermy, silver clips on the vessels, or by the application of patches of Surgicel or muslin compressed against the bleeding areas under pieces of lintine (which are then removed).

Extrinsic tumours which compress the neural structures from without, such as meningiomas, pituitary tumours, craniopharyngiomas and acoustic neuromas, are first incised and then gutted with either the sucker, pituitary rongeurs or the diathermy cutting loop. This permits the collapsed tumour capsule to be gently dissected away from the surrounding brain. Exposure of basal extrinsic tumours, such as acoustic neuromas, requires preliminary mobilisation of the overlying cerebral structures which are then gently held out of the way by fixed brain retractors, the brain being protected by layers of wet lintine beneath the retractors.

Even if an intracranial tumour such as a glioma cannot be completely removed, the *internal decompression* provided by debulking it and removing any non-evocative region of the adjacent brain may be sufficient to provide a prolonged relief of symptoms. An *external decompression* provided by the removal of an overlying bone flap may give temporary relief of the symptoms of raised intracranial pressure even if the tumour is left, but will eventually lead to a distressing herniation of the intracranial contents through the bone defect.

PITUITARY TUMOURS AND HYPOPHYSECTOMY

Suprasellar tumours and pituitary tumours with large suprasellar extensions are approached by a frontal craniotomy. The craniotomy is made on the right side so as not to interfere with the dominant cerebral hemisphere. The right frontal lobe is mobilised with division of the right olfactory nerve and is held upwards by fixed retractors to reveal the diaphragma sellae and the overlying optic nerves and chiasm. If these structures are involved by the tumour, they can then be freed under direct vision.

For the removal of small pituitary tumours confined within the sella, or for a hypophysectomy (i.e. removal of the pituitary gland, as in disseminated carcinoma of the breast) a transethmoidal or transphenoidal approach is now preferred. These are smaller operations than the subfrontal approach; they have lower mortality and morbidity rates and permit a faster postoperative recovery. They also provide a direct view of the intrasellar contents. These routes are not appropriate, however, if the lesion involves the optic nerves or chiasm.

The *transethmoidal* approach to the sella is through a medial orbital incision. The nasolacrimal duct is identified and preserved, the plane between the orbital fascia and the bony medial wall of the orbit is opened up, and the globe of the eye is retracted laterally. This allows a wide ethmoidectomy to be fashioned, and this is carried back into the sphenoid sinus. The position within the skull is checked with the image intensifier, the floor of the sella is drilled away, and the sellar contents are exposed by opening the sellar dura with the cutting diathermy. The *transphenoidal* approach to the sella is in the midline. The tip of the nose is retracted upwards and the sella is approached between the retracted folds of medial nasal mucosa after removal of the nasal septum and vomer.

Both approaches to the sella from below carry a risk of postoperative cerebrospinal fluid rhinorrhoea and meningitis. All operations on or near the pituitary gland should be 'covered' by large doses of corticosteroids. Maintain careful postoperative observation of the fluid balance as

diabetes insipidus (usually transient) is a common postoperative sequel.

OPERATIONS FOR TRIGEMINAL NEURALGIA

Relief of trigeminal neuralgia is proportional to the degree of damage inflicted on the trigeminal sensory root behind the Gasserian Ganglion. Total section of the sensory root produces a permanent remission but at the expense of total trigeminal sensory loss, including the cornea. Slight trauma to the root or partial section may produce prolonged remission of the neuralgia with little or no sensory loss. Section or avulsion of peripheral branches of the trigeminal nerve gives only brief and unsatisfactory relief of neuralgia.

Absolute alcohol or phenol in glycerine may be injected percutaneously to damage the sensory root. The needle is passed through the foramen ovale from just above and lateral to the angle of the mouth, under X-ray control. Recently, the use of these agents has been largely superseded by inserting a thermal probe through a hollow needle to carry out controlled thermocoagulation of the root.

Open division of the trigeminal sensory root may be carried out by one of two routes. The root may be exposed in Meckel's Cave by an extradural dissection along the floor of the middle fossa, while the overlying temporal lobe is retracted upwards, protected by its dura. Alternatively, the root may be exposed in the posterior fossa, where it travels between the pons and the entrance to Meckel's Cave. Whichever route is used, it is normal to spare the fibres subserving corneal sensation, otherwise there is a risk of postoperative corneal ulceration.

SUBARACHNOID HAEMORRHAGE

In 75% of cases this is caused by a berry aneurysm and in 5% of cases by an intracranial angioma (arteriovenous malformation). In the remaining 20% of cases, full cerebral angiography reveals no causative lesion, and in this group of patients the risk of recurrent haemorrhage is minimal.

Where a cause is found, the aim of operation is to prevent further bleeding. The risk of a second haemorrhage, which is fatal in 60% of cases, is greatest in the first few weeks after the presenting bleed, but very early surgery is attended by a very high mortality and morbidity rate. Most neurosurgeons now prefer to wait for 7–10 days before operating, thus allowing any cerebral vasospasm provoked by the original haemorrhage to subside.

Most aneurysms arise from the divisions of the Circle of Willis at the base of the brain. The base of the brain is gently retracted with fixed retractors, and using the operating microscope the aneurysm is dissected free from adjacent structures so that its neck can be defined and clipped. If the configuration of the aneurysm does not permit clipping, its wall may be reinforced by layers of muslin or by fast-setting methyl macrylate. With some types of aneurysm which cannot be tackled directly, the risk of rebleeding may be lessened by reducing the intra-aneurysmal pressure by ligation of the common carotid artery.

In most cases the only effective treatment of an angioma is total excision. The malformation is dissected away from adjacent normal brain. Its arterial feeders must be clipped and divided before dealing with any draining veins. Where there is no surgical access, the malformation may be obliterated by plastic emboli injected through an intra-arterial catheter.

REPAIR OF DEFECTS IN THE SKULL VAULT

Bone defects in the skull vault left by trauma or previous operation only require later repair if they are disfiguring or are so large as to leave the intracranial contents unprotected. To minimise the risk of infection, defer the repair for at least 6 months.

The defect is exposed by a scalp flap placed so that its edges are well clear of the defect. The defect may be covered by a premoulded titanium or tantalum plate, or by titanium strips. Holes in the metal permit it to be sutured to the surrounding pericranium. Alternatively, after the scalp flap has been reflected a methyl macrylate plate may be moulded to fit the defect and held in place by thick braided silk sutures. The sutures are passed through drill holes in the plate and the surrounding bone, after the bone edge round the defect has been cleared of tissue.

AFTERCARE FOLLOWING INTRACRANIAL SURGERY

1. Do not give opiate analgesics. Besides depressing the conscious level and thus interfering with postoperative assessment of the patient, they may also depress respiration and cause intracranial pressure to rise by retention of carbon dioxide. Cranial wounds are not very painful, and codeine phosphate in a dose for adults of 30–60 mg intramuscularly every 4 hours provides adequate analgesia.

2. The consequences of infection of an intracranial wound are so serious that broad-spectrum antibiotic therapy is a wise precaution. Start the antibiotic parenterally at the time of operation and continue it for 5 days postoperatively.

3. If there has been any injury to the cerebral cortex, give prophylactic anticonvulsants. Start the anticonvulsant by intravenous injection during the operation. Continue it

postoperatively for 3 months and then discontinue it if the patient has been free of seizures. Suitable regimes are: for adults, phenytoin 150 mg b.d.; for teenagers, phenytoin 100 mg bd; and for children aged 3–10 phenytoin 50 mg b.d.

4. Sometimes status epilepticus follows intracranial surgery. The safest and most effective way to stop it is with intramuscular paraldehyde, 10 ml for a teenager or adult, 5 ml for a child aged 3–10. Intravenous diazepam is both ineffective and dangerous, for it may seriously depress respiration and cause rising intracranial pressure.

5. The commonest complication of an intracranial operation is cerebral compression from bleeding or oedema at the operation site. The symptoms of this occurrence are three-fold: first, a steady deterioration of the conscious level; second, the appearance and progression of a focal neurological deficit appropriate to the site of compression. Thus compression of the left temporal lobe will give rise to dysphasia and a weakness of the right arm. Compression of the ipsilateral third nerve may give rise to a fixed dilated pupil on the side of the compression. Lastly, there will be a rise in blood pressure and a fall in the pulse rate. By the time these last features appear, cerebral compression will have reached an advanced stage.

To detect cerebral compression close observation should be kept on the patient in the early postoperative period. The following observations should be recorded by the nurse in attendance: conscious level (the most important parameter, which should be described in detail), the degree and extent of limb movements, the size, symmetry and reactions of the pupils, and the pulse and blood pressure. These observations should be performed every half-hour for the first 12 hours after operation and then, if the patient's condition is quite stable, they may be decreased to one-hourly for the next 12 hours. If there is anything to suggest cerebral compression, the patient must be taken back to theatre and the wound re-explored without delay.

6. Other complications such as wound infection or thrombo-embolism are rare after neurosurgical operations. In general, if a patient survives the first 24 hours after operation, his subsequent course is likely to be trouble-free.

7. Mobilise the patient from bed as soon as possible. This will generally be on the first postoperative day. Mobilisation will lessen any postoperative periorbital or facial swelling.

8. Since intracranial operations do not give rise to ileus, free oral or nasogastric feeding can be started within 24 hours. The intravenous drip can be taken down as soon as it is certain that no intravenous agents such as blood or mannitol will be required.

9. If the scalp has been closed in two layers, the skin sutures can be removed at 5 days from supratentorial incisions and at 7 days in the case of posterior fossa incisions.

Further reading

Jennett W B 1977 An introduction to neurosurgery, 3rd edn. Heinemann, London

Jennett B, Teasdale G 1981 Management of head injuries. Davis, Philadelphia

Northfield D W C 1973 The surgery of the central nervous system. Blackwell, Oxford

Rintoul R F 1985 Farquharson's textbook of operative surgery, 7th edn. Churchill Livingston, Edinburgh

Symon L 1979 Operative surgery: neurosurgery. Butterworths, London

Oral and dental surgery

Operations in and around the mouth may present difficulties to the surgeon unaccustomed to working in this area. The oral cavity is small and dark and surrounded by a sensitive, mobile tissue coated with a slimy material. Many important anatomical structures are contained in a small area. In a conscious patient, the tongue may constantly get in the way and if the operation is prolonged, the patient may inadvertently close his mouth at an inopportune moment.

This chapter is limited to oral surgical procedures which a general surgeon may need to perform when an appropriately trained colleague is not available. The advice of an oral surgeon should be sought where possible.

GENERAL PRINCIPLES OF ORAL SURGERY

PREPARE

1. Make sure you have good illumination.
2. Arrange for adequate suction apparatus.
3. Make sure your assistant is efficient and can anticipate.

ANAESTHESIA

1. Most minor procedures can be carried out using local analgesia, such as tooth extraction, biopsy, removal of salivary calculi and suturing of lacerations. Local anaesthetics are available in 2 ml glass cartridges, the most common of which contain 2% lignocaine with adrenaline. These cartridges fit into a syringe with a disposable needle.

In the upper jaw, deposit 1.5 ml of solution over the apex of the offending tooth on the buccal side and about 0.5 ml on the palatal side. In the lower jaw, a similar technique may suffice for the anterior teeth. For posterior teeth, an inferior dental and lingual nerve block is required at the lingula of the mandible, along with a long buccal nerve block at the anterior edge of the ramus of the mandible. Regional nerve block can also be used in the maxilla. Refer to appropriate literature before attempting these blocks.

The depth of analgesia may not be sufficient in the presence of inflammation but can be increased by depositing a few drops of anaesthetic solution into the periodontal membrane of the tooth.

2. General anaesthesia is often preferable in the treatment of children and nervous adults, or on the rare occasion where there is a history of allergy to local analgesics and in the presence of an extensive abscess. The anaesthetic should be maintained through a nasal endotracheal tube. Insert a moist pack into the oro-pharynx to prevent the inhalation of blood and debris during the treatment. Remember to remove the pack at the end of the operation. Separate the jaw with a prop or gag and stabilize the head in a rubber ring or horseshoe. The lips are easily scuffed when operating because of the drying effects of the anti-cholinergic drugs used in premedication so keep them moist or lightly coated with petroleum jelly.

HAEMOSTASIS

Post-extraction haemorrhage is often due to torn or unsupported mucosa.

1. Remove excess clot.
2. Suture tightly across the socket. Repair lacerations.
3. Apply pressure with a gauze pad for ten minutes.
4. If bleeding continues, press a resorbable haemostatic material (e.g. oxidised cellulose) into the socket. Thrombin

or Russell's viper venom on gelatin sponge can also be used but is more difficult to manipulate.

5. Medical reasons for prolonged bleeding must be treated according to their cause, e.g. haemophilia, thrombocytopenia or hepatic cirrhosis.

6. Control secondary haemorrhage with pressure and treat the infection with antibiotics (systemic and/or local) and hydrogen peroxide mouthwashes.

SUTURING

1. Use a half circle, 22 mm needle with a reverse cutting edge.

2. Sutures can be 000 braided silk or catgut. Silk is easy to use but must be removed. Catgut is suitable for mucoperiosteum but rapidly becomes untied on mobile mucosa such as tongue, lip and cheek. Polyglycolic acid and polyglactin remain intact in the mouth for 3–4 weeks but have sharp irritating knots and ends. Nylon must be removed and is uncomfortable.

3. Use a needleholder with a ratchet and avoid dropping the needle into the pharynx.

4. Insert the needle into the mucosa 3–5 mm from the edge, taking greater care on the more friable lingual edge.

5. The mucosal edges can rarely be approximated over a socket without excessive removal of bone. If you wish to apply even tension, insert a mattress suture.

6. Tie knots with the needleholder rather than fingers. This is easier if the tail of the suture material is kept short.

7. Remove sutures after 5–7 days.

AFTERCARE

1. During the healing period, there may be constant discomfort and anxiety as the mouth continues to be used for eating, swallowing, salivation and speaking. Mild analgesics usually suffice to control the pain. Aspirin mixture, used as a gargle, makes the swallowing more comfortable. Ice packs applied to the skin for the first 4–6 hours reduce the swelling and subsequent discomfort.

2. A soft diet may be required for the first few days because the patient has difficulty in opening the mouth wide and has reduced power when chewing.

3. Patients who have had their fractured jaws wired together require special care in the early postoperative hours to avoid inhalation of vomit. Keep wire cutters by the bedside and show the nurses which wires to cut in an emergency. Ensure that the stomach is empty and administer an anti-emetic such as prochlorperazine or metoclopramide. Vomiting is more common after oral surgery because swallowed blood is irritant to the stomach.

TOOTH EXTRACTION

Appraise

This procedure is indicated by
1. Large cavity in painful tooth
2. Loose tooth due to periodontal infection
3. Alveolar abscess.

Prepare

1. Extraction forceps — three pairs are usually sufficient (Figs. 34.1, 2 & 3) although many more specialised forceps are available.

2. Elevators (levers). They are used to remove broken roots or to loosen teeth before using forceps. If elevators are used with excessive force, the jaw may be fractured.

3. Tooth extraction may vary enormously in difficulty and the removal of roots can be unexpectedly complicated. Ideally, take a radiograph before removing the tooth. This displays unfavourable root patterns and latent pathology.

Action

1. The patient is usually seated but may be supine.
2. Use local or general anesthesia.
3. Stand in front of patient for all extractions, except for those on lower right (if you are right handed) when the ideal position is behind the patient's right shoulder.
4. Place the blades of the forceps on the buccal and lingual aspects of the tooth and push them *under* the gum as far as they will go along the root.

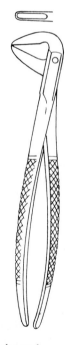

Fig. 34.1 Forceps for mandibular teeth

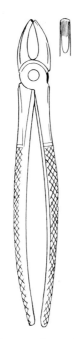

Fig. 34.2 Forceps for maxillary anterior teeth

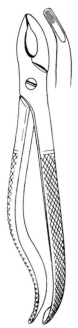

Fig. 34.3 Forceps for maxillary posterior teeth

5. Grip the tooth and move it so as to expand the socket.

6. Deliver the tooth in the direction of the weakest wall — generally the buccal.

7. Squeeze the socket with your fingers to reduce the dead space, and give the patient a gauze pad to bite on until the clot has formed.

8. Instruct the patient to avoid interfering with the clot for 24 hours. After this, the patient should frequently bathe the wound with warm saline until healing occurs.

9. Small broken roots can be left. Attempt to remove large superficial roots using fine forceps or elevators. Patients with unerupted or impacted wisdom teeth are best referred to a specialist.

10. If they become infected, see below for treatment.

JAW INFECTIONS

DENTAL ABSCESS

Once pus has escaped from bone, its direction of spread is influenced by gravity and muscle attachments. Antibiotics are usually given unless the tooth can be removed before fluctuation has occurred. Radiographs should be taken.

Action

1. Prior to fluctuation, remove the root. Antibiotics are rarely required.

2. When the tooth is partly erupted, cauterising the gum flap with an acid, such as chromic or trichloracetic will help to reduce infection. A sharp upper wisdom tooth may traumatize the cheek or the gum over a lower tooth. The removal of the upper is usually simple and gives relief of pain until the more complex lower can be extracted.

3. When fluctuation is present in the mouth, remove the tooth if accessible, and incise the swelling in the buccal sulcus or palate to release pus which has not emptied into the socket.

4. Pus around the muscles of mastication produces trismus and prevents easy access to posterior teeth. This usually presents as a sub-mandibular abscess.

5. Under endotracheal anaesthesia, incise the skin of the neck at the most dependant point of the swelling and parallel to the lower border of the mandible. Extend the wound by blunt dissection, then using Hilton's method, open up the loculi. Pass a pair of sinus forceps to the full depth of the cavity. Open the jaws of the forceps and remove them to enlarge the opening. Repeat this manoeuvre in a plane at right angles to the original. In large cavities, the septae can be broken down with a finger. Insert a drain for 24–48 hours. If the abscess is extensive, pass the drain from the skin through the abscess cavity and into the mouth through the lingual mucosa, lateral to the sub-mandibular duct. Draw it out of the mouth and fix it to the other end of the drain. Remove the diseased tooth when the acute phase is over.

CELLULITIS

Ludwig's angina is the bilateral involvement of the sublingual and sub-mandibular spaces and the cervical fascial planes by cellulitis. It is usually caused by streptococcal infection.

Action

1. Administer penicillin which produces rapid improvement in early cases.

2. In established infection, it may be necessary to make multiple superficial incisions of the skin of the neck to relieve pressure on the glottis.

3. If the source of infection is accessible, remove it. If dyspnoea is likely, perform a tracheostomy.

OSTEOMYELITIS OF THE JAW

This condition is rarely seen in a well-nourished population. The maxilla is not usually involved after infancy. Most patients respond to long-term treatment with antibiotic therapy.

Action

1. In the acute phase, expose the lateral cortex of the mandible through a sub-mandibular incision. Remove the cortex with a dental drill. If a large drill is not available, make multiple perforations and prise off segments with a chisel. Remove loose sequestra. Insert drains and close the wound.

2. In the chronic stage, expose the outer cortex of the mandible and dissect out the inferior alveolar neurovascular bundle. Remove the area of involved bone in a block and plan to graft the defect at a later date.

FACIAL SINUS

Appraise

A sinus on the face, such as the chin, cheek or naso-labial fold may be caused by a low-grade dental infection. Multiple or recurring sinuses may indicate actinomycosis. Clinical and radiographic examination usually shows the tooth involved.

Action

1. Remove the tooth in early cases.
2. Excise the sinus with an ellipse of skin if it is retracted. A small sinus can be encouraged to heal by cauterising the track with a crystal of silver nitrate.

BENIGN LUMPS IN THE MOUTH
EPULIS

An epulis, which is a swelling on the gum, contains giant cells and tends to recur and invades bone. Excise it with a wide base, including if necessary the contiguous teeth. Exclude parathyroid pathology.

BONE LESIONS

Exostoses can usually be left unless there is a sudden alteration in size or if they interfere with the fitting of a denture.

1. Reflect a mucoperiosteal flap, taking care over the lump where the mucosa may be very thin.

2. Remove the bone with a 5 mm chisel. Remember that the floor of the nose may dip down into a large torus palatinus.

3. Re-suture the flap, removing any excess soft tissue to reduce dead space and possible re-ossification of the haematoma.

SOFT TISSUE LUMPS

These include mucous cysts and fibro-epithelial polyps.

1. Excise the lump with an ellipse of mucosa. Attempted enucleation of a mucous cysts usually ruptures it. This makes it difficult to remove completely and it tends to recur.

2. Keep the excised area to a minimum when it is under the edge of a denture or this becomes more ill-fitting. File the denture down in this region to prevent pressure and recurrence.

CYSTS

Appraise

1. Cysts of the jaws may be single or multiple, related to teeth or apparently separate lesions within the bones. Multilocular radiolucencies may indicate an ameloblastoma. Multiple radiolucencies suggest neoplasm.

2. Treat them by excision or marsupialisation. Excision or enucleation is preferred where the cyst is small, unilocular or if follow-up care is difficult. Marsupialisation is useful in large multilocular cysts involving important structures but requires the help of a technician and frequent follow-up afterwards.

Action

Excise

1. Make a subcrestal incision with relieving incisions at either end. These incisions should be over sound bone and should include periosteum.

2. Raise a mucoperiosteal flap. If the cyst has perforated bone dissect the flap free from the cyst without bursting it.

3. If necessary, remove sufficient bone to allow access to the cyst.

4. Enucleate the cyst carefully. It may be attached near the roots of teeth. Beware of nearby normal anatomical structures such as the inferior alveolar neurovascular bundle, the maxillary antrum or the nasal cavity.

5. Suture the flaps back in position over bone.

6. Send *all* specimens for histological examination. Keratin-producing cysts often recur. Some tumours produce cystic spaces.

7. Teeth involved in a cyst are often best removed but can be saved by means of an apicectomy operation.

Marsupialize

1. Incise and reflect a flap as above.

2. Remove bone over the cyst to create as large an opening as possible (Fig. 34.4).

3. Excise part of the cyst for histology examination.

4. Trim the cyst lining and mucoperiosteal flap to the bone margin and suture them together (Fig. 34.5).

5. Carefully remove the cyst contents by suction and insert ribbon gauze soaked in Whitehead's varnish, flavine emulsion, or a bismuth iodoform paraffin paste.

6. Replace the pack after 10–14 days. When the edges have healed, replace the packing with a bung made from gutta percha or acrylic. The bung can be attached to a denture and is gradually reduced in size as the cyst shrinks.

7. Keep the cavity clean by syringing it with water.

8. A dentigerous (follicular) cyst contains the crown of a tooth. Occasionally it is possible to marsupialise the cyst to allow the tooth to erupt. If this is not feasible, remove the tooth and enucleate the cyst.

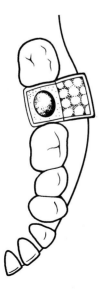

Fig. 34.4 Cyst displayed

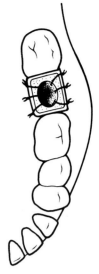

Fig. 34.5 Superficial part of cyst removed to expose contents

NON-DENTAL CYSTS

Inclusion cysts in the midline of the maxilla and globulo-maxillary cysts just lateral to the midline do not involve teeth, but may displace or be displaced by the roots. These cysts tend to recur and are difficult to enucleate completely.

AMELOBLASTOMA

When an ameloblastoma has been diagnosed early and is still small, it can be removed by intra-oral excision biopsy. Excise the lesion with 1 cm of apparently healthy bone. If possible, leave the lower border to help maintain a normal appearance. If the tumour has not been fully excised, wide resection is necessary.

Radical resection

1. Mandible. Make a submandibular incision, extending from the midline to the mandibular condyle. Divide the mandible with a Gigli saw. Use a bone graft from hip or rib to repair the defect. Wire the graft to the remainder of the mandible and immobilise the jaws for 6 weeks.

2. Maxilla. Remove palatal bone and expose the antrum. Initially, fill the defect with gauze soaked in an antiseptic. Later replace it with an acrylic prosthesis attached to a denture.

ORO-ANTRAL FISTULA

Appraise

1. This frequently follows tooth extraction but normally closes spontaneously. More commonly it follows when a root is accidently pushed into the antrum.

2. There are two routine approaches to closure of the fistula, buccal or palatal.

3. A small fistula may heal spontaneously if covered by a denture or plastic base plate. Similarly the suture line can be protected postoperatively with a plate provided the edge does not dig into the mucosa which has been stretched from the cheek.

BUCCAL FLAP

1. Excise the epithelial tract with a surround of muco-periosteum. A rim of bone must be visible on the palatal edge of the fistula.

2. Raise a broad based buccal flap of mucoperiosteum (Fig. 34.6).

3. Incise the periosteum above the level of the sulcus. This allows the flap to stretch (Fig. 34.7).

4. Lay the flap over the fistula and trim the edge if necessary.

5. Suture the edges, using vertical mattress sutures on the palate. Place the suture line over bone (Fig. 34.8).

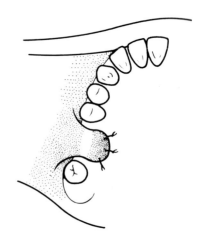

Fig. 34.8 Flap advanced and sutured on sound bone

PALATAL FLAP

1. Excise the fistula.

2. Raise a palatal flap. Avoid damage to palatal artery at the base of the flap (Fig. 34.9).

3. Turn the flap and suture it to the buccal mucoperiosteum ensuring the suture line is over bone (Fig. 34.10).

4. Cover the bare area of bone with ribbon gauze soaked in Whitehead's varnish. Suture the pack in place for 10–14 days.

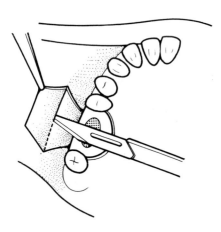

Fig. 34.6 Fistula tract excised and buccal flap raised

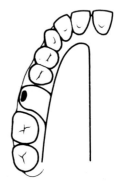

Fig. 34.9 Outline of palatal flap and its relation to the fistula

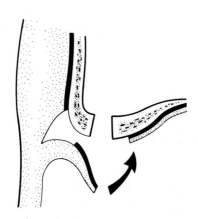

Fig. 34.7 Periosteum incised above sulcus

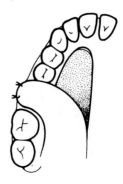

Fig. 34.10 Palatal flap sutured in position

FACIAL FRACTURES

Facial injuries involve the nose, maxilla, zygoma and mandible. Fractures of the nose are dealt with in Chapter 35.

IMMEDIATE TREATMENT

1. Respiratory. Posterior and downward displacement of the maxilla and blockage of the nose with blood clot causes respiratory distress. Pull the maxilla forward with a finger hooked around the back of the palate.

Bilateral fracture of the body of the mandible may result in lack of support of the tongue which falls back against the pharynx if the patient lies on his back. Place the patient in the tonsillar position, that is, lying on the side with the upper leg bent and the head extended. If necessary, insert a tongue stitch to pull the bulk of the tongue forward.

Remove foreign bodies, such as broken teeth or dentures from the mouth and pharynx. Severe facial injuries in an unconscious patient generally require an elective tracheostomy.

2. Haemorrhage. Bleeding from facial injuries may appear severe but is rarely life-threatening. If there are signs of shock, check other injured sites such as ruptured internal organs and fractured limbs. Control persistent bleeding from the nose with posterior nasal packs.

3. Fractures of the skull and other bones are often associated with facial injuries. Carry out appropriate observations and treatment as soon as possible.

Assess

1. Site of fracture or fractures. Mandibular fractures are often bilateral.
2. Type of fracture. Most fractures through the tooth-bearing areas are compound.
3. Number and position of teeth, and any wear facets.
4. Proximity of fracture line to apex of tooth.
5. Presence of cerebrospinal fluid leak from nose or ear.
6. Complications due to fracture, such as diplopia and trismus.
7. Presence and site of skin lacerations.

Appraise

1. If the teeth meet correctly, the mandibular fractures are probably reduced.
2. Maxillary fractures should be splinted to the skull, or zygomatic arches if they are intact.
3. Maintain fixation for 3 weeks for the maxilla and 4–6 weeks for the mandible.
4. Remove teeth if they are in the line of the fracture.
5. Give appropriate antibiotics.

6. Treat the patient under general anaesthesia unless the displacement is minimal.

MANDIBLE

Fix

1. *Barrel bandage.* This is used only as a temporary measure before the patient can get correct treatment. The bandage should be non-stretch material. Apply it to hold the lower jaw against the upper and not to pull the chin backwards (Fig. 34.11). Allow adequate space for easy observation of the pupils and lips.

2. *Eyelet wiring.* Use this when there are sufficient occluding teeth. Stretch soft stainless steel wire of 0.5 mm diameter by 10%. Twist 15 cm of wire round the shaft of a dental burr to form a loop in the middle of the wire. Pass the two ends between adjacent teeth so that the eyelet is on the buccal side. Separate the ends and pass them around each tooth. Thread one end through the eyelet and twist off with the other. The wire should be between the gum margin and the most bulbous part of the tooth (Fig. 34.12). When sufficient wires have been placed in both jaws and on all fragments, place the teeth in occlusion. Hook the tie wires through pairs of eyelets in each jaw. Place the twisted ends of the wires so that the ends cannot irritate the lips or cheeks (Fig. 34.13).

3. *Arch bars.* This is an alternative to eyelets especially when there are missing teeth. Commercially prepared bars are available with loops or cleats attached. Cut a sufficient length of bar and apply it to all the teeth in one jaw. The loops point towards the roots of the teeth. Fix the bar to the jaws with loops of wire twisted round each tooth and the bar. Carry out a similar procedure in the other jaw. It may be necessary to reduce the fracture before carrying out the final tightening. Place the teeth in occlusion and twist loops of wire around the opposing loops of the arch bars (Fig. 34.14).

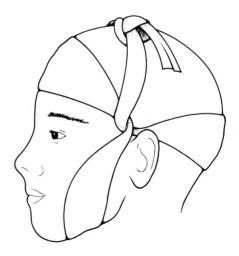

Fig. 34.11 Barrel bandage

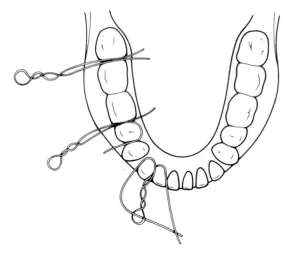

Fig. 34.12 Steps in the placement of eyelet wires

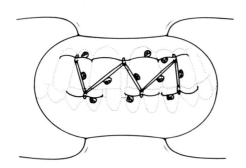

Fig. 34.13 Eyelet wires and intermaxillary wires in place

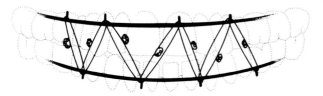

Fig. 34.14 Arch bars and intermaxillary fixation

4. *Upper border wiring.* Use this method when the posterior fragment is unstable, particularly after extraction of a tooth in the fracture line. Incise along the alveolar crest over fracture and raise a buccal mucoperiosteal flap. Drill holes 5 mm from fracture line, in each fragment, through the buccal cortex into the socket. Access may be difficult. Pass a length of pre-stretched 0.5 mm wire through the holes to form a loop. Twist the ends together and tuck the end into the anterior hole (Fig. 34.15). Suture the flap and apply intermaxillary fixation, such as eyelet wiring or arch bars.

5. *Lower border wiring.* This is stronger than upper border wiring and is useful in comminuted fractures. If a conveniently placed laceration is not available, make an incision in the neck 3 cm long, parallel to the lower border of the mandible and a finger breadth below it. This reduces

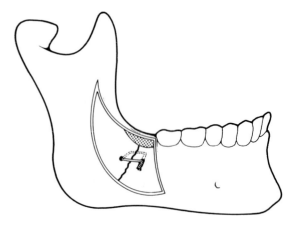

Fig. 34.15 Upper border interosseous wire inserted through tooth socket

the risk of damage to the mandibular branch of the facial nerve. Look for the facial artery where it emerges from the submandibular gland to curve round the lower border of the mandible. Raise the periosteum on either side of the fracture after incising along the lower border of the jaw. Place a metal retractor on the lingual side of the mandible and drill holes through the mandible, one hole in each fragment. Avoid drilling through the inferior alveolar neurovascular bundle. After reducing the fracture, pass a 0.5 mm wire through the holes to form a loop or make a sling in the form of a figure '8' at the lower border. Tuck the twisted ends into the holes and close the wound in layers (periosteum, platysma, skin). Apply intermaxillary fixation (Fig. 34.16).

6. *Plating.* This is useful in edentulous patients or occasionally in dentate patients when it is desireable to leave the jaws free to move. The approach is as for lower border wiring. Position the fragments and place a meta-carpal plate across the fracture. Drill holes in the bone and insert screws. Fix the end screws first. The drill size must match that of the screws and all instruments should be of the same metal to avoid electrolytic action. The plate must

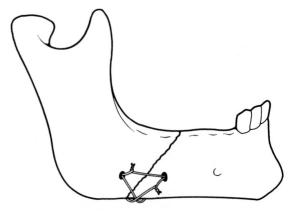

Fig. 34.16 Lower border interosseous wires. Loop and figure '8' pattern

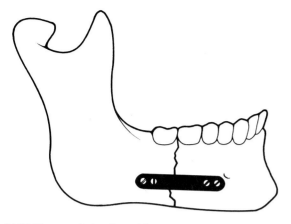

Fig. 34.17 Metacarpal plate in position across mandibular fracture

be flush against the bone (Fig. 34.17). In atrophic mandibles, the plate can be applied external to the periosteum to minimise the damage to an already compromised blood supply. Close the wound in layers.

7. *Gunning splints.* Use these for edentulous patients. Obtain the help of a dental technician. The splints are made from impressions of the patient's mouth or from dentures if available. The splints or dentures are wired to the jaws after reducing the fractures. Pass the wires with an awl which has a hole near the trocar point or through a lumbar puncture needle (Fig. 34.18). Take care not to let the wire enter the fracture or damage the submandibular ducts.

8. *Silver cast cap splints.* These are individually prepared splints which fit over the teeth. The aid of a skilled dental technician is required.

MAXILLA

Reduce

1. Reduction of the fracture may be difficult because of impaction of the bones and oedema. Special disimpaction forceps are available.

2. After disimpaction, fix the teeth in occlusion with eyelets, arch bars or splints. By applying pressure under the mandible, reduce the fracture between the maxilla and skull. Inadequate reduction results in a concave profile which is difficult to correct.

Fix

1. *Plaster of Paris headcap.* This is cheap and easy to use but tends to move. It is easiest to apply with the patient sitting. Place a length of tubular gauze over the head. Apply plaster bandages to the skull above the eyebrows and below the occiput. Various wire loops can be embedded in the plaster before it sets. Trim the tubular gauze. Use the wire loops to support the jaws by means of rods and joints (Fig. 34.19).

2. *Halo frame.* This is easy to use, versatile and firm. The modern version is made of a light alloy, is horse-shoe shaped and has many holes to which the rods and joints may be fixed. Fix the halo to the skull with four screws whose points just engage the outer cortex of the skull (Fig. 34.20).

3. *Internal fixation.* A laboratory technician is not required. Using an awl or lumbar puncture needle, pass a loop of wire round the zygomatic arch and into the mouth in the molar region. Pass one end through an eyelet or round a cleat on splints or arch bar in either jaw and twist with the other end (Fig. 34.21).

4. *Pins or bone screws.* Pins can be drilled into the bone and used to attach rods and joints to provide fixation. Insert the pins through stab incisions using a hand drill with a low gear ratio. The common sites used are the lateral

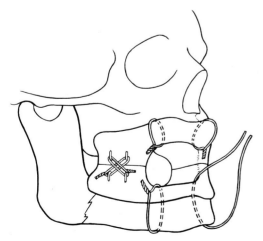

Fig. 34.18 Gunning splints fixed to jaws

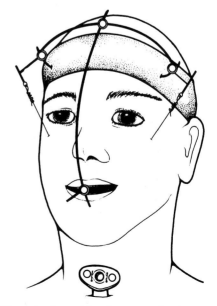

Fig. 34.19 Plaster headcap with rods connected to jaws

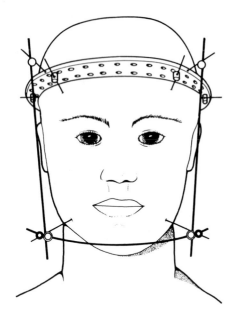

Fig. 34.20 Halo frame fixed to skull and connected to jaws

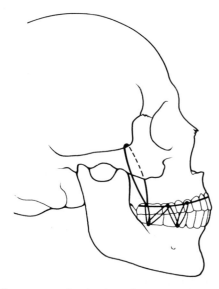

Fig. 34.21 Circumzygomatic wires looped round arch wire

ends of the superciliary ridges. Use a guide tube and a conventional drill bit to start the hole to prevent slipping and damage to nearby structures. Attach the pins by rods and joints to splints in the mouth, or pins in the mandible (Fig. 34.22).

5. *Kirschner wire*. Use where speed rather than accuracy is required. The maxilla is reduced and transfixed by the Kirschner wire passed from one intact zygomatic bone to the other. Avoid piercing the anaesthetist's nasal endotracheal tube.

Aftercare

1. Administer prophylactic antibiotics in compound fractures around the mouth.

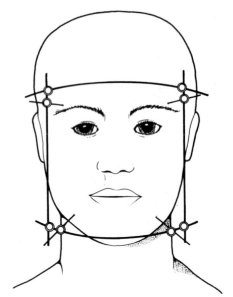

Fig. 34.22 Supra-orbital pins connected to pins in mandible

2. Before applying intermaxillary fixation, remove the anaesthetist's throat pack.

3. Patients with intermaxillary fixation need close supervision postoperatively in case they inhale vomit. Keep wire cutters by the bedside and instruct nursing staff in their use. Give anti-emetics at the end of the general anaesthetic.

4. Elastic bands are safer than wires for intermaxillary fixation but need frequent replacement.

5. Give fluid or semi-fluid diet. Six small meals are easier to take than three large ones.

6. Keep the mouth clean with mouthwashes and a small toothbrush.

ZYGOMATIC COMPLEX (MALAR)

These are best treated within a week of injury but allow excessive periorbital oedema to subside first.

Access

1. Use Gillie's temporal approach. Make a 2.5 cm incision in the hairline between the main branches of superficial temporal vessels. Cut nearly parallel to the zygomatic arch.

2. When glistening temporalis fascia is reached, incise it carefully to avoid damage to the temporalis muscle.

3. Slide Howarth's periosteal elevator under the fascia until it is beneath the zygomatic arch. No resistance should be felt until the arch is reached.

Action

1. Exchange the Howarth for a Bristow's elevator or one of the modifications, and lift the displaced bone with an

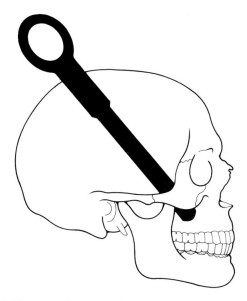

Fig. 34.23 Elevator under zygomatic arch

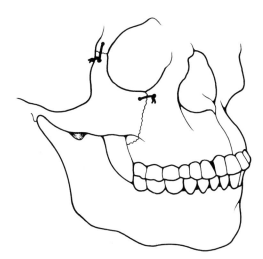

Fig. 34.24 Interosseous wires in orbital margin fractures

upwards and outwards motion. A slight forward rotation may also help. Do not lever against the middle cranial fossa. The bone usually jams into place with a click (Fig. 34.23).

2. Suture the skin.

3. Mark the affected cheek and instruct nurses not to lay the patient on that side.

Difficulty?

1. Instability

(a) Support the bone with interosseous wires inserted across the fractures in the fronto-zygomatic and infra-orbital regions. Insert these wires through small incisions in the eyebrow and lower eyelid respectively. Protect the eye when drilling the holes (Fig. 34.24).

(b) Similar support can be provided by inserting a pack into the antrum through a Caldwell Luc approach. Before packing, check the floor of the orbit for loose

spicules which might be displaced upwards into the optic nerve. The pack is usually 2.5 cm ribbon gauze soaked in Whitehead's varnish, BIPP or flavine emulsion. Remove it after 2 weeks.

2. In blow-out fractures where the orbital contents are trapped in the fracture, or have prolapsed into the antrum, the patient may display marked diplopia with unequal pupil levels. Correct this with an antral pack or preferably, with a Silastic sheet inserted under the globe through an incision in the lower eyelid. Check that there is full movement of the globe at the end of the operation.

ZYGOMATIC ARCH

Action

1. Use Gillies approach, as above (see p. 614).

2. Intra-oral approach. Make an incision over the zygomatic buttress, insert a lever under the arch, and elevate it. Check the reduction with a finger inserted through the incision and under the arch.

Further reading

Archer W H 1975 Oral surgery. Saunders, Philadelphia
Guralnick W C 1968 Textbook of oral surgery. Churchill Livingstone, London
Haglund J, Evers H 1975 Local anaesthesia in Dentistry, 2nd edn. Trycheri AB I Lundbladh, Sweden
Howe G L 1971 Minor oral surgery, 2nd edn. Wright, Bristol

Howe G L 1974 The extraction of teeth, 2nd edn. Wright, Bristol
Roberts D H, Sowray J H 1970 Local analgesia in dentistry. Wright, Bristol
Rowe N L, Williams J Ll 1985 Maxillofacial injuries. Churchill Livingstone, Edinburgh

Ear, nose and throat surgery

MYRINGOTOMY

Once the main therapy for acute suppurative otitis media, this is now rarely necessary as an emergency. General anaesthesia is essential, and no modern otologist would wish to proceed without an operating binocular microscope. If you are not trained in otology and there is no microscope, use a good otoscope with a new battery, and examine the patient's *normal* ear in a careful and leisurely way. Memorize the depth, angulation and general form of his normal meatus and drumhead, so that when you turn to the diseased ear you can better interpret what you see. The red bulging drum obliterates its own landmarks and inflammatory oedema spreads into the meatal roof and posterior wall. Every tool should be cherished and cutting tools must be sharp. The best myringotome is disposable and has never been used before. Do not try to use anything with a blunted edge and a turned-over point.

Action

1. Incise the convexity of the bulging membrane from below upwards (Fig. 35.1) making a slit of 3–5 mm vertically behind the malleus handle (if only it were visible!).
2. Mucoid pus emerges. Take a swab for culture. Use a very fine-tipped sucker gently to empty the middle ear but do not 'poke about' so as to risk dislocation of the ossicles. Leave a ribbon gauze wick soaked in gentamicin and hydrocortisone eardrops in the meatus for 24 hours.

Difficulty?

1. Babies have a short meatus, and a very obliquely placed drum membrane. Intensify the antibiotics, and send for an otologist unless you are very sure where to place the incision.
2. Wax must be carefully removed under the anaesthetic using suction. Do not abrade the meatal wall, which can bleed freely and so obstruct your view.
3. A narrow meatus means a small speculum must be used, with consequently greater difficulty of orientation.

Some operations are unneccesary, many can wait, and the vast majority call more for acumen and jugment beforehand, than for special skills in their performance. Every surgeon, of whatever experience or distinction, should reflect deeply before undertaking an operation for the first time. If it is an operation he has not even watched being done, his burden of responsibility is extreme. With today's increasing specialization within surgery practical training has become narrower, and it is more and more necessary to respect the skills of other disciplines. If a case presents a challenge outside the surgeon's personal experience but the operative techniques are familiar to him, he is equipped for the task, and may proceed properly if no more qualified colleague is available. If these conditions are not met, it may be wiser to accept the role of general practitioner and to temporise intelligently as a good but isolated general practitioner would. In this spirit a mature surgeon, lacking ENT training and with no ENT colleague at hand, may under pressure of unusual circumstances find the following operative surgical notes helpful.

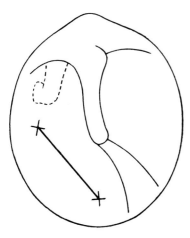

Fig. 35.1 Normal tympanic membrane (right ear). The line X–X indicates the incision for myringotomy in acute suppurative otitis media.

'SECRETORY' OTITIS MEDIA

This condition is not an emergency, not painful, and needs only a 'pinprick' to normalize the middle-ear pressure and allow the yellow watery fluid to escape from the drum — most adult patients can tolerate this without anaesthesia. Press the point of the myringotome gently through the membrane just below the umbo. If fluid does not run out spontaneously, tilt the patient's head towards the affected ear, and have him inflate the middle ear by Valsalva's manoeuvre.

An otologist will require the microscope, suction, and general anaesthesia for difficult cases.

FOREIGN BODY IN THE EAR

Action

1. Most occur in children. Animate intruders (e.g. insects) are an emergency because of pain. Fill the ear with olive oil (to asphyxiate the animal) and then syringe with water at body temperature to remove it.

2. Inanimate foreign bodies may yield to gentle syringing, but those which occlude, or nearly occlude, the meatus need instrumental extraction. *Never* try it unless you have fine equipment and the patient's complete confidence and cooperation. The child retreating in fear is wiser than he knows, and wiser than the doctor who thinks that *'force majeure'* will win the day.

3. If the child is tranquil and trusting, talk him along while you tickle his ear with a harmless instrument. When he has relaxed, touch the foreign body with a fine probe to confirm its shape and texture. Look for a graspable edge — if you can apply a very fine Hartmann's crocodile forceps accurately there is no further problem.

Difficulty?

1. If the object is smooth and rounded (e.g. a bead) do *not* apply forceps — they will certainly fail to grasp, and will push the foreign body deeper into the meatus. Disasters still happen because doctors push foreign bodies through the drum, ossicular chain, facial nerve and labyrinth.

2. The safest way to remove an occluding foreign body is under general anaesthesia. Use magnification, and the largest speculum the meatus will take. Insinuate a stapedectomy hook below the object (unless there is an obvious space above it), turn the hook to engate it, and ease it outwards by rolling or sliding until it is delivered.

3. *Golden rules*:
(a) Do nothing which pushes the foreign body medially.
(b) Pass hooks or probes anteroinferiorly, where the obliquity of the tympanic membrane allows deeper insertion without injury.

CORTICAL (SIMPLE) MASTOIDECTOMY

Because of its rarity today this is no longer within the province of the 'occasional' operator. Nonetheless it can be lifesaving, and in some geographical areas may have to be done whether or not an otologist is available.

Access

1. Make an incision firmly down to bone, parallel to and 1 cm behind the retro-auricular skin fold. Start above the pinna and end at the mastoid tip.

2. Elevate the periosteum backwards, and anteriorly to expose the suprameatal triangle. Identify the posterior meatal wall, but do not dissect the skin lining off the bone.

3. Push the temporal muscle upwards. Insert a mastoid retractor (Fig. 35.2).

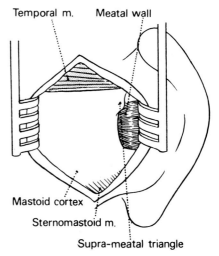

Fig. 35.2 Cortical mastoidectomy. Exposure of the bony field (right ear).

Action

1. Use hammer and gouge to cut out adjoining demi-lunes of mastoid cortex until the infected air cells are opened. Send pus for culture.

2. Enlarge the opening in the mastoid immediately behind and above the meatus, but leave the cortical shell of the bony meatus intact. One air cell leads to another. Saucerize and deepen the bone cavity with oblique shallow gouge strokes. In a triangle, bounded by dura above, sigmoid sinus behind and below and external meatus anteriorly, the mastoid antrum is found at a depth of about 2 cm (Fig. 35.3).

3. The penalty of inexperience is facial palsy. Unless you really know the temporal bone intimately do not attempt a complete mastoidectomy. Merely by opening and draining the mastoid you have solved the immediate problem.

4. Stitch a corrugated drain into the lower end of the wound and intensify antibiotic cover (including sulphonamides). The operation can be revised expertly at leisure if the cure is less than complete.

Pitfalls

Incomplete mastoidectomies had a bad reputation in pre-antibiotic times. If you elect for less than a clear exenteration of all infected cells, you must be all the more vigilant, post-operatively, not to miss intracranial spread of infection. Complications may be dangerously masked by antibiotics.

REMOVAL OF NASAL FOREIGN BODY

Appraise

Any young child with unilateral nasal discharge, obstruction or bleeding, must be suspected of a self-inserted

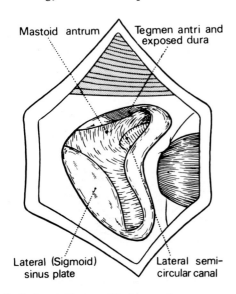

Fig. 35.3 Cortical mastoidectomy. The bony cavity.

Mastoid antrum

Tegmen antri and exposed dura

Lateral (Sigmoid) sinus plate

Lateral semi-circular canal

foreign body. If the discharge smells foul the diagnosis is certain. Expect to find screwed-up fragments of paper, vegetable matter, plastic or metal beads, or plastic sponge.

Prepare

1. As with aural foreign bodies, it is essential to have the child's cooperation, a graspable foreign body, the right tools for the job and clear visibility (headlight, and skill with nasal speculum). If any of these are lacking, general anaesthesia and a specialist are required.

2. Oral intubation is essential. The anaesthetist should be asked not to inflate the lungs with a face mask — this could force a nasal foreign body backwards.

3. Alternative positions:
(a) The tonsillectomy position and use of a Boyle Davis gag provide the surest safeguard against losing a difficult foreign body backwards. If it slips into the nasopharynx it will stay there by gravity while you are getting ready a mirror and suitable forceps for retrieval.
(b) Instead you may choose to have a firm oropharyngeal pack around the tube, relying on this to entrap the foreign body should the latter slip backwards. Have the head of the table raised so that you can look along the floor of the nose.

4. Use fine forceps if the object is graspable. Otherwise use a small hook, pass it above the foreign body, and ease the object downwards and forwards for delivery. *Full visibility throughout* is essential.

REMOVAL OF NASAL POLYPI

Appraise

If polypi completely obstruct both sides of the nose, and the patient cannot be transferred to the care of an ENT surgeon, it may be justifiable to relieve nasal occlusion by avulsion of the polypi.

Essential preconditions are:
(a) You must be proficient with a headlight in the inspection of deep cavities.
(b) General anaesthesia with orotracheal tube and pack.
(c) Availability of Luc's and Tilley-Henckel forceps (a snare is optional).

Action

1. First paint the nasal lining with 1 : 1000 adrenaline and wait a few minutes for vasoconstriction. Grasp and avulse all of the soft, grey pedunculated polypi. Allow your forceps to feel before they bite and pull, so that no bony structures are removed. The inferior and middle turbinates must be respected, though a rhinologist may decide to remove part or all of the latter. Similarly, you should not

allow yourself to be drawn into an ethmoidectomy, which if done inexpertly may lead to orbital or intracranial complications.

2. When the airways have been re-established, pack the nasal cavities gently but completely with vaseline ribbon gauze (2.5 cm wide) to prevent postoperative bleeding.

Aftercare

1. Antibiotics should be given for seven days. The packs must removed 24 hours after surgery.

2. Inspect the nose every two or three days for incipient adhesions. Prevent these by using a probe to break down any persistent bridge of fibrin between septum and lateral nasal wall.

CALDWELL-LUC ANTROTOMY

Appraise

Inspection of the interior of the maxillary antrum is mandatory, even without ENT specialist skills, in the following circumstances.

1. On suspicion of malignant disease (for assessment and biopsy).

2. For antral foreign body (e.g. dental root lost during extraction, or metal from shrapnel or gunshot).

3. For repositioning of bony fragments after zygomatic or orbital (blow-out) fractures. The reduction may be supported by packing the antrum with ribbon gauze soaked in vaseline or Whitehead's varnish.

4. Other indications for Caldwell-Luc's operation may be postponed indefinitely in the absence of an ENT surgeon.

5. Never perform this operation in the presence of acute sinusitis.

Action

1. General anaesthetic is essential, with orotracheal tube and pharyngeal pack. Infiltrate the submucosa of the canine fossa with 1 per cent lignocaine and 1 : 200 000 adrenaline (2–5 ml).

2. Correct retraction is crucial. Have the angle of the mouth drawn laterally and the upper lip pulled upwards. Hajek's retractors are the best. Incise the mucosa of the canine fossa horizontally 1 cm above the gingival margin, starting 1 cm lateral to the midline and extending for 4 cm laterally and backwards below the zygoma (Fig. 35.4).

3. Elevate the periosteum from the incision upwards, and reinsert the retractors beneath it. The bony canine fossa is thus exposed. Take care not to approach the infraorbital foramen too closely, otherwise intractable neuralgia may ensue.

4. Use hammer and gouge to enter the antrum and then

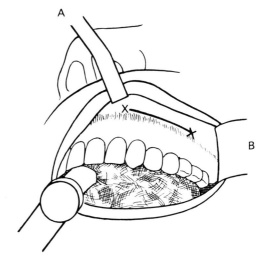

Fig. 35.4 Left Caldwell-Luc antrotomy. Retraction of upper lip (A, B) and incision (X–X).

enlarge the bony opening with punch forceps to about 2 cm in diameter. Send pus for culture, remove any foreign body and strip away any grossly diseased mucosal lining (Fig. 35.5).

5. *Antrostomy.* In most cases, and in all where chronic infection is present, an antrostomy opening is made by removing the antronasal wall beneath the inferior turbinate. Use a gouge, just above the floor of the antrum, and about 2 cm posterior to the most anterior extent of the sinus cavity. Enlarge the hole with punch forceps to about 2 cm by 1 cm and incise the nasal mucosa thus exposed (from its deep surface) to make a flap hinged below. Fold the flap downward on to the floor of the antrum. Confirm that a curved probe passed through the nostril and under the inferior turbinate will enter the antrum easily (Fig. 35.6).

Closure

1. If there is no bleeding, finish the operation with two or three plain catgut stitches to the sublabial incision.

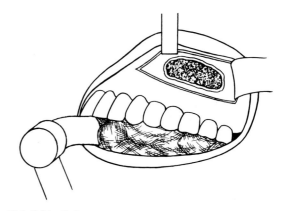

Fig. 35.5 Caldwell–Luc antrotomy. Retractors under mucoperiosteum; canine fossa opened into antral cavity.

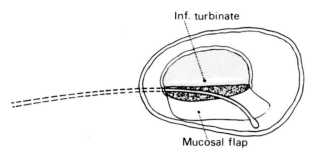

Fig. 35.6 Caldwell-Luc antrotomy. The counter-opening (antrostomy) into the nasal cavity.

2. If haemostasis requires it, pack the antrum before closure with lubricated 2.5 cm ribbon gauze. Bring the end through the antrostomy, under the turbinate and out through the nostril. Remove this pack 24 hours later.

EXCISION OF UPPER JAW TUMOURS

These may arise from oral or antral mucosa, dental structures, or from bone. They may be benign or malignant. Unless the lesion is obviously noninvasive, preliminary biopsy is essential. For most malignant tumours radiotherapy is indicated, either as curative treatment or as a preliminary to surgical excision.

1. Localized benign tumours are easily removed by a simple soft tissue excision, from the oral cavity, or from the maxillary antrum by Caldwell-Luc's approach. No special deescription is necessary.

2. 'Benign' tumours which are locally invasive (pleomorphic adenoma, adamantinoma) require wide excision to prevent inexorable progression, as do frankly malignant lesions.

PALATAL FENESTRATION WITH ALVEOLECTOMY

1. Mark out an incision with diathermy, cutting down to bone, in the buccal, alveolar and palatal mucosal so as to encompass the tumour with a margin of healthy tissue. Use gouge or chisel to cut clearly through bone in the line of the incision, so that from every aspect the maxillary sinus is entered, and the 'specimen' is free in the mouth (Fig. 35.7).

2. Often the excision must include the maxillary tuberosity. If so, drive an osteotome vertically upwards behind the tuberosity for about 1.5 cm to split the posterior antral wall forwards away from the pterygoid process. Medially the hard palate may be removed up to or even beyond the midline if necessary (Fig. 35.8).

3. Coagulate bleeding points, after packing the cavity firmly for a few minutes. Now you can see into the antrum

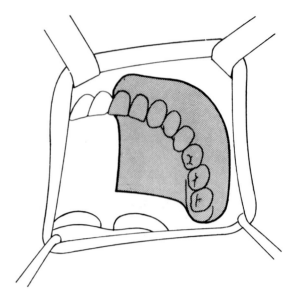

Fig. 35.7 Palatal fenestraction with alveolectomy. Incision (cuffed orotracheal tube and a pharyngeal gauze pack are essential).

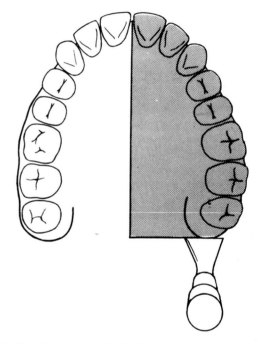

Fig. 35.8 Use of osteotome behind tuberosity.

(Fig. 35.9). Remove any suspicious-looking tissues, and label specimens carefully so that any areas of malignant extension (e.g. cheek or pterygoid fossa) can be identified for future reference.

4. Filling the hole in the mouth. The surgical defect in the palate can be packed with 2.5 cm ribbon gauze soaked in vaseline or Whitehead's varnish. It is better, with collaboration of dental colleagues, to take an immediate impression of the cavity and upper jaw from which a definitive prosthesis will later be made. Having taken this

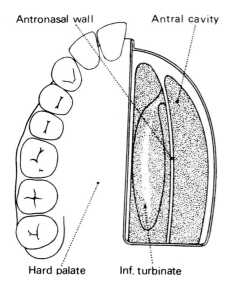

Fig. 35.9 Operative cavity after palatal fenestration with alveolectomy.

impression, you can with advantage complete the operation by fitting a gutta-percha 'bung' to the patient's own upper denture. This is an immediate aid to haemostasis (in lieu of packing). In the longer term it will keep food out of the cavity, and support the cheek until the definitive acrylic prosthesis has been made and fitted 7–10 days later.

5. Skin grafting the cavity. The gutta-percha bung will carry a splint skin graft to line the raw areas of the cavity. There is little to gain by grafting limited excisions (partial maxillectomies) but after total maxillectomy (see below) a graft is well worth considering.

6. Intracavitary irradiation. If the operative findings and histological reports show that excision of a malignant growth was inadequate, and if preoperative radiotherapy precludes further external irradiation, the prosthesis can be 'loaded' with radioactive material. The placement and dosage of such radioactivity *must always* be the work of a skilled radiotherapist.

TOTAL MAXILLECTOMY

Appraise

Malignant tumours, not radiosensitive, approaching the roof of the antrum or the ethmoidal air cells.

Access

1. Begin the incision just below the outer canthus of the eye and incise horizontally, parallel to the edge of the lower lid, until the nose is reached. Turn downwards at a right angle, cutting firmly down to the frontal process of maxilla. Carry the incision into the fold between the ala and the cheek, and then below the ala to the midline. From here, divide all layers of the upper lip, vertically, in the midline (Fig. 35.10).

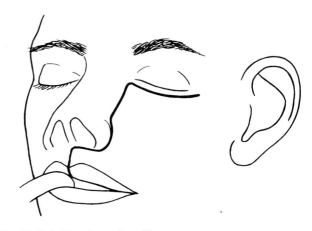

Fig. 35.10 Incision for total maxillectomy.

2. Turn the lip laterally and dissect the soft tissues of the cheek off the maxilla. Watch out for extension of growth into the cheek.

Action

Refer to the dried skull (Fig. 35.11).

1'. Elevate the periosteum of the floor and medial wall of the orbit.

2. Divide the frontal process of the maxilla with bone cutters or osteotome, cutting from the nasal aperture towards the orbit.

3. Divide the zygoma by a Gigli saw threaded into the

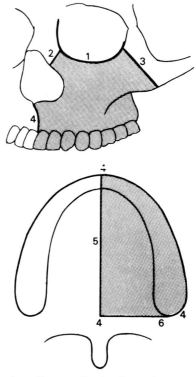

Fig. 35.11 Total maxillectomy. Freeing the specimen.

orbit, through the inferior orbital fissure, and out again below the zygomatic arch. If you fear that this might cut across the zygomatic extension of the tumour, bring the saw out above the arch, and divide the latter slightly further back by a second saw cut.

4. Use cutting diathermy in the mouth to incise between the central incisors, backwards just lateral to the midline of the hard palate, and then laterally along the posterior border of the hard palate and behind the maxillary tuberosity.

5. Divide the hard palate anteroposteriorly with an osteotome in the line of the mucosal incision, keeping just to one side of the nasal septum. A good alternative is the Gigli saw threaded behind the hard palate and brought out through the nose and mouth.

6. Drive an osteotome vertically upwards for 1.5 cm behind the tuberosity, and then use it as a lever gently to loosen the maxilla in a forward direction (see Fig. 35.8).

7. Grasp and rock the maxilla with Lion forceps until it breaks away from the ethmoid, its only remaining attachment. Remove it, and pack the cavity.

8. Haemostasis. Look for bleeding from maxillary vessels in the pterygoid fossa. Diathermy will suffice.

Extension of operation

1 In most cases it is wise to remove the entire ethmoidal system on the affected side with Henckel's or other nibbling forceps, up to the skull base, and back to the sphenoid.

2. If growth has invaded the orbit you must remove the entire orbital contents. *Never* embark on a maxillectomy without the patient's permission to do this if necessary.

3. If there is a major extension into the cheek it is a debatable question whether an attempt at curative surgery is justified. If you do go in, a wide margin of healthy face must be excised around the growth.

Closure

1. When you have closed the facial incision (take especial care to align the lip margins accurately), fill the cavity exactly as described on page 620.

2. Skin grafting is well worth while to accelerate healing of the cavity walls.

MANIPULATION OF FRACTURED NOSE

Realignment of displaced nasal bones is a purely cosmetic operation. Nonetheless, the nose is so dominant in our psyche and our culture that almost every female (of any age) and a majority of males under the age of fifty insist fervently that a deformed nose must be straightened. Doctors must insist upon the earliest possible opportunity to perform this social duty, because after the lapse of about two weeks it is exceedingly difficult, sometimes impossible, to realign the fragments satisfactorily.

Action

1. In the clinic, with no formality other than courtesy and gentleness, it is sometimes possible to straighten the nose by digital pressure, easing the bony skeleton back into the midline. A click will be felt as the fragments move.

2. Should this fail, general anaesthesia is necessary. *Never* be tempted to try a 'sniff of gas' or a 'shot of pentothal'. Bleeding, possibly massive, into the airway can convert a minor problem into a fatality. Formal anaesthesia, with cuffed endotrached tube and oropharyngeal pack, is mandatory.

3. First attempt manual reduction, pressing with your thumbs against the more prominent of the nasal bones. If this succeeds, over-reduce the fracture, and then mould the mobilized fragments into the desired symmetry.

4. Should this fail, insert one blade of a Walsham's forceps into the nostril and grasp the more prominent nasal bone. Rotate and displace it outward so as to free the depressed bone of the opposite side. Now grasp the latter with (the other-handed) Walsham's forceps and turn it laterally also. The nasal fragments are now mobile and can be centralized with digital moulding.

5. If the septum is displaced, or the bridgeline depressed, pass the blades of Asche's forceps into the nostrils, grasp the septum, and bring it into the midline, while lifting up the bridgeline.

6. In all these manoeuvres only the minimum force necessary must be used. Often the nasal mucosa will be torn, and then bleeding may be a nuisance, even requiring nasal packing.

7. Splinting the nose. If the reduced fracture is stable it is better not to cover it with a splint. Grossly comminuted, unstable fractures need a plaster of Paris splint secured by adhesive strapping across the forehead and cheeks. Mould the splint (and the nose underneath it) while the plaster is setting. Leave it on for at least ten days.

FOREIGN BODIES IN THE THROAT

Appraise

Fish bones lodge at any level, more substantial fragments (chicken, rabbit and chop bones) usually stick in the post-cricoid region or upper oesophagus. Rarely occluding foreign bodies (sweets, meat bolus) can cause airway obstruction — an emergency — or sudden death. Dentures (often broken) impact in the midoesophagus. A stricture, benign or malignant, may predetermine sudden oesophageal obstruction by a small bolus, such as a pea or piece of potato.

Action

1. Inspect the throat minutely, using a headlight and tongue depressor. Look for the tip of a buried fish bone in the tonsil or tongue. Use a fine pair of angled forceps, and the greatest delicacy, to grasp and remove the bone.

2. If direct examination proves negative, use a laryngeal mirror (as in indirect laryngoscopy) to examine the back of tongue and laryngopharynx. A bone in these sites can often be retrieved *under visual control* with angled forceps. Have the patient hold his own tongue as far out as possible (grasping it with a gauze swab). Use your left hand for the mirror and right hand for the forceps. You must see the forceps closing on the foreign body accurately. Blind lunges are not permissible under any circumstances.

3. If mirror examination shows a foreign body deep in the pyriform fossa or postcricoid space, *or* if X-ray shows it in the hypopharynx or upper oesophagus, direct endoscopy under general anaesthetic is mandatory. An endotracheal cuffed tube and muscle-relaxant drugs are required. Use a laryngoscope or short oesophagoscope and suitable forceps to bring the offending object into its lumen. Take care not to push a sharp object through the visceral wall. Try to rotate it so that its most traumatic aspect is disimpacted, and will either trail harmlessly, or be inside the endoscope, during withdrawal.

4. Special difficulties. Do not attempt the removal of a denture bearing sharp hooks from the oesophagus. Consultation with a thoracic surgeon is essential because in some cases it will be safer for the patient to have every facility for thoracotomy and oesophagotomy arranged beforehand.

INCISION OF QUINSY (PERITONSILLAR ABSCESS)

Appraise

Although well documented in traditional lore, this is a rare procedure nowadays. Most peritonsillar infections are minimized, if not quickly cured, by systemic antibiotics. Most early cases should be treated by massive dosage of broad-spectrum drugs, and reviewed after 24–36 hours. If the swelling is not then subsiding, and if a fluctuant peritonsillar abscess is evident, incision will be beneficial.

Action

1. Inject local anaesthetic (2 ml) into the palatal mucosa at the intersection of a horizontal line through the base of the uvula with a vertical line along the anterior faucial pillar. Allow at least five minutes for it to take effect.

2. Press a small knife (e.g. Bard-Parker 15) backwards through the mucosa to a depth of 1–2 cm (Fig. 35.12). When pus gushes out, widen the track with sinus forceps. Take a swab for culture.

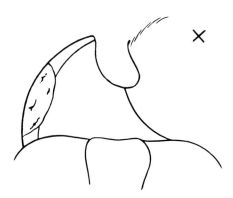

Fig. 35.12 Quinsy. X shows the point of incision.

INCISION OF RETROPHARYNGEAL ABSCESS

Appraise

As a cause of acute illness with respiratory obstruction in infants and toddlers, this abscess tends to be lateralized to one side. In older victims the abscess may be truly prevertebral, strictly midline and tuberculous in nature, secondary to vertebral caries. In the latter case treatment is primarily nonsurgical.

Incision of a pyogenic abscess in a young child or infant is required if, in spite of massive antibiotic treatment, respiratory obstruction threatens life.

Action

Lateralized pyogenic abscess

1. Incision through the pharyngeal mucosa may be appropriate, but death may result from inhalation of pus. Traditionally, therefore, general anaesthesia has been condemned, and incision through the mouth of the totally and forcibly restrained infant advised.

2. Modern techniques and skills, when available, commend general anaesthesia and intubation, with peroral needle aspiration of the abscess contents.

RELIEF OF UPPER AIRWAY OBSTRUCTION

Appraise

1. Lives are saved by practicality and common sense. Smashed face and jaws, laryngeal trauma and impacted foreign body, with or without bleeding in the throat or vomiting, require fast and effective attention to the mechanical impediment. Comatose cases require confirmation of a clear airway and assisted respiration — mouth-to-mouth, Ambi bag, intubation or mechanical respirator.

2. The principles are — remembering that asphyxia is fatal —

(a) Identify the cause of obstruction.

(b) Eliminate it, or

(c) Pass a tube through or past it, or

(d) Get below it by laryngotomy or tracheotomy.

If (a), (b) and (c) are sensibly deployed the heroics of laryngotomy or 'crash' tracheotomy should rarely if ever be called for. They are only briefly described here.

LARYNGOTOMY

1. Lie the patient on his back and extend his neck.

2. Make a horizontal stab incision between the cricoid and thyroid cartilages. Press the blade backwards until you feel the point enter the airway and air begins to hiss in and out with respiration through the wound (Fig. 35.13).

3. With no loss of time, remove the knife and insert a small metal tube, curved downwards, inside the tracheal lumen. A correctly designed laryngotomy tube is flattened somewhat, so as to lie neatly between the cartilages, but if none is available *any* type of tube, metal, rubber or plastic — even unsterile — is permissible if it maintains the airway.

4. Improvised tubes are difficult to keep in a correct position and must therefore be manually held until such time as a stable airway has been established.

5. Follow-up: unless the cause of acute asphyxia is quickly curable (e.g. removal of impacted foreign body, or angioneurotic oedema), perform an elective tracheostomy within 48 hours and close the laryngotomy incision.

'CRASH' TRACHEOTOMY

1. Laryngotomy is almost always to be preferred. *Very rarely* (e.g. if a subglottic lesion precludes laryngotomy and defies intubation even with a rigid bronchoscope) the trachea must be opened at speed. The patient's neck must be held in extension and strictly centred. Give your strongest assistant this task. Oxygen by face mask will sometimes give the patient a few more minutes.

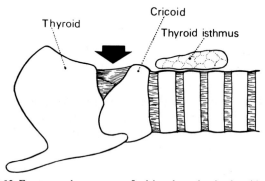

Fig. 35.13 Emergency laryngotomy. Incision through cricothyroid membrane.

2. Cut vertically from the Adam's apple in the midline to the suprasternal notch. Deepen the incision with two or three more strokes between the strap muscles and feel the first tracheal ring with your left index finger.

3. The next stroke divides the thyroid isthmus. Bleeding will be profuse, but if you have assistants holding retractors in the wound, with swabbing or suction, you may be able to see the anterior tracheal wall. Decide quickly whether you have time to clamp major bleeding points before incising the trachea vertically through the second, third and fourth rings.

4. Put a tube into the trachea, and then control the worst of the bleeding. Use suction with a soft, fine catheter through the tube to retrieve blood which has already been sucked into the trachea.

5. Subsequent decisions and procedures will depend upon the cause of the obstruction and the patient's general condition. Respiration and pulse must be carefully monitored during and for several hours after such a crisis. Be ready to give assisted respiration and/or cardiac resuscitation.

ELECTIVE TRACHEOSTOMY

In many ways this procedure is an easy one, by definition done at leisure in proper theatre conditions on an anaesthetized, intubated patient. Respiratory and circulatory functions are stabilized. The patient has had proper preparation and explanation of what needs to be done.

Action

1. You may indulge in the cosmetic luxury of a horizontal skin crease incision placed halfway between the cricoid and the suprasternal notch.

2. Separate the pretracheal muscles and divide the thyroid isthmus between clamps. Pretracheal vessels just below the cricoid may need diathermy. Oversew the raw edges of the thyroid isthmus and clean the anterior tracheal wall.

3. In a bloodless field cut out a 1 cm disc centred on the third or fourth ring (Fig. 35.14). Insert your selected tube (plain metal, e.g. Jackson's, or cuffed plastic if assisted respiration is intended) and close the skin incision loosely around it.

4. *Variation*: many surgeons make an inverted U-shaped tracheal incision, hingeing the flap downwards and forwards to be stitched to the lower edge of the skin incision. This is claimed to facilitate postoperative tube-changing (or reinsertion after accidental tube displacement). With proper postoperative care the advantages are minimal, however, and some have objected to the method on the grounds that respiratory tracheal movements can cause a tracheal tear if the windpipe is rigidly fixed to the skin.

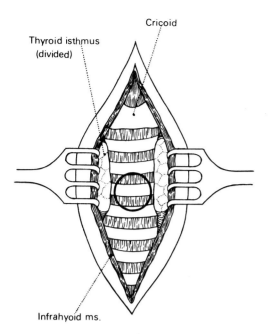

Thyroid isthmus
(divided)

Cricoid

Infrahyoid ms.

Fig. 35.14 Elective tracheostomy.

LARYNGEAL OPERATIONS FOR CANCER

Appraise

Curative operations (as distinct from biopsy and palliative tracheostomy) are nowadays essentially 'salvage' procedures required when radiotherapy has failed. They are practised more frequently in places where radiotherapy services are inadequate. There are operative techniques of partial laryngectomy (supraglottic partial laryngectomy, hemi-laryngectomy, etc.) but unless you are a highly trained specialist in such work you would be wise to limit your repertoire to the following.

(a) Laryngofissure for carcinoma limited to the anterior half of one vocal cord.
(b) Total laryngectomy for more extensive growths (with *en bloc* neck dissection if operable lymph node metastases are present).

LARYNGOFISSURE

Never embark upon this operation without the patient's consent for total laryngectomy, lest the extent of growth proves at operation to be beyond the scope of simple cordectomy.

Action

1. Incise vertically in the midline from the hyoid bone to the suprasternal notch. Separate the strap muscles, divide the thyroid isthmus and create a tracheostoma through the second, third or fourth tracheal rings. At this point the anaesthetist must withdraw his peroral endotracheal tube, and continue anaesthesia through a cuffed tube (under the drapes) inserted directly into the trachea through the lower end of the surgical wound. You now have *exclusive* access to the larynx (Fig. 35.15a).

2. Cut the thyroid cartilage in the midline. If it is calcified a small handsaw will be necessary. Retract the cartilage to either side and dissect the perichondrium off the outer and inner surfaces on the side of the growth. Remove the cartilage widely on this side, as far back as the oblique line. Open the larynx from below (through the cricothyroid membrane), cutting the mucosa upwards through the anterior commissure. You now have the growth and affected cord isolated and in view (Fig. 35.15b).

3. If you can remove a clear centimetre of normal tissue all around the tumour without encroaching on the arytenoid, do so. Straight and acutely angled scissors are all you need to cut backwards above and below the cord, and vertically across it behind the carcinoma (Fig. 35.15c).

4. Take especial care to perfect haemostasis, using diathermy. Stitch the external perichondrium together and close the wound, leaving in a cuffed tracheostomy tube. Insert a nasogastric feeding tube.

5. *Postoperative care* is especially vital to protect the lower respiratory tract, because the operation compromises the protective functions of the laryngeal sphincters. Antibiotics and tube feeding are essential, as well as a meticulous tracheobronchial toilet. After a few days small sips of fluid are allowed and increased as function returns with healing. As soon as the situation is stable (during the second week usually) the feeding tube is removed and the tracheostoma is allowed to close.

LARYNGECTOMY

Access

Incision: a U-shaped flap is best for most cases. The limbs follow the anterior borders of the sternomastoids, downwards from hyoid level, and join each other horizontally 3 cm above the sternum. If an intended cordectomy (see above) becomes a laryngectomy, make a transverse incision at the level of the hyoid to convert the initial midline approach into a T-shaped incision (Fig. 35.16).

Action

1. 'Skeletonize' the larynx: retract each sternomastoid in turn, and dissect and divide the inferior bellies of the omohyoids, and the sternohyoid and sternothyroid muscles. Divide the thyroid isthmus in the midline (Fig. 35.17).

2. On the side of the growth, leave the thyroid gland attached to the larynx for removal. Locate, ligate and cut

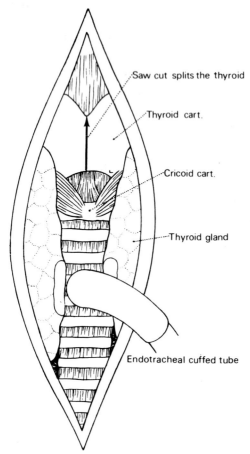

a

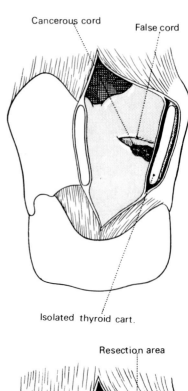

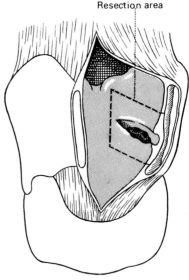

c

Fig. 35.15 Laryngofissure. (a) Approach. (b) Opening the larynx. (c) Excision of malignant disease.

the middle and inferior thyroid veins, and the superior and inferior thyroid arteries (Fig. 35.18).

3. On the healthy side, separate the thyroid gland (for preservation) from the larynx and trachea. Ligate and divide the superior laryngeal vessels as they pierce the thyrohyoid ligament. Here you will see and divide also the internal branch of the superior laryngeal nerve.

4. On both sides, incise the inferior constrictor muscle fibres close to their insertion into the thyroid cartilage. Push the cut muscle fibres backwards out of harm's way.

5. The airway: at some stage the anaesthetist's tube must be moved from the mouth into the future tracheostoma so that the larynx can be finally removed. Now is the best time. Cut across the interval between the third and fourth ring and place one or two sutures between the lower edge of the skin incision and the anterior wall of the distal part of the trachea. Allow the peroral tube to be withdrawn and a new cuffed tube to be placed through the wound into the lower trachea. Now the larynx is exclusively your own.

6. *Excision*. Remove the hyoid bone and larynx from above. Cut the muscular and ligamentous attachments along the upper border of the hyoid. Deepen the dissection until the mucosa of the vallecula is opened. Grasp the

epiglottis with tissue forceps and pull it forwards. Use scissors to cut the mucosa downwards on either side, keeping close to the laryngeal inlet, medial to the already skeletonized thyroid cartilage. Holding the nearly freed larynx forwards you can now complete the mucosal incision, transversely, just below the arytenoid cartilages (Fig. 35.19). The specimen is finally released by blunt dissection of the cricoid lamina off the pharynx and upper oesophagus, and by completing the transection of the posterior tracheal wall in line with the earlier opening described in (5) above.

7. *Repair*. Pass a nasogastric feeding tube, guiding it into the oesophageal lumen with forceps. Sew up the hole in the pharynx with inverting sutures. The closure is transverse across the base of the tongue, and vertical below this. Be meticulous in making a watertight repair. Next protect

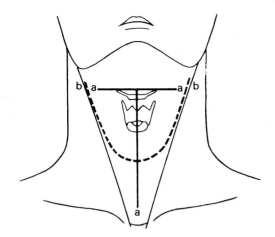

Fig. 35.16 Alternative laryngectomy incisions.

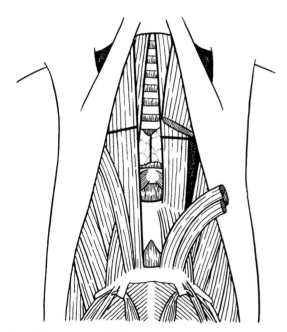

Fig. 35.17 Laryngectomy: division of the strap muscles and thyroid isthmus.

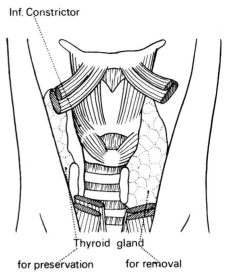

Fig. 35.18 Laryngectomy: 'skeletonizing' the larynx.

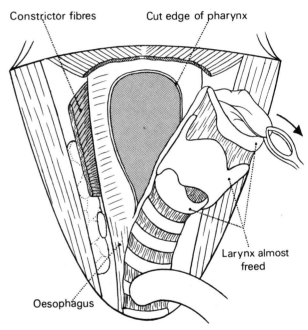

Fig. 35.19 Laryngectomy: delivering the larynx.

the closure by stitching together over it the divided edges of the inferior constrictors, and suture them above to the lingual muscles (Fig. 35.20).

Closure

The skin incision must be sutured, with drainage on both sides. Approximate the skin edges very accurately to the tracheal stump with stout non-absorbable sutures.

2. Remove the anaesthetic tube, suck out tracheal secretions (you should not have let any blood get past the cuff) and insert a plastic or metal laryngectomy tube (e.g. Moure's). Constant negative pressure drainage is used with tubular drains (e.g. 'Redivac') to keep the skin flaps from lifting.

3. Postoperatively, broad-spectrum antibiotics and tube feeding should continue for eight to ten days. Normal swallowing of liquids is then allowable, and a rapid return to normal diet encouraged if there is no fistula. Oesophageal voice is developed with the aid of speech therapy.

PHARYNGEAL OPERATIONS FOR CANCER

Appraise

As with laryngeal cancer, various excisional techniques exist aimed at conservation of function. Unless you are

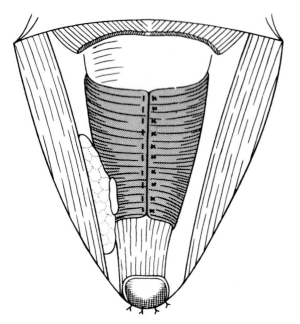

Fig. 35.20 Laryngectomy: the pharynx closed and constrictors sutured.

specifically trained and well experienced do not attempt partial pharyngectomies such as lateral pharyngotomy, or postcricoid excisions without laryngectomy. Most pharyn-geal growths are more extensive than they appear to be, and if radiotherapy is unavailable, or has failed, the choice is usually between purely palliative treatment and phar-yngolaryngectomy. This formidable mutilation has an appallingly low success rate (around 15%). If the patient is fit for surgery, try to move him to a centre specializing in this work.

Preparation for transfer

If respiratory obstruction threatens, an elective tracheos-tomy is wise. Afterwards wait several days before moving the patient between hospitals. In most cases a nasogastric feeding tube is necessary. Avoid gastrostomy as this would interfere with later mobilization of the stomach (one poss-ible method of 'one-stage' repair).

Further reading

Ballantyne J, Groves J 1979 Diseases of the ear, nose and throat, 4th edn. Butterworths, London

Hall I S, Colman B H 1976 Diseases of the nose, throat and ear, 11th edn. Churchill Livingstone, Edinburgh

Rob C, Smith R 1976 Operative surgery, 3rd edn, volumes on Ear and Nose and Throat. Butterworths, London

Ophthalmology

INTRODUCTION

The procedures described here are semi-expert but do not require extraordinary technical skills. Appraisal of particular cases which might indicate the need for these procedures is likely to take place without the full examination facilities available to the ophthalmologist. On the other hand, they would be undertaken by the non-specialist only in emergency circumstances; these indications will perforce be obvious even on unsophisticated examination.

PREPARE

Many of the procedures described in this chapter can be carried out with small instruments available in a general surgical theatre. Ideally, however, a selection of special instruments will render these eye operations easier to perform.

1. *Lid specula*: right and left, guarded, to keep the eyelashes away.

2. *Forceps*: plain (Moorfields); 1 in 2 (Lister's); 1 in 2 fine (Jayle's or St Martin's); 2 in 3 fixation forceps; iris forceps (Barraquer's).

3. *Scissors*: straight iris scissors; blunt-nosed straight and curved or spring conjunctival scissors; corneal scissors; De Wecker's iris scissors.

4. *Knives*: Graefe knife; Bard Parker handles with 11 and 15 blades.

5. *Needle holder*: coarse (Silcock's); fine (Barraquer's).

6. *Sutures*: black silk 3/0, 4/0, 6/0; virgin silk 8/0; plain catgut 4/0 and 6/0; plain collagen 6/0. All these are available on atraumatic needles.

7. *Muscle hooks*.

8. *Iris repositors*.

REMOVING AN EYE

Appraise

The main indications for removal of an eye are irreparable injury with loss of sight, total or near total, severe pain in an already blind eye, or neoplasms as for example, a choroidal malignant melanoma too large for local radiotherapy.

There are two surgical approaches, enucleation and evisceration. In the former the eyeball is removed from within Tenon's capsule, the sheet of connective tissue beneath the conjunctiva which covers both the eye and the insertion into it of the ocular muscles. In evisceration (p. 635), the eyeball is not removed as a whole but the structural wall, the sclera, is left in situ, the contents being removed; access is obtained by removing the cornea. Evisceration is usually reserved for blind eyes with obvious gross intraocular infection.

ENUCLEATION

Assess

Decide how sophisticated an operation you are going to do. A general anaesthetic is usual, but in severely ill patients, local anaesthesia, including a retrobulbar injection, may be adequate.

Action

1. Sit at the head of the table and put in an eye

speculum to separate the lids. Most specula are sprung. Keep the lids about 20 mm apart by tightening the screw.

2. Carry out a peritomy by first opening the conjunctiva close to the edge of the cornea. Pick up a fold at 6 o'clock on the corneal dial (Fig. 36.1) with plain forceps (Moorfields) and cut it with sharp pointed scissors. Undermine both away from the cornea and towards the left (if you are right-handed), keeping close to the cornea. Cut the conjunctiva close to this edge, undermine some more and proceed snipping right round the cornea. The conjunctiva should now be free from the globe (Fig. 36.2) and sufficiently undermined backward for you to explore and open Tenon's capsule. This is best done in the lower nasal quadrant, below the medial rectus muscle. If Tenon's is thick you may *not* be able to see the muscles at all at this stage. If you have opened the correct part of Tenon's capsule you will expose the sclera. This is a lustrous blue-grey colour, and you should satisfy yourself that you are really down to it by cutting away any other loose fascial planes, e.g. episcleral tissue, that can be picked up.

3. Next expose and cut off the extraocular muscles, starting with the medial rectus. Take a muscle hook and pass it upwards through the opening in Tenon's, with its blunt point against the sclera deep to this muscle. Test that you have caught the muscle by pulling the hook anteriorly, when it will be stopped short at the insertion and will then move the whole eye. With the point above the level of the muscle, rotate the hook so as to tent Tenon's capsule (Fig. 36.3). Cut down on this and then brush back Tenon's with a small swab so as to expose a length of the muscle tendon. Cut this off with blunt-nosed scissors, 3–5 mm behind the insertion.

4. Through the gap in Tenon's capsule above the medial rectus, pass a hook laterally to engage the superior rectus and cut this off, using the same steps described for the

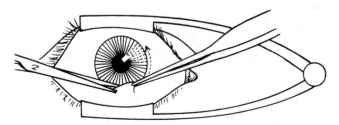

Fig. 36.1 Enucleation: opening the conjunctiva.

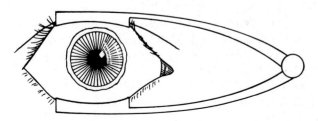

Fig. 36.2 Enucleation: conjunctiva freed.

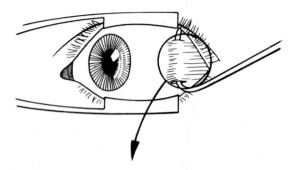

Fig. 36.3 Enucleation: tenting Tenon's capsule.

medial; then carry on round to the lateral and the inferior recti. Cut off the tendons of the superior, lateral and inferior recti flush with the globe instead of leaving a stump attached to the globe as was done with the medial rectus.

5. If you have any idea where the inferior and superior oblique muscles are and can be found, divide them. Usually, however, no formal search need be made for them as they can be dealt with as the globe is removed.

6. Once the rectus muscles have been dissected from the globe, test whether the globe rotates freely by grasping the stump of the medial rectus. If it does not do so, explore backwards beneath Tenon's with blunt-nosed scissors and divide any structures that resist the rotation.

7. Next, dislocate the globe forwards. Loosen the screw on the eye speculum and, holding it so as to keep it about 25 mm apart, press it back towards the apex of the orbit (i.e. towards the floor). The eyeball should now come forward with something of a jerk; its equator will be in front of the plane of the speculum. Now slightly close the speculum and tighten its screw so that the globe is kept in its forward dislocated position. This stretches its remaining attachments, making it easier to divide them.

8. Divide the optic nerve. There are special scissors for this: any short, but tough, blunt-nosed scissors, preferably slightly curved, will do. First rotate the globe outwards by grasping the stump of the medial rectus with two in three fixation forceps. Probe the region of the optic nerve (which cannot be seen) by passing the points of closed scissors from the nasal side to where it ought to be and moving up and down to feel the cord-like structure. Do this two or three times to make sure of its location. Now withdraw the scissors about 5 mm, open the blades widely enough to flank the nerve, then advance the blades to engage it, making sure you are far enough in to section the nerve with one cut. In order to avoid too flush a section of the nerve or, even worse, an amputation of the posterior pole of the eye, the scissors while in position embracing the nerve should be dipped about 15° so that the tips of the blades go slightly deeper into the orbit. In this position close the blades, boldly cutting through the nerve.

9. The globe will now come forward very easily. Trim away from it any remaining attachments — oblique

muscles, posterior ciliary vessels, etc. — allowing it to be removed completely.

10. Bleeding is usually brisk at this stage so proceed immediately to pack the socket with gauze wrung out in hot saline. Keep two or three fingers pressure on this for one minute. Inspect it then and reapply a fresh pack and pressure until bleeding stops. Direct haemostasis is virtually never needed. While applying pressure, inspect the enucleated eye for completeness of removal especially in the region of the optic nerve. In the most unsophisticated enucleation, simply put on some antibiotic powder, line the conjunctival sac with tulle gras, cover the lids similarly and apply a pressure dressing — two eyepads and a crêpe bandage. The deeper pad should be folded double.

Suturing the conjunctiva

Do this if it worries you not to; always do it, however, if you implant anything in the orbit (see below). Use continuous 6/0 plain catgut or collagen, either in a continuous keyhole or over-and-over pattern; tie at each end.

Orbital implants

Modify your technique as follows.

1. Put sutures into each of the rectus muscles before cutting them off the globe. If it is intended to use an implant to which the muscles will actually be attached, use 4/0 catgut. If the implant is simply a ball (glass or plastic) then use 4/0 black silk.

2. The sutures should be 'whipped' so as to give a better grip of the tendons (Fig. 36.4).

3. In all cases where an implant is to be used, dissect back under Tenon's capsule to make a definite layer which can be sutured over the front of the implant.

4. If a ball is to be used, after removing the eye and securing reasonable haemostasis, put the implant in and lift up the muscles by their silk sutures. Then sew a purse-string suture of 4/0 catgut to close Tenon's capsule over the ball and include the muscle tendons in the purse-string. Remove the black silk sutures. Finally close the conjunctiva as a separate layer with 6/0 catgut or collagen.

5. If the muscles are to be attached to the implant, do

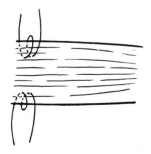

Fig. 36.4 Suturing the rectus muscles when using an implant.

this and then pull Tenon's capsule forward to cover it; it should have been dissected well enough not to be under much tension. Sew up Tenon's capsule using a continuous 6/0 catgut or collagen suture for both, starting with Tenon's right to left and then coming through to the conjunctiva proceeding left to right.

PROTECTING THE EYE: TARSORRHAPHY

Stitching the lids together may be done either centrally, which of course obscures vision, or laterally where the protection given is due to the shortening and consequent narrowing of the palpebral fissure. Central tarsorrhaphy is reserved for severe proptosis, particularly associated with advanced dysthyroid eye disease when inability to close the lids (lagophthalmos) is a serious danger to the covering of the cornea, or when ulceration is actually present. This type of tarsorrhaphy is also done when severe or protracted ulceration occurs for other reasons, for example in a numb cornea.

In milder dysthyroid disease and ectropion of the lower lid, especially that occurring in facial palsy, a lateral tarsorrhaphy will suffice.

Assess

1. First decide if a tarsorrhaphy proper is really necessary. Strapping the lids closed may well suffice if the protective covering is required for a short period only.

2. If strapping looks to be insufficient, a temporary tarsorrhaphy may be performed, sutures being inserted as detailed below but without denuding the surfaces of the lid margins.

Action

1. In all cases use local anaesthesia with amethocaine 1% drops to the conjunctiva and 1 per cent xylocaine infiltration into the lid substance both subcutaneously and subconjunctivally.

2. In tarsorrhaphy proper, raw surfaces of the lid margins are prepared. The easiest way to do this is simply to divide the lid into anterior and posterior layers through the 'grey line' (Fig. 36.5). This is the midline of the edge of the lid between the roots of the eyelashes in front and the mouths of the meibomian glands behind. The trouble is that in many patients it does not exist as a defined line, and when preparing the lid it is important to keep away from the roots of the lashes as this could distort them and lead to their growing inwards.

3. Start with the lower lid. Hold it up vertically with toothed forceps while an assistant holds it up with similar forceps some way along. Sink the blade (no. 15 BP) of a scalpel in about 3–4 mm through the grey line in the plane

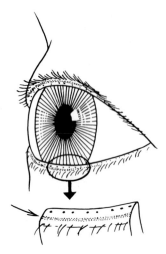

Fig. 36.5 Tarsorrhaphy.

of the lid, and take the cut the required length along the lid. If the initial stretch of lid grasped by yourself and your assistant is not long enough, both of you move along and continue the incision. Deal similarly with the upper lid opposite the raw area in the lower. In a lateral tarsorrhaphy make sure the two raw areas are continuous round the outer canthus.

4. Now put the sutures in (Fig. 36.6). Use double-armed 4/0 black silk and pass the needle through the bore of a 3 mm length of rubber tube so as to prevent it cutting out. Grasp the edge of the lower lid with one blade of the toothed forceps in the raw area in the lid margin, the other in the substance of the lid 3–4 mm from the margin. Enter the needle through the skin 4 mm from the lid margin and come out in the raw area. Now grasp the upper lid similarly and pass this needle through the raw area and out on the skin 4 mm from the lid margin. Repeat this procedure with the other needle, entering the skin of the lower lid about 4 mm laterally or medially from the entry of the first.

5. Now pass one needle through a second similar piece of rubber tube and either tie it or, according to the length of lid closure required, put in as many more of these mattress sutures as are indicated.

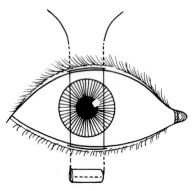

Fig. 36.6 Tarsorrhaphy: inserting the sutures.

6. Before tying, wipe away any clot from the raw edge of the lids. Do not buckle the lids when tying; moderately firm apposition is all that is needed as postoperative swelling will add further tension.

7. Put on antibiotic ointment and bandage the eye over paraffin gauze and a pad only if bleeding has been excessive. Uncover the next day. Inspect again in a week and remove the sutures after two weeks.

EYELID INJURIES

Lacerations heal well, but there are important points to remember.

1. If the lid margin is involved, try to appose the edges as accurately as possible. Use 4/0 silk for the skin but try to insert a fine suture of 6/0 or 7/0 silk through the lid margin itself. Enter the needle one side through the grey line 2 to 3 mm from the cut edge, emerging in the latter a similar distance down the cut and then in reverse through the other edge. After tying the suture, leave the ends 3 cm long and strap them down, then check that they do not abrade the cornea.

2. If the lids are widely split, suture the tarsal plate before the skin is tackled. Do this with interrupted 6/0 collagen or catgut; put the sutures in every 3 mm so that the knots are anteriorly placed in the substance of the lid, *not* facing backwards where they will be uncomfortable and again may abrade the cornea.

3. In cases where the inner third of the lower lid is lacerated, call in the experts immediately. Restoration of continuity of a possibly divided lower lacrimal canaliculus is too specialized a procedure to be covered here.

4. Massive loss of the substance of the lids may give rise to an immediate problem of ocular (particularly corneal) protection. A protective contact lens may be indicated. Immediate plastic procedures may be advisable if possible, finishing with some form of tarsorrhaphy or even a purse-string conjunctival flap to protect the cornea.

INJURIES OF THE GLOBE

LACERATIONS

1. *Conjunctiva.* Leave small cuts (less than 5 mm) alone. Suture larger ones under local anesthesia with 6/0 interrupted collagen at 4-mm intervals, removing any prolapsed Tenon's capsule if excessive, or burying it.

2. *Cornea and sclera.* Insert a speculum, and find and remove foreign bodies. Glass from windscreens is especially difficult. Put a drop of fluorescein in the eye; it may help to show small particles as well as corneal epithelial loss.

3. For removal of metal foreign bodies, see page 634, but always get a lacerated eyeball X-rayed as a matter of

routine. If obvious foreign bodies are present in the anterior chamber, attempt to remove them with the finest small-bladed forceps (do this only during a procedure for a lacerated cornea).

4. Cut off any prolapsed iris, ciliary body, lens remnants or vitreous. Pick them up with iris forceps and withdraw a little in an attempt to free them from an incarcerated position in the wound. Make a (De Wecker's) scissors cut to remove the tissue, flush with the plane of the globe at the site of the penetration. Gently reposit any further matter remaining in the wound using an iris repositor. Incarcerated material without actual external prolapse had best be left alone in emergency circumstances, particularly if the anterior chamber is not lost.

Closure

1. Closure of the wound can be of varying difficulty. Clean lacerations of less than 5 mm need not be dealt with other than by toilet as just described.

2. It cannot be expected that the general surgeon will always wish to undertake the minutiae of direct corneal or scleral suture. If this process is undertaken, however, it is important to remember that the sutures must be in the substance of the tissue and not through it (see Fig. 36.7); use magnification, if available, to ensure this. Enter and emerge about 1–1.5 mm from the wound edge. Grasp each edge lightly with the finest toothed forceps you have (e.g. Jayle's or finer). Use 8/0 virgin silk and keep the sutures in a line perpendicular to the wound. In suturing scleral wounds it may be necessary to dissect the conjunctiva back from the edge.

3. It may, however, be considered unwise to attempt direct suture, either because of lack of experience or because the wound is too irregular. In such cases, and particularly if the anterior chamber is shallow or absent, proceed to cover the wound with a conjunctival flap. In a corneal wound, for example, carry out a partial peritomy (see p. 630). Thus if, for example, the wound is in the 4 o'clock meridian, cut the conjunctiva at the limbus from 1 to 7 o'clock in the lower left half of the globe (Fig. 36.8). However, if it is possible to choose the origin and direction of the flap, remember that the upper and temporal conjunctiva is the loosest and easiest to mobilize. Under-

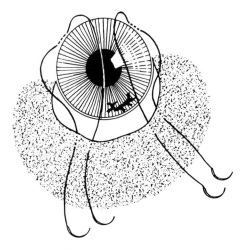

Fig. 36.8 Conjunctival flap.

mine the conjunctiva so freed back for at least 15 mm. Insert one needle of a double-armed 6/0 black silk suture in the paralimbal connective tissue at 8 o'clock and, using a second suture, do the same at 12 o'clock.

4. To put these sutures in you must try to get a reasonable bite without going right through the sclera into the eye. A 2 mm track should be aimed for, parallel to and 1 mm from the lumbus. To steady the eye use a fine toothed forceps (Jayle's) to grasp the episcleral tissue close to where you are going to put in the suture.

5. Now put the two arms of one suture through the edge of the freed conjunctiva at an appropriate place and repeat with the other suture. Figure 36.8 indicates suitable insertion points. Tie each suture while an assistant, using two pairs of plain forceps, pulls the edge of the flap well over the site of the penetration. If the penetration is central, it should still be possible to cover it in this way. An alternative is to peritomize all the conjunctiva at the corneoscleral junction and to put in a purse-string suture of 6/0 black silk; considerable undermining of the conjunctiva is, of course, essential.

6. Finally, give a subconjunctival injection of framycetin 250 mg in 0.5 ml of water. The injection should be supplemented with Mydricaine, if available. Use a fine needle (20 gauge) and give the injection by passing the needle tangentially through the conjunctiva in a horizontal direction 1 cm back from the limbus in the quadrant opposite to that of the penetrating injury.

BLUNT INJURIES

Evacuation of hyphaema

This procedure, a paracentesis of the anterior chamber, is *very rarely* indicated, as a hyphaema is invariably treated conservatively to begin with. Accordingly, paracentesis should only be undertaken in the following rare circum-

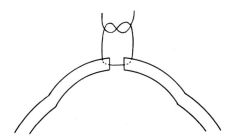

Fig. 36.7 Corneal and scleral sutures.

stances; the anterior chamber is *full* of blood, there is a considerable rise in the intraocular pressure which is unresponsive to Diamox and oral glycerol over a three-day period, and finally, the patient is in severe pain.

2. Anaesthetize the eye with 4% cocaine drops given at five-minute intervals. A general anaesthetic is not necessary. Insert an eye speculum; use a Graefe knife if available, otherwise a Bard Parker scalpel with a no. 11 blade. Grasp the medial rectus muscle with a two in three forceps and *lift* the eye ceilingwards gently, so as to fix its position. Hold the knife like a pencil and steady your hold by placing the fourth and fifth fingers on the temple. Pass the tip of the blade through the cornea 2 mm inside the limbus (corneoscleral junction) with the plane parallel to that of the *iris* (which cannot be seen, so this is presumptive), but in any case keep in the plane of the limbal 'ring' (the corneoscleral junction) (Fig. 36.9). Enter at 3 or 9 o'clock on the corneal dial.

2. The tip of the knife can be seen passing through the cornea but, once inside, it may disappear in blood; do not push on any further than 2 mm once this happens. Withdraw the knife gently but rapidly in its own plane. If done properly, nothing will escape from the anterior chamber even if the ocular tension is very high.

3. Now press gently on the posterior (peripheral) lip of the incision and some blood-stained aqueous should escape. Do not press for longer than a second at a time to begin with, as a very rapid drop in the eye pressure may start the bleeding again. Repeat this until there is some evidence of clearing of the anterior chamber, but it is not necessary to persist until all blood has been evacuated. Put in antibiotic ointment, remove the speculum and pad the eye.

4. In some cases very little may come out as the anterior chamber may contain a solid clot. A urokinase irrigation may be tried but this is probably too speculative a procedure for the general surgeon.

5. Paracentesis is also a standard emergency procedure for arrest of the retinal circulation (central retinal artery occlusion) and should be carried out within two to three hours of the onset. Here a much more rapid evacuation of the clear normal aqueous humour is called for.

Ruptured globe

A totally disrupted eyeball may require enucleation either

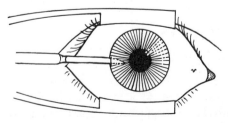

Fig. 36.9 Evacuation of hyphaema. Fixation of globe not shown.

immediately or within a few days of the injury, and the same applies to badly lacerated and collapsed eyes. The decision to do so must always be taken with the possibility in mind of the dreaded complication of sympathetic ophthalmia. Smaller posterior ruptures with some preservation of function may be indicated by a deep anterior chamber and chemosis from loss of the vitreous. Although an ophthalmic surgeon may consider exploration of some cases, it would probably be advisable for the general surgeon to manage such cases conservatively, as many will go to the bad whatever is done and some will do well on non-surgical management.

FOREIGN BODIES

1. *Intraocular foreign bodies.* These require specialist intervention; the important thing for the general surgeon is to recognize the possibility of the condition, which is particularly likely to be missed where the entry wound is small and the initial disturbance minimal. Here the history of something going into the eye, especially while hammering and chiselling, and the absence of a foreign body on superficial inspection should prompt an X-ray of the orbit. Most small intraocular foreign bodies are sterile, and once the condition is recognized no harm will accrue from delay until dealt with in more favourable conditions. If large, a foreign body may cause a penetrating injury that needs to be dealt with in itself.

2. *Subtarsal foreign bodies.* Remove these by everting the upper eyelid. Have a cotton-wool swab to hand *before* starting. Ask the patient to look down and to keep doing so. Grasp the upper lid lashes with the thumb and forefinger of one hand and pull the lid down and forwards. With an orange stick press the upper edge of the tarsal plate downwards (some 4 mm from the lid margin) and then lift the lashes so as to rotate the lid over the orange stick, which pushes the tarsal plate down and under the lid margin at the same time.

Once the eyelid is everted, keep hold of the lashes and press them against the eyebrow, instructing the patient the while to keep looking down. Remove the orange stick and use the hand released to remove the foreign body with the cotton-wool swab. Return the lid to its normal position by withdrawing both hands and asking the patient to look up.

3. *Corneal foreign bodies.* If you suspect the foreign body to be deep in the cornea, do not tackle it yourself, as manipulation may push it into the anterior chamber.

To remove superficial corneal foreign bodies, first anaesthetize the eye. A good light focussed on the cornea is essential.

Very superficial foreign bodies may be brushed off by a cotton-wool swab. Embedded foreign bodies require to be needled out. Insert a 17 gauge disposable needle tangentially to the cornea to get behind the foreign body — in other words do not go directly for it, enter the cornea a little to the side. Lever the foreign body out. Sometimes rust is left behind; attempt to pick it out, but do not try too hard. If the rust is slight and milk chocolate in colour, leave it; it will disappear itself. If it is darker, however, get as much out as comes easily. More may need to be removed after a period of a few days' softening up.

Pad the eye after putting in an antibiotic ointment. Put in a mydriatic according to the degree of manipulation, i.e. very easy removal, no mydriatic; moderately easy, homatropine 2 per cent drops; very difficult, atropine 1 per cent drops. See the patient the next day.

BURNS

1. *Chemical burns.* The immediate treatment is removal of any matter mechanically and, particularly, copious irrigation using any harmless fluid to hand. Do not hunt for specific antidotes. Antibiotic/steroid ointments are applied as well as atropine if the cornea is involved, and the conjunctival fornices should be kept patent to prevent symblepharon by twice-daily rodding with a glass rod. Always admit patients with lime burns for observation as the effects may be delayed.

2. *Thermal burns.* Those affecting the lids are treated as skin burns elsewhere, but problems of ocular protection may arise.

INFECTIONS AROUND THE EYE

Pyogenic infections

1. Incision should be avoided wherever possible, but in conditions where extreme tense swelling due to pus is causing severe pain the surgical maxim of 'where there's pus, let it out' is obeyed.

2. This situation arises in the lids (styes and more particularly infected meibomian cysts), in the lachrymal apparatus (acute dacryocystitis), and very rarely for a pointing orbital cellulitis. Whenever possible incise lid abscesses from the inner aspect. Anaesthetize the lid (see tarsorrhaphy, p. 631). Evert it (Fig. 36.10) and incise at right angles to the lid margin through the tarsal plate. Do *not* curette any meibomian granulations such as would be done for a non-infected cyst.

3. For acute dacryocystitis a local anaesthetic may not be necessary if it is obviously pointing. Incise from below the inner palpebral ligament down and out for 15 mm parallel to the orbital margin.

4. A drain is not necessary.

5. Infections of the eyeball itself may be localized, as for example a pyogenic corneal ulcer, or widely disseminated, as when a metastatic infection lodges in the choroid, spreading thence to the vitreous and all parts of the eye.

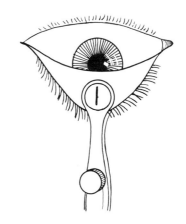

Fig. 36.10 Everting the lower lid, with a chalazion clamp.

6. A corneal ulcer may perforate and require a conjunctival flap to cover it and help it to heal. It may also be accompanied by pus in the anterior chamber (hypopyon) which if unresponsive to intense local and systemic chemotherapy may require evacuation by paracentesis.

7. Severe desctructive infection or endophthalmitis is treated by chemotherapy and steroids systemically and locally; failure to control it may require removal of the eye.

EVISCERATION

1. Destruction of vital internal structures by infection and loss of vision is an indication for evisceration, rather than enucleation where there is (an exaggerated) danger of the infection spreading via the subarachnoid space following severing of the optic nerve.

2. Insert a speculum and then proceed to cut off the cornea. This may be difficult if the eye is very soft, following, say, the perforation of an infected corneal ulcer. The simplest method is to fix the eye with toothed forceps on a rectus muscle insertion and then to cut through the periphery of the cornea circumferentially over a 5 mm length by progressively deepening a scalpel incision. Use the belly of a Bard Parker 15 blade.

3. Once the anterior chamber has been entered cut right round the edge of the cornea with corneal scissors, if available, or any narrow-bladed, blunt-nosed scissors to hand.

4. Having topped the eye, scoop out all its contents — lens, iris and retina as well as the humours. It is important to do this thoroughly. A special scoop is available, but a large and not-too-sharp curette will do as well. End by wrapping gauze round it to wipe away all the uveal remnants. Inspect the cavity to make sure that all you have left is sclera.

5. Finally, pack the socket with paraffin gauze, apply pad and bandage. Dress in 48 hours. No suture is required.

GLAUCOMA

Paracentesis is rarely indicated these days, but has some small part to play in the secondary glaucoma which may arise as a result of blood in the anterior chamber (p. 633).

In some intractable cases of secondary glaucoma associated with uveitis it also has a place.

In primary acute closed angle glaucoma it can again be used until more specialist aid is available, but in most cases the pressure can be lowered adequately, if temporarily, by Diamox, miotic drops and osmotic agents. For this reason, classical iridectomy for glaucoma is hardly ever employed as an emergency procedure. Should it be necessary, however, the following is a simple technique.

GLAUCOMA IRIDECTOMY

1. General anaesthesia is advisable. If local anesthesia is used, a retrobulbar xylocaine injection is essential.

2. Insert a speculum. Put two drops of 1 : 1000 adrenaline in the eye and wait for some blanching of the conjunctiva to occur before proceeding.

3. Put in a superior rectus stitch. Grasp the tendon with 1 in 2 forceps (Lister's) and pass a 4/0 black silk suture through it, avoiding catching the sclera (or penetrating it!) in so doing.

4. Turn down a conjunctival flap at the 12 o'clock position (Fig. 36.11) Grasp the conjunctiva about 5 mm from the limbus. Pick up conjunctiva only. To facilitate this a subconjunctival injection of 0.25 ml of xylocaine 1% and adrenaline may be given first to balloon it. Using blunt-nosed scissors cut an incision about 12 mm long concentric with the limbus. Undermine downwards and slightly laterally to clear the sclera down towards the cornea. Hold the flap of conjunctiva gently downwards and forwards, finally clearing the limbal tissues with sharp dissection, using sharp pointed scissors and also using the latter closed to obtain about 7–8 mm of bared sclera not more than 1 mm from clear cornea.

5. Enter the anterior chamber using a Bard Parker (no. 15 blade) to produce a linear incision about 5 mm long concentric with the limbus. Cut with the belly of the blade

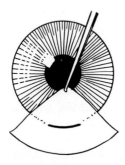

Fig. 36.11 Glaucoma iridectomy: turning down the conjunctival flap

initially, keeping its plane perpendicular to the sclera. Several strokes are usually necessary. Err on the cautious side with the pressure you exert, as you do not want the aqueous to spurt out as the anterior chamber is entered (Fig. 36.11).

6. As you enter the anterior chamber, a little aqueous only should escape from one point of the depths of the wound. Wait a few seconds before opening the depths of the wound to its full length. Do this by turning the scalpel over and using it with the back edge tangential to the globe.

7. The iris will almost certainly be prolapsing into and through the wound by this time. Try to avoid cutting it while enlarging the wound. Grasp the iris with iris forceps close to one end of the wound. Pull it out about 3 mm and cut off that pillar flush with the wound using de Wecker's scissors. Still holding the half abscissed piece of iris, tear it horizontally so that it remains attached only at the other end of the wound. Pull this out 3 mm again and cut it off flush as for the other pillar.

8. Using an iris repositor, clear the wound of iris remnants. Avoid touching the lens by keeping this instrument parallel to the plane of this iris; as you watch its tip in the anterior chamber, ensure it remains anterior to the pillar of the iris.

9. If the attack of glaucoma has been of long duration, say untreated for 5 days or more modify 7 and 8 as follows:- After tearing horizontally the half-abscised piece of iris, cut it off 2–3 mm away from the globe and leave that pillar incarcerated in the wound. This forms an 'iris inclusion' which may function as a drainage valve if the iridectomy alone in insufficient to restore the ocular pressure to normal.

10. Sew up the conjunctival flap with 6/0 collagen. Put in 1% atropine and antibiotic drops. Pad the eye over paraffin gauze and cover with a cartella shield.

RELIEF OF PAIN

Intractable glaucoma with severe pain is one example of the blind, painful eye, and for this sort of glaucoma some relief may be given by a retrobulbar alcohol injection if removal of the eye is impracticable.

RETROBULBAR ALCOHOL INJECTION

1. Put 1.5 ml of 1 per cent xylocaine wiht 1 : 200 000 adrenaline in a 2 ml syringe and fit a retrobulbar needle.

2. Sterilize the skin of the lower lid after determining the site of entry of the needle, which should be the lower outer angle of the bony orbit.

3. With the patient lying down, ask him to his eyes open and to look up over the top of the head and to the opposite

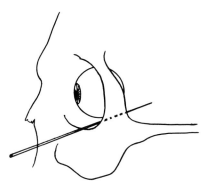

Fig. 36.12 Retrobulbar alcohol injection.

side — i.e. for the left eye look over the top and to the right.

4. Insert the needle through the skin in the intended direction, which is backwards, and slightly medially and upwards (Fig. 36.12). There is a tendency to avoid getting too close to the globe for fear of penetrating it; but if you keep too far away, you will miss the muscle cone which you want to penetrate through the stretched Tenon's capsule between the lateral and inferior recti.

5. Inject very slightly as you go in. You will probably feel resistance when Tenon's is about to be penetrated and you may see the eye roll slightly down and out at this point. Be resolute and push on; the eye will resume its former position. Inject the bulk of the local. When it has had time to work there will be some relief of pain.

6. Now leave the needle in place and detach the syringe. Draw up 1 ml of 75% alcohol and after an interval of one minute inject this through the retrobulbar needle still *in situ*. Withdraw needle and syringe.

7. Warn the patient that relief may not be very long-lasting (it does, however, often last months), and also warn of the possibility of ptosis of the upper lid, which again may not be permanent.

NEOPLASMS

The commonest important ocular neoplasms affect the lids and the uveal tract.

Small benign lesions of the lid

These can be removed by cautery excision under local anaesthetic.

Larger benign and malignant lesions of the lid

1. Careful consideration is needed before deciding upon the surgical approach. The size of the lesion and its position in relation to the lid margins are important. With malignancies the tissue to be removed must include at least 3 mm beyond the visible margin of the lesion.

2. For larger lesions away from the lid margin, excision and rearrangement of local skin flaps may suffice. Alternatively a free graft of skin from the contralateral upper lid is very helpful. The prior injection of local anaesthetic to distend the skin ensures that the area removed will be adequate and that closure of the donor site will be easy.

3. For lesions of the lid margin a 'V' excision is best, always provided that the gap can be simply closed by direct suture. If this is under too much tension, closure may be facilitated by an outer canthal incision so that the lateral portion of the lid can be more easily approximated. This type of procedure is also helpful as a simple method of shortening the lower lid for senile ectropion. Local anaesthesia is all that is required.

4. The V excised should be at least 2 cm in height with its nasal edge vertical, the other being angled towards it. Closure is effected in two layers as described in the section on lid injuries (p. 632).

5. Major reconstructive surgery of the eyelids is beyond the scope of this section. Intraocular malignancies are again a matter for the specialist, but the general principle applies that for lesions of any size (which to the nonspecialist means any degree of obviousness) enucleation is indicated.

Further reading

King J H, Wadsworth J A C et al 1981 An atlas of ophthalmic surgery 3rd edn. Lippincott, Philadelphia

Rice T S, Michels R G, Stark W J 1984 Rob and Smith's operative surgery: ophthalmic surgery 4th edn. Butterworths, London

Späeth G L (1982) Ophthalmic surgery: principles and practice. W.B. Saunders, Philadelphia

Index